Allergens and Allergen Immunotherapy

Sixth Edition

Allergens and Allergen Immunotherapy

Subcutaneous, Sublingual, and Oral

Sixth Edition

Edited by

Richard F. Lockey, MD, MS
Distinguished University Health Professor
Professor of Medicine, Pediatrics & Public Health
Joy McCann Culverhouse Chair of Allergy and Immunology
Director, Division of Allergy and Immunology
Department of Internal Medicine
University of South Florida Morsani College of Medicine
Tampa, Florida

Dennis K. Ledford, MD
Professor of Medicine & Pediatrics
Mabel & Ellsworth Simmons Professor
University of South Florida Morsani College of Medicine
Department of Internal Medicine
Chief, VA Section of Allergy/Immunology
James A. Haley Veterans' Hospital
Tampa, Florida

With the editorial assistance of Ms. Geeta Gehi, Administrative Specialist, Division of Allergy and Immunology, Department of Internal Medicine, University of South Florida Morsani College of Medicine, Tampa, Florida

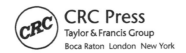

CRC Press
Taylor & Francis Group
Boca Raton London New York

CRC Press is an imprint of the
Taylor & Francis Group, an **informa** business

CRC Press
Taylor & Francis Group
6000 Broken Sound Parkway NW, Suite 300
Boca Raton, FL 33487-2742

First issued in paperback 2021

© 2020 by Taylor & Francis Group, LLC
CRC Press is an imprint of Taylor & Francis Group, an Informa business

No claim to original U.S. Government works

ISBN-13: 978-0-8153-8221-8 (hbk)
ISBN-13: 978-1-03-217327-6 (pbk)
DOI: 10.1201/9781351208994

Library of Congress Cataloging-in-Publication Data

Names: Lockey, Richard F., editor. | Ledford, Dennis K., 1950- editor.
Title: Allergens and allergen immunotherapy : subcutaneous, sublingual, and oral / [edited] by Richard F. Lockey, Dennis K. Ledford.
Description: Sixth edition. | Boca Raton : CRC Press/Taylor and Francis Group, [2020] | Includes bibliographical references and index. |
Summary: "The Sixth edition of Lockey and Ledford's Allergens and Allergen Immunotherapy continues to provide comprehensive coverage of all types of allergens and allergen vaccines, providing clinicians the essential information they need to accurately diagnose and manage all allergic conditions"-- Provided by publisher.
Identifiers: LCCN 2019045411 (print) | LCCN 2019045412 (ebook) | ISBN 9780815382218 (hardback) | ISBN 9781351208994 (ebook)
Subjects: MESH: Hypersensitivity--therapy | Allergens--immunology | Allergens--therapeutic use | Immunotherapy
Classification: LCC RC588.I45 (print) | LCC RC588.I45 (ebook) | NLM QW 900 | DDC 616.97/06--dc23
LC record available at https://lccn.loc.gov/2019045411
LC ebook record available at https://lccn.loc.gov/2019045412

Visit the Taylor & Francis Web site at
http://www.taylorandfrancis.com

and the CRC Press Web site at
http://www.crcpress.com

Dedicated to the past and present faculty and staff of the Division of Allergy and Immunology, Department of Internal Medicine, University of South Florida Morsani College of Medicine and James A. Haley Veterans' Hospital, founded 1973

Contents

SECTION III Immunotherapy techniques: Production, preparation, and administration of allergen immunotherapy

Preface

Welcome! This is the sixth edition of *Allergens and Allergen Immunotherapy: Subcutaneous, Sublingual and Oral*, the first edition of which was published in 1991. The first edition contained 13 chapters and the sixth, 38 chapters. The authors of these chapters are literally a Who's Who in the world of allergy and immunology, in particular, allergens and allergen immunotherapy. The book now addresses all forms of immunotherapy currently in use in clinical practice, including subcutaneous, sublingual, and oral.

What's new in this edition? Some topics have been combined into single chapters, and some were deleted. Other subjects added include chapters on aeroallergen sampling; local mucosal allergic diseases; manufacturing pollen, fungal, arthropod, mammalian, and food extracts; and biologic immunomodulators to treat allergic diseases. Chapter 5, entitled "Immunologic Response to Various Forms of Allergen Immunotherapy," authored by Umit Murat Sahiner and Stephen R. Durham, is extraordinarily informative regarding the mechanisms responsible for immunotherapy's efficacy. The book continues to be divided into five sections.

Section I, Basic Concepts: These chapters detail the history of allergen immunotherapy, definitions, immunologic responses, and knowledge about allergen nomenclature, so critical to the understanding of the formulation of an allergen vaccine.

Section II, Allergens: This section describes inhaled, ingested, and injected allergens relevant to immunotherapy. The major and minor allergens and their cross-reactivity with other allergens are discussed. Biologic and immunologic characteristics of allergens are included.

Section III, Immunotherapy Techniques: This subdivision covers details of the manufacturing and standardization of allergen extracts and vaccines for the diagnosis and treatment of allergic diseases and indications for their use.

Section IV, Clinical Application of Allergen Immunotherapy and Biological Therapy for Allergic Diseases: This section addresses adherence and cost-effectiveness of subcutaneous, sublingual, and oral immunotherapy as well as new biologics available to treat allergic diseases. It also discusses unproven forms of immunotherapy.

Section V, Recognition, Management, and Prevention of Adverse Effects of Allergen Immunotherapy: These chapters explain how to minimize, recognize, and treat adverse effects, including systemic allergic reactions (anaphylaxis). Instructions and consent forms for allergen immunotherapy are included.

What are the strengths of this sixth edition? First, it is the most detailed book written on allergens and allergen immunotherapy in the world; second, experts wrote each chapter; third, the editors have spent a great deal of time making sure that the topic is completely covered; and fourth, it provides practical information for the clinician to prescribe allergen immunotherapy. The editors believe that all allergists/immunologists who use allergen immunotherapy should read this book and keep it in their library as a reference.

The understanding of allergens and allergen immunotherapy has come a long way. Richard F. Lockey (RFL) was introduced to the specialty of allergy and immunology by his father, Stephen D. Lockey, Jr., MD, who practiced as an allergist beginning in the late 1940s in Lancaster, Pennsylvania. RFL was formally trained as an allergist/immunologist at the University of Michigan, Ann Arbor, Michigan, from January 1968 to December 1969. Dennis K. Ledford (DKL) was introduced to the same specialty while working as a resident with Phillip Lieberman, MD, at the Center for Health Sciences, University of Tennessee, Memphis, Tennessee, in 1979. He subsequently trained in allergy and immunology at the University of South Florida Morsani College of Medicine and James A. Haley VA Hospital, Tampa, Florida, from July 1983 to June 1985.

The whole field of immunotherapy has been revolutionized since the mid-twentieth century. It is now used not only to treat allergic diseases but also neurologic, autoimmune, cancer, and many other diseases. Think of what has occurred since the first well-designed, controlled trials by Lowell, Franklin, Norman, and others who followed. The World Health Organization published a monograph on allergen immunotherapy in 1998 entitled "WHO Position Paper—Allergen Immunotherapy: Therapeutic Vaccines for Allergic Diseases" edited by Drs. Jean Bousquet, RFL, and Hans-Jorgen Malling. It was the first document summarizing the evidence that supports the use of allergen immunotherapy to treat allergic diseases. Subsequently, sublingual, and oral immunotherapy have been proven effective and are now in clinical use. Oral immunotherapy is now used to treat food allergy, an epidemic that affects up to 8% of pediatric subjects in some parts of the world. Other forms of therapy, such as epicutaneous immunotherapy, application of modified allergens, and use of adjuvants or immunomodulators are under development.

The future, not only to treat but also to prevent allergic diseases, appears to be very promising. Perhaps, rather than altering the course of these diseases, it will be possible to prevent them in a cost-effective manner. The members of the specialty of allergy and immunology can be very proud that allergen immunotherapy was the first form of immunotherapy used to alter and downregulate immune responses that cause allergic diseases. It is a great honor and pleasure for the two editors to have worked with so many wonderful colleagues throughout the world to bring this book to fruition. Read and enjoy what helps define the specialty of allergy and clinical immunology. The editors are confident that the application of the information contained in this book will improve the health of patients with allergic diseases throughout the world.

We would like to acknowledge the late Samuel C. Bukantz, MD, the founding father of the Division of Allergy and Immunology, Department of Internal Medicine, University of South Florida Morsani College of Medicine, and the first Section Chief of Allergy and Immunology, James A. Haley VA Hospital. He coedited the first several editions of this book, and his expertise, intelligence, and hard work are still apparent in this edition. He is profoundly missed by all who knew him.

The editors are extraordinarily grateful to Ms. Geeta Gehi, who is our editorial assistant. She has been absolutely essential in completing all of these later editions. We also thank Ms. Peggy Hales, director of our administrative team, for her invaluable assistance.

Richard F. Lockey, MD, MS
Dennis K. Ledford, MD

Editors

Richard F. Lockey, MD, MS, director of the Division of Allergy and Immunology, Department of Internal Medicine, and professor of Medicine, Pediatrics and Public Health, was named the Joy McCann Culverhouse Chair in Allergy and Immunology at the University of South Florida Morsani College of Medicine, Tampa, Florida, in 1997. He is a tenured physician and in 2007 was honored to receive the additional title of University of South Florida Distinguished Health Professor. He joined the faculty in 1973 at which time he also became a staff member at the James A. Haley Veterans' Hospital, where he was chief of the Section of Allergy and Immunology until 2017. He is board certified in both internal medicine and in allergy and immunology.

The Division of Allergy and Immunology, Department of Internal Medicine, is a widely recognized treatment, teaching, and research facility in the field of allergy, asthma, and clinical immunology. For example, at different times in the history of the division, up to five division faculty have been named as "best doctors" in America. Through the efforts of Lockey, the division is now endowed with more than US$14 million dedicated to teaching and research. The faculty in the division work in the state-of-the-art Joy McCann Culverhouse Airway Disease Research Center, devoted to developing long term treatments and even a cure for allergic and immunologic diseases and asthma. In addition, the division's Joy McCann Culverhouse Airway Disease Research Center's Clinical Research Unit has participated in many of the major drug innovations for the treatment of allergic and immunologic diseases and asthma over the past 40 or more years. The division has approximately 50 members consisting of nine physicians, some of whom are also basic scientists, and four PhDs, devoted to basic research. Four clinician scientists are in the Division of Allergy and Immunology, Department of Pediatrics, at the University of South Florida Morsani College of Medicine, Tampa, Florida, and the Johns Hopkins/All Children's Hospital, St. Petersburg, Florida. The division is supported by 11 affiliated physicians who interact with the division regularly and help with the teaching and research programs.

Lockey received his undergraduate degree from Haverford College, Haverford, Pennsylvania, in 1961, and received a medical degree from Temple University School of Medicine, Philadelphia, Pennsylvania, in 1965, where he was a member of the Alpha Omega Alpha National Medical Honor Society. After completing his internship in medicine at Temple University School of Medicine in 1966, he finished his residency in internal medicine in December 1968 and fellowship in allergy and immunology at the University of Michigan, Ann Arbor, Michigan, in December 1970, where he also attended the University of Michigan Rackham Graduate School and received a master's degree in internal medicine this same year. He was a Major in the U.S. Air Force during the Vietnam War and served as Chief of Allergy and Immunology at Carswell Air Force Base, Fort Worth, Texas, from 1970 to 1972.

Widely published, Lockey has authored, coauthored, or edited over 750 scientific and review articles and book chapters, 17 books, and 20 monographs. He has published and coauthored articles in *Nature, JAMA,* and the *New England Journal of Medicine.* He has been an invited speaker on more than 450 occasions for both national and international scientific conferences and has served on the editorial boards of many peer-reviewed journals. In 1987, he edited a special edition for the *Journal of the American Medical Association, Primer on Allergic and Immunologic Diseases.* He was a coeditor of the first American College of Physicians and American Academy of Allergy, Asthma and Immunology *Medical Knowledge Self-Assessment Program (MKSAP) in Allergy and Immunology,* published in 1992. He is a fellow of the American Academy of Allergy, Asthma and Immunology and a past fellow of the American College of Chest Physicians and the American College of Physicians. He also is a past member of the American Thoracic Society, European Academy of Allergy and Clinical Immunology, Clinical Immunology Society, American College of Occupational and Environmental Medicine, European Thoracic Society, and the American Medical Association. He is a current member of the Florida Allergy, Asthma and Clinical Immunology Society, of which he is a past president. In 1992, Lockey received a "Certificate of Appreciation" from the Florida Medical Association in addition to being featured with Drs. Samuel C. Bukantz and Robert A. Good, mentors and colleagues, on the cover of the June/July 1996 special issue of *The Journal of the Florida Medical Association.*

Professional honors include serving as president of the American Academy of Allergy, Asthma and Immunology (1992–1993); director of the American Board of Allergy and Immunology from 1993 to 1998, the organization that oversees and examines physician candidates for certification as specialists in allergy/immunology; and the Board of the World Allergy Organization (WAO) from 1995 to 2016. He served as the WAO President from January 2010 until December 2012. The organization represents approximately 35,000 allergists/immunologists from over 100 countries throughout the world. He has also served as an associate on two World Health Organization committees, one on the *Prevention of Allergies and Asthma* and the other, *Allergic Rhinitis and Its Impact on Asthma.* He was also a coeditor of a third project, the *WHO Position Paper, Allergen Immunotherapy: Therapeutic Vaccines for Allergic Diseases,* published in 1998. He was the editor of the World Allergy Organization *WEB-Page* and the World Allergy Organization *E-MAIL News and Notes* from 2004 to 2009, which served all physicians, in particular, allergists/immunologists throughout the world.

Included among the numerous distinctions Lockey has received are the Alumni Achievement Award, Temple University School of Medicine, Philadelphia, Pennsylvania, and McCaskey High School, Lancaster, Pennsylvania, and listings in many *Who's Who in the World* and as an outstanding medical specialist in *Town and Country* magazine. He has also received an award for Outstanding Leadership in Chapter Development and Patient Support from the National Asthma and Allergy Foundation of America, an appreciation award from the Asthma and Allergy Foundation of America, Florida Chapter, and the Team Physician Award for his services as a volunteer physician for the University of South Florida Athletic Department. He received a Special Recognition Award in 1993 and Distinguished Service Award in 1999 from the American Academy of Allergy, Asthma and Immunology.

In 2008, he was awarded the Distinguished Clinician's Award from this same organization. He was awarded the Florida Academy of Sciences Medal for the year 2000, presented for outstanding work in scientific research, activities in the dissemination of scientific knowledge, and service to the community. He received the University of South Florida Distinguished Service Award in 2001. In the year 2006, Lockey received the Distinguished Visiting Professor Award from the Faculty of Medicine at the Catholic University of Cordoba, Argentina, and was also made an Honorable Member of the Latin-American Society of Allergy Asthma and Immunology. He is an honorary member of other societies. He was awarded the Southern Medical Society Dr. Robert D. and Alma W. Moreton Original Research Award in 2012. In 2018, he received the Distinguished Eagle Scout Award from the Boy Scouts of America, the highest honor bestowed by this organization. He was also inducted into the University of South Florida Robert A. Good Honor Society this same year. In 2019, he was honored by the American Academy of Allergy, Asthma and Immunology (AAAAI), which established the AAAAI Foundation and Richard F. Lockey, MD, MS, FAAAAI University of South Florida Lectureship and Faculty Development Award. The $250,000 generated for this award were donated by colleagues, both present and past, for which he is extremely grateful.

As director of the Division of Allergy and Immunology, Lockey has helped train over 100 MDs in the specialty program of allergy and immunology and approximately 40 postgraduate PhDs or MDs from various parts of the world in clinical and basic research. Most of them have assumed leadership positions in science and medicine in their respective communities or countries. He continues to spend equal amounts of time caring for patients, in basic and clinical research, and teaching at the University of South Florida Morsani College of Medicine and its affiliated hospitals. He is married to Carol Lockey and has two children, Brian Christopher Lockey and Keith Edward Lockey, and is blessed with five grandchildren, Olivia, Benjamin, William, Nicholas, and Matthew.

Dennis K. Ledford, MD, was born and grew up in East Tennessee and was valedictorian of his high school class.

He attended college at the Georgia Institute of Technology, Atlanta, Georgia. He graduated magna cum laude with a degree in chemical engineering and was selected for membership in Tau Beta Pi, the engineering honor society. He received his medical degree from the University of Tennessee Center for Health Sciences. Ledford is a member of Alpha Omega Alpha Medical Honor Society (AOA), being selected as a third-year student at the University of Tennessee, and he received the outstanding student of medicine award, graduating first in his class. He remained in Memphis for the completion of his internal medicine residency and served as chief medical resident for Dr. Gene Stollerman at the City of Memphis Hospitals. A fellowship in rheumatology and immunology followed at New York University and Bellevue Hospital in New York. A fellowship in allergy and immunology at the University of South Florida completed his education. Ledford remained in Tampa at the University of South Florida (USF), joining the faculty and achieving the rank of professor of medicine in 2000. He received the honor of being named the USF Morsani College of Medicine Mabel and Ellsworth Simmons Professor of Allergy in 2012. He is actively involved in the pediatric and internal medicine allergy/immunology training programs and established and was the prior program director of the program in Clinical and Laboratory Immunology at the University of South Florida.

Ledford has contributed in a variety of areas to the USF Morsani College of Medicine. He is the past president of the medical faculty, serving from 2012 to 2013. He has served on the medical student selection committee and was chair of the committee for two separate terms. He was honored with the Distinguished Service Award by the university in 2018.

Ledford received the outstanding teacher award from the USF medical house staff, the outstanding medical volunteer of the year in Hillsborough County, and the Governors Community Service Award from the American College of Chest Physicians. He has served on the American Board of Allergy and Immunology as secretary/treasurer and leader of the maintenance of certification initiative. He is a past president of the Florida Allergy Asthma and Immunology Society. Ledford was a member and vice-chair of the Residency Review Committee for Allergy/Immunology of the American Council of Graduate Medical Education. He has previously served as associate editor of the *Journal of Allergy and Clinical Immunology*, editorial board member for the *Annals of Allergy, Asthma and Immunology*, and *Journal of Allergy and Clinical Immunology: In Practice*, and is a past contributing editor for *Allergy Watch*. He is a contributor to *UpToDate*.

Ledford has served the American Academy of Allergy, Asthma and Immunology (AAAAI) in a number of capacities. He was a prior governor of the Southeast Region of the State Local and Regional Allergy Societies of the AAAAI and chair and member of several committees. He has been a member of the board of directors and was president of the AAAAI from 2011 to 2012. He served on numerous task forces for the AAAAI and as chair of the International Collaboration in Asthma Allergy and Immunology. Ledford is the past chair of the steering committee for the Allergy, Asthma, and Immunology Education and Research Trust, currently known as the AAAAI Foundation. He received the Outstanding Clinician Award from both the American Academy of Allergy, Asthma and Immunology and the World Allergy Organization.

Ledford works with the division's faculty in managing academic associates in allergy, asthma, and immunology, is chief of the section of allergy and immunology at the James A. Haley VA Hospital, and has been selected as one of *America's Best Doctors* consecutively for more than 25 years. Clinical responsibilities occupy the majority of his time, but he has developed research interests in severe, steroid-dependent asthma, allergen characterization, the association of gastroesophageal reflux disease and upper airway disease, and eosinophilic esophagitis. Ledford has been the principal investigator in more than 25 and coinvestigator in more than 180 clinical trials, authoring or coauthoring more than 150 publications. He has been married to Jennifer S. Ledford for 45 years and is blessed with three children, Keith, Michael, and Robert, and 11 grandchildren, Madelyn, Andrew, Isaiah, Ian, Lukas, Kaila, Annika, Grant, Ethan, Miles, and Parker.

Contributors

Babak Aberumand
Department of Medicine
Queen's University
Kingston, Ontario, Canada

Mübeccel Akdis
Swiss Institute of Allergy and Asthma Research (SIAF)
Davos, Switzerland

Andrew S. Bagg
University of Central Florida College of Medicine
and
Allergy Asthma Specialists
Orlando, Florida

Diego Bagnasco
Department of Internal Medicine
University of Genoa
Genoa, Italy

David I. Bernstein
Division of Immunology, Allergy, and
  Rheumatology
University of Cincinnati College of Medicine
Cincinnati, Ohio

Jonathan A. Bernstein
Department of Internal Medicine
University of Cincinnati College of Medicine
Cincinnati, Ohio

Whitney Block
Sean N. Parker Center for Allergy and Asthma Research
  at Stanford University
and
Department of Medicine
Stanford University
Stanford, California

Heimo Breiteneder
Institute of Pathophysiology and Allergy Research
Medical University of Vienna
Vienna, Austria

Jennifer L. Bridgewater
Division of Bacterial Parasitic and Allergenic Products
Office of Vaccines Research and Review
Center for Biologics Evaluation and Research
U.S. Food and Drug Administration
Silver Spring, Maryland

Paloma Campo
Allergy Unit
IBIMA–Hospital Regional Universitario de
  Málaga, UMA
Málaga, Spain

Giorgio Walter Canonica
Department of Internal Medicine
University of Genoa
Genoa, Italy
and
Asthma and Allergy Unit
Humanitas Clinical and Research Center
Humanitas University
Rozzano, Italy

Luis Caraballo
Allergy and Immunology
Institute for Immunological Research
University of Cartagena
Cartagena, Colombia

Thomas B. Casale
Department of Internal Medicine
University of South Florida Morsani College of Medicine
Tampa, Florida

Miguel Casanovas
Inmunotek S.L.
Alcalá de Henares, Spain

Martin D. Chapman
INDOOR Biotechnologies, Inc.
Charlottesville, Virginia

Seong H. Cho
Department of Internal Medicine
University of South Florida Morsani College of Medicine
Tampa, Florida

Rosa Codina
Allergen Sciences and Consulting
Lenoir, North Carolina
and
Division of Allergy and Immunology
University of South Florida Morsani College of Medicine
Tampa, Florida

Sheldon G. Cohen (Deceased)
National Institute of Allergy and Infectious Diseases
National Institutes of Health
Bethesda, Maryland

Linda Cox
Department of Medicine
Nova Southeastern University
Fort Lauderdale, Florida

Jennifer A. Dantzer
Pediatric Allergy and Immunology
Johns Hopkins University School of Medicine
Baltimore, Maryland

Natalie A. David
Center for Biologics Evaluation and Research
U.S. Food and Drug Administration
Silver Spring, Maryland

Richard D. deShazo
University of Mississippi Medical Center
Jackson, Mississippi

Stephen R. Durham
National Heart and Lung Institute
Imperial College
and
Asthma UK Centre in Allergic Mechanisms of Asthma
London, United Kingdom

Motohiro Ebisawa
Department of Allergy
Clinical Research Center for Allergology and Rheumatology
Sagamihara National Hospital
Kanagawa, Japan

Ibon Eguiluz-Gracia
Allergy Unit
IBIMA–Hospital Regional Universitario de Málaga, UMA
Málaga, Spain

Anne K. Ellis
Allergy Research Unit
Kingston General Health Research Institute
and
Department of Biomedical and Molecular Sciences
and
Department of Medicine
Queen's University
Kingston, Ontario, Canada

Robert E. Esch
School of Natural Sciences
Lenoir-Rhyne University
Hickory, North Carolina

Richard Evans III (Deceased)
Department of Pediatrics
Northwestern University Medical School and Division of Allergy
Children's Memorial Hospital
Chicago, Illinois

Jennifer E. Fergeson
Department of Internal Medicine
University of South Florida Morsani College of Medicine
James A. Haley VA Hospital
Tampa, Florida

Eva Abel Fernández
Research and Development Department
Inmunotek S.L.
Madrid, Spain

Enrique Fernández-Caldas
Inmunotek S.L.
Madrid, Spain
and
Division of Allergy and Immunology
University of South Florida Morsani College of Medicine
Tampa, Florida

Fatima Ferreira
Department of Biosciences
University of Salzburg
Salzburg, Austria

Lauren Fine
Nova Southeastern University
Kiran C. Patel College of Allopathic Medicine
Davie, Florida

David Fitzhugh
Allergy Partners of Chapel Hill
Chapel Hill, North Carolina

Gabriele Gadermaier
Department of Biosciences
and
Christian Doppler Laboratory for Biosimilar
    Characterization
University of Salzburg
Salzburg, Austria

David B.K. Golden
Johns Hopkins University
Baltimore, Maryland

Rick Goodman
Food Allergy Research and Resource Program
University of Nebraska–Lincoln
Lincoln, Nebraska

Miles Guralnick
Independent Scholar (now actively retired)

Robert G. Hamilton
Department of Medicine
Johns Hopkins University School of Medicine
Baltimore, Maryland

Michael Hauser
Department of Biosciences
University of Salzburg
Salzburg, Austria

Donald R. Hoffman
Department of Pathology and Laboratory Medicine
Brody School of Medicine at East Carolina University
Greenville, North Carolina

Christian Gauguin Houghton
ALK A/S
Hørsholm, Denmark

Victor Iraola
Research and Development Department
Inmunotek S.L.
Madrid, Spain

Stephen F. Kemp
University of Mississippi Medical Center
Jackson, Mississippi

Jonathan Kilimajer
Medical Department
Inmunotek S.L.
Madrid, Spain

Te Piao King
Rockefeller University
New York, New York

Mike Kulis
Department of Pediatrics
University of North Carolina at Chapel Hill
Chapel Hill, North Carolina

Jørgen Nedergaard Larsen
ALK A/S
Hørsholm, Denmark

Dennis K. Ledford
Department of Internal Medicine
University of South Florida Morsani College of Medicine
James A. Haley VA Hospital
Tampa, Florida

Estelle Levetin
Department of Biological Science
University of Tulsa
Tulsa, Oklahoma

Richard F. Lockey
Division of Allergy and Immunology
Department of Internal Medicine
University of South Florida Morsani College of Medicine
Tampa, Florida

Henning Løwenstein
Henning Løwenstein ApS
Fredensborg, Denmark

Josh D. McLoud
Department of Biological Science
University of Tulsa
Tulsa, Oklahoma

Rafael I. Monsalve
Research and Development Department
ALK–ABELLO
Madrid, Spain

Ulrich Müller-Gierok (Retired)
Wabern, Switzerland

Kari C. Nadeau
Sean N. Parker Center for Allergy and Asthma Research
   at Stanford University
and
Department of Medicine
and
Department of Pediatrics
Stanford University
Stanford, California

Harold S. Nelson
National Jewish Health
and
University of Colorado Denver School
   of Medicine
Denver, Colorado

Hendrik Nolte
ALK, Inc.
Bedminster, New Jersey

John Oppenheimer
Department of Medicine
University of Medicine and Dentistry of New Jersey
   (UMDNJ–Rutgers)
Newark, New Jersey
and
Pulmonary and Allergy Associates
Summit, New Jersey

Ricardo Palacios
Diater, S.A.
Madrid, Spain

Giovanni Passalacqua
Department of Internal Medicine
University of Genoa
Genoa, Italy

Shiven S. Patel
Department of Internal Medicine
University of South Florida Morsani College
   of Medicine
James A. Haley VA Hospital
Tampa, Florida

Anusha Penumarti
Department of Pediatrics
University of North Carolina at Chapel Hill
Chapel Hill, North Carolina

Fernando Pineda
Diater, S.A.
Madrid, Spain

Lisa Pointner
Department of Biosciences
University of Salzburg
Salzburg, Austria

Anna Pomés
Department of Basic Research
INDOOR Biotechnologies, Inc.
Charlottesville, Virginia

Leonardo Puerta
University of Cartagena
Cartagena, Colombia

Ronald L. Rabin
Division of Bacterial Parasitic and Allergenic Products
Office of Vaccines Research and Review
Center for Biologics Evaluation and Research
U.S. Food and Drug Administration
Silver Spring, Maryland

Matthew Rawls
Allergy Research Unit
Kingston General Health Research Institute
and
Department of Biomedical and Molecular Sciences
Queen's University
Kingston, Ontario, Canada

Carmen Rondón
Laboratorio de Investigación
Hospital Civil
Malaga, Spain

Marja Rytkönen-Nissinen
Department of Clinical Microbiology
Institute of Clinical Medicine
University of Eastern Finland
Kuopio, Finland

Tara V. Saco
Department of Internal Medicine
University of South Florida Morsani College
  of Medicine
Tampa, Florida

Umit Murat Sahiner
National Heart and Lung Institute
Imperial College
Hacettepe University School of Medicine
London, United Kingdom
and
Pediatric Allergy Department
Hacettepe University School of Medicine
Ankara, Turkey

Vanitha Sampath
Sean N. Parker Center for Allergy and Asthma Research
  at Stanford University
and
Department of Medicine
Stanford University
Stanford, California

Sakura Sato
Department of Allergy
Clinical Research Center for Allergology
  and Rheumatology
Sagamihara National Hospital
Kanagawa, Japan

Coby Schal
Department of Entomology and Plant Pathology
North Carolina State University
Raleigh, North Carolina

Mohamed H. Shamji
National Heart and Lung Institute
Imperial College
and
Asthma UK Centre in Allergic Mechanisms of Asthma
London, United Kingdom

Sayantani B. Sindher
Sean N. Parker Center for Allergy and Asthma Research
  at Stanford University
and
Department of Medicine
Stanford University
Stanford, California

Jay E. Slater
Center for Biologics Evaluation and Research
U.S. Food and Drug Administration
Silver Spring, Maryland

Andrew M. Smith
Allergy Associates of Utah
Murray, Utah

Ozge Soyer
Pediatric Allergy Department
Hacettepe University School of Medicine
Ankara, Turkey

Jeffrey Stokes
Washington University School of Medicine
St. Louis, Missouri

Farnaz Tabatabaian
Department of Internal Medicine
University of South Florida Morsani College
  of Medicine
Tampa, Florida

Haig Tcheurekdjian
Allergy/Immunology Associates, Inc.
Mayfield Heights
and
Department of Medicine and Pediatrics
Case Western Reserve University
Cleveland, Ohio

Mark W. Tenn
Allergy Research Unit
Kingston General Health Research Institute
Kingston, Ontario, Canada

Abba I. Terr
Department of Medicine
University of California San Francisco Medical Center
San Francisco, California

Stephen J. Till
Asthma UK Centre in Allergic Mechanisms of Asthma
and
Division of Asthma, Allergy and Lung Biology
King's College London, School of Medicine
Guy's Hospital
London, United Kingdom

Manuel Lombardero Vega
ALK S.A.
Madrid, Spain

Loida Viera-Hutchins
Tanner Clinic
Murray, Utah

Hari M. Vijay
VLN Biotech, Inc.
Ottawa, Ontario, Canada

Tuomas Virtanen
Department of Clinical Microbiology
Institute of Clinical Medicine
University of Eastern Finland
Kuopio, Finland

Dana V. Wallace
Department of Medicine
Nova Southeastern University College of Allopathic Medicine
Fort Lauderdale, Florida

Michael Wallner
Department of Biosciences
University of Salzburg
Salzburg, Austria

Richard W. Weber
Department of Medicine
National Jewish Health
Denver, Colorado

Emma Westermann-Clark
University of South Florida Morsani College
   of Medicine
Tampa, Florida

Sabrina Wildner
Department of Biosciences
and
Christian Doppler Laboratory for Biosimilar
   Characterization
University of Salzburg
Salzburg, Austria

Robert A. Wood
Pediatrics and International Health
and
Pediatric Allergy and Immunology
Johns Hopkins University School of Medicine
Baltimore, Maryland

SECTION I

Basic concepts

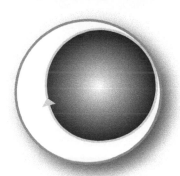

1 Historical perspectives of allergen immunotherapy

David Fitzhugh
Allergy Partners of Chapel Hill

Sheldon G. Cohen*
National Institutes of Health

Richard Evans III*
Children's Memorial Hospital

CONTENTS

1.1 IMMUNITAS

The term *immunitas* is derived from the Latin adjective *immunis* or its noun form *immunitas,* which means exemption—that is, freedom from cost, burden, tax, or obligation.

Original usage of the term pertained to the inferior Roman class of plebeians, artisans, and foreign traders who—deprived of religious, civil, and political rights and advantages of the patrician *gentes*—were immune to taxation, compulsory military service, and civic obligations and functions. After 294 BC, with the transition of the monarchy to the Roman Republic, *immunitas* defined special privileges (e.g., exemptions from compulsory military service and taxation granted by the Roman Senate to sophists, philosophers, teachers, and public physicians). In later years, common use of the Anglicized descriptor immunity continued to have legal relevance. In the Middle Ages, church property and clergy were granted immunity from civil taxes. In 1689, the English Bill of Rights formalized parliamentary immunity protecting members of the British Parliament from liability for statements made during debates on the floor. In France, a century later, a 1790 law prevented arrests

---

* Deceased.

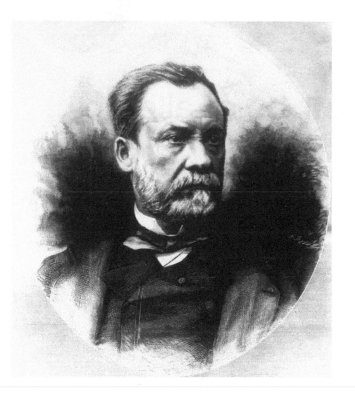

Figure 1.1 Louis Pasteur, ScD (1822–1895). Founding director of the Institut Pasteur, Paris. (Courtesy of the National Library of Medicine.)

of a member of the legislature during periods of legislative sessions without specific authorization of the accused member's chamber.

The first medically relevant usage of the term appears to be that of the Roman poet Lucan (Marcus Annaeus Lucanus, AD 39–65) in *Pharsolia* while referring to the "immunes" of members of the North African Psylli tribe to snakebite. In the scientific literature with definitive medical usage, the term appeared in an 1879 issue of London's *St. George's Hospital Reports (IX:715)*: "In one of the five, instances … the apparent immunity must have lasted for at least two years, that being the interval between the two diphtheritic visitation." The following year the descriptor found a place in medical terminology with Pasteur's (Figure 1.1) report of his seminal work on attenuation of the causal agent of fowl cholera, noting the "(induction) of a benign illness that immunizes (Fr. Immunise) against a fatal illness" [1].

1.2 IMMUNITY THROUGH INTERVENTION

Anthropological records reveal that from the earliest times that humans sought to understand the factors that made for well-being, there were attempts to intervene to prevent deviations from health and well-being. Healers of antiquity, priest-doctors, secular sorcerers, medicine men, and practitioners of folk medicine all played influential roles. In the ancient cradles of civilization—Mesopotamia, Babylonia, Assyria, and Egypt—magic and mystic methods were created to ward off divine and cosmic-directed afflictions mediated through spirits and demons with tools of intervention such as incantations, rituals, sacrifices, amulets, and talismans. In the biblical era of the Old Testament, freedom from disease and affliction (which were believed to be divine punishment for sin) was sought through the

power of prayer and left in the hands of rabbis who took on the dual role of a healer. In sixth-century BC India, preventive practice became synonymous with following the enlightened morality teachings of Gautama Buddha (566?–c. 480 BC). To herbs and dietary manipulations critical for maintaining health and preventing disease and promoting balance between internal yin and yang forces, ancient China added physical methods. To drain off yin or yang excesses, procedures employed insertion of needles (acupuncture) and heat-induced blistering (moxibustion at organ-related skin points along channels of vital flow). According to the tenets originating in classical Greece—with the writings of Hippocrates (460–370 BC)—and extended in Roman medicine by Claudius Galen (AD 130–200), it was the four internal humors (blood, phlegm, yellow bile, and black bile) that were the determinants of health and disease. Their pathogenetic imbalances could be corrected by preventively draining off excesses of the humors through interventions of bleeding, blistering (by cupping), sweating (by steam baths), purging, and inducing expectoration and emesis.

Regarding pestilence, the observation that survivors of an epidemic were spared from being stricken during return waves of the same illness was described by the ancient historians Thucydides (c. 460–400 BC) (Figure 1.2) [2], who described the plague of Athens,

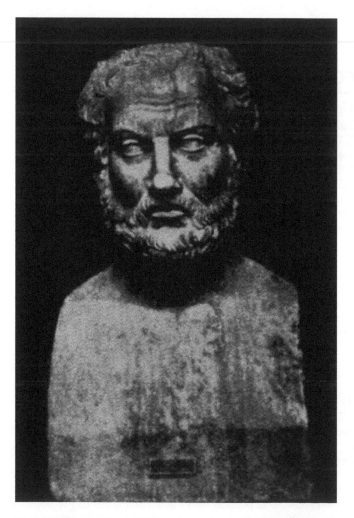

Figure 1.2 Thucydides (c. 460–400 BC). Greek historian. (From Gordon BL. *Medicine throughout Antiquity*, 1949. Courtesy of F.A. Davis Company, Philadelphia, PA.)

and Procopius of Byzantine (c. AD 490–562), who wrote about the plague of Justinian that struck the Mediterranean ports and coastal towns. First attempts to duplicate this natural phenomenon appeared in the eleventh century, when Chinese itinerant healers developed a method to prevent contraction of potentially fatal smallpox. These healers were able to deliberately induce a milder transient pox illness through the medium of a dried powder prepared from the material recovered from a patient's healing skin pustules and blown into a recipient's nostrils. The practice disseminated along China–Persia–Turkey trade routes ultimately reached Europe and the American colonies following communications with England during 1714–1716 by Timoni, a Constantinople physician [3], and Pylorini, the Venetian counsel in Smyrna (Izmir) [4]. Although effective in reducing susceptibility and incidence in epidemic attack, variolation presented difficulties; inoculations sometimes resulted in severe, even fatal, primary illness, and recipients could serve as sources of transmittable infection until all active lesions healed. A solution to the problem was found in the investigations of Jenner (Figure 1.3), the English rural physician who in 1795 reported a new benign method to prevent smallpox by inducing a single pustule of a related, but different, skin disease, cowpox (vaccinia, from the Latin word *vaccinus* meaning pertaining to a cow)—a lesion resembling smallpox only in appearance. From its name, the procedure became known as vaccination [5].

Jenner's carefully designed protocols carried out in 1796 stimulated experimental leads and raised a number of pertinent questions for future investigators: (1) Were disease-producing and protective (antigenic) qualities interdependent and equivalent? (Jenner had noted that some stored, presumably deteriorated, pox material did not evoke a vaccination lesion; however, he was unable to ascertain whether it still was capable of providing a protective effect.) (2) Could two different agents share the ability to induce identical protective responses? (Jenner believed vaccination succeeded because smallpox and cowpox were different manifestations of the same disease.) (3) Could the same agent induce protection against disease and tissue injury? (Jenner's description of the appearance of a local inflammatory lesion after revaccination provided the earliest documentation of hypersensitivity phenomena as a function of the immune response.)

Koch and Pasteur's early endeavors to develop preventive vaccines were innovative giant steps in establishing immunization as an efficacious measure in disease prevention; they also served as models for later developments of allergen immunotherapy.

Pasteur's use of attenuated microorganisms as vaccines in fowl cholera and sheep anthrax demonstrated that specific antigenic immunizing potential was not impaired by decreasing virulence of a bacterium [6]. Later studies by Salmon and Smith [7] with heat-killed vaccines indicated that immunogenicity also did not require antigen viability.

Some unfortunate outcomes of early immunotherapeutic ventures temporarily hindered the future of immunotherapy with allergens. Koch was premature in introducing injectable preparations of glycerol extracts of tubercle bacilli cultures for the treatment of tuberculosis. His error revealed that violent systemic reactions could result from injection of antigens that acted as specific challenges in delayed hypersensitivity states [8]. Pasteur's rabies vaccine met with enthusiastic success, but antigens of the rabbit spinal cords, used as culture medium for the aging rabies virus, also induced simultaneous production of antinervous tissue antibodies and adverse autoimmune neurologic reactions [9].

Practical approaches to immunization in the Western world might have had an earlier beginning had cognizance been taken of a centuries-old practice in Egypt. Dating back to antiquity, snake charmers in the temples—and later religious snake dancers among native Southwest American Indians—had found the key to protection from the danger of their craft. Beginning with self-inflicted bites from young snakes as sources of small amounts of venom, and progressing to repetition by large snakes led to tolerant outcomes of otherwise potentially fatal challenges. However, it was not until 1887 that Sewall's (Figure 1.4) experimental inoculation of rattlesnake venom in an animal model introduced appreciation and development of antitoxins [10].

The discovery of diphtheria exotoxin [11] spurred the practice of inducing antitoxins in laboratory animals and their therapeutic use by passive immunization [12]. The fact that the resultant antitoxins evolved into therapeutically effective agents was because of Ehrlich's (Figure 1.5) studies on the chemical nature of antigen-antibody reactions and applications to biological standardization [13]. Further, the methods by which antitoxins were obtained enabled early stages of development of allergen immunotherapy [14]. Subsequently, development of severe life-threatening hypersensitivity reactions following injection of the antibodies in serum proteins of the actively immunized horse [15] created a virtually insurmountable obstacle in later attempts to initiate a therapy for hay fever by passive immunization [14].

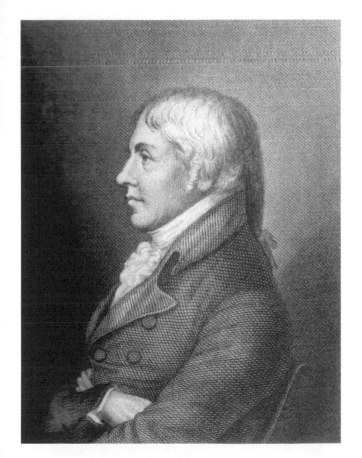

Figure 1.3 Edward Jenner, MD (1749–1823). Practicing physician in Cheltenham, rural England. (Courtesy of the National Library of Medicine.)

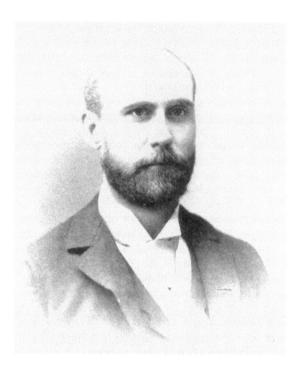

Figure 1.4 Henry Sewall, MD, PhD (1855–1936). Professor and chairman, Department of Physiology, University of Michigan. (From Webb GB, Powell D, *Henry Sewall, Physiologist and Physician*, 1946. Courtesy of Johns Hopkins, Johns Hopkins University Press, Baltimore, MD.)

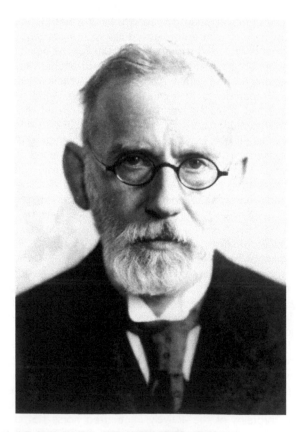

Figure 1.5 Paul Ehrlich, MD (1854–1915). Founding director of the Institute for Experimental Therapy, Frankfurt, Germany. (Courtesy of the National Library of Medicine.)

1.3 GENESIS OF ALLERGEN IMMUNOTHERAPY

Discoveries in the field of immunity gave rise to another pioneering area of study within the newly established discipline, and the introduction of immunologically based therapies for infectious diseases soon followed. The impact of widening applications of immunotherapy was largely responsible, in the first half of the nineteenth century, for the evolution of allergy as a separate segment of medical practice. The forerunner of this relationship occurred in 1819, when Bostock, a London physician, precisely described his own personal experience and classical case history of hay fever [16]. This landmark account of allergic disease was recorded only 23 years after Jenner's controlled demonstration of the ability of inoculation with cowpox to prevent smallpox [2].

Some 70-odd years after Bostock's report, Wyman identified pollen as the cause of autumnal catarrh in the United States [17]. A year later, Blackley published confirmatory descriptions on the basis of self-experimentation, which established that grass pollen was the cause of his seasonal catarrh, which was noninfective [18]. He also made the first investigational reference to allergen immunotherapy when he repeatedly applied grass pollen to his abraded skin areas, but without resultant diminution of local cutaneous reactions or lessened susceptibility.

In 1900, Curtis reported that immunizing injections of watery extracts of certain pollens appeared to benefit patients with coryza and/or asthma caused by these pollens [19]. Dunbar (Figure 1.6) then attempted to apply the principle of passive immunization developed with diphtheria and tetanus antitoxin to the preventive treatment of human hay fever. He tried using "pollatin," a horse and rabbit antipollen antibody preparation. As a powder or an

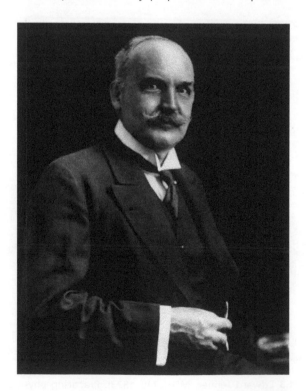

Figure 1.6 William Dunbar, MD (1863–1922). Director of the State Hygienic Institute, Hamburg. (Courtesy of the Hygienisches Institute, Hamburg, Germany.)

ointment, it was developed for instillation in and absorption from the eyes, nose, and mouth and as pastille inhalational material for asthma [13]. Subsequent attempts to immunize with grass pollen extracts were abandoned because of severe systemic symptoms induced by excessive doses. Dunbar's associate, Prausnitz, had failed to diminish either the mucous membrane reactions or symptom manifestations of hay fever after "thousands" of ocular installations of pollen "toxin" [14]. Dunbar then attempted immunization with pollen toxin-antitoxin (T-AT) neutralized mixtures—a technique that had been used with bacterial exotoxins (e.g., tetanus and diphtheria) [20].

While Dunbar's anecdotal reports of success could not be duplicated, the discovery of anaphylaxis formed a new concept of immunity and its relevance to immunotherapy. In 1902, Portier and Richet described anaphylactic shock and death in dogs that were under immunization with toxins from sea anemones [21]. Four years later, these exciting and provocative animal experiments were followed by reports of sudden death in humans after the injection of horse serum antitoxins and of exhaustive protocols with experimental animals that implicated anaphylactic shock as the likely mechanism [22]. Smith made similar observations while standardizing antitoxins, which prompted Otto to refer to the findings as the "Theobald Smith Phenomenon" [23].

Wolff-Eisner applied the concept of hypersensitivity to a conceptual understanding of hay fever [24]. Further, anaphylactically shocked guinea pigs were discovered to have respiratory obstruction because of contraction and stenosis of bronchiolar smooth muscle that resulted in air trapping and distension of the lungs [25], similar to the characteristic pulmonary changes in human asthma. This finding led Meltzer to conclude that asthma was a manifestation of anaphylaxis [26]. The role of the anaphylactic guinea pig as a suitable experimental model for the study of asthma was further enhanced by Otto's demonstration that animals that recovered from induced anaphylactic shock became temporarily refractory to a second shock-inducing dose [27]. Additionally, Besredka (Figure 1.7) and Steinhardt discovered that repeated injections of progressively larger, but tolerable, doses of antigen eventually protected sensitized guinea pigs from anaphylactic challenge [28]. These results suggested that a similar injection technique might successfully desensitize the presumed human counterpart disorders of asthma and hay fever.

Investigational pursuit of active immunization for hay fever was soon begun in the laboratories of the Inoculation Department at St. Mary's Hospital in London, where Wright had provided the setting for interaction with visiting European masters of microbiology and immunology, giving his students the opportunity to learn about the "new immunotherapy." Wright's enthusiasm was reflected in his frequent prediction that "the physician of the future may yet become an immunisator" [29].

Noon (Figure 1.8), Wright's assistant, following Dunbar's concept, also believed that hay fever was caused by a pollen "toxin." To accomplish active immunization, he initiated clinical trials in 1910 with a series of subcutaneous injections of pollen extract doses calculated on a pollen-derived weight basis (Noon unit), and thus introduced preseasonal immunotherapy. Noon's observations provided the following (still pertinent) guidelines: (1) a negative phase of decreased resistance develops after initiation of injection treatment; (2) increased resistance to allergen challenge, measured by quantitative ophthalmic tests, is dose dependent; (3) the optimal interval between injections is 1–2 weeks; (4) sensitivity may increase if injections are excessive or too frequent; and (5) overdoses may

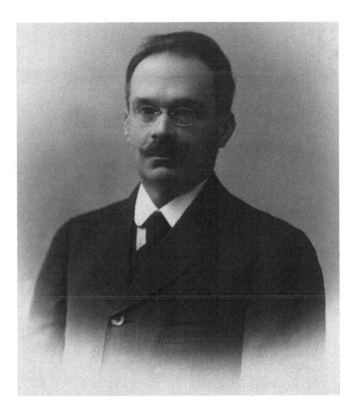

Figure 1.7 Alexandre Besredka, MD (1870–1940). Pasteur Institute, Paris. (Courtesy of the National Library of Medicine.)

induce systemic reactions [30]. Noon's work was continued by his colleague, Freeman (Figure 1.8), who in 1914 reported results of the first immunotherapeutic trial of 84 patients treated with grass pollen extracts during a 3-year period. The protocols lacked adequate controls, but successful outcomes were recorded with acquired immunity lasting at least 1 year after treatment was discontinued [31]. A cluster of related reports indicated that other clinical studies of immunization of hay fever patients by others had been underway, concurrently and independently [31–35].

Clinical and investigative aspects of this new modality were expanded with the beginnings of pioneering allergy clinics. The first in 1914 was started at the Massachusetts General Hospital by Joseph L. Goodale (Figure 1.9), a rhinologist introduced to immunology at Robert Koch's Berlin Institute for Infectious Diseases. Francis Rackemann subsequently joined Goodale as clinic codirector. The next year, I. Chandler Walker (Figure 1.10) initiated a clinic at Peter Bent Brigham Hospital, and in 1918, Robert A. Cooke (Figure 1.11) initiated a clinic at New York Hospital.

With the growing appreciation of pollens as allergens, the concept of pollen "toxin" faded, and the objective of immunotherapy took on a new meaning. Cooke, at a 1915 meeting at the New York Academy of Medicine, added his summary of favorable result—in a majority of 140 patients treated with pollen extracts [36]—to the series of 45 patients reported from Chicago by Koessler [34]. Developments during the next 10–15 years were characterized by an eagerness to accept a continuing stream of favorable reports and adopt an arbitrary and relatively unquestioned technique of immunization therapy. A number of factors influenced the widespread use of this therapeutic method.

The scratch test introduced by Schloss in 1912 [37] was popularized by Walker [38] and by Cooke [36], who introduced the

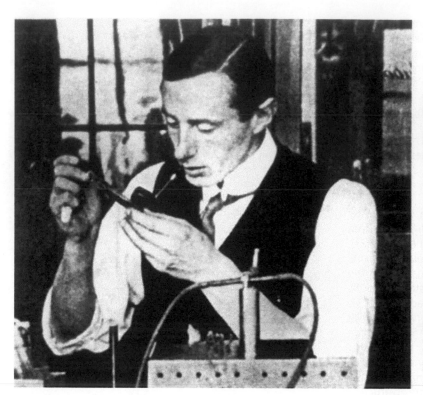
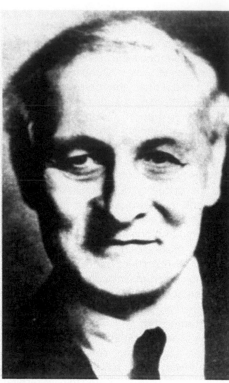

Figure 1.8 Leonard Noon, 1877–1913 (left) and John Freeman, 1877–1962 (right). Immunologists on staff, Inoculation Department, St. Mary's Hospital, London. (Courtesy of the College of Physicians of Philadelphia.)

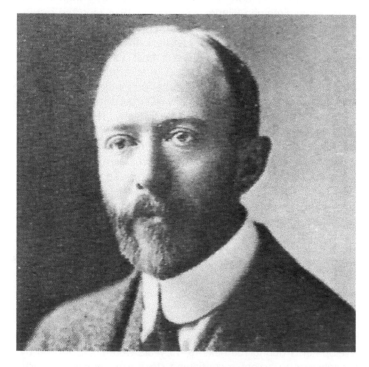

Figure 1.9 Joseph L. Goodale (1868–1957). Rhinolaryngologist and associate surgeon in otolaryngology at Massachusetts General Hospital. In 1949, by bringing hay fever patients into the hospital throat clinic for systematized study and treatment provided the nucleus for the first allergy clinic founded in the United States. (Courtesy of Robert L. Goodale, MD.)

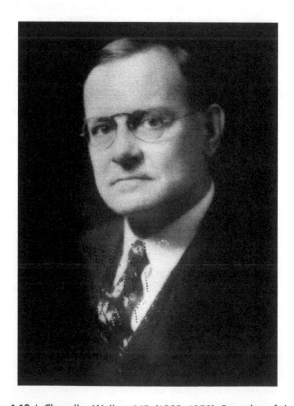

Figure 1.10 I. Chandler Walker, MD (1883–1950). Founder of the first allergy clinic in the United States, at Peter Bent Brigham Hospital, Boston; Department of Medicine, Harvard Medical School. (Courtesy of Frederick E. Walker.)

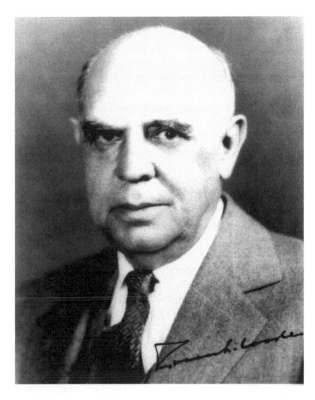

Figure 1.11 Robert A. Cooke, MD (1880–1960). Founding director of the Institute of Allergy, Roosevelt Hospital, New York. (Courtesy of the National Library of Medicine.)

intracutaneous skin test technique in 1915. These new diagnostic techniques obviated the need for the more limited ocular test site and permitted practical identification of a wide variety of allergenic substances that might be useful in treatment.

Development of methods of extracting allergenic fractions from foods and airborne and environmental materials was extensively pursued by Wodehouse and Walker (Figure 1.10) at the Peter Bent Brigham Hospital in Boston [39,40] and by Coca at a newly established Division of Immunology of New York Hospital [41]. A variety of injectable materials became available for the treatment of allergic patients whose problems were not exclusively seasonal.

Botanists identified and collected pollens of regional indigenous trees, grasses, and weeds, and developed methods for aerobiological sampling to provide the information and technology essential for specific diagnosis [42–46].

Hospital and clinic sections devoted to diagnosis and treatment of allergic disorders [47] were established. Immunization procedures were extended and applied to the treatment of asthma. With favorable results recorded in the treatment of seasonal asthmatic manifestations by pollen immunization, similar benefits were sought for chronic asthma by injections of extracts of perennial allergens and bacterial vaccines [38,48,49].

Medications capable of relieving allergic and asthmatic manifestations were relatively unavailable. During those early years, only epinephrine and atropine were mentioned as primary therapeutic agents and iodide, acetyl salicylate, anesthetic ether, morphine, and cocaine and their derivatives (with cautious qualifications) as secondary medications [50]. The pharmacologic action of ephedrine, with its limited value, was not defined until 1924 by Chen and Schmidt [51].

The strong leadership of Cooke and the dedication of Coca provided opportunities for training, experience, and structured courses on preparation and use of allergenic vaccines [52]. From these endeavors, an increasing number of clinics were seeded in the U.S. cities [53].

Rapid dissemination and application of the newly developed methods for identification of specific agents of hypersensitivity and desensitization therapy for hay fever and asthma patients engendered a new set of problems and questions complicating logical approaches well into the 1940s [53]. The era of grant-supported full-time institutional-based academic and research positions in allergy and clinical immunology was then still some three to four decades away. Meanwhile, awaiting definition through research-generated data, there developed a wide variability in ideas, criteria for indications, usage of materials, and methods and design of injection treatment plans. Adding to the complexity, Storm van Leeuwen in 1924 introduced a role for airborne mold spores as allergens after a comprehensive study of the seasonal pollen problem [54]. Thommen (Figure 1.12) formulated a set of postulates that offered rational guidelines for the assessment of specific tree, grass, and weed species in the etiology of hay fever and as a source of immunotherapeutic agents [55]: (1) The pollen must contain an excitant of hay fever. (2) The pollen must be anemophilous (i.e., wind borne) as regard to its mode of pollination. (3) The pollen

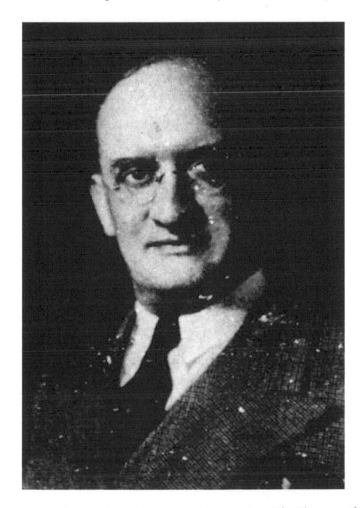

Figure 1.12 August A. Thommen, MD (1892–1943). Director of Allergy Clinic, New York University College of Medicine, New York. (Courtesy of New York Public Library.)

must be produced in sufficiently large quantities. It is characteristic of wind-pollinated flowers in general that they produce pollen in far greater quantities than flowers, which are insect pollinated. (4) The pollen must be sufficiently buoyant to be carried to considerable distances. (5) The plant producing the pollen must be widely and abundantly distributed.

Principles of preseasonal pollen desensitization were then applied to the treatment of patients with year-round reactions with vaccines of a variety of perennial allergens that had given positive skin reactions. Of these, house dust as an agent was described by Kern in 1921 [56] and its role became increasingly recognized as an important environmental allergen in respiratory disease. The high prevalence of positive skin tests to dust vaccines initiated a widespread use of stock and autogenous house dust vaccines for injection treatment of perennial rhinitis and asthma. Although there often was insufficient evidence to define the allergenic activity of house dust, a positive skin test alone—without differentiation of irritant properties of test materials—was frequently accepted as indication for its use. Some confusion in differentiating house dust-sensitive disease from nonallergic chronic respiratory disease led Boatner and Efron to develop a "purified" house dust vaccine with the objective of increasing the diagnostic significance of a positive skin test to house dust [57].

There was an obvious need to develop suitable guidelines for efficacious injection treatment methods with a minimum of untoward constitutional reactions. Progress depended on the availability of vaccines of uniform strength and stability. Cooke attempted to bypass the problems of variations in allergenic activity of different pollen batches (because of seasonal plant growth factors and/or inadequate storage of collected pollen) by using an assay of total nitrogen content in standardization, although he did note that total nitrogen and allergenic activity were not identical [58,59]. Subsequently, with a collaborating chemist, Stull, he developed and championed a unit on the basis of measurement of protein nitrogen content as a more accurate representation of residual stable activity of allergenic fractions [59].

Early treatment programs were developed by trial and error, and efficacy varied accordingly. In general, skin test reactivity was used for the determination of starting doses, their increments, and frequency of administration. Perennial rhinitis and asthma mandated uninterrupted treatment schedules, but the superiority of perennial versus preseasonal plans for treatment of hay fever could not be settled by impressions and anecdotal reports. Modifications of schedule were devised for applying the principle of desensitization within compressed time frames. Pollen extract injections were given in small daily doses when initiated after seasonal symptoms had already begun [60]. An intensive schedule of daily injections was required if initiated within 2 weeks of the anticipated seasonal onset [61,62]. Other modes and variations for pollen desensitization were described in 1921–1922 [63–67]: (1) daily nasal and throat sprays with atomized vaccines [63], (2) pollen-containing ointments applied to the nasal mucosa [64], (3) oral administration [65], (4) intracutaneous injections [66], and (5) a full-cycle return to Blackley's attempt 50 years earlier by contact at needle-puncture or skin-abraded sites [67].

1.4 EARLY DEVELOPMENTAL YEARS

In 1931, the (Western) Association for the Study of Allergy and the (Eastern) Society for the Study of Asthma and Allied Conditions established a Joint Committee of Survey and Standardization that achieved one objective by the mid-1930s: approval of medical school and hospital allergy clinics to meet the guidelines for allergy training developed by the committee [68]. However, the committee was unable to define standards for methods and materials. A lack of correlation was noted between skin test results and allergic manifestations in too many patients. Also, the committee believed that proper standardization must await the isolation and purification of etiologically responsible components of allergen vaccine such as accomplished by Heidelberger and Avery in isolating and purifying the specific soluble substances (capsular polysaccharide) of the pneumococcus [69].

In 1992, Cooke reported that cutaneous reactivity was not eliminated in patients receiving injection treatments for asthma or allergic conditions owing to horse and rabbit dander and serum. This contrasted with desensitization that accomplished complete inactivation of antibody action in animal models of anaphylaxis. Cooke, perceiving that the differences were functions of different mechanisms, referred to the beneficial effects of allergen injections rather as a result of hyposensitization than due to neutralization or desensitization [70]. This concept was confirmed in 1926 by Levine and Coca [71] and Jadassohn [72], both of whom found clinical improvement and allergen activity to be independent of effect, if any, on skin-sensitizing (reaginic) antibody. Levine and Coca's study also demonstrated that a rapid (two- to fourfold) increase in serum reaginic antibody sometimes followed allergen injections. This finding helped to explain some paradoxical observations in treatment programs that had been designed to lessen specific hypersensitivities. For example, (1) severe constitutional reactions followed small increments or even repeated the previously well-tolerated dosage, especially in early stages of injection schedules [73]; (2) local tolerance diminished even with reduced vaccine dosage; and (3) symptoms of the treated allergic disorder might increase rather than decrease.

In 1930, Freeman introduced "rush desensitization" in which injections of pollen vaccines were given at 1.5- to –2-hour intervals over a daily 14-hour period, under close observation and in a hospital setting [74]. Since the benefits to be derived were generally believed to be outweighed by the danger of severe reactions, rush desensitization found little receptivity in the United States.

In 1935, Cooke's group, relocated in a new Department of Allergy at New York's Roosevelt Hospital, presented evidence in favor of a protective serum factor induced by injection treatments [75]. Further, the transferable nature of the factor was indicated by Loveless's report that blood transfusions from ragweed-sensitive donors treated with pollen vaccine injections conferred equivalent beneficial effects on untreated ragweed-sensitive recipients during the hay fever season [76]. This finding provided the lead for extended investigation centered at the target tissue cell level.

The ability of posttreatment serum to inhibit reactions between serum-containing reaginic antibody and corresponding pollen allergen at passively sensitized cutaneous test sites by the technique of Prausnitz and Kustner (P-K test reaction) [76] was attributed to the effects of "blocking antibody" induced by injection treatment [77]. Demonstration, in specifically treated patients, of coexistent, characteristically different—sensitizing and blocking—antibodies provided both the technique and stimulus for continuing the study of hyposensitization phenomena. Additionally, relevant contributions by Cooke and associates included demonstrations of (1) production of the inhibiting factor (blocking antibody) by nonallergic individuals as a function of normal immune responsiveness [75], (2) specificity of blocking antibody activity and its relationship to the pseudoglobulin serum factor [77], and (3) decreases in serum reagin titers after long-term allergen immunotherapy [78].

Fortuitously, in 1955, the impetus to search for alternative explanations coincident with the emergence of the National Institute of Allergy and Infectious Diseases (NIAID), a body within the National Institutes of Health, spurred the establishment of the requisite resources to support relevant research endeavors. In an early project, Vannier and Campbell undertook pertinent immunochemical studies on the allergenic fraction of house dust [79]. A lead project, on the basis of a large multicenter collaborative study, later focused on the characterization of other allergens, and a working group was organized under Campbell's chairmanship. Ragweed was the selected prototype for initial investigation by subcommittees for chemistry, animal testing, and clinical trials. The subsequent isolation of the major allergenic fraction of ragweed pollen, designated as antigen E, provided the first quantifiable reagent for standardization of skin test and treatment extracts [80].

1.5 BACTERIAL VACCINES

A belief that nasopharyngeal bacterial flora were involved in the pathogenesis of the common cold led to a study in London in which Allen developed a respiratory bacterial vaccine [81]. The possibility that the immunizing effect of such an autogenous preparation might be of value in the treatment of respiratory illnesses other than the common cold led to its application to hay fever. The introduction, in 1912–1913, of bacterial vaccines for the management of seasonal rhinitis was integrated with an attempt to ameliorate nasopharyngeal and paranasal sinus infection as presumed factors in hay fever [82]. Morrey reasoned that a nasal mucosa strengthened by bacterial vaccination would be resistant to the effects of whatever irritants were responsible for hay fever [83]. Lowdermilk, in 1914, followed up both reports and utilized both Noon's pollen toxin and Allen's bacterial vaccine formulations in his introduction of immunotherapy [35].

Goodale's report of skin test reactions to bacterial preparations in vasomotor rhinitis [84] was followed by great interest in putative relationships between bacteria and asthma [85,86]. Walker, in popularizing the scratch test, extended the technique to a number of bacterial species along with pollens, perennial inhalants, and foods, and introduced autogenous vaccines into the treatment of asthma [86,87]. The groundwork for adopting the concept of bacterial allergy was already in place. It focused on demonstrations of (1) induced sensitization to bacteria in guinea pig models of anaphylaxis [88] and (2) skin test and systemic reactivity to bacterial products associated with active infection (e.g., tuberculin) [89].

Further clinical relevance was provided by Rackemann's classic study, which defined intrinsic asthma [90] as a subset in patients with infective asthma, eosinophilia, and family backgrounds of extrinsic allergic diseases—a disorder later characterized by Cooke as presumptively immunologically mediated [91]. Subsequent studies of treatment programs demonstrated lack of specificity of positive scratch, intracutaneous, and subcutaneous test reactions to bacterial preparations [92], as well as lack of specific or enhanced efficacy of autogenous over stock bacterial vaccines [93]. Although the concept of desensitization or hyposensitization mechanisms as responsible for beneficial effects in infective asthma was put aside, respiratory bacterial vaccines continued to occupy a prominent place in clinical practice. Cooke related respiratory tract infection, especially chronic sinusitis, to asthma, and exacerbations of asthmatic symptoms

to incremental overdoses of bacterial vaccine. On the basis of his experiences, he was a strong proponent of immunotherapy with autogenous vaccines as adjuvants for prevention of recurrences after removal of focal infection, particularly from the paranasal sinuses and upper respiratory tract [94].

Respiratory bacterial vaccines became entrenched immunotherapeutic agents. The first report of controlled trials, however, did not appear until 1955 [95], but within the next 4 years, publication of two additional studies followed [96,97]. Each failed to find efficacy for bacterial vaccines in attempts to prevent or treat asthma that was demonstrably related to respiratory infection. Following these reports, subsequent critical observations, and the diminishing influence of the earlier investigators whose uncontrolled impressions had influenced the clinical scene, respiratory bacterial vaccines slowly fell out of favor.

1.6 CLINICAL TRIALS

A new initiative cut to the heart of the accepted role of allergen immunotherapy when Lowell—whose in-depth experience and analytical probing added credibility to his position—heralded the need for sound investigation to meet the requirements of statistical significance [98]. A valid and unbiased evaluation of results of allergen immunotherapy, especially of pollenosis, was not available because controls for the many variables of periodic disease were found lacking in published trials. Sample sizes were too limited for tests of significance, and inconsistent seasonal, climatic, environmental, and biologically fluctuating factors had not been subjected to adequately controlled study.

"Controlled" studies presented during the preceding 10 years [99–101] were all found to be flawed. Reliance on historical features had not been replaced by placebo controls; double blinding of both subject and evaluator had not been followed; a single test group often consisted of pretreatment and newly entered patients; and comparable groups had not always been balanced for equivalent sensitivities (e.g., by skin test titrations). Lowell and Franklin then performed a double-blind trial of treatment of allergic rhinitis because of ragweed sensitivity. They reported that patients receiving injections of ragweed pollen vaccine had fewer symptoms and lower medication scores than a control group. The beneficial effect was specific for ragweed, and the effect diminished in varying degrees within 5 months after discontinuing treatments [102]. The following year, Fontana et al. reported that any beneficial effect of hyposensitization therapy in ragweed hay fever in children was indistinguishable from differences likely to occur in untreated controls [103]. Their study, however, looked only for the presence or disappearance of symptoms, rather than at comparable degrees of severity [104].

Immunotherapy gained credibility with the introduction of new evaluatory measurements (i.e., symptom index score and the *in vitro* measure of leukocyte histamine release) [105], especially in children [106].

1.7 ANTIGEN DEPOTS

During the late 1930s, allergen vaccines were modified in an effort to decrease the frequency of injections. Depot-like immunogenic materials were prepared to provide a slow, continuous release of allergen from injection sites. The first attempt used ground raw pollen suspended in olive oil [107]. Because particulate bacterial vaccines and modified toxoid proved to be effective immunogens, soluble pollen allergen vaccines were converted to particulate suspensions by alum precipitation and alum adsorption [108,109]. Other modifications included acetylation, heat, and formalin treatment [109]; precipitation by tannic [110] and hydrochloric acids [111]; and a mixture with gelatin [112]. Of these, only alum-adsorbed pollen extracts gained any popularity. Treatment of hay fever with an emulsified allergen vaccine was introduced by Naterman, who in 1937 emulsified a pollen extract with lanolin and olive oil [113]. Thirteen years later, he suspended grass and ragweed pollen tannate in peanut oil with aluminum monostearate [114]. Malkiel and Feinberg, encouraged by evidence of slow absorption from new penicillin-in-oil depot formulations, prepared extracts of ragweed in sesame oil–aluminum monostearate. With these, however, they were unable to avoid constitutional reactions, while failing to reduce the severity of symptoms [115]. Furthermore, other investigators detected increased titers of neutralizing antibody in treated patients without clinical benefit, thus casting doubt on the clinical relevance of "blocking" antibody [116,117].

Clinical trials with repository therapy, initiated by Loveless in 1947 [76], gave highly favorable results as reported 10 years later [119]. This stimulated the first major departure from conventional injection treatment schedules. Loveless, firmly believing that successful treatment was a function of induced "blocking" antibody, aimed her protocols at maintaining the highest possible humoral levels of blocking antibody. She was convinced that the threshold of conjunctival responses to graded local challenges was a valid measure of systemic sensitivity and that suppression of both depended on the generation of neutralizing factor. Although there were no data to equate desired results with those reported for influenza vaccine [120], she used the depot medium that Freund and McDermott had developed [121] as an immunogen adjuvant in experimental animal models. A large dose of pollen vaccine, calculated as the cumulative total that would be given in the course of a conventional preseason schedule, was emulsified in oil with an emulsion stabilizer, and administered as a single intramuscular injection [76,119]. A number of anecdotal reports by Brown spoke of "thousands" of uniformly successful results of treatment with emulsified vaccines of pollen and other airborne allergens [122]. However, adverse reactions consisting of late formation and persistence of nodules, sterile abscesses, and granulomata, and a potential for induction of delayed hypersensitivity to injected antigens were found inherent in emulsion therapy. Furthermore, subsequent controlled studies failed to confirm significant therapeutic effectiveness [123–125]. Finally, emulsion therapy was discontinued after a report that mineral oil and mineral oil adjuvants induced plasma cell myelomas in a certain strain of mice [126], and the U.S. Food and Drug Administration (FDA) did not approve the repository emulsion for therapy.

1.8 ORAL ROUTE TO TOLERANCE AND DESENSITIZATION

Possibilities for inducing protection by feeding on causative agents date back to stories of poisons in antiquity. In the first century BC, Mithradates VI (131–63 BC) (Figure 1.13), King of Pontus in Asia Minor, noted that ducks who fed on plants known to be poisonous to humans did not manifest any apparent ill effects. Applying

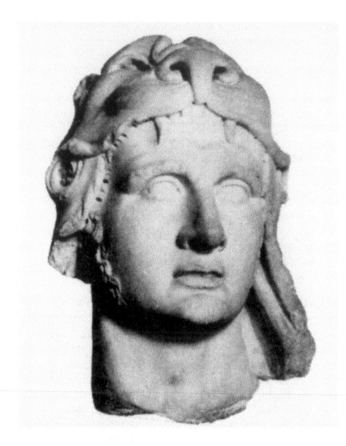

Figure 1.13 Mithradates VI Eupator (c. 131–63 BC), King of Pontus in Asia Minor. (Courtesy of the Musee de Louvre, Paris.)

this observation, he incorporated ducks' blood in an antidote he attempted to develop against poisons—an early concept of passive immunization. Further, in preparing himself for the ever-present possibility of a palace revolt, Mithradates VI sought to gain immunity from poisoning by swallowing small amounts of poison—particularly toadstool toxins—in gradually increasing doses [127]. So successful was the outcome of his experiments that he later failed to achieve attempted suicide by ingesting large doses of the same poison [128]. For many subsequent centuries, the technique of gaining tolerance or active immunity through incremental dosage schedules continued to be known as mithradatising.

The renowned Greek physician Claudius Galen (AD 130–200), who practiced in Rome, had noted that snake venoms taken by mouth were devoid of the systemic toxic actions effected by snake bites [129]. According to folklore, this knowledge allowed snake charmers of the classic Greco-Roman era to acquire protection against potentially fatal bites by drinking from serpent-infested water that contained traces of their venoms [130]—a less traumatic method than seeking protection through self-inflicted bites.

Moving to a more recent era and the beginning of the scientific study of immunity, in 1891 Ehrlich provided experimental evidence of orally achieved toxin tolerance in mice by feeding them the toxins ricin and abrin [131]. Then germane to delayed hypersensitivity, in 1946 Chase demonstrated an inhibiting effect of prior feeding [132]. The earliest recorded journal item of clinical relevance was noted in a description of plant-induced allergic contact dermatitis in 1829 [133]. In his discussion, Dakin reported that chewing poison ivy leaves, both as prevention and cure, was recommended by some "good meaning, marvelous, mystical physicians," despite adverse side effects—eruption, swelling, redness, and intolerable itching around the verge of the anus. It was also a practice seen among native North Americans (Indians), who chewed and swallowed the juice of early shoots as a preventive measure against the development of poison ivy dermatitis during ensuing summer months [134]. Apparently, this method had been found to be of some value since it was used in rural areas and by park workers and was considered an example of effective homeopathic autotherapy [135]. A novel modification reported partial immunity after drinking milk from cows deliberately fed poison ivy in grass mixtures [136].

The first move to explain the procedure that originated in folk medicine in terms of immune phenomena began with the approach of Strickler in 1918. Although unable to demonstrate circulating blood antibodies in patients affected by poison ivy and poison oak dermatitis, Strickler postulated the likely pathogenesis to be a form of "tissue immunity" to the plant toxins. Believing the mechanism to be similar to that of hay fever, he introduced adaptation of desensitization for treatment and prevention of the plant-related contact dermatitis with extracts of the alcohol-soluble leaf fraction given by intramuscular injection [137]. The following year, Schamberg introduced an oral approach to prophylactic desensitization using incremental drop doses of a tincture of *Rhus toxicodendron* [138]. Strickler's follow-up report 3 years later indicated favorable acceptance of intramuscular injection, oral methods, and a combination of both [134]. Although trials during subsequent years supported this early usage [139], there were differing reports varying from only short-term immunizing effects [140] to lack of either clinical benefit [141] or increased tolerance [142].

Despite divergence of opinion, the oral method of preventive therapy remained popular for 50-some years. Alcohol and acetone extracts in vegetable oils were prepared from a variety of plant-source polyhydric phenols (e.g., the *Rhus* ivy-oak-sumac group, primula, geranium, tulip, and chrysanthemum). In 1940, Shelmire expanded the spectrum of plant sources of delayed hypersensitivity by identifying ether-soluble fractions of pollens responsible for producing allergic contact dermatitis through airborne exposure. These were distinct from water-soluble pollen albumins implicated in the immediate hypersensitivity phenomenon of hay fever. Through Shelmire's work, preparations of specific pollen oleoresins were then made available for oral desensitization [143].

Proponents in the 1940s and 1950s based their belief in the validity of desensitization methods for plant contact dermatitis on the concept of cell-associated "antibody" to chemical haptens in the pathogenesis of delayed cutaneous hypersensitivity. However, there were complicating problems in the nature of induced dermatitis at locally injected or previously involved distal sites, exacerbations of existing lesions, stomatitis, gastroenteritis, anal pruritus, and dermatitis from mucous membrane contact with oral preparations. Additionally, in the face of a lack of convincing evidence of efficacy, the practice gradually faded from popular usage.

On a parallel track, a similar thought was being given to treatment of another group of allergic disorders that Coca in 1923 characterized as atopic—hay fever, asthma, and eczema. The first case record of desensitization to an allergenic food came from England in 1908, with Schoffield's report of successful reversal of severe egg-induced asthma, urticaria, and angioedema in a 13-year-old boy by the daily feedings of egg in homeopathic doses [144]. Three years later, Finzio, in Italy, reported similar success with cow's milk in infants [145]. Shortly thereafter, favorable results of trials of desensitization to foods in children were reported in the United States by Schloss—in a study that coincidentally established practicability of the scratch test in hypersensitivity [37]—and in a study by Talbot [146]. Owing to possible anaphylactic reactions to only a minute amount of an allergenic food in an exquisitely sensitive individual, Pagniez and Vallery-Radot in 1916 pre-fed patients with food digests consisting predominantly of peptones. Theoretically, these foods were reduced in allergenicity by the treatment process but retained immunogenic specificity [147,148]. Acceptance of oral food desensitization plans declined with later negative experiences [149,150].

The first use of an orally administered pollen-related preparation appeared in the homeopathic literature of 1890 with the description of "ambrose," a tincture of fresh flower heads and young shoots, recommended for the treatment of hay fever [151]. Impressed by an experience in which asthma caused by inhalation of ipecac was prevented with drop doses of syrup or tincture of ipecac, Curtis explored a like possibility in hay fever. In 1900—in conjunction with introduction of flower and pollen vaccines—he noted preliminary efficacious results with tincture and fluid extracts of ragweed flowers and pollen taken by mouth [19]. Touart later reported varying responses in six patients given enteric-coated tablet triturates of grass and ragweed pollen [65]. In 1927, Black demonstrated that large doses of orally administered ragweed extract effectively lowered nasal threshold responses to inhalational challenges [153] but later reported a large series of patients with results less favorable than could be expected after injection treatments [154]. Urbach attempted to bypass distressing gastrointestinal symptoms following ingestion of pollen vaccines by advocating oral administration of specific pollen digest peptones (propetan) [155]. Since collection of pollen supplies was difficult, Urbach prepared peptone derivatives of blossoms of trees, grasses, and grass seeds for use as orally administered allergens [156]. Passive transfer experiments by Bernstein and Feinberg calculated that more than a pound of raw pollen would be required orally to reach a circulating antigen concentration obtained by injection of maximally tolerated doses of pollen vaccine [157]. Also, a multicenter, collaborative, placebo-controlled study conducted later confirmed the lack of efficacy of this method [158].

1.9 DRUGS AND BIOLOGICAL PRODUCTS

The purported effectiveness of oral desensitization to foods was soon applied to drug hypersensitivity, and a report of successful oral desensitization of a malaria patient with anaphylactic hypersensitivity to quinine appeared in the French literature [159]. When the allergenic character of pharmaceutical and biological products derived from plant and animal sources became increasingly evident, attempts were made to desensitize reactive patients who otherwise would be deprived of essential specific therapy. An early problem was treatment of the horse-sensitive patient with horse antidiphtheria or antitetanus antiserum [160]. The cautious injections of horse dander vaccine offered some measure of protection after long-term treatment [161]. However, the potential for anaphylaxis resulting from the large volumes of therapeutic antisera required was too great. Even a minute dose could cause a fatal reaction [162], and early trials had failed to accomplish desensitization [163,164].

Success was achieved in use of dried and pulverized ipecacuanha plant root for treatment of ipecac-sensitive asthmatic pharmacists and physicians and of beef or pork insulin for desensitization injection of sensitive diabetes patients who required insulin replacement therapy [165,166].

Freeman's method of "rush inoculation" with pollen vaccines [74] was not generally accepted. However, the principle was effectively applied in treating drug hypersensitivities requiring prompt resumption of therapy, such as with insulin to control diabetes [167] and penicillin when required as the essential antibiotic to control a specific and severe infection [168]. This procedure probably induced transient anaphylactic desensitization, as first demonstrated in the guinea pig [28], or by a mechanism of hapten inhibition [169]. Over 40–50 years, a number of publications have affirmed effective desensitization to pharmaceutical products responsible for hypersensitivity reactions [170–172].

1.10 INSECT ANTIGENS

In classical Greece of the fourth century BC, the philosopher-biologist Aristotle, who had written extensively on the life history, types, and behavior patterns of bees, in his *Historia Animalia* noted their ability to sting large animals to death—even one as large as a horse. Yet it was recognized that beekeepers in the course of their work could be repeatedly or periodically stung without ill effect. No attempt was made to duplicate this observed natural phenomenon until the early years of the twentieth century, when the possibility of ameliorating insect hypersensitivity was provided by the description of favorable responses to injection treatments with extracts of gnats [173] and bees [174]. Hyposensitization to other species was also explored using mosquito [175] and flea [176] extracts. Some failed attempts were not understood until the acquisition of knowledge that delayed (cell-mediated) hypersensitivity and biochemistry of inflammation were the responsible mechanisms.

Whether hypersensitivity-induced states owed their reduction to the raising of blocking antibodies or to later defined mechanisms of regulatory control of IgE production, elements of cell-mediated immunity did not lend themselves to comparable diminishing effects sought in allergen immunotherapy for immediate hypersensitivity disorders.

Fine hairs and epithelial scales shed by swarming insects were also identified as airborne allergens responsible for conjunctivitis, rhinitis, and asthma, which could be managed by hyposensitization [177,178]. Benson reported extensive studies of *Hymenoptera* allergy and hyposensitization with whole-body vaccine. Efficacy of treatment was demonstrated for anaphylactic sensitivity to the venom of stings and for inhalant allergy to body parts and emanations incurred by exposed beekeepers [179]. Hyposensitization therapy employed whole-body vaccines until Loveless—based on her discovery and definition of neutralizing (blocking) factor as therapeutically responsible for the efficacy of pollen hyposensitization in hay fever—sought the same objective for the *Hymenoptera*-anaphylactically sensitive patient. She then introduced several variations: (1) use of isolated contents of dissected venom sacs in conventional hyposensitization schedules, (2) single-repository immunization with venom emulsified in oil adjuvant, (3) "rush" desensitization, and (4) deliberate controlled stinging with captured wasps to ascertain establishment and maintenance of a protective state [180,181]. Later studies confirmed the far greater efficacy of venom allergens (Chapter 18).

1.11 NONSPECIFIC IMMUNOTHERAPY

Attempts were made to duplicate the benefits of specific hyposensitization by altering, initiating, or regulating immune system functions through injections with a variety of nonspecific antigens (e.g., typhoid and mixed coliform vaccines, cow's milk, snake venom, soybean, and creation of a sterile fixation abscess with injection of turpentine) [182,183]. It was thought that repeated injections of small doses of protein-digested peptones might evoke subclinical anaphylactic mechanisms with resultant desensitization to a multiplicity of allergens [184].

Another global approach employing the administration of autogenous blood visualized that injected (autohemato- and autoserotherapeutic) samples contained absorbed causative allergens in quantities too small to produce an attack, yet sufficiently minutely antigenic to induce tolerance [185].

Another indirect approach considered possible benefits that might be derived from attempted hyposensitization responses to antigens to which specific sensitization resulted from past infection but were concurrently inactive and unrelated to the etiology of asthma. Two such agents—tuberculin [186] and the highly reaginic and anaphylactic antibody-inducing extract of *Ascaris lumbricoides* [187]—were given to correspondingly positive skin test reactors according to conventional hyposensitization schedules.

If unable to accomplish specific hyposensitization, therapy attempted to neutralize the alleged mediator of allergic reactions (i.e., histamine). Histamine "desensitization" was first introduced in 1932 for treatment of cold urticaria in the expectation that daily incremental injections would achieve correspondingly increased degrees of tolerance to histamine and thereby diminish allergic symptoms [188]. Enzymatic destruction of released histamine in urticaria and atopic dermatitis was then attempted with parenteral or oral administration of histaminase [189]. An immune-mediated blocking of histamine was postulated through injections of a histamine-linked antigen ([histamine-azo-depreciated horse serum] hapamine) to induce antihistamine antibodies [190]. While some of these modalities were initially encouraging, later studies failed to confirm their benefit. Favorable symptomatic improvements of empirical but nonspecific treatment designed to modulate immune functions could not be determined without controlled clinical trials. The use of these agents fell by the wayside as new scientific knowledge of allergy mechanisms was acquired [191].

1.12 UPDATE FOR THE FIFTH EDITION

Allergen immunotherapy used to treat allergic diseases for over 100 years both defines and distinguishes the specialty and practice of allergy and clinical immunology [201]. While much of the initial work in the therapeutic application of allergen immunotherapy was by necessity, empiric, enormous scientific strides have been made in the last 15 years in both the clinical delivery of such therapy and most crucially, the molecular mechanisms by which it actually works. This historical perspective offers a fascinating window into the past and the many dedicated scientists and clinicians leading up to Noon and Freeman and their landmark study and those who have subsequently refined the practice of allergen immunotherapy. However, in these final paragraphs, a look to the future and a review of advances of the past one-and-a-half decades, with particular attention to the mechanistic underpinnings of allergen immunotherapy, molecularly modified allergens, and alternative allergen immunotherapy delivery, are necessary. Many of these advances are made possible by the explosion of robust genomic, molecular, and informatics technologies, which have become an integral part of biomedical research.

Allergen immunotherapy was thought to be clinically effective for many years before a thorough understanding of the mechanisms that underlie its efficacy was achieved. One of the earliest insights into the possibility of allergen desensitization was the proposal of specific IgG "blocking antibodies" put forth by Robert A. Cooke in 1935 [202]. Twenty years later, Cooke and his colleagues confirmed in ragweed-treated patients via electrophoretic mobility studies that this factor was γ-globulin [203]. While the blocking antibody concept fell out of favor for a time, it, once again, has been convincingly demonstrated by other investigators, including Stephen Durham and his colleagues, that induction of IgG4 is an important part of the humoral response in grass allergen immunotherapy [204]. Though unproven, induction of allergen-specific IgG4 likely allows allergen capture prior to binding mast cell and basophil-bound IgE. Beyond the blocking antibody concept, however, the regulatory T cell is also implicated as a central event in the induction of allergen tolerance to allergen immunotherapy. These regulatory T cells produce two critical immunosuppressant cytokines, IL-10 and TGF-β. Akdis and colleagues first recognized the fundamental importance of IL-10, which Chen and colleagues extended by demonstrating that TGF-β is required for the FOXP3-mediated conversion of naïve $CD4^+$ $CD25^-$ T cells into the $CD24^+$ $CD25^+$ regulatory T-cell type [205,206]. The regulatory T-cell induction also causes a skewing toward a Th1 versus a Th2 response commonly associated with atopic phenotypes. Both the reemergence of the importance of the blocking antibody IgG4 and the central role of the regulatory T-cell response are important milestones in the understanding of how to induce a tolerogenic state in allergic individuals.

In addition to the enhanced understanding of the mechanisms of allergen immunotherapy, a proliferation of novel immunomodulatory strategies for allergen-specific immunotherapy has occurred over the past several decades. One emerging method is to modulate the innate immune system synchronously with allergen-specific changes via linking pollen extracts to toll-like receptor (TLR) agonists. This approach has been attempted with both TLR4 and TLR9 agonists, though neither has gone beyond early phase trials due to difficulties with adverse events or study design issues [207,208]. Recombinant allergens have been used either as a mixture in a pilot study in grass-allergic patients or as a single fusion protein encompassing multiple major allergens expressed in a mouse model of *Hymenoptera* allergy [209,210]. At the present time, there are no licensed conjugated or recombinant allergens available for clinical use, though the previously mentioned strategies show promise. Finally, the use of omalizumab, a monoclonal anti-IgE antibody, has been applied in the initiation phase of allergen immunotherapy for allergic rhinitis. This approach demonstrated a decrease in the frequency of systemic reactions [211].

Novel immunotherapy delivery approaches represent yet another area of active investigation. Paramount among these is the development and refinement of sublingual immunotherapy (SLIT). The use of SLIT to treat allergic diseases dates back to the beginning of the twentieth century; however, dose-response studies were never performed, leading to suboptimal doses and ineffective therapy, as demonstrated in a variety of different early studies on sublingual immunotherapy [212]. Over the past two decades, this form of therapy has been revitalized. In 1998, the World Health Organization paper, "Allergen immunotherapy: therapeutic vaccines for allergic diseases" included the statement "Sublingual (swallow) immunotherapy may be indicated in pollen and mite induced rhinitis" [213]. Subsequently in 2009, the World Allergy Organization published a position paper on SLIT, which indicated that SLIT therapy was safe and clinically effective after a review of over 60 controlled trials, the majority of which were monomeric therapy to either grass or dust mite [214]. Most of the studies quoted in this paper were not appropriately configured for the subjects studied. However, several high-quality and appropriately controlled studies are now published, which achieve statistical significance [215–217].

It should be noted that while SLIT has been an accepted part of the practice of allergy in Europe and in other parts of the world for the last decade, regulatory approval by the FDA is still pending. SLIT for other applications such as food allergy is still investigational at this point, though it is an active area of research. In addition, several groups have demonstrated that intralymphatic injection of allergen as well as transdermal delivery of allergens may offer novel routes to achieve clinical improvement in atopic patients more rapidly than traditional schedules via either the subcutaneous or sublingual routes [218–220].

This historical perspective offers an opportunity to reflect on the personalities of forbears in the specialty as they sought to apply and understand allergen immunotherapy used to treat their patients with atopic diseases. Molecular, genomic, and bioinformatics technologies hold vast promise not only in treating allergic diseases but also in preventing them. This history of allergen immunotherapy honors those many clinicians, some named, many unnamed, who devoted their careers to the study of allergen immunotherapy and to the improvement of patients with allergic diseases.

1.13 UPDATE FOR THE SIXTH EDITION

There are a number of new immunotherapy modalities that merit discussion since this history chapter was last published. These include sublingual immunotherapy (SLIT) for environmental allergens, oral immunotherapy (OIT) as a therapeutic option for food allergy, and the increasing number of biologics that antagonize specific molecular pathways of allergic and immunologic diseases.

There are four SLIT products that now have regulatory approval in the United States. Two are directed against grass pollen (Grastek, ALK-Abello, Hørsholm, Denmark, 2014; Oralair, Stallergenes Greer, Boston, Massachusetts, 2014); one against ragweed pollen (Ragwitek, ALK-Abello, Hørsholm, Denmark, 2014); and the last a dust mite–specific product (Odactra, ALK-Abello, Hørsholm, Denmark, 2017). All are formulated as sublingual tablets that dissolve under the tongue, versus the aqueous format of SLIT that has been used off-label and is still used in the United States. Difficulties with liquid SLIT include the deficiency of adequate dose-ranging studies and the fact that extrapolating from European data is difficult, given the widely varying allergen contents of available extracts [221]. SLIT efficacy has been demonstrated in numerous studies, and the U.S. regulatory approval of these products is a welcome endorsement of this treatment modality. However, a problem for these products is that the U.S. allergic versus the European allergic subject is usually polysensitized, somewhat restricting the utility of single allergen SLIT. Nevertheless, this remains an option for atopic subjects with one dominant allergen sensitivity or for whom there may be practical or logistical impediments to subcutaneous immunotherapy.

OIT for the desensitization of food-allergic subjects is now beginning to reach an inflection point in the United States and offers an active treatment beyond food avoidance. As of 2018, more than 2000 patients have been treated by 68 clinicians practicing OIT in the United States [118]. A typical protocol involves a standard escalation regimen on the "day 1" visit, usually given over several hours, to achieve a final subthreshold dose that does not induce a systemic allergic reaction, for instance, 2 mg of peanut protein. Thereafter, patients are dosed at a fixed daily dose at home and usually return to the clinic for an "updose" every 1–2 weeks. OIT is generally well tolerated, but it is essential that other allergic conditions, such as allergic rhinitis and asthma, be appropriately under control prior to beginning or continuing this therapy. Serious systemic allergic reactions are rare, occurring and requiring epinephrine in 1:1000 OIT doses as reported in a peanut OIT protocol [195]. There are dosing parameters that significantly decrease the rate of reaction, such as ensuring that OIT is not taken on an empty stomach, avoiding physical activity for several hours following the dose, and avoiding dosing with an illness, particularly with a fever [118]. Initiating OIT in an allergy clinic requires a substantial commitment by the physician and other healthcare professionals, since the clinic personnel have to prepare the foods for precise on-site dosing. It also requires 24/7 physician availability and a dedicated nursing staff in the clinic. Some clinics pursue multiple food OIT simultaneously, but it is more common to complete OIT for one food prior to beginning the same process for another food. OIT can be extremely helpful for patients and parents committed to a more active approach to food allergy management. An FDA Advisory Committee approved a standardized peanut protein powder developed by Aimmune Therapeutics in September 2019 (www.aimmune.com). However, it is not yet commercially available [152].

Finally, while this text is devoted to allergen-specific immunotherapy, it is impossible to ignore the changing landscape to treat asthma, particularly severe asthma, and other atopic diseases using available biologics. While these medications do not block selective allergens per se, they target the allergic pathway and interrupt the allergic cascade. Thus, they most properly are immunomodulatory agents. Omalizumab (Genetech, South San Francisco, California), which targets IgE, was approved in 2003 to treat severe allergic asthma and in 2014 for severe refractory chronic urticaria. Several anti-IL-5 therapies have also been approved, including mepolizumab (GlaxoSmithKline, Brentford, United Kingdom, 2015), benralizumab (AstraZeneca, Cambridge, United Kingdom, 2017), and reslizumab (Teva, Petah Tikva, Israel, 2016). All three IL-5 targeting biologics are indicated primarily for the eosinophilic phenotype of asthma. The most recent addition is dupilumab, which targets both IL-4 and IL-13 by blocking the IL-4 α-receptor subunit. Dupilumab (Regeneron Pharmaceuticals, Tarrytown, New York) gained approval for atopic dermatitis in 2016 and for allergic asthma in 2018.

1.14 CONCLUDING COMMENTS

In this review of the evolution of allergen immunotherapy (Table 1.1) as a method introduced into clinical medicine almost a century ago, two retrospective considerations are particularly noteworthy. The first relates to the several decades of trial and error, recorded observations, and transition from loosely conducted trials to controlled clinical investigative protocols. Relevant knowledge of the value of allergen immunotherapy was not advanced much beyond appreciation that varied approaches helped some treated patients, some of the time, to variable degrees. Establishing a requisite informational base still looks to (1) epidemiologic studies of a scope and design to provide in-depth understanding of the natural history of asthma and allergic disease and (2) large-scale clinical trials from which to construct critical criteria for exact indications, and use of materials and methods by which immunotherapeutic regimens can be properly evaluated.

Second is the awareness of the enormous impact and influence that allergen immunotherapy had on the launching, development, and continuation of allergy as a medical specialty. For 40–50 years following the original description of skin test and hyposensitization techniques, these modalities served as the mainstays of allergy when there was little else to offer in the way of adequate and feasible management. So, arbitrary patterns of allergen immunotherapy had been implanted firmly in clinical practice that only recently was an internationally representative effort made to sort out bias and unproven impressions from verifiable fact, and an attempt made to reach consensus [191].

This review, then, leaves allergen immunotherapy with a major question: With the advent of newer, effective, symptom-relieving pharmacologic agents and new relevant knowledge on chemical mediators of inflammation, were the empirical aspects of allergen immunotherapy perpetuated beyond justification? At the same time, this consideration leaves the history of allergen immunotherapy in the midstream of new technologies in molecular biology, informational advances, and research opportunities. Current interests and activities in the design of modified antigens of enhanced efficacy, immunochemical characterization and standardization of allergen vaccines, and definition of responsible immune mechanisms and targeted responses ultimately may provide answers to questions pursued by a century of pioneering research in biomedical science—particularly immunochemistry and cellular immunology—and clinical investigation. Later chapters deal with many of these relevant advances.

SALIENT POINTS

1. Although "injection treatments" with pollen vaccines were introduced into clinical practice in the early 1900s, development of the method is rooted in the genesis and evolution of immune function dating back to antiquity. An appreciation of allergen immunotherapy viewed in this historical context follows.

2. Immunity, as a naturally occurring phenomenon, was recognized as early as the fifth century BC, with the observation that those who recovered from epidemic illness during the plague of Athens were not similarly stricken a second time [2].

3. By applying the principles of nature, prototypical methods introduced the phenomenon of induced immunity as a result of deliberate exposure to causative agents: (1) tolerance to plant poisons by ingestion of subtoxic doses (Mithradates VI, 63 BC) and (2) protection from smallpox by contact with material recovered from disease lesions (variolation; eleventh-century Chinese healers).

4. Modification of variolation introduced methods for inducing immunity with reduced risk by inoculations of (1) biologically related agents of mild disease (vaccination [4]), (2) nonpathogenic attenuated microorganisms [1], and (3) killed bacteria [7]. In spite of being a relatively harmless procedure, inoculation demonstrated a potential for producing inflammatory effects concurrent with immunity (later defined as sensitization mechanisms).

Table 1.1 Pioneering highlights along the pathway to the development and understanding of allergen immunotherapy

Time	Observation/finding	Credit
430 BC	First recorded perception of immunity; recovery from plague-endowed protection from repeated attacks.	Thucydides
63 BC	Oral tolerance: method derived from repetitious ingestion of incremental, minute, and subtoxic doses of plant poisons [127].	Mithradates VI
1712–1776	Variolation: an ancient Oriental method, introduction of induced active immunity [2,3].	Emanuel Timoni, Giacomo Pilorini
1798	Vaccination: immunity induced through biologically related inoculum [4].	Edward Jenner
1880–1884	Immune responses not dependent on pathogenicity [1] or viability [7] of inocula.	Louis Pasteur, Daniel Salmon, and Theobald Smith
1880	Conceptual method for exhausting susceptibility to hay fever by repeated application of pollen to abraded skin [18].	Charles Blackley
1897	Immunizing method derived from inoculation series of minute sublethal doses of rattlesnake venom [10].	Henry Sewall
1890	Passive immunization with tetanus and diphtheria antitoxins; introduction of therapeutic antisera [12].	Shibasaburo Kitasato and Emil von Behring
1891–1907	Adverse outcomes: hypersensitivity disorders mediated by immunizing agents. Severe nonantibody reactions to biological product of disease agent tuberculin [89]; systemic cell-mediated delayed hypersensitivity.	Robert Koch
	Anaphylaxis; immediate hypersensitivity mechanism [21].	Paul Portier and Charles Richet
	Systemic foreign serum sickness [14] and local tissue reaction (Arthus phenomenon) [192]; antigen-antibody complex mechanism.	Clemens von Pirquet and Béla Schick; Maurice Arthus
1897	Standardization of diphtheria antitoxin; introduction of concept of biological standardization with application to immunogens and antisera [13].	Paul Ehrlich
1903	Conceptual immunization for hay fever with grass pollen "toxin" (proteid isolate) and foreign species antisera [13].	William Dunbar
1907–1913	Protection against anaphylactic challenges: animal models. "Antianaphylaxis": transient desensitization following recovery from anaphylactic shock because of temporary depletion of anaphylactic antibody [127].	Richard Otto
	Temporary protection (desensitization) induced by repeated subanaphylactic doses of antigen through neutralization or exhaustion of anaphylactic antibody [28]. "Masked anaphylaxis," partial refractory state: antigen prevented from reaching the shock tissue by excess of circulating anaphylactic antibody [193].	Alexandre Besredka Richard Weil
1911–1914	First reported successful immunization against grass pollen "toxin" for hay fever [30,31].	Leonard Noon and John Freeman
1917–1919	"Injection treatments" for desensitization expanded to allergens beyond pollens [38].	I. Chandler Walker
1917	Development of techniques for extraction of allergens: availability of expanded testing and treatment reagents made available [39,40].	Roger P. Wodehouse
1919	Oral tolerance to plant oil-soluble fraction agent of contact dermatitis: derivative modification of Native American preventive practice of chewing "poison ivy" shoots [134,137].	Jay Schamberg
1921	Differentiation between antibodies involved in states of hypersensitiveness and desensitization: anaphylactic antibody, precipitin, and atopic regain [194].	Arthur Coca and Ellen Grove
1922	"Desensitization" by the procedure of Besredka in an anaphylactic animal model not attainable in human hypersensitiveness objective of hyposensitization [70].	Robert A. Cooke

(Continued)

Table 1.1 (*Continued*) Pioneering highlights along the pathway to the development and understanding of allergen immunotherapy

Time	Observation/Finding	Credit
1922	Constitutional reactions from hyposensitization injection treatments: cause, nature, and prevention [73].	Robert A. Cooke
1922	Identification of house dust as a ubiquitous allergen: expanded scope of hyposensitization programs for the treatment of perennial rhinitis and asthma [49].	Robert A. Cooke
1926	Increase in serum reaginic antibodies following hyposensitization injection treatments explaining the nature of reactions to injections of pollen vaccines [196].	Philip Levine and Arthur Coca
1932	Arbitrary incorporation of bacterial vaccines in hyposensitization treatments influenced by the concept of immunologic mechanism in infective asthma [91].	Robert A. Cooke
1933	Laboratory technique of assay of allergenic vaccines: protein nitrogen unit standardization for guide to hyposensitization schedule [197].	Arthur Stull and Robert A. Cooke
1935	Identification of blocking antibody as a product of hyposensitization treatment: its chemical and immunologic differentiation and inhibiting action on atopic reagin + allergen [75].	Robert A. Cooke and Arthur Stull
1937	Guideline for prevention of precipitin-mediated serum disease by desensitization: contraindication in the presence of coexisting atopic reagins to foreign species antisera [198].	Louis Tuft
1940	Depot allergenic vaccines for delayed absorption: alum adsorption [109].	Arthur Stull, Robert A. Cooke, and William Sherman
1947–1957	Repository adjuvant therapy with single injection of water-in-oil emulsified vaccine [76,119].	Mary Loveless
1956	Desensitization to anaphylactic challenge of stinging insect venom [180].	Mary Loveless
1962	Desensitization to anaphylactic drug hypersensitivity in penicillin model explained by hapten-inhibition mechanism.	Charles Parker and Herman Eisen
1967–1987	Identification and assay of immunoglobulin E as the reaginic antibody [199] and function of a cytokine, IL-4, in its synthesis [200]; presenting new vistas for exploring applications of cellular and molecular immunologic phenomena to allergen immunotherapy through regulatory control of IgE.	Kimishiga and Teruko Ishizaka; William Paul

5. Demonstration of protection of an animal model from lethal snake venom by inoculation series of sublethal doses [10] provided the introductory approach to the development of methods for immunization against microbial toxins and identification of the antibody product, antitoxin, in blood serum [12].

6. Systemic shock reaction of anaphylaxis—discovered as an adverse effect of immunization [21]—provided animal models for the study of hypersensitivity as an aberrant immune phenomenon [22]; particularly relevant was the challenged-sensitized guinea pig whose respiratory manifestations suggested a counterpart expression of human hay fever and asthma. Discovery of refractory state following recovery from shock—attributed to temporary depletion of anaphylactic antibody [23]—led to the development of the method of "desensitization" by repeated injections of incremental tolerated doses of antigens [28].

7. In the erroneous belief that seasonal hay fever was caused by grass pollen toxin, serial injections of pollen solutions—designed to induce immunity by production of serum antitoxin—introduced the concept of allergen immunotherapy [30,31]. This method was subsequently defined as an approach to reverse sensitization to pollen proteins and expanded in scope by employing vaccines derived from a variety of airborne seasonal and perennial allergens [39,40].

8. Serum factors associated with hypersensitivity and desensitization treatments were differentiated as skin-sensitizing antibody (ssa) and precipitating antibody (pa), respectively [194]. Detection of concurrent induction of pa and increase in levels of ssa—identical with naturally occurring atopic disease reagins—following injections of allergen vaccines accounted for local and constitutional reactions associated with therapy [71].

9. Desensitization, as effected in animal anaphylactic models, when recognized as not attainable in allergen immunotherapy, aimed at the objective of inducing diminished (hypo) sensitization [70]. Studies of antibody raised by allergen-hyposensitizing injections demonstrated its chemical properties and its "blocking" of reactions of skin-sensitizing (reaginic) antibodies with allergens to explain putative responsible immune mechanisms [75].

10. Demonstrated adjuvant effect of allergen vaccine incorporated in oil-in-water emulsion [76] had the inherent potential for inducing plasma cell neoplastic proliferation as a function of hyperimmunization [126] and was thus contraindicated in allergen immunotherapy.

11. Desensitization of anaphylactic drug reactivity (e.g., penicillin and insulin) was accomplished by a special rush protocol of immunotherapeutic injections designed to affect the mechanism of hapten inhibition [169].

ACKNOWLEDGMENTS

In the search and collection of original source material, we drew heavily on the resources of the National Library of Medicine (NLM) and the archival and special collections of the NLM History of Medicine Division (HMD). For valued interactions and expert assistance graciously extended by information specialists of the Library Reference Section and HMD staff, our many thanks and special appreciation. We also gratefully acknowledge and thank Patricia E. Richardson, NIAID editorial assistant, for dedicated technical skills and assistance in the assembly and organization of materials from which this chapter was constructed.

REFERENCES

1. Pasteur L. De l'attenuation du virus du cholra des poules. *C R Acad Sci III* 1880; 91: 673.
2. Thucydides. Chapter 47. In Smith CF, trans. *The Peloponesian War—Book 2*, Volume 2. Cambridge, MA: Harvard University Press, 1958: 54.
3. Timoni E. A letter containing the method of inoculating the small pox; practiced with success at Constantinople. *Philos Trans R Soc London* 1714; 339: 72.
4. Pylarinum J. Nova et tuta Variolas per Transplantatonem Methodus, nuper inventa et in ufurn tracta. *Philos Trans R Soc London* 1716; 347: 393.
5. Jenner E. *An Inquiry into the Causes and Effects of the Variolae*. London: Sampson Low, Soho, 1798.
6. Pasteur L, Chamberland C, Roux E. Compte Rendu Sommaire des experiences faites a' Pouilly-le-Fort, pres' Melun, sur la vaccination charboneusse. *C R Acad Sci III* 1881; 92: 1378.
7. Salmon DE, Smith T. On a new method of producing immunity from contagious diseases. *Proc Biol Soc Wash* 1884/1886; 3: 29.
8. Koch R. Forsetzung der Muttheilungen über ein Hermittel gegen Tuberculose. *Dtsch Med Wochenschr* 1891; 9: 101.
9. Pasteur L. Method pour prevenir la rage apres' morsure. *C R Acad Sci III* 1885; 101: 765.
10. Sewall H. Experiments on the preventive inoculation of rattlesnake venom. *J Physiol* 1887; 8: 205.
11. Roux PPE, Yersin AEJ. Contribution à l'etude de la diphterie. *Ann Inst Pasteur* 1889; 2: 629.
12. von Behring EA, Kitasato S. Ueber das zustandekommen der diphtherie-immunitat und der tetanusimmunitat bei thieren. *Dtsch Med Wochenschr* 1890; 16: 1113.
13. Ehrlich P. Die Wertbestimmung des Diphtherieheislserums. *Klin Jb* 1897; 6: 299.
14. Dunbar WP. The present state of our knowledge of hay-fever. *J Hyg* 1902; 13: 105.
15. von Cesenatico P, Peter C, Schick B. *Die Serumkrankheit*. Vienna: F. Deutch, 1905.
16. Bostock J. Case of periodical affection of the eyes and chest. *Med Chir Trans* 1819; 10: 161.
17. Wyman M. *Autumnal Catarrh*. Cambridge, MA: Hurd and Houghton, 1872.
18. Blackley CH. *Hay Fever: Its Causes, Treatment, and Effective Prevention*. London: Balliere, 1880.
19. Curtis HH. The immunizing cure of hay fever. *Med News* 1900; 77: 16.
20. Park WH. Toxin-antitoxin immunization against diphtheria. *J Am Med Assoc* 1922; 79: 1584.
21. Portier P, Richet C. De l'action anaphylactique de certains venins. *CR Soc Biol* 1902; 54: 170.
22. Rosenau MJ, Anderson JF. A study of the cause of sudden death following the injection of horse serum. In: *Hygienic Laboratory Bulletin 29*. Washington, DC: Government Printing Office, 1906.
23. Otto R. Das Theobald Smithsche phenomenon der serum-veberfindlichkeit. In: Gendenkschr FD, editor. *verstorb Generalstabsarzt*, Volume 1. Berlin: von Leuthold, 1906: 153.
24. Wolff-Eisner A. *Das Heufieber*. Munchen: J. F. Lehman, 1906.
25. Auer J, Lewis PA. The physiology of the immediate reaction of anaphylaxis in the guinea pig. *J Exp Med* 1910; 12: 151.
26. Meltzer SJ. Bronchial asthma as a phenomenon of anaphylaxis. *J Am Med Assoc* 1910; 55: 1021.
27. Otto R. Zur frage der serum-ueberempfindlichkeit. *Munch Med Wochenschr* 1907; 54: 1664.
28. Besredka A, Steinhardt E. De l'anaphylaxie et de l'antianaphylaxie vis-a-vis due serum de cheval. *Ann Inst Pasteur* 1907; 21: 117, 384.
29. Colebrook L. *Almoth Wright. Provocative Doctor and Thinker*. London: William Heinemann Medical Books, 1954: 61.
30. Noon L. Prophylactic inoculation against hay fever. *Lancet* 1911; 1: 1572.
31. Freeman J. Vaccination against hay fever; report of results during the last three years. *Lancet* 1914; 1: 1178.
32. Clowes GHA. A preliminary communication on certain specific reactions exhibited in hay fever cases. *Proc Soc Exp Biol Med* 1913; 10: 70.
33. Lowdermilk RC. Personal communication to Duke WW. In: Duke WW, editor. *Allergy. Asthma, Hay Fever, Urticaria and Allied Manifestations of Reaction*. St. Louis, MO: Mosby, 1925: 222.
34. Koessler KK. The specific treatment of hayfever by active immunization. *Ill Med J* 1914; 24: 120.
35. Lowdermilk RC. Hay-fever. *J Am Med Assoc* 1914; 63: 141.
36. Cooke RA. The treatment of hay fever by active immunization. *Laryngoscope* 1915; 25: 108.
37. Schloss OM. A case of allergy to common foods. *Am J Dis Child* 1912; 3: 341.
38. Walker IC. Studies on the sensitization of patients with bronchial asthma (Study series III–XXXVI). *J Med Res* 1917: 35–37.
39. Wodehouse RP. Immunochemical study and immunochemistry of protein series. *J Immunol* 1917; 11: VI. cat hair, 227; VII. horse dander, 237; VIII. dog hair, 243.
40. Wodehouse RP. Study IX. Immunochemical studies of the plant proteins: Wheat seed and other cereals. *Am J Botany* 1917; 4: 417.
41. Coca AF. Studies in specific hypersensitiveness. XV. The preparation of fluid extracts and solutions for use in the diagnosis and treatment of the allergies, with notes on the collection of pollens. *J Immunol* 1922; 7: 163.
42. Goodale JL. Preliminary notes on the anaphylactic skin reactions exacted in hay fever subjects by the pollen of various species of plants. *Boston Med Surg J* 1914; 171: 695.
43. Goodale JL. Pollen therapy in hay fever. *Boston Med Surg J* 1915; 173: 42.

44. Wodehouse RP. *Hay Fever Plants*. Waltham, MA: Chronica Botanica, 1945.
45. Durham OC. The contribution of air analysis to the study of allergy. *J Lab Clin Med* 1925; 13: 967.
46. Unger L, Harris MC. *Stepping Stones in Allergy*. Minneapolis, MN: Craftsman Press, 1975: 75.
47. Cohen SG. Firsts in allergy. *N Engl Reg Allergy Proc* 1983; 4: 309; 1984; 5: 48; 5: 247.
48. Cooke RA. Protein sensitization in the human with special reference to bronchial asthma and hay fever. *Med Clin North Am* 1917; 1: 721.
49. Cooke RA. Studies in specific hypersensitiveness. New etiologic factors in bronchial asthma. *J Immunol* 1922; 7: 147.
50. Duke WW. *Allergy, Asthma, Hay Fever, Urticaria and Allied Manifestations of Reaction*. St. Louis, MO: C. V. Mosby, 1925: 237–241.
51. Chen KK, Schmidt CF. The action of ephedrine, the active principle of the Chinese drug MaHuang. *J Pharmacol Exp Ther* 1924; 24: 192.
52. Cohen SG. Firsts in allergy: IV. The contributions of Arthur F. Coca, M. D. (18751959). *N Engl Reg Allergy Proc* 1985; 6: 285.
53. Cohen SG. The American Academy of Allergy, an historical review. *J Allergy Clin Immunol* 1976; 64: 322–466.
54. Storm van Leeuwen W. Bronchial asthma in relation to climate. *Proc R Soc Med* 1924; 17: 19.
55. Thommen AA. Etiology of hay fever: Studies in hay fever. *N Y State J Med* 1930; 30: 437.
56. Kern RA. Dust sensitization in bronchial asthma. *Med Clin North Am* 1921; 5: 751.
57. Boatner CH, Efron BG. Studies with antigens. XII. Preparation and properties of concentrates of house dust allergen. *J Invest Dermatol* 1942; 5: 7.
58. Cooke RA. Human sensitization. *J Immunol* 1916; 1: 201.
59. Stull A, Cooke RA, Tenant J. The allergen content of protein extracts; its determination and deterioration. *J Allergy* 1933; 4: 455.
60. Thommen AA. The specific treatment of hay fever. In: Coca AF, Walzer M, Thommen AA, editors. *Asthma and Hay Fever in Theory and Practice*. London: Balliere, Tindall, & Cox, 1931: 757–774.
61. Bernton HS. Plantain hay fever and asthma. *J Am Med Assoc* 1925; 84: 944.
62. Kahn IS, Grothaus EM. Studies in pollen sensitivities. *Med J Rec* 1925; 121: 664.
63. MacKenzie GM. Desensitization of hay fever patients by specific local application. *J Am Med Assoc* 1922; 78: 787.
64. Caulfield AHW. Desensitization of hay fever patients by injection and local application. *J Am Med Assoc* 1922; 79: 125.
65. Touart MD. Hay fever; desensitization by ingestion of pollen protein. *N Y Med J* 1922; 116: 199.
66. Phillips EW. Relief of hay fever in intradermal injections of pollen extracts. *J Am Med Assoc* 1922; 79: 125.
67. Le Noir P, Richet C Jr. Renard. Skin test for anaphylaxis. *Bull Soc Med Hop* 1921; 45: 1283 (abstr); *J Am Med Assoc* 1921; 77: 1770.
68. American Academy of Allergy, report of the Joint Committee on Standards. *J Allergy* 1935; 6: 408.
69. Heidelberger M, Avery OT. The soluble specific substance of pneumococcus. *J Exp Med* 1924; 40: 301.
70. Cooke RA. Studies in specific hypersensitiveness, IX. On the phenomenon of hyposensitization (the clinically lessened sensitiveness of allergy). *J Immunol* 1922; 7: 219.
71. Levine P, Coca A. Studies in hypersensitiveness. XX. A quantitative study of the interaction of atopic reagins and atopen. *J Immunol* 1926; 11: 411; XXII. On the nature of alleviating effect of the specific treatment of atopic conditions. *J Immunol* 1926; 11: 449.
72. Jadassohn W. Beitrage zun idosynkrasie problem. *Klin Wochenschr* 1926; 5: 1957.
73. Cooke RA. Studies in specific hypersensitiveness. III. On constitutional reactions: The dangers of the diagnostic, cutaneous test and therapeutic injection of allergens. *J Immunol* 1922; 7: 119.
74. Freeman J. Rush inoculation with special reference to hay fever treatment. *Lancet* 1930; 1: 744.
75. Cooke RA, Barnard JH, Hebald S, Stull A. Serological evidence of immunity with coexisting sensitization in a type of human allergy (hay fever). *J Exp Med* 1935; 62: 733.
76. Loveless MH. Application of immunologic principles to the management of hay fever, including a preliminary report on the use of Freund's adjuvant. *Am J Med Sci* 1947; 214: 559.
77. Cooke RA, Loveless M, Stull A. Studies on immunity in a type of human allergy (hay fever): Serologic response of non-sensitive individuals to pollen injections. *J Exp Med* 1937; 66: 689.
78. Sherman WB, Stull A, Cooke RA. Serologic changes in hay fever cases treated over a period of years. *J Allergy* 1940; 11: 225.
79. Vannier WE, Campbell DH. The isolation and purification of purified house dust allergen fraction. *J Allergy* 1959; 30: 198.
80. King TP, Norman PS. Isolation studies of allergens from ragweed pollen. *Biochemistry* 1962; 1: 709.
81. Allen RW. The common cold: Its pathology and treatment. *Lancet* 1908; 172: 1589.
82. Farrington PM. Hay fever. *Memphis Med J* 1912; 32: 381.
83. Morrey CB. Vaccination with mixed cultures from the nose in hay fever. *J Am Med Assoc* 1913; 61: 1806.
84. Goodale JL. Preliminary notes on skin reactions excited by various bacterial proteins in certain vasomotor disturbances of the upper air passages. *Boston Med Surg J* 1916; 174: 223.
85. Walker IC. Studies on the sensitization of patients with bronchial asthma to bacterial proteins as demonstrated by the skin reaction and the methods employed in the preparation of those proteins. *J Med Res* 1917; 35: 487.
86. Walker IC. The treatment with bacterial vaccines of bronchial asthmatics who are not sensitive to proteins. *J Med Res* 1917; 37: 51.
87. Walker JW, Adkinson J. Studies on *Staphylococcus pyogenes, aureus, albus* and *citreus* and on *Micrococcus tetragenous* and *M. catarrhalis. J Med Res* 1917; 35: 373 (subsequent articles in this series appeared in 35: 391, 36: 293).
88. Kraus R, Doerr R. Uber bacterienanaphylaxie. *Wien Klin Wochenschr* 1908; 21: 1008.
89. Koch R. Fortsetzung der muttheilungen uber ein Heilmittel gegen Tuberculose. *Dtsch Med Wochenschr* 1891; 9: 101.
90. Rackemann FM. A clinical study of one hundred and fifty cases of bronchial asthma. *Arch Intern Med* 1918; 22: 552.
91. Cooke RA. Infective asthma: Indication of its allergic nature. *Am J Med Sci* 1932; 183: 309.
92. Walzer M. Asthma. In Coca AF, Walzer M, Thomen AA, editors. *Asthma and Hay Fever in Theory and Practice*. Springfield, IL: Charles C. Thomas, 1931: 260–261.
93. Hooker SB, Anderson LM. Heterogeneity of streptococci isolated from sputum with active critique on serological classification of streptococci. *J Immunol* 1929; 16: 291.

94. Cooke RA. Infective asthma with pharmacopeia. In: Cooke RA, editor. *Allergy in Theory and Practice*. Philadelphia, PA: W.B. Saunders, 1947: 151–152.

95. Frankland AW, Hughes WH, Garrill RH. Autogenous bacterial vaccines in the treatment of asthma. *Br Med J* 1955; 2: 941.

96. Johnstone DE. Study of the value of bacterial vaccines in the treatment of bronchial asthma associated with respiratory infections. *Am J Dis Child* 1957; 94: 1.

97. Helander E. Bacterial vaccines in the treatment of bronchial asthma. *Acta Allergy* 1959; 13: 47.

98. Lowell FC. American academy of allergy presidential address. *J Allergy* 1960; 31: 185.

99. Brun E. Control examination of specificity of specific desensitization in asthma. *Acta Allergol* 1949; 2: 122.

100. Frankland AW, Augustin R. Prophylaxis of summer hay-fever and asthma: Controlled trial comparing crude grass-pollen extracts with isolated main protein component. *Lancet* 1954; 1: 1055.

101. Johnstone DE. Study of the role of antigen dosage in treatment of pollenosis and pollen-asthma. *Am J Dis Child* 1957; 94: 1.

102. Lowell FC, Franklin W. A double blind study of the effectiveness and specificity of injection therapy in ragweed hay fever. *N Engl J Med* 1965; 273: 675.

103. Fontana VC, Holt LE Jr, Mainland D. Effectiveness of hyposensitization therapy in ragweed hay fever in children. *J Am Med Assoc* 1967; 195: 109.

104. Lowell FC, Franklin W, Fontana VJ et al. Hyposensitization therapy in ragweed hay fever. *J Am Med Assoc* 1966; 195: 1071 (lett).

105. Norman PS, Winkenwerder WL, Lichtenstein LM. Immunotherapy of hay fever with ragweed antigen F: comparisons with whole pollen extracts and placeboes. *J Allergy* 1968, 42. 93.

106. Sadan N, Rhyne MB, Mellits ED et al. Immunotherapy of pollenosis in children. Investigation of the immunologic basis of clinical improvement. *N Engl J Med* 1969; 280: 623.

107. Sutton C. Hay fever. *Med Clin North Am* 1923; 7: 605.

108. Zoss AR, Koch CA, Hirose RS. Alum-ragweed precipitate: Preparation and clinical investigation; preliminary report. *J Allergy* 1937; 8: 829.

109. Stull A, Cooke RA, Sherman WB et al. Experimental and clinical studies of fresh and modified pollen extracts. *J Allergy* 1940; 11: 439.

110. Naterman H. The treatment of hay fever by injections of suspended pollen tannate. *J Allergy* 1941; 12: 378.

111. Rockwell G. Preparation of a slowly absorbed pollen antigen. *Ohio State Med J* 1941; 37: 651. 26 Cohen and Evans.

112. Spain W, Fuchs A, Strauss M. A slowly absorbed gelatin-pollen extract for the treatment of hay fever. *J Allergy* 1941; 12: 365.

113. Naterman HL. The treatment of hay fever by injections of pollen extract emulsified in lanolin and olive oil. *N Engl J Med* 1937; 218: 797.

114. Naterman HL. Pollen tannate suspended in peanut oil with aluminum monostearate in the treatment of hay fever. *J Allergy* 1950; 22: 175.

115. Malkiel S, Feinberg SM. Effect of slowly absorbing antigen (ragweed) on neutralizing antibody titer. *J Allergy* 1950; 21: 525.

116. Gelfand HH, Frank DE. Studies on the blocking antibody in serum of ragweed treated patients. II. Its relation to clinical results. *J Allergy* 1944; 15: 332.

117. Alexander HL, Johnson MC, Bukantz SC. Studies on correlation of symptoms of ragweed hay fever and titer of thermostable antibody. *J Allergy* 1948; 19: 1.

118. Wasserman RL, Jones DJ, Windom HH. Oral immunotherapy for food allergy The FAST perspective. *Ann Allergy Asthma* 2018; 121: 272–275.

119. Loveless MH. Repository immunization in pollen allergy. *J Immunol* 1957; 79: 68.

120. Henle W, Henle G. Effect of adjuvants of vaccination of human beings against influenza. *Proc Soc Exp Biol Med* 1945; 59: 179.

121. Freund J, McDermott K. Sensitization to horse serum by means of adjuvants. *Proc Soc Exp Biol Med* 1942; 49: 548.

122. Brown EA II. The treatment of ragweed pollenosis with a single annual emulsified extract injection. *Ann Allergy* 1958; 16: 28 through XI.

123. Feinberg SM, Rabinowitz HI, Pruzanski JJ et al. Repository antigen injections. *J Allergy* 1960; 31: 421.

124. Sherman WB, Brown EB, Karol ES et al. Respository emulsion treatment of ragweed pollenosis. *J Allergy* 1962; 33: 473.

125. Arbesman CE, Reisman RE. Hyposensitization therapy including repository: A double blind study. *J Allergy* 1964; 35: 12.

126. Potter M, Boyce ER. Induction of plasma cell neoplasms in strain BALB/c mice with mineral oil and mineral oil adjuvants. *Nature* 1962; 193: 1086.

127. Pliny. *Pliny Natural History*. Book 15, Volume 7. In Jones WHS, trans. Cambridge, MA: Harvard University Press, 1956: 139.

128. Appian. Chapter 16. *Appian's Roman History*. Book 12. In White H, trans. Cambridge, MA: Harvard University Press, 1962: 453.

129. Galen. De Temperamentis. Coxe JR. *Writing of Hippocrates and Galen (epitomized from the Original Latin Translation)*. Philadelphia, PA: Lindsay and Blakiston, 1846: 493.

130. Pliny. In: Urbach L, Gottlieb I'M, editors. *Allergy*. New York: Grune & Stratton, 1943. 252.

131. Ehrlich P. Experimentelle intersuchungen uber immunitat. *Dsch Med Wochenschr I. Uber ricin* 1891; 17: 976; *II. Uber abrin.* 1891; 17: 1218.

132. Chase MW. Inhibition of experimental drug allergy by prior feeding of the sensitizing agent. *Proc Soc Exp Biol Med* 1946; 61: 257.

133. Dakin R. Remarks on a cutaneous affliction produced by certain poisonous vegetables. *Am J Med Sci* 1829; 1: 98.

134. Strickler A. The toxin treatment of dermatitis venenata. *J Am Med Assoc* 1921; 77: 910.

135. Duncan CH. Autotherapy in ivy poisoning. *J Am Med Assoc* 1916; 104: 901.

136. Diffenbach WW. Treatment of ivy poisoning. *South Cal Pract* 1917; 32: 91.

137. Strickler A. The treatment of dermatitis venenata by vegetable toxins. *J Cutan Dis* 1918; 36: 327.

138. Schamberg JF. Desensitization against ivy poisoning. *J Am Med Assoc* 1919; 73: 1213.

139. Blank JM, Coca AF. Study of the prophylactic action of an extract of poison ivy in the control of *Rhus* dermatitis. *J Allergy* 1936; 7: 552.

140. Molitch M, Poliakoff S. Prevention of dermatitis venenata due to poison ivy in children. *Arch Derm Syph* 1936; 33: 725.

141. Bachman LC. Prophylaxis of poison ivy: Use of an almond oil extract in children. *J Pediatr* 1938; 12: 31.

142. Sompayrac LM. Negative results of *Rhus* antigen treatment of experimental ivy poisoning. *Am J Med Sci* 1938; 195: 361.

143. Shelmire B. Contact dermatitis from vegetation. Patch testing and treatment with plant oleoresins. *South Med* 1940; 38: 337.

144. Schoffield AT. A case of egg poisoning. *Lancet* 1908; 1: 716.

145. Finzio G. Anaf. familiare per il latte di mucca. Tentativie di terapia antianaf. *Pediatria* 1911; 19: 641.

146. Talbot FB. Asthma in children, III. Its treatment. *Long Island Med J* 1917; 11: 245.

147. Pagniez P, Vallery-Radot P. Etude physiologique et therapeutique d'un cas d'urticaire geante. Anaphylaxie et anti-anaphylaxie alimentaires. *Nouv Presse Med* 1916; 24: 529.

148. Luithlen F. Ueberempfindlichkeit und ernahrungstherapie. *Wien Med Wschnsehr* 1926; 76: 907.

149. Rowe AH. Desensitization to foods with reference to propeptanes. *J Allergy* 1931; 3: 68.

150. Rowe AH. *Food Allergy. Its Manifestation and Control and the Elimination Diets, A Compendium.* Springfield, IL: Charles C Thomas, 1972: 71.

151. Wrightman HB, discussion of Iliff EH, Gay LN. Treatment with oral ragweed pollen. *J Allergy* 1941; 12: 601.

152. The PALISADE Group of Clinical Investigators, Vickery BP, Vereda A, Casale TB et al. AR101 oral immunotherapy for peanut allergy. *NEJM* 2018; 379: 1991–2001.

153. Black JH. The oral administration of pollen. *J Lab Clin Med* 1927; 12: 1156.

154. Black JH. The oral administration of ragweed pollen. *J Allergy* 1939; 10: 156.

155. Urbach E. Desensibilisiering pollen ullergischer individuen auforalem wege mittels art-spezitischer pollenpeptone. *Klin Wochenschr* 1931; 10: 534.

156. Urbach E. Die biologiche behandlung des henfiebers. *Munchen Med Wchnschr* 1937; 84: 488.

157. Bernstein TB, Feinberg SM. Oral ragweed pollen therapy clinical results and experiments in gastrointestinal absorption. *Arch Intern Med* 1938; 62: 297.

158. Feinberg SM, Foran FL, Lichtenstein ML. Oral pollen therapy in ragweed pollinosis. *J Am Med Assoc* 1940; 115: 231.

159. Heran J, Saint-Girans F. Un cas d'anaphylaxie a la quinine chez un paludeen intolerance absolus et urticaria. Antianaphylaxie par voie gastrique. *Paris Med* 1917; 7: 161.

160. Goodale JL. Anaphylactic reactions occurring in horse asthma after the administration of diphtheria antitoxin. *Boston Med Surg J* 1914; 170: 837.

161. Feinberg SM. *Allergy in Practice.* Chicago, IL: Year Book Publishers, 1946: 536.

162. Boughton TH. Anaphylactic deaths in asthmatics. *J Am Med Assoc* 1912; 73: 1912.

163. Kerley CG. Accidents in foreign protein administration. *Arch Pediatr* 1917; 34: 457.

164. Tuft L. Fatalities following injection of foreign serum; report of unusual case. *Am J Med Sci* 1928; 175: 325.

165. Widal F, Abrami P, Joltrain E. Anaphylaxie a l'ipeca. *Presse Med* 1922; 32: 341.

166. Jeanneret R. Desensitization in insulin urticaria. *Rev Med Suisse Rom* 1929; 49: 99 (Abstr J Am Med Assoc 1929; 92: 2197).

167. Corcoran AC. Note in rapid desensitization in a case of hyper-sensitiveness to insulin. *Am J Med Sci* 1938; 196: 357.

168. Reisman RE, Rose NR, Witebsky E et al. Penicillin allergy and desensitization. *J Allergy* 1962; 33: 178.

169. Parker CW, Shapiro J, Kern M, Eisen HN. Hypersensitivity to penicillenic acid derivatives in human beings with penicillin allergy. *J Exp Med* 1962; 115: 821.

170. O'Donovan WJ, Klorfajn I. Sensitivity to penicillin: Anaphylaxis and desensitization. *Lancet* 1946; 2: 444.

171. Peck SM, Siegel S, Bergamini R. Successful desensitization in penicillin sensitivity. *J Am Med Assoc* 1947; 134: 1546.

172. Crofton J. Desensitization to streptomycin and P. A. S. *Br Med J* 1953; 2: 1014.

173. Freeman J. Toxic idiopathies; the relationship between hay and other pollen fevers, animal asthmas, food idiosyncrasies, bronchial and spasmodic asthma, etc. *Proc R Soc Med* 1920; 13: 129.

174. Braun LIB. Notes on desensitization of a patient hypersensitive to bee stings. *South Afr Med Rec* 1925; 23: 408.

175. Benson RL. Diagnosis and treatment of sensitization to mosquitoes. *J Allergy* 1936; 8: 47.

176. McIvor BC, Cherney LS. Studies in insect bite desensitization. *Am J Trop Med* 1941; 21: 493.

177. Parlato SJ. A case of coryza and asthma due to sand flies. *J Allergy* 1929; 1: 35.

178. Figley KD. Asthma due to May fly. *Am J Med Sci* 1929; 178: 338.

179. Benson RL, Semenov H. Allergy in its relation to bee sting. *J Allergy* 1930; 1: 105.

180. Loveless MH, Fackler WR. Wasp venom allergy and immunity. *Ann Allergy* 1956; 14: 347.

181. Loveless MH. Immunization in wasp-sting allergy through venom-repositories and periodic insect stings. *J Immunol* 1962; 89: 204.

182. Walzer M. Asthma. In: Coca AF, Walzer M, Thommen AA, editors. *Asthma and Hay Fever in Theory and Practice.* London: Balliere, Tindall & Cox, 1931: 297–304.

183. Feinberg SM. *Allergy in Practice.* Chicago, IL: Year Book Publishers, 1946: 544–553.

184. Auld AG. Further remarks on the treatment of asthma by peptone. *Br Med J* 1918; 2: 49.

185. Kahn MH, Emsheimer HW. Autogenous defibrinated blood in the treatment of bronchial asthma. *Arch Intern Med* 1916; 18: 445.

186. Storm Van Leewuen W, Varekamp H. On the tuberculin treatment of bronchial asthma and hay fever. *Lancet* 1921; 2: 1366.

187. Brunner M. In: Coca AF, Walzer M, Thommen AA, editors. *Asthma and Hay Fever in Theory and Practice.* London: Balliere, Tindall & Cox, 1931: 301–302.

188. Bray GW. A case of physical allergy: A localized and generalized allergic type of reaction to cold. *J Allergy* 1932; 3: 367.

189. Laymon CW, Cumming H. Histaminase in the treatment of urticaria and atopic dermatitis. *J Invest Dermatol* 1939; 2: 301.

190. Sheldon JM, Fell N, Johnson JH et al. A clinical study of histamine azoprotein in allergic disease: A preliminary report. *J Allergy* 1941; 13: 18.

191. Thompson RA, Bousquet J, Cohen SG et al. Current status of allergen immunotherapy. Shortened version of World Health Organization/International Union of Immunological Societies Working Group Report. *Lancet* 1989; 1: 259.

192. Arthus M. Injections repetees de serum de cheval chez le lapin. *CR Soc Biol (Paris)* 1903; 55: 817.

193. Weil R. The nature of anaphylaxis and the relations between anaphylaxis and immunity. *J Med Res* 1913; 27: 497.

194. Coca AF, Grove EF. Studies in hypersensitiveness XII. A study of the atopic reagins. *J Immunol* 1925; 10: 445.

195. Wasserman RL, Hague AR, Pence DM et al. Real-world experience with peanut oral immunotherapy: Lessons learned from 270 patients. *J Allergy Clin Immunol Pract* 2014; 2(1): 91–96.

196. Levine P, Coca AF. Studies in hypersensitiveness XXII. On the nature of the alleviating effect by the specific treatment of atopic conditions. *J Immunol* 1926; 11: 449.

197. Stull A, Cooke RA, Tenant J. The allergen content of pollen extracts: Its determination and deterioration. *J Allergy* 1933; 4: 455.

198. Tuft L. *Clinical Allergy*. Philadelphia, PA: Saunders, 1937: 739.

199. Ishizaka K, Ishizaka T. Identification of gamma-E antibodies as a carrier of reaginic antibody. *J Immunol* 1967; 99: 1187.

200. Paul W, Ohara J. B-cell stimulatory factor-I/interleukin 4. *Ann Rev Immunol* 1987; 5: 429.

201. Fitzhugh D, Lockey RF. History of immunotherapy: The first 100 years. *Immunol Allergy Clin N Am* 2011; 31: 149–157.

202. Cooke RA, Barnard JH, Hebald S, Stull A. Serologic evidence of immunity with coexisting sensitization in a type of human allergy (hay fever). *J Exp Med* 1935; 62: 733–750.

203. Cooke RA, Menzel AE, Kessler WR, Myers PA. The antibody mechanisms of ragweed allergy; electrophoretic and chemical studies. I: The blocking antibody. *J Exp Med* 1955; 101: 177–196.

204. James LK, Bowen H, Calvert RA et al. Allergen specificity of IgG(4)-expressing B cells in patients with grass pollen allergy undergoing immunotherapy. *J Allergy Clin Immunol* 2012; 130: 663–670.

205. Akdis CA, Blesken T, Akdis M et al. Role of interleukin 10 in specific immunotherapy. *J Clin Invest* 1998; 102: 98–106.

206. Chen W, Jin W, Hardegen N et al. Conversion of peripheral CD41CD25-naive T cells to CD41CD251 regulatory T cells by TGF-β induction of transcription factor Foxp3. *J Exp Med* 2003; 198: 1875–1886.

207. McCormack PL, Wagstaff AJ. Ultra-short-course seasonal allergy vaccine (Pollinex Quattro). *Drugs* 2006; 66: 931–938.

208. Creticos PS, Schroeder JT, Hamilton RG et al. Immunotherapy with a ragweed-toll-like receptor 9 agonist vaccine for allergic rhinitis. *N Engl J Med* 2006; 355: 1445–1455.

209. Klimek L, Schendzielorz P, Pinol R, Pfaar O. Specific subcutaneous immunotherapy with recombinant grass pollen allergens: First randomized dose-ranging safety study. *Clin Exp Allergy* 2012; 42: 936–945.

210. Karamloo F, Schmid-Grendelmeier P, Kussebi F et al. Prevention of allergy by a recombinant multi-allergen vaccine with reduced IgE binding and preserved T cell epitopes. *Eur J Immunol* 2005; 35: 3268–3276.

211. Casale TB, Busse WW, Kline JN et al.; Immune Tolerance Network Group. Omalizumab pretreatment decreases acute reactions after rush immunotherapy for ragweed-induced seasonal allergic rhinitis. *J Allergy Clin Immunol* 2006; 117: 134–140.

212. Golbert T. Controversies. In: Lockey RF, editor. *Allergy. Allergy and Clinical Immunology*. Garden City, NY: Medical Examination Publishing, 1979: 1119–1162.

213. Bousquet J, Lockey RF, Malling H-J. WHO position paper-allergen immunotherapy: Therapeutic vaccines for allergic diseases. *Allergy* 1998; 53(Suppl 44): 1069–1088.

214. Canonica GW, Bousquet J, Casale T et al. Sublingual immunotherapy: World Allergy Organization position paper 2009. *Allergy* 2009; 64(Suppl 91): 1–59.

215. Durham SR, Emminger W, Kapp A et al. Long-term clinical efficacy in grass pollen-induced rhinoconjunctivitis after treatment with SQ-standardized grass allergy immunotherapy tablet. *J Allergy Clin Immunol* 2010; 125: 131–138.

216. Marogna M, Spadolini I, Massolo A, Canonica GW, Passalacqua G. Long-lasting effects of sublingual immunotherapy according to its duration: A 15-year prospective study. *J Allergy Clin Immunol* 2010; 126: 969–975.

217. Dahl R, Kapp A, Colombo G et al. Efficacy and safety of sublingual immunotherapy with grass allergen tablets for seasonal allergic rhinoconjunctivitis. *J Allergy Clin Immunol* 2006; 118: 434–440.

218. Senti G, PrinzVavricka BM, Erdmann I et al. Intralymphatic allergen administration renders specific immunotherapy faster and safer: A randomized controlled trial. *Proc Natl Acad Sci USA* 2008; 105: 17908–17912.

219. Hylander T, Latif L, Petersson-Westin U, Cardell LO. Intralymphatic allergen-specific immunotherapy: An effective and safe alternative treatment route for pollen-induced allergic rhinitis. *J Allergy Clin Immunol* 2013; 131: 412–420.

220. Senti G, Freiburghaus AU, Kundig TM. Epicutaneous/transcutaneous allergen-specific immunotherapy: Rationale and clinical trials. *Curr Opin Allergy Clin Immunol* 2010; 10: 582–586.

221. Nelson HS. Current and future challenges of subcutaneous and sublingual allergy immunotherapy for allergists in the United States. *Ann Allergy Asthma* 2018; 121: 278–280.

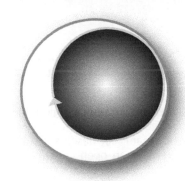

2 Aeroallergen sampling

Estelle Levetin and Josh D. McLoud
University of Tulsa

CONTENTS

2.1 INTRODUCTION

The atmosphere contains a tremendous diversity of bioaerosols including viruses, bacteria, fungal spores, and pollen; many of these can impact the health of humans, other animals, or plants [1–3]. In indoor environments, the air also includes a variety of bioaerosols, which can also impact health. Consequently, aerobiology and bioaerosols are of interest to researchers in many fields such as medicine (especially allergy), plant pathology, veterinary medicine, epidemiology, and public health.

For allergists, the best known and the most widely studied outdoor bioaerosols are pollen and fungal spores. Allergists have used the data on airborne pollen and spores to aid in the diagnosis and treatment of patients. They have also used the information to develop pollen calendars for their geographic areas, to study the effects of pollen exposure on patient symptoms, and to assess clinical trials [4–8]. In allergy-related research, aerobiological data are widely used to describe and predict atmospheric pollen or spore concentration in an effort to help those sensitive to aeroallergens. Aeroallergens currently are monitored throughout the world with 879 operating stations that are part of a regional or national network [8]. In addition, many active individual stations are not affiliated with an organized network. Indoor environments are usually sampled for fungal spores, as well as for dust mite, cat, dog, and cockroach allergens [9,10].

Researchers have used various devices to study the bioaerosol composition of the atmosphere for over 150 years. The early history of air sampling and the development of the field of aerobiology have been considered in several publications [1,2]. This chapter focuses on methods of interest to the allergy community, including traditional methods as well as modern approaches for both sampling and analysis.

2.2 TRADITIONAL METHODS: GRAVITY SAMPLING

The simplest methods of air sampling are passive methods that rely on gravity to collect pollen, fungal spores, and other bioaerosols onto various substrates. Common examples include exposing a greased microscope slide or an open Petri dish containing culture medium to the outdoor atmosphere or indoor air for a given period of time. This method cannot quantify concentrations of bioaerosols and is also biased toward larger or heavier pollen and spore types, which have a greater sedimentation rate. As a result, captured bioaerosols may not represent airborne taxa and abundance [11].

Although the limitations of gravity sampling are widely recognized [11,12], this method has been commonly used for long-term sampling in both outdoor and indoor environments. Tauber traps have been frequently used by geologists to examine pollen influx within a region; the trap consists of a glass container covered by a lid with a 5 cm central opening [13]. The lid is aerodynamically designed to avoid the turbulence that would be caused by an open container, thereby mimicking natural pollen deposition into sediments [14]. Analyses of pollen collected by Tauber traps are performed by microscopic analysis. Aerobiologists have used Tauber traps for long-term studies of allergenic pollen, often in remote regions [15–17]. Levetin et al. [13] compared the pollen types registered by Tauber traps and a volumetric sampler in Tulsa, Oklahoma. The authors found a strong correlation ($r = 0.914$, $p < .0001$) between the pollen influx data from the Tauber traps and the pollen index (cumulative sum of average daily concentration) registered by a Burkard volumetric sampler over a 12-month period. The results indicate that both samplers reflect the local anemophilous vegetation, although there were variations in the prevalence of individual pollen types recorded by each method.

In indoor environments, settled dust has been widely used as a surrogate for sampling airborne bioaerosols, especially for fungal spores [18–22]. Various studies that compared dust sampling to air sampling showed conflicting results, with some showing fungal spores recovered from dust samples reflecting airborne fungi and others showing that different taxa dominate air samples versus dust samples [18,19]. Collected dust is normally sieved to remove large particles. The fine dust is then cultured for fungal identification, with the results expressed as colony-forming units per gram of dust. Instead of culturing, DNA can be extracted from the dust or from Tauber traps and molecular methods used for fungal or pollen identification [22–24]. Immunoassays can also be performed on settled dust to determine levels of fungal, dust mite, cockroach, cat, and other indoor allergens [9,10].

2.3 TRADITIONAL METHODS: VOLUMETRIC SAMPLING

Numerous instruments are used to actively collect airborne particles from a known volume of air [25–27], and new instruments are constantly being developed. Lindsley et al. provide a complete list of current sampling equipment [25]. Data resulting from volumetric samplers can provide atmospheric concentrations of the bioaerosols under study. Volumetric samplers capture particles from the airstream by various methods, including impaction, filtration, impingement, cyclonic separation, and electrostatic precipitation (Table 2.1) [11].

2.3.1 Impaction samplers

The most widely used volumetric samplers are impaction samplers. These instruments separate particles from the airstream due to the inertia of the particles, resulting in particle impaction on a solid surface or an agar surface. Impaction sampler efficiency is based on particle size and density as well as the sampler design, and all samplers of this type have size cut points below which sampling efficiency decreases. This means that particles larger than the cut point will impact on the collection surface, while smaller particles remain in the airstream. Rotating arm impactors and suction impactors are widely used in aeroallergen sampling.

2.3.1.1 ROTATING ARM IMPACTORS

The rotating arm impactor was initially developed in the 1950s [28], and over several decades various models were created. These impactors have arms that rotate at high speeds, generally 2400 rpm, thereby accelerating the sampling surface. The sampling rate is 120 liters of air per minute, and particles entrained in the air may impact on the sampling surface during rotation. The samplers can be run continuously for short periods of time or set for intermittent sampling. In the early models, adhesive tapes were mounted on the arms; after sampling, the tapes were removed and examined microscopically. The current models used by the allergy community are intermittent samplers that generally run on a 10% duty cycle for 1 minute out of every 10 minutes. Particles are collected onto two short, acrylic rods. When the instrument cycles on, the rods are extended as the sampling head begins rotating. The leading edge of each rod is coated with silicon grease. The rods usually are changed daily. For analysis, the rods are placed into grooves within a specially designed microscope slide and stained with Calberla's pollen stain. Rods are examined with a microscope for pollen and spore identification, and the atmospheric concentrations are determined based on the number of particles and the collection times.

Pollen and large fungal spores are efficiently sampled with rotating arm impactors; however, the efficiency decreases for particles smaller than 10 μm. Many smaller spores fail to impact on the rods and remain in the airstream. As a result, calculated total fungal spore concentrations underrepresent various spore types such as basidiospores, small ascospores, and *Penicillium* and *Aspergillus* conidia [29]. Sampling efficiency may also decrease over time if the sampling surface becomes overloaded. In areas with high concentrations of pollen and spores or high particulate levels, a 5% duty cycle can help to avoid overload.

Rotating arm impactors are used for aeroallergen research [4,6,30,31]; in addition, these samplers have been widely used in plant pathology to study the dispersal of fungal pathogens in the field [32–34]. Sampler models currently available include the Rotorod Sampler, which is manufactured by IQVIA (https://www.pollen.com/help/rotorod) and the GRIPS-99M and GRIPST-2009 impactors that are manufactured by Aerobiology Research Laboratories (https://www.aerobiology.ca/).

2.3.1.2 SUCTION SAMPLERS: SLIT IMPACTORS

In suction impactors, a vacuum pump draws air into the instrument through one or more inlets or nozzles, and the bioaerosols, which separate from the airstream, are collected on various types of surfaces. There are many types of suction impactors, and only the most widely used devices are described here. These can be categorized as slit impactors for analysis of total spores and pollen and sieve impactors for culture-based sampling.

Slit impactors are used to collect airborne pollen and spores onto a solid substrate for microscope analysis; these instruments are often referred to as spore traps. Slit impactors are available as stationary instruments for continuous pollen and spore monitoring outdoors and as small portable devices for indoor investigations.

The Hirst-type spore trap is the most widely used instrument for the analysis of airborne pollen and fungal spores by aeroallergen sampling networks [8] and by independent investigators. This type of sampler was originally designed by James Hirst [35] as an instrument for plant pathologists to efficiently monitor

Table 2.1 Commonly used bioaerosol samplers

Sampling technology	Sampler name	Collection medium	Analysis methods
Rotating arm impactors	Rotorod sampler	Greased acrylic rods	Microscopy
	GRIPS samplers	Greased acrylic rods	Microscopy
Slit impactors: Hirst-type spore traps	Burkard 7-day spore traps	Greased tape or greased slide	Microscopy, immunoassays, molecular biology
	Lanzoni VPPS	Greased tape or greased slide	Microscopy, immunoassays, molecular biology
Slit impactors: Portable spore traps	Burkard continuous recording air sampler	Greased slide	Microscopy, immunoassays, molecular biology
	Allergenco MK-3	Greased slide	Microscopy, immunoassays, molecular biology
	Burkard personal sampler	Greased slide	Microscopy, immunoassays, molecular biology
	Buck BioSlide	Greased slide	Microscopy, immunoassays, molecular biology
	Air-O-Cell cassette	Sampling matrix	Microscopy
	Allergenco-D cassette	Sampling matrix	Microscopy
	Cyclex-d cassette	Sampling matrix	Microscopy
	Micro-5 cassette	Sampling matrix	Microscopy
Sieve impactors	Andersen 6-stage and 2-stage samplers	Agar plates	Culturing, molecular biology
	Andersen N-6 sampler	Agar plate	Culturing, molecular biology
	Other N-6-type sieve impactors	Agar plate	Culturing, molecular biology
	BioCassette	Agar plate	Culturing, molecular biology
Filter sampling	Various filter cassettes	Filter	Microscopy, culturing, immunoassays, molecular biology
	Button personal sampler	Filter	Microscopy, culturing, immunoassays, molecular biology
Light scattering	KH-3000-01	None	Automated sampler
Image analysis	BAA500	Greased disc	Automated sampler, microscopy for validation
Light scattering and fluorescence	Rapid-E	Optional slide	Automated sampler, microscopy for validation

airborne fungal spores. Current spore traps based on the Hirst design are available from Burkard Manufacturing Co. Ltd. (http://burkard.co.uk/) and Lanzoni, S.r.l. (https://www.lanzoni.it/). These instruments are generally supplied with a 7-day sampling head to permit continuous sampling.

Air is drawn into the spore trap through a 14 mm × 2 mm orifice at 10 L/min by a pump located at the base of the instrument (Figure 2.1). The cut point size for the standard orifice is 3.7 μm; this means that all but the smallest spores are efficiently captured by these spore traps [11]. A wind vane attached to the sampler ensures that the orifice is oriented into the wind. Particles entering through the orifice with sufficient inertia impact on a greased plastic (Melenex) tape, which is supported on a drum driven by a 7-day clock. The clock moves the impaction surface beneath the orifice

at 2 mm/h, and the tape makes a 360° revolution over 7 days. The sampler drum is changed each week; the tape is detached and subsequently cut into seven 48 mm segments representing the 7 days. For microscope analysis, the tape segments are fixed onto microscope slides. Glycerin jelly mounting medium containing basic fuchsin is added to stain pollen grains and make the slides semipermanent.

Once the mounting medium has solidified, the slides can be analyzed by microscopy. Pollen grains are normally counted at a magnification of ×400, while fungal spores are counted with an oil immersion objective for a total magnification of ×1000. Various counting methods can be used to analyze the slides including one to four longitudinal traverses down the 48 mm length of the tape segment or 12 transverse traverses across the tape

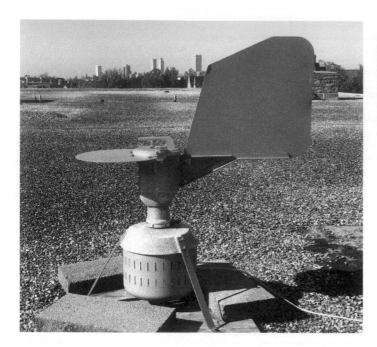

Figure 2.1 Hirst-type (Burkard) volumetric spore trap. This slit impactor can be equipped with a sampler head to sample for 7 days or 24 hours.

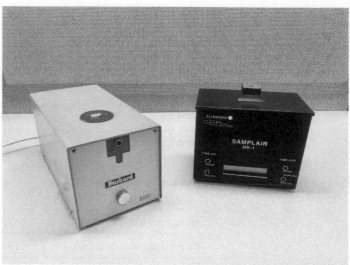

Figure 2.2 Burkard continuous recording air sampler (left) and Allergenco sampler (right). These portable slit impactors can collect bioaerosols onto a greased microscope slide for up to 24 hours. The Burkard instrument samples continuously, while the Allergenco can collect up to 24 discreet samples.

segment [36–40]. Because the sampler drum moves at 2 mm/h, time-discriminate analysis is possible. As a result, many investigators use the 12-transverse traverse method to determine counts at 4 mm intervals, which provides bioaerosol data for every 2 hours. Microscope counts are converted to atmospheric concentrations of enumerated pollen and fungal spores. In addition to microscopy, tape segments can be analyzed by immunoassays or by molecular methods.

A 24-hour sampling head, which permits direct sampling onto a greased microscope slide, is available for Hirst-type spore traps. This head contains a slide-holding carriage that moves the slide beneath the orifice. The slide is changed daily, stained, and analyzed by microscopy as described earlier. This alternate head is used by many investigators in the allergy community who want to make airborne pollen and spore concentrations available to their patients on a daily basis. An interchangeable orifice is also available for the Burkard spore trap to increase sampling efficiency. The cut size for this orifice is 2.17 μm, which increases the sampling efficiency for very small spores.

Portable spore traps are used for indoor air sampling as well as for specific, outdoor applications. The Burkard continuous recording air sampler (http://burkard.co.uk/) is designed for operation for 6, 12, or 24 hours (Figure 2.2). Air is drawn in through a slit on the top at 10 L/min, and particles are impacted on a microscope slide that moves beneath the orifice. The Allergenco MK-3 (https://www.emssales.net/) is a similar sampler that permits monitoring over time; it can collect up to 24 separate air samples on a single microscope slide (Figure 2.2). This sampler can be programmed for the sampling and inactive intervals. The standard setting collects a 10-minute air sample each hour; however, the programming can be easily adjusted for shorter or longer intervals. The flow rate of the Allergenco MK-3 is 15 L/min, and the particle cut point size is 2.5 μm.

A number of portable devices are designed to collect a single sample over a short period of time, typically from 5 to 15 minutes.

The Burkard personal sampler (http://burkard.co.uk/) is a small cylindrical spore trap containing a pump within the unit (Figure 2.3). A 14 mm × 1 mm slit orifice is situated at the top of the sampler, and air is aspirated at 10 L/min with a particle cut point of 2.5 μm. Bioaerosols and other particulates are impacted as a single trace on a standard greased microscope slide. The Buck BioSlide (http://www.apbuck.com/shop/) also collects a single sample on a greased microscope slide. The flow rate of the sampling pump is adjustable from 10 to 20 L/min, and sampling time can be programmed for a 1-, 2-, 5-, or 10-minute collection period.

A variety of single-use sampling cassettes are also available for collecting air samples. These impactors require a calibrated external pump and impact bioaerosols on a solid matrix (Figure 2.3). After sampling, the cassette is opened, and the impaction surface is

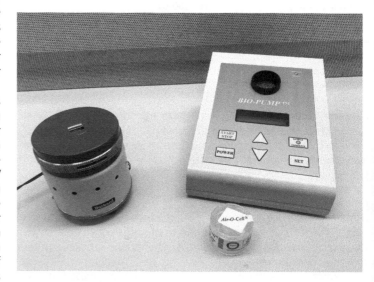

Figure 2.3 Burkard personal sampler and Air-O-Cell cassette with pump. These portable slit impactors collect a single air sample and generally operate for 5–10 minutes.

mounted on a microscope slide and analyzed by microscopy. Widely used sampling cassettes include Air-O-Cell (https://www.zefon.com/), Allergenco D, Cyclex-D, and Micro 5 (https:// www.emssales.net). Air-O-Cell cassettes have a 1.1 mm × 14.5 mm slit orifice and require a pump with 15 L/min capacity. The cut-size is approximately 2.5 μm. Other cassettes differ in the orifice design, flow-rate requirements for the external pump, and particle cutoff diameter [25].

2.3.1.3 SUCTION SAMPLERS: SIEVE IMPACTORS

Sieve impactors are used to collect airborne fungal spores or bacteria from outdoor or indoor environments for culturing. Airborne particles are drawn in through multiple holes and impact directly onto agar plates [11]. The original impactor of this type was a six-stage Andersen cascade impactor [41]. Each stage contains an open Petri dish with culture medium, and the cover plate for each stage has a sieve with 400 holes. The diameter of the holes decreases from 1.18 mm in stage 1 down to 0.25 mm in stage 6, and the particle cut size decreases as well from 7 μm down to 0.65 μm for stage 6. One- and two-stage models are also manufactured (https://www.thermofisher.com). The one-stage model (Figure 2.4), which consists of the sixth stage (N-6) from the original cascade impactor, is widely used in aerobiology research and has provided a wealth of data on culturable airborne fungi from both indoor and outdoor environments [42–45]. After the expiration of the patent, Andersen-type samplers have been produced by various other companies. A disposable version of the single-stage model, called the BioCassette device (https://www.emlab.com/), combines the sieve impactor and the Petri dish into a single unit. A study compared the BioCassette with a single-stage Andersen sampler and found no significant difference between total culturable fungi and *Penicillium* concentrations [46]. These sieve impactors all require an external pump capable of flow rates of 28.3 L/min. Sampling times generally range from 1 to 5 minutes. Many other types of sieve impactors are also available [11,25]. They differ in the number of openings in the sieve plate, the flow rate, and the optimum sampling time; some models even contain a sampling pump within the unit.

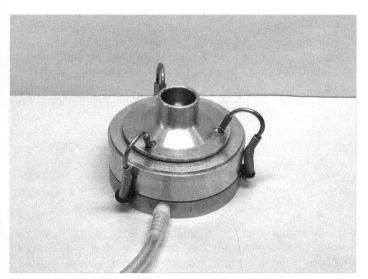

Figure 2.4 Anderson N-6 sampler. This sieve impactor is designed to collect particles onto an agar surface in an open Petri dish. A sieve plate with 400 holes is situated beneath the inlet cone.

After sampling Petri dishes are incubated, the colonies are counted and identified by microscopic examination. Concentrations are calculated and expressed as colony-forming units per cubic meter of air. When sieve impactors are used, more than one viable spore may pass through a single opening on the sieve plate, and these would likely be inaccurately counted as a single colony [25,27]. A positive-hole correction factor is used to adjust for multiple impactions.

Limitations of sieve impactors relate to culture-based sampling in general [47,48]. Not all fungi grow in culture; others may not grow on the culture medium used or under the incubation conditions applied. Other fungi may grow but not produce spores under the culture conditions used; these mycelial colonies cannot be identified by morphology. Diverse spore types are generally collected during air sampling, but standard culturing methods are biased toward fast-growing species. Last, some fungal spores may have lost viability, although they may still retain allergenic properties. As a result, culture-based sampling may not represent the total diversity of spores present in the atmosphere.

2.3.2 Filter samplers

Filter sampling traps bioaerosols and other particles as the airstream passes through a fibrous or porous matrix [2,11,25]. Samplers range from small cassettes used for personal exposure to larger devices that can process hundreds of liters of air every minute [49–52].

Disposable filter cassettes are the most frequently used method to assess personal exposure to allergens or other particulates in occupational settings [25,53]. Most filter cassettes are preloaded by the manufacturer with a single sterile filter in a standard diameter, such as 25, 37, or 47 mm. Cassettes have a single circular orifice and are worn by workers, typically in proximity to the nose and mouth. An external pump is required and is usually attached to the worker's belt. Pumps typically operate at low flow rates of 2–4 L/min to allow for sampling for multiple hours without overloading the filter.

A range of filter media and a range of pore sizes are available in cassettes; choice of filter types depends on the particulates to be sampled and the method of analysis to be used [11,25]. Sampling efficiency is quite high but influenced by the filter type and pore size. Cellulose ester filters are commonly used for microscopic analysis of fungal spores since they become transparent with mounting media. In fact, the 25 mm cellulose ester filters can be easily mounted on a standard microscope slide. For immunoassays, cassettes with polytetrafluoroethylene (PTFE) filters are normally utilized since the sample can easily be eluted from the filter. PTFE filters can also be processed for molecular analysis of bioaerosols. Several filter types can be used for culturing collected fungal spores or bacteria [54]; however, a limitation of filter sampling is desiccation of microorganisms over long sampling times.

Several reusable filter samplers are available [54], with the button personal sampler the most versatile (https://www.skcinc.com/catalog/index.php?cPath=400000000_401000000_401000200). The button sampler has a porous hemispheric inlet with numerous, 381 μm diameter orifices (Figure 2.5). This type of inlet improves particle collection across the filter and is insensitive to wind direction [55,56]. Therefore, this instrument can be used for both indoor and outdoor sampling.

Filter sampling is not generally used for routine outdoor monitoring of pollen and spores; however, the method has been used in a variety of studies to detect specific allergens in the

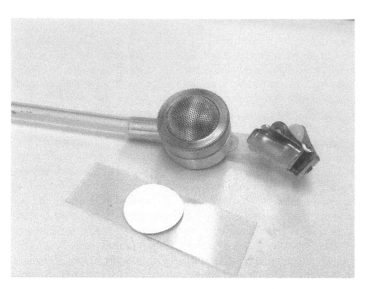

Figure 2.5 Button personal sampler. This reusable sampler holds small filters. It can be used outdoors or indoors and can also be attached to a worker's clothing for occupational exposure assessment.

atmosphere. Schäppi et al. [57] used a high-volume cascade sampler with filters to collect daily airborne Bet v 1 allergens detected with a monoclonal antibody-based enzyme-linked immunosorbent assay (ELISA). They found that allergen levels significantly correlated with airborne *Betula* pollen concentrations; however, during days with light rain, there were dramatic increases in concentrations of Bet v 1 in respirable particles. Brito et al. [49,50] used a high-volume filter sampler for the collection of daily grass allergens [49] and Ole e 1 allergens [50] identified with ELISA assays using pooled patient sera. In both studies, allergen levels significantly correlated with the respective airborne pollen concentrations and with patient symptoms. Filter sampling has also been used for the molecular detection of bioaerosols [51,52].

In addition to the use of filters directly for air sampling, Barnes et al. [58] analyzed furnace filters from 56 homes to indirectly examine airborne allergen abundance within homes. The authors analyzed the dust accumulated on the return side of furnace filters using both cultures for viable fungi and immunoassays for Fel d 1, Can f 1, Mus m 1, Der f 1, Der p 1, and Bla g 2, as well as antigens from *Alternaria alternata, Aspergillus fumigatus, Cladosporium herbarum,* and *Penicillium notatum.* The authors detected significant immunoassay levels of all allergens and cultured a variety of fungi.

2.3.3 Other samplers

There are a number of other types of sampling instruments used in bioaerosol research including cyclone samplers, impingement samplers, and electrostatic precipitators. In cyclone samplers, the airstream is drawn into a cylinder through a tangential inlet and follows a downward spiral through the cylinder [2,25,27]. The inertia of particles larger than the particle cut-size causes them to hit the walls of the cyclone and then drop to the bottom of the cylinder. Following the downward spiral, the airstream reverses and comes up through the center of the cylinder and out through an exit at the top. In several cyclone samplers, a detachable 1.5 mL microcentrifuge tube is at the bottom end of the cylinder, and bioaerosols and other particles collect there. External pumps for the

cyclone samplers vary from small pumps with low flow rates for personal sampling to larger pumps with high flow rates. Many types of cyclone samplers are available with some models collecting dry samples and others collecting into a liquid. Cyclone samplers may be paired with filters; larger particles are collected by the cyclone, and fine particles remain in the airstream and are subsequently collected by filtration. A variety of analytical methods can be used following cyclone sampling, with immunologic assays or molecular detection methods the most common.

Impingement samplers separate particles from the airstream using inertia; however, unlike impactors, the particles deposit into a collection fluid, not a solid surface. Air is drawn into the sampler through a nozzle using an external pump. The end of the nozzle is submerged in the liquid, and bioaerosols from the airstream are dispersed in the bubbling liquid [2,11]. The collection fluid is frequently a dilute buffer; however, surfactants may be added to ensure spores form a suspension [27]. Collection into liquid avoids the risk of desiccation, which can occur when fungal spores or bacteria are collected by other methods [12,25]. However, evaporation of the collection fluid can occur during prolonged sampling. This tends to limit sampling to 1 hour or less. Also, reentrainment of collected bioaerosols can occur when bubbles burst at the surface of the liquid [12]. Bioaerosols collected by liquid impingers can be analyzed by various methods including microscopy, culturing, immunoassays, and molecular biology.

In electrostatic precipitators, air is drawn into the sampler, and entrained particles are electrically charged. These charged particles are then subjected to an electrostatic field that deposits the particles on a collection plate [11,26]. The particles are subsequently extracted from the collection surface and available for analysis by various techniques.

2.4 MODERN METHODS: MOLECULAR ANALYSIS OF BIOAEROSOLS

Although microscopy and culturing remain useful tools for pollen and spore identification, neither method can identify all bioaerosols. In viable sampling methods, many fungi cannot be grown in culture at all; other fungi do not grow on common laboratory culture media or under standard incubation conditions [48]. When air samples are analyzed by microscopy, some fungi lack distinctive morphologic features for even genus-level identification. For example, *Penicillium* and *Aspergillus* conidia are generally grouped together as *Penicillium/Aspergillus*-type spores, and many basidiospores can only be identified to phylum level as basidiospores [12]. Also, some pollen types can only be identified to family level by microscopy; these include pollen in the grass family (Poaceae), nettle family (Urticaceae), and cedar family (Cupressaceae) [59].

Molecular methods of analysis can resolve these identification issues. These methods can be used to analyze a variety of air samples including those collected by gravity, impaction, filtration, impingement, cyclonic separation, and electrostatic precipitation. When sieve impactors are used for viable sampling, molecular methods can be used to identify unknown colonies or to confirm the identification based on morphologic analysis. For about 25 years, molecular methods have been used for identifying bioaerosols. This section describes some of the widely used molecular methods and provides just a few of the many examples of their applications in aerobiology.

2.4.1 Polymerase chain reaction

The polymerase chain reaction (PCR) is an indispensable tool for molecular identification. This technique amplifies a segment of DNA extracted from an organism or from an environmental sample resulting in large quantities of that DNA segment. PCR requires the use of primers, short, 20-base segments of DNA, that hybridize to the beginning and end of the DNA segment of interest. The primers can be highly specific targeting a single species or more general targeting large groups of organisms such as families or classes. With species-specific primers, only the DNA from that one species would be amplified, thereby confirming the identification of that species in the sample. Once the DNA has been amplified, it can be visualized, quantified, sequenced, or undergo additional analyses [60].

The first molecular aerobiology experiments used conventional (also referred to as endpoint) PCR for the detection of viral and microbial DNA. In 1991 Saksena et al. [61] identified viral DNA in passively collected air samples. Alvarez et al. [62] compared PCR detection with culture-based methods to detect aerosolized *Escherichia coli* and determined that PCR detection was more sensitive than culture-based methods. Subsequently, Alvarez et al. [63] developed improved methods for PCR use with bioaerosol samples and detected *E. coli* and/or *Shigella* spp. in outdoor samples.

Wakefield [64] tested spore trap air samples for the presence of *Pneumocystis carinii* f. sp. *hominis*. To verify that the 267 base-pair PCR product was from *P. carinii* f. sp. *hominis,* it was cloned into plasmids and sequenced. Calderon et al. [65] developed a nested-PCR assay to detect *Penicillium roqueforti* conidia in a wind tunnel trial using a rotating arm impactor and Hirst-type sampler. Nested PCR enhances the specificity of the PCR by using a second set of primers, and the resulting assay had a detection limit of 10 spores. The same lab also developed a nested-PCR assay for the plant pathogens *Leptosphaeria maculans* and *Pyrenopeziza brassicae* [66] with the same detection limit. The authors identified DNA from these pathogens in air samples collected with a Hirst-type spore trap situated near infected oilseed rape crops. The specificity, sensitivity, and reduced processing time of PCR methods, compared to culture-based methods, have been advantageous in screening air samples for specific organisms.

PCR products can also be used for the identification of unknown bioaerosols; however, this requires extensive processing of the amplified PCR products [24,51,67]. The PCR product must be cloned, analyzed by restriction fragment length polymorphism, and sequenced. Following sequencing of the gene, identification is made through a BLAST search.

2.4.2 Quantitative polymerase chain reaction

The development of real-time or quantitative PCR (qPCR) has allowed for the quantification of pollen, fungal spores, and other organisms in the environment in contrast to the qualitative assessment provided by endpoint PCR [68,69]. In qPCR the DNA product is monitored during the amplification process using a sequence-specific fluorescent probe or a fluorescent DNA-binding dye [70,71]. As new DNA is synthesized during the amplification process, the fluorescence is detected. For quantification, the threshold cycle (Ct value) for each sample is calculated; this is the amplification cycle at which the fluorescent threshold is exceeded. The DNA concentration of the sample is determined by comparing the Ct value to the Ct values of a standard curve [71].

Numerous studies have used qPCR to quantify airborne microorganisms and pollen [72–76]. Haugland et al. [72] developed a quick and accurate qPCR assay to detect indoor fungal concentrations of *Stachybotrys chartarum*. Their assay was robust and sensitive, detecting several different strains of *S. chartarum* with a two-cell limit of detection. Makino et al. [73] quantified *Bacillus anthracis* from air samples collected on a nitrocellulose filter. The qPCR assay was able to quantify the bacterium with the limit of detection at one cell. Schweigkofler et al. [74] developed a qPCR assay for *Fusarium circinatum*, a fungal pathogen on pine trees; this assay was able to rapidly quantify the amount of inoculum, which had settled on filters at two sites with infected pines. Zeng et al. [75] quantified *Cladosporium* conidia from indoor and outdoor filter-collected air samples using a qPCR assay. They tested the specificity of their assay against a mock community of 10 common airborne fungi.

Longhi et al. [76] carried out the first published studies using qPCR assays for quantifying pollen grains. The authors developed qPCR assays for many common allergenic pollen types and tested these with pollen suspension. For three of the pollen types, *Betula pendula, Ostrya carpinifolia,* and *Parietaria officinalis,* they compared quantification of pollen suspensions by microscopy and qPCR assays. The data showed no significant differences in quantities determined by the two methods. The authors also showed it was possible to extract DNA from pollen on a simulated Hirst-type air sample tape manually spread with various pollen types.

Mohanty et al. [77] identified and quantified *Juniperus* pollen grains to species level from 105 air samples from a Hirst-type spore trap using a qPCR assay. *Juniperus* is a member of the Cupressaceae, and the pollen can only be identified to the family level. The authors developed species specific primers for three Cupressaceae species that naturally occur in Oklahoma: *Juniperus virginia, J. ashei,* and *J. pinchotii.* The pollen concentrations estimated by the qPCR assays significantly correlated with Cupressaceae pollen concentrations determined by light microscopy. Additionally, they identified an overlap in the pollination seasons between *Juniperus pinchotii* and *J. ashei* in the fall and between *J. ashei* and *J. virginiana* in late winter by using species-specific primers. This work was especially important due to the highly allergenic nature of *J. ashei* pollen.

Like the Cupressaceae, pollen in the Poaceae can only be determined to the family level by microscopy. Ghitarrini et al. [78] laid the foundation for refining the pollen season for major allergenic grass species by establishing techniques for molecular identification of Poaceae taxa from a Hirst-type spore trap. They developed assays specific for *Dactylis glomerata, Phleum pretense, Festuca arundinacea,* and *Poa pratensis* as well as an assay for all members of the subfamily Pooideae. Although qPCR species-specific assays failed to amplify pollen directly from the air samples, the primers did show amplification of air samples in a nested PCR assay. In addition, the qPCR primers for the Pooideae successfully amplified pollen from spore trap samples.

These studies show that qPCR assays can successfully assess the concentration of specific airborne fungal spores and pollen. The method is relatively quick and less labor-intensive since neither culturing nor microscopy is required.

2.4.3 Next-generation sequencing

Next-generation sequencing (NGS) has become widely used over the past few decades for many applications, including for the identification and quantification of bioaerosols and other environmental samples. NGS is a general term used to describe several different sequencing technologies, which are often referred to as high-throughput sequencing [79,80]. These include Illumina sequencing, 454 pyrosequencing, Ion Torrent sequencing, and others. A detailed description of the different NGS platforms is beyond the scope of this chapter. These technologies are similar in that they sequence millions of small DNA fragments simultaneously. Subsequently, bioinformatic analyses are used to piece the fragments together. NGS determines DNA sequences more quickly and with less cost than previous sequencing, creating a revolution in genomics.

NGS is frequently used for metagenomic analysis—the study of the genetic material of all organisms from an environmental sample [81]. The aim of metagenomics is to characterize the microbial diversity and ecology of a specific environment, including atmospheric samples. NGS results yield operational taxonomic units (OTUs), clusters of similar DNA sequences for a particular marker gene, generally the 16S rRNA gene for bacteria, ITS gene for fungi, and 18S rRNA gene for other eukaryotes. The sequence similarity is commonly defined at 97%, and OTUs may designate a species, a genus, or other taxonomic level. Unlike qPCR, prior knowledge of the organisms present and prior development of species-specific primers are not needed.

Peay and Bruns [82] investigated spore dispersal of basidiomycete fungi using 454 pyrosequencing. Bioaerosols were collected in multiple sedimentary traps with samples harvested approximately monthly. DNA was extracted from the collected material, and a preliminary PCR step used primers that were specific for members of the Basidiomycota. This step restricted the subsequent NGS to members of that phylum. Results from the pyrosequencing showed that between 50 and 100 basidiomycete species were detected in the spore traps during each sampling period. Overall, the authors were able to assign the OTUs to 381 genera of basidiomycetes and 128 families, with the 20 most common genera accounting for 72% of all sequences.

Dannemiller et al. [52] used 454 pyrosequencing and qPCR to characterize the airborne fungi from Rehovot, Israel, using filter sampling. There were 10 sampling periods, most of which were 3 days long. DNA was extracted from a portion of each filter, and the ITS region of the rRNA gene was amplified by PCR prior to pyrosequencing. Sequence reads were identified by BLAST searches; overall, sequencing produced 2488 OTUs. Quantitative PCR analysis was also performed for total fungi and for select taxa. The NGS showed a highly diverse community of airborne microorganisms. The qPCR concentrations for four fungal taxa significantly correlated with adjusted NGS results for these taxa.

Keller et al. [83] performed NGS as well as microscopy on 16 mixed pollen samples, which consisted of pollen grains collected by honeybees and solitary bees. NGS pollen abundance was significantly correlated with abundance determined by microscopy. However, the authors found that NGS resulted in more taxa identified to genus level and to species level when compared to light microscopy.

Kraaijeveld et al. [84] developed a protocol for the identification of airborne grass pollen to genus level using the Ion Torrent NGS platform. The authors extracted DNA from 3 days of air samples collected with a Hirst-type spore trap and also from a control sample of six known grass pollen species. PCR was used to amplify a portion of the chloroplast gene *trnL* from the extracted DNA, and the PCR products were sequenced with the Ion Torrent platform. Following BLAST searches of the air sample sequences, the number of matches for a given genus or family closely correlated with the data from microscopy. In the control mixture of known grasses, four of grass pollen genera were correctly identified with 100% sequence similarity; however, the BLAST search could not identify the remaining two species with certainty.

Núñez et al. [85] investigated the use of a Hirst-type spore trap for the metagenomic analysis of bacteria, fungi, and pollen. Air samples analyzed included 3 weeks from December and 1 week in July. Melinex tape used on the sampler drum was split longitudinally prior to sampling with one-half used for Illumina Mi-Seq NGS and the other for microscopy. DNA was extracted from one-half of each weekly spore trap tape and amplified using universal primers specific for bacteria, fungi, and plants prior to sequencing. NGS revealed a high diversity of airborne bacteria, fungi, and pollen. When results were compared to microscopy for pollen and fungi, the sequencing results revealed greater discrimination in identified taxa. For example, as expected, all grass pollen was identified as Poaceae pollen using microscopy; however, 17 species of grass pollen were identified by NGS.

The studies described show the value of NGS in aerobiological research. These technologies allow for the identification of a large diversity of organisms from environmental samples, including aeroallergens and pathogens. As sequencing costs continue to decrease, NGS may provide a valuable alternative or supplement to microscopy.

2.5 MODERN METHODS: AUTOMATED AND REAL-TIME SAMPLING

The sampling techniques and analysis methods described earlier have been widely used to identify airborne pollen and spores. Unfortunately, none of these techniques or methods can provide real-time analysis of bioaerosols. Pollen levels currently available online or through mass media are, at best, data that represent the previous day's collections. In addition, these traditional sampling methods require considerable time and expertise for the microscopic analysis of collected air samples [86]. To overcome this time lag, many investigators have developed pollen or spore forecasts to estimate current and future pollen levels [39,87–90]. However, even the best forecasting models only provide an estimate of exposure based on meteorological conditions and plant phenology. For allergists and their patients, knowledge of current (real-time) exposure levels would be valuable [91].

Since the 1990s, researchers in several countries have been working on the development of automated and real-time sampling instruments, and great strides have been made in recent years [91–100]. Today, several instruments are available that can sample, identify, and quantify airborne pollen with the results available electronically. Other instruments are in the development stage. A number of these devices have been tested at the MeteoSwiss research facility in Payerne, Switzerland, where a range of monitoring devices and Hirst-type samplers are available (Figure 2.6). The monitors described here are those that are currently utilized in one or more national monitoring networks.

The KH-3000-01 developed by Yamatronics Corporation, Japan (http://www.yamatronics.com) is a laser particle counter and was one of the first real-time pollen monitors developed. Air is drawn into the device through an inlet at 4.1 L/min, and particulates pass through the beam of a 780 nm semiconductor laser [92,93]. The

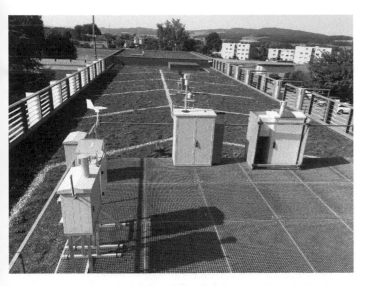

Figure 2.6 MeteoSwiss research site in Payerne, Switzerland, with four real-time samplers. (Left) Two KH-3000-1 samplers from Yamatronics. (Center) A Rapid-E from Plair. (Right) A Poleno prototype from Swisens. In the background are two Hirst-type spore traps used as reference samplers. (Photo courtesy of Dr. Bernard Clot, MeteoSwiss.)

resulting light scattered from particles is detected for both forward and side scatter, and these data are transmitted to a computer along with the number of particles detected. The intensity of scattered light relates to the particle size; therefore, the data also provide information on the pollen size, in the range of 25–38 μm. This instrument has been especially useful for detecting concentrations of *Cryptomeria japonica* (Japanese cedar) and *Chamaecyparis obtusa* (Japanese cypress) pollen, the major aeroallergens in Japan. Since 2008, the Ministry of Environment (MOE) in Japan has developed a network of 120 KH-3000-01 real-time pollen monitors throughout the country, and hourly pollen information is available to the population on the MOE website [8,93,94]. One limitation of this device is the inability to distinguish pollen from nonbiological particulates in the same size range [92].

The Hund BAA-500 (https://www.hund.de/en/) is an automated monitor that combines pollen collection with microscopy and image analysis to determine pollen identification in near real time [95,96]. The instrument draws in air at 1000 L/min and particulates with an aerodynamic diameter greater than 11 μm are deposited on a disc with a sticky surface. After a sampling period of 1–3 hours, the disc is mechanically moved toward an automated microscope equipped with a CCD camera for digital imaging. Pollen counts are based on image processing, and the identification is based on neural network algorithms. The results are transmitted to the pollen network and reported online. Depending on the length of the sampling period, the BAA500 pollen monitor can provide from 8 to 24 pollen reports each day. Oteros et al. [96] compared the results of the automated identification to the manual identification of the same samples. Results showed that the BAA500 correctly recognized over 77% of the pollen. However, some taxa such as *Salix* were not identified correctly, and rare pollen types were identified as unknown. The authors also compared the results from BAA500 monitor with those from a Hirst-type sampler run simultaneously and positioned approximately 5 m apart. Results showed highly signification correlations for airborne pollen concentrations from both instruments. Although there were significant correlations,

some pollen types were collected in different quantities by the two devices. There are currently six BAA500 monitors operating in Germany [8] with additional ones to be added.

The Rapid-E [97] is the latest version of a real-time bioaerosol detection instrument from Plair SA (http://www.plair.ch/). This monitor, originally referred to as Plair PA-300, is an all optical real-time detector with an hourly resolution [91]. Air is drawn into the device at 2 L/min, and each particle initially passes through the beam of infrared lasers. Two photodetectors record the light scattering, which characterizes the particle size and surface features. An ultraviolet laser then excites each particle inducing fluorescence of bioaerosols. The fluorescent spectrum and duration are detected, and these metrics are distinct for different pollen types. Using the fluorescence and light scattering data, machine-learning algorithms automatically determine the pollen identity [91]; the concentrations of the identified pollen are available online. Fluorescent-based monitors can also measure air pollutants; therefore, the online system also reports PM1, PM2.5, PM10, and total particulates [97]. An added feature of Rapid-E is the ability to collect airborne bioaerosols and other particles on filters, which can be used for quality control of real-time data. The Rapid-E is currently in use in several European countries.

In addition to the instruments previously described, many other real-time monitors are either available or in development, including Swisens Poleno (https://swisens.ch/) [98], WIBS (http://www.dropletmeasurement.com/) [99], and Pollen Sense (https://pollensense.com/) [100]. There is growing interest in these instruments by aerobiological networks around the world for multiple reasons: counting and identification are accomplished in real time, few consumables are needed, extensive training is not required, and there is potential to locate monitors in areas where no traditional counting stations are available. Although real-time monitoring is becoming a reality, it does not mean that traditional approaches to air sampling will stop. Real-time systems are still developing and are not currently able to identify new and rare pollen grains or most spore types. The most advanced instruments are only able to identify about 20 pollen types and far fewer fungal spore types. Also, the cost of these real-time monitors may limit their use, especially for individual clinicians. Nevertheless, these automatic devices expand the repertoire of techniques available for bioaerosol monitoring and help determine exposure risk and improve the accuracy of pollen and spore forecasting.

SALIENT POINTS

1. Bioaerosols are a significant component of the atmosphere as well as indoor air. Many bioaerosols impact human health causing infectious or allergic diseases, and air sampling is a valuable tool to estimate exposure to these organisms.
2. Slit impactors, rotating-arm impactors, and sieve impactors are widely used, traditional sampling instruments for routine monitoring of the outdoor atmosphere and indoor environments. Microscopy and culturing are the analytical methods most commonly used with these instruments.
3. Within the past 20 years, molecular methods such as polymerase chain reaction (PCR), quantitative PCR (qPCR), and Next-generation sequencing (NGS) have greatly increased our understanding of bioaerosol diversity both outdoors and indoors.
4. Real-time and automated air sampling instruments have also been developed in recent decades. Although still under

development, these instruments can sample, quantify, and identify many bioaerosols automatically and report the data electronically in real time.

5. Traditional sampling approaches in combination with these new sampling instruments and analytical techniques will continue to expand our knowledge of bioaerosols and their impact on human health.

REFERENCES

1. Gregory PH. *The Microbiology of the Atmosphere*, 2nd ed. New York, NY: Halstead Press, 1973.
2. Lacey ME, West JS. *The Air Spora: A Manual for Catching and Identifying Airborne Biological Particles*. Dordrecht, the Netherlands: Springer, 2007.
3. Amato P, Brisebois E, Draghi M et al. Main biological aerosols, specificities, abundance, and diversity. In: Delort AM, Amato P, editors. *Microbiology of Aerosols*. Hoboken, NJ: John Wiley & Sons, 2018.
4. Geller-Bernstein C, Portnoy JM. The clinical utility of pollen counts. *Clin Rev Allergy Immunol* 2019;57:340–349.
5. Darrow LA, Hess J, Rogers CA, Tolbert PE, Klein M, Sarnat SE. Ambient pollen concentrations and emergency department visits for asthma and wheeze. *J Allergy Clinic Immunol* 2012; 130(3): 630–638.
6. Silverberg JI, Braunstein M, Lee-Wong M. Association between climate factors, pollen counts, and childhood hay fever prevalence in the United States. *J Allergy Clinic Immunol* 2015; 135(2): 463–469.
7. Sun X, Waller A, Yeatts KB, Thie L. Pollen concentration and asthma exacerbations in Wake County, North Carolina, 2006–2012. *Sci Total Environ* 2016; 544: 185–191.
8. Buters JT, Antunes C, Galveias A et al. Pollen and spore monitoring in the world. *Clin Transl Allergy* 2018; 8(1): 9.
9. Chapman MD, Tsay A, Vailes LD. Home allergen monitoring and control–improving clinical practice and patient benefits. *Allergy* 2001; 56(7): 604–610.
10. Salo PM, Wilkerson J, Rose KM et al. Bedroom allergen exposures in US households. *J Allergy Clin Immunol* 2018; 141: 1870–1879.
11. Grinshpun SA, Buttner MP, Mainelis G, Willeke K. Sampling for airborne microorganisms. In Yates MV, Nakatsu CH, Miller RV, Pillai SD, editors. *Manual of Environmental Microbiology*, 4th ed. Washington, DC: American Society of Microbiology Press, 2016: 3.2.2.1–3.2.2.17.
12. Scott JA, Summerbell RC, Green BJ. Detection of indoor fungi bioaerosols. In: Aden OCG, Samson RA, editors. *Fundamentals of Mold Growth in Indoor Environments and Strategies for Healthy Living*. Wageningen, the Netherlands: Wageningen Academic, 2011: 353–379.
13. Levetin E, Rogers CA, Hall SA. Comparison of pollen sampling with a Burkard Spore Trap and a Tauber Trap in a warm temperate climate. *Grana* 2000; 39(6): 294–302.
14. Moore PD, Webb JA, Collinson ME. *Pollen Analysis*, 2nd ed. Oxford, UK: Blackwell, 1991.
15. Ranta H, Sokol C, Hicks S, Heino S, Kubin E. How do airborne and deposition pollen samplers reflect the atmospheric dispersal of different pollen types? An example from northern Finland. *Grana* 2008; 47(4): 285–296.
16. van der Knaap WO, van Leeuwen JF, Svitavská-Svobodová H et al. Annual pollen traps reveal the complexity of climatic control on pollen productivity in Europe and the Caucasus. *Veg Hist Archaeobot* 2010; 19(4): 285–307.
17. Latorre F, Romero EJ, Mancini MV. Comparative study of different methods for capturing airborne pollen, and effects of vegetation and meteorological variables. *Aerobiologia* 2008; 24(2): 107–120.
18. Frankel M, Timm M, Hansen EW, Madsen AM. Comparison of sampling methods for the assessment of indoor microbial exposure. *Indoor Air* 2012; 22(5): 405–414.
19. Chew GL, Rogers C, Burge HA, Muilenberg ML, Gold DR. Dustborne and airborne fungal propagules represent a different spectrum of fungi with differing relations to home characteristics. *Allergy* 2003; 58(1): 13–20.
20. Madsen AM, Matthiesen CB, Frederiksen MW et al. Sampling, extraction and measurement of bacteria, endotoxin, fungi and inflammatory potential of settling indoor dust. *J Environ Monitor* 2012; 14(12): 3230–3239.
21. Adams RI, Tian Y, Taylor JW, Bruns TD, Hyvärinen A, Täubel M. Passive dust collectors for assessing airborne microbial material. *Microbiome* 2015; 3(1): 46.
22. Green BJ, Lemons AR, Park Y, Cox-Ganser JM, Park JH. Assessment of fungal diversity in a water-damaged office building. *J Occup Environ Hyg* 2017; 14: 285–293.
23. Barberán A, Ladau J, Leff JW et al. Continental-scale distributions of dust-associated bacteria and fungi. *P Natl Acad Sci USA* 2015; 112: 5756–5761.
24. Leontidou K, Vernesi C, De Groeve J, Cristofolini F, Vokou D, Cristofori A. DNA metabarcoding of airborne pollen: New protocols for improved taxonomic identification of environmental samples. *Aerobiologia* 2018; 34(1): 63–74.
25. Lindsley WG, Green BJ, Blachere FM et al. Sampling and characterization of bioaerosols. In: Ashley K, O'Connor PF, editors. *NIOSH Manual of Analytical Methods*. 5th ed. Cincinnati, OH: National Institute for Occupational Safety and Health, 2017.
26. Amato P, Brisebois E, Draghi M et al. Sampling techniques. In: Delort AM, Amato P, editors. *Microbiology of Aerosols*. Hoboken, NJ: John Wiley & Sons, 2018.
27. West JS, Kimber RB. Innovations in air sampling to detect plant pathogens. *Ann App Biol* 2015; 166(1): 4–17.
28. Perkins, WA Leighton PA. The Rotorod sampler. *Second Semi-Annual Report* No. CML 186, Aerosol Laboratory 1957: 1–60.
29. Solomon WR, Burge HA, Boise JR, Becker M. Comparative particle recoveries by the retracting Rotorod, rotoslide, and Burkard spore trap sampling in a compact array. *Int J Biometeor* 1980; 24: 107–116.
30. Murray MG, Galán C, Villamil CB. Airborne pollen in Bahía Blanca, Argentina: Seasonal distribution of pollen types. *Aerobiologia* 2010; 26(3): 195–207.
31. Peel RG, Kennedy R, Smith M, Hertel O. Relative efficiencies of the Burkard 7-Day, Rotorod and Burkard Personal samplers for Poaceae and Urticaceae pollen under field conditions. *Ann Agr Env Med* 2014; 21(4): 745–752.
32. McCartney HA, Fitt BD, Schmechel D. Sampling bioaerosols in plant pathology. *J Aerosol Sci* 1997; 28: 349–364.
33. Aylor DE, Schmale III DG, Shields EJ, Newcomb M, Nappo CJ. Tracking the potato late blight pathogen in the atmosphere using unmanned aerial vehicles and Lagrangian modeling. *Ag Forest Meteorol* 2011; 151: 251–260.
34. Techy L, Schmale III DG, Woolsey CA. Coordinated aerobiological sampling of a plant pathogen in the lower atmosphere using two autonomous unmanned aerial vehicles. *J Field Robot* 2010; 27(3): 335–343.
35. Hirst J. An automatic volumetric spore trap. *Ann Appl Biol* 1952; 39: 257–265.

36. Kapyla M, Penttinen A. An evaluation of the microscopic counting methods of the tape in Hirst-Burkard pollen and spore trap. *Grana* 1981; 20: 131–141.

37. Comtois P, Alcazar P, Neron D. Pollen count statistics and its relevance to precision. *Aerobiologia* 1999; 15: 19–28.

38. Sterling M, Rogers C, Levetin E. An evaluation of two methods used for microscopic analysis of airborne fungal spore concentrations from the Burkard Spore Trap. *Aerobiologia* 1999; 15: 9–18.

39. Howard LE, Levetin E. Ambrosia pollen in Tulsa, Oklahoma: Aerobiology, trends, and forecasting model development. *Ann Allergy Asthma Immunol* 2014; 113: 641–646.

40. Galán C, Smith M, Thibaudon M et al.; EAS QC working group. Pollen monitoring: Minimum requirements and reproducibility of analysis. *Aerobiologia* 2014; 30(4): 385–395.

41. Andersen AA. New sampler for the collection, sizing, and enumeration of viable airborne particles. *J Bacteriol* 1958; 76(5): 471–484.

42. Shelton BG, Kirkland KH, Flanders WD, Morris GK. Profiles of airborne fungi in buildings and outdoor environments in the United States. *Appl Environ Microbiol* 2002; 68(4): 1743–1753.

43. Levetin E, Shaughnessy R, Fisher E, Ligman B, Harrison J, Brennan T. Indoor air quality in schools: Exposure to fungal allergens. *Aerobiologia* 1995; 11(1): 27–34.

44. Garrett MH, Rayment PR, Hooper MA, Abramson MJ, Hooper BM. Indoor airborne fungal spores, house dampness and associations with environmental factors and respiratory health in children. *Clin Exp Allergy* 1998; 28(4): 459–467.

45. Rosenbaum PF, Crawford JA, Anagnost SE et al. Indoor airborne fungi and wheeze in the first year of life among a cohort of infants at risk for asthma. *J Expo Sci Env Epid* 2010; 20(6): 503.

46. Gallup D, Purves J, Burge H. A disposable sampler for collecting volumetric air samples onto agar media. *J Allergy Clin Immunol* 2004; 113: S138.

47. Macher JM. Positive-hole correction of multiple-jet impactors for collecting viable microorganisms. *Am Ind Hyg Assoc J* 1989; 50(11): 561–568.

48. Lee T, Grinshpun SA, Martuzevicius D, Adhikari A, Crawford CM, Reponen T. Culturability and concentration of indoor and outdoor airborne fungi in six single-family homes. *Atmos Environ* 2006; 40(16): 2902–2910.

49. Brito FF, Gimeno PM, Carnés J et al. Grass pollen, aeroallergens, and clinical symptoms in Ciudad Real, Spain. *J Investig Allergol Clin Immunol* 2010; 20(4): 295–302.

50. Brito FF, Gimeno PM, Carnés J et al. *Olea europaea* pollen counts and aeroallergen levels predict clinical symptoms in patients allergic to olive pollen. *Ann Allergy Asthma Immunol* 2011; 106(2): 146–152.

51. Fröhlich-Nowoisky J, Pickersgill DA, Després VR, Pöschl U. High diversity of fungi in air particulate matter. *Proc Natl Acad Sci USA* 2009; 106(31): 12814–12819.

52. Dannemiller KC, Lang-Yona N, Yamamoto N, Rudich Y, Peccia J. Combining real-time PCR and next-generation DNA sequencing to provide quantitative comparisons of fungal aerosol populations. *Atmos Environ* 2014; 84: 113–121.

53. Soo JC, Monaghan K, Lee T, Kashon M, Harper M. Air sampling filtration media: Collection efficiency for respirable size-selective sampling. *Aerosol Sci Tech* 2016; 50(1): 76–87.

54. Wang CH, Chen BT, Han BC et al. Field evaluation of personal sampling methods for multiple bioaerosols. *PLOS ONE* 2015;10(3): e0120308.

55. Aizenberg V, Reponen T, Grinspun SA, Willeke K. Performance of Air-O-Cell, Burkard, and Button samplers for total enumeration of airborne spores. *Am Ind Hyg Assoc J* 2000; 61: 855–864.

56. Adhikaria A, Martuzeviciusa D, Reponen T. Performance of the Button personal inhalable sampler for the measurement of outdoor aeroallergens. *Atmos Environ* 2003; 37: 4723–4733.

57. Schäppi GF, Suphioglu C, Taylor PE, Knox RB. Concentrations of the major birch tree allergen Bet v 1 in pollen and respirable fine particles in the atmosphere. *J Allergy Clinic Immunol* 1997; 100(5): 656–661.

58. Barnes CS, Allenbrand R, Mohammed M et al. Measurement of aeroallergens from furnace filters. *Ann Allergy Asthma Immunol* 2015; 114(3): 221–225.

59. Lewis WH, Vinay P, Zenger VE. *Airborne and Allergic Pollen of North America*. Baltimore, MD: John Hopkins University Press, 1983.

60. Jenkins FJ. Basic methods for the detection of PCR products. *Genome Res* 1994; 3(5): S77–S82.

61. Saksena NK, Dwyer D, Barre-Sinoussi F. A "Sentinel" technique for monitoring viral aerosol contamination. *J Infect Dis* 1991; 164(5): 1021–1022.

62. Alvarez AJ, Buttner MP, Toranzos GA et al. Use of solid-phase PCR for enhanced detection of airborne microorganisms. *Appl Environ Microbiol* 1994; 60(1): 374–376.

63. Alvarez AJ, Buttner MP, Stetzenbach LD. PCR for bioaerosol monitoring: Sensitivity and environmental inference. *Appl Environ Microbiol* 1995; 61(10): 3639–3644.

64. Wakefield AE. DNA sequences identical to *Pneumocystis carinii* f. sp. *carinii* and *Pneumocystis carinii* f. sp. *hominis* in samples of air spora. *J Clin Microbiol* 1996; 34(7): 1754–1759.

65. Calderon C, Ward E, Freeman J, McCartney HA. Detection of airborne fungal spores sampled by rotating-arm and Hirst-type spore traps using polymerase chain reaction assays. *Aerosol Sci* 2002; 33: 283–296.

66. Calderon C, Ward E, Freeman J, Foster SJ, McCartney HA. Detection of airborne inoculum of *Leptosphaeria maculans* and *Pyrenopeziza brassicae* in oilseed rape crops by polymerase chain reaction (PCR) assays. *Plant Pathol* 2002; 51: 303–310.

67. Pashley CH, Fairs A, Free RC, Wardlaw AJ. DNA analysis of outdoor air reveals a high degree of fungal diversity, temporal variability, and genera not seen by spore morphology. *Fungal Biol* 2012; 116(2): 214–224.

68. Zhou G, Whong WZ, Ong T, Chen B. Development of a fungus-specific PCR assay for detecting low-level fungi in an indoor environment. *Mol Cell Probes* 2000; 14: 339–348.

69. Wu Z, Wang XR, Blomquist G. Evaluation of PCR primers and PCR conditions for specific detection of common airborne fungi. *J Environ Monit* 2002; 4: 377–382.

70. Heid CA, Stevens J, Livak KJ, Williams PM. Real time quantitative PCR. *Genome Res* 1996; 6(10): 986–994.

71. Rittenour WR, Hamilton RG, Beezhold DH, Green BJ. Immunologic, spectrophotometric and nucleic acid based methods for the detection and quantification of airborne pollen. *J Immunol Methods* 2012; 383(1–2): 47–53.

72. Haugland RA, Vesper SJ, Wymer LJ. Quantitative measurement of *Stachybotrys chartarum* conidia using real time detection of PCR products with the TaqMan fluorogenic probe system. *Mol Cell Probes* 1999; 13:329–340.

73. Makino SI, Cheun HI, Watarai M, Uchida I, Takeshi K. Detection of anthrax spores from the air by real-time PCR. *Lett Appl Microbiol* 2001; 33: 237–240.

74. Schweigkofler W, O'Donnell K, Garbelotto M. Detection and quantification of airborne conidia of *Fusarium circinatum*, the causal agent of pine pitch canker, from two California sites by using a real-time PCR approach combined with a simple spore trapping method. *Appl Environ Microbiol* 2004; 70(6): 3512–3520.

75. Zeng QY, Westermark SO, Rasmuson-Lestander A, Wang XR. Detection and quantification of *Cladosporium* in aerosols by real-time PCR. *J Environ Monit* 2005; 8: 153–160.

76. Longhi S, Cristofori A, Gatto P, Cristofolini F, Grando MS, Gottardini E. Biomolecular identification of allergenic pollen: A new perspective for aerobiological monitoring. *Ann Allergy Asthma Immunol* 2009; 103: 508–514.

77. Mohanty RP, Buchheim MA, Levetin E. Molecular approaches for the analysis of airborne pollen: A case study of *Juniperus* pollen. *Ann Allergy Asthma Immunol* 2017; 118(2): 204–211.

78. Ghitarrini S, Pierboni E, Rondini C et al. New biomolecular tools for aerobiological monitoring: Identification of major allergenic Poaceae species through fast real-time PCR. *Ecol Evol* 2018; 8(8): 3996–4010.

79. Shendure J, Ji H. Next-generation DNA sequencing. *Nat Biotechnol* 2008; 26(10): 1135–1145.

80. Goodwin S, McPherson JD, McCombie WR. Coming of age: Ten years of next-generation sequencing technologies. *Nat Rev Genet* 2016; 17(6): 333–351.

81. Cuadros-Orellana S, Leite LR, Smith A et al. Assessment of fungal diversity in the environment using metagenomics: A decade in review. *Fungal Genomics Biol* 2013; 3: 110.

82. Peay KG, Bruns TD. Spore dispersal of basidiomycete fungi at the landscape scale is driven by stochastic and deterministic processes and generates variability in plant-fungal interactions. *New Phytologist* 2014; 204: 180–191.

83. Keller A, Danner N, Grimmer G et al. Evaluating multiplexed next-generation sequencing as a method in palynology for mixed pollen samples. *Plant Biol* 2015; 17: 558–566.

84. Kraaijeveld K, De Weger LA, Garcia MV et al. Efficient and sensitive identification and quantification of airborne pollen using next-generation DNA sequencing. *Mol Ecol Resour* 2015; 15: 8–16.

85. Núñez A, de Paz GA, Ferencova Z et al. Validation of the Hirst-type spore trap for simultaneous monitoring of prokaryotic and eukaryotic biodiversity in urban air samples by NGS. *Appl Environ Microbiol* 2017; 83: e00472–e00417.

86. Huffman J, Santarpia J. Online techniques for quantification and characterization of biological aerosols. In Delort AM, Amato P, editors. *Microbiology of Aerosols*. Hoboken, NJ: John Wiley & Sons, 2018.

87. Levetin E, Van de Water PK. Pollen count forecasting. *Immunol Allergy Clin North Am* 2003; 23(3): 423–442.

88. Scheifinger H, Belmonte J, Buters J et al. Monitoring, modelling and forecasting of the pollen season. In: Sofiev M, Bergmann K-C, editors. *Allergenic Pollen: A Review of the Production, Release, Distribution and Health Impacts*. Dordrecht, the Netherlands: Springer, 2013.

89. Nowosad J, Stach A, Kasprzyk I et al. Forecasting model of *Corylus, Alnus*, and *Betula* pollen concentration levels using spatiotemporal correlation properties of pollen count. *Aerobiologia* 2016; 32(3): 453–468.

90. Liu X, Wu D, Zewdie GK et al. Using machine learning to estimate atmospheric *Ambrosia* pollen concentrations in Tulsa, OK. *Environ Health Insights* 2017; 11: 1–10.

91. Crouzy B, Stella M, Konzelmann T, Calpini B, Clot B. All-optical automatic pollen identification: Towards an operational system. *Atmos Environ* 2016; 140: 202–212.

92. Kawashima S, Clot B, Fujita T, Takahashi Y, Nakamura K. An algorithm and a device for counting airborne pollen automatically using laser optics. *Atmos Environ* 2007; 41(36): 7987–7993.

93. Kawashima S, Thibaudon M, Matsuda S et al. Automated pollen monitoring system using laser optics for observing seasonal changes in the concentration of total airborne pollen. *Aerobiologia*. 2017; 33(3): 351–362.

94. Watanabe K, Ohizumi T. Comparability between Durham method and real-time monitoring for long-term observation of Japanese cedar (*Cryptomeria japonica*) and Japanese cypress (*Cryptomeria obtusa*) pollen counts in Niigata Prefecture, Japan. *Aerobiologia*. 2018; 34: 257–267.

95. Heimann U, Haus J, Zuehlke D. Fully automated pollen analysis and counting: The pollen monitor BAA500. *Proceedings OPTO 2009* 2009; 125–128.

96. Oteros J, Pusch G, Weichenmeier I et al. Automatic and online pollen monitoring. *Int Arch Allergy Immunol* 2015; 167(3): 158–166.

97. Kiseleva S. Examining the particulates. *Meteorol Technol Int* 2018; September: 138–140.

98. Niederberger E, Abt R, Burch P, Zeder Y. First experiences with the newly-developed Swisens Pollen Monitor. *The 2018 WMO/CIMO Technical Conference on Meteorological and Environmental Instruments and Methods of Observation (CIMO TECO-2018)*. Amsterdam, the Netherlands: WMO, 2018.

99. O'Connor DJ, Healy DA, Hellebust S, Buters JT, Sodeau JR. Using the WIBS-4 (Waveband Integrated Bioaerosol Sensor) technique for the on-line detection of pollen grains. *Aerosol Sci Tech* 2014; 48(4): 341–349.

100. Bunderson LD, Allan N, Lambson K, Lucas RW. Evaluation of pollen images captured by an automated near-real-time pollen collection device. *Ann Allergy Asthma Immunol* 2015; 115: A49.

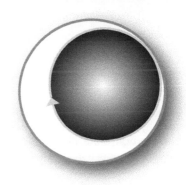

3 Definition of an allergen (immunobiology)

Lauren Fine

Nova Southeastern University Kiran C. Patel College of Allopathic Medicine

CONTENTS

3.1 INTRODUCTION

A variety of terms are used to define the substance that stimulates an atopic or allergic reaction. In the context of a general immunologic reaction, the triggering substance is called an antigen. An antigen is any substance that induces a state of sensitivity and/or resistance as a result of coming into contact with appropriate tissues of an animal body, usually by presentation to a lymphocyte [1,2]. The observed sequence; exposure to substance, latency period, and manifestation of substance-specific immune response upon reexposure to a substance is characteristic of immunologic memory and indicates that B cells and/or T cells are involved.

Allergens are defined in terms of the immune response to them. In 1923, Coca and Cooke coined the word *atopy* to describe a specific type of sensitized state. Subsequently, atopy has been further defined as an adverse immune reaction triggered by an allergen, due to production of immunoglobulin E (IgE) [1]. The term *allergen* defines the antigenic substance that induces the production of specific IgE antibodies. Routes of exposure to allergen include inhalation, ingestion, tactile contact, and injection. Interestingly, not all individuals have a demonstrable IgE response to common allergens, which may reflect the complexity of the allergic phenotype. A genetic basis for atopic predisposition has been recognized for nearly a century. The response to an allergen is influenced by the interplay of multiple factors: characteristics of the host (including genetic susceptibility), the environment, and

physical properties of the allergen itself. New research suggests that perinatal exposure and epigenetic changes that occur before birth or even at conception may also influence atopy [3,4]. Although we choose to define an allergen as an antigen that will induce and interact specifically with IgE, not all antigens will become an allergen in any given individual. The question therefore arises as to whether all antigens can be allergens under the proper conditions [1]. Why one individual is allergic to a particular allergen and a genetically similar atopic family member is not is likely the result of genetics, environment, and epigenetic changes. A series of investigations of allergy-prone families found that although the tendency to be sensitive to allergens was inherited, the antigens to which they were allergic appeared to be completely random. Clinically there was no correlation between the types of specific allergen sensitivity seen in the mother or father versus the children. Although any antigen may fulfill the structural criteria to be an allergen, not all antigens produce a clinical allergic response in all individuals, likely the result of the interaction of genes and environment [5].

Gell and Coombs separated immunologic reactions into four different types. Type I is immediate and IgE mediated. Allergenic proteins that cause type I reactions may also cause type II, III, and IV reactions, and vice versa. While most allergens are proteins, certain carbohydrate allergens can cause immediate and delayed allergic reactions. For example, exposure to a mammalian, nonprimate α-galactose-1,4-galactose carbohydrate moiety via a tick bite may sensitize an individual. Should that individual who now has circulating specific-IgE against the α-galactose-1,4-galactose carbohydrate moiety ingest beef, lamb, or pork containing the same carbohydrate, he or she may develop delayed anaphylaxis 4–8 hours after ingestion [6]. These observations demonstrate a blurring of the distinct categories created by Gell and Coombs as well as the definition of an allergen. Immunologic reactions and allergens are not easily characterized [7,8].

3.2 ALLERGIC ATOPIC REACTIONS AND INFLAMMATION (INCLUDING PATHOLOGY)

Clinical symptoms that result from allergic reactions may vary from those of rhinitis (sneezing, nasal discharge, and nasal congestion) and asthma or reversible airway obstruction (coughing, wheezing, chest tightness, and/or shortness of breath) to certain forms of urticaria, eczema, angioedema, and anaphylaxis. Inflammation is an important feature of these conditions as summarized earlier; it is a dynamic process that consists of cytological and histological reactions that occur in tissues in response to injury or abnormal stimulation. For example, vibration, pressure, and other physical stimulation can trigger non-IgE-mediated mast cell degranulation and result in an inflammatory cascade similar to that seen in IgE-mediated mast cell degranulation. Therefore, patients may manifest symptoms identical to IgE-mediated allergic reactions by indirect stimulation of mast cell degranulation.

Once sensitization to an allergen begins, the potential for inflammation has been set. Upon reexposure to the allergen, the immune system is further activated, resulting in greater inflammation. This immunologic reaction is what ultimately creates the clinical picture of allergy and atopy. Allergic reactions result from the involvement and interactions of a variety of cell types, ranging from monocytes and macrophages to T cells and B cells involved in the development of the specific immune reaction, to the granulocytic cells of the myeloid series (i.e., mast cells, eosinophils, neutrophils, and platelets). The interactions of all these cells are of importance in the inflammatory response. In a sensitized individual, reexposure to an allergen involves the interaction of the allergen with its specific IgE, which is attached to the surface of mast cells and basophils by the FcϵRI receptor. Once the allergen binds to and cross-links IgE molecules, the receptor is activated. The mast cell degranulates via downstream pathways and releases preformed mediators such as histamine, serotonin, tumor necrosis factor (TNF), as well as tryptase and other proteases. Newly synthesized leukotrienes, prostaglandins, platelet-activating factor, cytokines, and chemokines are also subsequently released [9]. Mast cell mediators regulate the functions of various organ systems, such as the vascular and pulmonary systems, by acting on multiple cells, such as the endothelium, smooth muscle cells, neurons, and epithelial cells including goblet cells [10]. The acute symptoms of allergic reactions, such as sneezing, wheezing, and urticaria may be due to the release of mediators such as histamine from the mast cells, whereas the chronic symptoms, such as bronchial inflammation, may be explained by eosinophil-mediated tissue damage. T cells of the T_H2 type produce interleukin-4 (IL-4) and IL-5, of which interleukin-5 (IL-5) potentiates the terminal differentiation and activation of eosinophils. Basic proteins, together with the platelet-activating factor and leukotrienes secreted by eosinophils, probably also contribute to chronic symptoms in allergic reactions.

The nature of the immune reaction to an allergen and the resulting clinical picture are dependent on many steps that are influenced by host and environmental factors such as properties of the allergen, route of exposure, as well as genetic controls. Therefore, as a result of the interaction of the allergen and antibody in a sensitized individual, a variety of cells and humoral components are activated, which results in inflammation. The difference between allergy and all other inflammatory processes lies in the types of cells and molecules causing the inflammation. In the case of allergy, the cause of inflammation is an aberrant humoral response to foreign molecules, usually involving specific IgE [11]. The tendency to produce IgE is likely a product of the environment in which the antigen was presented to the antigen-presenting cell (APC). If antigen presentation occurs in the environment of Th2 cytokines, this will induce production of IgE by plasma cells. In contrast, if the antigen is presented in the environment of Th1 cytokines, such as in the case of intracellular pathogens, the result is most likely to be production of IgG and IgM antibodies rather than IgE. In the former situation, subsequent exposure of the antigen, now an allergen, to IgE results in the allergic response outlined earlier. In allergic inflammation, the release of IL-5 by activated mast cells leads to the production, maturation, recruitment, differentiation, survival, and activation of eosinophils [12].

Eosinophilic disease may be IgE mediated, but the two are not always coincident. Although eosinophils are commonly seen as a result of antibody-allergen interactions, they may also be seen in nonallergic disease. Two therapeutic strategies reduce inflammation by targeting either IL-5 or IgE in asthmatics, each resulting in a reduction in exacerbation rates. Anti-IL-5 therapy reduces sputum and peripheral eosinophil counts in a range of asthma phenotypes. The most significant reductions in exacerbation rates are in those with eosinophilic asthma versus those with an alternative phenotype. Similarly, the anti-IgE antibody omalizumab significantly reduces exacerbation rates in IgE-mediated asthma. The ability of anti-IL-5 to reduce asthma exacerbation rates in a range of clinical phenotypes highlights the fact that eosinophilic inflammation and IgE-mediated inflammation are independent, although often coincident, processes [12,13]. Therefore, defining and identifying phenotypic differences in allergic disease could help to better target the development and implementation of optimal pharmaceutical interventions.

3.3 PROPERTIES OF AN ALLERGEN/ ANTIGEN/IMMUNOGEN

An operationally defined allergen shows immunogenicity (a capacity to establish a state of sensitivity and/or stimulate the formation of corresponding antibody) and also reacts specifically with those antibodies [1]. Typically, proteins are more immunogenic than carbohydrates. Because of their size, haptens (low molecular weight compounds, such as drugs) are not immunogenic in and of themselves but do possess antigenic epitopes [1]. In the proper context, such as may exist after a hapten has covalently bound to a larger protein, the hapten-protein complex is taken up and processed by an APC. The allergenic epitope of the hapten-protein complex is presented in the context of a MHC (cell surface antigens of the major histocompatibility complex). This results in the production of antibody specific for that allergenic epitope. In atopic immune responses, the antigen eliciting an immune response is termed an *allergen*. In order for the immune system to respond to an allergen, the allergen must be recognized as foreign. Thus, a molecule might function as an allergen in one organism but not in another simply because one organism recognizes it as foreign and the other does not. This chapter is primarily concerned with molecules recognized as antigens by the humoral system of humans, specifically those with the ability to induce an allergic, or IgE-mediated, response.

Normally, protein allergen recognition by both T and B cells is required for elicitation of humoral immunity. B-cell recognition and specific antibody response are directed toward a unique surface region of the allergen. B-cell epitopes are conformational and generally have a surface area of 500–1000 Å [2,14,15]. The antibody's antigen-binding region, composed jointly by variable regions of the light and heavy chains, is called the *paratope* and forms a tightly fitting complementary surface with the antigen's epitope. The juxtapositioning of charges and hydrophobic areas within the epitope and paratope releases the free energy for the binding reaction. The precise fit of the two surfaces excludes most of the water, tightening the complex [16]. The surface of an antigen represents a quilt of putative epitopes although the number of those putative dominant epitopes varies with the affected subject or situation [17]. Because the antibody is directed toward a specific epitope, whether linear or conformational, that antibody will recognize another allergen if it expresses the same or a very similar epitope. This is the basis for observed cross-reactivity among antigens [18]. The prediction of allergen cross-reactivity has mainly been based on protein homology (i.e., linear sequence data), although bioinformatics are being used successfully to identify cross-reactive allergens [19]. The structure and position of dominating epitopes are defined for an increasing number of protein antigens [14]. Although it may seem intuitive that structurally similar allergens should have the potential for allergenicity, this is not the case. Certain homologous proteins, such as those in peanut and soybean, do not have equal allergenic properties. The variability may be due to differences in the amino acid side chains. For example, arginine, glutamine, and tyrosine have large side chains that are more easily recognized by the immune system and more commonly induce an allergic response [20].

Consideration must be given to the function of antibodies both in general and in interaction with allergens. Any isotype, whether IgA, IgM, IgG, or IgE, in an individual may recognize the same epitopes [21]. However, the effector function of each of these antibodies differs greatly depending on the isotype. The most important feature of an antibody is its ability to recognize an allergen and to form a complex with its target epitope. In the case of an antibody formed against an allergen, the cellular antibody arms an antibody receptor situated on effector cells, such as mast cells, and the allergen cross-links the receptors. In order for cross-linking to occur, an allergen must carry at least two suitably separated epitopes, which allows the molecule to form a bridge between two antibodies, thereby potentially triggering the intracellular response [18]. Some purified allergens produce antibodies targeted against three to four dominant epitopes within the molecule [21,22]. From a receptor aggregation point of view, a favorable topography of epitopes would probably contribute to the potency of an allergen. One might argue that the necessity of a high-affinity antibody, in combination with the limited number of antibodies that can be produced by the human immune system, would restrict the number of antigens that may become allergens. In an atopic individual, the affinity of specific IgE toward an allergen is exceptionally high. However, another individual may develop IgG, IgM, or IgA, but not

IgE, with a high affinity toward that same allergen. The fact that other isotypes may have a high affinity toward the same antigen as IgE demonstrates that high affinity alone is not sufficient for the development of atopy. In fact, high affinity is not even required for an atopic reaction to occur. For example, in clinically atopic individuals who are skin test negative, lower-affinity antibodies may still produce allergic reactions [23].

While affinity is correlated to the ability to cross-link receptors, and high affinity is correlated with the likelihood of atopic reactions, affinity does not seem to be the limiting factor in characterizing the potency of an allergen. New evidence suggests that the closer the proximity of IgE-binding sites on allergens, the greater is the influence on strength of the reaction within the immune or effector cell. This may be due to an influence on the shape of the immune complex of allergen and antibody on the surface of the effector cell [24]. It is unknown how small an allergen can be while maintaining the allergenic property of cross-linking antigen receptors. It is likely, however, that the probability of finding an allergenic protein is lessened at lower molecular weights. The necessity of link formation between two separate epitopes might also induce a lower limit in molecular weight, as crowding on small surfaces could limit cross-linking activity. However, challenging the lower limits of molecular weight is Amb a 5, a relatively small (2500 MW) protein with at least three epitopes [21]. In order for a protein to be allergenic, it must elicit T-cell-dependent responses and be able to provide at least two, preferably three or four, spatially separated epitopes [25]. This establishes a potential lower molecular weight limit and raises the question of whether the majority of T-cell-dependent antigens have the potential to become allergens.

The sea of molecules acting as allergens is organized and named according to a schema proposed by the World Health Organization/International Union of Immunological Societies (WHO/IUIS). The molecules are labeled by the first three letters of the genus and the first letter of the species from which they are isolated, and then by an Arabic numeral indicating the sequence of isolation. Der p 1 is the first isolate from *Dermatophagoides petronyssinus*, a house dust mite. The distinction between major and minor allergens is a functional classification; a major antigen is one to which greater than 50% of allergic patients react. Allergens are generally proteins, glycoproteins, or lipoproteins of plant or animal origin. Many of the major allergens (including those from mites, some animal danders, pollens, insects, and foods) have been cloned and sequenced [26]. For many of these, the three-dimensional structure is now known by direct visualization via crystallography or has been modeled, i.e., the structure is inferred on the basis of sequence homology with other antigens. It does not appear that these molecule types can be divided into allergic/atopic or nonallergic/nonatopic on an *a priori* structural basis [27]. Allergens are derived from proteins with a variety of biological functions, including proteases, pathogenesis-related proteins, seed storage proteins, ligand-binding proteins, lipid transfer proteins, calcium-binding proteins, and other structural proteins; *in toto*, they have been identified as coming from more than 180 distinct protein families, and the list continues to grow [28]. However, the majority of the plant and animal allergens are clustered within just a few of these families. Classification of allergens into groups with structural similarity may help predict cross-reactivity or may provide other useful information [18]. For example, biological function, such as the proteolytic enzyme allergens of dust mites, may directly influence the development of IgE responses (i.e., via direct cleavage of CD23 from the B-cell surface, thus inhibiting negative feedback regulation) [25]. This same antigen might directly initiate inflammatory responses in the lung through allergen presentation by an APC to a T cell and subsequent development of IgE. IgE may later bind directly with the dust allergen and lead to the inflammatory response and bronchoconstriction associated with asthma via a different pathway. An antigen's intrinsic structural or biological properties may also influence the extent to which it persists in the indoor and outdoor environments or retains its allergenicity while within the digestive tract [28]. In the future, structural biology and proteomics may enable the identification of motifs, patterns, and structures of clinical and immunologic significance.

3.4 ALLERGEN: ROUTE AND AMOUNT OF EXPOSURE

Exposure to allergen is typically necessary to develop an IgE-mediated immune response. The skin and mucosal surfaces present in upper and lower respiratory tracts, gastrointestinal (GI) tract, genital tract, and mammary glands are the body's barriers to encounters with allergens and other environmental factors. The presence of these barriers safeguards the internal milieu by excluding foreign items. First, they act as physical barriers and thus prevent penetration of high molecular weight antigen. Schneeberger reported that the molecular weight cutoff above which nasal and alveolar membranes are impermeable is between 40,000 and 60,000 daltons [29]. In addition, skin and mucosal barriers are some of the first sites of contact with the innate and adaptive immune systems, both of which work in concert to defend the body from foreign pathogens.

The adaptive system exhibits specificity for its target antigens. It is based primarily on the antigen-specific receptors on the surfaces of the T and B lymphocytes [30]. The antigen-specific receptors of the adaptive response are assembled by somatic rearrangement of germline gene elements to form both intact T-cell receptors and B-cell antigen-specific receptors (Ig). The adaptive mucosal immune system involves two main tissue systems: (1) mucosa-associated lymphoid tissues (MALTs) within the gut such as the pharyngeal lymphoid ring, Peyer patches, and isolated lymphoid follicles; and (2) the scattered foci of lymphocytes within the mucosal immune system consisting of intraepithelial lymphocytes and the *lamina propria* [31]. IgA is the main mucosal antibody, present primarily within the lungs and gut [32]. The organized mucosal tissues play an important role in the inductive stage of an immune response. The mucosal surfaces of the upper and lower respiratory tracts and the GI tract are important routes of allergen entry for development of allergic sensitization, but they also represent key sites for initiation of non-IgE responses [33].

Once encountered, the amount/dose of exposure, duration, as well as modulating substances are a few of the many environmental factors that influence the type of response to an allergen. Dust mite allergen is variably allergenic, depending on the presence of other substances. Allergens appear to induce IgE production at relatively low doses [27]. The mean adult annual dosage of individual allergenic components is estimated to be in the nanogram range. The ambient exposure level of mite allergen for an average subject in a temperate climate is approximately 100 pg/m³. House dust with mite content >2 μg mite/gm dust is associated with sensitization in children [34]. Clinical studies suggest that the duration of exposure

needed for IgE sensitization to occur in an individual varies depending on the type of exposure. For example, IgE-mediated responses to parasitic allergens may take only days, while it may take months of exposure to perennial allergens and years of exposure to seasonal allergens for one to develop IgE against these proteins. Low levels of lipopolysaccharide (LPS), which is found in dust, may favor a Th2 response, whereas high levels of LPS may favor a Th1 response [35]. LPS binds to the toll-like receptor 4 (TLR4), which associates with MD-2 to allow for TLR4 signaling [36]. Interestingly, dust mite (Der p 2) can also signal through the TLR4 receptor by acting as a functional mimic of MD-2 [37].

3.5 ALLERGIC SENSITIZATION

The innate and adaptive immune systems work together to protect an organism from foreign substances that may possess a diverse collection of potentially pathogenic mechanisms. Though the innate and adaptive immune responses differ in their mechanisms of action, synergy between them is essential for a fully effective immune response [38]. The innate system is the first line of host defense; it sets the stage for the development of an adaptive response to the allergen.

Antigens (regardless of their allergenic properties) can be broadly divided based on whether or not they require T-cell help when eliciting a humoral response. The thymus-independent pathway allows direct activation of antigen-specific B-cell clones, thus eliminating the need for a T-cell epitope. Most bacterial, sugar-based (carbohydrate) antigens belong to this class [39]. Protein antigens, including allergens, are thymus dependent; this means that to act as antigen and trigger a humoral, antibody-based response, the molecule has to be able to first interact and activate antigen-specific T cells.

With the exception of superantigens, T cells are unable to bind to allergen in the absence of antigen presentation. The T-cell receptor (TCR) is restricted to recognizing allergenic peptides displayed in the context of molecules of the MHC [40]. MHC I genes are located on chromosome 6. All nucleated cells as well as platelets are capable of presenting allergen and activating the adaptive response via MHC class I. Dendritic cells, macrophages, and B cells play a major role in the innate response and also act as professional APCs via both MHC class I and II [41]. Macrophages phagocytose exogenous foreign substances such as allergens, bacteria, parasites, or toxins in the tissues, and then migrate via chemotactic signals to T-cell-enriched draining lymph nodes [2]. During migration, dendritic cells undergo a maturation process in which they lose phagocytic capacity and develop an increased ability to communicate with T cells. This maturation process is dependent on signaling through pattern recognition receptors, such as the members of the TLR family [42]. Lysosome-associated enzymes digest phagocytosed proteins into smaller peptides, which are loaded into the antigen-binding clefts of MHC class II molecules for display (i.e., as "T-cell epitopes"). MHC class II molecules bind peptides that are 10–30 amino acids long with a core region of 13 amino acids containing primary and secondary anchor residues. On the APC surface, the MHC-peptide antigen complexes are available for recognition by any naïve CD4+ T cell passing through the lymph node. CD4+ helper T lymphocytes release immune response mediators and play an important role in establishing and maximizing the capabilities of the adaptive immune response. Several different subtypes of CD4+ T cells can be activated by professional APCs, with each type of T cell being specially equipped to deal with different foreign substances, whether allergenic, bacterial, viral, or toxins [43]. The type of T cell activated, and therefore, the type of response generated, depends in part on the context in which the antigen is first encountered by the APC [44].

When a naïve T_H0 cell contacts an antigen and is stimulated through its antigen receptor, it begins to polarize along a lineage-determining developmental pathway [2,44]. T_H1, T_H2, T_H17, and T-regulatory [Tr1] cells all develop from the same naïve T_H0 cell, under the influence of genetic and environmental factors acting at the level of antigen presentation (Figure 3.1a). The predominance of specific cytokines in the microenvironment of the responding T_H0 cell is an important modulatory factor in this process. Signals through contact molecules and cytokine receptors elicit a complex series of molecular interactions. These interactions culminate in the binding of lineage-specific transcription factors to multiple regulatory elements in the genetic promoters, and subsequent activation of a differentiation pathway. Following activation, naïve T_H0 cells differentiate toward the T_H2 pathway in response to IL-4, which activates STAT6. Activation of STAT6 results in induction of GATA-3 and production of the T_H2 cytokines IL-4, IL-5, and IL-13 [44–46]. The molecular mechanisms of these pathways involve cross-talk on the level of the transcription factors: GATA-3 not only increases transactivation of the IL-4 locus promoter but also inhibits production of interferon gamma (IFN-γ); T-bet interferes with T_H17 cells and directly blocks GATA-3 while binding to its own targets [47]. For the T_H1, T_H2, and T_H17 lineages, the differentiation process includes a cascade of events that results in genetic imprinting—reorganization of the histone/chromatin structure so that the determined T-cell polarization is subsequently maintained [15,16,48]. A sketch of the various T-helper subsets and the cytokines thought to be key for induction and maintenance of their polarization is presented in Figure 3.1a.

As previously mentioned, early IL-4 production favors T_H2 polarization. In contrast, IFN-γ and IL-12 in the absence of IL-4 promote T_H1 polarization. While the source of IL-4 produced in the beginning of the immune response is not fully understood (the naïve T_H0 cells themselves, mast cells, basophils, natural killer T cells), both IL-12 and the IFNs responsible for T_H1 polarization are produced during innate immune responses [48]. For example, many bacteria and viruses contain one or more components able to interact with the TLRs present on dendritic cells and NK cells. IL-12 and IFN are among the cytokines released as a consequence of that activation. It is likely that T_H2 priming can occur either as a default pathway in the absence of TLR signaling or through currently unidentified T_H2-activating receptors. Although T_H2 cells are characterized, defining the properties of allergen-specific T cells is difficult in humans because of their low frequency within the T-cell repertoire.

Primary sensitization may occur in predisposed naïve individuals on their initial encounter with an allergen. The cellular and molecular pathways that lead to sensitization are quite similar to those that lead to a future recognition reaction in sensitized people; however, the cellular participants are probably different. The cells recruited for the sensitization response involve the naïve cell population, as memory cells are involved in the response to subsequent allergen exposure. Furthermore, heavy chain isotype switching and affinity maturation increase with repeated exposures to protein antigens/allergens. For some purified allergens, the antibody response is predominantly against three to four dominant epitopes [21]. In a sensitized individual, both IgG and IgE can be produced in response to a single epitope [11]. The rough outline of the process that leads

to production of IgE antibody is sketched in Figure 3.1b. The process is similar for other subtypes of antibody production as well, except that different cytokines are involved.

Most people, both atopic and nonallergic, mount a vigorous response to antigens, utilizing all subclasses of immunoglobulins except IgE [1]. Atopic individuals mount the same response as nonatopic individuals but with the addition of an IgE response. The major difference in immune antibody response to antigen and allergen is consequently quite narrowly localized. The additional production of high-affinity IgE is directed to the dominant epitopes of the antigen. The epitopes seem to be the same as those recognized by other antibody classes. However, the effector functions of the antibodies differ as a result of antibody binding to isotype-specific receptors, thereby leading to downstream intracellular signaling.

There is intrinsically very little in the structure of antigens that determines whether they will become allergens or not. All antigens, and therefore all allergens, are presented by APCs as short peptide sequences [27]. Interestingly, the conformation in which an allergen is presented to IgE molecules can affect not only whether a clinical allergic reaction will result, but also the severity of the reaction. Certain known allergens, especially food allergens, may induce allergic responses through either linear or conformational epitopes, the former of which generally induce less-severe allergic reactions than the latter [49]. Children with IgE-mediated allergy to the conformational epitopes of certain foods such as milk or egg often gain tolerance over the first few years of their life. In contrast, children with IgE-mediated allergy to linear, or sequential, epitopes, such as those that commonly cause peanut allergy, usually do not develop tolerance. Children with egg or milk allergy may also tolerate baked food products, which is likely due to the loss of conformational epitopes as the protein is denatured during the cooking process [50]. It has been suggested that sensitization to peanut protein may occur through dermal exposure [51]. New studies such as the Learning Early about Peanut Allergy (LEAP) study have suggested that early GI exposure to peanut protein, as early as 4 months of age, may prevent the development of IgE-mediated peanut allergy, coincident with an increase in peanut-specific IgG4 levels [52]. Consequently, whether a molecule is an "antigen" or an "allergen" probably ultimately is determined by the individual's genetics, circumstances, and the immunologic environment in which the presentation takes place [53]. The environment and timing of exposure are easily modifiable, but genetics are not. Future research may lead to better understanding of the best combination of conditions under which to expose our immune systems to various allergens to increase the likelihood of creating the desired phenotypic outcome.

3.6 GENETIC FACTORS MODULATING THE IMMUNE RESPONSE TO ALLERGENS

The atopic immune response is a complex reaction involving genetic as well as environmental factors (Figure 3.2). The evidence for genetic factors influencing the different phenotypes of atopy have consisted of familial disease clustering, increased prevalence in first-degree relatives, and increased concordance in monozygotic twins compared to dizygotic twins [1,54–56]. Genetic investigations to determine where the genes are located have used many approaches including forward genetics, candidate genes, genome screens, fine mapping, and functional genomics using statistical linkage and association analysis. The candidate gene studies are hypothesis

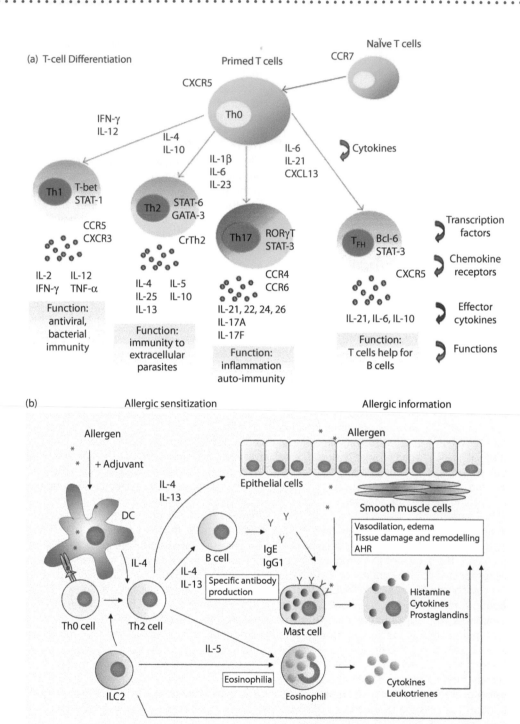

Figure 3.1 (a) T-helper cells of various subsets are thought to develop from the same naïve T_H0 cell under the influence of both genetic and environmental factors acting at the level of antigen presentation [66]. (b) Production of IL-4 results in polarization toward a T_H2 phenotype and is associated with structural changes and the production of allergen-specific IgE [67,68].

driven, and the results are easy to interpret. Although they can detect genes with modest effect size, they are limited to what we know and cannot discover novel genes or pathways and require linkage dissociation (LD) between markers and causal variants. They are selected for a particular gene or set of genes based on its biological plausibility or suspected role in the phenotype of interest. More than 1000 papers have been published with candidate genes studies examining asthma and related phenotypes, identifying more than 100 genes reviewed elsewhere [57]. Genome-wide linkage studies can discover novel genes and pathways. They require relatively few genetic markers, do not rely on LD between markers and causal variants, and can detect genes harboring rare risk variants. Disadvantages include the requirement of families, poor resolution, and low power to detect genes with modest effects.

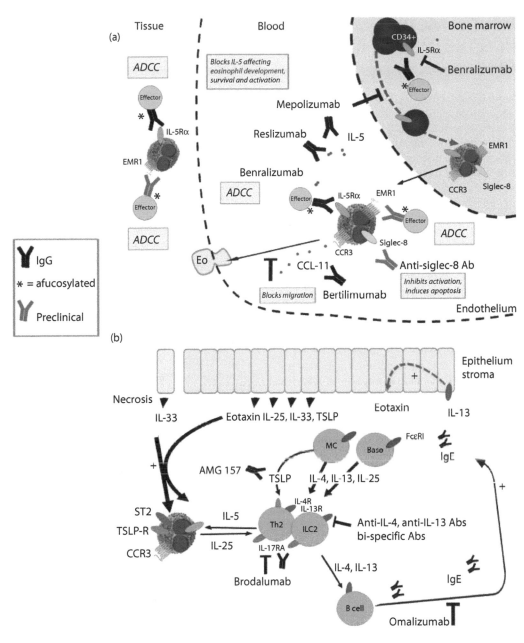

Figure 3.2 Mechanism of action of anti-IL5 therapies [6]. (ADCC, antibody-dependent cell-mediated cytotoxicity; AMG, Amgen; Bas0, basophil; CCR3, chemokine receptor 3; CCL11, eosinophil chemotactic protein and eotaxin-1; EMR1, human epidermal growth factor [EGF]-like module containing mucin-like hormone receptor 1; IL5-Rα, IL-5 receptor alpha; MC, mast cell; Siglec-8, sialic acid-binding immunoglobulin-like lectin; TSLP, thymic stromal lymphopoietin.)

The number of genome-wide association studies (GWASs) that link chromosomal regions to increased risk of asthma and atopy or related phenotypes continues to grow rapidly (Figure 3.4). The genes identified in these studies include ORMDL3, IL1RL1, TSLP, IL33, SMAD3 and at least eight more for asthma, 11q13 for allergic rhinitis, and FLG and at least 12 more for atopic dermatitis [57]. The numerous genome-wide linkage, candidate genes, and GWASs have resulted in an increasing list of genes implicated in asthma susceptibility and pathogenesis. Many have divided the list into several broad functional groups. These groups are epithelial barrier function, environmental sensing, cell signaling, T-cell function/Th2-mediated cell response, and control of gene transcription and apoptosis, among others. Unfortunately, although as of 2015 there were over 120 genes reported to be associated with atopy, no major susceptibility genes for asthma or atopy had been identified. It is likely that the development of atopy is due to a complex interaction of genes and environment, and the probability of identifying single genetic defects that lead directly to a particular atopic disease is becoming increasingly lower. The importance of the gene-environment interaction in the formation of atopic phenotypes becomes even more complex as epigenetics are considered [58]. Much work remains to be done in understanding the effect of the interaction between genes and between genetic factors and environmental risk and exposure [56,57].

3.7 ENVIRONMENTAL FACTORS MODULATING THE IMMUNE RESPONSE TO ALLERGENS

The influence of environmental factors, including pets, endotoxin, viruses, smoke, and pharmacologic agents, on the expression of genes and the ultimate clinical phenotype is being investigated and will be important in understanding the genetic basis of asthma and atopy. Even though there is a genetic predisposition to atopy, environmental factors probably modulate the effect, causing either tolerance or susceptibility [56,59–62].

Not only might the genes we inherit influence our response to the environment, but the environment has the potential to influence the expression of our genes, which may then interact further with the environment. Epigenetic studies examine heritable changes in phenotype or gene expression caused by mechanisms other than changes in the underlying DNA sequence, hence the name *epigenetic*. Environmental factors may cause epigenetic changes that produce an inheritable atopic phenotype. In this way, epigenetics may explain the increasing prevalence of atopy in developed countries, which cannot be explained by change in genetic sequence alone [54,56,59,60]. There is evidence that methyl donors in the maternal diet may increase the risk of developing food allergy in children. Later in life, the use of a multivitamin may reduce the risk of developing food allergy through similar mechanisms. At birth there is a skew toward a Th2 phenotype which may or may not persist, depending on environmental exposures. The typical shift to a Th1 phenotype

occurs through increased methylation of the IL-4 gene and loss of methylation at IFN-γ regulatory regions in Th1 cells. Inhalation of environmental toxins may affect methylation of IL-4 and IFN-γ promoter regions and alter IgE levels. Environmental factors can cause change that may persist long after exposure and lead to augmentation or modification of the immune response and phenotype. Epidemiologic studies support the idea that the allergic inflammation phenotype is influenced by environmental factors. With epigenetics, environmental factors may increase or may reverse aberrant gene expression profiles associated with different disease states. Allergic tendencies may therefore be influenced by classic genetic changes or epigenetic changes involving immune function, such as T-helper cell differentiation.

The environment must be of major importance in the increasing prevalence of atopy since expression of the atopic phenotype occurs as a result of complex interplay between genetic and environmental factors. Western living conditions, allergens, air pollution such as smoke and diesel fumes, and microbial exposure all may impact the immune system, and together influence an individual's risk for becoming atopic. The *hygiene hypothesis* postulates that reduced early childhood exposure to farm animals, microbes, and endotoxin or other microbial products, due to a combination of smaller family size, improved living standards, higher personal hygiene, changes in infant diet, and early life increased use of antibiotics, might result in increased risk for developing atopic disease. It was based on observations, many of which have not been consistently confirmed. These observations include an inverse relationship between some infections and atopic parameters, and children who grow up in a farming environment may have less asthma (atopic

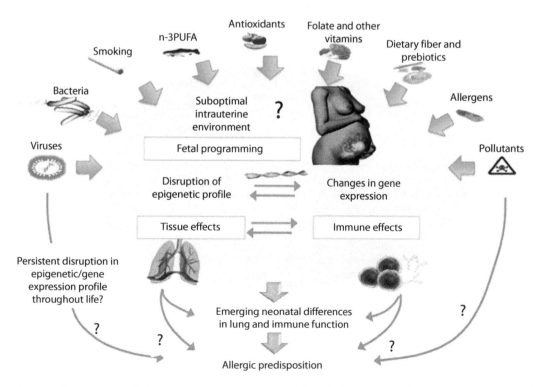

Figure 3.3 Environmental influences on early immune programming: an epigenetic perspective [7]. This illustrates the environmental factors that have been implicated as potential immune modifiers during early development in the prenatal and/or postnatal periods.

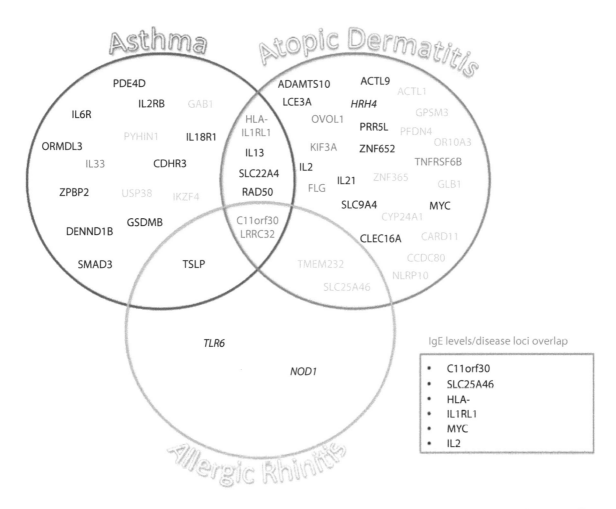

Figure 3.4 Candidate genes in atopy [57]. Venn diagram illustrating genes identified through genome-wide association studies as associated with the allergic diseases asthma, atopic dermatitis, and allergic rhinitis. Genes highlighted in black identify those discovered in Caucasian populations, with italics defining promising genes that nearly achieved genome-wide significance. Genes highlighted in blue identify those genes discovered in non-Caucasian populations, while those in red identify those genes discovered in both Caucasian and populations of other ancestry. The Venn diagram includes genes identified through genome-wide association studies. The diseases included are asthma, atopic dermatitis, and allergic rhinitis. (Black = genes identified in Caucasian populations; blue = genes identified in non-Caucasian populations; red = genes identified in both Caucasians and other ancestry; *italic* = genes showing promise in association with disease.)

sensitization, asthma, "hay fever") than children of the same age and living in the same communities, but not growing up on a farm. Along the same lines, the use of probiotics during pregnancy influences the expression of TLR-related genes in the placenta and fetal gut and in cord-blood cytokine expression [58]. Therefore, the probiotic environment in which the fetus develops may influence the future immunologic response to allergen. Acute respiratory infection such as respiratory syncytial virus (RSV) may increase the likelihood of developing an atopic profile by way of increased IL-4, IL-13, activation of Th2 memory cells, and the upregulation of FcεR1 [58]. In contrast, the presence of certain pathogens such as *Helicobacter pylori* may reduce the development of allergy [63]. In addition to increasing the risk of atopy, the environment has the potential to augment allergic responses in individuals with known atopy. For example, exposure to diesel fuel exhaust increases airway eosinophils, IL-5, and eosinophilic cationic protein [64]. Likewise, in atopic children, exposure to diesel exhaust particles

increases the risk of developing asthma and of increased airway hyperresponsiveness to house dust mite, possibly through the accumulation of allergen-specific Th2/Th17 cells in the lungs [65]. The risk of developing food allergy, such as peanut allergy, may also be augmented by transdermal exposure to peanut protein in house dust. Those individuals who have an impaired dermal barrier due to preexisting atopic dermatitis are at increased risk of developing peanut allergy. All of these examples demonstrate the complexity of the environment's impact on the immunologic, specifically atopic, response to an allergen. Environmental factors may enhance either sensitization or normalization (Figure 3.3). However, exactly which type of immune response will be favored is very complex and is determined by an interaction of both genes and environment. Although many genes and genetic patterns have been linked to atopy, it is likely that many genetic and environmental factors and mechanisms influencing atopy have yet to be discovered (Table 3.1).

Table 3.1 Candidate genes of atopy and allergy

Type	Examples
Cytokines influencing atopic phenotype	
Eosinophil growth-, activation-, and apoptosis-inhibiting factors	IL-5, IL-3, GM-CSF, CCL11, CCL5
Mast-cell growth factors	IL-3, IL-9, IL-10, SCF, TGF-β
Histamine-releasing factors	CCL2 (MCP-1), CCL7 (MCP-3), CCL5
IgE isotype switch factors	IL-4, IL-13
Inhibition of IgE isotype switch	IFN-γ, IL-12, IL-18, IL-23
Lipoxygenase pathway metabolism	5-LO, 5-LO–activating peptide, leukotriene C4 synthase
Proinflammatory cytokines	IL-1α, IL-1β, TNF-α, IL-6
Anti-inflammatory cytokines	TNF-β, IL-10, IL-1Rα
Receptors	
Antigen receptors	T-cell receptors (α/β, γ/δ), B-cell receptor (IG, κ/λ light chains)
IgE receptor	FceRI β chain, FceRII (CD23)
Cytokine gene receptors	IFN-γR β chain IL-1R, IL-4R, TNF receptors, common γ-chain
Adhesion molecules	VLA-4, VCAM-1, ICAM-1, LFA-1
Corticosteroid receptor	Grl-hsp90
Neurogenic receptors	β2-Adrenergic, cholinergic receptors
Nuclear transcription factors	GATA-3, T-bet, NF-κB, IκB, NFAT, Stat-1/2, Stat-4, Stat-6
Other molecules of importance	
MHC and antigen processing	HLA class I and II molecules, TAP-1 and -2, LMP
Cell signaling	CTLA-4, CD28, JAK1
Barriers and other defense	SPINK5, Clara cell protein 16, Endothelin 2

Abbreviations: CCL, chemokine ligand; GM-CSF, granulocyte-macrophage colony-stimulating factor; HLA, human leukocyte antigen; hsp, heat shock protein; ICAM, intercellular adhesion molecule; IFN, interferon; IL, interleukin; LFA, lymphocyte function-associated antigen; LMP, large multicatalytic proteosome; LO, lipoxygenase; MHC, major histocompatibility complex; SCF, stem cell factor; TAP, transporter associated with antigen processing; TNF, tumor necrosis factor; VCAM, vascular cell adhesion molecule; VLA, very late antigen.

SALIENT POINTS

1. Atopy is clinically defined is an inflammatory condition resulting from an allergen producing an adverse immune reaction.
2. Allergens/antigens have two properties: (1) immunogenicity (i.e., the capacity to stimulate the formation of the corresponding antibody and/or a state of sensitivity); and (2) the ability to react specifically with those antibodies. The two properties are not always associated.
3. Allergens are antigens that induce the production of an IgE-specific antibody that on future exposure will interact with the inducing antigen.
4. From the chemical standpoint, there is little to differentiate allergens from other antigens.
5. There are four restrictions for a molecule to become an allergen: (1) it must possess a surface to which the antibody can form a complementary surface; (2) it must have an amino acid sequence in its backbone able to bind the MHC II alleles of the responding individual; (3) it must have a reduced energy state when bound with the antibody to ensure interaction at low concentrations of allergen and antibody; and (4) it must form at least two epitopes in order to act as a bridge to link two IgE molecules.
6. The nature of the immune reaction to an allergen is dependent on many steps influenced by host and environmental factors.
7. Genetic factors include multiple genes regulating non-epitope-specific factors, such as those on chromosome 5q, as well as those that are allergen epitope specific, including genes in the MHC on chromosome 6.
8. The duration, route, and allergen exposure, as well as other modulating pollutants, are a few of the environmental factors that influence the type of response to an allergen.
9. Gene-environment interactions such as epigenetics may play an important role in the response to an allergen, and the effects of these interactions may be inheritable without a change in the genetic sequence.

DEFINITIONS

Antigens are substances that have immunogenicity. By binding to a T-cell receptor, they lead to T-cell activation and/or production of antibodies with which the antigen reacts.

Allergens are a subclass of antigens that stimulate the production of and combine with the IgE subclass of antibodies.

Haptens are substances that are not immunogenic in/or themselves (cannot stimulate humoral response without the help of carrier substances) but can combine specifically with antibody once it is formed.

Immunogens are substances that stimulate specific immune response such as the production of an antibody.

B-cell epitopes are specific surface areas on an antigen toward which the specificity of a single antibody is directed.

T-cell epitope is a proteolytic antigenic fragment (approximately 13 amino acids long) displayed by MHC; MHC-restricted recognition is required for activation of antigen-specific T cells.

T-Helper cell 2 (TH2) profile is a specific pattern of effector molecules, of which IL-4 and IL-5 are dominant, derived from activated T cells.

T-Helper cell 1 (TH1) profile is a specific pattern of effector molecules, where INF-γ is dominant, derived from activated T cells.

T-Helper cell 17 (TH17) profile is a specific pattern of effector molecules, of which the pro-inflammatory cytokine IL-17 is dominant, derived from activated T cells.

REFERENCES

1. Blumenthal MN, editor. *Genetics of Allergy and Asthma: Methods for Investigative Studies*. Vol. 10. New York: Marcel Dekker, 1997: pp. 392.
2. Abbas AK. *Cellular and Molecular Immunology*. 2017.
3. Illi S, Weber J, Zutavern A et al. Perinatal influences on the development of asthma and atopy in childhood. *Ann Allergy Asthma Immunol* 2014; 112(2): 132–139.e1.
4. Sabounchi S, Bollyky J, Nadeau K. Review of environmental impact on the epigenetic regulation of atopic diseases. *Curr Allergy Asthma Rep* 2015; 15(6).
5. Jackola DR, Liebeler CL, Blumenthal MN, Rosenberg A. Random outcomes of allergen-specific responses in atopic families. *Clin Exp Allergy* 2004; 34(4): 540–547.
6. Commins SP, Satinover SM, Hosen J et al. Delayed anaphylaxis, angioedema, or urticaria after consumption of red meat in patients with IgE antibodies specific for galactose-α-1,3-galactose. *J Allergy Clin Immunol* 2009; 123(2).
7. Wilson JM, Schuyler AJ, Schroeder N, Platts-Mills TAE. Galactose-α-1,3-galactose: Atypical food allergen or model IgE hypersensitivity? *Curr Allergy Asthma Rep* 2017; 17(1).
8. Calnan CD, Gell PG CR. In: Davis F, editor. *Clinical Aspects of Immunology*. Philadelphia, PA, 1963.
9. Theoharides TC, Valent P, Akin C. Mast cells, mastocytosis, and related disorders. *N Engl J Med* 2015; 373(2): 163–172.
10. Kunder CA, John ALS, Abraham SN, Dc W. Mast cell modulation of the vascular and lymphatic endothelium review article mast cell modulation of the vascular and lymphatic endothelium. *Blood* 2011; 118(20): 5383–5393.
11. Boyce JA, Bochner B, Finkelman FD, Rothenberg ME. Advances in mechanisms of asthma, allergy, and immunology in 2011. *J Allergy Clin Immunol* 2012; 129(2): 335–341.
12. Patterson MF, Borish L, Kennedy JL. The past, present, and future of monoclonal antibodies to IL-5 and eosinophilic asthma: A review. *J Asthma Allergy* 2015; 8: 125–134.
13. Solèr M, Matz J, Townley R et al. The anti-IgE antibody omalizumab reduces exacerbations and steroid requirement in allergic asthmatics. *Eur Respir J* 2001; 18(2): 254–261.
14. Wilson IA, Stanfield RL. Antibody-antigen interactions: New structures and new conformational changes. *Curr Opin Struct Biol* 1994; 4(6): 857–867.
15. López-Torrejón G, Díaz-Perales A, Rodríguez J et al. An experimental and modeling-based approach to locate IgE epitopes of plant profilin allergens. *J Allergy Clin Immunol* 2007; 119(6): 1481–1488.
16. Davies DR, Padlan EA, Sheriff S. Antibody-antigen complexes. *Annu Rev Biochem* 1990; 59(1): 439–473.
17. Jemmerson R. Epitope mapping by proteolysis of antigen-antibody complexes. In: Morris GE, editor, *Epitope Mapping Protocols*. 1996: 97–108.
18. Aalberse RC. Assessment of allergen cross-reactivity. *Clin Mol Allergy* 2007; 5. doi:10.1186/1476-7961-5-2.
19. Negi SS, Braun W. Cross-react: A new structural bioinformatics method for predicting allergen cross-reactivity. *Bioinformatics* 2017; 33(7): 1014–1020.
20. Han Y, Lin J, Bardina L et al. What characteristics confer proteins the ability to induce allergic responses? IgE epitope mapping and comparison of the structure of soybean 2S albumins and Ara h 2. *Molecules* 2016; 21(5). doi:10.3390/molecules21050622.
21. Kim KE, Rosenberg A, Roberts S, Blumenthal MN. The affinity of allergen specific IgE and the competition between IgE and IgG for the allergen in Amb a V sensitive individuals. *Mol Immunol* 1996; 33(10): 873–880.
22. Pierson-Mullany LK, Jackola DR, Blumenthal MN, Rosenberg A. Characterization of polyclonal allergen-specific IgE responses by affinity distributions. *Mol Immunol* 2000; 37(10): 613–620.
23. Pierson Mullany LK, Jackola DR, Blumenthal MN, Rosenberg A. Evidence of an affinity threshold for IgE-allergen binding in the percutaneous skin test reaction. *Clin Exp Allergy* 2002; 32(1): 107–116.
24. Gieras A, Linhart B, Roux KH et al. IgE epitope proximity determines immune complex shape and effector cell activation capacity. *J Allergy Clin Immunol* 2016; 137(5): 1557–1565.
25. Mita H, Yasueda H, Akiyama K. Affinity of IgE antibody to antigen influences allergen-induced histamine release. *Clin Exp Allergy* 2000; 30(11): 1583–1589.
26. Chapman MD, Pomés A, Breiteneder H, Ferreira F. Nomenclature and structural biology of allergens. *J Allergy Clin Immunol* 2007; 119(2): 414–420.
27. Aalberse RC. Structural biology of allergens. *J Allergy Clin Immunol* 2000; 106(2): 228–238.
28. Pomés A, Chruszcz M, Gustchina A et al. 100 Years later: Celebrating the contributions of x-ray crystallography to allergy and clinical immunology. *J Allergy Clin Immunol* 2015; 136(1): 29–37.e10.
29. Schneeberger EE. The permeability of the alveolar-capillary membrane to ultrastructural protein tracers. *Ann NY Acad Sci* 1974; 221(1): 238–243.
30. Pancer Z, Cooper MD. The evolution of adaptive immunity. *Annu Rev Immunol* 2006; 24(1): 497–518.
31. Janeway CJ, Travers P, Walport M, Shlomchik M. *Immunobiology: The Immune System in Health and Disease*, 5th ed. New York, NY: Garland Publishing, 2001: 101–103.

32. Woof JM, Ken MA. The function of immunoglobulin A in immunity. *J Pathol* 2006; 208(2): 270–282.

33. Strober W, Fuss IJ, Blumberg RS. The immunology of mucosal models of inflammation. *Annu Rev Immunol* 2002; 20: 495–549.

34. Platts-Mills TAE, de Weck AL, Aalberse RC et al. Dust mite allergens and asthma—A worldwide problem. *J Allergy Clin Immunol* 1989; 83(2 Part 1): 416–427.

35. Tan AM, Chen H-C, Pochard P, Eisenbarth SC, Herrick CA, Bottomly HK. TLR4 signaling in stromal cells is critical for the initiation of allergic Th2 responses to inhaled antigen. *J Immunol* 2010; 184(7): 3535–3544.

36. Rakoff-Nahoum S, Paglino J, Eslami-Varzaneh F, Edberg S, Medzhitov R. Recognition of commensal microflora by toll-like receptors is required for intestinal homeostasis. *Cell* 2004; 118(2): 229–241.

37. Platts-Mills TAE, Woodfolk JA. Allergens and their role in the allergic immune response. *Immunol Rev* 2011; 242(1): 51–68.

38. Kabelitz D, Medzhitov R. Innate immunity—Cross-talk with adaptive immunity through pattern recognition receptors and cytokines. *Curr Opin Immunol* 2007; 19(1): 1–3.

39. Rijkers GT, Sanders LA, Zegers BJ. Anti-capsular polysaccharide antibody deficiency states. *Immunodeficiency* 1993; 5(1): 1–21.

40. Rudolph MG, Stanfield RL, Wilson IA. How TCRS bind MHCS, peptides, and coreceptors. *Annu Rev Immunol* 2006; 24(1): 419–466.

41. Guermonprez P, Valladeau J, Zitvogel L, Théry C, Amigorena S. Antigen presentation and T cell stimulation by dendritic cells. *Annu Rev Immunol* 2002; 20(1): 621–667.

42. Gay NJ, Gangloff M, Weber AN. Toll-like receptors as molecular switches. *Nat Rev Immunol* 2006; 6(9): 693–698.

43. Kemper C, Atkinson JP. T-cell regulation: With complements from innate immunity. *Nat Rev Immunol* 2007; 7(1): 9–18.

44. Murphy KM, Reiner SL. The lineage decisions of helper T cells. *Nat Rev Immunol* 2002; 2(12): 933–944.

45. Weaver CT, Hatton RD, Mangan PR, Harrington LE. IL-17 family cytokines and the expanding diversity of effector T cell lineages. *Annu Rev Immunol* 2007; 25: 821–852.

46. Hwang ES, Szabo SJ, Schwartzberg PL, Glimcher LH. T helper cell fate specified by kinase-mediated interaction of T-bet with GATA-3. *Science* 2005; 307(5708): 430–433.

47. Ansel KM, Djuretic I, Tanasa B, Rao A. Regulation of T_H2 differentiation and Il4 locus accessibility. *Annu Rev Immunol* 2006; 24(1): 607–656.

48. Chang S, Aune TM. Dynamic changes in histone-methylation "marks" across the locus encoding interferon-gamma during the differentiation of T helper type 2 cells. *Nat Immunol* 2007; 8(7): 723–731.

49. Steckelbroeck S, Ballmer-Weber BK, Vieths S. Potential, pitfalls, and prospects of food allergy diagnostics with recombinant allergens or synthetic sequential epitopes. *J Allergy Clin Immunol* 2008; 121(6): 1323–1330.

50. Baker MG, Sampson HA. Phenotypes and endotypes of food allergy: A path to better understanding the pathogenesis and prognosis of food allergy. *Ann Allergy Asthma Immunol* 2018; 120(3): 245–253.

51. Fox DE, Lack G. Peanut allergy. *Lancet* 1998; 352(9129): 741.

52. Du Toit G, Roberts G, Sayre PH et al. Randomized trial of peanut consumption in infants at risk for peanut allergy. *N Engl J Med* 2015; 372(9): 803–813.

53. Berker M, Frank LJ, Geßner AL et al. Allergies—A T cells perspective in the era beyond the T_H1/T_H2 paradigm. *Clin Immunol* 2017; 174: 73–83.

54. March ME, Sleiman PM, Hakonarson H. The genetics of asthma and allergic disorders. *Discov Med* 2011; 11(56): 35–45.

55. Ober C, Yao TC. The genetics of asthma and allergic disease: A 21st century perspective. *Immunol Rev* 2011; 242(1): 10–30.

56. Blumenthal MN. Genetic, epigenetic, and environmental factors in asthma and allergy. *Ann Allergy, Asthma Immunol* 2012; 108(2): 69–73.

57. Portelli M, Hodge E, Sayers I. Genetic risk factors for the development of allergic disease identified by genome-wide association. *Clin Exp Allergy* 2015; 45(1): 21–31.

58. Campbell DE, Boyle RJ, Thornton CA, Prescott SL. Mechanisms of allergic disease—Environmental and genetic determinants for the development of allergy. *Clin Exp Allergy* 2015; 45(5): 844–858.

59. Vercelli D. Remembrance of things past: HLA genes come back on the allergy stage. *J Allergy Clin Immunol* 2012; 129(3): 846–847.

60. Bach JF. The biological individual—The respective contributions of genetics, environment and chance. *Comptes Rendus—Biol* 2009; 332(12): 1065–1068.

61. Tan THT, Ellis JA, Saffery R, Allen KJ. The role of genetics and environment in the rise of childhood food allergy. *Clin Exp Allergy* 2012; 42(1): 20–29.

62. Liu AH, Leung DYM. Renaissance of the hygiene hypothesis. *J Allergy Clin Immunol* 2006; 117(5): 1063–1066.

63. Arnold IC, Hitzler I, Müller A. The immunomodulatory properties of *Helicobacter pylori* confer protection against allergic and chronic inflammatory disorders. *Front Cell Infect Microbiol* 2012; 2: 10.

64. Carlsten C, Blomberg A, Pui M et al. Diesel exhaust augments allergen-induced lower airway inflammation in allergic individuals: A controlled human exposure study. *Thorax* 2016; 71(1): 35–44.

65. Brandt EB, Biagini Myers JM, Acciani TH et al. Exposure to allergen and diesel exhaust particles potentiates secondary allergen-specific memory responses, promoting asthma susceptibility. *J Allergy Clin Immunol* 2015; 136(2): 295–303.e7.

66. Yu SL, Kuan WP, Wong CK, Li EK, Tam LS. Immunopathological roles of cytokines, chemokines, signaling molecules, and pattern-recognition receptors in systemic lupus erythematosus. *Clin Dev Immunol* 2012; 2012. doi:10.1155/2012/715190.

67. Barranco P, Phillips-Angles E, Dominguez-Ortega J, Quirce S. Dupilumab in the management of moderate-to-severe asthma: The data so far. *Ther Clin Risk Manag* 2017; 13: 1139–1149.

68. Spacova I, Ceuppens JL, Seys SF, Petrova MI, Lebeer S. Probiotics against airway allergy: Host factors to consider. *Dis Model Mech* 2018; 11(7): dmm034314.

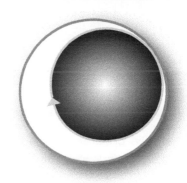

4 Allergen nomenclature

Heimo Breiteneder
Medical University of Vienna

Rick Goodman
University of Nebraska–Lincoln

Martin D. Chapman and Anna Pomés
INDOOR Biotechnologies, Inc.

CONTENTS

4.1 HISTORICAL INTRODUCTION

The history of allergen nomenclature dates to the time when extracts of allergen sources were fractionated using a variety of classical biochemical separation techniques, and the active (most allergenic) fraction was usually named according to the whim of the investigator. In the 1940–1950s, attempts were made to purify pollen and house dust allergens, using phenol extraction, salt precipitation, and electrophoretic techniques. In the 1960s, ion exchange and gel filtration media were introduced, and ragweed "antigen E" was the first allergen to be purified [1]. This allergen was named as such by King and Norman because it was one of five precipitin lines (labeled A–E) that reacted with rabbit polyclonal antibodies to ragweed in Ouchterlony immunodiffusion tests. Following purification, precipitin line E, or "antigen E" was shown to be a potent allergen. Later, Marsh, working in Cambridge, England, isolated an important allergen from ryegrass (*Lolium perenne*) pollen and used the name "Rye 1" to indicate that this was the first allergen purified from this species [2,3]. In the 1970s, many allergens were purified from ragweed, ryegrass, insect venoms, and other sources. The field was led by the laboratory of the late Dr. David Marsh, who had moved to the Johns Hopkins University, Baltimore, Maryland. At Hopkins, the ragweed allergens Ra3, Ra4, Ra5, and Ra6, and the ryegrass allergens Rye 2 and Rye 3 were isolated and used for immunologic and genetic studies of hay fever [4–6]. At the same time, Ohman identified Cat-l, the major cat allergen [7]. Elsayed purified allergen M from codfish [8,9].

The state of the art in the early 1970s was reviewed in a seminal book chapter by Marsh in *The Antigens* (Michael Sela, editor), which described the molecular properties of allergens, the factors that influenced allergenicity, the immune response to allergens, and immunogenetic studies of IgE responses to purified pollen allergens [10]. That chapter provided the first clear definition of a "major" allergen, which Marsh defined as a highly purified allergen that induced immediate skin test responses in more than 90% of allergic individuals, in contrast to a "minor" allergen, to which less than 20% of patients reacted with skin test responses. Today, a major allergen is generally regarded as one to which more than 50% of patients with an allergy to its source react, although that is typically considered as a measurement of IgE binding rather than the biological reaction as measured by skin test or by clinical symptoms [11].

With the introduction of crossed immunoelectrophoresis (CIE) and crossed radioimmunoelectrophoresis (CRIE) for allergen identification by Løwenstein and colleagues in Scandinavia, there was a tremendous proliferation of the number of antigenic proteins and CIE/CRIE peaks identified as allergens. Typically, 10–50 peaks could be detected in a given allergen source based on reactivity with rabbit polyclonal antibodies or IgE antibodies [6,11–13]. These peaks were given a multitude of names such as Dp5, Dp42, or Ag12. Inevitably, the same allergens were referred to by different names in different laboratories e.g., mite antigen P1 was also known as Dp42 or Ag12. It became clear that a unified nomenclature was urgently needed.

4.1.1 Three men in a boat

The origins of the systematic allergen nomenclature can be traced to a meeting among David Marsh (at that time, Johns Hopkins University, Baltimore, Maryland), Henning Løwenstein (at that time, University of Copenhagen, Denmark), and Thomas Platts-Mills (at that time, Clinical Research Centre, Harrow, United Kingdom) on a boat ride on Lake Constance (Bodensee), Konstanz, Germany, during the 13th Symposium of the Collegium Internationale Allergologicum in July 1980 [14]. The idea was to develop a systematic allergen nomenclature based on the Linnaean binominal nomenclature for naming all living things, with added numerals to indicate different allergens from the same source. It was decided to adopt a system whereby the allergen was named based on the first three letters of the genus and the first letter of the species (both in italics) followed by a Roman numeral to indicate the allergen in the chronological order of purification. Thus, ragweed antigen E became *Ambrosia artemisiifolia* allergen I or *Amb a* I, and Rye 1 became *Lolium perenne* allergen I or *Lol p* I.

An Allergen Nomenclature Sub-Committee was formed under the auspices of the World Health Organization and the International Union of Immunological Societies (WHO/IUIS), and criteria for including allergens in the systematic nomenclature were established. These included strict criteria for biochemical purity, as well as criteria for determining the allergenic activity of the purified protein. A committee chaired by Marsh, and including Henning Løwenstein, Thomas Platts-Mills, Te Piao King (Rockefeller University, New York), and Larry Goodfriend (McGill University, Canada), prepared a list of allergens that fulfilled the inclusion criteria and established a process for investigators to submit names of newly identified allergens. The original list, published in the *Bulletin* of the WHO in 1986, included 27 highly purified allergens from grass, weed, and tree pollens and from house dust mites [15].

The systematic allergen nomenclature was quickly adopted by allergy researchers and proved to be a great success. It was logical, easily understood, and readily assimilated by allergologists and other clinicians who were not directly involved with the details of allergen immunochemistry. The nomenclature and allergen designations, such as *Der p* I, *Fel d* I, *Lol p* I, and *Amb a* I, were used at scientific meetings and in the literature, and expanded rapidly to include newly isolated allergens.

4.2 REVISED ALLERGEN NOMENCLATURE

4.2.1 Allergens

The widespread use of molecular cloning techniques to identify allergens in the late 1980s and 1990s led to an exponential increase in the number of allergens described. Many allergen nucleotide sequences were obtained by cDNA cloning or polymerase chain reaction (PCR) amplification, and it soon became apparent that the use of Roman numerals was unwieldy, e.g., *Lol p* I through *Lol p* XI [16,17]. Moreover, the use of italics to denote a purified protein was inconsistent with the nomenclature used in bacterial genetics and the human leukocyte antigen system, where italicized names denote a gene product and regular typeface indicates expressed proteins. In 1994, the allergen nomenclature was revised so that the allergen designation was shown in regular type. Arabic numerals replaced the Roman ones. Thus, *Amb a* I, *Lol p* I, and *Der p* I of the original 1986 nomenclature are now referred to as Amb a 1, Lol p 1, and Der p 1 in the current nomenclature, which has been published in several scientific journals [18–20]. The first house dust mite allergen was purified by Chapman and Platts-Mills in 1980 [21]. The cDNA sequence that encoded the protein was described in 1988 [22,23]. The white-faced hornet venom protein Dol m 5 was characterized by Hoffman [24] and then cloned as a cDNA by Fang et al. in 1988 [25]. The cDNA clone encoding the first allergen of birch pollen, Bet v 1, was obtained by Breiteneder et al. in 1989 [26].

4.2.1.1 INCLUSION CRITERIA

A key part of the systematic WHO/IUIS allergen nomenclature is that the allergen should satisfy biochemical criteria, which define the molecular structure of the protein, and immunologic criteria, which define its importance as an allergen. Originally, the biochemical criteria were based on establishing protein purity, e.g., by sodium dodecyl sulfate polyacrylamide gel electrophoresis (SDS-PAGE), isoelectric focusing (IEF), or high-pressure liquid chromatography (HPLC), and physicochemical properties including molecular weight, pI (isoelectric point), and N-terminal amino acid sequence [18]. With few exceptions, the full nucleotide sequence and amino acid sequence is required. An outline of the inclusion criteria is shown in Table 4.1. A more detailed list of requirements for the inclusion of an allergen in the WHO/IUIS allergen nomenclature can be found in the allergen submission form (http://www.allergen.org/submission. php). An important aspect of these criteria is that the submission information should provide an unambiguous description whereby other investigators can identify the same allergen and perform comparative studies. Originally, allergens were characterized following purification from the natural source using monospecific or monoclonal antibodies to identify the allergen. Allergens or antibodies were provided to other researchers for verification. With improved technical methods, nucleotide and amino acid sequencing provides unambiguous data to identify the protein, which is then tested for allergenicity [27–30].

The second inclusion criterion involves demonstrating that the purified allergen has allergenic activity, both *in vitro* and *in vivo*. It is important to screen a panel of serum samples from allergic

Table 4.1 Criteria for including allergens in the WHO/IUIS nomenclature

1. The molecular and structural properties should be clearly and unambiguously defined, including:
   - Purification of the allergenic natural or recombinant protein to (near) homogeneity.
   - Verification of the presence of the protein in the natural allergen source.
   - Determination of nucleotide and/or amino acid sequence
   - Determination of molecular weight and isoelectric point.

Additional optional information:
   - Determination of the glycosylation pattern.
   - Production of monospecific or monoclonal antibodies to the allergen.

2. The importance of the allergen in causing IgE responses should be defined by:
   - Proving a prevalence of IgE reactivity. Preferably with more than 5% of allergic subjects testing positive or IgE binding from at least five patients, although rare allergens can be positive with fewer subjects.

Additional optional information:
   - Demonstration, where possible, of comparable IgE antibody-binding activity between the recombinant and the natural allergen (e.g., by inhibition assays).
   - Testing serum IgE binding of individual serum samples from a large population (preferably at least 50 individual patients allergic to the same allergen source) to understand actual prevalence of a specific allergy.
   - Demonstration of allergenic activity of the purified allergen by skin testing or histamine release assays which are negative when using control subjects or sera.
   - Investigating whether depletion of the allergen from an allergenic extract (e.g., by immunoabsorption) reduces its IgE-binding activity.

patients to establish the prevalence of IgE reactivity. Ideally, 50 or more sera should be screened, although an allergen can be included in the nomenclature if the prevalence of IgE reactivity is greater than 5% or if the allergen elicits IgE responses in as few as five patients. Alternatively, a smaller number of highly selected allergic subjects can be used to test IgE binding, depending on the clinical criteria demonstrating allergic reactions and on the frequency of subjects with symptoms (e.g., in cases of occupational allergies or uncommon exposures).

Several methods for measuring IgE antibodies to specific allergens *in vitro* are available. These methods originally included radio-allergosorbent test (RAST)–based assays and radioimmunoassays using labeled allergens. Immunoblotting was frequently used and remains one of the most specific and useful techniques for specificity of IgE binding, especially when used in inhibition assays to compare recombinant and natural allergens [31]. Additional techniques were developed that include enzyme-linked immunosorbent assay (ELISA) and fluorescent enzyme immunoassay (FEIA). ELISA systems allow large numbers of sera to be screened for allergen-specific IgE by either coupling the allergen directly to a solid support or by using a capture monoclonal antibody (mAb) to bind the allergen. Serum IgE antibodies bind to the immobilized allergen and are detected with biotinylated anti-IgE [32]. One of the current methods for quantitative IgE measurement by FEIA is the ImmunoCAP. A streptavidin-CAP assay, a variation of the ImmunoCAP, uses biotinylated allergens and allows IgE antibodies to specific allergens to be measured by FEIA [33,34].

More recently, static or suspension microarray systems have also been developed that enable simultaneous measurement of IgE antibodies to multiple allergens. These new technologies are based on chips, beads, or biosensors, and they have the advantage of using small volumes of sera [35–40].

Microarrays provide a profile of IgE responses to specific allergens. One commercial test uses a static allergen array on allergen-coated glass slides to measure IgE antibodies in sera to over 100 purified natural or recombinant allergens at the same time. Results of microarray assays are as sensitive as FEIA with allergen extracts, but the microarray requires only 30 µL of serum [35,41–43]. Arrays that measure IgE antibodies to over 150 allergens have been recently developed in the MEDALL study [44]. Fluorescent multiplex suspension array technology has been developed using allergens that are covalently coupled to polystyrene microspheres [36–38]. Array technologies are especially suited to large population surveys or birth cohorts for monitoring IgE responses to multiple allergens and for pediatric studies where sera are often in short supply.

Demonstrating that a protein has allergenic activity *in vivo* is important, especially since many allergens are now produced as recombinant molecules before the natural allergen is purified (if ever). Several mite, cockroach, and fungal allergens (e.g., *Aspergillus*, *Alternaria*, and *Cladosporium*) have been defined solely using recombinant proteins, and it is unlikely that much effort will be directed to isolating their natural counterparts. Ideally, the allergenic activity of recombinant proteins should be confirmed *in vivo* by quantitative skin testing or *in vitro* by histamine release assays with basophils and appropriate allergic sera. Skin testing studies were carried out using a number of recombinant allergens, including Bet v 1, Asp f 1, Bla g 4, Bla g 5, Der p 2, Der p 5, and Blo t 5 [28,45–47]. The recombinant proteins showed potent allergenic activity and gave positive skin tests at the picogram level.

4.2.1.2 RESOLVING AMBIGUITIES IN THE NOMENCLATURE

The allergen nomenclature system is based on the Linnaean genus and species names, and some of those share the same first three letters of the genus and/or the first letter of the species name. Consequently, some unrelated allergens would receive the same allergen designation: *Candida* allergens could be confused with dog allergens (*Canis domesticus*); there are multiple related species of *Vespula* (Vespid) allergens; and *Periplaneta americana* (American cockroach) allergens need to be distinguished from *Persea americana* (avocado) allergens. These ambiguities were overcome by adding a further letter to either the genus or species name. Examples are Cand a 1 for *Candida albicans* allergen 1 and Can f 1 for dog (*Canis familiaris*) allergen 1; Ves v 1 or Ves vi 1, to indicate *V. vulgaris* or *V. vidua* allergens, respectively. The genus *Prunus* is now listed with five different species (Pru p: *P. persica* for peach, Pru ar: *P. armenica* for apricot, Pru av: *P. avium* for sweet cherry; Pru d: *P. domestica* for European plum, and Pru du: *P. dulcis* for almond). Per a 1 or Pers a 1 now represent the respective cockroach or avocado allergen.

4.2.1.3 THE BIOLOGY OF ALLERGENS

Many allergens have biochemical names that describe their biological function and were assigned before the allergen nomenclature was conceived. Examples include egg allergens (ovomucoid and ovalbumin), insect allergens (phospholipases and hyaluronidases), and tropomyosins from shrimp, mite, and cockroach. Sequence homology searches have assigned allergens to particular protein families and have provided important clues to their biological function. To some extent, allergens segregate among protein families according to whether they are indoor allergens, outdoor allergens, plant or animal food allergens, or injected allergens:

- *Indoor allergens* (e.g., animal dander; fecal particles from mites and cockroaches; mold spores): proteolytic enzymes (serine and cysteine proteases), lipocalins (ligand-binding proteins), tropomyosins, albumins, protease inhibitors [28,48]. An example for allergenic cysteine proteases, Der p 1 and Der f 1, is shown in Figure 4.1.
- *Outdoor allergens* (e.g., pollens from grasses, trees, and weeds; mold spores): plant pathogenesis-related (PR-10) proteins, pectate lyases, β-expansins, calcium-binding proteins (polcalcins), defensin-like proteins, trypsin inhibitors [27,29,49]. An example for a PR-10 allergen, Bet v 1, is shown in Figure 4.2.
- *Plant or animal food allergens* (e.g., fruits, vegetables, nuts, seeds, milk, eggs, shellfish, fish): nonspecific lipid transfer proteins, profilins, seed storage proteins (i.e., 7S-globulins, 2S-albumins), ovalbumins, lysozymes, thaumatin-like proteins, lactoglobulins, caseins, tropomyosins, parvalbumins [50–52]. Examples for allergenic proteins from peanut, fish, hen's egg, and fruits are shown in Figure 4.3.
- *Injected allergens* (e.g., insect venoms and some therapeutic proteins): phospholipases, hyaluronidases, pathogenesis-related proteins [53,54].

Allergens belonging to these protein families have biologic functions that are important to the organism that is the allergen source. Proteolytic enzymes are involved in digestion, tropomyosins and parvalbumins in muscle contraction, and profilins in actin polymerization. The group 1 mite allergens are cysteine proteases and are involved in digestion (Figure 4.1). The mouse lipocalin allergen, Mus m 1, is produced in the liver of male mice, secreted in large amounts in the urine, and serves to mark the territories of male mice [55]. The cockroach allergen Bla g 4, a lipocalin homolog, is produced in accessory glands of the male reproductive system and is speculated to bind pheromones [56,57]. Crystallographic studies showed that Bet v 1, a plant pathogenesis related (PR-10) protein, contains a hydrophobic pocket (Figure 4.2) that could function as

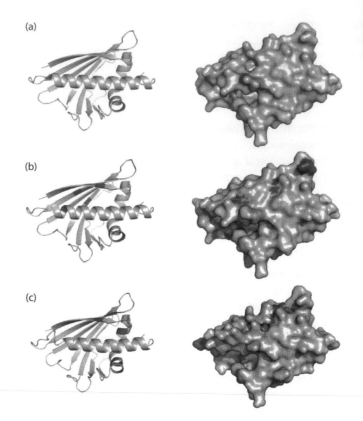

(a)

(b)

(c)

Figure 4.2 X-ray molecular structures of Bet v 1 variants that differ in IgE-binding capacity. Molecules are shown in ribbon (left) and surface (right) representations, and residues that differ from Bet v 1.0101 are indicated in red (or black for the black-and-white figure). (a) Bet v 1.0101 (= Bet v 1a); Protein Data Bank code: 4A88; high IgE-binding capacity [62]. (b) Bet v 1.0106 (= Bet v 1j); PDB code 4A8U; high IgE-binding capacity [62]. (c) Bet v 1.0107 (= Bet v 1 l); PDB code 1FM4; low IgE-binding capacity [58].

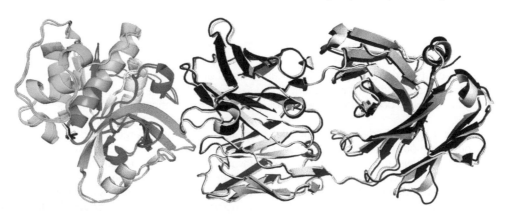

Figure 4.1 X-ray crystal structures of Der p 1 and Der f 1, each in complex with the cross-reactive monoclonal antibody 4C1. The allergens are colored from blue in the *N*-terminus to red in the *C*-terminus. The cysteines in positions 31 for Der p 1 and 32 for Der f 1 (shown as white and black sticks, respectively) are essential for catalysis. The Fabs of the mAb 4C1 are indicated in white and black ribbons for the Der p 1 and Der f 1 complexes, respectively (Protein Data Bank codes 3RVX and 3RVV, respectively) [63].

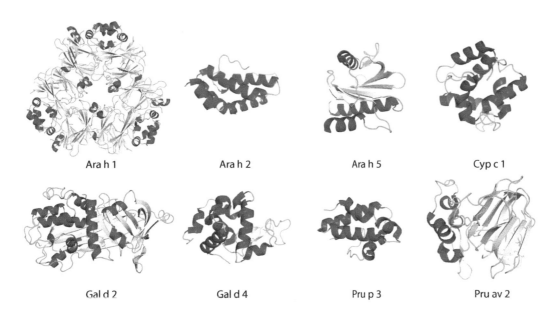

Figure 4.3 Molecular structures of food allergens. 7S globulin Ara h 1 (PDB code 3S7I), 2S albumin Ara h 2 (3OB4), profilin Ara h 5 (4ESP), parvalbumin Cyp c 1 (4CPV), ovalbumin Gal d 2 (1OVA), lysozyme Gal d 4, nsLTP Pru p 3 (2ALG), and thaumatin-like protein Pru av 2 (2AHN). Ribbon representations with secondary structural elements (α-helices in red, β-sheets in yellow, and loops in green) are shown.

a carrier for presumably multiple hydrophobic ligands such as plant steroids or flavonols [58,59].

In the allergy literature, it is preferable to use the systematic allergen nomenclature. In other contexts, such as comparisons of biochemical activities or protein structure, it may be appropriate or more useful to use the biochemical names. A selected list of the allergen nomenclature designations and biochemical names of inhalant, food, and venom allergens is shown in Table 4.2. There are 92 three-dimensional allergen structures in the Structural Database of Allergenic Proteins (http://fermi.utmb.edu/SDAP/). Publications in 2014 and 2015 list more than 250 x-ray crystal or nuclear magnetic resonance structures belonging to more than 105 allergenic proteins [60,61]. The Database of Allergen Families, AllFam (http://www.meduniwien.ac.at/allfam/), shows that allergens are found in 216 domains of the currently defined 16,306 protein families in the Pfam protein families database (https://pfam.xfam.org/). Thus, allergens are represented by a 1.3% of the Pfam domains, yet they represent a fair degree of diversity at both the structural and biological levels. Such diversity is likely to preclude the existence of a few common structural features, e.g., amino acid sequence motifs or protein structures, which predispose proteins to act as allergens [27,30].

4.2.2 Isoallergens, isoforms, and variants

Originally, isoallergens were broadly defined as multiple molecular forms of the same allergen, sharing extensive antigenic (IgE) cross-reactivity. The revised nomenclature defines an isoallergen as an allergen from a single species, sharing similar molecular size, identical biological function, and 67% or more amino acid sequence identity [8]. A two-digit number, following the dot after the number given to the allergen, designates the isoallergen. Some allergens, which were previously included in the nomenclature as separate entities, share extensive sequence identity and some antigenic cross-reactivity but were named independently as they do not meet all the criteria to be classified as isoallergens. Examples include Lol p 2 and Lol p 3 (65% identity) and Amb a 1 and Amb

a 2 (65% identity). In some cases, two allergen designations were fused into isoforms of the same allergen number (e.g., Amb a 2 was revised as an isoform of Amb a 1 in 2012). The first two numbers after the dot are used to designate isoallergens within an allergen type (e.g., Ara h 2.01 and Ara h 2.02 represent isoallergens of the 2S albumin of peanut).

The designation "Group" is still used by some authors to describe structurally related allergens from different species within the same genus, or from closely related genera. But in these cases, the levels of amino acid sequence identity can range from as little as 40% to ~90%. Similarities in tertiary structure and biologic function are also taken into account when describing allergen groups. Examples include the group 2 mite allergens (Der p 2, Der f 2 and Lep d 2, Gly d 2 and Tyr p 2) showing 40%–88% homology, and the group 5 ragweed allergens (Amb a 5, Amb t 5, and Amb p 5) showing ~45% identity. Allergens from the same groups sharing molecular structure may have common amino acids on the molecular surface that lead to antigenic cross-reactivity. The x-ray crystal structures of Der p 1 in complex with the murine mAb 4C1 and Der f 1 in complex with the same antibody illustrate the structural basis of cross-reactivity for these two mite group 1 allergens (Figure 4.1). The same group number cannot always be assigned to related homologous allergens, as illustrated for Ara h 2 that shares homology and fold with Ara h 6 and Ara h 7 (Figure 4.3), and for lipocalins among and within species (Mes a 1, Mus m 1, Phod s 1, Rat n 1, Equ c 1, Equ c 2, Can f 1, Can f 2, Can f 4, Can f 6, Bos d 2, Bos d 5, Cap v 1, Cap v 2, Cap v 3, Cap v 6, Ory c 1, Ory c 4, Bla g 4, Per a 4, Fel d 4). However, the WHO/IUIS Allergen Nomenclature Sub-Committee does not recognize a "Group" as a defined category.

The term "variant" or "isoform" is used to indicate allergen sequences that differ from each other by only a very limited number of amino acid substitutions (i.e., polymorphic variants of the same allergen). Typically, variants may be identified by sequencing several cDNA clones of a given allergen. Variants have been reported for Der p 1, Der p 2, Amb a 1, and Cry j 1. For the most prolific Bet v 1, 42 sequences have been deposited in the GenBank database.

Table 4.2 Molecular properties of common allergens

Source	Allergen	MW (kDa)	Homology/function
Inhalants			
Indoor			
House dust mite (*Dermatophagoides* *pteronyssinus*)	Der p 1	25	Cysteine protease[a]
	Der p 2	14	ML domain family member[a]
	Der p 3	30	Serine protease
Cat (*Felis domesticus*)	Fel d 1	36	Secretoglobin[a]
Dog (*Canis familiaris*)	Can f 1	25	Lipocalin
Mouse (*Mus musculus*)	Mus m 1	21	Lipocalin (territory marking protein)[a]
Rat (*Ratus norvegicus*)	Rat n 1	21	Pheromone-binding lipocalin[a]
Cockroach (*Blatella germanica*)	Bla g 2	36	Inactive aspartic protease[a]
Outdoor			
Pollen—Grasses			
Rye (*Lolium perenne*)	Lol p 1	28	β-Expansin
Timothy (*Phleum pratense*)	Phl p 5	32	Putative ribonuclease[a]
Bermuda (*Cynodon dactylon*)	Cyn d 1	32	β-Expansin
Pollen—Weeds			
Mugwort (*Artemisia vulgaris*)	Art v 1	28	Defensin-like protein[a]
Ragweed (*Ambrosia artemisiifolia*)	Amb a 1	38	Pectate lyase
Pollen—Trees			
Birch (*Betula verrucosa*)	Bet v 1	17	Pathogenesis-related protein[a]
Foods			
Cow's milk (*Bos domesticus*)	Bos d 5 (β-lactoglobulin)	18	Lipocalin[a]
Hen's egg (*Gallus domesticus*)	Gal d 1 (ovomucoid)	28	Trypsin inhibitor
Codfish (*Gadus callarias*)	Gad c 1	12	Caclium-binding muscle protein (parvalbumin)
Peanut (*Arachis hypogaea*)	Ara h 1	63	Vicilin seed storage protein[a]
Venoms			
Bee (*Apis mellifera*)	Api m 1	19.5	Phospolipase A_2[a]
Wasp (*Polystes annularis*)	Pol a 2	38	Hyaluronidase
European hornet (*Vespa crabro*)	Vesp c 1	34	Phospholipase A_1B
Fire ant (*Solenopsis invicta*)	Sol i 1	18	Phospholipase A_1B
Fungi			
Aspergillus fumigatus	Asp f 1	18	Cytotoxin (mitogillin)[a]
Alternaria alternata	Alt a 10	53	Aldehyde dehydrogenase
Latex			
Rubber tree (*Hevea brasiliensis*)	Hev b 1	14	Rubber elongation factor
	Hev b 2	34	β-1,3-glucanase

[a] Allergens with known three-dimensional structure.

Amino acid substitutions in variants might be relevant for antibody binding. A reduced IgE antibody binding of the Bet v 1 variant Bet v 1.0107 (Figure 4.2) has been described [58,62]. In other cases, as described for the anti-Der p 1 mAb 4C1 (Figure 4.1), antibody recognition might not be affected by sequence polymorphisms [63]. Isoallergens are denoted by the addition of two additional numerals after the dot. Numerals in positions 3 and 4 after the dot distinguish between allergen variants or isoforms.

One of the tasks of the WHO/IUIS Allergen Nomenclature Sub-Committee is a regular reevaluation and refinement of the sequence data deposited in the nomenclature database. Many allergens recorded in the WHO/IUIS allergen database were originally submitted with partial or missing sequence data. Subsequently, full sequences became available that revealed inconsistencies in allergen assignments. The Allergen Nomenclature Sub-Committee periodically screens and revises allergen designations. For example, the ragweed (*Ambrosia artemisiifolia*) pollen allergens Amb a 1 and Amb a 2 both belong to the pectate lyase family. Amb a 2 isoallergens showed 61%–70% sequence identity to Amb a 1 isoallergens and were hence renamed as Amb a 1.05 [64]. Entries for the larvae of the nonbiting midge *Chironomus thummi thummi* contained nine allergens (Chi t 1 to Chi t 9) with 16 variants, all of which are hemoglobin subunits with sequence identities between 28% and 99%. As Chi t 5 to Chi t 8 showed sequence identities greater than 50% to Chi t 3, they received new designations as Chi t 3 isoallergens [64]. This renaming was based on more detailed phylogenetic analyses of the proteins that showed a clear grouping of Chi t 5–8 with Chi t 3. The recommended 67% sequence identity for two allergens to be designated as isoallergens is only a guide.

The group 1 allergens from tree pollen have an unusually high number of isoallergens and variants. The major birch pollen allergen, Bet v 1, comprised a large number of isoallergens and variants recorded in the WHO/IUIS allergen database. Their sequences were grouped into two isoallergens: Bet v 1.01 with 14 variants and Bet v 1.02 with four variants [64]. Different variants of each isoallergen showed 91%–99% sequence identity, whereas identity between Bet v 1.01 and Bet v 1.02 sequences was 84%–89%. The group 1 allergens from hornbeam (*Carpinus betulus*), Car b 1, are classified into three isoallergens that show 74%–88% homology. Car b 1.01 has 13 variants, Car b 1.02 has one, and Car b 1.03 has two variants (http://www.allergen.org/). Four isoallergens of the hazel (*Corylus avellana*) allergen, Cor a 1, have been recorded. The isoallergens Cor a 1.01, 1.02, and 1.03 are pollen allergens. The isoallergen Cor a 1.04 has three variants that are nut allergens (http://www. allergen.org/).

Latex provides another example of distinctions in the nomenclature. The 20 kDa hevein precursor or prohevein, Hev b 6.01, gives rise to the most important 5 kDa latex allergen hevein, designated as Hev b 6.02. It is one of the two fragments derived from Hev b 6.01, the other being Hev b 6.03, the 14 kDa C-terminal fragment. This is one of the few examples where the two digits behind the dot were used to identify fragments derived from one protein rather than isoforms. Studies have also uncovered a prodigious number of isoforms among house dust mite group 1 and group 2 allergens. High-fidelity PCR sequencing of environmental isolates of dust mites revealed 23 isoforms of Der p 1 and 13 isoforms of Der p 2 [30]. Because isoforms differ by only a few amino acid residues, analysis of immunoreactivity to isoforms can be useful in defining antibody binding sites and T-cell epitopes on allergens [65].

4.3 NOMENCLATURE FOR ALLERGEN GENES AND RECOMBINANT OR SYNTHETIC PEPTIDES

In the revised nomenclature, italicized letters are reserved to designate genes coding for allergens. Two genomic allergen sequences have been determined for animal dander allergens: the cat allergen, Fel d 1 [66], and the mouse urinary allergen, Mus m 1 [67]. Fel d 1 has two separate genes encoding chain 1 and chain 2 of the molecule, which are designated *Fel d 1A* and *Fel d 1B*, respectively [30]. Genomic sequences of Bet v 1, Cor a 1, and an apple PR-10 family member, Mal d 1, have also been determined [68,69]. Mal d 1 is an example of an incomplete or nonsensitizing allergen, i.e., an allergen that can interact with preformed Bet v 1–specific IgE antibodies but is unable to induce the production of IgE. Thus, symptoms of the pollen food syndrome in birch pollen allergic patients who eat apples are due to IgE cross-reactivity between Bet v 1 (the primary sensitizer) and Mal d 1 (with which the anti-Bet v 1 IgE interacts). The subcommittee originally kept track of the gene sequences and had multiple variants of some allergen genes. However, in 2014 it was decided to stop designating gene names because many gene variants still encode the same amino acid sequences.

When recombinant allergens were first introduced, researchers often used the term *native allergen* to distinguish the natural protein from the recombinant allergen. However, because *native* has implications for protein structure (i.e., native conformation), it was decided that the term *natural allergen* should be used to indicate any allergen purified from natural source material. Natural allergens may be denoted by the prefix (n) to distinguish them from recombinant allergens, which are indicated by the prefix (r) before the allergen name (e.g., nBet v 1 and rBet v 1) in research publications or diagnostic test materials. Furthermore, the nomenclature system makes no distinction between recombinant allergens produced in bacterial, yeast, or mammalian expression systems.

Synthetic peptides are indicated by the prefix (s), with the particular peptide residues indicated in parentheses after the allergen name. Thus, a synthetic peptide encompassing residues 100–120 of Bet v 1.0101 would be indicated: sBet v 1.0101 (100–120). At such a detailed level, the nomenclature, while technically sound, begins to become cumbersome and rather long-winded for most purposes. There are also additional refinements to the nomenclature that cover substitutions of different amino acid residues within synthetic peptides. This aspect of the nomenclature (which is based on that used for synthetic peptides of immunoglobulin sequences) is detailed in the revised nomenclature document to which aficionados are referred for full details [19].

4.4 FUTURE PERSPECTIVES OF ALLERGEN NOMENCLATURE

4.4.1 Protein family membership

When the cDNA of the major birch pollen allergen Bet v 1 was published in 1989 as the first nucleotide sequence of a plant allergen [26], it became clear that this birch pollen protein belonged to a family of proteins. As more and more members of this family were discovered, the emerging superfamily of proteins, the Bet v 1–like superfamily, was

Table 4.3 Protein family membership and allergen designations

Allergen source	PR-10 family	Profilin family
Birch (*Betula verrucosa*)	Bet v 1	Bet v 2
Apple (*Malus domestica*)	Mal d 1	Mal d 4
Celery (*Apium graveolens*)	Api g 1	Api g 4
Kiwi (*Actinidia deliciosa*)	Act d 8	Act d 9
Peanut (*Arachis hypogaea*)	Ara h 8	Ara h 5
Soybean (*Glycine max*)	Gly m 4	Gly m 3

eventually named after Bet v 1 (Figure 4.2) [70]. Today, the Bet v 1-like superfamily of proteins contains 17 families and 37,376 member proteins from 3789 species distributed across all kingdoms of life (https://pfam.xfam.org/clan/CL0209). In general, the steadily increasing number of allergen sequences allows the study of the evolutionary biology of allergens [71] and the determination of their distribution into protein families [29,72]. The AllFam database (http://www.meduniwien.ac.at/allfam/) provides information about the protein family membership of allergens. Interestingly, all known allergens belong to only 1.3% of the 16,712 protein families described in version 31.0 (March 2017) of the Pfam database (http://pfam.sanger.ac.uk/ [73]).

Although the current official allergen nomenclature is directly linked to the source organism, it provides no information on the protein family membership of allergens. This is not surprising as the classification of allergens by protein family membership has only become available in more recent years, and its implications on allergen nomenclature were first discussed in 2008 [74]. Initially, the same allergen numbers were given to the same type of proteins, a procedure that could not be completely adhered to as the numbers of allergens rapidly increased. Hence, identical numbers could not be assigned to all Bet v 1 homologues or to the various profilins (Table 4.3). However, the grouping of allergens by protein families provides valuable information on possible cross-reactivities for researchers as well as for clinicians. Der p 1 from *Dermatophagoides pteronyssinus* and Der f 1 from *D. farinae* belong to the protein family of cysteine proteases. Both proteins are potent cross-reactive mite allergens. Chruszcz and colleagues located a common epitope on Der p 1 and Der f 1 (Figure 4.1) by determining the crystal structures of both natural allergens in complex with a monoclonal antibody [63] as well as allergen-specific epitopes [75,76].

Linking the allergen nomenclature database to a more specialized database, such as AllFam, can provide information on protein family memberships of allergens (Table 4.4). When the high-resolution structure of the *Alternaria alternata* allergen Alt a 1 became available, it revealed a new molecular structure [77]. Alt a 1 is a unique β-barrel composed of 11 β-strands and forms a butterfly-like dimer linked by a disulfide bond. This structure has no equivalent in the Protein Data Bank, and hence, Alt a 1 is the founding member of a new protein family.

4.5 WORLD HEALTH ORGANIZATION/ INTERNATIONAL UNION OF IMMUNOLOGIC SOCIETIES ALLERGEN NOMENCLATURE SUB-COMMITTEE

Allergens to be considered for inclusion in the nomenclature are reviewed by the WHO/IUIS Allergen Nomenclature Sub-Committee

(Table 4.5). The Sub-Committee is currently chaired by Richard Goodman (University of Nebraska–Lincoln) and includes 24 active members from all over the world and six members at large. The Sub-Committee meets annually at an international allergy/immunology meeting and discusses new proposals it has received during the year, together with any proposed changes or additions to the nomenclature and the database. The active members attend at least one meeting and review new allergen submissions. At-large Sub-Committee members were active in the past but now do not normally evaluate allergen submissions. The procedure for submitting candidate names for allergens to the Sub-Committee is straightforward [78]. Having purified the allergen, determined its sequence, and shown that it reacts with IgE from individuals who are allergic to its source, investigators should download the allergen submission form from the WHO/IUIS Allergen Nomenclature Sub-Committee website (http://www.allergen.org/submission.php) and send the completed form to the Sub-Committee prior to publishing articles describing the allergen. The Sub-Committee will provisionally accept the author's suggested allergen name or assign the allergen a name that is consistent with the Sub-Committee's practices, provided that the inclusion criteria are satisfied. The name will later be confirmed and posted on the website. Occasionally, the Sub-Committee resolves differences between investigators who may be using different names for the same allergen or disputes concerning the chronological order of allergen identification. These issues can normally be resolved by objective evaluation of each case. The Sub-Committee has provided submission guidelines concerning allergen nomenclature to all major, peer-reviewed allergy and immunology journals.

The WHO/IUIS Allergen Nomenclature Sub-Committee receives funding to support its activities from the IUIS; the American Academy of Allergy, Asthma and Immunology (AAAAI); and the European Academy of Allergy and Clinical Immunology (EAACI).

4.5.1 Allergen databases

The official website for the WHO/IUIS Allergen Nomenclature Sub-Committee is http://www.allergen.org. This site lists all allergens and isoforms that are recognized by the Sub-Committee and is updated on a regular basis. Over the past several years, a number of other allergen databases have been generated by academic institutions, research organizations, and industry-sponsored groups typically having a focus specific to their stated aims (Table 4.5). These sites naturally differ in their focus and emphasis but are useful sources of information about allergens. The Structural Database of Allergenic Proteins (SDAP) was developed at the Sealy Center for Structural Biology, University of Texas Medical Branch, and provides detailed structural data on allergens in the WHO/IUIS allergen nomenclature database, including sequence information, Protein Data Bank (http://www.rcsb.org/) files, and programs to analyze IgE antibody-binding epitopes. Amino acid and nucleotide sequence information is also compiled in the SWISS-PROT (https://www.ebi.ac.uk/uniprot/) and the National Center for Biotechnology Information (NCBI; http://www.ncbi.nlm.nih.gov/guide/all/) databases.

The Food Allergy Research and Resource Program (FARRP) database (http://AllergenOnline.org/) includes food, airway contact, and venom allergens and is intended as a sequence-driven risk assessment database with references based on peer-reviewed publications related to allergen characterization, IgE-binding, and allergenic activity. Since 2012, it also includes a celiac peptide and protein database. The InformAll database (http://research.bmh.manchester.ac.uk/informall/) provides extensive structural information related to important food allergens. However,

Table 4.4 Allergen databases

Database	Host	Curation	URL
WHO/IUIS Allergen Nomenclature Database, now partly supported by the EAACI and the AAAAI as well as IUIS and other funding sources	University of Nebraska Lincoln (2007–2017), now the European Academy of Allergy and Clinical Immunology	Expert panel reviews submissions of new allergens; the only body officially able to give allergen designations. Updated as new allergens are accepted.	http://www.allergen.org
SDAP, the Structural Database of Allergenic Proteins	University of Texas	Curated by host scientists with oversight by an expert review panel. Last updated in 2013.	http://fermi.utmb.edu/SDAP/sdap_ver.html
Allergen Online, an allergen sequence and information database	University of Nebraska, Food Allergy Research and Resource Programm (FARRP)	Reviewed by an expert panel headed by Richard Goodman, with annual database updates. Intended as an allergenic sequence risk assessment tool. Last updated March 2018.	http://Allergenonline.com
Allergome, an extensive knowledge database of molecular structures and publications designed to include data from multiple information sources and maintained by Adriano Mari	Allergy Data Laboratories, Latina, Italy	Curation is not defined, but rather it is based on "real-time" acquisition from NCBI and other sources, and is updated by Adriano Mari, updated every few days.	http://www.allergome.org
AllFam, a database that provides a classification of allergens into protein families using data from WHO/IUIS, AllergenOnline, and Pfam databases	Medical University of Vienna, Vienna, Austria	Curated by Christian Radauer with expert advice from Heimo Breiteneder and Merima Bublin. Last updated March 2017.	http://www.meduniwien.ac.at/allfam
AllerBase, a comprehensive allergen knowledgebase	Pune University, Pune, India, and Shiv Nadar University, Greater Noida, India	Curated by their authors and published in database, 2017, doi: 10.1093/database/bax066. Last updated March 24, 2018.	http://bioinfo.unipune.ac.in/AllerBase/Home.html
IEDB, an immune epitope database and analysis resource	Developed and maintained by the La Jolla Institute of Immunology, managed by Bjoern Peters, La Jolla, California.	Curated by the faculty and postdocs at La Jolla Institute of Immunology. Last updated September 16, 2018.	https:www.iedb.org

Table 4.5 The World Health Organization and International Union of Immunological Societies Allergen Nomenclature Sub-Committee (Status 2019)

Member	Function	Institution	City, State	Country
Richard E. Goodman, PhD	Chairman	University of Nebraska	Lincoln, NE	USA
Janet Davies, PhD	Vice Chair	Queensland University of Technology	Brisbane, Queensland	Australia
Anna Pomés, PhD	Secretary	INDOOR Biotechnologies, Inc.	Charlottesville, VA	USA
Gabriele Gadermaier, PhD	Treasurer	University of Salzburg	Salzburg	Austria
Thomas A. E. Platts-Mills, MD, PhD	Active Founding Member	University of Virginia	Charlottesville, VA	USA
Heimo Breiteneder, PhD	Committee Member	Medical University of Vienna	Vienna	Austria
Sanny K. Chan, MD, PhD	Committee Member	National Jewish Health	Denver, CO	USA
Maksymilian Chruszcz, PhD	Committee Member	University of South Carolina	Columbia, SC	USA
Christiane Hilger, Ph.D	Committee Member	Luxembourg Institute of Health	Luxembourg	Luxembourg
Thomas Holzhauser, PhD	Committee Member	Paul-Ehrlich-Institut	Langen	Germany
Alain Jacquet, PhD	Committee Member	Chulalongkorn University	Bangkok	Thailand
Uta Jappe, MD, MSc	Committee Member	Borstel Leibniz-Center for Medicine and Biosciences	Borstel	Germany
Jörg Kleine-Tebbe, MD, MSc	Committee Member	Allergy & Asthma Center Westend	Berlin	Germany
Jonas Lidholm, PhD	Committee Member	ThermoFisher Scientific	Uppsala	Sweden
Andreas Lopata, PhD	Committee Member	James Cook University	Townsville, Queensland	Australia
Vera Mahler, MD	Committee Member	Paul-Ehrlich-Institut	Langen	Germany
Geoffrey A. Mueller, PhD	Committee Member	National Institute of Environmental Health Sciences	Research Triangle Park, NC	USA
Andreas Nandy, PhD	Committee Member	ALLERGOPHARMA GmbH & Co. KG	Reinbek	Germany
Markus Ollert, MD	Committee Member	Centre de Recherche Public de la Santé	Luxembourg	Luxembourg
Christian Radauer, PhD	Committee Member	Medical University of Vienna	Vienna	Austria
Monika Raulf, PhD	Committee Member	Ruhr-University Bochum	Bochum	Germany
Edzard Spillner, PhD	Committee Member	Aarhus University	Aarhus	Denmark
Josefina Zakzuk Sierra, PhD	Committee Member	University of Cartagena	Cartagena de Indias	Colombia
Yuzhu Zhang, PhD	Committee Member	USDA, ARS, PWA, WRRC-PFR	Albany, CA	USA
Martin D. Chapman, PhD	Member at Large	INDOOR Biotechnologies, Inc.	Charlottesville, VA	USA
Jørgen N. Larsen, PhD	Member at Large	ALK A/S	Hørsholm	Denmark
Wayne R. Thomas, PhD	Member at Large	TVW Telethon Institute for Child Health Research	West Perth, Western Australia	Australia
Marianne van Hage, MD, PhD	Member at Large	Karolinska Institutet	Stockholm	Sweden
Ronald van Ree, PhD	Member at Large	University of Amsterdam	Amsterdam	The Netherlands
Stefan Vieths, PhD	Member at Large	Paul-Ehrlich-Institut	Langen	Germany

it has not been updated recently. The Allergome database (http://www.allergome.org/) provides regular updates on allergens, allergenic sources, and reactions from publications in the scientific literature. The AllFam database, which was developed based on allergen information in the Allergome database and the data on protein families from the Pfam database, contains all allergens with known sequences that can be assigned to at least one Pfam family. The database is maintained by Radauer and Breiteneder at the Medical University of Vienna and can be accessed at http://www.meduniwien.ac.at/allfam/.

The Immune Epitope Database and Analysis Resource (IEDB) is an inclusive immune epitope and prediction database maintained by the La Jolla Institute of Immunology in La Jolla, California (http://www.iedb.org) and funded by the National Institute of Allergy and Infectious Diseases (NIAID). The IEDB contains epitope and assay information related to infectious diseases, autoimmune and allergic diseases, and transplant/alloantigens for humans, nonhuman primates, mice, and other species. It also has information about T-cell, B-cell, MHC binding, and MHC ligand elution experiments, as well as predictive tools for MHC binding to class I and class II receptor types, and T- and B-cell epitopes [79,80]. The data in this database are curated primarily from the published literature and also include direct submissions from researchers involved in epitope discovery [80]. The IEDB does not have a comprehensive list of allergens, and the primary focus is the development of vaccines using scientific predictions of B-cell and T-cell epitopes. A description of a new database called "AllerBase" (http://bioinfo.net.in/AllerBase/Home.html) was published in 2017 [81] and reports to collect information and integrate it from the WHO/IUIS allergen nomenclature database, Allergome, AllergenOnline, GenBank, GenPept, UniProtKB, PDB, and PubMed looking for protein sequences, structures, IgE-binding epitopes, IgE antibody sequences, and IgE cross-reactivity. The article states that prediction tools for protein structure and epitopes are available and tested for validity.

4.6 CONCLUDING REMARKS

The three men in a boat did a remarkably good job. The use of the systematic allergen nomenclature has been extremely successful, has significantly enhanced research in the area, and continues to be revised and updated with remarkable changes in scientific methods and data related to proteins and allergy. The use of the generic terms *major* and *minor* allergen continues to evoke discussion. Relatively few allergens fulfill the criteria originally used by Marsh to define a major allergen (i.e., an allergen that causes IgE responses in 90% or more of allergic patients, such as Bet v 1, Fel d 1, Der p 2, Lol p 1) [10]. However, there are a large number of allergens that cause sensitization in more than 50% of patients, and Løwenstein used this figure of 50% to define major allergens in the early 1980s [6]. There are important questions that are hard to answer including which proteins in a given allergy source are the dominant sources of allergic reactions. For instance, peanut has major seed storage proteins that seem to cause most IgE binding and likely allergy including Ara h 1, Ara h 2, and Ara h 3, as well as a few other proteins. The major concentration on a mass basis shows Ara h 1 and Ara h 3 are extremely common at 10%–30% by mass, but they are large proteins. The 2S albumin Ara h 2 is also abundant based on mass at ~4% of the total protein, but when based on moles of protein and epitopes, it is a dominant source by abundance. It is also highly

stable under heating and digestion conditions [82,83]. Some other peanut proteins bind IgE and may cause some allergic reactions but are probably not important in eliciting food allergy [82,84]. Scientists like to describe their allergen as *major* because it is effective in promoting their research and carries some weight in securing research funding. The question continues to be "What defines a major allergen?" Demonstrating a high prevalence of IgE-mediated sensitization among subjects with clinical reactivity to the source material is a minimal requirement, given the increasing sensitivity of assays to detect IgE antibodies. The contribution of an allergen to the total potency of an allergen extract should be considered (e.g., by absorption studies), as well as the amount of IgE antibody directed against the allergen, compared to other allergens purified or cloned from the same source. Other criteria include whether the allergen induces strong T-cell responses and, for indoor allergens, whether it is a suitable marker of exposure in house dust and air samples. But most important is biological activity as demonstrated by direct challenge (unlikely to be performed), by specific IgE binding to pure proteins controlling for abundance relative to the source, and by basophil or skin prick test reactivity.

It is clear from many studies that some allergens play a preeminent role in causing immune responses in allergic individuals, are better marker proteins for immunologic, clinical, and epidemiologic studies, and are usually considered to be high-profile targets for allergy diagnostics and therapeutics. Table 4.6, which was developed together with Rob Aalberse (University of Amsterdam), lists the eight criteria for defining the properties' allergens that are clinically relevant. Examples of allergens that we consider to fulfill most of these criteria are as follows:

Mite	Group 1 and Group 2 (*Dermatophagoides* sp.) allergens
Animal	Fel d 1, Bos d 5, Bos d 9, Bos d 10, Bos d 11
Tree pollen	Bet v 1 (and structurally homologous allergens); Ole e 1
Grass pollen	Phl p 1, Phl p 5
Weed pollen	Amb a 1
Peanut	Ara h 1, Ara h 2, Ara h 3
Shellfish	Pen a 1 and other tropomyosins from shellfish
Insect allergens	Api m 1, Api m 2, Api m 5 (and homologous insect venom allergens)

Recombinant Bet v 1 and recombinant Phl p 5a were produced under Good Manufacturing Practice and recently established as reference standards in the European Pharmacopeia for the determination of the respective proteins both in natural allergen extracts as well as in recombinant allergen products [85]. The determination of the presence and concentrations of allergens are also widely used for environmental exposure assessments and for measuring the allergen content of vaccines. To this end, more well-defined purified allergen standards are being developed. In 2012, eight purified natural allergens were formulated into a single multiallergen standard containing the major allergens of mite, cockroach, cat, dog, mouse, and rat [86,87]. ELISA methods have been validated for the measurement of Bet v 1 and are expected to be approved by the European Pharmacopeia in 2019.

Table 4.6 Eight criteria for defining allergens that make a difference

1. A sensitization rate greater than 80% (>2 ng allergen-specific IgE/mL) in a large panel of allergic patients, with exclusion of the CCD (cross-reactive carbohydrate determinants).
2. A significant proportion of total IgE (greater than 10%) from a subject can be allergen-specific.
3. Removal of the allergen from the source material significantly reduces the potency of the extract.
4. Absorption of serum with purified allergen significantly reduces specific IgE to the allergen extract.
5. The allergen accounts for a significant proportion of the extractable protein in the source material.
6. The allergen can be used as a marker for environmental exposure assessment.
7. Both antibody and cellular responses to the allergen can be measured in a high proportion of patients allergic to the source material.
8. The allergen has been shown to be effective as part of an allergy vaccine.

For most purposes, allergists only need to be familiar with the nomenclature for allergens, rather than isoallergens, isoforms, peptides, and so on. As measurements of allergens in diagnostics and vaccines and assessments in environmental exposure are becoming a routine part of the care of allergic patients, allergists will need to understand more about the structure and functions of allergens and their abundance in allergenic sources as well as their ability to elicit reactions. The use of purified allergens in molecular diagnostics is quickly becoming adopted in Europe, and the EAACI has published a 250-page user's guide about molecular allergology in clinical practice [88]. Having a systematic nomenclature is essential to expand our knowledge of allergens and to underscore the development of innovative allergy diagnostics and therapeutics. The systematic allergen nomenclature is a proven success and is versatile enough to evolve with advances in molecular biology and proteomics that will continue to occur.

SALIENT POINTS

1. A systematic nomenclature for all allergens that cause disease in humans has been formulated by the Allergen Nomenclature Sub-Committee of the WHO and the IUIS.
2. Allergens are described using the first three or four letters of the genus, followed by one or two letters for the species, and an Arabic numeral to indicate the chronological order of allergen purification (e.g., *Dermatophagoides pteronyssinus* allergen 1 = Der p 1) or their protein family membership.
3. Allergens have to satisfy criteria of biochemical purity and criteria to establish their allergenic importance. It is important that the amino acid sequence of an allergen is defined without ambiguity and that allergenic activity is demonstrated in a population of allergic patients who are exposed to the allergen.
4. Modifications of the nomenclature are used to identify isoallergens, isoforms, allergen genes, recombinant allergens, and synthetic peptides. For examples, Bet v 1.01 is an isoallergen of Bet v 1, and Bet v 1.0101 is an isoform or variant of the Bet v 1.01 isoallergen.

ACKNOWLEDGMENTS AND DISCLAIMER

This chapter has reviewed the systematic WHO/IUIS allergen nomenclature as revised in 1994 through 2018. Other views expressed in the chapter are personal opinions and do not necessarily reflect the views of the WHO/IUIS Allergen Nomenclature Sub-Committee. Author HB wishes to acknowledge the support of the Austrian Science Fund (FWF) Doctoral Program MCCA W1248-B30. Author RG acknowledges the funding of research for AllergenOnline.org, and specific allergy and IgE-binding studies from a variety of company sources from studies focusing on allergy risk assessment. Research in this publication was supported in part by the National Institute of Allergy and Infectious Diseases of the National Institutes of Health under Award Number R01AI077653 (to AP and MDC). The content is solely the responsibility of the authors and does not necessarily represent the official views of the National Institutes of Health. The authors collectively thank the IUIS, EAACI, and AAAAI for providing financial support to the WHO/IUIS allergen nomenclature database in 2016–2018.

REFERENCES

1. King TP, Norman PS. Isolation studies of allergens from ragweed pollen. *Biochemistry* 1962; 1: 709–720.
2. Johnson P, Marsh DG. "Isoallergens" from rye grass pollen. *Nature* 1965; 206(987): 935–937.
3. Johnson P, Marsh DG. Allergens from common rye grass pollen (*Lolium perenne*). II. The allergenic determinants and carbohydrate moiety. *Immunochemistry* 1966; 3(2): 101–110.
4. Marsh DG, Bias WB, Santilli J, Jr., Schacter B, Goodfriend L. Ragweed allergen Ra5: A new tool in understanding the genetics and immunochemistry of immune response in man. *Immunochemistry* 1975; 12(67): 539–543.
5. Platts-Mills TA, Chapman MD, Marsh DG. Human immunoglobulin E and immunoglobulin G antibody responses to the "minor" ragweed allergen Ra3: Correlation with skin tests and comparison with other allergens. *J Allergy Clin Immunol* 1981; 67(2): 129–134.
6. Lowenstein H, King TP, Goodfriend L, Hussain R, Roebber M, Marsh DG. Antigens of *Ambrosia elatior* (short ragweed) pollen. II. Immunochemical identification of known antigens by quantitative immunoelectrophoresis. *J Immunol* 1981; 127(2): 637–642.
7. Ohman JL, Jr., Lowell FC, Bloch KJ. Allergens of mammalian origin. III. Properties of a major feline allergen. *J Immunol* 1974; 113(6): 1668–1677.
8. Elsayed SM, Aas K. Characterization of a major allergen (cod.) chemical composition and immunological properties. *Int Arch Allergy Appl Immunol* 1970; 38(5): 536–548.
9. Elsayed S, Bennich H. The primary structure of allergen M from cod. *Scand J Immunol.* 1975; 4(2): 203–208.
10. Marsh DG. Allergens and the genetics of allergy. In: Sela M, editor. *The Antigens. III.* New York, NY: Academic Press, 1975: 271–350.
11. Lowenstein H. Quantitative immunoelectrophoretic methods as a tool for the analysis and isolation of allergens. In: Kallos P, Waksman PH, de Weck AL, editors. *Progress in Allergy*, Vol. 25 Basel: Karger, 1978.

12. Lind P, Korsgaard J, Lowenstein H. Detection and quantitation of *Dermatophagoides* antigens in house dust by immunochemical techniques. *Allergy.* 1979; 34(5): 319–326.

13. Lowenstein H. Timothy pollen allergens. *Allergy.* 1980; 35(3): 188–191.

14. de Weck AL, Ring J. *CIA Collegium Internationale Allergologicum: History and Aims of a Special International Community Devoted to Allergy Research 1954–1996.* Munich: MMV Medizin Verlag, 1996.

15. Marsh DG, Goodfriend L, King TP, Lowenstein H, Platts-Mills TA. Allergen nomenclature. *Bull World Health Organ* 1986; 64(5): 767–774.

16. Scheiner O, Kraft D. Basic and practical aspects of recombinant allergens. *Allergy* 1995; 50(5): 384–391.

17. Thomas WR. Mite allergens groups I-VII. A catalogue of enzymes. *Clin Exp Allergy* 1993; 23(5): 350–353.

18. King TP, Hoffman D, Lowenstein H, Marsh DG, Plattsmills TAE, Thomas W. Allergen nomenclature. *B World Health Organ* 1994; 72(5): 797–806.

19. King TP, Hoffman D, Lowenstein H, Marsh DG, Platts-Mills TA, Thomas W. Allergen nomenclature. WHO/IUIS Allergen Nomenclature Subcommittee. *Int Arch Allergy Immunol* 1994; 105(3): 224–233.

20. King TP, Hoffman D, Lowenstein H, Marsh DG, Platts-Mills TA, Thomas W. Allergen nomenclature. *Allergy* 1995; 50(9): 765–774.

21. Chapman MD, Platts-Mills TA. Purification and characterization of the major allergen from *Dermatophagoides pteronyssinus*-antigen P1. *J Immunol* 1980; 125(2): 587–592.

22. Chua KY, Stewart GA, Thomas WR et al. Sequence analysis of cDNA coding for a major house dust mite allergen, Der p 1. Homology with cysteine proteases. *J Exp Med* 1988; 167(1): 175–182.

23. Thomas WR, Stewart GA, Simpson RJ et al. Cloning and expression of DNA coding for the major house dust mite allergen Der p 1 in *Escherichia coli. Int Arch Allergy Appl Immunol* 1988; 85(1): 127–129.

24. Hoffman DR. Allergens in *Hymenoptera* venom XIV: IgE binding activities of venom proteins from three species of vespids. *J Allergy Clin Immunol* 1985; 75(5): 606–610.

25. Fang KS, Vitale M, Fehlner P, King TP. cDNA cloning and primary structure of a white-face hornet venom allergen, antigen 5. *Proc Natl Acad Sci USA* 1988; 85(3): 895–899.

26. Breiteneder H, Pettenburger K, Bito A et al. The gene coding for the major birch pollen allergen Betv1, is highly homologous to a pea disease resistance response gene. *EMBO J* 1989; 8(7): 1935–1938.

27. Aalberse RC. Structural biology of allergens. *J Allergy Clin Immunol* 2000; 106(2): 228–38.

28. Chapman MD, Smith AM, Vailes LD, Arruda LK, Dhanaraj V, Pomes A. Recombinant allergens for diagnosis and therapy of allergic disease. *J Allergy Clin Immunol* 2000; 106(3): 409–418.

29. Radauer C, Breiteneder H. Pollen allergens are restricted to few protein families and show distinct patterns of species distribution. *J Allergy Clin Immunol* 2006; 117(1): 141–147.

30. Chapman MD, Pomes A, Breiteneder H, Ferreira F. Nomenclature and structural biology of allergens. *J Allergy Clin Immunol* 2007; 119(2): 414–420.

31. Kuehn A, Hilger C, Lehners-Weber C et al. Identification of enolases and aldolases as important fish allergens in cod, salmon and tuna: Component resolved diagnosis using parvalbumin and the new allergens. *Clin Exp Allergy* 2013; 43(7): 811–822.

32. Trombone AP, Tobias KR, Ferriani VP et al. Use of a chimeric ELISA to investigate immunoglobulin E antibody responses to Der p 1 and Der p 2 in mite-allergic patients with asthma, wheezing and/or rhinitis. *Clin Exp Allergy* 2002; 32(9): 1323–1328.

33. Erwin EA, Custis NJ, Satinover SM et al. Quantitative measurement of IgE antibodies to purified allergens using streptavidin linked to a high-capacity solid phase. *J Allergy Clin Immunol* 2005; 115(5): 1029–1035.

34. Glesner J, Filep S, Vailes LD et al. Allergen content in German cockroach extracts and sensitization profiles to a new expanded set of cockroach allergens determine *in vitro* extract potency for IgE reactivity. *J Allergy Clin Immunol* 2019; 143(4):1474–1481.

35. Canonica GW, Ansotegui IJ, Pawankar R et al. A WAO-ARIA-GA(2)LEN consensus document on molecular-based allergy diagnostics. *World Allergy Organ J* 2013; 6(1): 17.

36. Chapman MD, Wuenschmann S, King E, Pomes A. Technological innovations for high-throughput approaches to *in vitro* allergy diagnosis. *Curr Allergy Asthma Rep* 2015; 15(7): 36.

37. King EM, Vailes LD, Tsay A, Satinover SM, Chapman MD. Simultaneous detection of total and allergen-specific IgE by using purified allergens in a fluorescent multiplex array. *J Allergy Clin Immunol* 2007; 120(5): 1126–1131.

38. King EM, Filep S, Smith B et al. A multi-center ring trial of allergen analysis using fluorescent multiplex array technology. *J Immunol Methods* 2013; 387(1–2): 89–95.

39. Platt GW, Damin F, Swann MJ et al. Allergen immobilisation and signal amplification by quantum dots for use in a biosensor assay of IgE in serum. *Biosens Bioelectron* 2014; 52: 82–88.

40. Heffler E, Puggioni F, Peveri S, Montagni M, Canonica GW, Melioli G. Extended IgE profile based on an allergen macroarray: A novel tool for precision medicine in allergy diagnosis. *World Allergy Organ J* 2018; 11(1): 7.

41. Harwanegg C, Laffer S, Hiller R et al. Microarrayed recombinant allergens for diagnosis of allergy. *Clin Exp Allergy* 2003; 33(1): 7–13.

42. Wohrl S, Vigl K, Zehetmayer S et al. The performance of a component-based allergen-microarray in clinical practice. *Allergy* 2006; 61(5): 633–639.

43. Hiller R, Laffer S, Harwanegg C et al. Microarrayed allergen molecules: Diagnostic gatekeepers for allergy treatment. *FASEB J* 2002; 16(3): 414–416.

44. Skrindo I, Lupinek C, Valenta R et al. The use of the MeDALL-chip to assess IgE sensitization: A new diagnostic tool for allergic disease? *Pediatr Allergy Immunol* 2015; 26(3): 239–246.

45. Schmid-Grendelmeier P, Crameri R. Recombinant allergens for skin testing. *Int Arch Allergy Immunol* 2001; 125(2): 96–111.

46. Pauli G, Purohit A, Oster JP et al. Comparison of genetically engineered hypoallergenic rBet v 1 derivatives with rBet v 1 wild-type by skin prick and intradermal testing: Results obtained in a French population. *Clin Exp Allergy* 2000; 30(8): 1076–1084.

47. Barbosa MC, Santos AB, Ferriani VP, Pomes A, Chapman MD, Arruda LK. Efficacy of recombinant allergens for diagnosis of cockroach allergy in patients with asthma and/or rhinitis. *Int Arch Allergy Immunol* 2013; 161(3): 213–219.

48. Arruda LK, Vailes LD, Ferriani VP, Santos AB, Pomes A, Chapman MD. Cockroach allergens and asthma. *J Allergy Clin Immunol* 2001; 107(3): 419–428.

49. Gadermaier G, Dedic A, Obermeyer G, Frank S, Himly M, Ferreira F. Biology of weed pollen allergens. *Curr Allergy Asthma Rep* 2004; 4(5): 391–400.

50. Breiteneder H, Radauer C. A classification of plant food allergens. *J Allergy Clin Immunol* 2004; 113(5): 821–830; quiz 31.

51. Reese G, Schicktanz S, Lauer I et al. Structural, immunological and functional properties of natural recombinant Pen a 1, the major allergen of Brown Shrimp, *Penaeus aztecus. Clin Exp Allergy* 2006; 36(4): 517–524.

52. Vieths S, Scheurer S, Ballmer-Weber B. Current understanding of cross-reactivity of food allergens and pollen. *Ann N Y Acad Sci* 2002; 964: 47–68.

53. Henriksen A, King TP, Mirza O et al. Major venom allergen of yellow jackets, Ves v 5: Structural characterization of a pathogenesis-related protein superfamily. *Proteins* 2001; 45(4): 438–448.

54. King TP, Spangfort MD. Structure and biology of stinging insect venom allergens. *Int Arch Allergy Immunol* 2000; 123(2): 99–106.

55. Hurst JL, Payne CE, Nevison CM et al. Individual recognition in mice mediated by major urinary proteins. *Nature* 2001; 414(6864): 631–634.

56. Fan Y, Gore JC, Redding KO, Vailes LD, Chapman MD, Schal C. Tissue localization and regulation by juvenile hormone of human allergen Bla g 4 from the German cockroach, *Blattella germanica* (L.). *Insect Mol Biol* 2005; 14(1): 45–53.

57. Gore JC, Schal C. Cockroach allergen biology and mitigation in the indoor environment. *Annu Rev Entomol* 2007; 52: 439–463.

58. Markovic-Housley Z, Degano M, Lamba D et al. Crystal structure of a hypoallergenic isoform of the major birch pollen allergen Bet v 1 and its likely biological function as a plant steroid carrier. *J Mol Biol* 2003; 325(1): 123–33.

59. Seutter von Loetzen C, Hoffmann T, Hartl MJ et al. Secret of the major birch pollen allergen Bet v 1: Identification of the physiological ligand. *Biochem J* 2014; 457(3): 379–390.

60. Dall'antonia F, Pavkov-Keller T, Zangger K, Keller W. Structure of allergens and structure-based epitope predictions. *Methods* 2014; 66(1): 3–21.

61. Pomes A, Chruszcz M, Gustchina A et al. 100 Years later: Celebrating the contributions of x-ray crystallography to allergy and clinical immunology. *J Allergy Clin Immunol* 2015; 136(1): 29–37 e10.

62. Kofler S, Asam C, Eckhard U, Wallner M, Ferreira F, Brandstetter H. Crystallographically mapped ligand binding differs in high and low IgE binding isoforms of birch pollen allergen bet v 1. *J Mol Biol* 2012; 422(1): 109–123.

63. Chruszcz M, Pomes A, Glesner J et al. Molecular determinants for antibody binding on group 1 house dust mite allergens. *J Biol Chem* 2012; 287(10): 7388–7398.

64. Radauer C, Nandy A, Ferreira F et al. Update of the WHO/IUIS Allergen Nomenclature Database based on analysis of allergen sequences. *Allergy* 2014; 69(4): 413–419.

65. Piboonpocanun S, Malainual N, Jirapongsananuruk O, Vichyanond P, Thomas WR. Genetic polymorphisms of major house dust mite allergens. *Clin Exp Allergy* 2006; 36(4): 510–516.

66. Griffith IJ, Craig S, Pollock J, Yu XB, Morgenstern JP, Rogers BL. Expression and genomic structure of the genes encoding FdI, the major allergen from the domestic cat. *Gene* 1992; 113(2): 263–268.

67. Mudge JM, Armstrong SD, McLaren K et al. Dynamic instability of the major urinary protein gene family revealed by genomic and phenotypic comparisons between C57 and 129 strain mice. *Genome Biol* 2008; 9(5): R91.

68. Schenk MF, Gilissen LJ, Esselink GD, Smulders MJ. Seven different genes encode a diverse mixture of isoforms of Bet v 1, the major birch pollen allergen. *BMC Genomics* 2006; 7: 168.

69. Gao ZS, van de Weg WE, Schaart JG et al. Genomic cloning and linkage mapping of the Mal d 1 (PR-10) gene family in apple (*Malus domestica*). *Theor Appl Genet* 2005; 111(1): 171–183.

70. Radauer C, Lackner P, Breiteneder H. The Bet v 1 fold: An ancient, versatile scaffold for binding of large, hydrophobic ligands. *BMC Evol Biol* 2008; 8: 286.

71. Radauer C, Breiteneder H. Evolutionary biology of plant food allergens. *J Allergy Clin Immunol* 2007; 120(3): 518–525.

72. Jenkins JA, Griffiths-Jones S, Shewry PR, Breiteneder H, Mills EN. Structural relatedness of plant food allergens with specific reference to cross-reactive allergens: An *in silico* analysis. *J Allergy Clin Immunol* 2005; 115(1): 163–170.

73. Radauer C, Bublin M, Wagner S, Mari A, Breiteneder H. Allergens are distributed into few protein families and possess a restricted number of biochemical functions. *J Allergy Clin Immunol* 2008; 121(4): 847–852e7.

74. Breiteneder H. Protein families: Implications for allergen nomenclature, standardisation and specific immunotherapy. *Arb Paul Ehrlich Inst Bundesinstitut Impfstoffe Biomed Arzneim Langen Hess* 2009; 96: 249–254; discussion 54–6.

75. Osinski T, Pomes A, Majorek KA et al. Structural analysis of Der p 1-antibody complexes and comparison with complexes of proteins or peptides with monoclonal antibodies. *J Immunol* 2015; 195(1): 307–316.

76. Glesner J, Vailes LD, Schlachter C et al. Antigenic determinants of Der p 1: Specificity and cross-reactivity associated with IgE antibody recognition. *J Immunol* 2017; 198(3): 1334–1344.

77. Chruszcz M, Chapman MD, Osinski T et al. *Alternaria alternata* allergen Alt a 1: A unique beta-barrel protein dimer found exclusively in fungi. *J Allergy Clin Immunol* 2012; 130(1): 241–247e9.

78. Pomes A, Davies JM, Gadermaier G et al. WHO/IUIS allergen nomenclature: Providing a common language. *Mol Immunol* 2018; 100: 3–13.

79. Vita R, Overton JA, Greenbaum JA et al. The immune epitope database (IEDB) 3.0. *Nucleic Acids Res* 2015; 43(Database issue): D405–12.

80. Fleri W, Vaughan K, Salimi N, Vita R, Peters B, Sette A. The immune epitope database: How data are entered and retrieved. *J Immunol Res* 2017; 2017: 5974574.

81. Kadam K, Karbhal R, Jayaraman VK, Sawant S, Kulkarni-Kale U. AllerBase: A comprehensive allergen knowledgebase. *Database (Oxford)* 2017; 2017.

82. Chen X, Wang Q, El-Mezayen R, Zhuang Y, Dreskin SC. Ara h 2 and Ara h 6 have similar allergenic activity and are substantially redundant. *Int Arch Allergy Immunol* 2013; 160(3): 251–258.

83. Palmer GW, Dibbern DA, Jr., Burks AW et al. Comparative potency of Ara h 1 and Ara h 2 in immunochemical and functional assays of allergenicity. *Clin Immunol* 2005; 115(3): 302–312.

84. Palladino C, Breiteneder H. Peanut allergens. *Mol Immunol* 2018; 100: 58–70.

85. Vieths S, Barber D, Chapman M et al. Establishment of recombinant major allergens Bet v 1 and Phl p 5a as Ph. Eur. reference standards and validation of ELISA methods for their measurement. Results from feasibility studies. *Pharmeur Bio Sci Notes* 2012; 2012: 118–134.

86. Filep S, Tsay A, Vailes L et al. A multi-allergen standard for the calibration of immunoassays: CREATE principles applied to eight purified allergens. *Allergy* 2012; 67(2): 235–241.

87. Filep S, Tsay A, Vailes LD et al. Specific allergen concentration of WHO and FDA reference preparations measured using a multiple allergen standard. *J Allergy Clin Immunol* 2012; 129(5): 1408–1410.

88. Matricardi PM, Kleine-Tebbe J, Hoffmann HJ et al. EAACI molecular allergology user's guide. *Pediatr Allergy Immunol* 2016; 27(Suppl 23): 1–250.

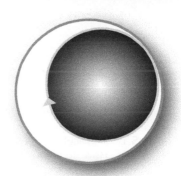

Immunologic responses to various forms of allergen immunotherapy

Umit Murat Sahiner
National Heart and Lung Institute, Imperial College
Hacettepe University School of Medicine

Mohamed H. Shamji
National Heart and Lung Institute, Imperial College
Asthma UK Centre in Allergic Mechanisms of Asthma

Sakura Sato
Sagamihara National Hospital

Ozge Soyer
Hacettepe University School of Medicine

Stephen J. Till
Asthma UK Centre in Allergic Mechanisms of Asthma
King's College London

Motohiro Ebisawa
Sagamihara National Hospital

Mübeccel Akdis
Swiss Institute of Allergy and Asthma Research (SIAF)

Stephen R. Durham
National Heart and Lung Institute, Imperial College
MRC and Asthma UK Centre in Allergic Mechanisms of Asthma

CONTENTS

5.1 INTRODUCTION

Allergen-specific immunotherapy (AIT) is the only treatment that leads to prolonged tolerance against allergens. Besides the classical AIT method, subcutaneous immunotherapy (SCIT), data about the immunologic mechanisms of sublingual immunotherapy (SLIT) are growing and show mostly similar immune regulation patterns compared to SCIT. In addition, studies of mucosal tolerance indicate the generation of T-regulatory cells and their cytokines by application of vaccines via sublingual, oral, and other mucosal routes. The induction of a tolerant state in peripheral T cells represents an essential step in AIT and peptide immunotherapy (PIT) [1]. Peripheral T-cell tolerance is mainly characterized by suppressed proliferative and cytokine responses against the major allergens. It is initiated by autocrine action of interleukin (IL)-10 and/or transforming growth factor-β (TGF-β), which are produced by the antigen-specific T-regulatory (Treg) cells. Tolerized T cells can be reactivated to produce either distinct Th1 or Th2 cytokine patterns, thus directing allergen-AIT toward successful or unsuccessful treatment. Treg cells directly or indirectly influence effector cells of allergic inflammation, such as mast cells, basophils, and eosinophils. In addition, there is accumulating evidence that they may suppress IgE production and induce IgG4 and IgA production against allergens. By the application of the recent knowledge in mechanisms of AIT, more rational and safer approaches are awaiting development for prevention and possibly cure of allergic diseases [2].

AIT is highly effective in appropriately selected patients with allergic disease. Whereas conventional vaccination strategies are employed to initiate and then boost immunologic memory, AIT subdues established pathological immune responses mediated by IgE and allergen-specific memory T cells through controlled exposure to the offending allergen. Since subcutaneous injection (SCIT) of sufficient native allergen to invoke immunoregulatory mechanisms can trigger unwanted IgE-mediated reactions, the amounts of allergen contained in injections are increased incrementally from low levels until a safe but sufficient maintenance dose is achieved. Patient selection is important, and the risk-benefit ratio must be assessed on an individual basis. The underlying mechanisms are important since they provide insight into the mechanisms of allergic disease and induction of clinical tolerance. In addition, AIT is allergen specific. This enables one to observe the effects of specific modulation of the immune response in a patient in whom the provoking factor (common aeroallergen or venom) is known. The effects of the allergen exposure may be observed during either experimental provocation in a clinical laboratory or natural environmental conditions. Similarly, the influence of immunotherapy on clinical, immunologic, and pathological changes may be observed under controlled conditions. This is in contrast to other immunologic diseases where the antigen is unknown and no antigen-specific treatment is available. SLIT has emerged as a viable clinical alternative to the traditional injection route. Several well-controlled studies have shown that it is clinically effective and induces clinical and immunologic tolerance.

AIT results in a rapid inhibition of allergen-challenged late responses, with a slower and proportionately smaller decline in early responses. Biopsies taken from skin and nasal mucosa reveal reductions in inflammatory cell numbers, including mast cells, basophils, and eosinophils. Around 6–8 weeks after starting weekly SCIT, updosing injections, increases occur in allergen-specific IgG, particularly of IgG4 isotype. These antibodies block IgE effector mechanisms including basophil histamine release and IgE-facilitated antigen presentation by dendritic cells (via FcεRI) and B cells (via FcεRII, CD23) to T cells. Induction of allergen-specific IgA is also observed, and these antibodies can induce monocytic cells to produce IL-10, an immunoregulatory cytokine. These humoral responses likely reflect modulation of allergen-specific T-cell responses. Immunotherapy modifies peripheral and mucosal Th2 responses to allergen in favor of Th1 cytokine, IL-10, and/or TGF-β production. Inducible T-regulatory cell (iTregs), in particular, IL-10 (T_{r1}) and TGF-β (Th3) cells, are detectable within a few weeks of the first injection. IL-10 favors B-cell production of IgG4 and inhibits mast cell, eosinophil, and T-cell responses (Figure 5.1). The mechanism leading to development of these cells has yet to be elucidated, though similar populations can be experimentally induced by tolerogenic dendritic cells (DCs).

While current treatment regimes are effective, refinement of immunotherapy both in terms of the efficacy and safety profile remains an important goal. Novel approaches being clinically tested include the combination of allergens with immunomodulatory adjuvants to potentiate responses. Two examples of adjuvants are bacterially derived, modified lipid compounds or CpG-rich immunostimulatory oligodeoxynucleotides that act through toll-like receptors (TLR) 4 and 9, respectively. Alternative strategies include the use of allergen-derived peptides or modified recombinant allergen vaccines. In addition, intralymphatic allergen-specific immunotherapy (ILIT), which directly delivers the allergen into inguinal lymph nodes, substantially shortens the duration of

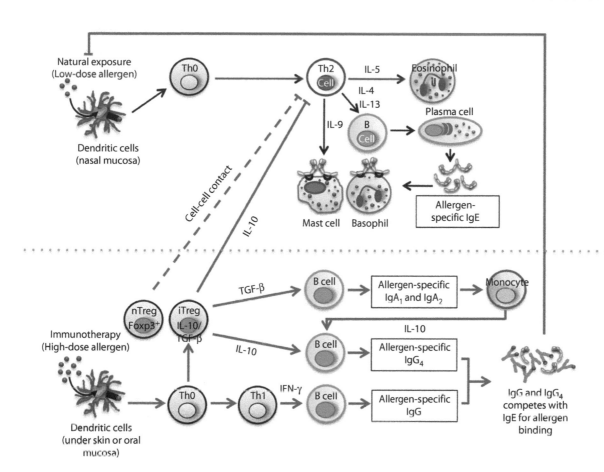

Figure 5.1 Immunologic mechanisms of subcutaneous allergen-specific immunotherapy are shown. Low-dose and repeated allergen exposure at mucosal surfaces in atopic individuals drive type I IgE-mediated allergic responses. High allergen dose through subcutaneous or sublingual route results in the shift of T-cell polarization from a T helper 2 (Th2) to a T helper 1 (Th1) response. This is accompanied by an increase in the ratio of Th1 cytokines (IFN-γ, IL-12) to Th2 cytokines (IL-4, IL-5, and IL-13). The induction of T-regulatory cells (inducible Treg cells [iTreg] and natural Treg cells [nTreg]) and cytokines such as IL-10 and TGF-β following immunotherapy play an important role in suppressing Th1 and Th2 responses and contribute to the induction of allergen-specific IgA$_1$, IgA$_2$, and in particular, IgG$_4$ antibodies with inhibitory activity. IgG$_4$ antibodies are able to suppress FcεRI and CD23-mediated IgE-facilitated allergen presentation and basophil histamine release. (Figure adapted with permission from Shamji MH, Durham SR. *Clin Exp Allergy* 2011; 41(9): 1235–1246.)

treatment. Low allergen doses are effective with ILIT resulting in reduced risk of systemic allergic reactions. Another approach is the repeated intradermal injection of extremely low doses of grass pollen extract (containing nanogram quantities of allergen). This strategy dramatically suppresses allergen-induced late cutaneous responses in an antigen-specific fashion and increases allergen-specific IgG levels [3]. The intradermal route directly targets DC populations with likely rapid access to regional lymphoid tissue. Whether or not this translates into clinical benefit during the pollen season is currently being tested. These novel interventions aim to maintain the beneficial effects of vaccines while minimizing the immediate IgE-dependent complications, which currently require SCIT to be conducted cautiously and under specialist supervision.

5.2 THE ALLERGIC RESPONSE

5.2.1 Early and late responses

Experimental allergen exposure in the nose, eyes, or bronchi leads to development of mast cell–dependent sneeze, itch, watery discharge, and bronchospasm, maximal at 15–30 minutes and resolving within 1–3 hours. This "early response" is triggered by activation of mast cells through cross-linking of allergen-specific IgE molecules pre-bound to high-affinity IgE receptors (FcεRI). The sequelae of this activation are the release of numerous preformed and newly synthesized mediators, including histamine, tryptase, TAME-esterase, bradykinin, leukotrienes (including LTC$_4$, LTD$_4$, and LTE$_4$), prostaglandins (including PGF$_{2a}$ and PGD$_2$ [specific for mast cells]), and platelet activating factor. These mediators collectively induce vasodilatation, increased vascular permeability, mucosal edema, increased mucus production from submucosal glands and goblet cells within the respiratory/gastrointestinal epithelium, and smooth muscle contraction in the lower respiratory tract [4].

In a subgroup of individuals, the early response resolves to be followed by a late response. Airflow obstruction is usually the predominant symptom of the late response in both upper and lower airways. A nasal allergen provocation test elicits nasal early and late responses within the nasal mucosa resulting in clinical symptoms, nasal airflow and resistance, and local inflammation. Similarly, skin challenge testing provokes cutaneous early and late responses with wheal and flare followed by late-onset localized edema and tenderness. Late responses are maximal at 6–12 hours after allergen challenge and resolve within 24 hours. The late response is characterized by recruitment of eosinophils, basophils, activated T cells, and DCs to the site of allergen exposure. These activated cells are a rich source of potentially pathogenic mediators such as Th2 cytokines (IL-4, IL-5, IL-9, and IL-13), which modulate inflammatory cell function and upregulate adhesion molecule expression and B-cell IgE synthesis. The immunopathologic changes in the mucosa during the late response are largely representative of those seen during "natural," prolonged allergen exposure (e.g., during the pollen season).

Eozinophilia and mast cell activation are directed by Th2 cells, and Th2 differentiation is dependent on the microenvironment and presence of local cytokines, which are produced as a result of interactions between epithelial cells, local DCs, innate lymphoid cells, and regional lymph nodes [4]. As the DCs are activated by epithelial-derived CCL2 and CCL 20, they migrate to regional lymph nodes and polarize naïve T cells to Th2 cells. DC migration is driven by IL-13 produced by ILC2 s and IL-4 produced by basophils [4] (Figure 5.2).

Innate lymphoid cells (ILCs) are defined as a novel subset of lymphoid cells that lack antigen-specific receptors and are divided into three different subgroups. ILC2s are under the control of transcription factor GATA-3, and once activated by epithelium-derived IL-25, IL-33, and thymic stromal lymphopoietin (TSLP), they produce type 2 cytokines IL-4, IL-5, and IL-13 [5,6]. ILC2s represent an important alternative source of type 2 cytokines and are likely to increase and maintain the local allergic inflammation. Recently, the role of ILC2s is defined in several diseases, such as allergic airway inflammation [7,8], allergic rhinitis [9], atopic dermatitis [10], and eosinophilic esophagitis [11].

5.2.2 Effects of allergen immunotherapy

AIT inhibits the late responses in the skin [12], nose [13], and lung [14], though it is not established that this effect is predictive of clinical efficacy. In comparison, the effect on the early response appears to be relatively modest and variable. For example, certain investigators describe only temporary inhibition of the early response in the skin [15] and no inhibition in the lung [14]. Within a group of house dust mite–sensitive children, suppression of the early skin response was predictive of prolonged suppression following discontinuation of treatment, though this requires confirmation in a prospective study [16]. The evolution of early and late response inhibition has

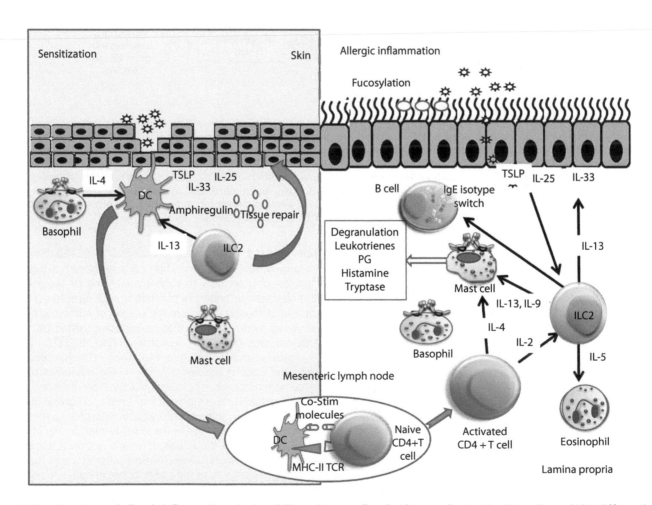

Figure 5.2 Sensitization and allergic inflammation. Eosinophilia and mast cell activation are directed by Th2 cells, and Th2 differentiation is dependent on the microenvironment and the presence of local cytokines, which are produced as a result of interactions between epithelial cells, local dendritic cells (DCs), innate lymphoid cells, and regional lymph nodes [4]. As the dendritic cells are activated by epithelial-derived CCL2 and CCL 20, they migrate to regional lymph nodes and polarize naïve T cells to Th2 cells. DC migration is driven by IL-13 produced by ILC2s and IL-4 produced by basophils.

been examined during a conventional grass pollen immunotherapy regime [17] (Figure 5.3). Remarkably, late responses to intradermal challenge testing are reduced 2 weeks into treatment, by which time patients had received less than 1% of the total cumulative allergen dose administered weekly during the 2-month updosing phase. In this same study, the decline in the sizes of early responses is proportionally much less but evolves slowly over a time frame more in keeping with clinical protection from symptoms [3].

(a) Immunotherapy regime

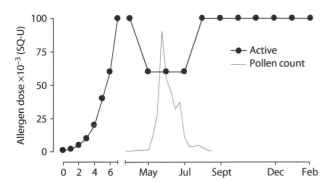

(b) Early-phase responses

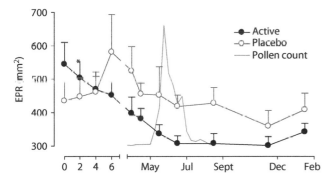

(c) Late-phase responses

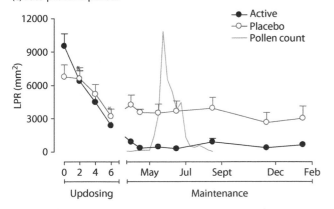

Figure 5.3 Time course analysis of clinical measurements during the first year of grass pollen immunotherapy with the dose of grass pollen allergen administered at each visit represented in the top panel. Early and late skin responses were assessed at 15 minutes and 24 hours following intradermal challenge with grass pollen allergen. Data are expressed as mean ± standard error. The green line represents pollen counts in London, United Kingdom. Asterisk indicates $p < .05$ versus pre-immunotherapy value. (Figure adapted with permission from Francis JN et al. *J Allergy Clin Immunol* 2008; 121(5): 1120–1125.e1122.)

5.3 EFFECTOR CELL RECRUITMENT

5.3.1 Mast cells and basophils

The initial mechanism of action seen on effector cells is mast cell and basophil desensitization [18]. The number of these cells decreases during AIT, and their thresholds for cytokine release increase with time. Early in the course of AIT, there is a decrease in peripheral blood basophil numbers and the release of basophil-derived cytokines, such as IL-4 and IL-13 [19]. Basal serum tryptase level, which is a marker of mast cell burden and mast cell function, decreases over time during AIT [20]. In patients with venom immunotherapy (VIT), the suppression of surface antigens on blood basophils was shown previously [21]. Besides the changes observed in basophil surface antigens, the amount of histamine released from basophils following sting challenges decreases in patients with VIT depending on their clinical reactivity [22]. The clinical response to VIT can be assessed in the flow-cytometric evaluation of CD63 expression, which is a basophil surface marker that measures degranulation of basophils during a basophil activation test [23]. A new method of functional assay that measures intracellular staining of phycoerythrin-conjugated diamine oxidase (DAO) has been validated for detecting the amount of histamine released from basophils. Following allergen stimulation, intracellular DAO levels decrease in proportion to the intracellular histamine released. This reduction was shown in patients treated with *Vespula* VIT, which is important for increasing the threshold for venom to induce an anaphylactic reaction in VIT patients [24]. Not only the preformed mediator release but also the production and release of newly generated mediators, such as leukotriene C4 in blood basophils in patients following VIT, decreases [25].

Following rush VIT, a decrease in T-cell expressed and secreted (RANTES) protein, IL-8, and monocyte chemoattractant protein 1 (MCP-1) production have been reported in peripheral blood mononuclear cell (PBMC) cultures at protein as well as mRNA levels [26].

During the early phases of AIT, the mechanisms that start desensitization are not fully understood. In 2010, Bussmann et al. performed a study on patients with rush VIT. They analyzed expression levels of different tolerogenic markers at protein and mRNA levels within the first 5 days of VIT. They observed a prominent degradation of tryptophan, which is linked to the suppression of T-cell responses and induction of tolerance; elevated ILT3 and ILT4, which are inhibitory receptors for monocytes, and IL-10 production of CD3+ T cells and monocytes followed by increased IL-10 serum levels, which is an important regulatory interleukin for the suppression of allergen-induced responses [27].

In studies with aeroallergens, AIT was shown to inhibit early and late-phase allergic responses at allergic tissue sites through the suppression of several cytokines and decreases in numbers of eosinophils, mast cells, and basophils [4]. This information indicates that allergen immunotherapy is effective at both systemic and local levels. Similar mechanisms are likely to apply to VIT.

Seasonal allergic rhinitis induced by grass pollen exposure is also associated with migration of tryptase-positive mast cells into the nasal mucosa, which may not be inhibited by SCIT [28]. Reexamination of mast cell numbers, using the c-kit/stem cell factor receptor transmembrane tyrosine kinase as a marker, subsequently revealed a recruitment of c-kit+ cells during the pollen season, which is suppressed by SCIT [29] (Figure 5.4). In the same study, nasal mucosal expression of mRNA encoding IL-9, a growth factor

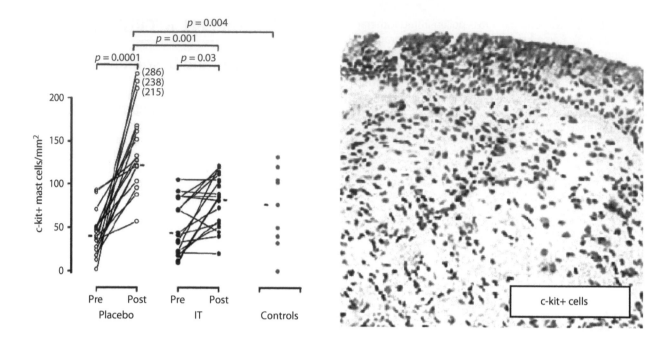

Figure 5.4 Effects of natural seasonal exposure to grass pollen and allergen immunotherapy on numbers of c-kit+ mast cells in the nasal mucosa. Nasal biopsies were collected outside the pollen season before immunotherapy ("pre") and during the peak of the pollen after immunotherapy or placebo treatment ("post"). As a further control, biopsies were also collected from a cohort of nonatopic subjects during the peak of the pollen season ("controls"). The right panel shows an example of a nasal biopsy section immunostained with a monoclonal antibody specific for c-kit. (Figure adapted with permission from Nouri-Aria KT et al. *J Allergy Clin Immunol* 2005; 116(1): 73–79.)

for mast cells, was also lower in AIT- or SCIT-treated patients. Using the 2D7 monoclonal antibody, basophils were examined in the nasal mucosa of SCIT-treated, grass pollen allergic subjects during grass season [28]. No effect of treatment was seen on basophil numbers in the lamina propria. However, basophil infiltration into the epithelium occurred in approximately 35% of placebo-treated patients with rhinitis but only 5% of immunotherapy patients. Thus, data suggest that AIT or SCIT may reduce the seasonal recruitment of both mast cells and basophils into the nasal mucosa.

5.3.2 Eosinophils

SCIT is also associated with reduced eosinophil recruitment into tissue after allergen challenge. For example, reductions in the cutaneous late response to grass pollen allergen provocation are accompanied by a trend for lower eosinophil numbers in skin biopsies [30]. Ragweed SCIT is also associated with lower eosinophil numbers in nasal lavage fluid collected during ragweed-induced nasal late responses [31]. In the nasal biopsy model, mucosal eosinophils were also examined after grass pollen immunotherapy. SCIT is associated with inhibition of eosinophil recruitment during the allergen-induced late response [32] and natural seasonal exposure [33]. In contrast, the available data suggest that mucosal neutrophil numbers are not affected by immunotherapy. The effect of SCIT on lower airway eosinophilia was also examined in subjects with birch pollen–induced seasonal asthma [34]. Bronchoalveolar lavage was examined for

eosinophils and eosinophil cationic protein (ECP) during the birch pollen season. SCIT-treated subjects develop less lung symptoms on exposure, with lower measurable bronchial hyperactivity, eosinophil counts, and ECP concentrations.

5.4 DENDRITIC CELL RESPONSES

SCIT enhances peripheral DC function [35]. SCIT increased DC TLR9-mediated innate immune function, which was diminished at baseline in allergic subjects. In this study, a robust innate immune response from isolated plasmacytoid dendritic cells (pDCs) was reestablished among HDM-allergic subjects undergoing AIT, resulting in a three- to fivefold increase in IFN-α production in response to CpG stimulation [35]. Additionally, the proportions of peripheral blood pDCs, but not myeloid DCs (mDCs), were significantly reduced after initiation of *Hymenoptera* venom–specific SCIT. This was associated with changes in the expression of function-associated surface molecules such as CD32, CD40, and TLR2 on DCs during treatment. Numeric and phenotypic changes of blood DCs may contribute to a suppression of allergic inflammatory response during SCIT [36]. For example, different populations of human DCs purified from peripheral blood could be "conditioned" *in vitro* to preferentially induce a population of regulatory T cells that on coculture inhibited allergen-driven Th2 responses. Proteomic and mass spectroscopy analysis of these conditioned human DCs identified two candidate proteins, namely, STAB1 and C1Q, that may be important factors inducing tolerogenic T-regulatory responses. These *in vitro* data were supported by preliminary *ex vivo* studies following grass pollen tablet sublingual immunotherapy where expression of these molecules was accompanied by a positive response to immunotherapy [37].

5.4.1 Innate lymphoid cells and allergen immunotherapy

In a study by Lao-Araya and colleagues, grass pollen immunotherapy suppressed seasonal increases in ILC2s in peripheral blood of patients compared to untreated controls [9]. There was a correlation between decreased ILC2s numbers and self-reported symptoms. Moreover, the proportion of IL-13+ ILC2s also decreased. In another study of seasonal asthmatic patients, Lombardi et al. could not show any changes in the number of ILC2s during immunotherapy, which was explained by nonseasonal measurements while patients were asymptomatic [38]. To date, there is no evidence that immunotherapy has any effect on epithelially derived cytokines such as IL-25, IL-33, and TSLP, which have regulatory effects on local type 2 inflammation and ILCs [4].

5.4.2 Histamine and histamine receptors and allergen-specific immunotherapy

During VIT, an early desensitization develops within days or even hours depending on the type of immunotherapy protocol used such as rush and ultrarush types of VIT. There is a decrease in basophil numbers, preformed mediators, and mediator release by time [24,39,40]. Among the four different types of histamine receptors, histamine receptor type 2 (HR2) plays important roles with the peripheral antigen tolerance [41]. Basophil suppression starts by the activation of HR2s. HR2 decreases allergen-induced FceRI-mediated basophil degranulation and mediator release [42]. HR2 is mainly involved in tolerogenic immune responses. It is upregulated in Th2 cells and both suppresses allergen-stimulated T-cell responses and increases IL-10 production in beekeepers [41], which induces the development of peripheral tolerance [25,43,44]. Histamine via HR2, induces IL-10 production by dendritic cells and Th2 cells [45]; increases the suppressive effect of TGF-b on T cells [46], and decreases IL-4 and IL-13 production which are the main Th2-type cytokines [47].

5.5 T- AND B-CELL RESPONSES

Considerable attention has focused on characterizing T-cell responses before and after AIT. These studies have led to two major mechanistic hypotheses: first, that deviation occurs of Th2 responses in favor of a Th0/Th1 phenotype (assumed to be less pathogenic); and second, that allergen-specific T-cell responses are suppressed by newly induced regulatory T cells or through inhibition of antigen presentation by IgG. The development of immune tolerance during AIT has been shown to be related to the modification of T- and B-cell responses [48]. A Th2 to Th1 shift occurs, and an increase in interferon gamma (IFN-γ) levels is observed parallel to the decrease in IL-4 and IL-13 in whole blood [49,50]. Th2 responses during AIT are reduced, and there is also an increase in Treg cell numbers

and functions [49,51]. Treg cells are divided into two subgroups as natural regulatory T (nTreg) cells, which are characterized by the transcription factor forkhead box P3 (FOXP3), and iTreg cells such as IL-10 producing T$_{r1}$ cells and TGF-b producing TH3 cells [52–54]. IL-10 plays an inhibitory role on B cells by blocking the B7/CD28 pathway. This results in a suppressive effect on dendritic cell maturation and in MHC class II and costimulatory ligand expressions [55]. TGF-β downregulates FceRI expression on Langerhans cells and also upregulates FOXP3 and RUNX and assists CTLA-4 expression on T cells [56,57].

A body of evidence suggests the induction of long-term immunologic and clinical tolerance after immunotherapy is associated with a delayed immune deviation of T-helper responses, usually in conjunction with a shift in the patterns of cytokine production from a Th2/0 toward Th1/0 profile [30,32,58–63], though no consistent pattern of change has emerged that is common to all studies. Many but not all *in vitro* studies of peripheral blood T cells from subjects following SCIT demonstrate reductions in proliferative and cytokine responses to allergen [56,64–66]. Potential reasons for these discrepancies include variations in laboratory methodology and lack of standardization of allergen extracts used for SCIT. Another possible explanation is that inhibition of *peripheral* T-cell proliferation and Th2 cytokine production is not required for SCIT efficacy, and these responses poorly reflect the critical immune interactions and responses in lymphoid and mucosal tissues.

AIT modifies the cytokine profile of T cells recruited into tissue [56,65]. Nasal mucosal biopsies from SCIT-treated subjects, performed during the allergen-induced late response to grass pollen, reveal increases in IFN-γ mRNA expressing cells [31]. The relevance of this finding is supported by the inverse correlation between numbers of IFN-γ mRNA+ cells and clinical symptoms. A potential inducer of IFN-γ expression by mucosal T cells is IL-12 [67], and there is evidence that this mechanism may be operative in grass pollen SCIT. Skin biopsies collected during the cutaneous late response were examined for IL-12 mRNA by *in situ* hybridization [68]. In SCIT, but not placebo-treated patients, there is concomitant late response suppression and enhanced IL-12 mRNA expression. The latter correlates directly with increased IFN-γ, and the principal source of IL-12 mRNA is the CD68+ macrophages. Similar studies demonstrate that SCIT significantly inhibits seasonal increases in IL-5 and IL-9 mRNA expressing cells in the nasal mucosa [28,32]. These studies underline the probable relevance of studying "end organ" immune responses rather than the peripheral blood, particularly for diseases induced by inhalant allergens such as grass pollen.

In beekeepers, IL-10-producing Treg cells inhibit the proliferation of PLA-specific effector T cells shortly after the start of bee venom season. This suppressive effect can be reversed by blocking CTLA-4, PD-1, and IL-10 receptors [41]. Additionally, induction of indoleamine 2,3-dioxygenase enzyme in dendritic cells, by the effect of Tregs, causes the transformation of inflammatory dendritic cells into regulatory dendritic cells [69]. In a similar manner, during VIT, T$_{r1}$-type Treg cell proliferation is prominent, and the antigen-specific proliferative and cytokine responses against the major bee venom allergen, the phospholipase A2 (PLA), have been significantly suppressed by the end of the first week of VIT [58]. The allergen-induced secretions of Th2 cytokines such as IL-4, IL-5, and IL-13 were abolished [70]. Treg cells can also suppress immune responses via cell-to-cell interactions besides IL-10 production.

The role of increased IL-10 levels in the development of a clinical and immunological tolerance during AIT is prominent. Blockage of IL-10 in PBMC reconstitutes the specific proliferative and cytokine responses. This situation can also be seen in beekeepers who have received multiple bee stings [58]. The presence of increased numbers of CD4+ CD25+ FOXP3+ Treg cells in the target organ, nasal mucosa, after grass pollen allergen immunotherapy suggests that Treg cells play an important role in the development of allergen-specific immune tolerance [71]. In a similar manner, VIT was found to be related to the progressive expansion of circulating CD4+ CD25+ FOXP3+ Treg cell numbers [72]. During all types of AIT, a deviation toward a regulatory/suppressor T-cell response has been reported [62]. In a study by Nasser et al., allergen-induced changes in cytokine mRNA and cellular profiles from cutaneous biopsies were compared before and 3 months after wasp VIT. There was a significant decrease in IL-4 mRNA and an increase in IL-10+ cells. Additionally, a trend toward an increase in IL-10 mRNA was also observed [73]. In another study by Schuerwegh et al., the effects of VIT on CD4+ CD8+ T lymphocytes were evaluated before VIT, at the end of 5-day semirush VIT, and at 6 months during VIT. A significant decrease in IL-producing CD4+ and CD8+ T-cell numbers, compared with cytokine-producing cells before VIT, was observed by the end of the 5-day semirush VIT. After 6 months of VIT, a higher amount of IL-2 and IFN-γ-producing CD4+ CD8+ T lymphocytes was found confirming a shift from Th2- to Th1-type immune deviation [50]. IL-10 serum levels began to increase from the second day of VIT [27], and on day 28 of treatment, a desensitized condition was seen in allergen-specific T cells associated with the direct suppressive effects of IL-10 [72].

5.5.1 T-follicular-helper cells and follicular regulatory T cells

T-follicular-helper (T_{FH}) cells are defined by the CXCR5+ surface receptor, and they help in B-cell maturation and immunoglobulin class-switching. CXCR5+ FoxP3+ Treg cells are a subset of Tregs, called follicular regulatory T (T_{FR}) cells, which are capable of suppressing T- and B-cell responses by migrating to germinal centers of lymph nodes [74,75]. A study by grass pollen immunotherapy has shown a significant decrease in memory T_{FH} cell numbers after immunotherapy [76]. Additionally, T_{FR} cells were found to produce more IL-10 compared to T_{FH} cells. The plasticity between T_{FH} and T_{FR} cells has been shown in the same study, suggesting that T_{FR} cells may play important roles in suppressing TH2 responses and allergen-specific IgE production during immunotherapy [76]. It is likely that similar T_{FR} and T_{FH} cell mechanisms are present during venom immunotherapy as in grass pollen immunotherapy.

Recently, IL-10-secreting allergen-specific Breg cells have been identified in bee venom tolerant beekeepers and VIT administered patients [77]. Breg cells are characterized as CD73− CD25+ CD71+ B cells, which are capable of suppressing bee venom–specific CD4+ T cells and producing allergen-specific IgG4 antibodies after bee VIT [77]. Additionally, Breg cells can show their inhibitory capacity by producing IL-35 and TGF-β [78]. Apart from Treg and Breg cells, IL-10-secreting natural killer regulatory cells have also been shown to suppress allergen-stimulated T-cell proliferation in humans and may be important in tolerance induction as other regulatory cell types [79].

5.5.2 How do immunotherapy vaccines induce IL-10 responses?

Identifying the mechanism by which SCIT induces IL-10 producing T cells could be important in the design of new vaccines. Murine models provide some insights. Nevertheless, important differences exist between SCIT administered to patients to modulate mature Th2 responses and animal models where the emphasis is on tolerizing regimes given before sensitization. Tolerizing animals by oral or intranasal exposure to ovalbumin prior to intraperitoneal sensitization induces IL-10 producing regulatory T cells [80,81]. In the intranasal tolerance model, induction of these T_{r1}-like cells is dependent on pulmonary lymph node dendritic cells expressing IL-10 and the costimulatory molecule ICOS ligand. Indeed, adoptive transfer of these dendritic cells or T_{r1} cells alone is sufficient to confer tolerance on the recipients [80,82]. Human peripheral blood pDCs stimulated with a TLR 9 agonist express ICOS ligand and induce differentiation of T_{r1} cells from naïve T cells in vitro [83]. Furthermore, cross-linking of the high-affinity IgE receptor (FcϵRI) on pDCs by allergen also induces IL-10 expression [84]. Although these mechanisms have not yet been directly implicated during SCIT, they do indicate that dendritic cells could induce T-cell responses following allergen vaccination.

5.6 ANTIBODY RESPONSES

5.6.1 Isotype changes

In atopic subjects, sensitization to environmental allergen is associated with increased concentrations of allergen-specific IgE in serum and also with locally detectable specific IgE in target organs. Initially AIT is associated with transient early increases in serum allergen-specific IgE (sIgE) levels, and then there is a decrease in sIgE over several years [85–87]. AIT is also associated with increases in allergen-specific IgA, IgG1, and IgG4 antibodies, which are called *blocking antibodies*. Studies with aeroallergens have shown significant increases in serum concentrations of blocking antibodies, up to 100 times in a time- and dose-dependent manner [4,88,89].

In SCIT-treated grass pollen allergic subjects, a transient increase in ryegrass pollen (Lol p 1, 2, 3, and 5)-specific IgE occurs during the pollen season and is followed by a gradual decrease over time [33]. SCIT in patients with hay fever is associated with transient early increases in allergen-specific IgE followed by blunting of seasonal increases in IgE antibody [90,91]. In a proportion of individuals who received birch pollen AIT, low concentrations of IgE antibodies specific to previously unrecognized allergen components of the vaccine were identified [86]. The clinical relevance of these new sensitizations is doubtful since they paralleled clinical improvement with no apparent adverse allergic responses.

The functional significance of the humoral response to AIT was first addressed in the 1930s by Cooke who demonstrated that transfer of sera from SCIT-treated patients inhibited allergic responses. From nasal lavage of AIT-treated patients, Platts-Mills and colleagues identified antibodies that inhibit in vitro histamine release from basophils [92]. Quantitative measurements of immunoreactive IgG subclasses in SCIT-treated patients revealed increases in allergen-specific IgG1 and IgG4 antibody concentrations in sera and in local target organs [62,93,94]. Changes in allergen-specific IgG2 and IgG3 are not significant [93]. Despite increased allergen-specific antibodies, many studies have failed to demonstrate a relationship between specific IgG1 and IgG4 antibody concentrations and clinical efficacy.

Several studies elucidate the possible functional relevance of these inhibitory/blocking allergen-specific IgG1 and IgG4 antibodies. Bet v1-specific IgG1 and IgG4 antibodies from SCIT-treated patients inhibited basophil histamine release in an antigen-specific fashion [93–97]. Bet v1–specific IgG1 and IgG4 antibodies could compete with Bet v1–specific IgE and prevent its interaction with Bet v1 allergen. In a murine model of allergy, the inhibitory activities of IgG were mediated via the FcγRIIb receptor. Incubation of IgE, allergen, and IgG immune complexes with mouse mast cells resulted in juxtaposition or coaggregation of the FcγRIIb and FcϵRI resulting in suppression of mast cell degranulation [98]. Additionally, inhibition of basophil histamine release occurred using a recombinant chimeric Fcγ-Fcϵ construct that potentiates FcγRIIb and FcϵRI coaggregation on human basophils *in vitro* [99]. This inhibitory effect was dependent on immunoreceptor tyrosine-based inhibitory motif (ITIM) phosphorylation, resulting in the activation of intracellular phosphatases that counterbalance the influence of immunoreceptor-based activation motifs (ITAMs) within the intracellular tail of the FcϵRIγ [100]. In contrast, in a human model [101,102], blockade of downstream signaling of FcγRIIb with monoclonal antibody directed against CD32 (FcγRIIb) did not block IgG-mediated inhibitory activity following birch pollen SCIT, which supports the mechanism of direct competition with IgE for allergen rather than a mechanism involving downstream inhibition of the IgE receptor signaling pathway as observed in the murine model.

Immunoglobulin isotype class switching, in particular, switching from IgE to IgG4, is dependent on Th2 cytokines (IL-4 and IL-13) and cognate interaction of CD40 on T-helper cells and CD40 ligand on B cells [103,104]. The induction of IL-10 following SCIT has a profound effect on isotype class switching. In the presence of IL-4, additional IL-10 induces preferential class switch in favor of IgG4 and suppresses both total and allergen-specific IgE responses [105,106]. A detailed time-course of IL-10 induction in patients treated with grass pollen–specific AIT revealed a significant increase in IL-10 production in parallel with suppression of late cutaneous responses and clinical responsiveness prior to IgG4 induction [17]. Therefore, immunoreactive IgG4 may be a surrogate biomarker of IL-10 induction [17,107].

Furthermore, elevated levels of allergen-specific IgA2 antibodies and polymeric (secretory) IgA2 occur following AIT. Passive sensitization of monocytes *in vitro* using purified polymeric IgA2 from IgA-containing sera, followed by cross-linking of IgA on monocytes by antigen or anti-IgA resulted in IL-10 production [68]. This indirect production of IL-10 from accessory cells may in turn favor isotype class switching in favor of IgG4 antibody production. These findings implicate a possible novel role for IgA antibodies in the induction of tolerance following AIT.

5.6.2 Effects on antigen presentation

In addition to blocking allergen binding by cell surface FcϵRI-bound IgE, IgG4 antibodies also inhibit formation of IgE-allergen complexes in solution. Formation of these multivalent complexes enhances and is required for IgE binding to low-affinity FcϵRII

(CD23) IgE receptors expressed by antigen presenting cells (APCs), including B cells, DCs, and monocytes. The low-affinity FcϵRII may facilitate these cells binding and processing low concentrations of allergen for presentation to T cells by HLA class II molecules.

In the 1990s, van Neerven and colleagues were the first to demonstrate that sera obtained from subjects following birch pollen–SCIT inhibited IgE-facilitated allergen presentation by B cells to allergen-specific T-cell clones, resulting in decreased T-cell proliferation and reduced Th2 cytokine production [108]. These findings were reproduced in a randomized, double-blind, placebo-controlled trial of grass pollen AIT [88]. Moreover, by using a simplified assay in which allergen-IgE complexes bound to FcϵRII on the surface of B cells were detected by flow cytometry (IgE-FAB), mixing studies demonstrated that the vigor of proliferative responses by T-cell clones reflected the binding of these complexes [109–111]. The increases in serum allergen-specific IgG4 following SCIT are associated with inhibitory/blocking activity for IgE-facilitated CD23-mediated allergen binding and presentation by B cells. This serum inhibitory activity co-purified with IgG4 but not IgA-containing fractions following affinity chromatography [88,112]. These findings suggest that IgG antibodies are involved in the underlying mechanisms of successful SCIT. Hence, the measurement of inhibition of IgE-facilitated allergen binding has been utilized as a potential surrogate marker of successful SCIT in several clinical trials [17,52,111,113–115].

An objection to the blocking antibody model is the weak correlation between allergen-specific IgG concentrations and the clinical response to AIT [114,115]. However, data from our group show that 2 years following discontinuation of grass-pollen immunotherapy, grass pollen allergen–specific IgG4 levels decline by approximately 80%, though functional blocking activity *in vitro* persists during this period, as does clinical remission (Figure 5.5). It is possible that a population of long-lived, high-avidity memory IgG$^+$ B cells selectively persist following SCIT withdrawal, perhaps due to ongoing low-dose natural antigen exposure.

A particular feature of allergen-specific AIT is the induction of long-term, antigen-specific tolerance, namely, persisting clinical benefit for several years after treatment is withdrawn [113]. These findings after 3 years grass pollen–SCIT have now been confirmed in a separate study after 2 years of blinded treatment and withdrawal [116]. Long-term clinical tolerance correlated with persistence of IgG-associated inhibitory activity against binding of IgE-allergen complexes to B cells, a surrogate of IgE-facilitated antigen presentation and activation of antigen-specific T cells [116]. In this study, IgG-associated inhibitory bioactivity, rather than absolute levels of IgG4 antibody, correlated with clinical tolerance, as reflected in sustained suppression of combined symptom and rescue medication scores 2 years after SCIT withdrawal. This suggests that the functional activity of blocking antibodies rather than their levels may be a more accurate measure of clinical efficacy and seems to correlate closely with long-term immune tolerance [4]. However, this may not be the case for bee venom immunotherapy, where although successful desensitization was accompanied by increases in both IgG4 and IgE-Inhibitory activity, both the elevated specific IgG4 levels and IgE-FAB inhibitory activity returned to baseline within months of discontinuation of VIT, and further follow-up revealed a more sustained decrease in venom-specific IgE levels [114] representing a putative alternative mechanism of prolonged protection following IgG withdrawal. This is also supported by the observation of low/absent IgE levels in tolerant beekeepers [117].

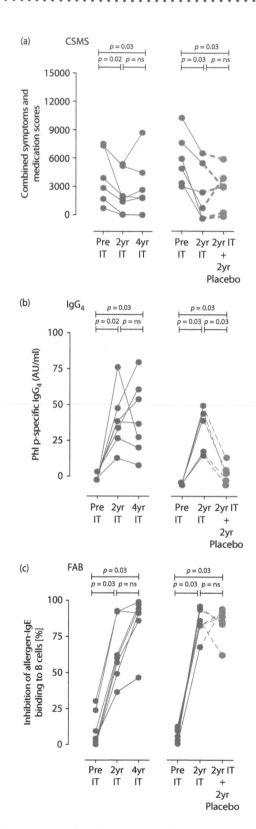

Figure 5.5 Long-term clinical improvement following discontinuation of immunotherapy is associated with persistent IgG-associated blocking activity but not total allergen-specific IgG4 antibodies. (a) Symptom and medication scores. (b) *Phleum pratense*–specific IgG4 antibodies measured by ELISA. (c) Serum inhibitory activity for allergen-IgE binding to B cells. FAB: Facilitated allergen binding (Figure adapted with permission from James LK et al. *J Allergy Clin Immunol* 2011; 127(2): 509–516.e501–505.)

5.7 POTENTIAL BIOMARKERS FOR MONITORING ALLERGEN IMMUNOTHERAPY

Although AIT is an effective and disease-modifying treatment modality, some patients do not respond to the therapy [52,113,118]. Also, from the perspective of personalized medicine, there is a clear need for clinical biomarkers that may play a paramount role in finding patients who are most likely to respond, when to stop treatment, how to predict relapse, and when to apply a booster treatment [4,119,120]. Biomarkers are defined as "indicators of normal biologic processess, pathogenetic processess and/or response to therapeutic or other interventions" [121]. To date, no biomarker predictive or indicative of clinical reponse has been identified and validated. Despite the presence of several candidate biomarkers, there are problems of standardization, reproducibility of the results and the definition of responders and nonresponders, and difficulties concerning complexity of the laboratory methods [4,119,120,122]. According to a recent task force report, candidate biomarkers of AIT can be grouped into seven domains (Table 5.1) [120]:

1. IgE (total IgE, specific IgE, and sIgE/total IgE ratio)
2. IgG-subclasses (sIgG1, sIgG4 including sIgE/IgG4 ratio)
3. Serum inhibitory activity for IgE (IgE-FAB and IgE-BF)
4. Basophil activation tests
5. Cytokines and chemokines
6. Cellular markers like T-regulatory cells, B-regulatory cells, and DCs
7. *In vivo* markers

Clinical surrogate markers, such as endpoint skin prick test titration to allergens, airway-specific and nonspecific hyperresponsiveness, and nasal or conjunctival challenges, have been assessed for their potential role in monitoring SCIT [123,124]. In an open, nonrandomized study in children sensitive to house dust mite (HDM), suppression of immediate skin test reactivity at 3 years of SCIT correlated with reduced relapse and the need for retreatment in the following 3 years after discontinuation of SCIT [125]. In blinded trials of grass pollen SCIT, Walker and colleagues demonstrated complete inhibition of seasonal increases in bronchial hyperresponsiveness, and Roberts and colleagues demonstrated significant reductions in allergen-induced cutaneous and conjunctival responses [123]. Although there are associations between clinical responses to grass pollen SCIT and clinical surrogates, convincing correlations with the magnitude of the clinical response in terms of reduced symptoms or improved quality of life are not available. This partially reflects the complexity and interdependency of the underlying mechanisms as well as the number of factors modulating target organ responsiveness, such as neurogenic influences and altered environmental effects.

The predictive value of the ratio of serum specific–IgE/total IgE for clinical outcomes was evaluated in a trial of grass pollen SCIT [126]. Subjects who received active treatment showed a transient increase in specific IgE followed by seasonal blunting of the expected increase. The ratio of serum specific–IgE/total IgE correlated with the clinical response to SCIT; however, this was not observed in another study of HDM-SCIT [125]. Thus, the usefulness of this ratio requires further evaluation. Although AIT is associated with early increases in the concentration of allergen-specific IgG4 blocking antibodies and delayed, modest reduction in allergen-specific IgE

Table 5.1 Clinical biomarkers to predict the clinical effect of allergen-specific immunotherapy [120,147]

Domain	Advantages	Disadvantages	References
1. IgE tIgE, sIgE, sIgE/tIgE	• Serum based • sIgE/tIgE (promising predictor of clinic response)	• Early rise of sIgE does not correlate with the clinical outcomes • No Validity of sIgE/tIgE	[68,113,116,125,126,148–153]
2. IgG and subclasses sIgG4, sIgE/sIgG4	• Serum based • sIgG4 shows allergen exposure • ISAC chip for sIgG4 is available	• Lack of clinical studies • Insufficient data with clinical correlation • Limited data on local antibody levels • sIgG4 levels	[54,88,93,94,116,150,151,154–160]
3. Serum Inhibitory activity IgE-FAB, IgE-BF, ELIFAB	• Serum based • High reproducibility for IgE-FAB	• IgE-BF no longer present • No data on IgE-FAB to predict responders • Clinical correlation data limited	[85,88,92,108,109,116,146, 150,154,161–166]
4. Basophil activation tests CD63, CD203c, CD107a DAO	• Shows Fc-γRI mediated *in vivo* response with basophil activation • Small amount of blood	• Variability in basophil activation responses • Difficulties in technique, standardization • Lack of basophil response in 5%–10% of the population	[24,88,161,167–175]
5. Cytokines and chemokines ECP, Eotaxin, Th2: IL-4, IL-5, IL-9, IL-13, IL-17 Th1: IFN-γ, IL-12 Treg: TGF-β, IL-10 CCR3, TARC, Tryptase	• Highlight the mechanisms of AIT • Serum levels may not represent the target organs	• No cytokine or chemokine identified to predict clinical response • Inconsistency of the results	[87,176–180]
6. Cellular biomarkers Tregs B regs Dendritic cells ILCs	• Tregs are important for the shift from Th2 to Th1 immune response • Bregs may be important in the mechanism of AIT • DC markers can be monitored by PCR	• Technical difficulties • No specific marker for T cells • No data for clinical correlation • Low frequency of Tregs and Bregs • DC markers shared with other cells	[9,37,71,111,175,181,182]
7. *In vivo* biomarkers SPT Conjunctival provocation tests Nasal provocation tests (NPT) Environmental challange chambers	• More standardized, avoid seasonal pollen variation • ECC: Accurate for time-course and dose-response studies • EMA recommends in proof-of concept and dose finding studies	• Conjunctival provocation test and NPT are not standardized • Allergens used for provocation tests need regulatory approval • ECC are expensive • Not accepted as primary endpoints in phase III clinical trials	[16,17,32,113,183–194]

Abbreviations: AIT, allergen immunotherapy; CCR3, C-C *chemokine* receptor type 3; DAO, diamine oxidase; ECP, eosinophilic cationic protein; ELIFAB, enzyme-linked immunosorbent-facilitated antigen-binding assay; IgE-BF, IgE blocking factor; IgE-FAB, IgE facilitated antigen binding; IFN-γ, interferon-gamma; ILCs, innate lymphoid cells; ISAC, ImmunoSolid Allergen Chip Assay; SPT, skin prick testing; TARC, *Chemokine* (C-C motif) ligand 17 (CCL17); TGF-β, transforming growth factor-beta.

antibody, these antibody levels do not correlate with clinical efficacy [90,125,127]. The antibody changes most frequently reported are an increase in specific IgG4 and reduction in specific IgE. Fractionated IgG4 antibodies in sera from patients treated with grass pollen SCIT are responsible for the *in vitro* inhibition of IgE-FAB binding to B cells [88]. This suggests a functional role of IgG4. Support for the functional role of specific-IgG in the beneficial effects of SCIT is provided by IgG4 inhibition of allergen-induced, IgE-dependent histamine release by basophils. These data suggest that specific IgG4 serves a blocking antibody function.

5.8 NOVEL IMMUNOTHERAPY STRATEGIES

Immunotherapy performed with modern vaccines is a relatively safe form of treatment in trained hands. However, administering native allergen to IgE-sensitized individuals can trigger both local and systemic reactions. SCIT regimes therefore tend to be cautious, involving numerous injections of gradually increasing allergen doses performed under specialist supervision. The aim for novel AIT strategies is to reduce the potential for IgE-mediated side effects while exposing patients to fewer injections and making fewer demands on health services.

5.8.1 Circumventing IgE-mediated side effects

The first category of novel therapies is based on the hypothesis that AIT works primarily through stimulating T cells at high antigen doses and that this directly leads to regulatory T-cell induction. This class of therapies is also based on the assumption that IgE-dependent mechanisms mediate AIT side effects but are not necessary for vaccine efficacy. Strategies tested include genetically modified allergen proteins with reduced IgE binding but intact T-cell epitopes. For example, recombinant fragments of major birch pollen allergen Bet v 1 have been generated with minimal allergenicity in cutaneous and nasal challenge models [128]. These recombinant proteins successfully induce Bet v 1-specific IgG1 and IgG4 responses that block basophil histamine release triggered by exposure to wild-type Bet v 1 [128]. Another approach is the use of allergen-derived peptides that stimulate T cells but cannot cross-link IgE. Overlapping peptides representing the cat allergen, Fel d 1, have been examined in small clinical studies with promising results [129,130].

Peripheral T-cell tolerance occurs following administration of synthetic Fel d 1 and Api m 1 peptide-based vaccine. These short peptides consist of a native sequence or sequence with amino acid substitutions and reduced IgE cross-linking activity. A mixture of a large number of short peptides resulted in induction of IL-10 and reduced IFN-γ, IL-4, and IL-13. T-cell proliferative responses were also reduced [131]. Induction of IL-10+ regulatory T cells may occur following PIT [131]. Isolated CD4+ T cells after PIT in cat-allergic, asthmatic patients actively suppressed allergen-specific proliferative responses of pretreatment CD4− PBMCs in coculture experiments [131]. Furthermore, in one study, PIT induced a linked epitope suppression of antigen-specific responses in allergic asthmatic subjects [132]. In a randomized, double-blind, placebo-controlled study of PIT consisting of a mixture of 12 Fel d 1 peptides, PBMC proliferative responses were assessed to each of 16 Fel d 1 peptides

(12 treatment peptides and 4 Fel d 1 peptides that were not included in the vaccine). Responses to all 12 treatment peptides were significantly reduced in the 16 cat-allergic patients receiving active treatment, but not in the 8 subjects receiving placebo. Th2 cell responses to the four nontreatment peptides were also significantly reduced in active but not placebo-treated subjects [132].

Anti-IgE therapy has the potential to inhibit IgE-facilitated antigen presentation, thereby possibly improving AIT efficacy while reducing the risk of anaphylaxis. In a randomized, double-blind, placebo-controlled trial, pretreatment with a humanized, anti-IgE monoclonal antibody (omalizumab) reduced the side effects in a rapid updosing (rush) protocol of ragweed SCIT [133]. The addition of omalizumab resulted in complete suppression of IgE-facilitated presentation that was accompanied by a fivefold reduction of the risk of anaphylaxis during the 1-day rapid updosing period [133,134]. This combination protocol may improve the convenience and compliance with SCIT while preserving safety and efficacy.

Some novel approaches such as allergen peptide-based molecules that target T- or B-cell epitopes that selectively induce allergen-specific IgG responses and recombinant hypoallergenic molecules will decrease the systemic side effects related to allergen immunotherapy [130,135,136].

5.8.2 Adjuvants

The second category of novel therapy is based on the use of adjuvants to potentiate the immunologic effects of vaccination with whole allergen proteins. Ideally, such adjuvants should not only potentiate Th2 to Th1 immune deviation but should also favor induction of regulatory T-cell responses. The type-B immunostimulatory phosphorothioate oligodeoxynucleotide 5′-TGACTGTAACGTTCGAGATGA (ODN-1018) was tested in ragweed-stimulated PBMC responses. ODN-1018 promotes Th1 cytokine and IL-12 responses at the expense of Th2 cytokine production. This activity could be further enhanced by conjugation of ODN-1018 with the major ragweed allergen, Amb a 1 [137]. A functionally similar type-B phosphorothioate oligodeoxynucleotide (ODN-2006) activates human pDCs through the TLR-9 and induces regulatory T cells [138]. A randomized, double-blind, placebo-controlled, phase 2 trial examined the effects of six weekly injections of the ODN-1018-Amb a 1 conjugate on ragweed-induced allergic rhinitis [139]. Treatment is associated with improvement in peak season nasal and quality of life symptom scores. However, this combination has failed at phase III trial [75]. Another clinically tested adjuvant is a derivative of monophosphoryl lipid A (MPL) from bacterial lipopolysaccharide. The structurally modified MPL acts through TLR-4 to induce IL-12 production and promote Th1 responses to allergen by human PBMC [140]. In a randomized, double-blind, placebo-controlled study, a vaccine containing MPL and tyrosine-absorbed glutaraldehyde-modified extracts of grass pollen (Pollinex Quattro) reduced hay fever symptoms and increased allergen-specific IgG when administered as four pre- and coseasonal injections [141].

5.8.3 Alternatives to subcutaneous immunotherapy

Studies demonstrate that AIT, which utilizes direct administration of the sensitizing allergen into lymph nodes, called ILIT, is effective and a potential alternative to SCIT. ILIT was well tolerated, and patient compliance was improved as compared with SCIT. ILIT resulted in a desirable immunologic response. The dose and the number of allergen injections were reduced, making ILIT safer and faster than other forms of AIT [142,143].

Epicutaneous allergen immunotherapy has also proved to be safer [144] than the classical SCIT despite the lack of knowledge to assess the clinical efficacy compared to other forms of AIT.

In a recent study by Slovick et al., intradermal grass pollen immunotherapy suppressed the skin late-phase responses; however, this resulted in worsening of the seasonal clinical symptoms and was ineffective [145].

In addition to guiding the development of novel treatment approaches, knowledge of AIT mechanisms is also likely to enable the development of effective biomarkers in order to predict patients who are likely to respond to AIT and to predict relapse following discontinuation. Measurement of the biological activity of "blocking" antibodies holds some promise [146]. The sublingual route is also emerging as an effective and safe alternative. Meanwhile, SCIT using standardized natural allergens remains the gold standard against which to test putative biomarkers and novel immunomodulatory approaches.

5.9 CONCLUSION

AIT is effective and induces long-lasting clinical tolerance that persists for years after discontinuation of treatment. AIT is accompanied by suppression of allergic inflammation in target organs and increases in "protective" blocking antibodies of the IgG, particularly IgG4 and IgA2 subclasses. These events are accompanied by a reduction and/or redirection of underlying allergen-specific Th2 cell-driven responses to the allergen(s) used for therapy. This suppression occurs within weeks or months as a consequence of the appearance of a population of regulatory T cells that exert their effects by mechanisms involving cell-cell contact, but also by release of immunomodulatory cytokines such as interleukin 10 (IL-10) (increases IgG4) and TGF-β (increases specific IgA). The more delayed-in-time appearance of antigen-specific Th1 responses and alternative mechanisms such as Th2 cell anergy and/or apoptosis may also be involved. A greater understanding of mechanisms has informed novel immunotherapy approaches, whereas the identification of predictive biomarkers for success of immunotherapy remains elusive.

SALIENT POINTS

1. Allergen-specific immunotherapy (AIT) is effective in selected patients with IgE-mediated disease.
2. Allergic disorders in humans are characterized by expression of Th2 cytokines including IL-4, IL-5, IL-9, and IL-13.
3. AIT inhibits allergen-induced early and late responses in the skin, nose, and lung.
4. AIT inhibits recruitment of mast cells, basophils, and eosinophils in target organs, including the nose and lung.
5. IL-10 has numerous anti-allergic properties and promotes IgG4 production by B cells. AIT induces IL-10 production in the nasal mucosa and peripheral blood. The dominant source is likely different populations of regulatory T cells, including induced peripheral, iTreg cells. Accessory cells such as monocytes and dendritic cells are additional sources of IL-10. IL-10 has numerous anti-allergic properties and promotes IgG4 production by B cells.
6. A potential mechanism of AIT involves immune deviation in favor of allergen-specific Th1 responses. Induction of IL-10+ Treg cells occurs within 3–6 months of initiating subcutaneous immunotherapy (SCIT), whereas immune deviation occurs later, at approximately 12 months.
7. AIT increases allergen-specific IgA and IgG, especially IgG4. IgG antibodies inhibit multiple effects of IgE *in vitro*, but the clinical importance is not established. Biomarkers predictive of clinical efficacy are desirable but not available.
8. Novel approaches of AIT include non-IgE-binding recombinant allergens, allergen-derived peptides, the combination of conventional vaccines with anti-IgE (omalizumab) or with bacterial-derived oligonucleotides; lipids acting through toll-like receptors (TLR) promote Th1 and Treg responses.

ACKNOWLEDGMENTS

Prof. Durham reports grants from ALK, Denmark; personal fees from Anergis, Switzerland; personal fees from Biomay, Austria; personal fees from Allergy Therapeutics, United Kingdom; personal fees from ALK, Horsholm, Denmark; and personal fees from Allergy Therapeutics, outside the submitted work. Dr. Sahiner has no conflict of interest.

REFERENCES

1. Akdis M, Akdis CA. Mechanisms of allergen-specific immunotherapy. *J Allergy Clin Immunol* 2007; 119(4): 780–791.
2. Fujita H, Meyer N, Akdis M, Akdis CA. Mechanisms of immune tolerance to allergens. *Chem Immunol Allergy* 2012; 96: 30–38.
3. Rotiroti G, Shamji M, Durham SR, Till SJ. Repeated low-dose intradermal allergen injection suppresses allergen-induced cutaneous late responses. *J Allergy Clin Immunol* 2012; 130(4): 918–924.e911.
4. Shamji MH, Durham SR. Mechanisms of allergen immunotherapy for inhaled allergens and predictive biomarkers. *J Allergy Clin Immunol* 2017; 140(6): 1485–1498.
5. Spits H, Artis D, Colonna M et al. Innate lymphoid cells—A proposal for uniform nomenclature. *Nat Rev Immunol* 2013; 13(2): 145–149.
6. Bal SM, Bernink JH, Nagasawa M et al. IL-1β, IL-4 and IL-12 control the fate of group 2 innate lymphoid cells in human airway inflammation in the lungs. *Nat Immunol* 2016; 17(6): 636–645.
7. Jia Y, Fang X, Zhu X et al. IL-13+ Type 2 innate lymphoid cells correlate with asthma control status and treatment response. *Am J Respir Cell Mol Biol* 2016; 55(5): 675–683.
8. Chen R, Smith SG, Salter B et al. Allergen-induced increases in sputum levels of group 2 innate lymphoid cells in subjects with asthma. *Am J Respir Crit Care Med* 2017; 196(6): 700–712.
9. Lao-Araya M, Steveling E, Scadding GW, Durham SR, Shamji MH. Seasonal increases in peripheral innate lymphoid type 2 cells are inhibited by subcutaneous grass pollen immunotherapy. *J Allergy Clin Immunol* 2014; 134(5): 1193–1195.e1194.
10. Saunders SP, Moran T, Floudas A et al. Spontaneous atopic dermatitis is mediated by innate immunity, with the secondary lung inflammation of the atopic march requiring adaptive immunity. *J Allergy Clin Immunol* 2016; 137(2): 482–491.

11. Doherty TA, Baum R, Newbury RO et al. Group 2 innate lymphocytes (ILC2) are enriched in active eosinophilic esophagitis. *J Allergy Clin Immunol* 2015; 136(3): 792–794. e793.

12. Pienkowski MM, Norman PS, Lichtenstein LM. Suppression of late-phase skin reactions by immunotherapy with ragweed extract. *J Allergy Clin Immunol* 1985; 76(5): 729–734.

13. Iliopoulos O, Proud D, Adkinson NF Jr. et al. Effects of immunotherapy on the early, late, and rechallenge nasal reaction to provocation with allergen: Changes in inflammatory mediators and cells. *J Allergy Clin Immunol* 1991; 87(4): 855–866.

14. Warner JO, Price JF, Soothill JF, Hey EN. Controlled trial of hyposensitisation to *Dermatophagoides pteronyssinus* in children with asthma. *Lancet* 1978; 2(8096): 912–915.

15. Walker SM, Varney VA, Gaga M, Jacobson MR, Durham SR. Grass pollen immunotherapy: Efficacy and safety during a 4-year follow-up study. *Allergy* 1995; 50(5): 405–413.

16. Des Roches A, Paradis L, Knani J et al. Immunotherapy with a standardized *Dermatophagoides pteronyssinus* extract. V. Duration of the efficacy of immunotherapy after its cessation. *Allergy* 1996; 51(6): 430–433.

17. Francis JN, James LK, Paraskevopoulos G et al. Grass pollen immunotherapy: IL-10 induction and suppression of late responses precedes IgG4 inhibitory antibody activity. *J Allergy Clin Immunol* 2008; 121(5): 1120–1125.e1122.

18. Sturm GJ, Varga EM, Roberts G et al. EAACI guidelines on allergen immunotherapy: *Hymenoptera* venom allergy. *Allergy* 2018; 73(4): 744–764.

19. Plewako H, Wosinska K, Arvidsson M et al. Basophil interleukin 4 and interleukin 13 production is suppressed during the early phase of rush immunotherapy. *Int Arch Allergy Immunol* 2006; 141(4): 346–353.

20. Dugas-Breit S, Przybilla B, Dugas M et al. Serum concentration of baseline mast cell tryptase: Evidence for a decline during long-term immunotherapy for *Hymenoptera* venom allergy. *Clin Exp Allergy* 2010; 40(4): 643–649.

21. Siegmund R, Vogelsang H, Machnik A, Herrmann D. Surface membrane antigen alteration on blood basophils in patients with *Hymenoptera* venom allergy under immunotherapy. *J Allergy Clin Immunol* 2000; 106(6): 1190–1195.

22. Eberlein-Konig B, Ullmann S, Thomas P, Przybilla B. Tryptase and histamine release due to a sting challenge in bee venom allergic patients treated successfully or unsuccessfully with hyposensitization. *Clin Exp Allergy* 1995; 25(8): 704–712.

23. Kucera P, Cvackova M, Hulikova K, Juzova O, Pachl J. Basophil activation can predict clinical sensitivity in patients after venom immunotherapy. *J Investig Allergol Clin Immunol* 2010; 20(2): 110–116.

24. Nullens S, Sabato V, Faber M et al. Basophilic histamine content and release during venom immunotherapy: Insights by flow cytometry. *Cytometry B Clin Cytom* 2013; 84(3): 173–178.

25. Jutel M, Muller UR, Fricker M, Rihs S, Pichler WJ, Dahinden C. Influence of bee venom immunotherapy on degranulation and leukotriene generation in human blood basophils. *Clin Exp Allergy* 1996; 26(10): 1112–1118.

26. Akoum H, Duez C, Vorng H et al. Early modifications of chemokine production and mRNA expression during rush venom immunotherapy. *Cytokine* 1998; 10(9): 706–712.

27. Bussmann C, Xia J, Allam JP, Maintz L, Bieber T, Novak N. Early markers for protective mechanisms during rush venom immunotherapy. *Allergy* 2010; 65(12): 1558–1565.

28. Wilson DR, Irani AM, Walker SM et al. Grass pollen immunotherapy inhibits seasonal increases in basophils and eosinophils in the nasal epithelium. *Clin Exp Allergy* 2001; 31(11): 1705–1713.

29. Nouri-Aria KT, Pilette C, Jacobson MR, Watanabe H, Durham SR. IL-9 and c-Kit+ mast cells in allergic rhinitis during seasonal allergen exposure: Effect of immunotherapy. *J Allergy Clin Immunol* 2005; 116(1): 73–79.

30. Varney VA, Hamid QA, Gaga M et al. Influence of grass pollen immunotherapy on cellular infiltration and cytokine mRNA expression during allergen-induced late-phase cutaneous responses. *J Clin Invest* 1993; 92(2): 644–651.

31. Furin MJ, Norman PS, Creticos PS et al. Immunotherapy decreases antigen-induced eosinophil cell migration into the nasal cavity. *J Allergy Clin Immunol* 1991; 88(1): 27–32.

32. Durham SR, Ying S, Varney VA et al. Grass pollen immunotherapy inhibits allergen-induced infiltration of CD4+ T lymphocytes and eosinophils in the nasal mucosa and increases the number of cells expressing messenger RNA for interferon-γ. *J Allergy Clin Immunol* 1996; 97(6): 1356–1365.

33. Wilson DR, Nouri-Aria KT, Walker SM et al. Grass pollen immunotherapy: Symptomatic improvement correlates with reductions in eosinophils and IL-5 mRNA expression in the nasal mucosa during the pollen season. *J Allergy Clin Immunol* 2001; 107(6): 971–976.

34. Rak S, Lowhagen O, Venge P. The effect of immunotherapy on bronchial hyperresponsiveness and eosinophil cationic protein in pollen-allergic patients. *J Allergy Clin Immunol* 1988; 82(3 Pt 1): 470–480.

35. Tversky JR, Bieneman AP, Chichester KL, Hamilton RG, Schroeder JT. Subcutaneous allergen immunotherapy restores human dendritic cell innate immune function. *Clin Exp Allergy* 2010; 40(1): 94–102.

36. Dreschler K, Bratke K, Petermann S et al. Impact of immunotherapy on blood dendritic cells in patients with *Hymenoptera* venom allergy. *J Allergy Clin Immunol* 2011; 127(2): 487–494.e481-483.

37. Zimmer A, Bouley J, Le Mignon M et al. A regulatory dendritic cell signature correlates with the clinical efficacy of allergen-specific sublingual immunotherapy. *J Allergy Clin Immunol* 2012; 129(4): 1020–1030.

38. Lombardi V, Beuraud C, Neukirch C et al. Circulating innate lymphoid cells are differentially regulated in allergic and nonallergic subjects. *J Allergy Clin Immunol* 2016; 138(1): 305–308.

39. Novak N, Mete N, Bussmann C et al. Early suppression of basophil activation during allergen-specific immunotherapy by histamine receptor 2. *J Allergy Clin Immunol* 2012; 130(5): 1153–1158.e1152.

40. Maintz L, Bussmann C, Bieber T, Novak N. Contribution of histamine metabolism to tachyphylaxis during the buildup phase of rush immunotherapy. *J Allergy Clin Immunol* 2009, 123(3): 701–703.

41. Meiler F, Zumkehr J, Klunker S, Ruckert B, Akdis CA, Akdis M. *In vivo* switch to IL-10-secreting T regulatory cells in high dose allergen exposure. *J Exp Med* 2008; 205(12): 2887–2898.

42. Cavkaytar O, Akdis CA, Akdis M. Modulation of immune responses by immunotherapy in allergic diseases. *Curr Opin Pharmacol* 2014; 17: 30–37.

43. Akdis CA, Jutel M, Akdis M. Regulatory effects of histamine and histamine receptor expression in human allergic immune responses. *Chem Immunol Allergy* 2008; 94: 67–82.

44. Jutel M, Akdis M, Akdis CA. Histamine, histamine receptors and their role in immune pathology. *Clin Exp Allergy* 2009; 39(12): 1786–1800.

45. Mazzoni A, Young HA, Spitzer JH, Visintin A, Segal DM. Histamine regulates cytokine production in maturing dendritic cells, resulting in altered T cell polarization. *J Clin Invest* 2001; 108(12): 1865–1873.

46. Osna N, Elliott K, Khan MM. Regulation of interleukin-10 secretion by histamine in TH2 cells and splenocytes. *Int Immunopharmacol* 2001; 1(1): 85–96.

47. Jutel M, Watanabe T, Klunker S et al. Histamine regulates T-cell and antibody responses by differential expression of H1 and H2 receptors. *Nature* 2001; 413(6854): 420–425.

48. Lesourd B, Paupe J, Thiollet M, Moulias R, Sainte-Laudy J, Scheinmann P. *Hymenoptera* venom immunotherapy. I. Induction of T cell-mediated immunity by honeybee venom immunotherapy: Relationships with specific antibody responses. *J Allergy Clin Immunol* 1989; 83(3): 563–571.

49. Mamessier E, Birnbaum J, Dupuy P, Vervloet D, Magnan A. Ultra-rush venom immunotherapy induces differential T cell activation and regulatory patterns according to the severity of allergy. *Clin Exp Allergy* 2006; 36(6): 704–713.

50. Schuerwegh AJ, De Clerck LS, Bridts CH, Stevens WJ. Wasp venom immunotherapy induces a shift from IL-4-producing towards interferon-γ-producing CD4+ and CD8+ T lymphocytes. *Clin Exp Allergy* 2001; 31(5): 740–746.

51. Tilmant L, Dessaint JP, Tsicopoulos A, Tonnel AB, Capron A. Concomitant augmentation of CD4+ CD45R+ suppressor/inducer subset and diminution of CD4+ CDw29+ helper/inducer subset during rush hyposensitization in *Hymenoptera* venom allergy. *Clin Exp Immunol* 1989; 76(1): 13–18.

52. Shamji MH, Ljorring C, Francis JN et al. Functional rather than immunoreactive levels of IgG4 correlate closely with clinical response to grass pollen immunotherapy. *Allergy* 2012; 67(2): 217–226.

53. Shamji MH, Ljorring C, Wurtzen PA. Predictive biomarkers of clinical efficacy of allergen-specific immunotherapy: How to proceed. *Immunotherapy* 2013; 5(3): 203–206.

54. Bohle B, Kinaciyan T, Gerstmayr M, Radakovics A, Jahn-Schmid B, Ebner C. Sublingual immunotherapy induces IL-10-producing T regulatory cells, allergen-specific T-cell tolerance, and immune deviation. *J Allergy Clin Immunol* 2007; 120(3): 707–713.

55. Jutel M, Akdis M, Blaser K, Akdis CA. Mechanisms of allergen specific immunotherapy—T-cell tolerance and more. *Allergy* 2006; 61(7): 796–807.

56. Chen W, Jin W, Hardegen N et al. Conversion of peripheral CD4+ CD25− naive T cells to CD4+CD25+ regulatory T cells by TGF-β induction of transcription factor Foxp3. *J Exp Med* 2003; 198(12): 1875–1886.

57. Klunker S, Chong MM, Mantel PY et al. Transcription factors RUNX1 and RUNX3 in the induction and suppressive function of Foxp3+ inducible regulatory T cells. *J Exp Med* 2009; 206(12): 2701–2715.

58. Akdis CA, Blesken T, Akdis M, Wuthrich B, Blaser K. Role of interleukin 10 in specific immunotherapy. *J Clin Invest* 1998; 102(1): 98–106.

59. Ling EM, Smith T, Nguyen XD et al. Relation of CD4+ CD25+ regulatory T-cell suppression of allergen-driven T-cell activation to atopic status and expression of allergic disease. *Lancet* 2004; 363(9409): 608–615.

60. Mobs C, Slotosch C, Loffler H, Jakob T, Hertl M, Pfutzner W. Birch pollen immunotherapy leads to differential induction of regulatory T cells and delayed helper T cell immune deviation. *J Immunol* 2010; 184(4): 2194–2203.

61. Gorelik L, Constant S, Flavell RA. Mechanism of transforming growth factor β-induced inhibition of T helper type 1 differentiation. *J Exp Med* 2002; 195(11): 1499–1505.

62. Jutel M, Akdis M, Budak F et al. IL-10 and TGF-β cooperate in the regulatory T cell response to mucosal allergens in normal immunity and specific immunotherapy. *Eur J Immunol* 2003; 33(5): 1205–1214.

63. Faith A, Richards DF, Verhoef A, Lamb JR, Lee TH, Hawrylowicz CM. Impaired secretion of interleukin-4 and interleukin-13 by allergen-specific T cells correlates with defective nuclear expression of NF-AT2 and jun B: Relevance to immunotherapy. *Clin Exp Allergy* 2003; 33(9): 1209–1215.

64. Gorelik L, Fields PE, Flavell RA. Cutting edge: TGF-β inhibits Th type 2 development through inhibition of GATA-3 expression. *J Immunol* 2000; 165(9): 4773–4777.

65. Karagiannidis C, Akdis M, Holopainen P et al. Glucocorticoids upregulate FOXP3 expression and regulatory T cells in asthma. *J Allergy Clin Immunol* 2004; 114(6): 1425–1433.

66. Fantini MC, Becker C, Monteleone G, Pallone F, Galle PR, Neurath MF. Cutting edge: TGF-β induces a regulatory phenotype in CD4+CD25− T cells through Foxp3 induction and down-regulation of Smad7. *J Immunol* 2004; 172(9): 5149–5153.

67. Oida T, Xu L, Weiner HL, Kitani A, Strober W. TGF-β-mediated suppression by CD4+ CD25+ T cells is facilitated by CTLA-4 signaling. *J Immunol* 2006; 177(4): 2331–2339.

68. Pilette C, Nouri-Aria KT, Jacobson MR et al. Grass pollen immunotherapy induces an allergen-specific IgA2 antibody response associated with mucosal TGF-β expression. *J Immunol* 2007; 178(7): 4658–4666.

69. Fallarino F, Grohmann U. Using an ancient tool for igniting and propagating immune tolerance: IDO as an inducer and amplifier of regulatory T cell functions. *Curr Med Chem* 2011; 18(15): 2215–2221.

70. Botturi K, Vervloet D, Magnan A. T cells and allergens relationships: Are they that specific? *Clin Exp Allergy* 2007; 37(8): 1121–1123.

71. Radulovic S, Jacobson MR, Durham SR, Nouri-Aria KT, Grass pollen immunotherapy induces Foxp3-expressing CD4+ CD25+ cells in the nasal mucosa. *J Allergy Clin Immunol* 2008; 121(6): 1467–1472.e1461.

72. Pereira-Santos MC, Baptista AP, Melo A et al. Expansion of circulating Foxp3+)D25bright CD4+ T cells during specific venom immunotherapy. *Clin Exp Allergy* 2008; 38(2): 291–297.

73. Nasser SM, Ying S, Meng Q, Kay AB, Ewan PW. Interleukin-10 levels increase in cutaneous biopsies of patients undergoing wasp venom immunotherapy. *Eur J Immunol* 2001; 31(12): 3704–3713.

74. Varricchi G, Harker J, Borriello F, Marone G, Durham SR, Shamji MH. T follicular helper (Tfh) cells in normal immune responses and in allergic disorders. *Allergy* 2016; 71(8): 1086–1094.

75. Sage PT, Sharpe AH. T follicular regulatory cells. *Immunol Rev* 2016; 271(1): 246–259.

76. Schulten V, Tripple V, Seumois G et al. Allergen-specific immunotherapy modulates the balance of circulating T_{fh} and T_{fr} cells. *J Allergy Clin Immunol* 2018; 141(2): 775–777. e776.

77. van de Veen W, Stanic B, Yaman G et al. IgG4 production is confined to human IL-10-producing regulatory B cells that suppress antigen-specific immune responses. *J Allergy Clin Immunol* 2013; 131(4): 1204–1212.

78. Rosser EC, Mauri C. Regulatory B cells: Origin, phenotype, and function. *Immunity* 2015; 42(4): 607–612.

79. Deniz G, van de Veen W, Akdis M. Natural killer cells in patients with allergic diseases. *J Allergy Clin Immunol* 2013; 132(3): 527–535.

80. Akdis CA, Joss A, Akdis M, Faith A, Blaser K. A molecular basis for T cell suppression by IL-10: CD28-associated IL-10 receptor inhibits CD28 tyrosine phosphorylation and phosphatidylinositol 3-kinase binding. *FASEB J* 2000; 14(12): 1666–1668.

81. Zhang X, Izikson L, Liu L, Weiner HL. Activation of CD25+ CD4+ regulatory T cells by oral antigen administration. *J Immunol* 2001; 167(8): 4245–4253.

82. Akbari O, Freeman GJ, Meyer EH et al. Antigen-specific regulatory T cells develop via the ICOS-ICOS-ligand pathway and inhibit allergen-induced airway hyperreactivity. *Nat Med* 2002; 8(9): 1024–1032.

83. Ito T, Yang M, Wang YH et al. Plasmacytoid dendritic cells prime IL-10-producing T regulatory cells by inducible costimulator ligand. *J Exp Med* 2007; 204(1): 105–115.

84. Novak N, Allam JP, Hagemann T et al. Characterization of FcεRI-bearing CD123 blood dendritic cell antigen-2 plasmacytoid dendritic cells in atopic dermatitis. *J Allergy Clin Immunol* 2004; 114(2): 364–370.

85. Shamji MH, Francis JN, Wurtzen PA, Lund K, Durham SR, Till SJ. Cell-free detection of allergen-IgE cross-linking with immobilized phase CD23: Inhibition by blocking antibody responses after immunotherapy. *J Allergy Clin Immunol* 2013; 132(4): 1003–1005.e1001–1004.

86. Gleich GJ, Zimmermann EM, Henderson LL, Yunginger JW. Effect of immunotherapy on immunoglobulin E and immunoglobulin G antibodies to ragweed antigens: A six-year prospective study. *J Allergy Clin Immunol* 1982; 70(4): 261–271.

87. Scadding GW, Calderon MA, Shamji MH et al. Effect of 2 years of treatment with sublingual grass pollen immunotherapy on nasal response to allergen challenge at 3 years among patients with moderate to severe seasonal allergic rhinitis: The GRASS Randomized Clinical Trial. *JAMA* 2017; 317(6): 615–625.

88. Wachholz PA, Soni NK, Till SJ, Durham SR. Inhibition of allergen-IgE binding to B cells by IgG antibodies after grass pollen immunotherapy. *J Allergy Clin Immunol* 2003; 112(5): 915–922.

89. Oefner CM, Winkler A, Hess C et al. Tolerance induction with T cell-dependent protein antigens induces regulatory sialylated IgGs. *J Allergy Clin Immunol* 2012; 129(6): 1647–1655.e1613.

90. Van Ree R, Van Leeuwen WA, Dieges PH et al. Measurement of IgE antibodies against purified grass pollen allergens (Lol p 1, 2, 3 and 5) during immunotherapy. *Clin Exp Allergy* 1997; 27(1): 68–74.

91. Lichtenstein LM, Ishizaka K, Norman PS, Sobotka AK, Hill BM. IgE antibody measurements in ragweed hay fever. Relationship to clinical severity and the results of immunotherapy. *J Clin Invest* 1973; 52(2): 472–482.

92. Platts-Mills TA, von Maur RK, Ishizaka K, Norman PS, Lichtenstein LM. IgA and IgG anti-ragweed antibodies in nasal secretions. Quantitative measurements of antibodies and correlation with inhibition of histamine release. *J Clin Invest* 1976; 57(4): 1041–1050.

93. Moverare R, Elfman L, Vesterinen E, Metso T, Haahtela T. Development of new IgE specificities to allergenic components in birch pollen extract during specific immunotherapy studied with immunoblotting and Pharmacia CAP System. *Allergy* 2002; 57(5): 423–430.

94. Gehlhar K, Schlaak M, Becker W, Bufe A. Monitoring allergen immunotherapy of pollen-allergic patients: The ratio of allergen-specific IgG4 to IgG1 correlates with clinical outcome. *Clin Exp Allergy* 1999; 29(4): 497–506.

95. Devey ME, Wilson DV, Wheeler AW. The IgG subclasses of antibodies to grass pollen allergens produced in hay fever patients during hyposensitization. *Clin Allergy* 1976; 6(3): 227–236.

96. Mothes N, Heinzkill M, Drachenberg KJ et al. Allergen-specific immunotherapy with a monophosphoryl lipid A-adjuvanted vaccine: Reduced seasonally boosted immunoglobulin E production and inhibition of basophil histamine release by therapy-induced blocking antibodies. *Clin Exp Allergy* 2003; 33(9): 1198–1208.

97. Garcia BE, Sanz ML, Dieguez I, de las Marinas MD, Oehling A. Modifications in IgG subclasses in the course of immunotherapy with grass pollen. *J Investig Allergol Clin Immunol* 1993; 3(1): 19–25.

98. Lambin P, Bouzoumou A, Murrieta M et al. Purification of human IgG4 subclass with allergen-specific blocking activity. *J Immunol Methods* 1993; 165(1): 99–111.

99. Daeron M, Malbec O, Latour S, Arock M, Fridman WH. Regulation of high-affinity IgE receptor-mediated mast cell activation by murine low-affinity IgG receptors. *J Clin Invest* 1995; 95(2): 577–585.

100. Zhu D, Kepley CL, Zhang K, Terada T, Yamada T, Saxon A. A chimeric human-cat fusion protein blocks cat-induced allergy. *Nat Med* 2005; 11(4): 446–449.

101. Kepley CL, Taghavi S, Mackay G et al. Co-aggregation of FcγRII with FcεRI on human mast cells inhibits antigen-induced secretion and involves SHIP-Grb2-Dok complexes. *J Biol Chem* 2004; 279(34): 35139–35149.

102. Ejrnaes AM, Svenson M, Lund G, Larsen JN, Jacobi H. Inhibition of rBet v 1-induced basophil histamine release with specific immunotherapy -induced serum immunoglobulin G: No evidence that FcγRIIB signalling is important. *Clin Exp Allergy* 2006; 36(3): 273–282.

103. Punnonen J, Aversa G, de Vries JE. Human pre-B cells differentiate into Ig-secreting plasma cells in the presence of interleukin-4 and activated CD4+ T cells or their membranes. *Blood* 1993; 82(9): 2781–2789.

104. Jabara HH, Loh R, Ramesh N, Vercelli D, Geha RS. Sequential switching from mu to epsilon via γ4 in human B cells stimulated with IL-4 and hydrocortisone. *J Immunol* 1993; 151(9): 4528–4533.

105. Agresti A, Vercelli D. Analysis of γ4 germline transcription in human B cells. *Int Arch Allergy Immunol* 1999; 118(2–4): 279–281.

106. Meiler F, Klunker S, Zimmermann M, Akdis CA, Akdis M. Distinct regulation of IgE, IgG4 and IgA by T regulatory cells and toll-like receptors. *Allergy* 2008; 63(11): 1455–1463.

107. Satoguina JS, Weyand E, Larbi J, Hoerauf A. T regulatory-1 cells induce IgG4 production by B cells: Role of IL-10. *J Immunol* 2005; 174(8): 4718–4726.

108. van Neerven RJ, Wikborg T, Lund G et al. Blocking antibodies induced by specific allergy vaccination prevent the activation of CD4+ T cells by inhibiting serum-IgE-facilitated allergen presentation. *J Immunol* 1999; 163(5): 2944–2952.

109. Wurtzen PA, Lund G, Lund K, Arvidsson M, Rak S, Ipsen H. A double-blind placebo-controlled birch allergy vaccination study II: Correlation between inhibition of IgE binding, histamine release and facilitated allergen presentation. *Clin Exp Allergy* 2008; 38(8): 1290–1301.

110. Pree I, Shamji MH, Kimber I, Valenta R, Durham SR, Niederberger V. Inhibition of CD23-dependent facilitated allergen binding to B cells following vaccination with genetically modified hypoallergenic Bet v 1 molecules. *Clin Exp Allergy* 2010; 40(9): 1346–1352.

111. Scadding GW, Shamji MH, Jacobson MR et al. Sublingual grass pollen immunotherapy is associated with increases in sublingual Foxp3-expressing cells and elevated allergen-specific immunoglobulin G4, immunoglobulin A and serum inhibitory activity for immunoglobulin E-facilitated allergen binding to B cells. *Clin Exp Allergy* 2010; 40(4): 598–606.

112. James LK, Bowen H, Calvert RA et al. Allergen specificity of IgG(4)-expressing B cells in patients with grass pollen allergy undergoing immunotherapy. *J Allergy Clin Immunol* 2012; 130(3): 663–670.e663.

113. Durham SR, Walker SM, Varga EM et al. Long-term clinical efficacy of grass-pollen immunotherapy. *N Engl J Med* 1999; 341(7): 468–475.

114. Varga EM, Francis JN, Zach MS, Klunker S, Aberer W, Durham SR. Time course of serum inhibitory activity for facilitated allergen-IgE binding during bee venom immunotherapy in children. *Clin Exp Allergy* 2009; 39(9): 1353–1357.

115. Ball T, Sperr WR, Valent P et al. Induction of antibody responses to new B cell epitopes indicates vaccination character of allergen immunotherapy. *Eur J Immunol* 1999; 29(6): 2026–2036.

116. James LK, Shamji MH, Walker SM et al. Long-term tolerance after allergen immunotherapy is accompanied by selective persistence of blocking antibodies. *J Allergy Clin Immunol* 2011; 127(2): 509–516.e501–505.

117. Varga EM, Kausar F, Aberer W et al. Tolerant beekeepers display venom-specific functional IgG4 antibodies in the absence of specific IgE. *J Allergy Clin Immunol* 2013; 131(5): 1419–1421.

118. Radulovic S, Wilson D, Calderon M, Durham S. Systematic reviews of sublingual immunotherapy (SLIT). *Allergy* 2011; 66(6): 740–752.

119. Kouser L, Kappen J, Walton RP, Shamji MH. Update on biomarkers to monitor clinical efficacy response during and post treatment in allergen immunotherapy. *Curr Treat Options Allergy* 2017; 4(1): 43–53.

120. Shamji MH, Kappen JH, Akdis M et al. Biomarkers for monitoring clinical efficacy of allergen immunotherapy for allergic rhinoconjunctivitis and allergic asthma: An EAACI Position Paper. *Allergy* 2017; 72(8): 1156–1173.

121. Food, Drug Administration HHS. International Conference on harmonisation; guidance on E15 pharmacogenomics definitions and sample coding; availability. *Fed Regist* 2008; 73(68): 19074–19076.

122. Shamji MH, Durham SR. Mechanisms of immunotherapy to aeroallergens. *Clin Exp Allergy* 2011; 41(9): 1235–1246.

123. Roberts G, Hurley C, Turcanu V, Lack G. Grass pollen immunotherapy as an effective therapy for childhood seasonal allergic asthma. *J Allergy Clin Immunol* 2006; 117(2): 263–268.

124. Benjaponpitak S, Oro A, Maguire P, Marinkovich V, DeKruyff RH, Umetsu DT. The kinetics of change in cytokine production by CD4 T cells during conventional allergen immunotherapy. *J Allergy Clin Immunol* 1999; 103(3 Pt 1): 468–475.

125. Eifan AO, Akkoc T, Yildiz A et al. Clinical efficacy and immunological mechanisms of sublingual and subcutaneous immunotherapy in asthmatic/rhinitis children sensitized to house dust mite: An open randomized controlled trial. *Clin Exp Allergy* 2010; 40(6): 922–932.

126. Di Lorenzo G, Mansueto P, Pacor ML et al. Evaluation of serum s-IgE/total IgE ratio in predicting clinical response to allergen-specific immunotherapy. *J Allergy Clin Immunol* 2009; 123(5): 1103–1110, 1110.e1101–1104.

127. Ewan PW, Deighton J, Wilson AB, Lachmann PJ. Venom-specific IgG antibodies in bee and wasp allergy: Lack of correlation with protection from stings. *Clin Exp Allergy* 1993; 23(8): 647–660.

128. Niederberger V, Horak F, Vrtala S et al. Vaccination with genetically engineered allergens prevents progression of allergic disease. *Proc Natl Acad Sci USA* 2004; 101(Suppl 2): 14677–14682.

129. Oldfield WL, Larche M, Kay AB. Effect of T-cell peptides derived from Fel d 1 on allergic reactions and cytokine production in patients sensitive to cats: A randomised controlled trial. *Lancet* 2002; 360(9326): 47–53.

130. Patel D, Couroux P, Hickey P et al. Fel d 1-derived peptide antigen desensitization shows a persistent treatment effect 1 year after the start of dosing: A randomized, placebo-controlled study. *J Allergy Clin Immunol* 2013; 131(1): 103–109.e101–107.

131. Verhoef A, Alexander C, Kay AB, Larche M. T cell epitope immunotherapy induces a CD4+ T cell population with regulatory activity. *PLOS Med* 2005; 2(3): e78.

132. Campbell JD, Buckland KF, McMillan SJ et al. Peptide immunotherapy in allergic asthma generates IL-10-dependent immunological tolerance associated with linked epitope suppression. *J Exp Med* 2009; 206(7): 1535–1547.

133. Klunker S, Saggar LR, Seyfert-Margolis V et al.; Immune Tolerance Network G. Combination treatment with omalizumab and rush immunotherapy for ragweed-induced allergic rhinitis: Inhibition of IgE-facilitated allergen binding. *J Allergy Clin Immunol* 2007; 120(3): 688–695.

134. Casale TB, Busse WW, Kline JN et al. Omalizumab pretreatment decreases acute reactions after rush immunotherapy for ragweed-induced seasonal allergic rhinitis. *J Allergy Clin Immunol* 2006; 117(1): 134–140.

135. Valenta R, Campana R, Focke-Tejkl M, Niederberger V. Vaccine development for allergen-specific immunotherapy based on recombinant allergens and synthetic allergen peptides: Lessons from the past and novel mechanisms of action for the future. *J Allergy Clin Immunol* 2016; 137(2): 351–357.

136. Ellis AK, Frankish CW, O'Hehir RE et al. Treatment with grass allergen peptides improves symptoms of grass pollen-induced allergic rhinoconjunctivitis. *J Allergy Clin Immunol* 2017; 140(2): 486–496.

137. Marshall JD, Abtahi S, Eiden JJ et al. Immunostimulatory sequence DNA linked to the Amb a 1 allergen promotes T(H)1 cytokine expression while downregulating T(H)2 cytokine expression in PBMCs from human patients with ragweed allergy. *J Allergy Clin Immunol* 2001; 108(2): 191–197.

138. Moseman EA, Liang X, Dawson AJ et al. Human plasmacytoid dendritic cells activated by CpG oligodeoxynucleotides induce the generation of CD4+CD25+ regulatory T cells. *J Immunol* 2004; 173(7): 4433–4442.

139. Creticos PS, Schroeder JT, Hamilton RG et al. Immunotherapy with a ragweed-toll-like receptor 9 agonist vaccine for allergic rhinitis. *N Engl J Med* 2006; 355(14): 1445–1455.

140. Puggioni F, Durham SR, Francis JN. Monophosphoryl lipid A (MPL) promotes allergen-induced immune deviation in favour of Th1 responses. *Allergy* 2005; 60(5): 678–684.

141. Drachenberg KJ, Wheeler AW, Stuebner P, Horak F. A well-tolerated grass pollen-specific allergy vaccine containing a novel adjuvant, monophosphoryl lipid A, reduces allergic symptoms after only four preseasonal injections. *Allergy* 2001; 56(6): 498–505.

142. Senti G, Prinz Vavricka BM, Erdmann I et al. Intralymphatic allergen administration renders specific immunotherapy faster and safer: A randomized controlled trial. *Proc Natl Acad Sci USA* 2008; 105(46): 17908–17912.

143. Senti G, Graf N, Haug S et al. Epicutaneous allergen administration as a novel method of allergen-specific immunotherapy. *J Allergy Clin Immunol* 2009; 124(5): 997–1002.

144. Senti G, von Moos S, Tay F et al. Epicutaneous allergen-specific immunotherapy ameliorates grass pollen-induced rhinoconjunctivitis: A double-blind, placebo-controlled dose escalation study. *J Allergy Clin Immunol* 2012; 129(1): 128–135.

145. Slovick A, Douiri A, Muir R et al. Intradermal grass pollen immunotherapy increases TH2 and IgE responses and worsens respiratory allergic symptoms. *J Allergy Clin Immunol* 2017; 139(6): 1830–1839.e1813.

146. Shamji MH, Wilcock LK, Wachholz PA et al. The IgE-facilitated allergen binding (FAB) assay: Validation of a novel flow-cytometric based method for the detection of inhibitory antibody responses. *J Immunol Methods* 2006; 317(1–2): 71–79.

147. Pfaar O, Bonini S, Cardona V et al. Perspectives in allergen immunotherapy: 2017 and beyond. *Allergy* 2018, 73(Suppl 104): 5–23.

148. Keskin O, Tuncer A, Adalioglu G, Sekerel BE, Sackesen C, Kalayci O. The effects of grass pollen allergoid immunotherapy on clinical and immunological parameters in children with allergic rhinitis. *Pediatr Allergy Immunol* 2006; 17(6): 396–407.

149. Durham SR, Yang WH, Pedersen MR, Johansen N, Rak S. Sublingual immunotherapy with once-daily grass allergen tablets: A randomized controlled trial in seasonal allergic rhinoconjunctivitis. *J Allergy Clin Immunol* 2006; 117(4): 802–809.

150. Didier A, Malling HJ, Worm M et al. Optimal dose, efficacy, and safety of once-daily sublingual immunotherapy with a 5-grass pollen tablet for seasonal allergic rhinitis. *J Allergy Clin Immunol* 2007; 120(6): 1338–1345.

151. Rolinck-Werninghaus C, Kopp M, Liebke C, Lange J, Wahn U, Niggemann B. Lack of detectable alterations in immune responses during sublingual immunotherapy in children with seasonal allergic rhinoconjunctivitis to grass pollen. *Int Arch Allergy Immunol* 2005; 136(2): 134–141.

152. Fujimura T, Yonekura S, Horiguchi S et al. Increase of regulatory T cells and the ratio of specific IgE to total IgE are candidates for response monitoring or prognostic biomarkers in 2-year sublingual immunotherapy (SLIT) for Japanese cedar pollinosis. *Clin Immunol* 2011; 139(1): 65–74.

153. Li Q, Li M, Yue W et al. Predictive factors for clinical response to allergy immunotherapy in children with asthma and rhinitis. *Int Arch Allergy Immunol* 2014; 164(3): 210–217.

154. Dahl R, Kapp A, Colombo G et al. Sublingual grass allergen tablet immunotherapy provides sustained clinical benefit with progressive immunologic changes over 2 years. *J Allergy Clin Immunol* 2008; 121(2): 512–518 e512.

155. Gomez E, Fernandez TD, Dona I et al. Initial immunological changes as predictors for house dust mite immunotherapy response. *Clin Exp Allergy* 2015; 45(10): 1542–1553.

156. Nelson HS, Nolte H, Creticos P, Maloney J, Wu J, Bernstein DI. Efficacy and safety of timothy grass allergy immunotherapy tablet treatment in North American adults. *J Allergy Clin Immunol* 2011; 127(1): 72–80.e71–72.

157. Wollmann E, Lupinek C, Kundi M, Selb R, Niederberger V, Valenta R. Reduction in allergen-specific IgE binding as measured by microarray: A possible surrogate marker for effects of specific immunotherapy. *J Allergy Clin Immunol* 2015; 136(3): 806–809 e807.

158. La Rosa M, Ranno C, Andre C, Carat F, Tosca MA, Canonica GW. Double-blind placebo-controlled evaluation of sublingual-swallow immunotherapy with standardized *Parietaria judaica* extract in children with allergic rhinoconjunctivitis. *J Allergy Clin Immunol* 1999; 104(2 Pt 1): 425–432.

159. Troise C, Voltolini S, Canessa A, Pecora S, Negrini AC. Sublingual immunotherapy in *Parietaria* pollen-induced rhinitis: A double-blind study. *J Investig Allergol Clin Immunol* 1995; 5(1): 25–30.

160. Bahceciler NN, Arikan C, Taylor A et al. Impact of sublingual immunotherapy on specific antibody levels in asthmatic children allergic to house dust mites. *Int Arch Allergy Immunol* 2005; 136(3): 287–294.

161. Shamji MH, Layhadi JA, Scadding GW et al. Basophil expression of diamine oxidase: A novel biomarker of allergen immunotherapy response. *J Allergy Clin Immunol* 2015; 135(4): 913–921.e919.

162. Nouri-Aria KT, Wachholz PA, Francis JN et al. Grass pollen immunotherapy induces mucosal and peripheral IL-10 responses and blocking IgG activity. *J Immunol* 2004; 172(5): 3252–3259.

163. Durham SR, Emminger W, Kapp A et al. SQ-standardized sublingual grass immunotherapy: Confirmation of disease modification 2 years after 3 years of treatment in a randomized trial. *J Allergy Clin Immunol* 2012; 129(3): 717–725.e715.

164. Petersen AB, Gudmann P, Milvang-Gronager P et al. Performance evaluation of a specific IgE assay developed for the ADVIA centaur immunoassay system. *Clin Biochem* 2004; 37(10): 882–892.

165. Reich K, Gessner C, Kroker A et al. Immunologic effects and tolerability profile of in-season initiation of a standardized-quality grass allergy immunotherapy tablet: A phase III, multicenter, randomized, double-blind, placebo-controlled trial in adults with grass pollen-induced rhinoconjunctivitis. *Clin Ther* 2011; 33(7): 828–840.

166. Corzo JL, Carrillo T, Pedemonte C et al. Tolerability during double-blind randomized phase I trials with the house dust mite allergy immunotherapy tablet in adults and children. *J Investig Allergol Clin Immunol* 2014; 24(3): 154–161.

167. Van Overtvelt L, Baron-Bodo V, Horiot S et al. Changes in basophil activation during grass-pollen sublingual immunotherapy do not correlate with clinical efficacy. *Allergy* 2011; 66(12): 1530–1537.

168. Buhring HJ, Streble A, Valent P. The basophil-specific ectoenzyme E-NPP3 (CD203c) as a marker for cell activation and allergy diagnosis. *Int Arch Allergy Immunol* 2004; 133(4): 317–329.

169. Knol EF, Mul FP, Jansen H, Calafat J, Roos D. Monitoring human basophil activation via CD63 monoclonal antibody 435. *J Allergy Clin Immunol* 1991; 88(3 Pt 1): 328–338.

170. Hennersdorf F, Florian S, Jakob A et al. Identification of CD13, CD107a, and CD164 as novel basophil-activation markers and dissection of two response patterns in time kinetics of IgE-dependent upregulation. *Cell Res* 2005; 15(5): 325–335.

171. Kepil Ozdemir S, Sin BA, Guloglu D, Ikinciogullari A, Gencturk Z, Misirligil Z. Short-term preseasonal immunotherapy: Is early clinical efficacy related to the basophil response? *Int Arch Allergy Immunol* 2014; 164(3): 237–245.

172. Aasbjerg K, Backer V, Lund G et al. Immunological comparison of allergen immunotherapy tablet treatment and subcutaneous immunotherapy against grass allergy. *Clin Exp Allergy* 2014; 44(3): 417–428.

173. Ceuppens JL, Bullens D, Kleinjans H, van der Werf J, Group PBES. Immunotherapy with a modified birch pollen extract in allergic rhinoconjunctivitis: Clinical and immunological effects. *Clin Exp Allergy* 2009; 39(12): 1903–1909.

174. Ebo DG, Bridts CH, Mertens CH, Hagendorens MM, Stevens WJ, De Clerck LS. Analyzing histamine release by flow cytometry (HistaFlow): A novel instrument to study the degranulation patterns of basophils. *J Immunol Methods* 2012; 375(1–2): 30–38.

175. Gueguen C, Bouley J, Moussu H et al. Changes in markers associated with dendritic cells driving the differentiation of either TH2 cells or regulatory T cells correlate with clinical benefit during allergen immunotherapy. *J Allergy Clin Immunol* 2016; 137(2): 545–558.

176. Plewako H, Holmberg K, Oancea I, Gotlib T, Samolinski B, Rak S. A follow-up study of immunotherapy-treated birch-allergic patients: Effect on the expression of chemokines in the nasal mucosa. *Clin Exp Allergy* 2008; 38(7): 1124–1131.

177. Makino Y, Noguchi E, Takahashi N et al. Apolipoprotein A-IV is a candidate target molecule for the treatment of seasonal allergic rhinitis. *J Allergy Clin Immunol* 2010; 126(6): 1163–1169.e1165.

178. Salmivesi S, Paassilta M, Huhtala H, Nieminen R, Moilanen E, Korppi M. Changes in biomarkers during a six-month oral immunotherapy intervention for cow's milk allergy. *Acta Paediatr* 2016; 105(11): 1349–1354.

179. Li H, Xu E, He M. Cytokine responses to specific immunotherapy in house dust mite-induced allergic rhinitis patients. *Inflammation* 2015; 38(6): 2216–2223.

180. Ciprandi G, De Amici M, Murdaca G, Filaci G, Fenoglio D, Marseglia GL. Adipokines and sublingual immunotherapy: Preliminary report. *Hum Immunol* 2009; 70(1): 73–78.

181. Boonpiyathad T, Meyer N, Moniuszko M et al. High-dose bee venom exposure induces similar tolerogenic B-cell responses in allergic patients and healthy beekeepers. *Allergy* 2017; 72(3): 407–415.

182. Doherty TA, Scott D, Walford HH et al. Allergen challenge in allergic rhinitis rapidly induces increased peripheral blood type 2 innate lymphoid cells that express CD84. *J Allergy Clin Immunol* 2014; 133(4): 1203–1205.

183. Agache I, Bilo M, Braunstahl GJ et al. *In vivo* diagnosis of allergic diseases—Allergen provocation tests. *Allergy* 2015; 70(4): 355–365.

184. Pfaar O, Demoly P, Gerth van Wijk R et al. Recommendations for the standardization of clinical outcomes used in allergen immunotherapy trials for allergic rhinoconjunctivitis: An EAACI Position Paper. *Allergy* 2014; 69(7): 854–867.

185. Position paper. Allergen standardization and skin tests. The European Academy of Allergology and Clinical Immunology. *Allergy* 1993; 48(14 Suppl): 48–82.

186. Bousquet J, Maasch H, Martinot B, Hejjaoui A, Wahl R, Michel FB. Double-blind, placebo-controlled immunotherapy with mixed grass-pollen allergoids. II. Comparison between parameters assessing the efficacy of immunotherapy. *J Allergy Clin Immunol* 1988; 82(3 Pt 1): 439–446.

187. Moller C, Bjorksten B, Nilsson G, Dreborg S. The precision of the conjunctival provocation test. *Allergy* 1984; 39(1): 37–41.

188. Sarandi I, Classen DP, Astvatsatourov A et al. Quantitative conjunctival provocation test for controlled clinical trials. *Methods Inf Med* 2014; 53(4): 238–244.

189. Scadding G, Hellings P, Alobid I et al. Diagnostic tools in rhinology EAACI position paper. *Clin Transl Allergy* 2011; 1(1): 2.

190. Senti G, Crameri R, Kuster D et al. Intralymphatic immunotherapy for cat allergy induces tolerance after only 3 injections. *J Allergy Clin Immunol* 2012; 129(5): 1290–1296.

191. Creticos PS, Marsh DG, Proud D et al. Responses to ragweed-pollen nasal challenge before and after immunotherapy. *J Allergy Clin Immunol* 1989; 84(2): 197–205.

192. Scadding GW, Calderon MA, Bellido V et al. Optimisation of grass pollen nasal allergen challenge for assessment of clinical and immunological outcomes. *J Immunol Methods* 2012; 384(1–2): 25–32.

193. Scadding GW, Eifan A, Penagos M et al. Local and systemic effects of cat allergen nasal provocation. *Clin Exp Allergy* 2015; 45(3): 613–623.

194. Rosner-Friese K, Kaul S, Vieths S, Pfaar O. Environmental exposure chambers in allergen immunotherapy trials: Current status and clinical validation needs. *J Allergy Clin Immunol* 2015; 135(3): 636–643.

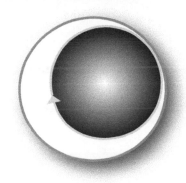

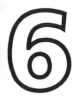 *In vivo* testing

Richard W. Weber
National Jewish Health

CONTENTS

6.1 INTRODUCTION

Diagnosis of allergic disorders, as with any other medical condition, relies primarily on the historical determination of the timing, duration, and triggering factors associated with the disorder. After making the history-based presumptive diagnosis, the healthcare professional will rely on a bioassay to collaborate the diagnosis. This may be useful when there is uncertainty about the primary trigger, and which other factors are less relevant confounders. In diagnosing certain allergic diseases, the issue becomes whether an *in vivo* test is preferable to an *in vitro* test. Historically, allergen skin tests were thought to be less costly, therefore providing a rationale for more extensive testing, as well as being more sensitive than the first-generation radioallergosorbent test (RAST) [1]. However, newer assays have closed the sensitivity gap. The strengths and weaknesses of *in vitro* allergen testing are discussed in Chapter 7.

6.2 IMMEDIATE HYPERSENSITIVITY CONJUNCTIVAL TESTING

Research on allergic diseases or IgE hypersensitivity performed early in the 1900s utilized the conjunctival test to assess the degree of sensitivity and response to therapy. The advantage and practicality

of using the skin versus the conjunctival test to determine clinical hypersensitivity became apparent: the introduction of miniscule amounts of allergen via a prick or puncture into the superficial layers of the epidermis resulted in a wheal surrounded by erythema, which was also called the flare. The reaction was easier to quantify than was conjunctival injection. However, the conjunctival challenge has seen a resurgence of popularity recently, especially in certain circumstances such as food hypersensitivity. In polysensitized individuals, it may clarify which allergen is responsible for symptoms, and in food allergic patients it may be a safer alternative to oral challenge [2,3]. Nonreactivity to conjunctival provocation tests after 4 weeks of sublingual immunotherapy was a good predictor of successful outcome [4]. The European Academy of Allergy and Clinical Immunology (EAACI) published a position paper providing guidelines for use of conjunctival allergen provocative testing in clinical practice [5].

6.3 IMMEDIATE HYPERSENSITIVITY SKIN TESTING

Those interested in the early history of "scratch" and a variety of different epicutaneous and intracutaneous skin testing may find descriptions of these tests in an older allergy textbook [6].

Table 6.1 Timing of cutaneous reactions [7]

Substance	Peak wheal (minutes)	Wheal duration (minutes)
Histamine	8–9	15
Compound 48/80	10–12	24–25
Allergen immediate	12–15	>30
Allergen late	180–360	360–720

Morphologically, a positive skin reaction to an allergen is similar to a positive skin test response to histamine. While other vasoactive substances are released with cutaneous mast cell degranulation associated with a positive skin test, the important role of histamine in the wheal and flare formation is supported by marked inhibition with the prior administration of antihistamines. Degrees of suppression of whealing range from 30% to 90%, depending on the relative potency of the antihistamine [7–9]. As delineated in Table 6.1, timing of the formation of the wheal differs among histamine, allergen, and pharmacologic mast cell degranulators such as surfactants or opiates. The histamine wheal size will peak in 8–10 minutes and resolve over the next 15 minutes. Allergen-induced wheals develop more slowly, peaking between 12 and 17 minutes and persisting much longer, taking over 30 minutes to resolve. Degranulating agents such as compound 48/80 or opiates peak in an intermediate time, 10–12 minutes, and persist for at least 20 minutes [7]. Diminution of the flare response usually indicates the presence of an inhibiting medication. Such a presence is routinely looked for by the placement of a histamine prick test. Variable concentrations of histamine have been used. Shtessel and Tversky have shown that suppression is less likely if a stronger versus a weaker concentration of histamine (1 versus 6 mg/mL) is used [10]. Following a large allergen-induced wheal and flare, some sensitive persons will develop late-phase cutaneous responses. These are characterized by a large, more diffuse induration of the skin test site that persists for 6–12 hours; it is entirely IgE mediated and does not involve IgG, as in the Arthus reaction [11].

The size of the wheal and flare is determined in part by the location of the test site. On the forearm, the volar surface is more sensitive than the dorsal, whereas the skin of the antecubital fossa is more sensitive than is the skin above the wrist. The back is more sensitive than the forearm, with allergen-induced reactions more prominent than histamine reactions: these observations may be due to differences in cutaneous mast cell density in one location versus the other [7,12]. Many practitioners have utilized a simple categorical 0–4+ ranking to record results. This method to record skin test results may not be uniform from one practice to another. If the categorical recording is used, the specific criteria for each category should be specified on the clinical report. The ideal technique is to outline the wheal and the flare with a pen and then perform a scotch-tape transfer onto a recording sheet. Although not practical for clinical practice, a computerized planimeter could be used to establish the exact surface area of the wheal and flare. Less desirable is to measure the longest diameter and the largest orthogonal diameter and record results in millimeters (see Figure 6.1a). Similar measurements can also be recorded for the flare [13].

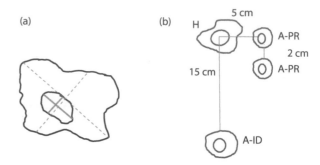

Figure 6.1 (a) Measurement of wheal and flare in millimeters: solid lines are longest wheal diameter and the orthogonal; dashed lines are longest flare diameter and the orthogonal. (b) Suggested distances between skin test sites to minimize false-positive reactions. (A-ID, allergen intradermal skin test site; A-PR, allergen prick skin test site; H, histamine positive control site.)

6.3.1 Epicutaneous allergen skin testing

Although previously referred to as a "scratch" test, this technique is more properly referred to as a "prick" or "puncture" skin test. Producing a scratch across the skin with a sharp instrument and applying a droplet of allergen extract at some point in its length produces variable results. Various applicators are used today for the prick or puncture tests. With the prick test, the instrument is dipped into the testing extract and the skin pricked. An alternative is to place a droplet of allergen extract on the skin, introduce the sharp point of the instrument through the droplet into the superficial epidermis at a 30°–45° angle, and then lift slightly (Figure 6.2). With proper technique, a very tiny portion of skin is elevated introducing approximately 3 μL of the testing extract [13]. This technique is attributed to Pepys, who used a small-gauge hypodermic needle. Modification of this technique became the current standard of care

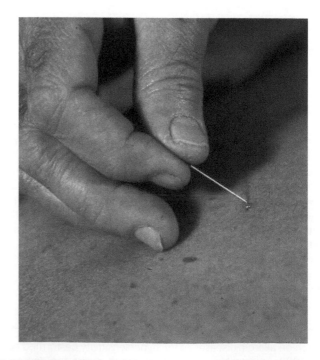

Figure 6.2 Prick test technique using a straight surgical needle.

[14]. Prick testing requires some training and repetition to master the technique and is more difficult to perform reproducibly than is the puncture method. In the puncture method, the instrument is held perpendicular to the skin and pressed through the droplet of extract into the epidermis. Several devices specifically designed for puncture testing have a short spike with a shoulder to prevent the tip from penetrating too deeply. Some devices also have the specific allergen extracts on the tip, eliminating the need to place a drop on the skin.

Numerous instruments are used for either prick or puncture skin testing: metal straight surgical needles, bifurcated smallpox needles, lancets, or bent needles; plastic rods with single spike points, bifurcated tips, or sawtooth circular edges; and multiheaded devices so that several tests can be applied simultaneously. Numerous comparative studies have been reported, since new devices are frequently introduced onto the market [15–20]. In general, single devices are superior to multiheaded devices in terms of precision, as determined by coefficient of variance, sensitivity, and patient acceptability. Multiheaded devices show greater intradevice variability, are more painful, result in more false positives, and tend to result in larger reactions than single devices (5 mm versus 3 mm) [15,19]. Zarei and colleagues evaluated a Greer Dermapik for prick skin testing in cat-allergic patients, using *in vitro* testing and nasal provocative challenge to establish true positivity [21]. Utilizing receiver operating characteristic (ROC) curves, a typical 3 mm wheal definition of positivity overestimated cat allergy, and a 6 mm wheal cutoff reliably distinguished those who were cat allergic from those who were not. The manufacturers of some puncture devices, which have a serrated edge at the end of the rod, recommend a twisting motion as well as downward pressure when doing the test. This form of testing is less than desirable since the twisting of the sawtoothed edges creates greater trauma, increasing the likelihood of false-positive results [18].

The reproducibility of prick skin tests is good. Almost 600 schoolchildren had prick tests to birch, grass, *Dermatophagoides pteronyssinus* dust mite, and cat performed three times at 11-month intervals [22]. The positive predictive value for continued positive tests ranged between 75.3% and 88.2%. The incidence of new positivity ranged between 3.2% and 4.3%.

6.3.2 Intracutaneous allergen skin testing

Intracutaneous or intradermal skin testing is performed using a small-gauge needle. Its advantages over epicutaneous testing are increased sensitivity and better reproducibility, especially if performed as recommended by the Committee on Standardization of the American College of Allergy, Asthma and Immunology [7,13]. A 0.1cc glass syringe with a 30-gauge needle with a metal plunger was used. It was held almost flat at 10° to the skin surface, bevel up. As soon as the opening of the needle disappeared into the skin, 0.02 mL of extract was injected and the needle then withdrawn. Ideally, this should result in approximately a 3 mm skin bleb. It is doubtful today that these recommendations are followed precisely by practitioners who perform such tests. In general, a disposable 1.0cc tuberculin-type plastic syringe is used with a half-inch 27-gauge needle. Comparative testing in the same individual shows that to obtain the same size wheal and flare as occurs with intracutaneous testing, a prick test using a 1000-fold greater concentration is necessary [23]. In comparison to the prick skin test,

the older technique of the scratch test, which introduced a greater amount of allergen extract into the epidermis, required 30- to 500-fold greater concentration of allergen to achieve a similar size wheal and flare to the intracutaneous skin test [6].

With greater sensitivity comes the risk of irrelevant or false positives. Curran and Goldman showed in a study of 100 individuals with no personal or family history of atopy that 5% reacted to scratch tests, while 9% reacted to intradermal tests [24]. Similarly, Lindblad and Farr showed that pollen extract intradermals using a concentration of 0.1 mg nitrogen/mL resulted in 35% positivity in 100 nonallergic and nonasthmatic subjects [25]. Six percent of glycerin in saline also resulted in a 16% false-positive rate. A dust extract without glycerin demonstrated a 50% positivity rate. However, at least 5% of this asymptomatic group had specific IgE demonstrated by the Prausnitz-Küstner passive transfer test. Nelson and colleagues demonstrated that the presence of a positive intradermal skin test in the face of a negative prick test was not associated with clinical symptomatology in a grass pollen nasal challenge study [26]. A position paper of the EAACI states that for potent pollen extracts, prick or puncture testing alone is indicated, and that intradermal testing for these extracts is not warranted [27]. Similarly, Wood and coworkers found that intradermal testing added little to the efficiency of prick skin testing and RAST testing to diagnose cat allergy [28]. While not documented, it is possible that intracutaneous testing may play a role in determining sensitivity in allergic individuals to less potent pollen, fungal, and epidermal extracts. The role of intracutaneous testing in *Hymenoptera* sensitivity and certain antibiotics, however, is established, where several concentration titrations are commonly used to determine the degree of sensitivity [29].

6.3.3 Confounding factors

Factors which may falsely augment or diminish skin test reactivity are listed in Table 6.2. Several reasons for false positive skin tests already have been discussed and include: a too concentrated intracutaneous extract; a too concentrated extract with additives such as glycerin; and use of an applicator device associated with traumatic, irritant reactions. A large reaction, whether to an allergen or to the positive histamine control, will increase the size of an adjacent skin test, presumably through the histamine "axon reflex" which causes substance P release with resultant vasodilatation (see Figure 6.3). Therefore, Voorhorst recommends that tests be applied at least 5 cm apart [7]. It is unclear from his discussion whether he felt this distance was necessary for prick, intradermal, or both types of skin tests. Tipton convincingly demonstrated that *Hymenoptera* venom intradermal tests placed on the upper arm could be falsely increased in size on the ipsilateral side by the histamine control when compared to intradermal tests of the same concentrations on the contralateral upper arm [30]. This occurred in spite of the fact that histamine control was at least 15 cm from the venom skin test site, suggesting that the histamine control should be placed a greater distance from intradermal skin tests. A distance of at least 2 cm between allergen prick tests, however, appears to be adequate based on data from Nelson and coworkers (see Figure 6.1b) [12].

Skin test reactivity to seasonal allergens fluctuates throughout the year. Reactivity to ragweed, elm, and Rocky Mountain juniper is greatest in October and remains unchanged to February, while histamine reactivity is greatest in October but decreases in other

Table 6.2 Confounding factors in allergen skin testing

Factor	Effect	Comment	Reference
High concentration	FP	Intracutaneous	[24,25]
Irritant additives	FP	Intracutaneous	[25]
Serrated puncture device	FP	5 mm positive rather 3 mm	[18]
Distance	FP	Histamine proximity to allergen: <5 cm to prick site and <15 cm to intradermal site	[7,13,30]
Season	+/–	Allergen reactivity increased postseason	[31]
Circadian rhythm	+/–	Conflicting reports of minor effects	[32,33]
Age	+/–	Decreased reactivity at extremes of age	[34–36]
Medication	FN	Antihistamine decreased immediate skin response, with differing effect on late-phase response; short-term corticosteroids have no effects on immediate reactivity, long-term corticosteroids diminish the response to mast cell degranulating agents	[7–9,37–41]
Commercial extracts	FN	Compared to fresh food extracts, commercial extracts may give negative results in evaluation of oral allergy syndrome	[42,43]

Abbreviations: +/–, equivocal; FN, false negative; FP, false positive.

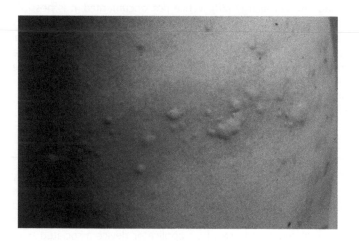

Figure 6.3 False-positive prick skin tests in a dermatomic distribution in response to a large medial wheal and flare.

seasons. Dust mite and cat sensitivity peaks in February [31]. To explain these results, the authors postulate a nonspecific priming effect, or a circannual rhythm unrelated to pollen exposure [31]. Skin test reactivity was reported in the 1960s to fluctuate with a circadian rhythm, and this was replicated in 1977 [32]. A study of 11 subjects shows that greater sensitivity occurs between 7 p.m. and 11 p.m., with the least sensitivity present at 7 a.m. Peaks for histamine, house dust, and grass pollens were all twice as great as the trough results. In 1989, another study performed with 20 adults and 20 children failed to reproduce these results [33]. The 8 a.m. and 4 p.m. duplicate testing with fivefold serial dilutions to ragweed and histamine revealed only a trend to larger morning means, without significant differences. The authors conclude that any circadian fluctuation was unlikely to produce meaningful differences during typical clinic hours.

The age of the subject also impacts both histamine and allergen responsiveness. Skin testing to common allergens in 331 subjects, drawn from a larger general population study, reveals that peak prevalence occurs in the 20- to 34-year-old age group and decreases with increasing age, somewhat mirroring the fall in total IgE levels associated with age [34]. Although total IgE was highest in the 9- to 19-year-old age group, the histamine responsiveness was lower in this age group, and allergen skin test positivity was mid-range between the other age groups. Seventy-eight infants from birth to age 24 months were compared to 30 adults with skin prick tests to histamine, codeine, and allergen extracts. Hyporesponsiveness to both histamine and codeine was found with infants, especially those under 6 months of age [35]. Positive allergen prick tests were present in some infants with a suggestive allergic history but tended to be in the 2–5 mm range. The same group assessed skin test reactivity using threefold dilutions of histamine in 365 subjects, ages 1–85 years [36]. Mean wheal size increased gradually throughout childhood, achieving a plateau between 15 and 50 years of age and then declining to a lower plateau after age 60 years.

The impact of antihistamines on immediate allergen skin test results has already been discussed [7–10]. The effect of histamine on the late-phase response is less clear. Bierman and associates found no inhibition of the late response by astemizole, a very potent less-sedating antihistamine that is no longer on the U.S. market [37]. Likewise, Zweiman and colleagues found cetirizine had no impact on either the gross appearance or the cellular infiltrate of the late-phase response [38]. However, Charlesworth and coworkers demonstrated that cetirizine causes a late 50% suppression of prostaglandin D2 production and a 75% reduction in eosinophil infiltration [39].

Short courses of oral corticosteroids, such as methylprednisolone for 1 week, do not suppress allergen, histamine, or compound 48/80 wheal sizes [40]. Long-term oral corticosteroids have a differential effect. In an age-matched controlled study, corticosteroids did not affect the histamine mean wheal diameters but did significantly decrease the size of codeine-induced wheal [41]. It is postulated that the vascular dilatory response to histamine is not affected but that cutaneous mast cells are either decreased in number or have suppressed releasability with prolonged corticosteroid therapy.

False-negative tests to commercial food skin testing extracts may occur in the evaluation of oral allergy syndrome (OAS), also termed pollen food syndrome. Ortolani and colleagues demonstrated that skin testing with fresh foods was preferable when testing with several fruits and vegetables in OAS [42]. Testing with fresh foods may utilize prick-prick/puncture-puncture testing, i.e., pricking the raw food with a test instrument and then pricking/puncturing the skin of the test subject with the same instrument. Alternatively, although less commonly, fresh food extracts are prepared by mixing the fresh food with a buffer and then removing the particulate before using as a test reagent. Rosen and associates also reported false-negative tests results to commercial food versus fresh food extracts, not only with OAS but in some cases of anaphylaxis [43]. These authors also commented that a large number of their patients who responded only to a fresh food extract did not respond to commercial extracts of peanut, walnut, Brazil nut, milk, egg, tuna, shrimp, and scallop, all of which are traditionally felt to contain nonlabile allergens. This report suggests that it is not appropriate to be completely confident with negative results with commercial extracts, especially when there is a history suggestive of clinical sensitivity.

6.3.4 Potency and standardized extracts in skin testing

The strength of allergen extracts used for *in vivo* tests depends on several factors: nature of the allergen source, extraction procedures, and storage conditions following extraction. Crude pollen extracts are mixtures of numerous allergenic and nonallergenic substances, and the relative concentrations of allergens will make some inherently more potent than others. Soil, climate, rainfall, as well as time and site of collection all affect relative potency. Preparation of extracts and standardization protocols for the United States and Europe are reviewed in Section III, Chapters 21–25, of this text .

The advent of commercially available, U.S. Food and Drug Administration (FDA)-approved, standardized extracts in the United States propelled studies to compare these to conventional weight/volume extractions. Adinoff and colleagues found that using a greater than 3 mm wheal as a positive result, cat prick tests with standardized extracts had a sensitivity of 0.90, a specificity of 0.90, and a diagnostic accuracy of 0.90 when compared to the history [44]. House dust mites, *Dermatophagoides pteronyssinus* and *Dermatophagoides farinae*, in standardized concentrations of 10,000 AU/mL resulted in positive skin tests in nonallergic subjects in 17% and 12%, respectively. The authors conclude that while cat and pollen standardized extract concentrations are suitable for diagnosis, perhaps full-strength house dust mite extracts were too potent for diagnostic skin testing [44]. Lavins and associates compared standardized extracts of white oak, timothy, Bermuda, Russian thistle, short ragweed, sagebrush, *Alternaria*, and cat with conventional weight/volume counterparts [45]. The standardized extracts were either FDA-approved or in-house standardized extracts by the extract manufacturer. The standardized extracts were tested in dilutions of 100,000, 10,000, and 1000 AU/mL. Conventional extracts were 1:10 or 1:20 w/v. The conventional wheal and flare area results, measured by computerized planimetry, generally fell between the 10,000 and 100,000 AU/mL concentration using the standardized extracts. When using a categorical ranking (0–4+), there are no differences in the number of 3+ or 4+ reactions between conventional and standardized extracts.

There is no consensus on the appropriate number of skin tests, either prick or intracutaneous, needed for the evaluation of uncomplicated allergic rhinitis. Constraints, however, may be placed by governmental regulatory agencies and by private medical insurance payers. The availability of specific allergen extracts for diagnosis and/or treatment may also be affected by the balance between production costs and clinical need. A report from Central China in 2017 suggested that testing with eight allergens (*Dermatophagoides pteronyssinus*, *D. farinae*, *Platanus*, *Artemisia*, *Cryptomeria*, *Blatella germanica*, *Humulus*, and *Alternaria*) was sufficient in identifying over 99% of sensitized patients [46]. A position paper from EAACI in 2018 recommended that in order to ensure the availability of high-quality allergen extracts, it would be necessary to establish active partnerships between manufacturers, appropriate scientific societies, consumer groups, and governmental authorities [47].

6.4 PROVOCATIVE ALLERGEN TESTING

Provocative allergen challenges, conjunctival, nasal, or bronchial, are utilized to confirm clinical diagnoses or to define the pathophysiology of immediate, delayed, and dual responses. Spector and Farr delineated indications for inhalation challenges that are listed in Table 6.3 [48]. Pepys and colleagues performed extensive challenges on a variety of agents including drugs, metals and other occupational substances, dust mites, molds, and pollens [49]. They characterized the timing of the onset, duration of the reactions, and response to appropriate treatment. The literature on bronchial challenge is extensive, and a review of this literature is beyond the scope of this chapter. However, there are aspects that need to be addressed.

6.4.1 Bronchial allergen provocation

Pepys demonstrated that a single inhalant allergen challenge resulting in both an immediate and delayed response could be attended by sequential nocturnal worsening of asthma for several nights [49]. Cockcroft and coworkers determined that nonspecific bronchial hyperreactivity, as determined by histamine inhalation, could be increased for up to a week following a single allergen challenge [50]. Further studies reveal that this increase in nonspecific reactivity occurs only in asthmatics with a late-phase response [51]. Additionally, the increase in histamine responsiveness did not occur

Table 6.3 Indications for allergen inhalation challenge [48]

1. Elucidation of the role of specific allergens in asthma
2. Means of comparison for other tests such as skin tests, *in vitro* tests, or new diagnostic methods
3. When skin tests cannot be performed
4. Evaluation of therapeutic effect of immunotherapy
5. Evaluation of new or specific allergens in pulmonary disease
6. Evaluation of treatment modalities and blocking agents
7. Convince the patient of cause-and-effect relationships

until the subject had experienced a late-phase reaction. Segmental bronchial allergen challenge in subjects with ragweed allergic rhinitis followed by bronchoalveolar lavage (BAL) 48 hours later reveals the pathophysiology of the late response [52]. Immediately after the ragweed instillation, there is an increase in histamine and tryptase, but no cellular infiltration. Forty-eight hours later, BAL shows large numbers of intact and degranulated eosinophils, as well as increased levels of major basic protein, eosinophil-derived neurotoxin, eosinophil cationic protein, and eosinophil peroxidase. Additionally, leukotriene C4 and IL-5, but not tryptase, are elevated. Similar to what is found with a nasal challenge, it appears that the immediate phase bronchial reaction is driven by mast cell degranulation, and that release of chemoattractants recruits inflammatory cells such as eosinophils to the site with subsequent degranulation and a more marked inflammatory response.

As pointed out by Spector and Farr, bronchial provocation may be necessary when skin tests cannot be performed, or to evaluate the effectiveness of therapeutic interventions [48]. However, Cockcroft and coworkers also showed that there is good correlation between cutaneous sensitivity to a tested allergen and the allergen PC_{20}, the provocative concentration of allergen necessary to induce a 20% drop in the FEV_1 [53]. Using multiple linear regression analysis, there was a high correlation between allergen PC_{20}, as a function of histamine PC_{20}, and cutaneous sensitivity to an allergen extract. Therefore, under typical conditions, the response to allergen bronchoprovocation can be predicted simply by knowing the degree of nonspecific bronchial hyperreactivity and the intensity of the skin test response to the allergen. This suggests that allergen bronchoprovocation is rarely necessary in clinical practice, with the exception of evaluating occupational respiratory disease, especially when the exact allergen inducing the disease may not be known or an appropriate skin test extract is not available (see Table 6.2). EAACI published a position paper in 2015 delineating indications and contraindications for bronchial, nasal, and conjunctival allergen provocation tests [2]. Additionally, the paper discussed advantages and disadvantages of using allergen challenge chambers.

6.4.2 Nasal allergen provocation

Nasal allergen provocation also is most often used as a research tool to document clinical relevance of sensitization or response to a therapeutic intervention. Extensive work on the immediate and late-phase nasal responses to both allergen and nonspecific irritants, such as cold air, was performed by a large research team at Johns Hopkins University, Maryland [55,56]. Their work elucidated the pathophysiology of the immediate phase response to allergen with recruitment of inflammatory cells and the differential cellular responses to the early and late-phase responses. As summarized by Walden and colleagues, nasal lavage after instillation of ragweed pollen in sensitized subjects demonstrates the immediate release of histamine, prostaglandin D_2 (PGD_2), kinins, and esterases, which was associated with increased sneezing [56]. Nine of 12 subjects had recurrence of symptoms 3–11 hours later after the initial single challenge. This was associated with an increase in histamine, kinins, and esterases, but not PGD_2. Since mast cells but not basophils produce PGD_2, these results support the fact that mast cells are crucial in the initial reaction but that the late-phase response is due to the influx of basophils and not the reactivation of mast

cells. Togias and coworkers also showed that even nonspecific irritants such as a cold air challenge resulted in a similar pattern of early and late-phase release of mediators [55]. The authors postulate that the cold air nasal challenge is analogous to the bronchial exercise challenge. The same group also demonstrated that topical corticosteroids attenuate the late-phase nasal response. In addition to assessing nasal lavage constituents, changes in nasal congestion can be monitored by peak nasal inspiratory flow [57].

Rondón and associates utilized nasal challenge with a battery of multiple allergens to evaluate presumed nonallergic rhinitis [58]. Patients were identified with suggestive histories, negative skin prick and serum-specific IgE tests, and reaction to nasal challenge [59]. The mechanism for this phenomenon is thought to be localized production of mucosal specific IgE as first reported by Huggins and Brostoff [60]. Rondón and coworkers demonstrated that simultaneous challenge with multiple allergen mixes was concordant with single allergen challenge [58]. Meta-analysis by Hamizan and colleagues of 46 studies concluded that local allergen sensitivity occurs in over 26% of patients initially considered nonallergic [61]. An EAACI position paper on standardization of nasal allergen challenges published in 2018 delineated indications and contraindications for challenge, techniques of exposure and assessment of results, as well as the risks of false-positive and false-negative outcomes [62]. In 2018, Pepper and Ledford reviewed aspects of nasal and ocular challenges, commenting that despite direct allergen challenges exposing subjects to higher than natural exposures, they are still helpful clinical and research tools [63]. Gotlib and associates commented on the asymmetric response to bilateral nasal allergen provocation and found that this was independent of the nasal cycle [64].

Nasal provocative challenge can also be used to assess the impact of nasal allergen exposure on adjacent structures. Rhinomanometry can be used to measure the degree of nasal obstruction. Evaluation of concomitant eustachian tube obstruction also can be done by sonotubometry, which measures the transmission of sound from the nares, posterior pharynx, through the eustachian tube into the ear [65]. Tympanic membrane motility can likewise be measured following challenge.

6.5 DELAYED HYPERSENSITIVITY SKIN TESTING

6.5.1 Patch testing

It is common to refer to antigens used for patch testing as allergens. However, this is erroneous since the term *allergen* usually is restricted to an immunogen that induces IgE. Allergic contact dermatitis is generally accepted to be secondary to a cellular immune injury mechanism, also referred to as Gell and Coombs type IV reaction. Delayed hypersensitivity patch testing is the preferred diagnostic assay. Batteries of small squares impregnated with validated concentrations of "contactants" are placed on normal skin (usually the back). They are removed 48–72 hours later, evaluated, and finally also interpreted 24–48 hours after removal [66]. Later time points may occasionally be used to determine a positive reaction, especially with metal hypersensitivity. The number of agents used for testing depends on regional differences. Total numbers may range from 28 items in the standardized European battery to over 70 in the North American Contact Dermatitis Group (NACDG) [66,67]. Typical screening patch testing in the United States utilizes a battery that was expanded from 24 to 36 items in 2013. However, the use of the shorter screening battery can miss up to a quarter of reactors induced by the 70-item panel, and an even larger panel can pick up additional reactions [67]. Regional differences are also seen in the selection of routine agents to be tested [68]. Individual agents suspected by history can be tested separately using small discs, such as Finn chambers (SmartPractice). Since these test materials are nonstandardized, there is a risk that an inappropriately strong concentration of the alleged contactant may result in a false-positive, irritant reaction. Duarte and colleagues repeated patch testing in 49 patients within an interval of 1–5 years [69]. They found that for moderate and strongly positive tests, positivity was maintained in 86% and 100%, respectively. Weak positives were negative on repeat testing in 65%, which suggests that weak positive results may not be reliable.

Patch testing has been investigated for a variety of clinical conditions including irritable bowel syndrome, eosinophilic enteropathies, and chronic idiopathic urticaria [70,71]. It is unclear and controversial whether delayed hypersensitivity testing is of value in these conditions.

Contact urticaria is defined as whealing, erythema, and pruritus developing within minutes after cutaneous or mucosal contact with the causative agent, usually clearing completely within 24 hours [72]. In distinction to delayed hypersensitivity reactions, these reactions are presumably IgE mediated. Raw foods are commonly incriminated, although similar reactions to chemicals, such as dyes in clothing, also can occur [73]. Patch testing may be negative or result in slow development of a wheal, whereas prick testing is frequently positive [74].

In a study of chronic summer prurigo in French children, 52% had a positive prick skin test to mosquito at 48 hours, compared to 7% positivity at 20 minutes [54]. In children with perennial prurigo, patch tests to *Dermatophagoides pteronyssinus* and *D. farinae* were positive at 48 hours in 45% and 40%, respectively.

6.6 CONCLUSION

In vivo testing to document allergic disease has a long history and remains valid in the present. Epicutaneous skin testing, whether done by a prick or puncture technique, is validated as reproducible and with good sensitivity, specificity, and accuracy. Intracutaneous (or intradermal) testing has good reproducibility and sensitivity, but due to that greater sensitivity, the likelihood of clinical irrelevance also is greater. With potent pollen extracts or standardized allergen extracts, intradermal positivity in the face of epicutaneous test negativity is unlikely to correlate with the clinical history or provocative challenge results. With allergen extracts that are less potent or less characterized, intradermal skin testing may have utility, though this is not delineated. Commercially available, standardized, allergen extracts do not produce skin test results appreciably different than conventional extracts. Thus, it is not necessary to adjust the assessment of what constitutes a meaningful response. The value of standardized extracts lies in the assurance that potency is consistent. Standardized house dust mite extracts should be tested at concentrations of 5000 AU/mL rather than 10,000 AU/mL.

Varying cutaneous regions of the body have differing sensitivity to histamine, allergens, and other mast cell degranulators. The placement of positive controls, like histamine, may affect the size of adjacent allergen test sites. This effect is greater for intradermal than for epicutaneous tests. Recommendations are that prick tests should be at least 5 cm and intradermal tests at least 15 cm from the positive control. Likewise, the distance between adjacent epicutaneous tests should be at least 2 cm, realizing that this distance is practical, but a large reaction may still falsely augment the size of adjacent tests. Negative confounders include concomitant medications, such as antihistamines or long-term topical or systemic corticosteroids, and extremes of age. The use of fresh food skin tests compared to only using commercial extracts decreases the likelihood of false-negative results when assessing oral allergy syndrome. Skin reactivity variation related to circadian rhythms or seasonality has little practical impact.

Nasal and bronchial allergen challenge studies are crucial to elucidate the pathophysiology of the immediate and late-phase allergic reactions. The timing of mediator increase and decrease delineates the role of resident and recruited cell types. With the exception of the evaluation of occupational exposures, allergen provocation challenges are primarily research tools but may have clinical utility, and following published guidelines, may be utilized in the clinical setting.

Delayed hypersensitivity skin testing, also known as patch testing, is the preferred method to evaluate contact dermatitis. It distinguishes true antigen-mediated allergic contact dermatitis from irritant dermatitis. Batteries of contactants whose concentrations are standardized and validated are placed simultaneously, removed after 48 hours, and evaluated immediately and 24–48 hours after removal. Occasionally, results may be evaluated at later time points as well, which may be more likely in assessing metal hypersensitivity. The larger the testing battery, the greater is the number of positive results found.

In vivo allergen testing continues to play a central role in the diagnosis of immediate and delayed hypersensitivity. In some cases, it merely supports the clinical impression derived from the clinical history. However, in some situations, the testing is crucial for the delineation of the causative agent.

SALIENT POINTS

- IgE-mediated inhalant, food, venom, and some antibiotic-induced allergic diseases can be confirmed with sensitivity, specificity, and accuracy utilizing epicutaneous and intracutaneous skin test techniques.
- Prick and puncture techniques with a variety of devices are reproducible methods to perform epicutaneous skin testing, while a tuberculin-type plastic syringe with ½-inch 27-gauge needle is commonly used for intracutaneous skin testing.
- Prick or puncture skin testing is all that is required for standardized allergen extracts and potent pollen extracts. In the face of negative epicutaneous testing, positive intradermal testing is not necessarily relevant to the clinical history, as demonstrated with grass and cat allergens.
- Epicutaneous skin tests should be placed at least 2 cm apart to avoid false-positive reactions due to adjacent large reactions.
- Histamine-positive controls should be at least 5 cm from adjacent epicutaneous tests and at least 15 cm from intradermal tests to avoid false positives.

- False-negative epicutaneous tests may occur, especially in evaluating oral allergy syndrome, if fresh food extracts are not utilized.
- Skin reactivity to both allergens and positive controls is diminished but not absent in infancy. Likewise, the skin is less reactive in the elderly.
- Nasal and bronchial allergen challenges have limited relevance in clinical practice and are primarily research modalities. The exceptions are their usefulness in assessing occupational allergy and "local mucosal allergy."
- Late-phase, IgE-dependent reactions, whether in the skin, nose, or bronchi, are due to the recruitment of inflammatory effector cells initiated by the release of cytokines and chemokines during the immediate allergic response.
- Delayed hypersensitivity skin testing (patch testing) with standardized and validated concentrations of contactants is the preferred technique to evaluate allergic contact dermatitis; the larger the battery, the more reactants are discovered.

REFERENCES

1. Norman PS, Lichtenstein LM, Ishizaka K. Diagnostic tests in ragweed hay fever. *J Allergy Clin Immunol* 1973; 52: 210–224.
2. Agache I, Bilò M, Braunstahl G-J et al. Position paper: *In vivo* diagnosis of allergic diseases—Allergen provocation tests. *Allergy* 2015; 70: 355–365.
3. Lindvik H, Lødrup Carlsen KC, Mowinckel P, Navaratnam J, Borres MP, Cerlsen KH. Conjunctival provocation test in diagnosis of peanut allergy in children. *Clin Exp Allergy* 2017; 47: 785–794.
4. Köther J, Mandl A, Allekotte S et al. Early nonreactivity in the conjunctival provocation test predicts beneficial outcome of sublingual immunotherapy. *Clin Transl Allergy* 2018; 8: 28–38.
5. Fauquert J-L, Jedrzejczak-Czechowicz M, Rondon C et al. Position paper: Conjunctival allergen provocation test: Guidelines for daily practice. *Allergy* 2017; 72: 43–54.
6. Walzer M, Thommen AA. Methods of testing for hypersensitiveness. In: Coca AF, Walzer M, Thommen AA, editors. *Asthma and Hay Fever in Theory and Practice.* Springfield, IL: Charles C. Thomas, 1931: 311–367.
7. Voorhorst R, van Krieken H. Atopic skin test reevaluated. I. Perfection of skin testing technique. *Ann Allergy* 1973; 31: 137–142.
8. Long WF, Taylor RJ, Wagner CJ et al. Skin test suppression by antihistamines and the development of subsensitivity. *J Allergy Clin Immunol* 1985; 76: 113–117.
9. Cook TJ, MacQueen DM, Wittig HJ et al. Degree and duration of skin test suppression and side effects with antihistamines: A double blind controlled study with five antihistamines. *J Allergy Clin Immunol* 1973; 51: 71–77.
10. Shtessel M, Tversky J. Reliability of allergy skin testing. *Ann Allergy Asthma Immunol* 2018; 120: 80–83.
11. Tipton WR. Evaluation of skin testing in the diagnosis of IgE-mediated disease. *Pediatr Clin N Amer* 1983; 30: 785–793.
12. Nelson HS, Knoerzer J, Bucher B. Effect of distance between sites and region of the body on results of skin prick tests. *J Allergy Clin Immunol* 1996; 97: 596–601.
13. Nelson HS. Diagnostic procedures in allergy. I. Allergy skin testing. *Ann Allergy* 1983; 51: 411–418.
14. Pepys J. Skin testing. *Br J Hosp Med* 1975; 14: 412–417.
15. Adinoff AD, Rosleniec DM, McCall LL et al. A comparison of six epicutaneous devices in the performance of immediate hypersensitivity skin testing. *J Allergy Clin Immunol* 1989; 84: 168–174.
16. Demoly P, Bousquet J, Manderscheid J-C et al. Precision of skin prick and puncture tests with nine methods. *J Allergy Clin Immunol* 1991; 88: 758–762.
17. Nelson HS, Rosloniec DM, McCall LL et al. Comparative performance of five commercial prick skin test devices. *J Allergy Clin Immunol* 1993; 92: 750–756.
18. Nelson HS, Laher J, Buchmeier A et al. Evaluation of devices for skin prick testing. *J Allergy Clin Immunol* 1998; 101: 153–156.
19. Carr WW, Martin B, Howard RS et al. Comparison of test devices for skin prick testing. *J Allergy Clin Immunol* 2005; 116: 341–346.
20. Masse MS, Granger Vallée A, Chiriac A et al. Comparison of five techniques of skin prick tests used routinely in Europe. *Allergy* 2011; 66: 1415–1419.
21. Zarei M, Remer CF, Kaplan MS et al. Optimal skin prick wheal size for diagnosis of cat allergy. *Ann Allergy Asthma Immunol* 2004; 92: 604–610.
22. Kuehr J, Karmaus W, Frischer T et al. Longitudinal variability of skin prick test results. *Clin Exp Allergy* 1992; 22: 839–844.
23. Indrajana T, Spieksma FT, Voorhorst R. Comparative study of the intracutaneous, scratch and prick tests in allergy. *Ann Allergy* 1971; 29: 639–650.
24. Curran WS, Goldman G. The incidence of immediately reacting allergy skin tests in a "normal" adult population. *Ann Int Med* 1961; 55: 777–783.
25. Lindblad JH, Farr RS. The incidence of positive intradermals reactions and demonstration of skin sensitizing antibody to extract of ragweed and dust in humans without history of rhinitis or asthma. *J Allergy* 1961; 32: 392–401.
26. Nelson HS, Oppenheimer J, Buchmeier A et al. An assessment of the role of intradermal skin testing in the diagnosis of clinically relevant allergy to timothy grass. *J Allergy Clin Immunol* 1996; 97: 1193–1201.
27. The European Academy of Allergology and Clinical Immunology. Position paper: Allergen standardization and skin test. *Allergy* 1993; 48(14 Suppl): 48–82.
28. Wood RA, Phipatanakul W, Hamilton RG et al. A comparison of skin prick tests, intradermal skin tests, and RASTs in the diagnosis of cat allergy. *J Allergy Clin Immunol* 1999; 103: 773–779.
29. Golden DBK. Diagnostic methods in insect allergy. In: Levine MI, Lockey RF, editors. *Monograph on Insect Allergy*, 4th ed. Pittsburgh: Dave Lambert Associates, 2003: 63–74.
30. Tipton WR. Influence of histamine controls on skin tests with Hymenoptera venom. *Ann Allergy* 1980; 44: 204–205.
31. Oppenheimer JJ, Nelson HS. Seasonal variation in immediate skin test reactions. *Ann Allergy* 1993; 71: 227–229.
32. Lee RE, Smolensky MH, Leach CS et al. Circadian rhythms in the cutaneous reactivity to histamine and selected antigens, including phase relationship to urinary cortisol excretion. *Ann Allergy* 1977; 38: 231–236.
33. Vichyanond P, Nelson HS. Circadian variation of skin reactivity and allergy skin test. *J Allergy Clin Immunol* 1989; 83: 1101–1106.
34. Barbee RA, Brown WG, Kaltenborn W et al. Allergen skin-test reactivity in a community population sample: Correlation with age, histamine skin reactions, and total serum immunoglobulin E. *J Allergy Clin Immunol* 1981; 68: 15–19.

35. Ménardo JL, Bousquet J, Rodière M et al. Skin test reactivity in infancy. *J Allergy Clin Immunol* 1985; 75: 646–651.

36. Skassa-Brociek W, Manderscheid J-C, Michel F-B et al. Skin test reactivity to histamine from infancy to old age. *J Allergy Clin Immunol* 1987; 80: 711–716.

37. Bierman CW, Maxwell D, Rytina E et al. Effect of H_1-receptor blockade on the late cutaneous reactions to antigen: A double-blind, controlled study. *J Allergy Clin Immunol* 1991; 87: 1013–1019.

38. Zweiman B, Atkins PC, Moskovitz A et al. Cellular inflammatory responses during immediate, developing, and established late-phase allergic cutaneous reactions: Effects of cetirizine. *J Allergy Clin Immunol* 1997; 100: 341–347.

39. Charlesworth EN, Kagey-Sobotka A, Norman PS et al. Effect of cetirizine on mast cell-mediator release and cellular traffic during the cutaneous late-phase reaction. *J Allergy Clin Immunol* 1989; 83: 905–912.

40. Slott RI, Zweiman B. A controlled study of the effect of corticosteroids on the immediate skin test reactivity. *J Allergy Clin Immunol* 1974; 54: 229–234.

41. Olson R, Karpink MH, Shelanski S et al. Skin reactivity to codeine and histamine during prolonged corticosteroid therapy. *J Allergy Clin Immunol* 1990; 86: 153–159.

42. Ortolani C, Ispano M, Pastorello EA et al. Comparison of results of skin prick tests (with fresh foods and commercial food extracts) and RAST in 100 patients with oral allergy syndrome. *J Allergy Clin Immunol* 1989; 83: 683–690.

43. Rosen JP, Selcow JE, Mendelson LM et al. Skin testing with natural foods in patients suspected of having food allergies: Is it a necessity? *J Allergy Clin Immunol* 1994; 93: 1068–1070.

44. Adinoff AD, Rosloniec DM, McCall LL et al. Immediate skin test reactivity to food and drug administration-approved standardized extracts. *J Allergy Clin Immunol* 1990; 86: 766–774.

45. Lavins BJ, Dolen WK, Nelson HS et al. Use of standardized and conventional allergen extracts in prick skin testing. *J Allergy Clin Immunol* 1992; 89: 658–666.

46. Wang J, Wu Y, Huang X, Zhu R. Eight aeroallergen skin test extracts may be the optimal panel for allergic rhinitis patients in Central China. *Int Arch Allergy Immunol* 2017; 173: 193–198.

47. Cardona V, Demoly P, Dreborg S et al. Position paper: Current practice of allergy diagnosis and the potential impact of regulation in Europe. *Allergy* 2018; 73: 323–327.

48. Spector S, Farr R. Bronchial inhalation challenge with antigens. *J Allergy Clin Immunol* 1979; 64: 580–586.

49. Pepys J, Hutchcroft BJ. Bronchial provocative tests in etiologic diagnosis and analysis of asthma. *Am Rev Respir Dis* 1975; 112: 829–859.

50. Cockcroft DW, Ruffine RE, Dolovich J et al. Allergen-induced increase in non-allergic bronchial reactivity. *Clin Allergy* 1977; 7: 503–513.

51. Cockcroft DW, Murdock KY. Changes in bronchial responsiveness to histamine at intervals after allergen challenge. *Thorax* 1987; 42: 302–308.

52. Sedgwick JB, Calhoun WJ, Gleich GJ et al. Immediate and late airway response of allergic rhinitis patients to segmental antigen challenge. *Am Rev Respir Dis* 1991; 144: 1274–1281.

53. Cockcroft DW, Ruffin RE, Frith PA et al. Determinants of allergen-induced asthma: Dose of allergen, circulating IgE antibody concentration, and bronchial responsiveness to inhaled histamine. *Am Rev Respir Dis* 1979; 120: 1053–1058.

54. Maridet C, Perromat M, Miquel J et al. Childhood chronic prurigo: Interest in patch tests and delayed-reading skin prick tests to environmental allergens. *J Allergy Clin Immunol* 2018; 141: 797–799.

55. Togias A, Naclerio RM, Proud D et al. Studies on the allergic and nonallergic nasal inflammation. *J Allergy Clin Immunol* 1988; 81: 782–790.

56. Walden SM, Proud D, Bascom R et al. Experimentally induced nasal allergic responses. *J Allergy Clin Immunol* 1988; 81: 940–949.

57. Boelke G, Berger U, Bergmann K-C et al. Peak nasal inspiratory flow as outcome for provocation studies in allergen exposure chambers: A GA²LEN study. *Clin Transl Allergy* 2017; 7: 33–43.

58. Rondón C, Campo P, Herrera R et al. Nasal allergen provocation test with multiple aeroallergens detects polysensitization in local allergic rhinitis. *J Allergy Clin Immunol* 2011; 128: 1192–1197.

59. Rondón C, Romero JJ, López S et al. Local IgE production and positive nasal provocative test in patients with persistent nonallergic rhinitis. *J Allergy Clin Immunol* 2007; 119: 899–905.

60. Huggins KG, Brostoff J. Local production of specific IgE antibodies in allergic rhinitis patients with negative skin tests. *Lancet* 1975; 2: 148–150.

61. Hamizan AW, Rimmer J, Alvarado R et al. Positive allergen reaction in allergic and nonallergic rhinitis: A systematic review. *Int Forum Allergy Rhinol* 2017; 7: 868–877.

62. Augé J, Vent J, Agache I et al. EAACI position paper on the standardization of nasal allergen challenges. *Allergy* 2018; 73: 1597–1608.

63. Pepper AN, Ledford DK. Nasal and ocular challenges. *J Allergy Clin Immunol* 2018; 141: 1570–1577.

64. Gotlib T, Samoliński B, Grzanka A. Effect of the nasal cycle on congestive response during bilateral nasal allergen provocation. *Ann Agric Environ Med* 2014; 21: 290–293.

65. Fireman P. Nasal provocative testing: An objective assessment for nasal and eustachean tube obstruction. *J Allergy Clin Immunol* 1988; 81: 953–960.

66. White JML. Patch testing: What allergists should know. *Clin Exp Allergy* 2011; 42: 180–185.

67. Warshaw EM, Belsito DV, Taylor JS et al. North American Contact Group patch test results: 2009–2010. *Dermatitis* 2013; 24: 50–59.

68. Chow ET, Avolio AM, Lee A et al. Frequency of positive patch test reactions to preservatives: The Australian experience. *Austalas J Dermatol* 2013; 54: 31–35.

69. Duarte I, Silva MdF, Malvestiti AA et al. Evaluation of the permanence of skin sensitization to allergens in patients with allergic contact dermatitis. *An Bras Dermatol* 2012; 87: 833–837.

70. Stierstorfer MB, Sha CT, Sasson M. Food patch testing for irritant bowel syndrome. *J Am Acad Dermatol* 2013; 68: 377–384.

71. Hession MT, Scheinman PL. The role of contact allergens in chronic idiopathic urticaria. *Dermatitis* 2012; 23: 110–116.

72. Wakelin SH. Contact urticaria. *Clin Exp Dermatol* 2001; 26: 132–136.

73. Davari P, Maibach HI. Contact urticaria to cosmetic and industrial dyes. *Clin Exp Dermatol* 2011; 36: 1–5.

74. Martínez de Lagrán Z, Ortiz de Frutos FJ, González de Arribas M et al. Contact urticaria to raw potato. *Dermatol Online J* 2009; 15: 14–16.

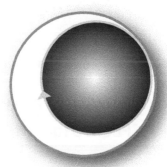

7 Serological (*in vitro*) and component testing methods in the diagnosis of human allergic disease

Robert G. Hamilton

Johns Hopkins University School of Medicine

CONTENTS

7.1 INTRODUCTION

The diagnosis of human allergic disease begins with a thorough clinical history and physical examination [1,2]. The probability for allergic disease, for example, IgE antibody-dependent immediate-type hypersensitivity, increases if the patient's history provides evidence that allergic symptoms have occurred in relationship to a known allergen exposure and there are objective signs of an allergic response based on a physical examination. However, the accuracy of the patient's history is not always reliable, because it depends on many factors, including their environment, demographics (e.g., age, family atopic history, social economic status), and the patient's ability to recognize symptoms. Thus, to confirm sensitization and verify the allergens that induce the alleged allergic response and facilitate management of the disease, a second level of the diagnostic algorithm guides clinicians to detect IgE antibody by either *in vivo* skin tests (see Chapter 6) or *in vitro* serological assays [3]. This chapter examines the current state of *in vitro* assays that are used to detect and quantify IgE antibodies in human serum. Extract-based allergosorbents are contrasted with newer reagents that use allergenic components. Assays are discussed for total serum IgE, mast cell tryptase, and precipitins that are less frequently performed but are useful to support the diagnosis and management of selected immunologic diseases. While the basophil mediator release, cell surface expression assays, and allergen-specific IgG/IgG4 assays rarely are used clinically, they are discussed in this chapter because of their extensive use in allergy research involving immunotherapy and in the documentation of an allergen extract's potency. Finally, inappropriate or unproven *in vitro* tests that are not useful in the diagnosis of human allergic disease are overviewed.

7.2 HISTORICAL EVOLUTION IN ALLERGEN-SPECIFIC IgE ANTIBODY ASSAYS

IgE was identified as the fifth human immunoglobulin isotype in 1967 [4,5]. By 1974, the first immunoassay for the detection of allergen-specific IgE antibody in human serum was introduced into clinical testing. The radioallergosorbent test (RAST) [6] involved the incubation of serum in individual test tubes with any of several hundred extracted allergens that were immobilized covalently onto cyanogen bromide-activated cellulose in the form of a paper disc. Following a buffer wash to remove unbound serum proteins, bound IgE antibody was detected with molar excess quantities of ^{125}I-labeled anti-human IgE. After a second buffer wash to remove unbound radiolabeled anti-IgE, the magnitude of the RAST's response (counts per minute bound) was detected in a gamma counter. The final assay response was shown to be proportional to the quantity of IgE bound and thus the quantity of allergen-specific IgE in the original serum. Measured levels of radioactivity were interpolated from an IgE anti-birch pollen reference serum dose response curve into arbitrary Phadebas relative units per milliliter or (PRU/mL).

While the general assay design of the RAST has withstood years of evolution, many diagnostic companies have produced allergen-specific IgE assays with different solid-phase matrices (plastic plates, microbeads, threads, nitrocellulose paper), coupling chemistries, labels (radioisotopes, enzymes, fluorophors), detection endpoints (counts per minute, colorimetry, fluorescence/luminescence intensity), calibration schemes, and reported units. One notable evolutionary event involved the Matrix by Abbott Laboratories [7]. In this assay, specific IgE was detected to a fixed number of immobilized airborne allergens ($n = 14$), and each was individually calibrated using a unique calibration serum. Experience with this assay led IgE antibody manufacturers to several conclusions that have shaped the design and general calibration system used in current state-of-the-art autoanalyzer-based assays. First, an assay like the Matrix that was designed to detect IgE antibody to a fixed panel involving only a limited number of aeroallergen specificities will not successfully compete with assays that are designed to detect IgE antibodies to over hundreds of clinically important aero-, food-, and injected-allergen specificities. Second, IgE antibody assays should not be designed so that each allergen specificity has its own unique calibration serum. This strategy of using a homologous reference serum for each allergen specificity, while consistent with the design of most clinically used immunoassays for drugs and hormones, is an impractical calibration strategy for IgE antibody assays. This strategy requires large quantities of serum from donor blood for each allergen specificity, which is often not available for most major and less prevalent IgE antibody specificities. Out of experience with the original RAST and Matrix was born the concept of interpolation of IgE antibody assay response levels from a heterologous (different) "universal" total serum IgE calibration curve that is traceable to a World Health Organization (WHO) IgE International Reference Preparation (IRP). Originally, the 75/502 IRP was used, but the current third IRP is the present reference reagent [3,8]. Use of heterologous interpolation of IgE antibody results from a total serum IgE "universal" calibration curve is technically permissible because solid-phase immunoassay technology allows test (allergen-specific IgE) and the heterologous (total IgE) calibrator portions of the assay to dilute out in parallel.

Current clinically used IgE antibody assays are performed using computer-controlled random access singleplex (individual allergen per analysis based) autoanalyzers that essentially eliminate intra-assay variability that can be associated with the technician and manual instrumentation. Automation also has led to more quantitative antibody measurements and remarkably consistent interlaboratory agreement for the methods that are performed in laboratories throughout the world [9]. Several manufacturers dominate the clinical IgE antibody market in North America: Thermofisher Scientific (previously Pharmacia/Phadia: ImmunoCAP) and Siemens Healthcare Diagnostics (Immulite). Hycor Biomedical is developing a new instrument called the NOVEOS that will replace their HyTech 288 and MCS EIA systems. These assays use a solid phase on which individual allergen extracts (and some component allergens) are immobilized (using different chemistries), an enzyme-labeled anti-IgE detection antibody (with different substrates and response measures), and interpolation of response data into antibody estimates from a total IgE calibration curve (with different adjustment schemes) in kilo units of allergen-specific IgE per liter (kUa/L). By 2008, the clinically reported analytical sensitivity of these IgE antibody autoanalyzers was formally reduced from 0.35 kUa/L, which was set based on clinical significance criteria, to 0.1 kUa/L, which was set based on their technically achievable analytical sensitivity. Presently, weakly positive IgE antibody levels between 0.1 and 0.35 kUa/L need to be interpreted by a specialist who knows the history of the patient, since the clinical relevance of positive allergen-specific IgE results in this range is undetermined. There is one study that used receiver operating characteristic curves to demonstrate that optimal diagnostic sensitivity and specificity for detecting allergic symptoms to cat and dog allergens in young adults were 0.12 and 0.2 kUa/L, respectively [10]. While the technical performance (intra-assay precision, interassay reproducibility, interdilutional parallelism, turnaround time) of the clinically used autoanalyzers is unsurpassed as a result of their computer-based automation, all three assays report different final IgE antibody levels for any given serum and allergen specificity [3,9,11,12]. Whether these different reported levels of allergen-specific IgE antibody are a result of the use of different allergen sources and coupling chemistries that produce divergent distributions of allergens on the assays' solid matrices or different methods of calibrating or adjusting the total IgE calibration curve for consistency remains to be determined.

More recent allergen-specific IgE antibody technologies include the multiplex assays such as chip-based microarrays using allergenic components and extracts that remain excellent research tools [13,14] and point-of-care lateral flow assays [15,16]. The Immuno-Solid Phase Allergen Chip or ISAC assay (ThermoFisher Scientific, Phadia Division, Uppsala, Sweden) is a current microarray that uses an activated chip on which 112 purified native or recombinant allergenic components are spotted in a triplicate matrix pattern. Human serum (40 µL) is layered over the circumscribed allergen-coated chip area and antibodies of any isotype if present bind. After a buffer wash, fluorescent-labeled anti-IgE detects bound IgE. Following a final buffer wash, the chip is scanned, and the level of bound fluorescence is interpolated into semiquantitative ISAC Unit (ISU) estimates of IgE antibody. Analytically, the ISAC's sensitivity approaches the singleplex autoanalyzers. The ISAC is particularly good at identifying antibody cross-reactivity between structurally similar inhalant and ingested allergens. Other IgE antibody-based microarray technologies involve a novel hydrogel biochip that uses 15 extracts and 6 component allergens [17], a multiple Luminex xMAP (Austin, Texas) based microarray for the detection of IgE antibody to a limited number of aeroallergens [18], and a surface plasmon resonance assay for IgE antibody to peanut Ara h 2 [19]. All of these microarray assays detect IgE to fixed panels of a limited number of allergen specificities. Moreover, they generate semiquantitative results; IgE binding in the assay is interfered with to different degrees by non-IgE-specific antibodies, and they have not been cleared by the U.S. Food and Drug Administration. Thus, they are considered research assays and not used clinically to evaluate patients.

The point-of-care assay was designed by Thermofisher Scientific (Phadia Division, Uppsala, Sweden) as a novel, handheld cassette in which a drop of whole blood flows in minutes with a fluid front across nitrocellulose strips impregnated with lines of either extract-based aeroallergens or food allergens (in separate cassettes). If IgE antibody is present, it binds to its respective allergen and is detected with colloidal gold labeled anti-IgE that subsequently migrates up the same nitrocellulose strips. As a primary care screening device, the aeroallergen-based lateral flow assay device is effective to obtain correct identification in 88.4%–97.6% of children with allergic sensitization, depending on the study [15,16]. However, because of its limited fixed allergen repertoire (the Matrix phenomenon, see earlier), less quantitative endpoint than the singleplex assays, lower analytical sensitivity than current autoanalyzers, and reimbursement constraints, the lateral flow device has not found active use among practicing clinicians.

7.3 SEROLOGY VERSUS SKIN TESTING FOR CONFIRMATION OF SENSITIZATION

The golden rule of diagnostic allergy testing is that the presence of allergen-specific IgE antibody as detected either in the skin or the blood does not make a diagnosis without the support of a clear clinical history [1,2]. In other words, the presence of specific IgE antibody is necessary as it confirms sensitization but is not alone sufficient to make the diagnosis without clinical evidence of allergic disease. Given this backdrop, by the 1970s when allergen-specific IgE antibody serology first became available to the practicing allergist [6], prick/puncture skin testing had been used diagnostically for over 300 years [20]. Skin testing's immediately available results in visual format for the patient to see, utility using crude allergen extracts, and relevancy as a biological response in the patient remain its most positive attributes. When skin testing and serology based detection of aeroallergen-specific IgE antibody were performed together in clinical studies using the historic RAST, this early assay was diagnostically less sensitive than prick/puncture skin tests [21–23]. Using manually performed RAST data (pre-IgE antibody autoanalyzer), the U.S. 2008 allergy diagnostic testing practice parameter states that "the precise sensitivity of immunoassays compared with prick/puncture skin tests has been reported to range from <50% to more than 90% with an average being approximately 70–75% for most studies" (Summary Statement 115, p. S44 [1]). In contrast to these past impressions, advances in solid-phase materials, anti-IgE conjugates, and autoanalyzer technology have maximized assay performance to the point where the diagnostic sensitivity and specificity (predictability) of current IgE antibody serology and prick/puncture skin tests should be considered comparable when both are objectively viewed against results of a controlled provocation test [2,24]. Intradermal skin testing is not favored in assessing sensitization to aeroallergens and food allergens because of its high false-positive rate, but it

continues to be indicated for the diagnosis of life-threatening Hymenoptera venom and drug allergy. In terms of standardization and reproducibility, the reagents and overall assay performance of the current IgE antibody singleplex autoanalyzers have surpassed that which are obtainable by prick/puncture or intradermal skin testing methodology using the majority of crude, nonstandardized allergen extracts [2,3,24–26]. Intradermal skin testing is used to diagnose Hymenoptera venom and drug allergy and remains somewhat controversial to test for aeroallergen sensitization when prick/puncture tests are negative [27]. I.D. tests are not useful to diagnose food allergy.

7.4 CLINICAL USE OF ALLERGEN-SPECIFIC IgE LEVELS

The qualitative presence of IgE antibody was principally used as verification of sensitization in support of a suspected allergy history in the early years of IgE measurements in serum. As assay methods became more quantitative and IgE antibody was reported in kUa/L units, there was increasing evidence that the actual level of IgE antibody could provide additional clinically useful information. Predictability of quantitative allergen-specific IgE levels became clinically useful with Sampson's studies of food allergy patients [28,29]. Children who had been referred for a food allergy evaluation were serologically evaluated for IgE antibodies to egg, milk, peanut, soy, wheat, and fish. A definitive diagnosis of food allergy was obtained using their history and by performing an oral food challenge. The authors reported levels of IgE antibody that in their pediatric atopic dermatitis population defined the relative probability of reacting to a food challenge. Both retrospective and prospective studies concluded that the need for oral food challenge could be reduced by quantitatively measuring food-specific IgE antibody levels in serum and applying predictive decision criteria [28,29].

In an attempt to replicate Sampson's observations, multiple other groups have performed similar IgE antibody versus food challenge studies and have reported different predictive confidence intervals for failing an oral food challenge. The differences in these reported predictive clinical decision levels are attributed to differences in the study subjects' degree and quality of sensitization (IgE antibody level, specificity, affinity, and IgE specific activity [30,31]), diet, demographics (especially age and geography), disease state (e.g., presence or absence of atopic dermatitis), and the challenge protocol and data analysis methods. As a result of the wide range of reported food-specific IgE antibody concentrations associated with a 95% probability of failing an oral food challenge, judicious care is needed when extrapolating a clinical significance to an individual with any quantitative measure of IgE antibody that is based on population-derived predictive probability values. While limited data also suggest a possible correlation between the magnitude of food allergen-specific IgE and the severity of a clinical reaction to the food [32], most data indicate that the magnitude of a food-specific IgE level in the blood does not predict the severity of the clinical reaction [33]. In terms of terminology, arbitrarily defined class levels and alternate scoring methods and the term "RAST" need to be eliminated from the clinician's vocabulary as kUa/L measures are reported by all the principal clinically used IgE antibody autoanalyzers, and these assays no longer use radioisotopes [3].

7.5 ALLERGENIC MOLECULES IN THE DIAGNOSTIC EVALUATION OF ALLERGIC DISEASE

While a limited number of purified "component" allergens among the drugs (e.g., penicillin, insulin) and foods (e.g., bovine serum albumin, ovalbumin) have been used in serological IgE antibody assays for years [3], the majority of allergosorbents in clinical use have employed physiologic "extracts" of biological materials. These extracts contain complex mixtures of allergenic molecules or components and some nonallergenic material. Advances in protein biochemistry and molecular biology technologies have fostered the emergence of the unique area referred to as "component-resolved diagnosis" or "molecular allergology" [34–36]. Extensive research has led to the identification of principal allergens among protein families with sequence and structural similarity for clinically important and structurally cross-reactive food, pollen, and venom specificities. Isolation methods for purification have been used to produce naturally occurring (native) allergens. Other allergenic molecules have been generated by recombinant DNA technology in a manner that they fold properly to maintain their immunoreactivity and allergenic epitopes, but they can lack modifications such as carbohydrate side chains if produced in *Escherichia coli* [37].

There are four reasons that molecular allergens are gradually becoming incorporated in diagnostic allergy testing, especially for polysensitized subjects [3,35,36]. For certain clinically important allergens that are underrepresented or missing in aqueous extracts, their use in supplementing the extract has led to improved analytical sensitivity of the assay. However, their use can also lead to potential concerns with the interpretation of IgE antibody results when there is interallergen cross-reactivity [38,39]. Molecular allergens also can enhance assay selectivity (analytical specificity) by providing information about sensitization to cross-reactive allergens, potential risks for serious systemic allergic reactions, and primary (species-specific) sensitization [35]. Finally, native and recombinant component allergens have been successfully applied to the ISAC chip-based microarray (Thermofisher Scientific/Phadia), which uses small quantities of serum and provides IgE antibody profiles to over 100 food and pollen allergens [13,14]. All of these technologic advances have allowed rapid, reproducible analysis of IgE antibodies to over 100 clinically important and often cross-reactive allergenic component specificities.

Despite the availability of IgE anti-allergenic component measurements using both established (singleplex) autoanalyzers and the chip-based multiplex microarray, component-resolved diagnosis has been slow to be adopted into clinical practice for multiple reasons. Many clinicians feel unprepared to interpret the vast amounts of IgE anticomponent results that are provided through microarray analysis. Allergist education on the clinical significance of cross-reactivity among structurally similar component allergens is improving. One group correlated different patterns of IgE antibody reactivity to allergen components in the ISAC assay with clinical disease states such as asthma, rhinoconjunctivitis, wheeze, and eczema [40]. They concluded that reasonable discrimination was possible using logistic regression and nonlinear statistical learning models, but improved threshold decision points and interpretation algorithms were needed to make "machine learning" of microarray component-specific IgE antibody data clinically useful. Another issue is the cost of microarray panel testing. The extent of reimbursement for IgE anticomponent testing using microarrays is marginal, and it varies widely by country, healthcare plan, and insurance company. Pediatric practices that focus on sensitization to foods may have a greater interest in microarray-based IgE anticomponent testing as it can elucidate food-pollen cross-reactivity [35,36]. Possibly most importantly, only for select specificities (e.g., peanut, hazelnut, and possibly egg and Hymenoptera venoms) do IgE anticomponent results add unique diagnostic information to that which is already provided by extract-based singleplex IgE antibody measurements. Since extract-based allergosorbents are generally considered "all allergen inclusive," they may be most useful in detecting IgE antibody to all the allergens (major and minor) of a given specificity and not just to selected major allergenic components.

Peanut (*Arachis hypogaea*) has emerged as one allergen specificity where component-resolved diagnosis can facilitate the diagnosis by distinguishing between sensitization that is caused by a genuine allergy or cross-reactivity. Component analysis may be particularly useful to diagnose peanut allergy since only approximately one-quarter of IgE antipeanut extract positive (sensitized) children using singleplex autoanalyzer analyses may actually have peanut-induced allergic reactions as judged by a failed oral peanut challenge [41]. Among the known peanut allergens, the presence of IgE anti-Ara h 2, often together with IgE anti-Ara h 1 and 3, provides indication of a genuine allergy [41,42]. A restricted IgE anti-Ara h 8 [Bet v 1 (birch pollen) homologue response from the PR10 allergen family] is a marker of cross-reactivity and an indicator of generally more mild symptoms, often restricted to the oral cavity [41,43]. Using retrospectively collected specimens, one group has reported that IgE anti-Ara h 2 levels above 1.63 kUa/L provide a diagnostic specificity for genuine peanut allergy of 100% with a diagnostic sensitivity of 70% [44]. If Ara h 1,2,3 specific IgE antibodies are undetectable, however, anaphylaxis may still occur if IgE antibodies specific for Ara h 6, which is structurally similar to Ara h 2, are present [45]. Other groups have confirmed the utility of component testing in the diagnosis of peanut allergy in different populations [46–49]. One American study shows that sensitization to individual peanut components (Ara h 1,2,3,8, and 9) can be dependent on the geographic location and the age of the individual [50].

Comprehensive overviews of the clinical significance of many of the clinically available allergenic components are presented elsewhere by either allergen group or by functional uniqueness or cross-reactivity families [35–37]. At present, the ISAC provides IgE antibody measurements to 112 allergenic components judiciously selected for inclusion due to their clinical importance to different regions of the world as being species/allergen group unique (Table 7.1 [aeroallergens], Table 7.2 [food allergens], and Table 7.3 [venom and latex allergens]) or effective markers of allergenic cross-reactivity (Table 7.4). The cross-reactive allergen families that are covered by the ISAC-112 include the tropomyosins, serum albumins, nonspecific lipid transfer proteins, group 10 pathogenesis-related proteins (also known as the Bet v 1 homologues), and the profilins.

Possibly the most elegant and systematic prospective application of ISAC component-resolved analyses is reported by O'Nell et al. [51]. Swedish babies with an atopic history ($n = 46$) or no family history of atopy ($n = 21$) were studied by providing an allergy history and undergoing prick/puncture skin tests and ISAC serology for temporal changes in their IgE anti-allergen component profiles at 3, 6, 9, and 18 months and 6 and 18 years of age. The "allergy march" from food to aeroallergen sensitivity was studied. Each child displayed a unique sensitization fingerprint with one of four distinct patterns. Group 1 comprised 40% of the study population that did not reveal any IgE antibody response.

Table 7.1 Aeroallergen components in serological IgE antibody assays[a]

Grass Pollen	
Bermuda grass (*Cynodon dactylon*)	Cyn d 1: Expansin-CCD bearing protein
Timothy grass (*Phleum pratense*)	Phl p 1: Expansin-CCD bearing protein
	Phl p 2: Unknown function
	Phl p 4: Berberine bridge enzyme
	Phl p 5: Ribonuclease
	Phl p 6: Unknown function
	Phl p 7: Calcium-binding protein
	Phl p 11: Trypsin inhibitor
	Phl p 12: Profilin
Tree Pollen	
Alder (*Alnus glutinosa*)	Aln g 1: Ribonuclease
Birch (*Betula verrucosa*)	Bet v 1: PR10
	Bet v 2: Profilin
	Bet v 4: Polcalcin
	Bet v 6- Isoflavone reductase
Japanese cedar (*Cryptomeria japonica*)	Cry j 1: Pectate lyase
Cypress (*Cupressus arizonica*)	Cup a 1. Pectate lyase
Olive (*Olea europaea*)	Ole e 1: Trypsin inhibitor
	Ole e 7: Lipid transfer protein
	Ole e 9: Glucanase
Plane (*Platanus acerifolia*)	Pla a 1.0101: Invertase inhibitor
	Pla a 2: Polygalacturonase
Weed Pollen	
Common ragweed (*Ambrosia artemisiifolia*)	Amb a 1: Pectate lyase
Mugwort (*Artemisia vulgaris*)	Art v 1: Defensin
	Art v 3: Lipid transfer protein
Goosefoot/Lamb's quarters (*Chenopodium album*)	Che a 1: Trypsin inhibitor
Wall pellitory (*Parietaria judaica*)	Par j 2: Lipid transfer protein
Plantain/Ribwort (*Plantago lanceolata*)	Pla l 1: Trypsin inhibitor
Saltwort/Russian thistle (*Salsola kali*)	Sal k 1: Pectin methylesterase
Epidermal and Animal Proteins	
Cat (*Felis domesticus*)	Fel d 1: Uteroglobin
	Fel d 2: Albumin
	Fel d 4: Lipocalin
Cow (*Bos domesticus*)	Bos d 6: Albumin
Dog (*Canis familiaris/domesticus*)	Can f 1: Lipocalin

(*Continued*)

Table 7.1 *(Continued)* Aeroallergen components in serological IgE antibody assays[a]

	Can f 2: Lipocalin
	Can f 3: Albumin
	Can f 5: Arginine esterase
Horse (*Equus caballus*)	**Equ c 1:** Lipocalin
Mouse (*Mus musculus*)	**Mus m 1:** Lipocalin (prealbumin)
Microorganisms/Mold	
Alternaria alternata	**Alt a 1:** Unknown function
	Alt a 6: Glycolytic enzyme
Aspergillus fumigatus	**Asp f 1:** Ribonuclease
	Asp f 2: Fibrinogen-binding protein
	Asp f 3: Peroxisomal membrane protein
	Asp f 4: Unknown function
	Asp f 6: Glycolytic enzyme (Enolase)
Cladosporium herbarum (Hormodendrum)	**Cla h 8:** Mannitol dehydrogenase
Mites	
Blomia tropicalis	**Blo t 5:** Unknown function
Dermatophagoides farinae	**Der f 1:** Cysteine protease
	Der f 2: NPC2 family
Dermatophagoides pteronyssinus	**Der p 1:** Cysteine protease
	Der p 2: NPC2 family
	Der p 10: Muscle contraction protein
Storage mite (*Lepidoglyphus destructor*)	Lep d 2: NPC2 family
Insects	
Cockroach (*Blattella germanica*)	**Bla g 1:** Unknown function
	Bla g 2: Aspartic protease (inactive)
	Bla g 5: Glutathione-*S*-transferase

[a] Bold allergen components are available for IgE antibody testing of patient serum specimens.

Two children in this group with egg allergy and one with cat and dog allergy were missed by ISAC despite a positive history and prick/puncture skin tests. Group 2 comprised 4% of the children with a low-level response less than 2 ISU to an egg component before 1.5 year of age and no sensitization later in life. For these groups 1 and 2, ISAC component measurements did not provide any new, relevant information over extract-based singleplex serology or skin testing. In group 3, 18% of children expressed early IgE anti-egg and milk by 1.5 years of age, sometimes with IgE antibody to fish or storage protein from soy, peanut, or tree nuts. By 1.5 years or older, sensitization to aeroallergens such as pollen, animal dander, or mites became prevalent. The ISAC profile in this "early multiple food-aeroallergen sensitized group" was particularly useful to identify cosensitization due to cross-reacting allergens and identify unexpected allergen triggers prior to symptom development. The "late sensitized" (group 4) included 38% of children who expressed *no* sensitization to egg, milk, fish, soy, wheat, or peanut early in life but developed IgE antibodies to aeroallergens (pollen, mites, cat, or dog) by age 6 years or older. Some developed IgE anti-aeroallergen components that cross-reacted with food allergens (e.g., PR-10 protein family). Approximately half of group 4 produced IgE antibody to only one or two specificities (e.g., monosensitized to birch, grass, or cat). The other half develop sensitivities to multiple cross-reactive and specific components, where ISAC data provided novel and relevant diagnostic information that was not readily obtained from skin testing or the subject's clinical history. Thus, the assessment of allergic disease in approximately one-third of children of this study population with complex patterns of multiple sensitivities benefited from novel and clinically informative IgE

Table 7.2 Allergenic food components in serological IgE antibody assays*

Chicken Egg (*Gallus domesticus*)	
Egg white	**Gal d 1:** Ovamucoid
	Gal d 2: Ovalbumin
	Gal d 3: Conalbumin
	Gal d 4: Glycosyl hydrolase
Egg yolk	**Gal d 5:** Albumin
Cow's milk (*Bos domesticus*)	**Bos d 4:** α-Lactalbumin
	Bos d 5: β-Lactoglobulin
	Bos d 6: Albumin
	Bos d 8: Casein
	Bos d: Lactoferrin
Pig–Swine (*Sus scrofa*)	**Sus s-**
Fish (Cod) (*Gadus morhua*)	**Gad c 1:** Parvalbumin—calcium-binding protein
Carp (*Cyprinus carpio*)	**Cyp c 1:** Parvalbumin—calcium-binding protein
Fish (herring) parasite (*Anisakis simplex*)	**Ani s 1:** Serine protease inhibitor
Shrimp (*Penaeus monodon*)	**Pen a 1:** Tropomyosin
	Pen m 2: Arginine kinase
	Pen m 4: Calcium-binding protein
Nuts and Seeds	
Cashew nut (*Anacardium occidentale*)	**Ana o 2:** Legumin-like protein
	Ana o 3: 2S albumin
Brazil nut (*Bertholletia exelsa*)	**Ber e 1:** 2S albumin
Hazelnut (*Corylus avellana*)	**Cor a 1:** Ribonuclease
	Cor a 8: Lipid transfer protein
	Cor a 9: 11S globulin
	Cor a 14: 2S albumin
Walnut (*Juglans* spp.)	**Jug r 1:** 2S albumin
	Jug r 3: Lipid transfer protein
	Jug r 2: 7S vicilin-like globulin
Sesame (*Sesamum indicum*)	**Ses i 1:** 2S albumin
Legumes	
Peanut (*Arachis hypogaea*)	**Ara h 1:** Glycinin—seed storage
	Ara h 2: Conglutin—trypsin inhibitor
	Ara h 3: Glycinin—seed storage
	Ara h 6: Conglutin—2S albumin
	Ara h 8: PR10
	Ara h 9: Lipid transfer protein

(Continued)

Table 7.2 (*Continued*) Allergenic food components in serological IgE antibody assays*

Soy (*Glycine max*)	**Gly m 4: PR10**
	Gly m 5: 7S vicilin
	Gly m 6: 2S albumin
Cereals	
Buckwheat (*Fagopyrum esculentum*)	**Fag e 2: 2S albumin**
Wheat (*Triticum aestivum*)	**Tri a 14: Lipid transfer protein**
	Tri a 19.010 (gliadin, gluten)
Fruit	
Green kiwi/gooseberry (*Actinidia deliciosa*)	**Act d 1: Actinidin—cysteine protease**
	Act d 5: Kiwellin
	Act d 8: PR10
Peach (*Prunus persica*)	**Pru p 1: PR10—ribonuclease**
	Pru p 3: Lipid transfer protein
	Pru p 4: Actin-binding protein
Apple (*Malus domestica*)	**Mal d 1: PR10—ribonuclease**
Papaya (*Carica papaya*)	**Car p 1: Cysteine protease**
Pineapple	**Ana c 2: CCD-bearing cysteine protease**
Vegetables	
Celery (*Apium graveolens*)	**Api g**

Note: Bold allergen components are available for IgE antibody testing of patient serum specimens.

antibody patterns provided by the multiplex chip-based allergen component ISAC. Application of allergen component-based IgE antibody analyses to the diagnostic algorithm for allergic disease can be expected to grow with more education, proof-of-concept research studies that lead to clearance by regulatory agencies, and the availability of insurance reimbursement. At present, IgE anti-peanut and hazelnut component measurements using singleplex IgE antibody assays are useful adjunct testing to routine IgE anti-peanut and hazelnut allergen extract analyses [35,36,49,51,52].

7.6 OTHER ANALYTES MEASURED AND TESTS PERFORMED IN THE DIAGNOSTIC ALLERGY LABORATORY

A number of other serological tests including total serum IgE, mast cell tryptase, precipitins, and the basophil-based mediator release assays have utility in the diagnosis of selected allergic diseases.

7.6.1 Total serum IgE

The total IgE concentration in serum is highly age dependent; thus, interpretation of total IgE levels needs to be made in relation to an age-adjusted nonallergic reference population [3,35,53]. Moreover,

the wide overlap of total serum IgE levels between otherwise healthy atopic and nonatopic populations diminishes the diagnostic predictive value of quantitative total serum IgE levels. Thus, a low or normal total serum IgE value does not eliminate the possibility of IgE-mediated disease. Elevated age-adjusted levels of total serum IgE are common in individuals with parasitic infections, and they are diagnostic for hyper-IgE (Job syndrome) and allergic bronchopulmonary aspergillosis when there is also a positive IgE anti-*Aspergillus* serology. Possibly the most common current rationale for total serum IgE measurements is verification that the patient's IgE level is in the range (30–700 kU/L) that is acceptable for omalizumab (humanized anti-IgE) therapy. From an analytical point of view, the College of American Pathologists proficiency data verify that equivalent total serum IgE levels are accurately and reproducibly measured by any of the clinically used autoanalyzers (Abbott Architect c System; Hycor Biomedical: Total IgE EIA; Thermofisher Scientific/Phadia: ImmunoCAP Systems; Roche: Cobas; and Siemens Healthcare Diagnostics: ADVIA Centaur, Immulite and Dimension Vista). This excellent interlaboratory agreement is achieved because all the assays are calibrated against the same WHO IgE reference preparation [3,8,9,54].

7.6.2 Mast cell tryptase

Tryptase is a serine esterase that resides in mast cell granules as four noncovalently linked and enzymatically active subunits, each 31–38 kd. It is stored in association with heparin at concentrations of 10–35

Table 7.3 Allergenic venom and occupational components in serological IgE antibody assays

Hymenoptera venoms	
Honeybee (*Apis mellifera*)	**Api m 1: Phospholipase A2**
	Api m 4: Melittin (hemolysin)
	Api m 10: Unknown function
Yellow jacket (*Vespula vulgaris*)	**Ves v 5: Antigen 5**
Paper wasp (*Polistes dominulus*)	**Pol d 5: Antigen 5**
Natural rubber latex	
Hevea brasiliensis	**Hev b 1: Rubber elongation factor**
	Hev b 3: Small rubber particle protein
	Hev b 5: Unknown
	Hev b 6.01: Hevein-like
	Hev b 6.02: Chitin-binding protein
	Hev b 8: Actin-binding protein—profilin
	Hev b 11: Chitinase
Occupational Allergens	
α-Amylase (*Aspergillus oryzae*)	**Asp o 21: Amylase**
Gliadin	**Gliadin**
Alkalase (*Bacillus* spp.)	**Alkalase**

Note: Bold allergen components are available for IgE antibody testing of patient serum specimens.

picograms per resting mast cell in connective tissue throughout human skin and the respiratory and digestive tracts. When released from heparin, it degrades into its monomers and loses enzymatic activity [55]. Basophils contain 300- to 700-fold less tryptase; thus, the primary source of tryptase in human serum is believed to be the mast cell. Two forms of tryptase (α and β) are produced. α-Pro-tryptase is continually secreted into blood by all mast cells as an inactive proenzyme along with unprocessed β-pro-tryptase. Under acid conditions, β-pro-tryptase is converted to a mature monomer and then assembled into an active "mature β-tryptase tetramer," which is stabilized by heparin. Most tryptase detected in the blood of normal individuals is composed of α and pro-β forms, and these become elevated in individuals with mastocytosis [56]. In contrast, mature β-tryptase is released in parallel with prestored histamine and other newly generated vasoactive mediators following mast cell degranulation associated with anaphylaxis. Cumulative α and pro-β tryptase levels are considered indicators of total mast cell number and are estimated by subtracting the level of mature β-tryptase from the total tryptase level as measured in serum by immunoassay [57]. The levels of mature β-tryptase in blood generally reflect the magnitude of mast cell activation.

Analytically, tryptase is intentionally converted to its monomeric enzymatically inactive form. The total serum level of mast cell tryptase is then measured in a noncompetitive fluorescent enzyme immunoassay that uses a capture monoclonal antibody that binds both the α-pro-tryptase and mature β-tryptase [57]. Serum levels of total tryptase in healthy (nondiseased) individuals range from 1 to 10 ng/mL (average 5 ng/mL). Systemic mastocytosis should be suspected if baseline serum total tryptase levels exceed 20 ng/mL. Quantification of mature β-tryptase is accomplished with a solid-phase noncompetitive immunoassay that uses a mature β-tryptase-specific capture monoclonal antibody. However, since the β-tryptase-specific antibody reagent weakly cross-reacts with α-protryptase, high levels of α-protryptase in serum may result in falsely lower levels of mature β-tryptase as a result of competitive inhibition. Mature β-tryptase levels less than 1 ng/mL are found in blood of healthy individuals and levels greater than 1 ng/mL indicate mast cell activation. Insect sting–induced systemic anaphylaxis can result in mature β-tryptase levels greater than 5 ng/mL by 30–60 minutes after the sting, which then declines with a biological half-life of approximately 2 hours [58]. Optimal blood collection is 0.5–4 hours following the initiation of a suspected mast cell–mediated systemic allergic reaction [59]. Mature β-tryptase levels greater than 10 ng/mL in a postmortem blood specimen provide evidence for anaphylaxis as a probable cause of death. Finally, *Hymenoptera* sting–induced reaction severity increases with baseline total tryptase levels. This indicates that the mast cell load may be partially responsible for the observed increased tendency for more severe allergic reactions and importantly that elevated baseline tryptase levels may serve as a predictor for severe allergic sting reactions [60].

7.6.3 Basophil mediator release and flow cytometry assays

A good correlation exists between *in vitro* basophil mediator release to allergens and prick/puncture skin test and serological measures of specific IgE antibody [61,62]. Despite its unquestioned use in research and qualification of allergen extracts used in diagnosis and treatment, the basophil mediator (histamine and leukotriene C4 [LTC4]) release assay and its flow cytometry equivalent, which measures surface marker expression, are rarely used clinically in the routine diagnosis of human allergic disease. Basophil mediator release assays are also useful as an *in vitro* model for the study of triggering mechanisms of effector cells (basophils and mast cells). In its most basic form, peripheral blood leukocytes are isolated from a donor and incubated with varying concentrations (e.g., 3- to 10-fold dilutions) of allergen extract or antihuman IgE as a positive control. Histamine or LTC4 release is measured in the supernatant by enzymatic, radiometric, or spectrophotofluorometric or immunoassay techniques [62–64]. Alternatively, the upregulation of expressed surface proteins (e.g., CD45, CD63, CD69, and CD203c) is monitored by flow cytometry following the activation of basophils by the addition of allergen [64,65]. Its limited use in the diagnostic laboratory results from its expense, time-consuming nature, and logistic challenges associated with the need for fresh blood (less than 24 hours old). Basophil mediator release assays are particularly useful in clarifying discrepancies between skin test and serological IgE antibody test results.

Analytically, there are technical challenges to the optimization and validation of basophil-based assays. If endotoxin-free whole blood can be delivered to the laboratory within 24 hours, it is preincubated with buffer containing varying concentrations of allergen and often IL3 that modifies the extent of mediator release or CD64/CD203c upregulation. Crude allergen extracts are often toxic to basophils, and so allergen preparations need to be qualified for basophil assay use. Criteria for defining positive results vary with

Table 7.4 Cross-reactive food aeroallergen families in serological IgE antibody assays

Tropomyosin: Actin-binding muscle protein that regulates actin mechanics in muscle contraction	
Anisakis-Herring worm (*Anisakis simplex*)	Ani s 3
German cockroach (*Blattella germanica*)	Bla g 7
Dust mite (*Dermatophagoides pteronyssinus*)	Der p 10
Shrimp (*Penaeus monodon*)	Pen m 1
Serum Albumin: Protein in blood that functions to transport fats and fatty acids to muscle tissue	
Cow (*Bos domesticus*)	Bos d 6
Dog (*Canis familiaris*)	Can f 3
Horse (*Equus caballus*)	Equ c 3
Cat (*Felis domesticus*)	Fel d 2
Nonspecific Lipid Transfer Proteins: Conserved plant proteins that function to shuttle phospholipids and other fatty acids between cell membranes	
Peanut (*Arachis hypogaea*)	Ara h 9
Hazelnut (*Corylus avellana*)	Cor a 8
Walnut (*Juglans* spp.)	Jug r 3
Peach (*Prunus persica*)	Pru p 3
Mugwort (*Artemisia vulgaris*)	Art v 3
Olive pollen (*Olea europaea*)	Ole e 7
Plane tree (*Platanus acerifolia*)	Pla a 3
Pathogenesis-Related Proteins: PR10 Family (Bet v 1 homologues)—Ribonuclease	
Birch (*Betula verrucosa*)	Bet v 1
Hazel pollen (*Corylus avellana*)	Cor a 1.010
Hazelnut (*Corylus avellana*)	Cor a 1.040
Apple (*Malus domesticus*)	Mal d 1
Peach (*Prunus persica*)	Pru p 1
Soybean (*Glycine max*)	Gly m 4
Peanut (*Arachis hypogaea*)	Ara h 8
Kiwi (*Actinidia deliciosa*)	Act d 8
Celery (*Apium graveolens*)	Api g 1
Profilin: An actin-binding protein involved in the dynamic turnover and restructuring of the actin cytoskeleton	
Birch (*Betula verrucosa*)	Bet v 2
Natural rubber latex (*Hevea brasiliensis*)	Hev b 8
Mercury (*Mercurialis annua*)	Mer a 1
Timothy grass (*Phleum pratense*)	Phl p 12
Thaumatin-Like Protein	
Green kiwi (*Actinidia deliciosa*)	Act d 2
Carbohydrate Cross-Reactive Determinants	
Bromelain (pineapple)	MUXF3

Note: Bold allergen components are available for IgE antibody testing of patient serum specimens.

different simulating allergen lots and sources. Platelet adherence on basophils can create false-positive results in the flow-based CD63 basophil assay. Details of the assay design and protocols, methods of optimizing reagent concentrations and qualifying allergen preparations, strategies for quality control and data analysis, and strengths and pitfalls of the various assay formats are presented in detail elsewhere [61–67].

7.6.4 Precipitating IgG antibodies (precipitins)

The precipitin assay remains one of the earliest immunologic tests and provides useful information about high-level precipitating IgG antibodies that can induce hypersensitivity pneumonitis (extrinsic allergic alveolitis). Hours after inhalation of mold or bird droppings containing dust, a hypersensitivity reaction can occur involving the lung interstitium and terminal bronchioles [68]. Precipitin antibodies to cow's milk proteins also have been implicated in chronic respiratory symptoms (cough, wheezing, nasal congestion, dyspnea) in infants who have radiologic evidence of pulmonary infiltrates [69]. The Ouchterlony or double-diffusion assay involves pipetting antigen (extract) and antibody (control or patient's serum) in adjacent wells in an agarose gel. As they diffuse toward each other, precipitin lines that indicate optimal antibody-antigen cross-linking at equivalence can be visualized, especially when specific IgG antibodies are high. Quality control is performed with known positive polyclonal antisera for each antigen. The precipitating antibodies or precipitins can be detected in the serum of nearly all ill patients but also in the serum of as many as 50% of asymptomatic individuals who have been exposed to the relevant organic dusts [68]. Immunoassays for IgG antibody to the appropriate organic dust antigens may be less useful clinically because they are too analytically sensitive. Precipitin assays are currently available with specificities for the thermophilic actinomyces (*Micropolyspora faeni*, *Thermoactinomyces vulgaris*, and *T. candidus*), *Aspergillus* antigens (*A. fumigatus*, *A. niger*, *A. flavus*), pigeon serum, *Aureobasidum pullulans*, and fecal particles from chickens, parakeets, a variety of exotic household birds (cockatiel, Amazon), and cow's milk for assessment of the Heiner syndrome [69] in infants.

7.6.5 Allergen-specific IgG/IgG4

Clinically successful immunotherapy is almost always accompanied by an elevation in allergen-specific IgG "blocking" antibodies [70], often of the subclass 4 [71,72]. A serological marker such as allergen-specific IgG antibody has been sought to guide individualization of the immunotherapy dose and the frequency of injections to maximize protective effects of the treatment. An early report involving venom immunotherapy showed that the highest rate of allergic reactions following inadvertent stings (26%) occurred in venom immunotherapy treated patients who had both a venom-specific IgG antibody level less than 3 μg/mL and fewer than 4 years of venom immunotherapy [73]. However, quantitative measurements of allergen-specific IgG and IgG4 antibodies have been disappointing as they rarely correlate with objectively observed clinical changes during and after immunotherapy. Other assays of functional inhibitory IgG4 antibodies that examine the ability of IgG antibodies to compete with IgE and inhibit IgE-allergen complex formation are reportedly more effective surrogates of clinical response to immunotherapy [74]. IgG antibodies measured with the CD23-dependent IgE-facilitated allergen binding (IgE-FAB) assay

block IgE-mediated facilitated allergen presentation and IgE-mediated basophil activation. However, access to these measurements is limited since few laboratories perform the IgE-facilitated allergen binding assay as technically described elsewhere [75].

7.7 UNPROVEN ALLERGY LABORATORY TESTS

There are two categories of laboratory tests offered for the diagnosis of allergic disease for which there is no evidence of diagnostic validity [1,76,77]. The first group includes procedures that possess an obscure theoretical basis, and they suffer from poor reproducibility and an absence of technical and clinical validation that is needed to justify their use. Among these tests are bioresonance, electroacupuncture, iridology, hair analysis, applied kinesiology, and the antigen leukocyte antibody test (ALCAT). The ALCAT involves pipetting a drop of white blood cell rich buffy coat or whole blood onto an unstained glass slide that has been precoated with a dried allergen extract. Changes in cell morphology such as increases in the white blood cell diameter, vacuolation, or crenation are used as an indication of a positive test and evidence of allergy to the food. The ALCAT is currently marketed by Cell Science Systems (Deerfield Beach, Florida), which now sells an automated liquid handling system (ROBOCat II) that employs electronic particle counting and sizing to examine changes in electrical resistance, which occur by a blood cell that is suspended in a conductive liquid as it transverses a small aperture. Reports state that the ALCAT is not supported by research, is not a reliable medical diagnostic test, and is not a suitable guide for therapeutic decisions [76,77].

The second group of inappropriate tests produces valid results, but they provide a misleading interpretation that has no objective utility in the diagnosis of allergic disease. Lymphocyte proliferation tests with food extracts and assays for food antigen–specific IgG or IgG4 antibodies are examples. The later analyses stem from a 1982 report in which monoclonal antibodies specific for human IgG4 were reported to induce histamine release from human basophils *in vitro* [78]. This has led to some clinical laboratories that measure antigen-specific IgG4 antibodies for the evaluation of food and aeroallergy and intolerance. In 1992, we verified that this *in vitro* basophil phenomenon results from IgG4 anti-IgE autoantibodies bound to IgE (IgG-IgE complexes) on the surface of basophils, which can be activated to release histamine when incubated with human IgG4-specific monoclonal antibodies [79]. Antigen-specific IgG and IgG4 antibodies can be viewed as a marker of exposure to foreign components that are recognized by the immune system. Objective data indicate that serological testing of IgG or IgG4 antibodies specific for food and airborne antigens is irrelevant and is not useful in the diagnostic workup of a patient with suspected food or respiratory allergy or intolerance [80]. Results of these unproven tests do not permit the separation of healthy from diseased individuals, whether it is for food intolerance, allergy, or other diagnoses.

SALIENT POINTS

1. The technology for quantitatively and reproducibly measuring allergen-specific IgE antibody has matured with computer-driven autoanalyzers, and application of these measurements to the diagnosis of allergic disease is constantly evolving with new clinical research studies.

2. Allergen extract–based allergosorbents and singleplex autoanalyzers will remain the primary sources of reagents and analytical methods used by diagnostic allergy laboratories to confirm sensitization (allergen-specific IgE antibody positivity) to support a clinical history driven allergy diagnosis.

3. Component peanut and hazelnut allergens are useful adjuncts to extract-based IgE antibody analyses. Other component allergen-based IgE antibody measurements can be used to identify clinically relevant pollen–food cross-reactivities in complex, multiply sensitized individuals.

4. Microarrays using purified and recombinant allergens and basophil-based IgE analyses will continue to be used in select research projects. As cost decreases, multiplex chip-based systems using component allergens may become more prominent; however, point-of-care panel-based IgE antibody tests will not likely surface as major diagnostic allergy assays.

5. Total serum IgE, tryptase, and precipitins can be performed to clarify the suitability of a patient for omalizumab therapy or to support the diagnosis of anaphylaxis or hypersensitivity pneumonitis.

6. Better serological surrogates of immunotherapy efficacy than allergen-specific IgG/IgG4 levels are needed. Leading the list is the CD23-dependent IgE-facilitated allergen binding assay shown to block IgE-mediated facilitated allergen presentation. To be useful, however, it needs to be configured into an assay that routine clinical immunology laboratories can readily perform.

7. Ultimately, successful implementation of diagnostic allergy laboratory IgE antibody test measurements depends on optimal interpretation by knowledgeable clinicians using the patient's clinical history as a final arbiter in making the diagnosis of allergic disease [2,81].

ABBREVIATIONS

Ara h 1,2,3,8,9	Peanut (*Arachis hypogaea*) allergenic components
Bet v 1	Group 1 allergen from birch pollen (*Betula verrucosa*)
CAP	College of American Pathologists
IgE	Immunoglobulin E
ISAC	Immunosorbent allergen chip
IU	International unit of IgE that is equivalent to approximately 2.4 ng of IgE
ISU	ISAC units of IgE antibody
kUa/L	Kilo international units of allergen-specific IgE antibody
LTC4	Leukotriene C4
PRU	Phadebas RAST units
RAST	Radioallergosorbent test (for allergen-specific IgE)
WHO	World Health Organization

ACKNOWLEDGMENTS

The author wishes to recognize Dr. Adriano Mari and the Allergome as the sources of some of the information in this chapter related to components allergens.

REFERENCES

1. Bernstein IL, Li JT, Bernstein DI et al. Allergy diagnostic testing: An updated practice parameter. *Ann Allergy Asthma Immunol* 2008; 100(Suppl 3): S1–S148.

2. Adkinson NF Jr, Hamilton RG. Clinical history-driven diagnosis of allergic diseases: Utilizing *in vitro* IgE testing. *J Allergy Clin Immunol Pract* 2015; 3: 871–876.

3. Hamilton RG, Matsson PNJ, Adkinson NF Jr et al. *Analytical Performance Characteristics, Quality Assurance, and Clinical Utility of Immunological Assays for Human Immunoglobulin E Antibodies of Defined Allergen Specificities*. ILA20, 3rd ed. Wayne, PA: Clinical and Laboratory Standards Institute, 2017. (https://clsi.org).

4. Ishizaka K, Ishizaka T. Physiochemical properties of reaginic antibody. I. Association of reaginic activity with an immunoglobulin other than gamma A or gamma G globulin. *J Allergy* 1967; 37: 169–172.

5. Johansson SGO, Bennich H. Immunological studies of an atypical (myeloma) immunoglobulin. *Immunology* 1967; 13: 381–394.

6. Wide L, Bennich H, Johansson SGO. Diagnosis by an *in vitro* test for allergen specific IgE antibodies. *Lancet* 1967; 2: 1105–1109.

7. Ownby DR, Adkinson NF, Hamilton RG et al. Multi-centre comparison of ABBOTT MATRIX Aero to Pharmacia Standard RAST, Modified RAST and skin prick/puncture tests. *Eur J Clin Chem Clin Biochem* 1994; 32: 631–637.

8. Thorpe SJ, Heath A, Fox B, Patel D, Egner W. The Third International Standard for serum IgE: International collaborative study to evaluate a candidate preparation. *Clin Chem Lab Med* 2014; 52: 1283–1289.

9. Hamilton RG. Proficiency survey based evaluation of clinical total and allergen-specific IgE assay performance. *Arch Path Lab Med* 2010; 134: 975–982.

10. Linden CC, Misiak RT, Wegienka G et al. Analysis of allergen specific IgE cut points to cat and dog in the Childhood Allergy Study. *Ann Allergy Asthma Immunol* 2011; 106: 153–158.

11. Wood RA, Segall N, Ahlstedt S et al. Accuracy of IgE antibody laboratory results. *Ann Allergy Asthma Immunol*. 2007; 99: 34–41.

12. Wang J, Godbold JH, Sampson HA. Correlation of serum allergy (IgE) tests performed by different assay systems. *J Allergy Clin Immunol* 2008; 121: 1219–1224.

13. Hiller R, Laffer S, Harwanegg C et al. Microarrayed allergen molecules: Diagnostic gatekeepers for allergy treatment. *FASEB J* 2002; 16: 414–416.

14. Hamilton RG. Microarray technology applied to human allergic disease. *Microarrays (Basel)* 2017; 6.

15. Sarratud T, Donnanno S, Terracciano L et al. Accuracy of a point-of-care testing device in children with suspected respiratory allergy. *Allergy Asthma Proc* 2010; 31: 11–17.

16. Diaz-Vazquez C, Torregrosa-Bertet MJ, Carvajal-Urueña I et al. Accuracy of ImmunoCAP(R) Rapid in the diagnosis of allergic sensitization in children between 1 and 14 years with recurrent wheezing: The IReNE study. *Pediatr Allergy Immunol*. 2009; 6: 601–609.

17. Smoldovskaya O, Feyzkhanova G, Arefieva A et al. Allergen extracts and recombinant proteins: comparison of efficiency of *in vitro* allergy diagnostics using multiplex assay on a biological microchip. *Allergy Asthma Clin Immunol*. 2016; 12: 9.

18. King EM, Vailes LD, Tsay A et al. Simultaneous detection of total and allergen-specific IgE by using purified allergens in a fluorescent multiplex array. *J Allergy Clin Immunol* 2007; 120: 1126–1131.

19. Joshi AA, Peczuh MW, Kumar CV, Rusling JF. Ultrasensitive carbohydrate-peptide SPR imaging microarray for diagnosing IgE mediated peanut allergy. *Analyst* 2014; 1399: 5728–5735.

20. Harper DS, Avenberg KM. *"First Datable Skin Test Under Medical Auspices was Conducted by Pierrre Borel in 1656"* Excerpted from Footnotes in Allergy. Uppsala, Sweden: Pharmacia Press, 1980: 57.

21. Norman PS, Lichtenstein LM, Ishizaka K. Diagnostic tests in ragweed hay fever: A comparison of direct skin tests, IgE antibody measurements and basophil histamine release. *J Allergy Clin Immunol* 1973; 52: 210–224.

22. Perera MG, Bernstein IL, Michael JG et al. Predictability of the radioallergosorbent test (RAST) in ragweed pollenosis. *Am Rev Respir Dis* 1975; 111: 605–610.

23. Paula G, Bessot JC, Thierry R et al. Correlation between skin tests, inhalation tests, and specific IgE in a study of 120 subjects allergic to house dust and *Dermatophagoides pteronyssinus*. *Clin Allergy* 1977; 7: 337–346.

24. Wood RA, Phipatanakul W, Hamilton RG et al. A comparison of skin prick/puncture tests, intradermal skin tests and RASTS in the diagnosis of cat allergy. *J Allergy Clin Immunol* 1999; 103: 773–779.

25. McCann WA, Ownby DR. The reproducibility of the allergy skin test scoring and interpretation by board-certified/board-eligible allergists. *Ann Allergy Asthma Immunol* 2002; 89: 368–371.

26. Szefler SJ, Wenzel S, Brown R et al. Asthma outcomes: Biomarker. *J Allergy Clin Immunol* 2012; 129: S9–S23.

27. Ledford DK, Lockey RF. Controversies in allergy: Intradermal aeroallergen skin testing. *JACI-InPract* 2018; 6: 1863–1865.

28. Sampson HA, Ho DG. Relationship between food-specific IgE concentrations and the risk of positive food challenges in children and adolescents. *J Allergy Clin Immunol* 1997; 100: 444–451.

29. Sampson HA. Utility of food-specific IgE concentrations in predicting symptomatic food allergy. *J Allergy Clin Immunol* 2001; 107: 891–896.

30. Christensen LH, Holm J, Lund G et al. Several distinct properties of the IgE repertoire determine effector cell degranulation in response to allergen challenge. *J Allergy Clin Immunol* 2008; 122: 298–304.

31. Hamilton RG, MacGlashan DW Jr, Saini SS. IgE antibody specific activity in human allergic disease. *Immunol Res* 2010; 47: 273–284.

32. Benhamou AH, Zamora SA, Eigenmann PA. Correlation between specific immunoglobulin E levels and the severity of reactions in egg allergic patients. *Pediatr Allergy Immunol* 2008; 19: 173–179.

33. Sicherer SH, Morrow EH, Sampson HA. Dose-response in double-blind, placebo-controlled oral food challenges in children with atopic dermatitis. *J Allergy Clin Immunol* 2000; 105: 582–586.

34. Lidholm J, Ballmer-Weber BK, Mari A et al. Component resolved diagnostics in food allergy. *Curr Opinion Allergy Clin Immunol* 2006; 6: 234–240.

35. Kleine-Tebbe J, Jakob T, editors. *Molecular Allergy Diagnostics: Innovation for a Better Patient Management*. Cham, Switzerland: Springer International Publishing, 2017.

36. Matricardi PM, Kleine-Tebbe J, Hoffmann HJ et al. EAACI molecular allergology user's guide. *Pediatr Allergy Immunol* 2016; 27(Suppl 23): 1–250.

37. Blank S, Bilò MB, Ollert M. Component-resolved diagnostics to direct in venom immunotherapy: Important steps towards precision medicine. *Clin Exp Allergy* 2018; 48: 354–364.

38. Andersson K, Ballmer-Weber BK, Cistero-Bahima A et al. Enhancement of hazelnut extract for IgE testing by recombinant allergen spiking. *Allergy* 2007; 62: 897–904.

39. Sicherer SH, Dhillon G, Laughery KA, Hamilton RG, Wood RA. Caution: The Phadia hazelnut ImmunoCAP (f17) has been supplemented with recombinant Cor a 1 and now detects Bet v 1-specific IgE, which leads to elevated values for persons with birch pollen allergy. *J Allergy Clin Immunol* 2008; 122: 413–414.

40. Prosperi MC, Belgrave D, Buchan I, Simpson A, Custovic A. Challenges in interpreting allergen microarrays in relation to clinical symptoms: A machine learning approach. *Pediatr Allergy Immunol* 2014; 25: 71–79.

41. Nicolaou N, Poorafshar M, Murray C et al. Allergy or tolerance in children sensitized to peanut: Prevalence and differentiation using component-resolved diagnostics. *J Allergy Clin Immunol* 2010; 125: 191–197.

42. Flinterman AE, Van Hoffen E, den Hartog Jager CF et al. Children with peanut allergy recognize predominantly Ara h 2 and Ara h 6, which remains stable over time. *Clin Exp Allergy* 2007; 37: 1221–1228.

43. Mittag D, Akkerdaas J, Ballmer-Weber BK et al. Ara h 8, a Bet v 1 homologous allergen form peanut, is a major allergen in patients with combined birch pollen and peanut allergy. *J Allergy Clin Immunol* 2004; 114: 1410–1417.

44. Eller E, Brindslev-Jensen C. Clinical value of component-resolved diagnosis in peanut allergic patients. *Allergy* 2013; 68: 190–194.

45. Asarnoj A, Glaumann S, Elfstrom L et al. Anaphylaxis to peanut in a patient predominantly sensitized to Ara h 6. *Int Arch Allergy Immunol* 2012; 159: 209–212.

46. Pedrosa M, Boyano-Martínez T, García-Ara MC et al. Peanut seed storage proteins are responsible for clinical reactivity in Spanish peanut-allergic children. *Pediatr Allergy Immunol* 2012; 23: 654–659.

47. Dang TD, Tang M, Choo S et al. Increasing the accuracy of peanut allergy diagnosis by using Ara h 2. *J Allergy Clin Immunol* 2012; 129: 1056–1063.

48. Ebisawa M, Movérare R, Sato S et al. Measurement of Ara h 1-, 2-, and 3-specific IgE antibodies is useful in diagnosis of peanut allergy in Japanese children. *Pediatr Allergy Immunol* 2012; 23: 573–581.

49. Flores Kim J, McCleary N, Nwaru B, Stoddart A, Sheikh A. Diagnostic accuracy, risk assessment, and cost-effectiveness of component-resolved diagnostics for food allergy: A systematic review. *Allergy*. 2018; 73: 1609–1621.

50. Valcour A, Jones JE, Lidholm J, Borres MP, Hamilton RG. Sensitization profiles to peanut allergens across the United States. *Ann Allergy Asthma Immunol* 2017; 119: 262–266.

51. Onell A, Hjalle L, Borres MP. Exploring the temporal development of childhood IgE profiles to allergen components. *Clin Translational Allergy* 2012; 2: 24–30.

52. Datema MR, van Ree R, Asero R et al. Component-resolved diagnosis and beyond: Multivariable regression models to predict severity of hazelnut allergy. *Allergy* 2018; 73: 549–559.

53. Hamilton RG. Human immunoglobulins. In: O'Gorman MRG, Donnenberg AD, editors. *Handbook of Human Immunology*. 2nd ed. Boca Raton, FL: CRC Press, 2008: 63–106.

54. College of American Pathologists. In: Diagnostic Allergy (SE) Survey, participants summary, SE-cycle A-2018, Northfield, IL.

55. Schwartz, LB, Bradford TR. Regulation of tryptase from human lung mast cells by heparin. Stabilization of the active tetramer. *J Biol Chem* 1986; 261: 7372.

56. Schwartz LB. Diagnostic value of tryptase in anaphylaxis and mastocytosis. *Immunol Allergy Clin North Am* 2006; 26: 451.

57. Enander I, Matsson P, Andesson AS et al. A radioimmunoassay for human serum tryptase released during mast cell activation. *J Allergy Clin Immunol* 1990; 85: 154.

58. Van der Linden PW, Hack CE, Poortman J et al. Insect sting challenge in 138 patients: Relation between clinical severity of anaphylaxis and mast cell activation. *J Allergy Clin Immunol* 1992; 90: 110.

59. Schwartz LB, Yunginger JW, Miller J et al. Time course of the appearance and disappearance of human mast cell tryptase in the circulation after anaphylaxis. *J Clin Invest* 1989; 83: 1551.

60. Ruëff F, Przybilla B, Biló MB et al. Predictors of severe systemic anaphylactic reactions in patients with Hymenoptera venom allergy: Importance of baseline serum tryptase. *J Allergy Clin Immunol* 2009; 124: 1047–1054.

61. Nolte H, Schiltz PO, Kruse A et al. Comparison of intestinal mast cell and basophil histamine release in children with food allergic reactions. *Allergy* 1989; 44: 544–565.

62. Van Rooyen C, Anderson R. Assessment of determinants of optimum performance of the CAST-2000 ELISA procedure. *J Immunol Methods* 2004; 288: 1–7.

63. Siraganian RP. Automated histamine analysis for in vitro allergy testing. II. Correlation of skin test results with *in vitro* whole blood histamine release in 82 patients. *J Allergy Clin Immunol* 1977; 59: 214.

64. Maly FE, Marti-Wyss S, Blumber S et al. Mononuclear blood cell sulpholeukotriene generation in the presence of interleukin 3 and whole blood histamine release in honeybee and yellow jacket venom allergy. *J Invest Allergy Clin Immunol* 1997; 7: 217–224.

65. MacGlashan D. Autoantibodies to IgE and FcεRI and the natural variability of spleen tyrosine kinase expression in basophils. *J Allergy Clin Immunol.* 2019; 143: 1100–1107.

66. Bochner BS, Sterbinsky SA, Saini SA et al. Studies of cell adhesion and flow cytometric analyses of degranulation, surface phenotype and viability using human eosinophils, basophils and mast cells. *Methods* 1997; 13: 61–68.

67. Schroeder JT. Biology of basophils. In: Adkinson NF Jr, Bochner BS, Busse WW, Holgate ST, Lemanske RF Jr, Simons FER, editors. *Middleton's Allergy: Principles and Practice. 7th ed., Chapter 20. Maryland Heights, MO: Mosby Elsevier* 2009: 329–340.

68. Fink JN, Zacharisen MC. Hypersensitivity pneumonitis. In: Adkinson NF Jr, Yunginger JW, Busse WW et al., editors. *Middleton's Allergy: Principles and Practice. 6th ed. St. Louis, MO: Mosby,* 2003: 1373.

69. Moissidis I, Chaidaroon D, Vichyanond P et al. Milk-induced pulmonary disease in infants (Heiner syndrome). *Pediatr Allergy Immunol* 2005; 16: 545–552.

70. Lichtenstein LM, Norman PS, Winkenwerder WL. A single year of immunotherapy of ragweed hay fever: Immunologic and clinical studies. *Ann Intern Med* 1971; 75: 663.

71. James LK, Bowen H, Calvert RA et al. Allergen specificity of IgG(4)-expressing B cells in patients with grass pollen allergy undergoing immunotherapy. *J Allergy Clin Immunol* 2012; 130: 663–670.

72. Aalberse RC. The role of IgG antibodies in allergy and immunotherapy. *Allergy* 2011; 66(Suppl 95): 28–30.

73. Golden DBK, Lawrence ID, Hamilton RG et al. Clinical correlation of the venom-specific IgG antibody level during maintenance venom immunotherapy. *J Allergy Clin Immunol* 1992; 90: 386.

74. Shamji MH, Ljørring C, Francis JN et al. Functional rather than immunoreactive levels of IgG4 correlate closely with clinical response to grass pollen immunotherapy. *Allergy* 2012; 67: 217–226.

75. Shamji MH, Wilcock LK, Wachholz PA et al. The IgE-facilitated allergen binding (FAB) assay: Validation of a novel flow-cytometric based method for the detection of inhibitory antibody responses. *J Immunol Methods* 2006; 317: 71–79.

76. Kleine-Tebbe J, Herold DA. Inappropriate test methods in allergy. *Hautarzt* 2010; 61: 961–966.

77. Wüthrich B. Unproven techniques in allergy diagnosis. *J Investig Allergol Clin Immunol* 2005; 15: 86–90.

78. Fagan DL, Slaughter CA, Capra JD et al. Monoclonal antibodies to immunoglobulin G4 induce histamine release from human basophils *in vitro. J Allergy Clin Immunol* 1982; 70: 399–404.

79. Lichtenstein LM, Kagey-Sobotka A, White JM et al. Anti-human IgG causes basophil histamine release by acting on IgG-IgE complexes bound to IgE receptors. *J Immunol* 1992; 15: 3929–3936.

80. Stapel SG, Asero R, Ballmer-Weber BK et al. Testing for IgG4 against foods is not recommended as a diagnostic tool: EAACI Task Force Report. *Allergy* 2008; 63: 793–796.

81. Hamilton RG. Responsibility for quality IgE antibody results rests ultimately with the referring physician. (Invited Editorial). *Ann Allergy Asthma Immunol* 2001; 86: 353–354.

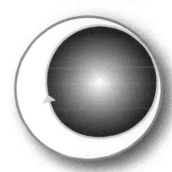

8 Nasal, bronchial, conjunctival, and food challenge techniques and epicutaneous immunotherapy of food allergy

Mark W. Tenn
Kingston General Health Research Institute

Matthew Rawls
Kingston General Health Research Institute
Queen's University

Babak Aberumand
Queen's University

Anne K. Ellis
Kingston General Health Research Institute
Queen's University

CONTENTS

8.1 INTRODUCTION

Allergen challenge is a tool that can be utilized by clinicians to diagnose allergic diseases. This technique administers an allergen of interest in a controlled and safe manner to assess allergic symptoms. The allergic disease in question will often dictate the route of exposure for the challenge. For example, when examining potential food allergies, an oral challenge involving ingestion of the allergen is typically selected. Allergen challenges may also be used to study allergic disease pathophysiology and biomarkers and to assess the efficacy of allergic medications or allergen-specific immunotherapies. This chapter focuses on the following allergen challenge techniques: nasal, bronchial, conjunctival, and oral food. Epicutaneous treatment of food allergy will also be reviewed (Table 8.1).

8.2 ALLERGIC RHINITIS AND NASAL ALLERGEN CHALLENGES

Allergic rhinitis (AR) is an upper airway disorder characterized by IgE-mediated inflammation of the nasal mucosa. After inhalation of sensitized allergens, AR patients experience nasal and ocular symptoms such as sneezing, nasal itching and congestion, rhinorrhea, and itchy/watery eyes [1,2]. In clinical practice, nasal allergen challenges (NACs) can serve as a diagnostic tool for AR. NACs can also be used to evaluate AR pathophysiology and AR medications such as intranasal corticosteroids and antihistamines. During NACs, allergen is directly delivered into the nasal cavity, producing an immediate allergic response. The subsequent sections that follow provide an overview of two different nasal challenge protocols along with the different methods of symptom assessments, allergen delivery, and implications.

8.2.1 Single-dose nasal challenge protocol

NACs can be performed using a single concentration, ideally of a standardized allergen extract, that induces clinical symptoms in most participants. These challenges typically occur during a single study visit and usually include three stages: baseline assessment, a control challenge, and the allergen challenge [3–5]. The first stage is the measurement of baseline nasal symptoms and nasal patency following acclimation to the study facility. To account for the preservatives in allergen extracts (e.g., glycerol or phenol), a control challenge is performed using the extract diluent or aqueous solution in which the allergen is prepared to exclude participants with nasal hyperreactivity [6]. An optional saline wash can be included to clean the nasal cavity prior to challenge. Approximately 10 minutes after the control challenge, clinical symptoms can be assessed. If no significant reactions were observed (i.e., symptoms are less than 50% of the positivity criteria), a bilateral NAC with the prespecified single allergen concentration is conducted with subjective and objective symptom assessments recorded 10–15 minutes postchallenge [3,4]. Bilateral challenges (i.e., both nostrils receive the allergen) are recommended to account for the parasympathetic reflex response of the opposite nasal cavity resulting in symptoms contralateral to the challenged nasal cavity [7]. Symptom assessment can also be repeated after an additional 10 minutes (25 minutes postchallenge) if a negative result was observed 15 minutes post-allergen challenge [3].

8.2.2 Titrated nasal challenge protocol

As an alternative to single-dose protocols, NACs can be performed using a series of increasing concentrations of allergen extract. Participants undergoing titrated allergen challenges receive different cumulative doses of the allergen depending on their symptom severity. Titrated NACs are completed during a single study visit with baseline

Table 8.1 Advantages and disadvantages of nasal, bronchoprovocation, ocular, and oral challenges

Route	Types of challenge	Advantages	Disadvantages
Nasal challenge	Nasal allergen challenges	• Use as a clinical tool for the diagnosis of allergic rhinitis • Use as a research tool for studying allergic rhinitis pathophysiology • Cost effective	• Allergen delivery method does not resemble natural outdoor allergen exposure
Bronchoprovocation challenge	Direct bronchoprovocation testing (e.g., with methacholine)	• High sensitivity for excluding an asthma diagnosis • Safe	• Small risk of severe bronchoconstriction during testing
	Indirect bronchoprovocation testing (e.g., with exercise, mannitol, allergens)	• High specificity to confirm an asthma diagnosis and accompanying trigger • Use as a research tool to study asthma	• Risk of anaphylaxis during testing • Can be time-consuming if testing is done in a titrated manner
Ocular challenge	Conjunctival allergen challenge	• Clinical diagnosis of allergic conjunctivitis • Useful for research of new anti-allergic ocular medications • Safe model	• Difficult for individuals who are uncomfortable with eye drops
Oral challenges	Open food challenge	• Food is eaten in a graded method, with 1–2 hours of observation between each step • A negative result confirms that the challenged food does not cause a reaction	• Largest potential of all oral food challenges (OFCs) for bias • Cost effective • Requires limited use of resources and time
	Single-blinded challenge	• Can use when there is potential for subjective symptoms to be reported • Can use a placebo • If the food is tolerated or there is evidence of objective symptoms, then a placebo challenge is not required	• Reliable • Does not exclude observer bias
	Double-blind placebo-controlled challenge	• Observer, patient, and dietician are blinded • Gold standard • Used for research purposes	• Patient and observer bias are minimized • Rigorous process
	Challenges to multiple foods	• Can be useful when the specific food cannot be determined from the clinical assessment, skin prick test, or allergen-specific serum IgE • Helpful when the patient is avoiding all related foods	• Potential for adverse reactions must be low • If positive, may be forced to avoid all foods that were mixed in the challenge if individual OFCs are not obtained • Potential for false-positives due to cross-reactivity between foods

assessments followed by control challenges [3–5]. Following a negative control challenge, participants receive a series of graded NACs with increasing concentrations of allergen extract. Clinical symptoms are assessed 10–15 minutes after each dose, and the titration is stopped once a positive response is observed (i.e., a predetermined threshold of clinical symptoms is reached) [8]. The starting allergen concentration is often approximately 1/100 of the allergen concentration required to induce a positive skin prick test (SPT) (3 mm wheal) or a general 1:1000 dilution from the stock extract concentration [4,9].

Both titrated and single-dose NACs can also be conducted together over two study visits [8,10]. Approximately 1–4 weeks after the allergen titration, participants can return to the study facility for a single-dose NAC using their qualifying allergen dose [8]. The qualifying allergen dose can be taken as the cumulative dose of all allergen concentrations received during the titrated NAC, or as the concentration that induced predefined clinical symptoms [8,10,11]. Clinical symptoms can then be assessed at regular time intervals extending up to 24 hours post-allergen challenge.

8.2.3 Subjective

There are multiple tools available for participants to subjectively rate the severity of their nasal and ocular symptoms. The visual analogue scale (VAS) was proposed by the Allergic Rhinitis and its Impact on Asthma (ARIA) guidelines as a method of grading the severity of nasal symptoms and congestion [1]. Participants are given a 10 cm long scale where they can indicate the severity of their symptoms as not bothersome (0 cm), mild (1–3 cm), moderate (4–7 cm), or extremely bothersome (8–10 cm) [12]. In the clinic, VAS is a highly sensitive tool in evaluating symptom severity in patients with symptomatic rhinitis [13]. The total nasal symptom score (TNSS) is recognized by the U.S. Food and Drug Administration as a self-reported composite score for the assessment of AR nasal symptoms. Compared to VAS, participants instead evaluate four individual nasal symptoms of nasal congestion, sneezing, nasal itching, and rhinorrhea using a Likert scale. For example, if a four-point scale is used, each individual nasal symptom can be scored between 0 (no symptoms) and 3 (severe symptoms) with TNSS ranging between 0 and 12 [8]. The Lebel and Linder symptom scores are two additional point scales that evaluate nasal and ocular symptoms. Compared to TNSS, the Lebel and Linder scales also quantify ocular symptoms and the amount of sneezing by each participant, for a maximum of 11 and 13 points, respectively [14,15].

8.2.4 Objective

Objective measurements complement subjective assessments of nasal symptom severity. Peak nasal inspiratory flow (PNIF) is a simple, cost-effective technique to measure nasal congestion following an NAC [11,16]. Participants are instructed to quickly and forcefully inhale through their nose while wearing a sealed mask over their nose and mouth. The resulting air flow measurements are in liters per minute (L/min) and strongly correlate with TNSS when the maneuver is performed correctly [8]. Also using a fitted mask, active anterior rhinomanometry (AAR) is an internationally recognized technique used to measure unilateral nasal airway resistance. During the procedure, both left and right nostrils are evaluated separately using a pressure probe. However, AAR cannot be performed if one of the two nostrils is blocked [17]. As an alternative, acoustic rhinomanometry (AcRh) can be used to evaluate nasal patency by detecting changes in nasal cavity volume. By using sound waves reflected in the nasal cavity, different cross-sectional areas (CSAs) can be measured before and after allergen challenge [18]. For example, CSA-2 is the CSA recorded at the second visible notch, corresponding to the level of the inferior turbinate head [4,18]. Finally, four-phase rhinomanometry (4PR) is another objective method used to evaluate nasal patency. This technique accounts for all four phases of the nasal breathing cycle (i.e., ascending and descending phases of both inspiration and expiration) [19].

8.2.5 Positive criteria

As described by the European Academy of Allergy and Clinical Immunology (EAACI) Task Force for the standardization of NAC protocols, both subjective and objective symptom assessments can be used when defining a positive NAC. For clearly positive responses, the task force recommends a measurement of 5.5 cm or greater using VAS, or an increase in five points or more in TNSS, Lebel, or Linder scores after allergen challenge [3]. Using objective assessments, a decrease of 40% or more in nasal airflow measured using PNIF or AAR (flow evaluated at 150 Pa) also indicates a clearly positive response. A decrease of at least 40% in CSA-2 using AcRh and an increase of at least 40% in logarithmic effective resistance using 4PR after allergen challenge indicates the same [3]. Both subjective and objective assessments can be used in combination to define a positive NAC. For example, when TNSS and PNIF were incorporated in the positive challenge criteria, qualifying participants demonstrated reproducible clinical changes between screening and challenge visits compared to the "TNSS only" or "PNIF only" groups [8].

8.2.6 Delivery methods and allergen preparation

How the allergen is delivered into the nose can impact the results of the NAC. The most common delivery method recommended by the EAACI Task Force is a pump-aerosol spray that can deliver 50–100 µL of allergen solution onto the anterior inferior turbinate. Although these devices are safe and easy to use, they carry a small risk of affecting the lower airways [3,4]. Alternative delivery methods include direct application of allergen onto the middle and inferior turbinate using a syringe, nose dropper, pipette, or paper disks/cotton saturated with allergen solution [4]. These methods require a higher level of control and can be difficult to perform. Finally, a nebulizer can be used to deliver allergen in powdered form. However, this method has a greater risk of depositing allergen into the lower airways [4].

Allergen extracts are often used when performing NACs. Commercial extracts are available for common environmental allergens (e.g., pollens, pet dander, house dust mite) and can be prepared as powders or glycerinated and aqueous (with phenol as a preservative) solutions [8,10,11,20,21]. However, extracts from different manufacturers are difficult to compare as several methods can be used to assess extract potency. For example, different concentration units can include standard quality units (SQ-U/mL), protein nitrogen units (PNU/mL), allergy units (AU/mL), and percentage weight/volume. The use of standardized units (e.g., the International System of Units) to quantify extract potency, such as microgram per milliliter (µg/mL) of major allergen, is suggested by many experts [3].

8.2.7 Implications

In addition to clinical practice, NACs are useful in evaluating the efficacy and mechanism of action of different AR medications, such as intranasal corticosteroids [22,23], antihistamines [24], and biologics [25]. More recently, NACs were used to evaluate the efficacy of two allergen-specific immunotherapy products targeting timothy grass and house dust mite allergens, respectively [26,27]. NACs can also be performed with smaller populations compared to ambient or natural allergen exposure [8,10]. Biologic sampling is facilitated with NAC. For example, nasal lavage and secretions, nasal scrapings, and peripheral blood samples can be collected following an NAC to study the allergic response and identify potential mediators as targets for therapy [11,28].

8.3 BRONCHOPROVOCATION TESTING

Asthma is a chronic lower airway inflammatory disorder characterized by reversible airway obstruction and airway hyperresponsiveness (AHR) [29,30]. Asthma symptoms include dyspnea (shortness of breath), chest tightness, wheezing, and coughing [30]. Exacerbations can be brought on by different triggers, such as cleaning products (irritant or occupational asthma), viral infection, and environmental allergens (allergic asthma). Subjects with asthma often require inhaled corticosteroids and bronchodilators to control symptoms [31–33].

The diagnosis of asthma is complex and requires a thorough patient history, physical examination, assessment of potential asthma triggers, and pulmonary lung function testing [30,34]. Asthma is a variable condition that obfuscates the value of a single spirometry assessment. Bronchoprovocation testing is a valuable tool in assessing the severity of airway responsiveness to a specific or nonspecific stimulant [35]. When negative, direct provocation testing with methacholine can help exclude an asthma diagnosis. In contrast, positive indirect provocation testing with physical or pharmacologic stimuli can help confirm an asthma diagnosis [36]. Provocation testing with allergen can also be used to investigate the pathophysiology of allergic asthma. The following sections discuss protocols commonly used during direct and indirect bronchoprovocation testing along with the selection of appropriate methacholine/allergen concentrations, delivery devices, and patient monitoring after testing.

8.4 DIRECT PROVOCATION TESTING WITH METHACHOLINE

Methacholine is a synthetic, cholinergic agonist that induces bronchoconstriction after inhalation by binding to surface muscarinic receptors on airway smooth muscle cells. Compared to healthy individuals, these cells are more responsive and contract at lower methacholine concentrations in asthma [30]. The degree of bronchoconstriction can then be quantified using spirometry. This section focuses on recent recommendations on bronchial challenge testing made by an International Task Force organized by the European Respiratory Society and the American Thoracic Society [35].

8.4.1 Inhalation protocol

A pretest questionnaire can be given to participants to screen for any contraindications to testing. Only a qualified technician or respiratory scientist should give instructions for the testing and perform the test. After inclusion and exclusion criteria are reviewed and informed consent is obtained, an optional physical examination of the lungs and chest can be performed prior to testing [35]. As recommended by the task force, methacholine challenge testing should not be performed if baseline forced expiratory volume (FEV_1) is less than 60% predicted for adults and children [35].

On the day of testing, all required material should be prepared and equipment (spirometer and nebulizer device) calibrated. The calculated concentrations of methacholine should be prepared and warmed to room temperature at least 30 minutes before testing [37]. Prechallenge spirometry is conducted to ensure participants are able to perform accurate and reproducible forced vital capacity (FVC) maneuvers to ensure the FEV_1 is greater than 55%–70% of predicted normal, and to establish a baseline FVC and FEV_1 (forced expiratory volume in 1 second) values. During the test, participants wear a nose clip and breathe in the lowest methacholine concentration aerosolized by the nebulizer. The task force recommends tidal breathing (i.e., restful or quiet breathing) of at least 1 minute with spirometry performed at 30 and 90 seconds postnebulization [35]. FEV_1 from acceptable FVC maneuvers is collected from each time point with the highest FEV_1 reported. If a less than 20% drop in FEV_1 is observed (20% drop calculated as $0.8 \times$ baseline FEV_1), the nebulizer is emptied, and the procedure is repeated with the next highest methacholine concentration. If a greater than 20% drop in FEV_1 is observed, the test is deemed positive, the procedure is terminated, and participants are given a fast-acting inhaled bronchodilator to reverse bronchoconstriction [35]. Spirometry can be done 5 minutes after administering the bronchodilator to ensure a return to baseline. The test results are typically reported as the provocative methacholine concentration required to cause a 20% drop in FEV_1 compared to baseline (PC_{20}). This calculation requires the last two methacholine concentrations used and the corresponding percentage (%) drops in FEV_1 from baseline [37].

Prior to giving the first methacholine concentration, a diluent step can be included in order to account for excessive AHR. Testing can continue if the postdiluent FEV_1 is within 10% of the baseline FEV_1. However, testing should not continue if a greater than 20% drop in postdiluent FEV_1 is observed [35]. Due to the cumulative effect of methacholine, the period of time between each concentration administered should also be kept constant. The task force recommends a maximum of three to four FVC maneuvers per concentration and a time interval of 5 minutes between concentrations [35].

8.4.2 Preparation of methacholine concentrations

Methacholine is prepared as a room temperature solution in sterile vials using sterile 0.9% saline (diluent). The solutions can be stored in the refrigerator until use. For methacholine challenges, the task force recommends an initial methacholine dose of 1–3 µg for participants with normal spirometry results and 1 µg for children and participants with highly sensitive airways [35,37]. Given the availability of different nebulizer devices, the methacholine concentration for the starting dose may need to be calculated based on the manufacturer's device specifications. For example, using the standard English Wright (EW) nebulizer with 2-minute tidal breathing, a starting concentration of 0.0625 mg/mL yields a dose of approximately 1.425 µg [35]. During challenge, the starting dose can be increased using doubling or quadrupling steps up to 16 mg/mL for a total of nine and five concentration steps, respectively.

8.4.3 Aerosol delivery devices and breathing methods

Two standard aerosol delivery methods are often used in methacholine challenge testing as recommended by the 1999

American Thoracic Society guidelines for methacholine and exercise challenge testing: the 2-minute tidal breathing method and five-breath dosimeter method [37]. The former uses a device capable of continuous nebulization (e.g., the EW nebulizer) with participants breathing in the aerosolized solution for 2 minutes before spirometry is performed. The latter uses a nebulizer that can generate aerosol when manually triggered (e.g., the DeVilbiss 646 nebulizer) or automatically when a specific inspiratory flow is reached by the participant. Using this method, participants inhale slowly and deeply from functional residual capacity up to total lung capacity over 5 seconds. The technician can trigger the device at the start of inhalation. Participants hold their breath for 5 seconds and then slowly exhale over another 5-second period. This is repeated for a total of five breath holds at each methacholine concentration with spirometry done after the fifth exhalation [37,38]. Compared to the doubling steps used in 2-minute tidal breathing, the five-breath dosimeter method uses quadrupling steps [37].

Due to the difficulty in finding standard EW and DeVilbiss 646 nebulizers, and the varying aerosol output rates and particle size distributions of modern devices, the task force recommends that methacholine challenge results be reported as the provocative dose of methacholine required to cause a 20% drop in FEV_1 (PD_{20}) instead of the PC_{20} [35]. PC_{20} values can vary depending on the nebulizer and inhalation protocol used. For example, in a randomized crossover study comparing two jet nebulizers, the breath-actuated AeroEclipse II nebulizer (20-second breathing protocol) yielded significantly lower methacholine PC_{20} values compared to the EW nebulizer (2-minute breathing protocol) in participants with asthma (0.79 versus 1.63 mg/mL, $P < .05$) [39]. In another crossover study with asthmatics, only the methacholine PD_{20} remained consistent across two different nebulizers and protocols with differing starting methacholine concentrations and inhalation times [40]. Calculating the PD_{20} is similar to calculating the PC_{20} and is dependent on the last two methacholine doses (in μg) and the corresponding percentage (%) drops in FEV_1 from baseline [35,40]. Compared to the concentrations used in calculating the PC_{20}, the formula for calculating the methacholine dose is based on the individual characteristics of the selected nebulizer (aerosol particle size and output rate) along with the methacholine concentration used, length of breathing, and respirable fraction [35].

8.5 INDIRECT PROVOCATION TESTING WITH PHYSICAL OR PHARMACOLOGIC STIMULI

Compared to methacholine, which directly binds to airway smooth muscle cells, indirect stimuli act through intermediate inflammatory and neuronal cells to induce bronchoconstriction. Stimuli such as exercise and mannitol facilitate airway water loss and increase the osmolarity of the airway surface liquid. This leads to the release of mediators such as leukotrienes and prostaglandins into the airways, resulting in bronchoconstriction during challenge [36,41]. In practice, direct challenges with methacholine have high sensitivity to exclude an asthma diagnosis, while indirect challenges have high specificity to confirm the presence of asthma along with identifying a potential trigger [36].

From recent recommendations made by the task force, exercise challenge testing can be used to determine the presence of exercise-induced bronchoconstriction in asthmatic patients [36]. Following

baseline spirometry, participants take part in vigorous exercise using a treadmill or cycle ergometer. The task force recommends a target minute ventilation of 60% of predicted maximum voluntary ventilation or a target heart rate greater than 85% of the predicted maximum should be reached within the first 2–3 minutes of testing and be maintained for 6 minutes thereafter [36]. Serial spirometry is then performed over the first 30 minutes after exercise. The challenge is deemed positive when a greater than 10% drop in FEV_1 from baseline is observed [36].

Indirect challenge testing with mannitol involves the delivery of increasing doses of dry powdered mannitol using a capsule-based inhaler device. The starting dose is typically 5 mg and is increased using doubling steps up to 320 mg [36]. Similar to the diluent step in methacholine challenges, a capsule without mannitol is first administered and participants are instructed to hold their breath for 5 seconds before resuming tidal breathing. The task force recommends two FVC maneuvers be performed 1 minute after the start of inhalation with the largest FEV_1 taken as baseline [36]. The procedure is then repeated with the starting dose of mannitol and the next largest dose thereafter until a positive response is obtained or a cumulative dose of 635 mg is reached, at which the test is stopped. The test is deemed positive when either a greater than 15% drop in FEV_1 from baseline or 10% drop in FEV_1 between two consecutive doses is observed [36]. In addition to supporting an asthma diagnosis, positive mannitol challenges can indicate the presence of eosinophilic airway inflammation [41,42]. For example, a recent study showed a significant positive correlation between AHR to mannitol and both submucosal and sputum eosinophils in a cohort of asthmatic individuals [43].

8.6 INDIRECT PROVOCATION TESTING WITH ALLERGEN: TYPES OF CHALLENGE PROTOCOLS

Allergic asthmatics can experience both an early-phase response and a late-phase asthmatic response 4–6 hours after allergen exposure [44]. Standardized bronchoprovocation testing with allergen can serve as a research tool to assess the biological mechanisms of these responses along with the evaluation of new asthma medications [45,46]. Allergen bronchoprovocation may also be useful clinically to establish a culprit allergen, e.g., occupational asthma. Similar to methacholine challenges, participants inhale specific concentrations of allergen extract aerosolized using a nebulizer. The resulting allergen-induced bronchoconstriction is monitored with spirometry. Examples of different protocols for allergen inhalation challenges are described next.

Allergen inhalation challenges can be performed in a titrated manner using a series of increasing (e.g., doubling steps) concentrations of allergen extract. Following a review of the inclusion and exclusion criteria and a baseline measurement of FEV_1 greater than 50%–60% of predicted normal, an initial screening challenge is performed to determine the allergen concentration required to cause an early phase asthmatic response (EAR), or a 20% drop in FEV_1 compared to baseline (APC_{20}). As with methacholine challenges, an optional diluent step is used to exclude participants with excessive or nonspecific AHR [47]. To begin, participants inhale the starting allergen concentration using the chosen nebulizer and breathing protocol (e.g., 2-minute tidal breathing or five-breath dosimeter method). FEV_1 is measured 10 minutes postnebulization, and the procedure is repeated with the next highest allergen concentration if a 20% decrease compared to baseline in FEV$_1$ is not observed. Once a 20% drop is observed, the challenge is terminated [47]. The challenge can also be stopped with a 15% decrease in FEV$_1$ [45]. A rapid-acting bronchodilator is administered to restore the FEV$_1$ to baseline. FEV$_1$ measurements can sequentially be performed at regular time intervals, often up to 7 hours postchallenge, to capture late-phase asthmatic responses [47]. A single-dose challenge can also be performed after the allergen titration [48]. Participants are challenged with the cumulative allergen dose that induced an EAR with spirometry performed thereafter. However, participants must be closely monitored due to the possibility of severe allergen-induced bronchoconstriction as a larger allergen dose is given at once instead of several doses over time [47].

Other challenge protocols include a chronic low-dose challenge model and segmental allergen challenges. The former includes challenging participants with low doses of the allergen daily over multiple weeks and is suggested to better reflect the natural course of allergic asthma [49,50]. The latter uses bronchoscopy to directly deliver the allergen into specific areas of the lung [51]. Using this method, participants can act as their own controls (i.e., diluent control and allergen can be delivered to the corresponding location of the right and left lung), and biological samples can be collected from tissue sites directly contacted by the allergen [52].

8.6.1 Preparation of allergen concentrations

Compared to methacholine challenges where 1–3 µg is the recommended starting dose for most participants, selecting a starting allergen concentration depends on the allergen concentration required to induce an EAR (i.e., APC$_{20}$). APC$_{20}$ depends on the severity of the participant's AHR and allergic sensitization [53,54]. The former can be assessed using methacholine or histamine bronchoprovocation and the latter with skin test endpoint titration where the lowest concentration required to induce a 2–3 mm wheal is determined [47,54]. APC$_{20}$ prediction equations have been developed using methacholine or histamine PC$_{20}$ and skin test endpoints [53–55]. It is considered safe to define the starting allergen concentration as three doubling concentrations less than the participant's calculated APC$_{20}$ [54].

8.7 COMMON CONTRAINDICATIONS, PARTICIPANT SAFETY, AND MONITORING AFTER CHALLENGES

Although bronchoprovocation testing with methacholine or allergen is considered safe, there is still a possibility of severe bronchoconstriction and/or allergen-induced anaphylaxis during challenge. Participants should always be monitored during and after the challenge to ensure breathing has returned to normal (i.e., FEV$_1$ ± 10% of baseline values) [35]. During allergen inhalation challenges, participants with positive allergen challenge responses should be monitored for at least 7 hours postexposure for possible late-phase asthmatic responses [47]. In cases of emergency, physicians or qualified personnel should be immediately available. Rescue medication such as bronchodilators and epinephrine should also be readily available [47].

As identified by the task force, common contraindications for bronchoprovocation testing include an inability to perform the inhalation protocol or reliably produce FVC maneuvers, airflow

limitations (e.g., FEV$_1$ less than 60% predicted), cardiovascular complications such as recent myocardial infarctions and uncontrolled hypertension, and recent eye surgeries [35,56]. For allergen inhalation challenges, common contraindications can also include a history of other immunologic disorders, cancers, a history of anaphylaxis or severe drug allergies, and the presence of severe or uncontrolled asthma [47].

8.8 ALLERGIC CONJUNCTIVITIS AND CONJUNCTIVAL ALLERGEN CHALLENGES

Allergic conjunctivitis is a symptomatic disorder of the eye that results from immunoglobulin E (IgE)–mediated mast cell degranulation initiating the release of histamine, cytokines, chemokines, and the recruitment of inflammatory cells. Common symptoms and signs of allergic conjunctivitis include ocular itching, tearing, redness, and chemosis, which is otherwise known as swelling of the conjunctiva. The conjunctiva is a thin, protective, mucosal membrane that covers the anterior sclera extending to behind the eyelids [57]. Allergic conjunctivitis symptoms are estimated to affect approximately 15%–20% of the population worldwide, with the United States reporting a prevalence of 40% [58,59]. Patients with allergic conjunctivitis often experience a reduced quality of life with a potential impact on daily activities such as reading, driving, and sleeping [60].

Conjunctival allergen challenge (CAC), also known as conjunctival allergen provocation test (CAPT), provides a model for safely evaluating the allergic inflammatory response to allergen placed on the conjunctival surface. Lyophilized extracts in diluent or saline may be used to provoke allergic conjunctivitis symptoms during a CAC [61]. During CAC, phenolic and glycerinated solutions should be avoided due to the potential risk of damaging the eye. A variety of environmental aeroallergens have been used for CAC. Some examples of allergens include Kentucky bluegrass, timothy grass, short ragweed, elm, birch, cat hair/dander, and dust mite [62–65]. CAC has also been used to investigate skin sensitizations and food allergies for latex, peanut, milks, and eggs [67–69]. According to EAACI guidelines for CAPT testing, there should be a minimum of 1 week between ocular allergen challenges [61].

8.9 CONJUNCTIVAL ALLERGEN CHALLENGE PROTOCOL

Although there are a variety of different techniques of ocular challenges, we focus on the ORA-CAC protocol established by Abelson et al. in 1990 [63]. The ORA-CAC model can be divided into three visits with variations depending on the goals of the CAC.

8.9.1 Visit 1

The intent of the first visit is to develop background information in order to identify and diagnose potential allergic conjunctivitis [63]. After obtaining written informed consent and demographic data, a medical history is collected to uncover possible allergens of interest. The physical examination is completed to ensure the participant does not have any physical abnormalities that may hinder the participant from safely undergoing an ocular challenge. Furthermore, ophthalmoscopic examination may be used to discover any ocular signs that are not consistent with allergic conjunctivitis such as corneal damage or dry eyes. Next, skin sensitization can be assessed using an SPT to allergens of interest. An SPT is a cost-effective technique to identify aeroallergen hypersensitivity with reported sensitivities ranging from 76% to 84% for aeroallergens in adults [66,67]. However, an SPT alone cannot definitively diagnose allergic conjunctivitis. After determining which allergens may be provoking ocular symptoms, a bilateral ocular allergen challenge may be performed by instilling 25 µL of saline (control) in one eye and 25 µL of allergen extract into the other eye [63]. Each solution is administered onto the inferior external quadrant of the bulbar conjunctiva [63]. Assessment of ocular symptoms may be performed at a variety of time intervals postchallenge. However, 15 minutes is commonly used to assess response [61–63]. If positive or qualifying criteria are not met, the allergen challenge may be repeated with a greater allergen concentration [61]. In research settings, nonallergic controls are challenged with the strongest dilution of an allergen extract to assess nonspecific, irritant reactions.

8.9.2 Visit 2

Participants return to assess the reproducibility of their allergic ocular symptoms during visit 2. All inclusion and exclusion criteria should be reevaluated along with baseline symptoms and signs. Participants are retested in both eyes with the allergen dilution used during the positive baseline challenge [63]. Nonallergic participants may also be challenged with the strongest dilution of allergen extract. Reproducibility of ocular signs and symptoms provides each participant with a baseline ocular response that may be useful when designing clinical trials to examine new medications for allergic conjunctivitis.

8.9.3 Visit 3

During visit 3, participants who have already verified allergic conjunctivitis and reproducibility may undergo a final bilateral ocular challenge. This visit follows a similar protocol as visits 1 and 2 with a physical examination, review of exclusion and inclusion criteria, and recording of baseline signs and symptoms. Participants may be excluded if significant symptoms are present that could compromise the response to allergen. The third visit provides the opportunity to examine ocular medication efficacy or other allergic conjunctivitis treatments such as immunotherapy [63]. Depending on the clinical trial design, intervention or placebo may be placed in either eye before or after allergen challenge using the previously qualified allergen dilution. The CAC model may be used to examine the duration of action or onset of treatment options.

8.9.4 Ocular symptom assessment

The traditional development of the CAC model proposed that clinical assessment of a positive challenge be measured using signs and symptoms of ocular itching, redness, tearing, lid swelling, and chemosis [63]. Total ocular symptom score (TOSS) measures these four symptoms on a four-point scale from 0 to 3 (0 = no symptoms, 1 = mild, 2 = moderate, 3 = severe symptoms warranting treatment).

However, not every participant may experience all symptoms when challenged. Ocular itching and redness are frequently used as primary responses in order to determine a positive allergic response. Itching and redness peak at approximately 3 and 15 minutes postchallenge, respectively [64,70]. Tearing and chemosis may also be objectively assessed. Chemosis can be examined by using a slit lamp, a tool that uses a bright light emitted through a long narrow opening, to determine if the conjunctivae are raised or ballooned. A score of five or greater using TOSS is considered a positive reaction following ocular challenge [61]. Alternatively, studies have used the validated five-stage Gronemeyer grading scale to measure the allergic response during a CAC [71,72]. For this method, stage 0 is an absence of a reaction, whereas stages 1 through 4 indicate progressively more severe signs and symptoms. Stage 1 indicates itching, ocular redness, and foreign-body sensation. Stage 2 adds tearing and vasodilation of conjunctiva bulbi to stage 1 signs and symptoms [71,72]. Next, stage 3 includes blepharospasm, erythema, and vasodilation of conjunctiva tarsi on top of stage 2 observations. Finally, stage 4 adds chemosis and lid swelling to stage 3 findings [71,72]. CAC that results in stage 2 or greater is considered a positive reaction.

8.9.5 Safety

The CAC model is regarded as a safe model for determining if an allergen can produce allergic conjunctivitis symptoms [63,73]. CAC is not recommended for patients who are pregnant or lactating, have uncontrolled diseases (asthma), and have systemic disorders such as heart and vascular diseases [61]. CAC is not recommended for drug allergy testing [61]. Potential adverse events are both systemic and local. Adverse events include bronchoconstriction, late-onset urticaria, one case of acute respiratory distress and wheeze (in a well-controlled asthmatic subject), periocular edema, eyelid swelling despite treatment, severe chemosis, severe ocular itching requiring an eyepatch, and one occurrence of anaphylaxis [61,73,74]. Based on these rare adverse events and a potential risk of anaphylaxis, CAC should always be performed by well-trained and experienced health professionals. An ophthalmologist or allergist on site is necessary when performing CAC. All participants should be monitored for 2 hours or until symptoms have subsided [61]. It is recommended by EAACI that participants leaving the facility have contact information for a medical professional and oral and/or topical antihistamines for possible late-phase reactions [61].

8.9.6 Implications

CAC may be used clinically to evaluate the relevance of an allergen causing allergic conjunctivitis. In particular, this model may be useful for diagnosis when there is an unclear history. CAC also has high specificity, positive predictive value, and negative predictive value for identifying allergic rhinitis due to sensitivity of aeroallergens such as *Dermatophagoides pteronyssinus* [62]. In addition, evidence suggests that CAC may be an alternative technique in the assessment of food allergies prior to oral challenge. In 2010, Kvenshagen et al. reported that regardless of wheal size and specific IgE, children with a negative CAC did not have a clinical IgE mediated food reaction during oral challenge [69]. Furthermore, all children who reacted with strong symptoms following CAC had a positive oral food challenge [69]. A subsequent study in 2017 supported this finding by demonstrating that 81 children with a positive CAC also had a positive response in a double-blind, placebo-controlled oral food challenge to peanut [68]. Likewise, no children with a negative CAC had a positive oral food challenge with a sensitivity and specificity for peanut allergy of 96% and 83%, respectively [68]. With increased research into this field, CAC could be a safe, preliminary step to support the identification of food allergy, particularly if patients or parents do not feel comfortable with oral food challenge.

8.10 FOOD ALLERGY AND ORAL FOOD CHALLENGES

Food allergy (FA) is defined as an adverse reaction arising from a specific immune response that occurs reproducibly on exposure to a given food or food additive [75,76]. These symptoms are triggered by exposure to food allergens, which are characterized as specific components of food, such as proteins and chemical haptens. These food allergens are recognized by allergen-specific immune cells and elicit immunologic responses leading to the adverse reaction. FA is increasing in prevalence in most countries, particularly in more affluent regions [75]. Despite its ability to negatively affect quality of life and to cause significant morbidity and even death, very limited options remain for treatment of FA. The mainstay of treatment is avoidance of the allergen, treatment of symptoms, and periodic rechallenge to verify the persistence of the FA [75,77]. However, new, emerging food immunotherapy options are promising.

8.11 DIAGNOSIS OF FOOD ALLERGY

Initial evaluation of a food allergy should begin with a thorough medical history and a focused physical examination [75]. Important considerations include the time between the development of symptoms and the ingestion of the suspected food, the quantity of the suspected food that caused the reaction, the frequency and reproducibility of the reaction, and the effect of extenuating circumstances, such as exercise [77]. The history and physical examination alone cannot confirm a diagnosis of FA [75]. An SPT with the food extract and allergen-specific serum IgE may help identify foods that potentially provoke an IgE-mediated, food-induced allergic reaction. However, these prerequisite tests are also not diagnostic of FA. In fact, specific IgE measurements do not always correlate with oral provocation tests [78].

Food elimination diets, whereby one or a few specific suspected foods are removed from the diet for a span of 1–2 weeks, can be helpful in identifying the culprit food, but elimination diet does not confirm the diagnosis of FA [78]. Oral food challenges (OFCs), whereby the allergen is ingested in incremental doses over time, are the gold standard for diagnosing FA [75,79]. There are three types of OFCs: open, single-blind, and double-blind, placebo-controlled (DBPC) [75,77]. The choice of challenge depends on the clinical assessment and the likely level of bias in interpreting the results [77,80].

8.12 INDICATIONS FOR AN ORAL FOOD CHALLENGE

An OFC may be indicated to confirm an adverse reaction to a suspected food based on the clinical assessment, SPT results, and/or allergen-specific IgE levels. Alternatively, an OFC can be used to

Box 8.1 Indications for an OFC

- To confirm an adverse reaction to a suspected food
- To identify a food that may have caused an adverse reaction
- To determine whether a known food allergy has resolved
- To determine the lowest threshold dose at which a food can cause an adverse reaction

determine whether a prior food allergy has resolved. For research purposes, an OFC can determine the lowest dose (i.e., threshold) at which a food can cause an adverse immunologic reaction. This is particularly useful in clinical trials (Box 8.1). A complete evaluation of the risk-benefit ratio should help determine whether to pursue an OFC [79–81]. Factors to consider are the patient's age, medical history, and previous adverse food reactions; the likelihood that the suspected allergic reaction was IgE or non-IgE mediated; SPT and serum food-specific IgE results; the type of food implicated; and the importance of the food in the diet. As many as 50% of challenges in patients with a suspected food reaction will be positive, and approximately 11% will be severe [79,80,82,83]. This information should be shared with a challenge subject and the family.

8.13 TYPES OF ORAL FOOD CHALLENGES

8.13.1 Open food challenge

An open OFC involves eating the challenged food in its natural form. The food is eaten in a graded method, starting with a very low amount, followed by a half-hour to 2-hour observation period after each step. The natural form of the food may be raw or prepared the way the patient normally eats the food [77,78,80]. In this scenario, the challenge is unblinded, in that the patient and the observer are aware of the food. In clinical practice, this procedure is used as a screening challenge as objective symptoms are anticipated and there is potential for a severe reaction, making a home challenge ill advised. OFC should only be used if likely bias is low, as it has the largest potential of all OFCs for bias [77,80]. A negative open OFC confirms that the challenged food does not cause a reaction. However, a positive result with subjective symptoms requires a further challenge that is blinded to confirm that this is a true reaction [77,80,82]. An open OFC is a reasonable starting challenge for the evaluation of an adverse reaction to a specific food as it is cost effective and requires limited use of resource and time [80,82].

8.13.2 Single-blind challenge

A single-blinded OFC uses the method of delivering the food in question via a masking vehicle or an opaque capsule to reduce bias. In this challenge, the patient is blinded to the food, but the observer knows the food is being tested. The decision to use a placebo depends on the potential for subjective symptoms to be reported [79,80]. A placebo can be used for either single-blind or DBPC challenges. If a placebo is not used, the patient is informed that food that is being tested may or may not be given during the challenge. If the patient tolerates the food or there is evidence of objective symptoms, then a placebo challenge is not required. Single-blinded OFCs tend to be reliable in the clinical setting; however, they are limited in that they do not exclude observer bias [79,80].

If a placebo is used, the food being challenged and the placebo should be administered at least 2 hours apart. It is imperative that the placebo and food being challenged do not differ in texture, smell, appearance, taste, and feel. If subjective symptoms are anticipated, repeated challenges with the placebo and active food may help to interpret the results. If subjective symptoms follow three doses of the test food but not the placebo, the challenge is considered positive [80]. If a negative single-blinded OFC is obtained, an open OFC should be done at least 2 hours thereafter with the food prepared the way the patient consumes and with normal portions [79,80,84].

8.13.3 Double-blind, placebo-controlled challenges

In a DBPC OFC, the food is prepared by someone other than the observer and test subject, often a dietician, who is not involved in administering or evaluating the patient during the challenge. The patient and the observer are unaware of when the test food is administered. Consequently, patient and observer bias are minimized. There is no set order in terms of administering the placebo or food in question. This form of challenge is deemed the "gold standard" when it comes to diagnosing FA [80]. However, DBPC OFC is a rigorous process and is often reserved for research purposes or select clinical cases [77,79,80,82].

8.14 CHALLENGES TO MULTIPLE FOODS

Open or single-blind OFCs may use more than one food on the same day, separated by at least 2 hours, if the concern for a delayed reaction is low. If the clinical assessment indicates that it was likely a delayed reaction, i.e., the reaction had occurred longer than 2 hours after the consumption of the food, multiple food challenges should not occur on the same day. If multiple OFCs are negative, then the patient should reintroduce the tested foods into their diet [80].

Some foods, such as tree nuts, fish, and shellfish, have a potential for cross-reactivity. An OFC to multiple foods during one session may be pursued, especially if the potential of having an adverse reaction is low. A mixed OFC may be attempted for patients who avoid all related foods such as the patient who had an adverse reaction to peanuts and avoids all tree nuts. The foods, in this case nuts, are mixed together and administered in one session. If the OFC is positive, then either further individual OFCs to each food to delineate the food allergen culprit or avoidance of all foods that were mixed in the challenge is recommended. A mixed OFC consisting of the entire meal may also be beneficial when the specific food cannot be determined from the clinical assessment, SPT, or allergen-specific serum IgE [80].

8.15 GENERAL CONSIDERATIONS FOR ORAL FOOD CHALLENGES

A detailed medication list from the patient should be obtained prior to any OFC, as there is a potential for certain medications to interfere with the interpretation of an OFC and mask symptoms. The patient should have discontinued antihistamines for at least five half-lives of the specific drug. Inhaled and topical steroids, calcineurin inhibitors, leukotriene antagonists, and β-agonists should be temporarily stopped or used at the lowest dose. Aspirin, nonsteroidal anti-inflammatory drugs (NSAIDs), angiotensin-converting enzyme inhibitors (ACEi), alcohol, proton pump inhibitors (PPIs), and antacids can also affect OFC results and should be stopped, if possible, before the challenge. β-Blockers can cause issues if anaphylaxis occurs and epinephrine is required [79,80]. If a patient is taking high-dose systemic corticosteroids or a biologic such as omalizumab, an OFC should not take place as these may impact interpretation of the food challenge result. Special consideration should be made to the patient's medical condition and its severity, as adjustments may be required [79].

The test subject ideally should fast for 4 hours before the OFC to ensure that the results are not confounded by other foods. Non-IgE-mediated reactions may require a longer fasting period [78]. Liquids and nonfatty snacks may be allowed in special circumstances [79]. Before starting the OFC, the subject's blood pressure, heart rate, respiratory rate, and oxygen saturation should be obtained, and any pertinent physical examination findings should be documented [80]. Challenges should occur in either a clinic that is equipped to handle anaphylaxis or a monitored hospital setting. A clinician, ideally an allergist and immunologist trained in managing acute allergic reactions including anaphylaxis, should observe the challenged subject [78–80]. Epinephrine, oxygen, antihistamines, β-agonists, corticosteroids, and intravenous fluids should be readily available for management of acute allergic reactions [79,85].

Determining the initial dose to use in an OFC can be challenging as lower doses and longer intervals between administering the food pose a risk of a false-negative result due to partial desensitization during the challenge [79,86], whereas, higher starting doses increase the likelihood for a severe reaction during the challenge. For immediate, IgE-mediated reactions, it is recommended that a challenge that utilizes a semilogarithmic schedule of 3, 10, 30, 100, 300, 1000, and 3000 mg of food protein administered at least at 20-minute intervals is used [79]. The time interval may be prolonged depending on the patient's history, especially in those reporting a delayed reaction. However, most acute, serious reactions occur within 15 minutes [78,80,82]. The patient should be reexamined before each dose is administered [80].

Challenges should be postponed if the patient has an unstable atopic disease such as asthma, atopic dermatitis, or allergic rhinitis, or has chronic urticaria. The challenge can be reconsidered when these conditions are better controlled and stable. Furthermore, challenges should not be conducted in patients that have chronic medical conditions that increase the risk of anaphylaxis such as unstable angina, dysrhythmias, and severe chronic lung disease. Pregnant patients should not undergo an OFC [79,80]. A convincing, recent (within several weeks) anaphylactic reaction to the food in question should also prompt deferring the OFC, in the opinion of most experts [80].

8.16 WHEN TO STOP AN ORAL FOOD CHALLENGE

A positive OFC is judged to result in a clinical reaction as determined by objective signs or symptoms. Conversely, a negative OFC is one in which no clinical reaction occurs. The involvement of two or more organ systems is a strong indication of a true, positive OFC. In nonverbal children, clues to the onset of a reaction may include ear picking, tongue rubbing, putting a hand in the mouth, or neck scratching, or a change in general demeanor such as becoming quiet, withdrawn, or assuming the fetal position. In older patients, clues to an impending severe reaction may include subjective symptoms of throat tightness or pruritus, nausea, abdominal pain, or general malaise. A positive OFC prompts observation for at least 2 hours postchallenge to ensure resolution. Patients with a clinical history of biphasic anaphylactic reactions to food should be observed longer (i.e., at least 6 hours). Following a positive OFC, patients should be provided with a self-injectable epinephrine device and educated on specific food avoidance. A negative OFC indicates that the food can be consumed safely and should be reintroduced into the diet [80].

An OFC should be stopped whenever objective symptoms of an allergic reaction are documented, and treatment should commence promptly. If subjective symptoms occur, a longer interval period of observation before administering the next dose is advisable. Severe symptoms, even without objective findings, may justify discontinuing OFC and initiating treatment. This can particularly be a problem in unblinded challenges.

8.17 FOOD ALLERGY AND EPICUTANEOUS IMMUNOTHERAPY

Given the increasing prevalence of food allergies, there is a great deal of interest in additional treatment of this debilitating condition beyond avoidance and elimination of the allergen in the diet [75,87]. One such method to treat food allergies is epicutaneous immunotherapy (EPIT) [88]. Unlike the other routes of allergen-specific immunotherapy (AIT), such as oral immunotherapy (OIT), sublingual immunotherapy (SLIT), and subcutaneous immunotherapy (SCIT), EPIT relies on altering the immune system through direct contact of the allergen with intact skin [88,89]. The allergen is contained in a soluble form in a skin patch that is applied to the skin; subsequently, the allergen is absorbed into the epidermis where there are numerous antigen-presenting cells [88,90]. The immune response is modified with minimal systemic effects.

8.17.1 Mechanism

The exact mechanism by which EPIT modulates the immune system is not completely understood. It is believed the production of regulatory T cells (Tregs) and suppression of mast cell and basophil reactivity results in a decrease in allergen-specific IgE and an increase in allergen-specific IgG4, shifting T-helper (Th) 2 responses to a Th1 phenotype. This chain of events is initially achieved by the uptake of the allergen in the skin by dendritic cells and Langerhans cells. Subsequently, the allergen is transported to the lymph nodes resulting in an increase in Tregs. Repeated allergen patch applications to the skin increase Tregs and reduce systemic allergen-specific immune responses. Induction of Tregs has also been observed in SCIT and SLIT, but the type of Tregs differs in the various forms

of immunotherapy [89,91,92]. Termination of EPIT does not affect immediately the suppressive activity of Tregs, and this may provide a sustained benefit [92].

As with other methods of AIT, the aim is to desensitize patients to a maintenance dose, which would increase the antigen threshold that can lead to an allergic reaction. The long-term clinical goal is remission after discontinuation, also known as sustained unresponsiveness [88].

8.17.2 Efficacy

The first case study of EPIT occurred in 1921 by Vallery Radot in which he administered horse allergen on scarified skin to reduce systemic allergic symptoms in patients allergic to horses [93]. Between the years of 1950 and 1960, French allergologists further investigated EPIT after applying drops of pollen and house dust mite allergen extract repeatedly to scarified skin of the volar forearm to improve hay fever [94,95]. This form of EPIT was successful and deemed safe, but it fell out of favor due to the discomfort associated with skin scarification that was achieved by using a needle to scratch the skin [96]. The disruption of the epidermis was thought to promote an increase in a pro-inflammatory immune response and consequently increase antigen uptake [97].

There is a revival of EPIT with the development of new epicutaneous delivery systems. Murine studies demonstrated that EPIT has comparable efficacy compared with SCIT in desensitization to peanut, ovalbumin, pollen, and house dust mite allergy [96]. These findings prompted further studies in humans. A randomized trial of EPIT containing 12 pollen extracts showed significant symptom improvement with minimal side effects in adult subjects with allergic rhinitis [98,99]. Similar findings were observed in a pediatric study [100].

Parallel to those studies, clinical trials looking at EPIT via Viaskin Patch (DBV Technologies SA, Paris, France) for the treatment of FA have produced some promising results. This form of patch utilizes the moisture from transepidermal water loss to increase the permeability of the stratum corneum and as a result increase allergen delivery across intact skin [90]. A DBPC pilot study of milk EPIT in children between the ages of 3 months to 15 years with milk allergy demonstrated clinical efficacy with a good safety profile over a 3-month period [101]. EPIT treatment of peanut allergy shows a modest treatment response, with higher responses among younger children, and higher adherence rates compared to other forms of immunotherapy [102–104]. Treatment longer than 12 months demonstrates an increase in the efficacy of EPIT, but sustained effects of EPIT are undefined [103].

8.17.3 Safety

EPIT is safe in comparison with other allergen-specific immunotherapies. There is no large systemic exposure to the allergen [89,90]. The result is a low risk of systemic reactions including anaphylaxis. Most clinical trials have noted only minor local reactions such as erythema, pruritus, edema, eczema, or urticaria at the site of or near to the patch. These local reactions were mild, well tolerated, and often self-resolving or responsive to oral antihistamines and topical corticosteroids. There were no severe, systemic reactions requiring epinephrine [101,104,105].

8.17.4 Summary

EPIT, at its infancy state, serves as a promising alternative to subcutaneous, sublingual, and oral forms of immunotherapy with the advantages of being needle free, easy to administer, and safe [106]. Clinical trials suggest that EPIT has a similar efficacy to that of SLIT and low-dose OIT but not to that of high-dose OIT in the treatment of FA. Further studies of EPIT are required to determine the optimal doses and protocols for long-term efficacy for various FAs. Interestingly, a difference in immunologic response to EPIT in older and younger subjects (aged 11 years and younger) has been noted, with the younger having a more successful response [105]. This age-dependent response along with the allergen dose in the patch, the number of patches administered, and the duration of each patch application are important considerations in determining the efficacy, safety, and side effects of future EPIT studies [107]. Furthermore, EPIT biomarkers as a surrogate of clinical efficacy and treatment outcome are currently lacking and should be explored [90].

8.18 SUMMARY OF ALLERGEN CHALLENGES

Allergen challenges can be utilized in clinical practice to diagnose allergic diseases such as AR, allergic asthma, allergic conjunctivitis, and food allergy. In a research setting, allergen challenges may also provide an opportunity to study pathophysiologic development of allergic diseases. In addition, allergen challenges may be used for clinical trials to evaluate the efficacy and mechanism of action for medications that attempt to alleviate allergic symptoms. NACs and bronchoprovocation challenges are utilized to examine AR and allergic asthma, respectively. CACs are performed to diagnose and study allergic conjunctivitis. OFCs are used to confirm a suspected food allergy. Regardless of the type of allergen challenge, it should be performed in a controlled environment to prevent exposure to other allergens, which may confound the result. Furthermore, a trained healthcare professional, ideally an allergist, should be available to monitor the challenge in a facility or hospital setting that is equipped to handle severe allergic reactions such as anaphylaxis. Overall, allergen challenges are a technique for confirming a suspected allergic response and provided a clinical model to study allergic diseases.

SALIENT POINTS

- Nasal allergen challenges and conjunctival allergen challenges are safe and reliable models that can be used to study the efficacy of anti-allergic medications for individuals with ocular and nasal allergies.
- Nasal allergen challenges are often performed using allergen extracts and either a single-dose or titrated challenge protocol.
- The pump-aerosol spray device is the most common method for intranasal allergen delivery. Alternative methods include syringes, nose drippers, pipetting, and paper disks/cotton saturated with allergen solution.
- Direct bronchoprovocation testing has a high sensitivity to exclude an asthma diagnosis. Indirect bronchoprovocation testing has a high specificity to confirm an asthma diagnosis.
- During bronchoprovocation testing, provocative dose calculations can be preferred over the provocative concentration due to their consistency across different nebulizers.

- Selection of a starting allergen concentration for allergen inhalation testing depends on both the severity of the participant's airway hyperresponsiveness (AHR) (measured via methacholine challenges) and degree of allergic sensitization (measured with skin test endpoint titration).
- Double-blind placebo-controlled food challenges are considered the "gold standard" in the diagnosis of food allergy. Other challenge methods include open food challenges and single-blind challenges (only the participant is blinded to the food).
- An increasing semilogarithmic schedule with each food protein amount given 20 minutes apart is recommended during oral food challenges.
- Epicutaneous immunotherapy is a safe and simple to administer therapeutic option that attempts to treat allergic symptoms by modulating the immune response through direct exposure of an allergen on intact skin.

REFERENCES

1. Bousquet J, Van Cauwenberge P, Khaltaev N, Aria Workshop Group, World Health Organization. Allergic rhinitis and its impact on asthma. *J Allergy Clin Immunol* 2001; 108(5 Suppl): S147–S334.
2. Keith PK, Desrosiers M, Laister T, Schellenberg RR, Waserman S. The burden of allergic rhinitis (AR) in Canada: Perspectives of physicians and patients. *Allergy Asthma Clin Immunol* 2012; 8(1): 7.
3. Augé J, Vent J, Agache I et al. EAACI Position paper on the standardization of nasal allergen challenges. *Allergy* 2018; 73(8): 1597–1608.
4. Dordal MT, Lluch-Bernal M, Sánchez MC et al. Allergen-specific nasal provocation testing: Review by the rhinoconjunctivitis committee of the Spanish Society of Allergy and Clinical Immunology. *J Investig Allergol Clin Immunol* 2011; 21(1): 1–12.
5. Campo P, Barrionuevo E, Eguiluz I, Salas M, Torres MJ, Rondón C. Nasal provocation tests with allergens: Just a research tool or suitable for everyday clinical practice? *Curr Treat Options Allergy* 2017; 4(1): 98–109.
6. Lluch-Bernal M, Dordal MT, Anton E et al. Nasal hyperreactivity: Nonspecific nasal provocation tests. Review by the Rhinoconjunctivitis Committee of the Spanish Society of Allergy and Clinical Immunology. *J Investig Allergol Clin Immunol* 2015; 25: 396–407.
7. Bachert C. Nasal provocation test: Critical evaluation. In: Ring J, Behrendt HD, editors. *New Trends in Allergy IV*. Berlin, Heidelberg: Springer-Verlag, 1997, pp. 277–280.
8. Ellis AK, Soliman M, Steacy L et al. The Allergic Rhinitis – Clinical Investigator Collaborative (AR-CIC): Nasal allergen challenge protocol optimization for studying AR pathophysiology and evaluating novel therapies. *Allergy Asthma Clin Immunol* 2015; 11: 16.
9. Loureiro G, Tavares B, Machado D, Pereira C. Nasal provocation test in the diagnosis of allergic rhinitis. In: Kowalski M, editor. *Allergic Rhinitis*. London: InTech, 2012, pp. 153–182.
10. Soliman M, North ML, Steacy LM et al. Nasal allergen challenge studies of allergic rhinitis: A guide for the practicing clinician. *Ann Allergy Asthma Immunol* 2014; 113(3): 250–256.
11. Scadding GW, Calderon MA, Bellido V et al. Optimisation of grass pollen nasal allergen challenge for assessment of clinical and immunological outcomes. *J Immunol Methods* 2012; 384: 25–32.

12. Bousquet J, Khaltaev N, Cruz AA et al. Allergic Rhinitis and its Impact on Asthma (ARIA) 2008 Update (in collaboration with the World Health Organization, GA2LEN and AllerGen). *Allergy* 2008; 63(Suppl 86): 8–160.
13. Demoly P, Bousquet PJ, Mesbah K, Bousquet J, Devillier P. Visual analogue scale in patients treated for allergic rhinitis: An observational prospective study in primary care: Asthma and rhinitis. *Clin Exp Allergy*. 2013 Aug; 43(8): 881–888.
14. Lebel B, Bousquet J, Morel A et al. Correlation between symptoms and the threshold for release of mediators in nasal secretions during nasal challenge with grass-pollen grains. *J Allergy Clin Immunol* 1988; 82: 869–877.
15. Linder A. Symptom scores as measures of the severity of rhinitis. *Clin Allergy* 1988; 18: 29–37.
16. Starling-Schwanz R, Peake HL, Salome CM et al. Repeatability of peak nasal inspiratory flow measurements and utility for assessing the severity of rhinitis. *Allergy* 2005; 60: 795–800.
17. Carney AS, Bateman ND, Jones NS. Reliable and reproducable anterior active rhinomanometry for the assessment of unilateral nasal resistance. *Clin Otolaryngol* 2000; 25: 499–503.
18. Gotlib T, Samoliński B, Grzanka A. Bilateral nasal allergen provocation monitored with acoustic rhinometry. Assessment of both nasal passages and the side reacting with greater congestion: Relation to the nasal cycle. *Clin Exp Allergy* 2005; 35: 313–318.
19. Vogt K, Jalowayski AA, Althaus W et al. 4-Phase-Rhinomanometry (4PR)--basics and practice 2010. *Rhinol Suppl* 2010; 21: 1–50.
20. Neighbour H, Soliman M, Steacy LM et al. The Allergic Rhinitis Clinical Investigator Collaborative (AR-CIC): Verification of nasal allergen challenge procedures in a study utilizing an investigational immunotherapy for cat allergy. *Clin Transl Allergy* 2018; 8: 15.
21. Chusakul S, Phannaso C, Sangsarsri S et al. House-dust mite nasal provocation: A diagnostic tool in perennial rhinitis. *Am J Rhinol Allergy* 2010; 24: 133–136.
22. Erin EM, Leaker BR, Zacharasiewicz AS et al. Single dose topical corticosteroid inhibits IL-5 and IL-13 in nasal lavage following grass pollen challenge. *Allergy* 2005; 60(12): 1524–1529.
23. Baroody FM, Shenaq D, DeTineo M, Wang J, Naclerio RM. Fluticasone furoate nasal spray reduces the nasal-ocular reflex: A mechanism for the efficacy of topical steroids in controlling allergic eye symptoms. *J Allergy Clin Immunol* 2009; 123(6): 1342–1348.
24. Deruaz C, Leimgruber A, Berney M, Pradervand E, Spertini F. Levocetirizine better protects than desloratadine in a nasal provocation with allergen. *J Allergy Clin Immunol* 2004; 113(4): 669–676.
25. Hanf G, Noga O, O'Connor A, Kunkel G. Omalizumab inhibits allergen challenge-induced nasal response. *Eur Respir J* 2004; 23(3): 414–418.
26. Scadding GW, Calderon MA, Shamji MH et al. Effect of 2 years of treatment with Sublingual Grass Pollen Immunotherapy on Nasal response to allergen challenge at 3 years among patients with moderate to severe seasonal allergic rhinitis: The GRASS randomized clinical trial. *JAMA* 2017; 317(6): 615–625.
27. Gunawardana NC, Zhao Q, Carayannopoulos LN et al. The effects of house dust mite sublingual immunotherapy tablet on immunologic biomarkers and nasal allergen challenge symptoms. *J Allergy Clin Immunol* 2018; 141(2): 785–788 e9.
28. Leaker BR, Malkov VA, Mogg R et al. The nasal mucosal late allergic reaction to grass pollen involves type 2 inflammation (IL-5 and IL-13), the inflammasome (IL-1β), and complement. *Mucosal Immunol* 2017; 10(2): 408–420.
29. Maslan J, Mims JW. What is Asthma? pathophysiology, demographics, and health care costs. *Otolaryngol Clin North Am* 2014; 47(1): 13–22.
30. Mathur SK, Busse WW. Asthma: Diagnosis and management. *Med Clin North Am* 2006; 90(1): 39–60.
31. Wenzel SE. Asthma phenotypes: The evolution from clinical to molecular approaches. *Nat Med* 2012; 18(5): 716–725.
32. Wenzel SE. Asthma: Defining of the persistent adult phenotypes. *The Lancet* 2006; 368(9537): 804–813.
33. Maestrelli P, Boschetto P, Fabbri LM, Mapp CE. Mechanisms of occupational asthma. *J Allergy Clin Immunol* 2009; 123(3): 531–542.
34. Yurdakul AS, Dursun B, Canbakan S, Cakaloğlu A, Capan N. The assessment of validity of different asthma diagnostic tools in adults. *J Asthma* 2005; 42(10): 843–846.
35. Coates AL, Wanger J, Cockcroft DW, Bronchoprovocation Testing Task Force: Kai-Håkon Carlsen et al. ERS technical standard on bronchial challenge testing: General considerations and performance of methacholine challenge tests. *Eur Respir J* 2017; 49(5).
36. Hallstrand TS, Leuppi JD, Joos G et al. ERS technical standard on bronchial challenge testing: Pathophysiology and methodology of indirect airway challenge testing. *Eur Respir J* 2018; 52(5).
37. Crapo RO, Casaburi R, Coates AL et al. Guidelines for methacholine and exercise challenge testing-1999. This official statement of the American Thoracic Society was adopted by the ATS Board of Directors, July 1999. *Am J Respir Crit Care Med* 2000; 161(1): 309–329
38. Wubbel C, Asmus MJ, Stevens G, Chesrown SE, Hendeles L. Methacholine challenge testing: Comparison of the two American Thoracic Society-recommended methods. *Chest* 2004; 125(2): 453–458.
39. El-Gammal AI, Killian KJ, Scime TX et al. Comparison of the provocative concentration of methacholine causing a 20% fall in FEV1 between the AeroEclipse II breath-actuated nebulizer and the wright nebulizer in adult subjects with asthma. *Ann Am Thorac Soc* 2015; 12(7): 1039–1043.
40. Dell SD, Bola SS, Foty RG, Marshall LC, Nelligan KA, Coates AL. Provocative dose of methacholine causing a 20% drop in FEV1 should be used to interpret methacholine challenge tests with modern nebulizers. *Ann Am Thorac Soc* 2015; 12(3): 357–363.
41. Leuppi JD. Bronchoprovocation tests in asthma: Direct versus indirect challenges. *Curr Opin Pulm Med* 2014; 20(1): 31–36.
42. Sverrild A, Porsbjerg C, Thomsen SF, Backer V. Diagnostic properties of inhaled mannitol in the diagnosis of asthma: A population study. *J Allergy Clin Immunol* 2009; 124(5): 928–932 e1.
43. Sverrild A, Bergqvist A, Baines KJ et al. Airway responsiveness to mannitol in asthma is associated with chymase-positive mast cells and eosinophilic airway inflammation. *Clin Exp Allergy* 2016; 46(2): 288–297.
44. Verstraelen S, Bloemen K, Nelissen I, Witters H, Schoeters G, Van Den Heuvel R. Cell types involved in allergic asthma and their use in in vitro models to assess respiratory sensitization. *Toxicol In Vitro* 2008; 22(6): 1419–1431.
45. Gauvreau GM, Arm JP, Boulet L-P et al. Efficacy and safety of multiple doses of QGE031 (ligelizumab) versus omalizumab and placebo in inhibiting allergen-induced early asthmatic responses. *J Allergy Clin Immunol* 2016; 138(4): 1051–1059.

46. Singh A, Shannon CP, Kim YW et al. Novel Blood-based Transcriptional Biomarker Panels Predict the Late-Phase Asthmatic Response. *Am J Respir Crit Care Med* 2018; 197(4): 450–462.

47. Diamant Z, Gauvreau GM, Cockcroft DW et al. Inhaled allergen bronchoprovocation tests. *J Allergy Clin Immunol* 2013; 132(5): 1045–1055 e6.

48. Taylor DA, Harris JG, O'Connor BJ. Comparison of incremental and bolus dose inhaled allergen challenge in asthmatic patients. *Clin Exp Allergy* 2000; 30(1): 56–63.

49. Leckie MJ. Chronic allergen challenge as an experimental model: necessary, significant or useful? *Clin Exp Allergy* 2000; 30(9): 1191–1193.

50. Gauvreau GM, Sulakvelidze I, Watson RM, Inman MD, Rerecich TJ, O'Byrne PM. Effects of once daily dosing with inhaled budesonide on airway hyperresponsiveness and airway inflammation following repeated low-dose allergen challenge in atopic asthmatics. *Clin Exp Allergy* 2000; 30(9): 1235–1243.

51. Julius P, Lommatzsch M, Kuepper M et al. Safety of segmental allergen challenge in human allergic asthma. *J Allergy Clin Immunol* 2008; 121(3): 712–717.

52. Carlsten C, Blomberg A, Pui M et al. Diesel exhaust augments allergen-induced lower airway inflammation in allergic individuals: A controlled human exposure study. *Thorax* 2016; 71(1): 35–44.

53. Cockcroft DW, Murdock KY, Kirby J, Hargreave F. Prediction of airway responsiveness to allergen from skin sensitivity to allergen and airway responsiveness to histamine. *Am Rev Respir Dis* 1987; 135(1): 264–267.

54. Cockcroft DW, Davis BE, Boulet L-P et al. The links between allergen skin test sensitivity, airway responsiveness and airway response to allergen. *Allergy* 2005; 60(1): 56–59.

55. Ravensberg AJ, van Rensen ELJ, Grootendorst DC et al. Validated safety predictions of airway responses to house dust mite in asthma. *Clin Exp Allergy* 2007; 37(1): 100–107.

56. Cooper BG. An update on contraindications for lung function testing. *Thorax* 2011; 66(8): 714–723.

57. Carr W, Schaeffer J, Donnefeld E. Treating allergic conjunctivitis: A once-daily medication that provides 24-hour symptom relief. *Allergy Rhinol (Providence)* 2016; 7(2): 107–114.

58. Riedi CA, Rosario NA. Prevalence of allergic conjunctivitis: A missed opportunity? *Allergy* 2009; 65(1): 131–132.

59. Singh K, Axelrod S, Bielory L. The epidemiology of ocular and nasal allergy in the United States, 1988-1994. *J Allergy Clin Immunol* 2010; 126(4): 779–783.

60. Sánchez MC, Fernández Parra B, Matheu V et al. Allergic conjunctivitis. *J Investig Allergol Clin Immunol* 2011; 21(Suppl 2): 1–19.

61. Fauquert JL, Jedrzejczak-Czechowicz M, Rondon C et al. Conjunctival allergen provocation test: Guidelines for daily practice. *Allergy* 2017; 72(1): 43–54.

62. Anantasit N, Vilaiyuk S, Kamchaisatian W et al. Comparison of conjunctival and nasal provocation tests in allergic rhinitis children with Dermatophagoides pteronyssinus sensitization. *Asian Pac J Allergy Immunol* 2013; 31(3): 227–232.

63. Abelson MB, Chambers WA, Smith LM. Conjunctival allergen challenge. A clinical approach to studying allergic conjunctivitis. *Arch Ophthalmol* 1990; 108: 84–88.

64. Gomes PJ, Ousler GW, Welch DL, Smith LM, Coderre J, Abelson MB. Exacerbation of signs and symptoms of allergic conjunctivitis by a controlled adverse environment challenge in subjects with a history of dry eye and ocular allergy. *Clin Ophthalmol* 2013; 7: 157–165.

65. Tagawa Y, Namba K, Nakazono Y, Iwata D, Ishida S. Evaluating the efficacy of epinastine ophthalmic solution using a conjunctivitis allergen challenge model in patients with birch pollen allergic conjunctivitis. *Allergol Int* 2017; 66(2): 338–343.

66. Almaliotis D, Michailopoulos P, Gioulekas D et al. Allergic conjunctivitis and the most common allergens in Northern Greece. *World Allergy Organ J* 2013; 6(1): 12.

67. Chelminska M, Niedoszytko M, Jassem E. Clinical value of conjunctival allergen challenge in diagnosing allergic conjunctivitis related to latex. *Int Arch Allergy Immunol* 2011; 154(2): 149–154.

68. Lindvik H, Lødrup Carlsen KC, Mowinckel P, Navaratnam J, Borres MP, Carlsen KH. Conjunctival provocation test in diagnosis of peanut allergy in children. *Clin Exp Allergy* 2017; 47(6): 785–794.

69. Kvenshagen BK, Jacobsen M, Halvorsen R. Can conjunctival provocation test facilitate the diagnosis of food allergy in children. *Allergol Immunophathol* 2010; 38: 321–326.

70. Spangler DL, Bensch G, Berdy GJ. Evaluation of the Efficacy of Olopatadine hydrochloride 0.1% ophthalmic solution and Azelastine hydrochloride 0.05% Ophthalmic solution in the conjunctival allergen challenge model. *Clinical Ther* 2001; 23: 1272–1280.

71. Gronemeyer U. Der konjunktivale Provokationstest. In: Fuchs E, Schulz KH, editors. *Manuale Allergologicum*. Deisenhofen: Dustri-Verlag, 1994.

72. Dogan S, Astvatsatourov A, Deserno TM, Bock F, Shah-Hosseini K, Michels A, Mösger R. Objectifying the conjunctival provocation test: Photography-based rating and digital analysis. *Int Arch Allergy Immunol* 2014; 163: 59–68.

73. Mourão EMM, Rosário NA. Adverse reactions to the allergen conjunctival provocation test. *Ann Allergy Asthma Immunol* 2011; 107(4): 373–374.

74. Ousler GW, Gomes PJ, Welch D, Abelson MB. Methodologies for the study of ocular surface disease. *Ocul Surf* 2005; 3(3): 143–154.

75. Boyce JA, Assa'ad A, Burks AW et al. Guidelines for the diagnosis and management of food allergy in the United States: Summary of the NIAID-sponsored expert panel report. *Nutr Res* 2011; 31(1): 61–75.

76. Sampson HA. IgE-mediated food intolerance. *J Allergy Clin Immunol* 1988; 81(3): 495–504.

77. Bock SA, Sampson HA, Atkins FM et al. Double-blind, placebo-controlled food challenge (DBPCFC) as an office procedure: A manual. *J Allergy Clin Immunol* 1988; 82(6): 986–997.

78. Niggemann B, Wahn U, Sampson HA. Proposals for standardization of oral food challenge tests in infants and children. *Pediatr Allergy Immunol* 1994; 5(1): 11–13.

79. Sampson HA, Gerth van Wijk R, Bindslev-Jensen C et al. Standardizing double-blind, placebo-controlled oral food challenges: American Academy of Allergy, Asthma & Immunology-European Academy of Allergy and Clinical Immunology PRACTALL consensus report. *J Allergy Clin Immunol* 2012; 130(6): 1260–1274.

80. Nowak-Wegrzyn A, Assa'ad AH, Bahna SL et al. Work Group report: Oral food challenge testing. *J Allergy Clin Immunol* 2009; 123(Suppl 6): S365–S383.

81. Perry TT, Matsui EC, Kay Conover-Walker M, Wood RA. The relationship of allergen-specific IgE levels and oral food challenge outcome. *J Allergy Clin Immunol* 2004; 114(1): 144–149.

82. Bindslev-Jensen C, Ballmer-Weber BK, Bengtsson U et al. Standardization of food challenges in patients with immediate

reactions to foods--position paper from the European Academy of Allergology and Clinical Immunology. *Allergy* 2004; 59(7): 690–697.

83. Sicherer SH, Morrow EH, Sampson HA. Dose-response in double-blind, placebo-controlled oral food challenges in children with atopic dermatitis. *J Allergy Clin Immunol* 2000; 105(3): 582–586.

84. May CD. Objective clinical and laboratory studies of immediate hypersensitivity reactions to foods in asthmatic children. *J Allergy Clin Immunol* 1976; 58(4): 500–515.

85. Joint Task Force on Practice P, American Academy of Allergy A, Immunology, American College of Allergy A, Immunology, Joint Council of Allergy A et al. The diagnosis and management of anaphylaxis: An updated practice parameter. *J Allergy Clin Immunol* 2005; 115(3 Suppl 2): S483–S523.

86. Niggemann B, Lange L, Finger A, Ziegert M, Muller V, Beyer K. Accurate oral food challenge requires a cumulative dose on a subsequent day. *J Allergy Clin Immunol* 2012; 130(1): 261–263.

87. Savage J, Johns CB. Food allergy: Epidemiology and natural history. *Immunol Allergy Clin North Am* 2015; 35(1): 45–59.

88. Kostadinova AI, Willemsen LE, Knippels LM, Garssen J. Immunotherapy - risk/benefit in food allergy. *Pediatr Allergy Immunol* 2013; 24(7): 633–644.

89. Dioszeghy V, Mondoulet L, Dhelft V et al. Epicutaneous immunotherapy results in rapid allergen uptake by dendritic cells through intact skin and downregulates the allergen-specific response in sensitized mice. *J Immunol* 2011; 186(10): 5629–5637.

90. Wang J, Sampson HA. Safety and efficacy of epicutaneous immunotherapy for food allergy. *Pediatr Allergy Immunol* 2018; 29(4): 341–349.

91. Akdis M, Akdis CA. Mechanisms of allergen specific immunotherapy: Multiple suppressor factors at work in immune tolerance to allergens. *J Allergy Clin Immunol* 2014; 133(3): 621–631.

92. Dioszeghy V, Mondoulet L, Dhelft V et al. The regulatory T cells induction by epicutaneous immunotherapy is sustained and mediates long-term protection from eosinophilic disorders in peanut-sensitized mice. *Clin Exp Allergy* 2014; 44(6): 867–881.

93. Vallery-Radot P, Hangenau J. Asthme d'origine equine. Essai de desensibilisation par des cutireactions repetees. *Bull Soc Med Hop Paris* 1921; 45: 1251–1260.

94. Pautrizel R, Cabanieu G, Bricaud H, Broustet P. [Allergenic group specificity & therapeutic consequences in asthma; specific desensitization method by epicutaneous route]. *Sem Hop* 1957; 33(22): 1394–1403.

95. Blamoutier P, Blamoutier J, Guibert L. [Treatment of pollinosis with pollen extracts by the method of cutaneous quadrille ruling]. *Presse Med* 1959; 67: 2299–2301.

96. Mondoulet L, Dioszeghy V, Ligouis M, Dhelft V, Dupont C, Benhamou PH. Epicutaneous immunotherapy on intact skin using a new delivery system in a murine model of allergy. *Clin Exp Allergy* 2010; 40(4): 659–667.

97. Wood LC, Jackson SM, Elias PM, Grunfeld C, Feingold KR. Cutaneous barrier perturbation stimulates cytokine production in the epidermis of mice. *J Clin Invest* 1992; 90(2): 482–487.

98. Senti G, Graf N, Haug S et al. Epicutaneous allergen administration as a novel method of allergen-specific immunotherapy. *J Allergy Clin Immunol* 2009; 124(5): 997–1002.

99. Senti G, von Moos S, Tay F et al. Epicutaneous allergen-specific immunotherapy ameliorates grass pollen-induced rhinoconjunctivitis: A double-blind, placebo-controlled dose escalation study. *J Allergy Clin Immunol* 2012; 129(1): 128–135.

100. Agostinis F, Forti S, Di Berardino F. Grass transcutaneous immunotherapy in children with seasonal rhinoconjunctivitis. *Allergy* 2010; 65(3): 410–411.

101. Dupont C, Kalach N, Soulaines P, Legoue-Morillon S, Piloquet H, Benhamou PH. Cow's milk epicutaneous immunotherapy in children: A pilot trial of safety, acceptability, and impact on allergic reactivity. *J Allergy Clin Immunol* 2010; 125(5): 1165–1167.

102. Jones SM, Agbotounou WK, Fleischer DM et al. Safety of epicutaneous immunotherapy for the treatment of peanut allergy: A phase 1 study using the Viaskin patch. *J Allergy Clin Immunol* 2016; 137(4): 1258–1261 e10.

103. Sampson HA, Shreffler WG, Yang WH et al. Effect of varying doses of epicutaneous immunotherapy vs Placebo on reaction to peanut protein exposure among patients with peanut sensitivity: A randomized clinical trial. *JAMA* 2017; 318(18): 1798–1809.

104. Jones SM, Sicherer SH, Burks AW et al. Epicutaneous immunotherapy for the treatment of peanut allergy in children and young adults. *J Allergy Clin Immunol* 2017; 139(4): 1242–1252 e9.

105. Sampson HA, Agbotounou W, Thébault C et al. Epicutaneous Immunotherapy (EPIT) is effective and safe to treat peanut allergy: A multi-national double- blind placebo-controlled randomized Phase IIb trial. *J. Allergy Clin. Immunol* 2015; 135(2): AB390.

106. Werfel T. Epicutaneous allergen administration: A novel approach for allergen-specific immunotherapy? *J Allergy Clin Immunol* 2009; 124(5): 1003–1004.

107. Senti G, von Moos S, Tay F, Graf N, Johansen P, Kundig TM. Determinants of efficacy and safety in epicutaneous allergen immunotherapy: Summary of three clinical trials. *Allergy* 2015; 70(6): 707–710.

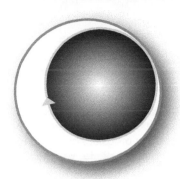

9 Local mucosal allergic disease

Ibon Eguiluz-Gracia and Paloma Campo
IBIMA–Hospital Regional Universitario de Málaga, UMA

Carmen Rondón
Plaza del Hospital Civil

CONTENTS

9.1 INTRODUCTION

Allergic rhinitis (AR) constitutes an important health problem worldwide [1]. This IgE-mediated chronic inflammatory disease negatively impacts patients' social life, school performance, and work productivity. Moreover, AR is a risk factor for allergic asthma [2]. Allergic rhinitis and asthma should not be considered two differentiated entities but the organ-specific expressions of a single condition. Thus, the term *allergic respiratory disease* (ARD) has been recently proposed to collectively refer to allergic rhinitis and asthma [3]. In most cases of ARD, the IgE sensitization to environmental allergens induces the onset of AR during childhood or adolescence. The disease naturally evolves toward clinical worsening, the development of new IgE sensitizations, and the association of comorbidities in other mucosal organs like the bronchi or the conjunctiva. Therefore,

ARD should be regarded as a chronic, lifelong respiratory disorder naturally progressing possibly to severe phenotypes [3].

The clarification of the immune mechanisms underlying ARD is crucial to develop effective therapies aiming not only to control the symptoms but also to prevent disease progression. In clinical practice, atopy is defined as the positivity of the tests to detect systemic allergen-specific IgE (sIgE): skin prick test (SPT) and/or serum sIgE. The diagnosis of ARD has classically relied on the confirmation of atopy by either test in a patient with a consistent symptom pattern [1,3]. Therefore, ARD has been historically regarded as an immunologic, systemic condition due to the presence of detectable free sIgE antibodies in serum or bound to the surface of skin mast cells. Nevertheless, the clarification of IgE immune responses demonstrates that this antibody isotype exerts its more prominent activities in mucosal tissues, and that the sIgE directed against environmental allergens is mainly synthetized at the mucosal level. These advances have reinforced the idea of ARD being mainly a "mucosal immune condition" whose systemic repercussions are merely reflecting the immune processes occurring in the airways [4].

In the last 15 years, evidence indicates that nasal allergen reactivity can occur in the absence of systemic atopy as detected by sIgE [5]. This evidence suggests that the synthesis of IgE at the mucosal level does not necessarily require a systemic component to become clinically relevant. These findings expand the concept of ARD and further identify the condition as a fundamentally mucosal disorder. Moreover, this observation has very important clinical implications, as it challenges the idea that classical tests for systemic atopy are sufficient for ruling out ARD.

In this chapter, the mucosal immune system of the airways is described, with special focus on B cells, antibody production, and IgE immune responses. Moreover, the role of mucosal IgE synthesis in the primary respiratory diseases within the allergic spectrum is analyzed. Finally, the epidemiology, natural evolution, diagnosis, and therapeutic options for local allergic rhinitis are thoroughly discussed.

9.2 MUCOSAL IMMUNE SYSTEM IN THE AIRWAYS

The main function of the human immune system is to protect the individual against pathogens. The immune system is also responsible for eliminating genetically damaged cells and thus protecting the organism from neoplastic disorders. The human immune system can be divided into an innate arm and an adaptive arm. The innate immune system appeared earlier in evolutionary development and is characterized by a fast but less diverse and less specific response. It comprises different cell types including macrophages, dendritic cells (DCs), mast cells, basophils, eosinophils, neutrophils, innate lymphoid cells, and natural killer T cells, together with humoral components such as the complement system. The adaptive immune system provides an antigen-specific response that requires multiple days to develop but persists in the form of immunologic memory. The adaptive immune system comprises T and B lymphocytes; the latter differentiate into antibody-producing cells (plasma cells). The two arms of the immune system usually act together, with an initial innate response that shapes the ensuing adaptive response. The mucosal immune system in the airways is composed of many different immune cell types (as described previously) that reside or traffic through the respiratory mucosa and lung parenchyma and the correspondent secondary lymphoid organs. The latter can be divided into the locoregional (cervical, paratracheal, parabronchial, and hilar) draining lymph nodes and the mucosa-associated lymphoid tissue (MALT), less prominent than in the gut but important in the airway immune response. The MALT in the respiratory tract is composed of the lymphoid tissue associated with Waldeyer ring (pharyngeal, tubal, palatine, and lingual tonsils) and the bronchus-associated lymphoid tissue (BALT). These structures are clusters of immune cells (T cells, B cells, macrophages, DCs) and, similar to lymph nodes, are the sites of induction of adaptive immune responses. The BALT is consistently found in children but tends to regress from adolescence [6], whereas the Waldeyer ring persists throughout adult life. Both lymph nodes and MALT possess efferent lymphatic vessels, but MALT lacks afferent lymphatics. This difference influences the arrival of antigens to the tissue [7]. Similar to the gut-associated lymphoid tissue, the BALT is populated with microfold (M) cells that can take up the antigens from the airway lumen and deliver them via transcytosis to BALT-resident DCs and lymphocytes [8].

9.2.1 B cells in the respiratory mucosa

The main role of B cells is to produce antibodies (also termed *immunoglobulins*), which are either soluble or membrane-bound molecules. Membrane antibodies are usually called B-cell receptors (BCRs) and determine the specificity of the B cell. An antibody molecule is composed of two identical heavy chains and two identical light chains. Soluble antibodies can be proteolytically broken down into two functionally different fragments: the Fab (antigen-binding) fragment and the Fc (crystallizable region) fragment. The Fab fragment possesses the highly variable regions of the antibody that specifically bind to the antigen, whereas the Fc fragment contains the region attaching to immune receptors and determining the effector properties of the antibody [9]. Differences in the Fc fragment of the antibodies determine the various isotypes of immunoglobulins: in humans IgG, IgA, IgM, IgE, and IgD [10]. B cells are generated in the bone marrow from lymphoid precursors that differentiate into pro-B cells. The next maturation steps involve the recombination of the genes for the V (variable), D (diversity), and J (joint) segments of the heavy chains followed by a similar V-J recombination of the light chains. These phenomena determine the antigen specificity of the B cell and give rise to IgM+ naïve B cells. The combination of the previous processes is called antigen-independent B-cell maturation and is followed by the migration of naïve B cells to the germinal centers (GCs) of secondary lymphoid organs (including those in the airways) where they reside [11]. The GCs are also populated by follicular DCs that retain unprocessed antigens for long periods of time [7]. Naïve B cells in GCs may take up these antigens and present them to T follicular helper (Tfh) cells in the context of MHC-II molecules. When a Tfh cell encounters its cognate antigen, it starts providing help to the presenting B cell to initiate its antigen-dependent maturation (GC reaction). Stimulated B cells initially produce antigen-specific IgM, but with the help of Tfh cells, most of them rapidly undergo isotype class switch recombination (CSR) [12] resulting in loss of IgM expression [13]. The process of CSR involves an exchange in the Fc portion of the heavy chains, thus altering the receptors the antibody can bind to and ultimately affecting its functional specialization [14]. During CSR, the DNA in the locus of the immunoglobulin heavy chain is rearranged to juxtapose distant DNA regions and to generate switch circles that are eliminated. These switch circles are isotype-specific and can be transiently detected. Class switch recombination is followed by the somatic hypermutation of the antibody in order to increase the affinity for its cognate antigen [5]. After mutations in the genes of the variable regions of their antibodies, B cells migrate from the dark zone to the light zone of the GC. In the light zone, mutated B cells are reexposed to their cognate antigens displayed by follicular DCs, and only those having increased affinity will continue their maturation (positive selection) (Figure 9.1) [13]. The processes of CSR and somatic hypermutation are affected by genes codifying enzymes such as *activation-induced cytidine deaminase* (AID), *recombination activating gene* (RAG) *1* (RAG1) or *2* (RAG2) [14]. After CSR and somatic hypermutation, activated IgG+ or IgA+ B cells exit the secondary lymphoid organs, enter the circulation, and differentiate into plasmablasts or memory B cells. Plasmablasts eventually migrate to the bone marrow or peripheral tissues (including the airway mucosa) and mature to long-lived plasma cells. Plasma cells provide protection by the sustained production of high-affinity antibodies, whereas memory B cells rapidly proliferate upon antigen reencounter [13].

(a)

(b)

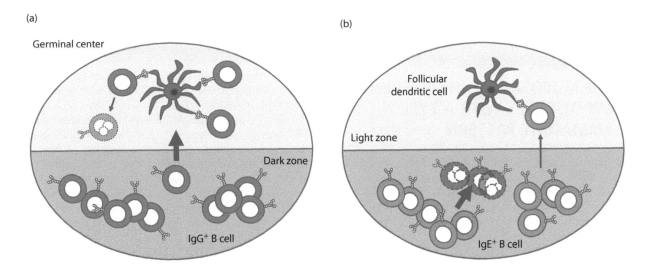

Figure 9.1 Differential germinal center reaction in IgE immune responses. (a) After somatic hypermutation, IgG+ or IgA+ B cells migrate at high rates from the dark zone to the light zone of the germinal centers. In the light zone, follicular dendritic cells reexpose B cells to their cognate antigens. Those cells not having increased their affinity die by apoptosis in the light zone, whereas the rest of the B cells continue their maturation process (positive selection). (b) Mutated IgE+ B cells do not efficiently traffic from the dark zone to the light zone. Therefore, most of them die by apoptosis in the dark zone of the germinal centers without being able to carry out the positive selection process.

9.2.2 Secretory IgA and IgD in the respiratory mucosa

The respiratory mucosa harbors a robust population of IgA-producing plasma cells, and IgA is the most abundant immunoglobulin isotype in the airways. A complex of two IgA molecules attached to a J (joining) chain is produced by plasma cells in the lamina propria of the mucosae [15]. This dimeric IgA is taken up by epithelial cells and transported by transcytosis to the luminal surface using the polymeric immunoglobulin receptor (pIgR). A complex formed by parts of pIgR and dimeric IgA, jointly called secretory IgA (SIgA), is cleaved from the membrane of epithelial cells and released into the lumen of the airways. Secretory IgA acts as a neutralizing antibody coating luminal microbes and limiting their contact with stromal and immune cells. IgD is also produced by some plasma cells in the nasal mucosa, and even though the nature of its receptor remains elusive, IgD is able to activate basophils in response to microorganisms commonly found in the nasal cavity [16].

9.2.3 Synthesis of IgE in the respiratory mucosa: A special case

The production of high-affinity IgE is tightly regulated at the molecular and cellular levels, resulting in serum concentrations that are several orders of magnitude lower than that of either IgG or IgA. On the other hand, the proportion of IgE in the airway mucosa is significantly higher than the peripheral blood. Of note, the human respiratory and intestinal mucosae host the largest populations of IgE-producing plasma cells [17].

Similar to the other isotypes, the generation of high-affinity sIgE requires the activation of the adaptive immune system. Class switch recombination to IgE (εCSR) in GC B cells has a stronger dependence on Tfh cell collaboration than the other isotypes [18]. The initiation of εCSR requires the interaction of CD40L expressed on GC B cells with CD40 induced on activated type 2 Tfh cells, which

also provide IL-4, the crucial inductor for the process [19]. Additional initiators of εCSR include the stimulation of a *proliferation-inducing ligand* (APRIL) and *toll-like receptor-4* (TLR4) on GC B cells by *B-cell activating factor* (BAFF) and LPS, respectively [20]. Globally, these stimuli activate the transcription factor STAT6, which induces the gene changes resulting in εCSR [19]. The differences between IgE and other immunoglobulin isotypes are even more pronounced for the affinity maturation process after CSR [21]. Switched IgE+ B cells cannot efficiently traffic to the light zone of the GCs in order to undergo their positive selection after somatic hypermutation [20]. The increased residence of IgE+ B cells in the GC dark zone results in increased apoptosis of IgE+ B cells and impaired formation of IgE+ memory B cells (Figure 9.1). These factors result in a reduced number of IgE+ memory B cells and inefficient affinity maturation of GC-derived IgE antibodies [22].

High-affinity IgE can be produced by IgG+ memory B cells in the mucosa following εCSR. This sequential εCSR (from IgM to IgG followed by IgG to IgE) generates a switch circle different from that of direct εCSR (from IgM to IgE) and probably represents an additional checkpoint for IgE production. The decreased production of high-affinity IgE seems to be a result of evolutionary pressure to reduce but not eliminate sIgE [18] (Figure 9.2). Even though the sequential εCSR in mice seems restricted to IgG+ memory B cells [22], in the airway mucosa of humans, CSR from IgA to IgE also has been reported [19]. Markers of sequential εCSR are detected in the mucosa of individuals with type 2 nasal inflammatory diseases [23]. Even though it is not clear whether mucosal εCSR is necessarily associated to GC-like structures, lymphoid aggregates are detected in the nasal mucosa of patients with chronic rhinosinusitis with nasal polyps (CRSwNP) [24]. Mucosal IgE can undergo luminal transcytosis through CD23 expressed on respiratory epithelial cells and thus is found in secretions [25]. Of note, sIgE is detected in the nasal secretions of patients with type 2 nasal inflammatory disorders [26]. In this regard, allergen-sIgE represents a much higher proportion of total IgE in the respiratory secretions than in the peripheral blood of patients with ARD, implying that local sIgE production is relevant for the sensitization of resident mast cells and for the local allergic reaction. The high-affinity, sIgE in the peripheral blood of allergic individuals might be produced more in the airway mucosa than in the secondary lymphoid organs [23] (Figure 9.2).

9.3 ROLE OF MUCOSAL IgE IN DIFFERENT AIRWAY DISEASES WITH A TYPE 2 INFLAMMATORY PATTERN

Since the discovery of IgE in the 1960s, investigators have sought the anatomic location of IgE-producing cells. As early as in the 1970s, several studies concluded that 70%–80% of human IgE was synthesized at the mucosal level [27] (Figure 9.2). The evidence of local IgE in the most relevant phenotypes of respiratory disease is summarized in the following sections.

9.3.1 Allergic rhinitis

Respiratory mucosa is a site of IgE production during allergic responses. In the 1970s, Tse et al. identified ragweed sIgE in the nasal secretions of individuals with AR [28]. Subsequently, Platts-Mills et al. measured grass sIgE in the nasal secretions of SPT+ subjects, and the authors showed that 90% of this sIgE was produced locally [29]. A study performed in the 1990s demonstrated that house dust mite (HDM) sIgE increases faster in the nasal secretions than in serum after natural allergen exposure [30]. A study analyzing turbinate mucosa from AR patients demonstrated the presence of IgE+ mast cells, plasma cells, and B cells [31]. Moreover, *de novo* production of IgE occurs in mucosal explants from AR subjects [32]. Somatic hypermutation and εCRS have been demonstrated in the nasal mucosa of AR patients [23], although GC formation has not been proven. In this regard, a study in AR subjects reported that natural pollen exposure induces changes in IgE repertoires that are suggestive of GC reactions, and that these changes are more apparent in the nasal mucosa than in peripheral blood [33]. Furthermore, the allergen exposure triggers a sequential εCSR (from IgG or from IgA) in the nasal mucosa of AR individuals [23]. As mentioned earlier, most serum IgE in AR patients may derive from the respiratory mucosa [34], and IgE-producing B cells and plasma cells are relatively more abundant in the nasal mucosa than in peripheral blood [31]. Importantly, the IgE produced locally in AR subjects [32] is sufficient, not only to saturate the sIgE receptor system on resident cells, but also to spill over into the bloodstream, sensitize circulating basophils and skin mast cells, and be found free in the peripheral blood (Figure 9.3) [4].

9.3.2 Local allergic rhinitis

Local allergic rhinitis (LAR) is characterized by rhinitis symptoms, absence of atopy (negative SPT and undetectable serum sIgE), and a nasal allergic response to aeroallergens [35]. The immunopathology of LAR is only partially understood. The nasal mucosa of LAR patients shows signs of type 2 inflammation including increased eosinophils and mast cells together with their activation markers: eosinophil cationic protein (ECP) and tryptase, respectively [36–38]. The clinical similarities between AR and LAR prompted studies to investigate the role of sIgE in the later condition. Brostoff and Huggins published the first report of sIgE in nasal secretions of nonatopic rhinitis patients

with a positive response to the nasal allergen challenge (NAC) [39]. Thereafter, Powe et al. reported the presence of grass and HDM sIgE in turbinate samples from 30% of nonatopic rhinitis patients [40]. More recently, several authors have demonstrated mucosal sIgE to different allergens (HDM, pollen, molds, epithelia) in both adult and pediatric LAR populations [36,37,41,42]. Studies from Rondón et al. reported the presence of grass and HDM sIgE in LAR patients out of the allergen season [36,37]. Interestingly, studies on the kinetics of inflammatory mediators in LAR showed a rapid and progressive increase in nasal sIgE concentration during the 24 hours post-NAC [37,38]. It is tempting to speculate that in LAR individuals the sIgE produced at the mucosal level may be sufficient to sensitize nasal effector cells but not to reach skin mast cells or to be detected in a free state in the blood (Figure 9.3). In support of this hypothesis, close to 50% of HDM-sensitized LAR individuals have positive IgE-mediated basophil activation test (BAT) responses, suggesting that the mucosal sIgE has gained access to the bloodstream (Figure 9.3) [43,44]. Additional indirect evidence suggesting a sIgE-mediated mechanism for LAR is the effectiveness of allergen immunotherapy (AIT) in 70% of LAR individuals despite the absence of positive SPT or *in vitro* sIgE [45–47]. Nevertheless, many aspects remain to be clarified as the proportion of LAR subjects with detectable nasal sIgE is highly variable but overall low [36,41,42]. Moreover, the mucosal synthesis of IgE in LAR patients has not been demonstrated. Some authors have proposed immunoglobulin free light chains (FLCs) as potential mediators of rhinitis in nonatopic patients [48]. In nonatopic individuals with type 2 nasal inflammatory conditions, higher levels of FLC (both κ and λ) occur both at the mucosa and peripheral blood as compared with healthy and atopic subjects or subjects with other types of nasal inflammation [49,50]. The FLCs are secreted by plasma cells in parallel with complete antibodies, and similar to sIgE can sensitize mast cells for activation [48] upon cross-linking by their cognate antigens. Nevertheless, no evidence has related FLCs to positive NAC responses or to LAR immunopathology [51]. In summary, even though indirect evidence suggests an IgE-mediated mechanism, further studies are warranted to elucidate the immunopathology of LAR.

9.3.3 Asthma

Asthma has been classified historically into allergic and nonallergic phenotypes, based on classical biomarkers such as SPT and serum sIgE. Nevertheless, several studies show that this dichotomy is not accompanied by a distinct inflammatory pattern, as multiple similarities exist in the bronchial infiltrate of allergic and nonallergic asthma [52,53]. Both phenotypes are characterized by the increased expression of IL-4, IL-5, IL-13, eotaxin-1, eotaxin-2, monocyte chemotactic proteins (MCP)-3 and -4, and CCR3, among other mediators [52,54]. Similar to rhinitis, mucosal IgE is suspected to play an important role in asthma, and there is ample evidence for local IgE synthesis in asthmatic patients regardless of their atopic status. Several studies demonstrate that nonatopic asthmatics display markers of εCSR and increased expression of FcεRI in the bronchial mucosa [53,55]. Interestingly, local IgE production may have a greater influence on the clinical outcomes of asthma than the systemic biomarkers of atopy [56]. Nevertheless, the specificity and affinity of mucosal IgE in asthma patients have not been sufficiently investigated, and it is unknown whether bronchial IgE can bind to environmental allergens as demonstrated for nasal IgE in AR and LAR individuals. Even though one study described

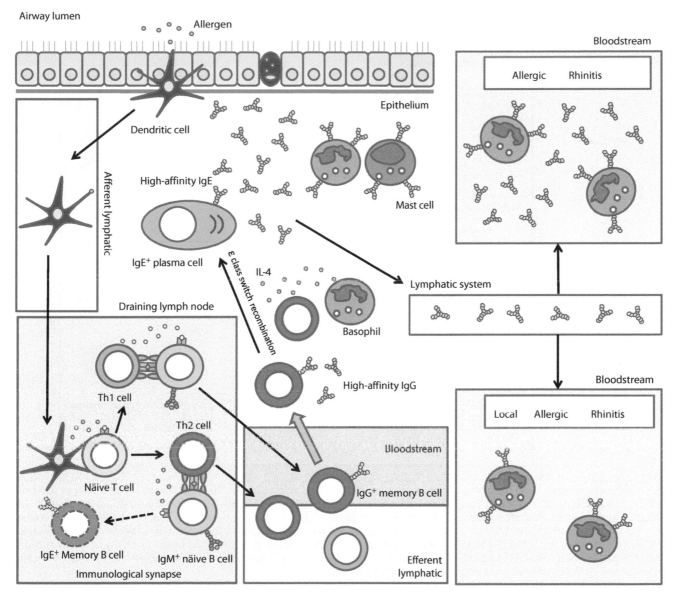

Figure 9.2 Mucosal synthesis of IgE in allergic rhinitis and local allergic rhinitis patients. Allergen-activated dendritic cells traffic through the lymphatic vessels to the germinal center of the draining lymph nodes. In that location, dendritic cells activate allergen-specific näive T cells to generate Th1 and Th2 cells. Th1 cells subsequently stimulate allergen-specific IgM+ näive B cells that undergo class switch recombination (CSR) to IgG and somatic hypermutation to give rise to IgG+ plasma cells (not shown) and IgG+ memory B cells. Allergen-specific Th1 and IgG+ B cells exit the lymphoid system through the efferent vessels and reach the bloodstream. Activated Th2 cells in the germinal centers also stimulate IgM+ näive B cells that underdo CSR to IgE. Nevertheless, IgE+ B cells cannot efficiently carry out their somatic hypermutation and die by apoptosis before exiting the germinal centers. Conversely, Th2 cells reach the bloodstream and extravasate at the lamina propria of the airway mucosa, together with Th1 cells (not shown) and IgG+ memory B cells. In the lamina propria, IgG+ memory B cells can undergo sequential CSR to IgE upon allergen reencounter (not shown) and stimulation with IL-4 provided by Th2 cells and basophils among other cells. This process results on the generation of IgE+ plasma cells releasing vast amounts of high-affinity IgE to the lamina propria. Mucosal IgE can bind FcεRI on resident basophils and mast cells and sensitize them for activation upon allergen reencounter. After saturating the receptor system of the mucosa, free IgE can reach the bloodstream through the lymphatic vessels. In the bloodstream, IgE binds first to FcεRI on circulating basophils. In allergic rhinitis patients, IgE saturates the receptor system of blood basophils and subsequently binds FcεRI on mast cells residing at the different peripheral tissues including the skin. Moreover, after saturating the receptor system on mast cells, IgE can be found at a free state in serum of allergic rhinitis patients. In individuals with local allergic rhinitis, IgE is sometimes sufficient to sensitize circulating basophils, but it is not enough to sensitize skin mast cells or to be found at a free state in serum.

functional HDM-sIgE in sputum samples from nonatopic asthmatics, the studied individuals failed to experience a positive bronchial allergen challenge. Therefore, the clinical relevance of neither the allergen nor the sIgE could be confirmed. Another study examining bronchial biopsies from atopic and nonatopic asthmatics showed that only atopic individuals had detectable bronchial sIgE [57]. In conclusion, even though εCSR can occur in the bronchial mucosa of all asthmatics regardless of their atopic status, the IgE involvement in the immunopathology of the nonatopic asthma phenotypes is not confirmed.

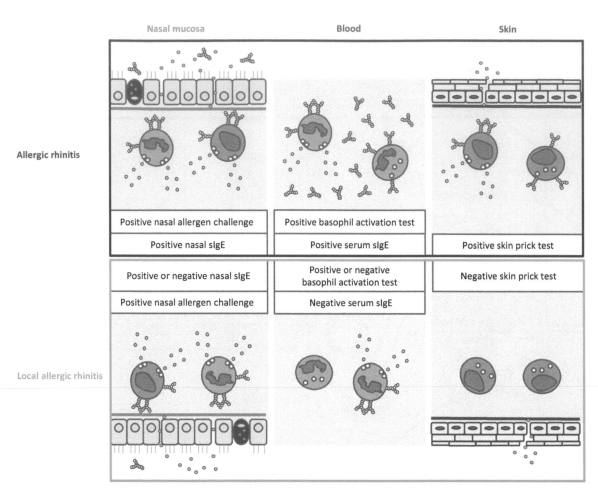

Figure 9.3 Diagnostic biomarkers in the allergic phenotypes of rhinitis. Allergic rhinitis (AR) is characterized by the positivity of skin prick test (SPT) and serum-specific (s)IgE. These two biomarkers are sufficient for diagnosis in many cases of AR. In AR individuals, the clinical relevance of an IgE sensitization can be accurately established by a nasal allergen challenge (NAC). The basophil activation test (BAT) and the nasal sIgE are positive in most cases of AR, even though they are not necessary for diagnostic purposes. By definition, patients who have local allergic rhinitis (LAR) test negative for both SPT and serum sIgE. The diagnosis of LAR is routinely established by the positivity of the NAC. Some LAR individuals have detectable nasal sIgE or positive BAT responses, and these tests can assist to reach the diagnosis. (Reprinted from Hospital Healthcare Europe 2019 with permission [http://hospitalhealthcare.com].)

9.3.4 Chronic rhinosinusitis with nasal polyps

Nasal inflammation in patients with chronic rhinosinusitis with nasal polyps (CRSwNP) is characterized by tissue eosinophilia and the production of large amounts of IgE. The local IgE in CRSwNP individuals can be produced in a polyclonal or in an allergen-specific manner [58]. Similar to AR, the local production of high-affinity IgE is triggered by the allergen, and the resulting sIgE can sensitize resident mast cells for subsequent activation [59]. On the other hand the generation of polyclonal IgE is induced by *Staphylococcus aureus* enterotoxins acting as superantigens, with the capacity to nonspecifically stimulate resident T and B cells [24,58]. This activation triggers a rapid εCSR and the release of polyclonal, low-affinity IgE without a proper somatic hypermutation process [60]. Both types of IgE compete for the binding to FcεRI receptors. Given its higher abundance, polyclonal IgE may act as a functional inhibitor of the sIgE-mediated activation of resident cells. This phenomenon explains why the local IgE level does not correlate with the atopic status in CRSwNP patients [61]. Moreover, high levels of FLCs able to mediate allergen-triggered mast cell activation have been described in CRSwNP [49].

9.4 CLINICAL IMPLICATIONS OF LOCAL ALLERGY: CASE OF LOCAL ALLERGIC RHINITIS

Local allergic rhinitis is defined by seasonal or perennial rhinitis symptoms, absence of systemic atopy, and a positive response to the NAC. Both LAR and AR patients share many clinical features. The diagnosis of LAR should be especially suspected in young, nonsmoking, nonatopic women, with moderate-to-severe, persistent, and perennial rhinitis [62]. LAR can also be present in children [41,42,63,64] and the elderly [65]. Several studies suggest that a few allergens trigger most cases of LAR; those mainly include HDM [36,38], grass and olive pollen [37,44], and *Alternaria alternata* [66]. Similar to AR, the mite *Dermatophagoides pteronyssinus* is the most common individual allergen inducing nasal reactivity in LAR patients. Comparing AR and LAR, the reactivity to *Alternaria alternata* is more frequent among LAR subjects, whereas pollens and animal dander are more frequent in AR individuals [62,67].

9.4.1 Epidemiology

Many studies suggest that LAR is an underdiagnosed entity, affecting individuals from different countries, ethnic backgrounds, and ages [35,68]. A recent, systematic review analyzed 46 studies including 3230 patients with different rhinitis phenotypes and 165 healthy controls. The review concluded that the prevalence of LAR among nonatopic patients with rhinitis was 24.7%, with a prevalence of 16.1% and 21% in pediatric and elderly populations, respectively [65,67]. Nevertheless, the studies included in this review displayed great heterogeneity in the NAC protocols, the selection criteria and age range of individuals, the allergens investigated, the methods to measure the nasal patency, and the cutoff point to determine NAC positivity [67]. All of these factors greatly limit direct comparisons among them and highlight the need for a multicenter study with uniform protocols and criteria to clarify the true prevalence of LAR.

9.4.2 Local allergic rhinitis in children

Allergic rhinitis is a common condition in children and increases with age, increasing from 3.4% at age 4 years to greater than 30% at age 18 years. Many studies suggest that a significant proportion of LAR subjects begin their symptoms during childhood. Several articles highlight the need of considering LAR as a major potential diagnosis in children with rhinitis [31,41,64,66,69]. Collectively, published literature includes approximately 300 nonatopic individuals, with ages ranging from 4 to 18 years and symptoms of

either perennial or seasonal rhinitis. The reported prevalence of a positive NAC in this population is highly variable (range 0–66.6%). Fuiano et al. [66] performed NAC with *Alternaria alternata* in 36 children and adolescents without systemic sIgE and found that 64% of them experienced positive responses. Another study from Thailand including 25 nonatopic patients aged 8–18 years did not find positive nasal response to HDM [69]. In conclusion, LAR is a relevant diagnosis to consider when evaluating nonatopic children and adolescents with rhinitis.

9.4.3 Natural evolution and quality of life

Shortly after the description of LAR, several investigators questioned the diagnosis as a "definitive" phenotype and suggested that the condition was a "temporary" form of rhinitis with ultimate development of atopy, systemic sIgE, and AR. The results of the first 10-year follow-up study including 194 LAR patients and 130 healthy controls who were evaluated on a yearly basis may help address this question (Figure 9.4). Interestingly, the rate of conversion to systemic atopy was low and comparable between LAR and control individuals (9.7% and 7.8%, respectively) [70,71]. During the 10 years of observation, the cases of severe rhinitis increased from 19% to 42%, and the prevalence of conjunctivitis and asthma-like symptoms increased in 12%. These changes were associated with a 100% increase in the number of visits to the emergency room due to suspected asthma attacks and a decrease in lung function as measured by FEV1 [70]. Moreover, 42% of patients reported a worsening of

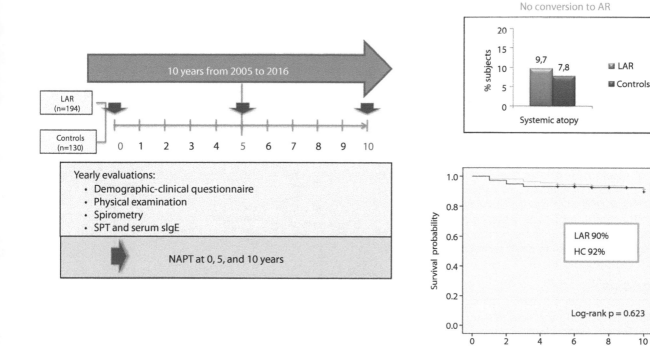

Figure 9.4 Natural evolution of local allergic rhinitis (LAR). The main results of 10-year follow-up study of a cohort of 194 LAR patients and 130 healthy controls confirmed LAR is an independent and well-defined rhinitis phenotype, with a low and similar rate of development of atopy compared to healthy controls (9.7% versus 7.8%, *p* = .623). Demographic-clinical questionnaire, physical examination, spirometry, skin-prick test, and serum determination of specific IgE were evaluated yearly. Additionally, nasal allergen challenge tests (NAPT) were performed at baseline, at fifth year of evolution, and at 10th year of evolution. (This figure is reprinted from Rondon C et al. Local allergic rhinitis is an independent rhinitis phenotype: the results of a 10-year follow-up study. *Allergy.* 2018 Feb;73(2):470–478.)

their disease and a negative impact of LAR on their health and quality of life [70]. These results suggest that LAR is a respiratory disease with a chronic course, a natural evolution toward clinical worsening, and an association with comorbidities in other mucosal organs [70]. A subanalysis of the evolution during the first 5 years of the same 10-year study yielded similar results [71]. Importantly, the increase in rhinitis severity and the onset of asthma-like symptoms occurred primarily during the first 5 years of observation, with a lower rate of worsening during the subsequent 5 years [70].

9.4.4 Comorbidities in other mucosal organs

9.4.4.1 BRONCHI

As described, the bronchial inflammatory infiltrate in nonatopic asthma resembles that of atopic asthma. Between 20% and 47% of LAR patients self-report asthma-like symptoms [62,70,71]. Moreover, the previously mentioned 10-year observational study describes a progressively increasing prevalence of asthma-like symptoms during the first 10 years of LAR. This increase is associated with a significantly higher proportion of patients requiring visits to the emergency room due to wheezing and dyspnea [70]. Nevertheless, the diagnosis of asthma in LAR patients is not confirmed in the published literature. In a recent communication including rhinitis patients with methacholine provocation-confirmed asthma, 53% of LAR subjects had a positive bronchial challenge with HDM and increased methacholine reactivity performed 24 hours after the bronchial challenge [72]. These observations suggest that a bronchial counterpart of LAR may exist, yet studies with larger cohorts are required to validate this observation. The existence of a "local allergic" asthma phenotype would also reinforce the idea of the unified airways and further expand the concept of ARD.

9.4.4.2 CONJUNCTIVA

Natural exposure to allergen [62] or NAC [62,68,73] can induce ocular symptoms suggestive of allergic conjunctivitis in many LAR individuals. The ocular symptoms are more frequent in pollen-reactive LAR individuals than in those reacting to HDM or molds [62]. Nevertheless, it is unknown whether the involvement of the conjunctiva in LAR subjects arises from a true ocular sensitization or from the activation of nasal-ocular reflexes. The conjunctival epithelium hosts a robust population of immune cells including mast cells [74]. Moreover, resident B cells from allergic conjunctivitis patients are able to produce functional sIgE [75]. Whether conjunctival sensitization in addition to nasal-ocular reflexes work synergistically in LAR patients to induce ocular symptoms is not sufficiently investigated.

9.4.5 Diagnosis

In many healthcare systems, the confirmation of atopy is the primary criterion for referral to allergy/immunology specialists. This unfortunate fact greatly limits the chances of LAR individuals to be evaluated by a specialist and to obtain an accurate diagnosis. Moreover, an allergological workup for rhinitis exclusively based on STP and serum sIgE [1,76] results in a significant rate of misdiagnosis, as it classifies the LAR individuals in the nonallergic rhinitis (NAR) phenotype. The implementation of NAC protocols in the diagnostic algorithms of rhinitis is usually necessary for the identification of LAR [77]. Because LAR worsens during the first 5 years [70,71],

the earlier identification of the trigger eliciting rhinitis is necessary to advise appropriate allergen avoidance measures and specific therapies. The recommended diagnostic algorithm of rhinitis is shown in Figure 9.5.

9.4.5.1 FIRST DIAGNOSTIC STEPS

Local allergic rhinitis should be considered in the differential diagnosis of most nonatopic individuals with rhinitis [78,79]. In the evaluation of rhinitis patients, a detailed clinical history should always be conducted, including the assessment of comorbidities such as ocular and bronchial symptoms. Other important aspects to investigate include the age at symptom onset, the urban/rural dwelling, the family history of atopy, or the history of tobacco use [62]. The clinical history should be followed by a thorough examination of the nasal cavity via nasal endoscopy (or computed tomography [CT] scan if needed) to assess for signs of chronic rhinosinusitis and other nasal disorders. Subsequently, the presence of atopy should be investigated by means of SPT and/or serum sIgE. If these tests are positive and the results are consistent with the clinical history, the patient can be accurately diagnosed with AR. When SPT and serum sIgE tests are negative, the response of the target organ to an allergen challenge is required for excluding LAR [78].

9.4.5.2 NASAL ALLERGEN CHALLENGE

The NAC is the recommended method to assess for the response of the nasal mucosa to allergen [22,62,78]. The NAC discriminates between allergen-triggered rhinitis (AR and LAR) and the nonallergic forms of the condition [80]. Before administering the allergen during a NAC, nasal hyperreactivity must be excluded by means of a saline challenge or other methods [81]. The NAC mimics the naturally

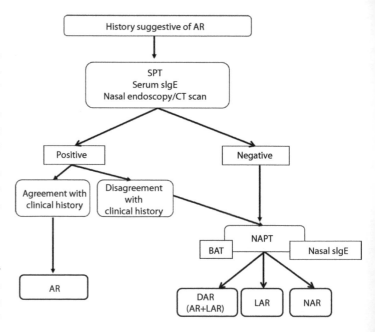

Figure 9.5 Diagnostic algorithm of rhinitis. (AR, allergic rhinitis; BAT, basophil activation test; CT, computed tomography; DAL, dual allergic rhinitis; LAR, local allergic rhinitis; NAPT, nasal allergen provocation test; NAR, nonallergic rhinitis; sIgE, specific immunoglobulin E; SPT, skin prick test.) (This figure is reprinted from P. Campo et al. Local allergic rhinitis: Implications for management. *Clin and Exp Allergy* 2018 Jun 14.)

occurring symptoms induced by allergen exposure in AR and LAR individuals. Due to its optimal sensitivity, specificity, reproducibility, and safety, the NAC is the diagnostic gold standard for LAR, yet it is a time-consuming technique requiring trained personnel. A strategy to shorten the diagnostic protocol is to perform consecutive NACs with up to four allergens on the same day [77]. Similar to AR, LAR subjects respond to allergenic proteins in addition to the whole allergenic extract (83% of LAR subjects reacting to olive tree pollen also reacted to *nOle e 1*) [44].

9.4.5.3 NASAL ALLERGEN-SPECIFIC IgE

In a subset of LAR subjects, sIgE can be detected in the nasal secretions. The sensitivity of this measurement depends on the technique used, but it is generally low. The quantification of sIgE in the nasal lavage has a sensitivity of 20%–40% but a specificity of greater than 90% [36,37]. Other techniques, like nasal brushing [82] or sinus packs [83], have proven useful in the detection of nasal sIgE, but these techniques need confirmation. A minimally invasive method using an automated immunoassay has been described for the detection of nasal sIgE in HDM-reactive LAR patients [84]. This method detects nasal sIgE by the direct application of the solid phase of a commercial ImmunoCAP to the mucosa of the head of the inferior turbinate. The technique has a sensitivity of 42.86% and a specificity of 100% for LAR diagnosis [84]. One of the main advantages of this method is that the crucial step of the immunoassay (the binding of the sIgE to the allergen) occurs in the nasal cavity, without processing of the sample.

9.4.5.4 BASOPHIL ACTIVATION TEST

The basophil activation test (BAT) investigates the allergen-triggered, IgE-mediated reactivity of peripheral basophils. When performed 24 hours after a NAC, the BAT has a sensitivity of 50% and 66% for the diagnosis of LAR due to HDM and olive pollen tree, respectively [43,44]. With both allergens specificity was greater than 90%. The pretreatment of basophils with the PI3K inhibitor wortmannin suppressed the positive BAT responses, thus confirming an IgE-mediated mechanism of basophil activation [43].

9.4.5.5 OTHER DIAGNOSTIC CONSIDERATIONS

The evidence of sIgE in LAR (either unbound in nasal secretions, or bound to the receptors on blood basophils) should be regarded as sensitization. The diagnosis of local allergy requires a consistent symptom pattern and/or positive NAC [5,68]. Some atopic subjects exclusively sensitized to seasonal pollens, as measured by SPT, experience perennial symptoms with or without seasonal exacerbation. This clinical scenario has been historically explained by the coexistence of AR and nasal hyperreactivity; but preliminary data from our group suggest that a subset of these subjects has a positive NAC with perennial allergens (primarily HDM and *Alternaria alternata*). We propose the term *dual allergic rhinitis* (DAR) for this phenotype, to reflect that both local and systemic allergic sensitization coexist in the same patient. We believe that the existing term *mixed rhinitis* is not appropriate for this condition, as it was coined to name the coexistence of allergic and nonallergic forms of rhinitis in the same individual.

In conclusion, the NAC is still the most reliable tool for LAR diagnosis, but it can be supported by the measurement of nasal sIgE and/or BAT.

9.4.6 Therapeutic options

The therapeutic goal in both AR and LAR is to control the disease and to prevent the onset of comorbidities. The first treatment step in LAR patients usually consists of health education, allergen avoidance measures, and standard reliever therapy such as oral antihistamines and intranasal corticosteroids, as recommended by the Allergic Rhinitis and its Impact on Asthma (ARIA) guidelines [1]. Allergen avoidance is not always feasible, and the symptomatic therapy does not control the disease in many cases. Moreover, none of those interventions alter the natural course of the disease [70,71]. Allergen immunotherapy (AIT) is an effective and safe treatment to control the symptoms of ARD. A 3-year cycle of AIT provides long-term protection after therapy discontinuation and is the only treatment option with disease-modifying effect, reducing the occurrence of asthma in AR patients [1,79,85].

9.4.6.1 SUBCUTANEOUS ALLERGEN IMMUNOTHERAPY FOR LOCAL ALLERGIC RHINITIS

The clinical and pathological similarities between AR and LAR prompted investigators to evaluate the effect of subcutaneous allergen immunotherapy (SCIT) on LAR individuals. The first approach was an observational study to compare the safety and efficacy of a 6-month, preseasonal SCIT treatment compared with symptomatic medication, in subjects with moderate-to-severe LAR due to grass pollen [86]. This study provided promising results, and subsequently, a 2-year randomized double-blind, placebo-controlled clinical trial (RDBPCCT) with *Dermatophagoides pteronyssinus* SCIT (DP-SCIT) [45], a 2-year RDBPCCT with *Phleum pratense* SCIT (Phleum-SCIT) [47], and a 2-year RDBPCCT with *Betula verrucosa* SCIT (Bet-SCIT) [46] were conducted (Figure 9.6). Overall, these trials have provided consistent evidence about the short-term beneficial effect of SCIT in LAR. The SCIT is associated with a significant decrease in rhinitis severity and an increase in medication-free days. The clinical improvement is evident after 6 months of treatment but increases further throughout the studies, with the greatest clinical benefit achieved at the end of the trials [45–47]. The three RDBPCCTs published to date show consistent and similar results [19,68,73]. The Phleum-SCIT study resulted in significant improvements in ocular symptoms, asthma control, and quality of life compared to placebo. In the three trials, SCIT also induced a significant, progressive, and dose-dependent increase in the concentration of allergen tolerated in the NAC, which was observed after only 3 months of treatment. Thirty percent, 50%, and 56% of LAR patients treated with 6-month grass-SCIT, 2-year DP-SCIT, and 2-year Phleum-SCIT, respectively [24,69,83] tolerated the maximum allergen concentration in the NAC. The SCIT produced a significant increase in serum sIgG4, starting after 6 months of treatment and progressing until the end of the studies. Therefore, it is tempting to speculate that in LAR individuals, SCIT induces IL-10-producing Tregs and IgG$_4$-producing Bregs [87] as was shown for AR patients. Nevertheless, the immunologic effects of SCIT in LAR and the associated response biomarkers need to be investigated in future studies. Furthermore, it is necessary to establish the long-term effect of AIT in LAR and to evaluate the impact, if any, on the development of comorbidities such as asthma. In summary, published literature supports the clinical efficacy of LAR for controlling the symptoms, increasing the allergen tolerance, and improving the quality of life in LAR patients.

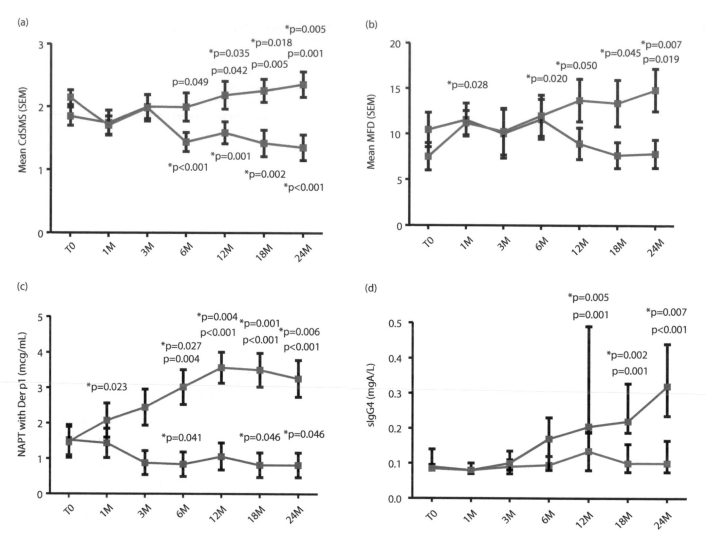

Figure 9.6 Clinical and immunologic effects of subcutaneous *Dermatophagoides pteronyssinus* specific immunotherapy (DP-SCIT) versus placebo in subjects with local allergic rhinitis. (a) Combined daily symptoms–medication score (CdSMS). (b) Medication-free days (MFDs). (c) Nasal tolerance to DP. (d) Serum levels of specific IgG4 (sIgG4) to DP (mgA/mL). Blue line: placebo group; red line: DP-SCIT group. (This figure is reprinted from Rondón C et al. Efficacy and safety of *D. pteronyssinus* immunotherapy in local allergic rhinitis: a double-blind placebo-controlled clinical trial. *Allergy.* 2016 Jul;71(7):1057-1061.)

9.4.6.2 OTHER TREATMENT OPTIONS

Besides the classical subcutaneous and sublingual routes, the intralymphatic, intradermal, or epicutaneous administration of allergen is also under investigation for ARD [88]. None of these routes of immunotherapy have been tested in LAR subjects. The efficacy of intranasal AIT was reported in a mouse model of allergic asthma [89]. Because LAR is defined by a localized immune response in the nasal mucosa, it would be interesting to develop intranasal AIT strategies for LAR and to compare their clinical and immunologic effects with those induced by SCIT. Omalizumab is an anti-IgE, humanized monoclonal antibody (mAb) approved for severe allergic asthma [90] and chronic urticaria [91]. Several asthma studies indicate a beneficial effect of omalizumab on the concomitant rhinitis [92]. Mepolizumb, reslizumab, and benralizumab are humanized mAbs directed against the IL-5 pathway [93]. These drugs are effective for eosinophilic asthma, but their effects on nasal allergy are unknown. Dupilumab is a human mAb targeting the IL-4/IL-13 pathway, approved for severe atopic dermatitis [94]

and asthma. Its role, if any, for other types of ARD is unknown. Omalizumab, mepolizumb, and dupilumab have promising results in CRSwNP. Even though cost-efficiency limits the use of biologicals for nasal allergy, it can be expected that some of these drugs may have a beneficial effects in LAR patients.

9.5 CONCLUSION

Most respiratory diseases are related to some extent to the dysregulation of the mucosal immune system in the airways. In the case of ARD, this relationship is especially relevant and apparent. Among the different components of the mucosal immune system, resident or trafficking B cells and plasma cells are responsible for the synthesis of immunoglobulins. Unlike IgG but similar to IgA, IgE primarily exerts its biological functions at the mucosal tissues. The production of this immunoglobulin isotype is tightly regulated by several checkpoints at different levels during the B-cell activation process. The production of IgE in the secondary lymphoid organs is limited and ineffective, but upon the appropriate stimuli, high-affinity IgE can be produced in the airways. In humans, the IgE produced in the airway mucosa can enter the peripheral blood and subsequently sensitize skin mast cells, thus producing SPT-positive results. Therefore, the mucosal synthesis of sIgE is a very relevant disease mechanism in atopic conditions like ARD, and in other nasal disorders with a type 2 inflammatory pattern like CRSwNP.

Growing evidence over 15 years indicates that nasal reactivity to allergens can occur in the absence of systemic atopy. Even though a multicenter, cross-sectional study is lacking, published literature suggests that LAR might account for a significant proportion of individuals previously diagnosed as nonallergic rhinitis. Yet the immunopathology of LAR remains to be defined, evidence indicates an IgE-mediated mechanism; namely, some subjects have detectable sIgE in nasal secretions and positive BAT responses, and SCIT is effective in the majority of LAR individuals. It is also necessary to study the long-term effects of SCIT in LAR, especially the effect of SCIT on the development of conjunctivitis and asthma. The concept of local allergy has important implications for the clinical management of individuals with rhinitis, as negative SPTs and/or serum sIgE do not exclude *per se* nasal reactivity to environmental allergens. The identification of LAR requires the implementation of NAC in the diagnostic algorithms for rhinitis, at least until the *in vitro* tests become ready for clinical practice. Local allergic rhinitis seems to worsen after diagnosis and is associated with the development of asthma and conjunctivitis. These observations suggest that an early diagnosis and initiation of specific therapies are crucial for controlling the symptoms and potentially for preventing the comorbidities.

SALIENT POINTS

1. The differential germinal center reaction of IgE-producing B cells determines a low frequency and insufficient affinity maturation of germinal center–derived IgE antibodies.
2. High-affinity IgE can be produced in the peripheral mucosal tissues following sequential class switch recombination of IgG-producing memory B cells. IgE mainly exerts its biological functions at the peripheral level through the binding to its specific receptors (FcεRI and CD23) on the surface of resident cells.
3. The mucosal synthesis of IgE is one of the main disease mechanisms of allergic rhinitis, allergic asthma, and chronic rhinosinusitis with nasal polyps, and might be also involved in the pathophysiology of local allergic rhinitis (LAR). Importantly, circulating IgE in the bloodstream of atopic patients is believed to derive from the mucosae with subsequent spillover through the lymphatic vessels.
4. Local allergic rhinitis is a new rhinitis phenotype defined by typical allergic rhinitis symptoms, absence of systemic atopy (negative skin prick test and serum allergen-specific IgE), and positivity of the nasal allergen challenge (NAC).
5. Local allergic rhinitis is a differentiated rhinitis phenotype that does not progress to systemic atopy over time. Patients with LAR suffer from a moderate-to-severe disease naturally evolving toward the clinical worsening and the association of comorbidities such as conjunctivitis and asthma.
6. The NAC is the gold standard for LAR diagnosis, as it displays optimal safety and reproducibility and excels in identifying the allergen triggers of rhinitis. The basophil activation test and the measurement of nasal allergen-specific IgE can assist the diagnosis.

7. Allergen immunotherapy has demonstrated to control the symptoms, reduce the need for rescue medication, increase the nasal tolerance to the allergen, and improve the quality of life of LAR patients while it is being administered.

REFERENCES

1. Bousquet J, Schunemann HJ, Samolinski B et al. Allergic Rhinitis and its Impact on Asthma (ARIA): Achievements in 10 years and future needs. *J Allergy Clin Immunol* 2012; 130: 1049–1062.
2. Shaaban R, Zureik M, Soussan D et al. Rhinitis and onset of asthma: A longitudinal population-based study. *Lancet* 2008; 372: 1049–1057.
3. Navarro AM, Delgado J, Muñoz-Cano RM, Dordal MT, Valero A, Quirce S; on behalf of the ARD Study Group. Allergic respiratory disease (ARD), setting forth the basics: Proposals of an expert consensus report. *Clin Transl Allergy* 2017; 18: 16.
4. Dullaers M, De Bruyne R, Ramadani F, Gould HJ, Gevaert P, Lambrecht BN. The who, where, and when of IgE in allergic airway disease. *J Allergy Clin Immunol* 2012; 129: 635–645.
5. Campo P, Eguiluz-Gracia I, Bogas G et al. Local allergic rhinitis: Implications for management. *Clin Exp Allergy* 2019; 49(1): 6–16.
6. Heier I, Malmstrom K, Sajantila A, Lohi J, Makela M, Jahnsen FL. Characterisation of bronchus-associated lymphoid tissue and antigen-presenting cells in central airway mucosa of children. *Thorax* 2011; 66: 151–156.
7. Girard JP, Moussion C, Förster R. HEVs, lymphatics and homeostatic immune cell trafficking in lymph nodes. *Nat Rev Immunol.* 2012; 12(11): 762–773.
8. Kraehenbuhl JP, Neutra MR. Epithelial M cells: Differentiation and function. *Annu Rev Cell Dev Biol* 2000; 16: 301–332.
9. Grossberg AL, Stelos P, Pressman D. Structure of fragments of antibody molecules as revealed by reduction of exposed disulfide bonds. *Proc Natl Acad Sci USA* 1962; 48: 1203–1209.
10. Schroeder HW, Jr., Cavacini L. Structure and function of immunoglobulins. *J Allergy Clin Immunol* 2010; 125: S41–S52.
11. Herzog S, Reth M, Jumaa H. Regulation of B-cell proliferation and differentiation by pre-B-cell receptor signalling. *Nat Rev Immunol* 2009; 9: 195–205.
12. Stavnezer J, Guikema JE, Schrader CE. Mechanism and regulation of class switch recombination. *Annu Rev Immunol* 2008; 26: 261–292.
13. Kurosaki T, Kometani K, Ise W. Memory B cells. *Nat Rev Immunol* 2015; 15: 149–159.
14. Klein U, Dalla-Favera R. Germinal centres: Role in B-cell physiology and malignancy. *Nat Rev Immunol* 2008; 8: 22–23.
15. Pabst O. New concepts in the generation and functions of IgA. *Nat Rev Immunol* 2012; 12: 821–832.
16. Chen K, Cerutti A. The function and regulation of immunoglobulin D. *Curr Opin Immunol* 2011; 23: 345–352.
17. Tada T, Ishizaka K. Distribution of γ E-forming cells in lymphoid tissues of the human and monkey. *J Immunol* 1970; 104: 377–387.
18. He JS, Narayanan S, Subramaniam S, Ho WQ, Lafaille JJ, Curotto de Lafaille MA. Biology of IgE production: IgE cell differentiation and the memory of IgE responses. *Curr Top Microbiol Immunol* 2015; 388: 1–19.
19. Wu LC, Zarrin AA. The production and regulation of IgE by the immune system. *Nat Rev Immunol* 2014; 14: 247–259.

20. Tong P, Wesemann DR. Molecular mechanisms of IgE class switch recombination. *Curr Top Microbiol Immunol* 2015; 388: 21–37.

21. He JS, Meyer-Hermann M, Xiangying D et al. The distinctive germinal center phase of IgE+ B lymphocytes limits their contribution to the classical memory response. *J Exp Med* 2013; 18: 2755–2771.

22. Xiong H, Dolpady J, Wabl M, Curotto de Lafaille MA, Lafaille JJ. Sequential class switching is required for the generation of high affinity IgE antibodies. *J Exp Med* 2012; 13: 353–364.

23. Cameron L, Gounni AS, Frenkiel S, Lavigne F, Vercelli D, Hamid Q. SεSμ and SεSγ switch circles in human nasal mucosa following *ex vivo* allergen challenge: Evidence for direct as well as sequential class switch recombination. *J Immunol* 2003; 171: 3816–3822.

24. Gevaert P, Nouri-Aria KT, Wu H et al. Local receptor revision and class switching to IgE in chronic rhinosinusitis with nasal polyps. *Allergy* 2013; 68: 55–63.

25. Palaniyandi S, Liu X, Periasamy S et al. Inhibition of CD23-mediated IgE transcytosis suppresses the initiation and development of allergic airway inflammation. *Mucosal Immunol* 2015; 8: 1262–1274.

26. Duan W, Croft M. Control of regulatory T cells and airway tolerance by lung macrophages and dendritic cells. *Ann Am Thorac Soc*, 2014; 11: S306–S313.

27. Tada T, Ishizaka K. Distribution of γ E-forming cells in lymphoid tissues of the human and monkey. *J Immunol* 1970; 104: 377–387.

28. Tse KS, Wicher K, Arbesman CE. IgE antibodies in nasal secretions of ragweed-allergic subjects. *J Allergy Clin Immunol* 1970; 46: 352–357.

29. Platts-Mills TA. Local production of IgG, IgA and IgE antibodies in grass pollen hay fever. *J Immunol* 1979; 122: 2218–2225.

30. Sensi LG, Piacentini GL, Nobile E et al. Changes in nasal specific IgE to mites after periods of allergen exposure-avoidance: A comparison with serum levels. *Clin Exp Allergy* 1994; 24: 377–382.

31. KleinJan A, Vinke JG, Severijnen LW, Fokkens WJ. Local production and detection of (specific) IgE in nasal B-cells and plasma cells of allergic rhinitis patients. *Eur Respir J* 2000; 15: 491–497.

32. Smurthwaite L, Walker SN, Wilson DR, Birch DS et al. Persistent IgE synthesis in the nasal mucosa of hay fever patients. *Eur J Immunol* 2001; 31: 3422–3431.

33. Wu YC, James LK, Vander Heiden JA et al. Influence of seasonal exposure to grass pollen on local and peripheral blood IgE repertoires in patients with allergic rhinitis. *J Allergy Clin Immunol* 2014; 134: 604–612.

34. Eckl-Dorna J, Pree I, Reisinger J et al. The majority of allergen-specific IgE in the blood of allergic patients does not originate from blood-derived B cells or plasma cells. *Clin Exp Allergy* 2012; 42: 1347–1355.

35. Rondón C, Eguiluz-Gracia I, Campo P. Is the evidence of local allergic rhinitis growing? *Curr Opin Allergy Clin Immunol* 2018; 18: 342–349.

36. Rondon C, Romero JJ, Lopez S et al. Local IgE production and positive nasal provocation test in patients with persistent nonallergic rhinitis. *J Allergy Clin Immunol* 2007; 119: 899–905.

37. Rondon C, Fernandez J, Lopez S et al. Nasal inflammatory mediators and specific IgE production after nasal challenge with grass pollen in local allergic rhinitis. *J Allergy Clin Immunol* 2009; 124: 1005–1011.e1.

38. Lopez S, Rondon C, Torres MJ et al. Immediate and dual response to nasal challenge with *Dermatophagoides pteronyssinus* in local allergic rhinitis. *Clin Exp Allergy* 2010; 40: 1007–1014.

39. Huggins KG, Brostoff J. Local production of specific IgE antibodies in allergic-rhinitis patients with negative skin tests. *Lancet* 1975; 2: 148–150.

40. Powe DG, Jagger C, Kleinjan A, Carney AS, Jenkins D, Jones NS. "Entopy": Localized mucosal allergic disease in the absence of systemic responses for atopy. *Clin Exp Allergy* 2003; 33: 1374–1379.

41. Zicari AM, Occasi F, Di Fraia M et al. Local allergic rhinitis in children: Novel diagnostic features and potential biomarkers. *Am J Rhinol Allergy* 2016; 30: 329–334.

42. Krajewska-Wojtys A, Jarzab J, Gawlik R, Bozek A. Local allergic rhinitis to pollens is underdiagnosed in young patients. *Am J Rhinol Allergy* 2016; 30: 198–201.

43. Gomez E, Campo P, Rondon C et al. Role of the basophil activation test in the diagnosis of local allergic rhinitis. *J Allergy Clin Immunol* 2013; 132: 975–976.e1–5.

44. Campo P, Villalba M, Barrionuevo E et al. Immunologic responses to the major allergen of *Olea europaea* in local and systemic allergic rhinitis subjects. *Clin Exp Allergy* 2015; 45: 1703–1712.

45. Rondon C, Campo P, Salas M et al. Efficacy and safety of *D. pteronyssinus* immunotherapy in local allergic rhinitis: A double-blind placebo-controlled clinical trial. *Allergy* 2016; 71: 1057–1061.

46. Bożek A, Kołodziejczyk K, Jarząb J. Efficacy and safety of birch pollen immunotherapy for local allergic rhinitis. *Ann Allergy Asthma Immunol* 2018; 120: 53–58.

47. Rondón C, Blanca-López N, Campo P et al. Specific immunotherapy in local allergic rhinitis: A randomized, double-blind placebo-controlled trial with *Phleum pratense* subcutaneous allergen immunotherapy. *Allergy* 2017; November 23.[Epub ahead of print].

48. Groot Kormelink T, Thio M, Blokhuis BR, Nijkamp FP, Redegeld FA. Atopic and non-atopic allergic disorders: Current insights into the possible involvement of free immunoglobulin light chains. *Clin Exp Allergy* 2009; 39: 33–42.

49. Groot Kormelink T, Calus L, De Ruyck N et al. Local free light chain expression is increased in chronic rhinosinusitis with nasal polyps. *Allergy* 2012; 67: 1165–1172.

50. Powe DG, Groot Kormelink T, Sisson M et al. Evidence for the involvement of free light chain immunoglobulins in allergic and nonallergic rhinitis. *J Allergy Clin Immunol* 2010; 125: 139–145.e1–3.

51. Rondon C, Canto G, Fernandez J, Blanca M. Are free light chain immunoglobulins related to nasal local allergic rhinitis? *J Allergy Clin Immunol* 2010; 126: 677; author reply, 8.

52. Humbert M, Durham SR, Ying S et al. IL-4 and IL-5 mRNA and protein in bronchial biopsies from patients with atopic and nonatopic asthma: Evidence against "intrinsic" asthma being a distinct immunopathologic entity. *Am J Respir Crit Care Med* 1996; 154: 1497–1504.

53. Humbert M, Grant JA, Taborda-Barata L et al. High-affinity IgE receptor (FcεRI)-bearing cells in bronchial biopsies from atopic and nonatopic asthma. 1996; 153: 1931–1937.

54. Humbert M, Ying S, Corrigan C et al. Bronchial mucosal expression of the genes encoding chemokines RANTES and MCP-3 in symptomatic atopic and nonatopic asthmatics: Relationship to the eosinophil-active cytokines interleukin (IL)-5, granulocyte macrophage-colony-stimulating factor, and IL-3. *Am J Respir Cell Mol Biol* 1997; 16: 1–8.

55. Takhar P, Corrigan CJ, Smurthwaite L et al. Class switch recombination to IgE in the bronchial mucosa of atopic and nonatopic patients with asthma. *J Allergy Clin Immunol* 2007; 119: 213–218.

56. Balzar S, Strand M, Rhodes D, Wenzel SE. IgE expression pattern in lung: Relation to systemic IgE and asthma phenotypes. *J Allergy Clin Immunol* 2007; 119: 855–862.

57. Pillai P, Fang C, Chan YC et al. Allergen-specific IgE is not detectable in the bronchial mucosa of nonatopic asthmatic patients. *J Allergy Clin Immunol* 2014; 133: 1770–1772.e11.

58. Bachert C, Zhang N, Holtappels G et al. Presence of IL-5 protein and IgE antibodies to staphylococcal enterotoxins in nasal polyps is associated with comorbid asthma. *J Allergy Clin Immunol* 2010; 126: 962–968.

59. Baba S, Kondo K, Toma-Hirano M et al. Local increase in IgE and class switch recombination to IgE in nasal polyps in chronic rhinosinusitis. *Clin Exp Allergy* 2014; 44: 701–712.

60. Van Zele T, Gevaert P, Holtappels G, van Cauwenberge P, Bachert C. Local immunoglobulin production in nasal polyposis is modulated by superantigens. *Clin Exp Allergy* 2007; 37: 1840–1847.

61. Gevaert P, Holtappels G, Johansson SG, Cuvelier C, Cauwenberge P, Bachert C. Organization of secondary lymphoid tissue and local IgE formation to *Staphylococcus aureus* enterotoxins in nasal polyp tissue. *Allergy* 2005; 60: 71–79.

62. Rondon C, Campo P, Galindo L et al. Prevalence and clinical relevance of local allergic rhinitis. *Allergy* 2012; 67: 1282–1288.

63. Fuiano N, Fusilli S, Passalacqua G, Incorvaia C. Allergen-specific immunoglobulin E in the skin and nasal mucosa of symptomatic and asymptomatic children sensitized to aeroallergens. *J Investig Allergol Clin Immunol* 2010; 20: 425–430.

64. Duman H, Bostanci I, Ozmen S, Dogru M. The relevance of nasal provocation testing in children with nonallergic rhinitis. *Int Arch Allergy Immunol* 2016; 170: 115–121.

65. Bozek A, Ignasiak B, Kasperska-Zajac A, Scierski W, Grzanka A, Jarzab J. Local allergic rhinitis in elderly patients. *Ann Allergy Asthma Immunol* 2015; 114: 199–202.

66. Fuiano N, Fusilli S, Incorvaia C. A role for measurement of nasal IgE antibodies in diagnosis of Alternaria-induced rhinitis in children. *Allergol Immunopathol (Madr)* 2012; 40: 71–74.

67. Hamizan AW, Rimmer J, Alvarado R et al. Positive allergen reaction in allergic and nonallergic rhinitis: A systematic review. *Int Forum Allergy Rhinol* 2017; 7: 868–877.

68. Rondon C, Campo P, Togias A et al. Local allergic rhinitis: Concept, pathophysiology, and management. *J Allergy Clin Immunol* 2012; 129: 1460–1467.

69. Buntarickpornpan P, Veskitkul J, Pacharn P et al. The proportion of local allergic rhinitis to *Dermatophagoides pteronyssinus* in children. *Pediatr Allergy Immunol* 2016; 27: 574–579.

70. Rondon C, Campo P, Eguiluz-Gracia I et al. Local allergic rhinitis is an independent rhinitis phenotype: The results of a 10-year follow-up study. *Allergy* 2018; 73(2): 470–478.

71. Rondon C, Campo P, Zambonino MA et al. Follow-up study in local allergic rhinitis shows a consistent entity not evolving to systemic allergic rhinitis. *J Allergy Clin Immunol* 2014; 133: 1026–1031.

72. Campo P, Antunez C, Rondon C et al. Positive bronchial challenges to *D. pteronyssinus* in asthmatic subjects in absence of systemic atopy. *J Allergy Clin Immunol* 2011; 127: AB6.

73. Campo P, Salas M, Blanca-Lopez N, Rondon C. Local allergic rhinitis. *Immunol Allergy Clin North Am* 2016; 36: 321–332.

74. Galletti JG, Guzman M, Giordano MN. Mucosal immune tolerance at the ocular surface in health and disease. *Immunology* 2017; 150(4): 397–407.

75. Leonardi A. Allergy and allergic mediators in tears. *Exp Eye Res* 2013; 117: 106–117.

76. Greiner AN, Hellings PW, Rotiroti G, Scadding GK. Allergic rhinitis. *Lancet* 2011; 378: 2112–2122.

77. Rondon C, Campo P, Herrera R et al. Nasal allergen provocation test with multiple aeroallergens detects polysensitization in local allergic rhinitis. *J Allergy Clin Immunol* 2011; 128: 1192–1197.

78. Campo P, Rondon C, Gould HJ, Barrionuevo E, Gevaert P, Blanca M. Local IgE in non-allergic rhinitis. *Clin Exp Allergy* 2015; 45: 872–881.

79. Papadopoulos NG, Bernstein JA, Demoly P et al. Phenotypes and endotypes of rhinitis and their impact on management: A PRACTALL report. *Allergy* 2015; 70: 474–494.

80. Rondon C, Bogas G, Barrionuevo E, Blanca M, Torres MJ, Campo P. Nonallergic rhinitis and lower airway disease. *Allergy* 2017; 72: 24–34.

81. Dordal MT, Lluch-Bernal M, Sanchez MC et al. Allergen-specific nasal provocation testing: Review by the rhinoconjunctivitis committee of the Spanish Society of Allergy and Clinical Immunology. *J Investig Allergol Clin Immunol* 2011; 21: 1–12; quiz.

82. Reisacher WR, Bremberg MG. Prevalence of antigen-specific immunoglobulin E on mucosal brush biopsy of the inferior turbinates in patients with nonallergic rhinitis. *Int Forum Allergy Rhinol* 2014; 4: 292–297.

83. Berings M, Arasi S, De Ruyck N et al. Reliable mite-specific IgE testing in nasal secretions by means of allergen microarray. *J Allergy Clin Immunol* 2017; 140: 301–303.e8.

84. Campo P, Del Carmen Plaza-Seron M, Eguiluz-Gracia I et al. Direct intranasal application of the solid phase of ImmunoCAP increases nasal specific immunoglobulin E detection in local allergic rhinitis patients. *Int Forum Allergy Rhinol* 2018; 8: 15–19.

85. Roberts G, Pfaar O, Akdis CA et al. EAACI guidelines on allergen immunotherapy: Allergic rhinoconjunctivitis. *Allergy* 2018; 73: 765–798.

86. Rondon C, Blanca-Lopez N, Aranda A et al. Local allergic rhinitis: Allergen tolerance and immunologic changes after preseasonal immunotherapy with grass pollen. *J Allergy Clin Immunol* 2011; 127: 1069–1071.

87. Shamji MH, Kappen JH, Akdis M et al. Biomarkers for monitoring clinical efficacy of allergen immunotherapy for allergic rhinoconjunctivitis and allergic asthma: An EAACI Position Paper. *Allergy* 2017; 72: 1156–1173.

88. Senti G, Kundig TM. Novel delivery routes for allergy immunotherapy: Intralymphatic, epicutaneous, and intradermal. *Immunol Allergy Clin North Am* 2016; 36: 25–37.

89. Corthesy B, Bioley G. Therapeutic intranasal instillation of allergen-loaded microbubbles suppresses experimental allergic asthma in mice. *Biomaterials* 2017; 142: 41–51.

90. Busse W, Corren J, Lanier BQ et al. Omalizumab, anti-IgE recombinant humanized monoclonal antibody, for the treatment of severe allergic asthma. *J Allergy Clin Immunol* 2001; 108: 184–190.

91. Maurer M, Metz M, Brehler R et al. Omalizumab treatment in patients with chronic inducible urticaria: A systematic review of published evidence. *J Allergy Clin Immunol* 2018; 141(2): 638–649.

92. Gibson PG, Reddel H, McDonald VM et al. Effectiveness and response predictors of omalizumab in a severe allergic asthma population with a high prevalence of comorbidities: The Australian Xolair Registry. *Intern Med J* 2016; 46: 1054–1062.

93. Farne HA, Wilson A, Powell C, Bax L, Milan SJ. Anti-IL5 therapies for asthma. *Cochrane Database Syst Rev* 2017; 9: CD010834.

94. Simpson EL, Bieber T, Guttman-Yassky E et al. Two phase 3 trials of dupilumab versus placebo in atopic dermatitis. *N Engl J Med* 2016; 375: 2335–2348.

SECTION II

Allergens: Inhalation, ingested, and injected

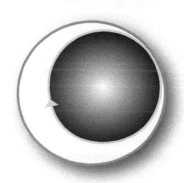

10 Tree pollen allergens

Rosa Codina
University of South Florida Morsani College of Medicine

Fernando Pineda and Ricardo Palacios
Diater, S.A.

CONTENTS

10.1 INTRODUCTION

IgE-mediated allergy affects more than 25% of the world's population, and proteins from pollen, mites, insects, and mammals are the most relevant causes of this disease [1]. Allergenic proteins from trees can be present in pollen, fruits, and seeds. Pollen released in great abundance during the flowering season of certain tree species represents a major trigger of respiratory manifestations of allergy (e.g., rhinoconjunctivitis and asthma), whereas fruits and seeds can elicit various symptoms of food allergy.

Trees recognized as relevant sources of pollen allergens belong to certain botanical orders, families, and genera with defined geographic distributions and flowering periods [2]. Allergenic tree species are generally wind-pollinated, whereas insect-pollinated trees rarely elicit an allergic response. This is mainly due to the fact that wind-pollinated trees release larger amounts of airborne pollen than those generated by insect-pollinated trees, and individuals sensitized to pollen require certain threshold levels of allergens to experience allergy symptoms [3,4].

In the temperate climatic zones on Earth, "flowering plants" (division Angiospermae), which include trees belonging to the order Fagales (e.g., birch, oak, alder, and hazel), represent the predominant allergenic sources. These zones are located in northern and central Europe, from North America to the Andes, northwest Africa, east Asia, and certain areas of Australia [1,2,5,6]. In Mediterranean countries and in areas with a Mediterranean climate, olive trees, which are members of the order Scrophulariales, are the most relevant sources of airborne allergens [7]. Other trees capable of inducing pollen allergy belong to two closely related plant families of the "nonflowering" plants (division Gymnospermae), the Families Cupressaceae (e.g., cypress and cedar) and Taxodiaceae (e.g., yew and Japanese cedar). Cupressaceae trees are relevant causes of pollinosis, especially in areas of the world with a mild climate, where up to 30% of atopic individuals might be sensitized to Cupressaceae pollen [8]. Japanese cedar (*Cryptomeria japonica*) is being recognized as the most common cause of seasonal allergy in Japan [9]. *Juniperus virginiana* (red cedar), which grows in particular areas of the United States, has been reported to be dispersed to distant areas from its original source [10].

Studies indicate that in subtropical and tropical climates, clinically relevant pollen allergens derive from trees such as *Peltophorum pterocarpum* (yellow gulmohar; order Fabales), *Dolichandrone platycalyx* (Nile trumpet tree; order Lamiales; subclass Asteridae), *Prosopis juliflora* (mesquite; order Fabales), and *Casuarina* spp. (Australian pine). However, the molecular structures of these allergens have not been fully elucidated to date [10,11] and might not be needed to produce safe and efficacious allergen extracts for diagnosis and allergen-specific immunotherapy.

The most clinically relevant, but not all, allergens of highly allergenic trees have been identified and characterized. Many of them have been cloned and produced as defined recombinant proteins, which can be used as tools to study the immunopathology of allergic diseases [12]. These defined proteins also form the basis for the development of novel strategies for diagnosis, treatment, and prevention of allergies [13,14]. While this approximation deserves many considerations, regulations often dictate what types of raw materials should be used to manufacture allergen extracts in different areas of the world.

Tree pollen allergens characterized to date represent predominantly low molecular weight intracellular proteins or glycoproteins [15]. Carbohydrate moieties may represent cross-reactive IgE epitopes occurring in tree pollen and several unrelated allergen sources but seem to have little clinical relevance [16,17].

The cross-reactivity observed among certain closely related tree species can be attributed to the structural and immunologic similarity of relevant cross-reactive allergens [18]. This finding implies that diagnosis and immunotherapy could be performed, at least theoretically, with a few cross-reactive marker allergens that harbor a large proportion of the cross-reactive epitopes [19]. This chapter presents a perspective regarding tree allergens, particularly in Europe.

10.2 TOPICS PERTAINING TO THIS CHAPTER

10.2.1 Taxonomy and distribution of allergenic trees

Among the 250,000 species described of pollen-producing plants, fewer than 100 are considered potent causes of pollen allergy [20]. Figure 10.1 shows the phylogenetic relationships among trees that are relevant sources of allergenic pollen and indicates that trees of both plant divisions, the Angiospermae ("flowering plants") and the Gymnospermae ("nonflowering plants"), have an impact on eliciting allergic symptoms in individuals sensitized to them. Knowledge about taxonomic relationships among trees is important because pollen of closely related families and genera often contain cross-reactive allergen molecules (e.g., order Fagales with the major birch pollen allergen, Bet v 1), which are not present in pollen from phylogenetically unrelated trees.

As previously mentioned, wind pollination appears to be a dispersion method for a tree pollen to affect a population. However, the critical parameter is whether pollen exposure occurs. Therefore, insect-pollinated trees can also be clinically relevant in particular populations, for example, in arborists and plant nursery workers.

Looking at the Plant Kingdom, several genera of the orders Fagales (e.g., birch, oak, alder, hazel, and beech), Scrophulariales (e.g., olive and ash), and Pinales (e.g., cypress, cedar) comprise the trees that produce the most allergenic pollen. Within these orders, pollen derived from birch, oak, olive tree, and cypress are the most relevant triggers of pollen allergy. However, other genera belonging to the orders mentioned have lesser allergenic potential, e.g., alder, hazel, and chestnut (from the order Fagales), privet (from the order Scrophulariales), and pine (from the order Pinales). Moreover, trees of the order Hamamelidales (e.g., plane trees) appear to be clinically relevant in southern Europe and Asia [21,22].

Ecological niches appropriated for particular plants to grow are often distributed over long or short distances; sometimes they

can be specific. Trees belonging to the order Fagales show distinct geographic distributions. For example, birch is prominent in various areas of Northern Europe and America. On the contrary, oak trees are abundant in warmer areas of the world. It is worth noting that oak species hybridize and speciate easily, and that a number of oak species prevail in particular locations; for example, in Florida [11,23].

Other plant orders include predominantly trees of low or uncertain importance in eliciting allergic symptoms at the population level. These are the orders Sapindales (e.g., maple tree) and Myrtales (e.g., gum tree, melaleuca). So far, little is known about the sensitizing potential of pollen allergens from trees belonging to the orders Juglandales (e.g., walnut), Fabales (e.g., acacia), and Salicales (e.g., willow, cottonwood) [24].

In the case of melaleuca (*Melaleuca* spp.), its low allergenic potential can be explained, at least partially, by the fact that this tree is not wind pollinated [25]. However, other less allergenic trees, like maples, acacias, and walnuts, are wind pollinated, which indicates that the sensitization potential of a plant cannot only be explained by the pollination method. It is interesting to note that the plant subclasses Hamamelidae and Asteridae not only comprise clinically relevant allergenic trees but also the most relevant allergenic weeds; for example, the genus *Parietaria* (from the order Urticales) and the genera *Artemisia* (mugwort) and *Ambrosia* (ragweed; order Asterales), which represent the most potent elicitors of weed pollen allergy in particular areas of the world. The subclass Rosidae includes trees (within the order Rosales) that are considered as the most relevant sources of allergenic fruits (e.g., apple, peach, and cherry).

Regarding the geographic distribution of allergenic trees, areas with a preferential occurrence of certain trees can be distinguished from areas with mixed vegetation. For example, subtropical areas such as those in the south of the United States often have unique vegetation, and the associated pollen sensitizes local populations [23].

The geographic distribution influences the sensitization profiles of allergic patients toward certain allergens [26]. Trees belonging to the order Fagales grow in temperate climatic zones and are abundant in Europe, northwest Africa, East Asia, and from North America to the Andes. In contrast, olive trees, the most allergenic trees of the order Scrophulariales, grow in Mediterranean countries and in areas with a Mediterranean climate of North and South Americas, South Africa, and Australia. These Mediterranean climatic zones are also the preferred areas of the most allergenic trees of the order Pinales, cypress and cedar, which grow in Mediterranean countries, Australia, New Zealand, North and South Americas, and parts of Asia. Ash, the other relevant pollen allergen source of the Scrophulariales, grows in middle Europe and North America, often in the same area as the Fagales trees.

Research that investigated the sensitization profiles of allergic patients has revealed interesting differences depending on geographic areas. For example, subjects allergic to birch pollen from the northern parts of Europe are mainly sensitized to the major birch pollen allergen, Bet v 1, which therefore may be considered as a genuine marker for birch sensitization [26]. By contrast, patients from the more southern parts of Europe appear positive in a birch pollen extract–based diagnostic test but when tested with pure recombinant allergens are more frequently positive to cross-reactive allergens (e.g., profilins and calcium-binding allergens). Therefore, it is likely that those patients are sensitized to these other allergen sources and, due to cross-reactivity, appear positive when tested with a birch pollen extract. An analogous study performed with recombinant *Parietaria* allergens [27] revealed similar results.

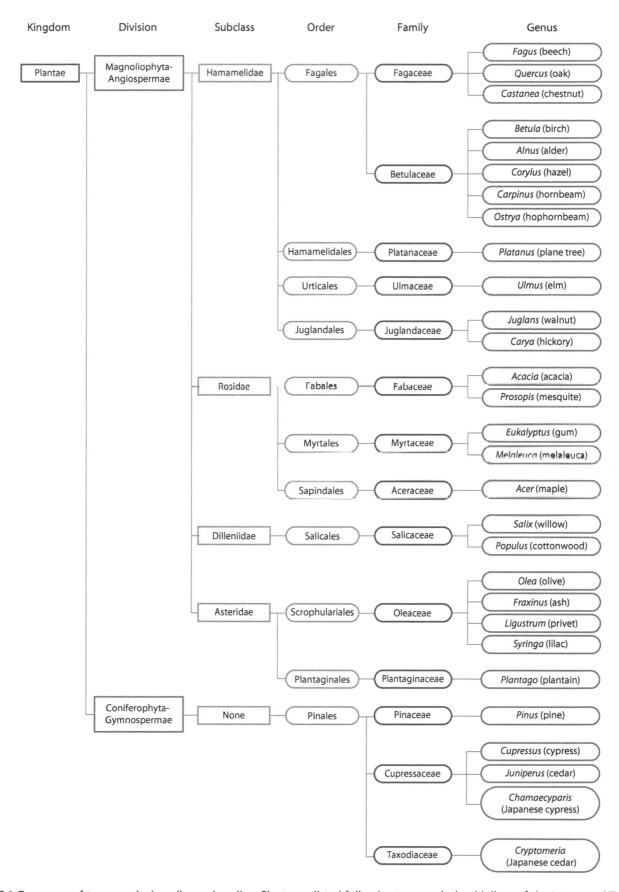

Figure 10.1 Taxonomy of trees producing allergenic pollen. Plants are listed following taxonomical guidelines of the Integrated Taxonomic Information System (https:// www.itis.gov).

10.2.2 Tree pollen identification

Pollen grains are the sperm cells from plants that contain the male reproductive genome. They deliver the genome to the female parts of the flower, where the process of fertilization takes place. Pollen grains are enclosed within an inner wall, the intine, and an outer wall, the exine, which protect the pollen from harmful environmental influences, such as desiccation and irradiation, during pollination. The outer wall consists of very elaborate, three-dimensional patterns and is interrupted by openings, called apertures. The number, distribution, and architecture of the apertures vary among plants and can be used to classify and identify pollen by microscopical analysis [28].

The collection of air samples and the analysis and identification of pollen are important for both physicians and patients (reviewed in Chapter 2). The allergist needs to know which species of allergenic pollen are present in the atmosphere, the number of allergenic pollen grains in each volume of air, and the time and spatial variations of concentrations of airborne allergenic pollen. Measurements of pollen loads during certain periods of the year permit prediction of allergen exposure, and such information distributed to allergic patients can help them to minimize exposure [29].

Examination of these sources, considering the atmospheric transportation of pollen, provides valuable parameters, because this information can be incorporated into weather forecasts, which can be used to minimize exposure to aeroallergens and result in the use of appropriate medications [30]. However, since there may be variations of the allergen contents in pollen grains, and because allergens are also released in pollen fragments and submicronic particles, it is important to measure and quantify not only the pollen grains but also the concentrations of the released allergenic molecules [31]. Other methods, including nucleic acid-based assays, to quantify pollen allergens are being developed (Figure 10.2).

A correlation between date of birth and sensitization to certain pollen species has been described. For example, children born in early spring and summer are more frequently sensitized to birch and grass pollen, respectively, than children born in other seasons [32,33]. There is also compelling evidence that sensitization to certain pollen species (e.g., birch) is more frequent in children exposed to heavy pollen loads early in life than in children who have experienced mild pollen exposure [34].

10.2.3 Cloning of tree pollen allergens

Diagnosis and specific immunotherapy of allergic diseases are currently performed with allergen extracts obtained by simple extraction procedures in aqueous buffers, due to mandatory regulations in many areas of the world. Whole allergen extracts have been used for years because they contain most, if not all, allergens present in the associated allergenic raw materials, and, in addition, their safety and efficacy have been demonstrated.

However, many attempts have been made to improve the quality of whole extracts derived from some sources because they may lack sufficient quantities of clinically relevant allergens, may contain nonallergenic materials, and also vary greatly regarding their composition [35,36]. Furthermore, now, it would be technically very challenging, due to various reasons, to purify all the major and minor allergens of a natural allergen source to obtain adequate, pure components for diagnosis and treatment applications. However, the application of molecular biology techniques has enabled the production of recombinant forms of the most relevant allergens from common allergen sources, mainly in Europe, but not in other areas of the world [37].

In principle, there are two strategies that can be applied to obtain cDNAs coding for allergens [38]. The first approach uses

(a)

(b)

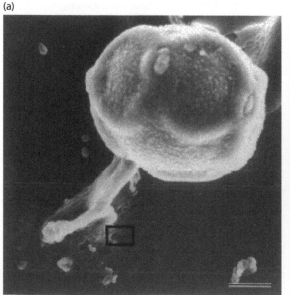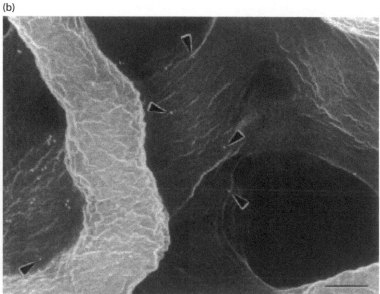

Figure 10.2 Humidity-induced release of allergens from abortively germinated alder pollen. Upon contact with rainwater, allergen-containing particles are liberated from ruptured pollen tubes. Field emission scanning electron micrographs after immunogold labeling for Aln g 1. The rectangle in (a) marks an area comparable to the area shown in higher magnification in (b). Bound Aln g 1–specific antibodies were detected with secondary antibodies coupled to colloidal gold particles, which appear as white dots (bars represent 5 μm in [a] and 0.25 μm in [b]). (The figure is reprinted with permission from [104].)

patients' specific IgE for the isolation of allergen-encoding cDNAs from expression cDNA libraries that have been constructed from the allergen source (Figure 10.3). For this approach, mRNA is isolated from the allergen source and converted into a cDNA by reverse transcription. Subsequently, this cDNA is inserted into a vector (usually a phage vector) suitable for construction of an expression cDNA library. After infection of appropriate host cells (usually *Escherichia coli* bacteria), clones expressing allergens can be located with patient's serum-specific IgE using immune-screening technology. DNA from the positive clones is then isolated, purified, and subjected to sequence analysis. The second approach for the isolation of allergen-encoding cDNAs involves DNA-based screening technologies (e.g., DNA-based screening of libraries, polymerase chain reaction [PCR], or reverse transcriptase-PCR [RT-PCR] strategies). Once allergen-encoding cDNAs have been obtained using either approach, they can be inserted into expression vectors, and highly purified recombinant allergens can be produced in large amounts (Figure 10.3).

The first cloning strategy has been used to produce a number of major and minor allergens from several genera belonging the orders Fagales and Scrophulariales, including those derived from birch (Bet v 1, Bet v 2, Bet v 3, Bet v 4, a birch actin-binding protein) and a calcium-binding protein from alder (Aln g 4) [38–42].

The second cloning strategy has been used successfully to clone other allergens belonging to the same orders [43–49], and in addition, from *Cryptomeria japonica*.

Using the second cloning strategy, oligonucleotides constructed according to a previously determined amino acid sequence of an allergen are applied either for PCR cloning or for screening of cDNA libraries. Cry j 1 and Cry j 2, the major allergens of Japanese cedar, were obtained by DNA-based screening of cDNA libraries [50,51]. On the basis of sequence similarity at the protein and nucleic acid level with the major birch pollen allergen, Bet v 1, an RT-PCR approach was used to isolate cDNAs coding for the major

allergens from apple, celery, and cherry (Mal d 1, Api g 1, and Pru av 1, respectively). These relevant food allergens were produced as recombinant proteins, and their cross-reactivity with Bet v 1 was demonstrated [52–54].

There are a variety of different expression systems available, which allow production of both glycosylated and nonglycosylated allergens, and thus, discrimination of IgE antibodies directed to protein or carbohydrate epitopes. The latter is useful to diagnose venom allergy but may also be helpful to diagnose pollinosis in the future [55].

Table 10.1 provides an overview of tree pollen allergens, their biological functions and characteristics. The spectrum of tree pollen and tree nut allergens has further been reviewed in several publications, and there are several allergen databases that are continuously updated when new allergens are identified [56].

The home page of the World Health Organization (WHO)/ International Union of Immunological Societies (IUIS) Allergen Nomenclature Subcommittee (http://www.allergen.org) summarizes the allergens that have been submitted to the allergen nomenclature subcommittee by researchers for approval and registration. The Structural Database of Allergenic Proteins (SDAP) from the University of Texas Medical Branch (https://fermi.utmb.edu/SDAP/) offers structural data about allergens. The Allergome database (http://www.allergome.org) represents a frequently updated and well-maintained allergen database that contains published allergen sequences and studies using allergen molecules. A useful summary of currently available allergen databases can be found in a review article by Mari [57]. Allergen Online (http://www.allergenonline.org/) provides access to an allergen list and sequence searchable database for the identification of allergenic proteins. Additionally, AllFam (http://www.meduniwien.ac.at/allfam/) is a useful database to obtain information about the classification of certain allergens into protein families. The rapid progress in the field of recombinant allergens in Europe indicates that perhaps most of the traditional

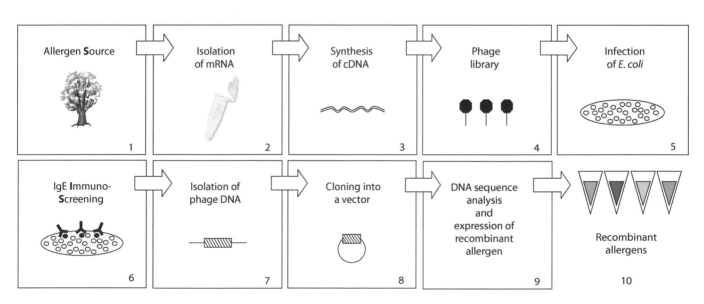

Figure 10.3 Cloning of tree pollen allergens and production of recombinant allergens. The different steps of the procedure, from mRNA isolation to the production of recombinant allergens, are displayed. The mRNA is isolated from the allergen source and converted into a cDNA, which is then ligated into a phage vector. Expression of the inserted cDNA is achieved after infection of *Escherichia coli* cells and allergen-expressing phage clones can be located with IgE antibodies from allergic patients using immunoscreening technology. After the isolation of phage DNA, allergen-encoding cDNAs can be inserted in suitable vector systems [8] and recombinant allergens can be produced in various host organisms (e.g., prokaryotic, eukaryotic organisms).

Table 10.1 Tree pollen allergens cloned and/or characterized to date

Species	Common name	Allergen	Function and similarity	MW (kDa)
Betula verrucosa	Birch	Bet v 1	Pathogenesis-related protein (PR10)	17
		Bet v 2	Profilin	15
		Bet v 3	Polcalcin-like protein (4 EF-hand)	24
		Bet v 4	Polcalcin	7–8
		Bet v 6	Phenylcoumaran benzylic ether reductase	35
		Bet v 7	Cyclophilin	18
		Bet v 8	Glutathione-*S*-transferase	27
Alnus glutinosa	Alder	Aln g 1	Pathogenesis-related protein, PR-10, Bet v 1 family member	18
		Aln g 4	Polcalcin	6–7
Corylus avellana	Hazel	Cor a 1	Pathogenesis-related protein, PR-10, Bet v 1 family member	17
		Cor a 2	Profilin	14
		Cor a 6	Isoflavone reductase homologue	35
		Cor a 8	Nonspecific lipid transfer protein type 1	9
		Cor a 9	11S seed storage globulin (legumin-like)	40
		Cor a 10	Luminal-binding protein	70
		Cor a 11	7S seed storage globulin (vicilin-like)	48
		Cor a 12	17 kDa Oleosin	17
		Cor a 13	14–16 kDa Oleosin	14–16
		Cor a 14	2S albumin	10
Carpinus betulus	Hornbeam	Car b 1	Pathogenesis-related protein, PR-10, Bet v 1 family member	17
Ostrya carpinifolia	Hop-hornbeam	Ost c 1	Pathogenesis-related protein, PR-10, Bet v 1 family member	17
Castanea sativa	Chestnut	Cas s 1	Pathogenesis-related protein, PR-10, Bet v 1 family member	22
		Cas s 5	Chitinase	32
		Cas s 8	Nonspecific lipid transfer protein type 1	12–13
		Cas s 9	Cytosolic class I small heat shock protein	17
Fagus sylvatica	Beech	Fag s 1	Pathogenesis-related protein, PR-10, Bet v 1 family member	17
Quercus alba	White oak	Que a 1	Pathogenesis-related protein, PR-10, Bet v 1 family member	17
Platanus acerifolia	London plane tree	Pla a 1	Invertase inhibitor	18
		Pla a 2	Polymethylgalacturonase	43
		Pla a 3	Lipid transfer protein	10
Platanus orientalis	Oriental plane	Pla or 1	Plant invertase/pectin methylesterase inhibitor	18
		Pla or 2	Polygalacturonase	42
		Pla or 3	nsLTP1	11
Olea europaea	Olive tree	Ole e 1	Common olive group 1	16
		Ole e 2	Profilin 1	15

(Continued)

Table 10.1 (Continued) Tree pollen allergens cloned and/or characterized to date

Species	Common name	Allergen	Function and similarity	MW (kDa)
		Ole e 3	Polcalcin	9
		Ole e 4		32
		Ole e 5	Superoxide dismutase [Cu-ZN]	16
		Ole e 6		9–10
		Ole e 7	Putative nonspecific lipid transfer protein	10
		Ole e 8	Polcalcin-like protein (4 EF-hands)	21
		Ole e 9	1 3-β-glucanase	46
		Ole e 10	X8 domain-containing protein	11
		Ole e 11	Pectin-methylesterase	39.4
		Ole e 12	Isoflavone reductase	37
		Ole e 13	Thaumatin	23
		Ole e 14	Polygalacturonase	46.5
		Ole e 15	Cyclophilin	19
Fraxinus excelsior	Ash	Fra e 1	Ole e 1-like protein family member	20
Ligustrum vulgare	Privet	Lig v 1	Ole e 1-like protein family member	20
Syringa vulgaris	Lilac	Syr v 1	Ole e 1-like protein family member	20
		Syr v 3	Polcalcin	8.9
Plantago lanceolata	English plantain	Pla l 1	Ole e 1–related protein	18
		Pla l 2	Profilin	15
Cryptomeria japonica	Japanese cedar	Cry j 1	Pectate lyase	41–45
		Cry j 2	Polymethylgalacturonase	45
Chamaecyparis obtusa	Japanese cypress	Cha o 1	Pectate lyase; Cry j 1-related	40.2
		Cha o 2	Polymethylgalacturonase; Cry j 2 related	46
Cupressus arizonica	Arizona cypress	Cup a 1	Pectate lyase; Cry j 1 related	43
Cupressus sempervirens	Italian cypress	Cup s 1	Pectate lyase; Cry j 1 related	43
		Cup s 2	PR5; thaumatin-like protein	34
		Cup s 3	Not known	14
Juniperus ashei	Mountain cedar	Jun a 1	Pectate lyase	43
		Jun a 2	Polygalacturonase	43
		Jun a 3	Thaumatin-like protein	34
Juniperus oxycedrus	Prickly juniper	Jun o 4	Polcalcin-like protein (4 EF-hand domains)	18
Juniperus virginiana	Eastern red cedar	Jun v 1	Pectate lyase	43
		Jun v 3	Thaumatin-like protein	34

Note: Allergenic molecules are listed according to their taxonomic orders (underlined). Allergen sources (species and common name) are designed according to the International Union of Immunological Societies Allergen Nomenclature Sub-Committee (WHO-IUIS).

whole allergen extracts could be replaced by recombinant allergens in the future because they cover the complete epitope repertoire of the extracts [58].

10.2.4 Biological functions and structural characteristics of tree pollen allergens

The application of molecular biology techniques to allergen characterization has permitted the determination of the molecular characteristics for the most common environmental allergens during the last decades [58]. The DNA and deduced amino acid sequences can be obtained by sequencing the allergen-encoding cDNAs and thus allow for comparisons with sequences deposited in databases. Using this approach, the biological functions of various allergens can be estimated. For example, the cDNA and the amino acid sequence of the major birch pollen allergen, Bet v 1, has a high level of sequence homology with a group of proteins that were identified to be upregulated when plants were wounded, infected, or subjected to stressful conditions. Accordingly, these proteins were designated as pathogenesis-related proteins (PR proteins) [59]. Although to date there are no definitive experimental data to support that the family of Bet v 1–related allergens contributes to the plant defense system, it is possible that they have protective functions, i.e., antimicrobial properties [59–60]. Other functions (e.g., RNAse activity and lipid carrier) have been claimed for the Bet v 1 allergen family based on *in vitro* experiments and structural data [59,61].

Numerous Bet v 1 homologous allergens have been identified to date in pollen from trees belonging to the order Fagales (e.g., Que a 1: white oak; Aln g 1: alder; Cor a 1: hazel; Car b 1: hornbeam; and Cas s 1: chestnut) (see http://www.allergen.org, http://www.meduniwien.ac.at/allfam/). Figure 10.4 displays the relationships among Bet v 1–related plant allergens on the basis of sequence identities, which indicate that almost all proteins contain cross-reactive IgE epitopes. However, it is also known that even birch pollen contains proteins with high sequence identity to Bet v 1

but without relevant allergenic activity [62]. The existence of these hypoallergenic Bet v 1 isoforms and nonallergenic proteins with high sequence homology to Bet v 1 demonstrates that sequence homology *per se* cannot predict with certainty whether a protein is allergenic or not [63]. The latter aspect is also relevant because it is impossible to predict with the allergenic potential of genetically modified plants exclusively based on sequence homologies of the transgene with genes code for known allergens [64].

Table 10.1 provides an overview of tree pollen allergens, grouped according to botanical classifications. Each of the different trees contains a spectrum of allergens. However, it appears that certain allergenic molecules occur in different tree species as proteins with significant sequence homology and cross-reactive epitopes. In general, it is possible to identify certain groups of cross-reactive allergens. For example, there are the Bet v 1–related allergens, Que e 1, Aln g 1, Cor a 1, Car b 1, Ost c 1, Fag s 1, and Cas s 1, that can be found in pollen from trees belonging to the order Fagales. These allergens are also expressed in the nuts of trees belonging to this same order and in fruits of unrelated trees belonging to the order Rosales (within the subclass Rosidae). Due to cross-reactivity, they might elicit symptoms of food allergy, particularly oral allergy syndrome, in pollen-allergic patients (Figure 10.5a).

A second group of highly cross-reactive allergens includes the profilins. These are actin-binding proteins, expressed in all eukaryotic cells, which link signal transduction processes with the reassembling of the cytoskeleton [39,66]. They are structurally conserved low molecular weight proteins (12–15 kDa) and represent probably the most widely distributed allergens described to date [39]. They include proteins from pollen of botanically unrelated plants (trees, grasses, weeds), for instance, birch pollen (Bet v 2) and olive pollen profilin (Ole e 2), as well as proteins from plant-derived foods (see Table 10.1 and Figure 10.5b).

The birch pollen allergens, Bet v 3 and Bet v 4 [40,41]; the alder pollen allergen, Aln g 4 [42]; as well as the olive pollen allergens, Ole e 3 [67] and Ole e 8 [68], belong to the group of calcium-binding proteins [69]. Sequence analysis of the cDNAs coding for these allergens revealed the presence of typical calcium-binding motifs (i.e., binding sites for calcium), termed EF-hands [70]. Bet

	Asparagus	Carrot	Celery	Tomato	Soybean	Pea	Medicago	Pear	Apricot	Cherry	Apple	Beech	Hornbeam	Alder	Hazel	Birch
Birch	39	38	40	47	49	54	55	58	60	59	66	69	79	81	83	100
Hazel	40	41	40	46	53	53	55	59	63	59	67	69	92	82	100	
Alder	41	39	40	40	50	50	52	55	61	57	64	67	79	100		
Hornbeam	39	42	40	46	51	51	56	56	62	58	66	68	100			
Beech	39	41	42	49	57	54	55	70	74	74	71	100				
Apple	39	40	45	47	50	51	54	70	79	76	100					
Cherry	37	40	43	49	55	51	51	84	76	100						
Apricot	37	44	50	50	53	51	52	73	100							
Pear	35	39	40	43	54	50	50	100								
Medicago	33	36	40	42	66	83	100									
Pea	29	33	39	39	70	100										
Soybean	34	37	40	41	100											
Tomato	43	32	40	100												
Celery	32	51	100													
Carrot	33	100														
Asparagus	100															

Figure 10.4 Sequence identities (%) among Bet v 1 homologous proteins from different sources.

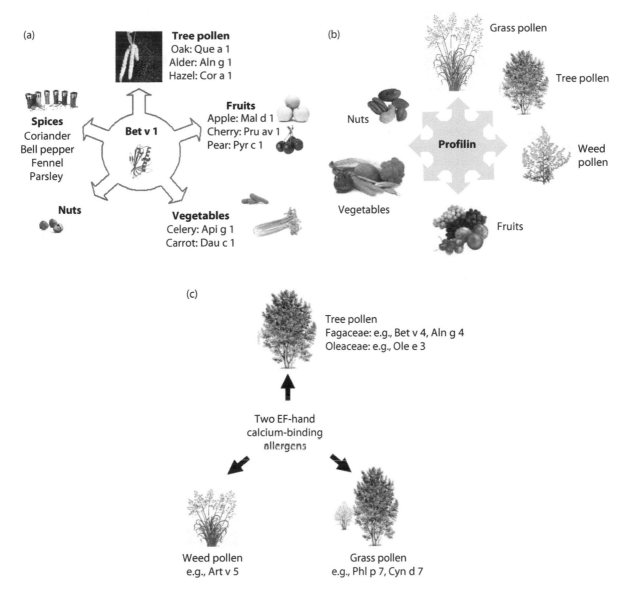

Figure 10.5 (a) Bet v 1 cross-reactive allergens can be found in pollen of trees belonging to the order Fagales as well as in fruits, vegetables, nuts, and spices. (b) Profilins, the most cross-reactive allergens described to date, typically present in pollen of botanically unrelated plants (trees, grasses, weeds) and in plant-derived foods (fruits, vegetables, nuts). (c) Two EF-hand calcium-binding allergens can be found in pollen from trees, grasses, and weeds.

v 3, an allergen mainly expressed in mature pollen [40], contains three EF-hands; the olive pollen allergen, Ole e 8; and the cypress pollen allergen, Jun o 4, contain four EF-hands [68,71]. Bet v 4, Aln g 4, and Ole e 3 contain two EF-hand calcium-binding motifs [41,72]. The calcium-binding allergens with two EF-hands have been found in a variety of pollen species from botanically unrelated trees, grasses, and weeds. They represent another family of highly cross-reactive allergens (Figure 10.5c).

It is important to note that calcium-binding allergens are predominantly expressed in pollen but not in other plant tissues and therefore are responsible only for pollen allergy, but not for food cross-reactivity. IgE inhibition experiments indicate that also there is extensive IgE cross-reactivity between members with different numbers of EF-hands [35,73]. IgE recognition of calcium-binding allergens is enhanced in the presence of calcium, and calcium binding causes a conformational change resulting in higher allergen

thermal stability of the allergens [35]. The calcium dependence of IgE binding suggests that patients are preferentially sensitized to the calcium-bound allergens [35].

The first three-dimensional structure of a two EF-hand allergen, namely, of the two EF-hand allergens from timothy grass (Phl p 7), has been resolved by x-ray crystallography. This analysis provides further insight into the structure and conformational changes of these highly cross-reactive allergens and suggests a ligand-binding function [74]. Profilin and two EF-hand pollen allergens, e.g., Ole e 2 and Ole e 3, could serve as markers of polysensitization [75].

Lipid transfer proteins (LTPs) are relevant plant food allergens with elevated allergenic activity [76]. They are highly conserved, low molecular weight proteins and are responsible for the transport of lipids across cell membranes. A high resistance to heat treatments and enzymatic digestion has been reported, and allergic reactions caused by LTPs are often associated with severe systemic symptoms [76].

LTPs are also present in pollen from trees and weeds [77], and patients can be sensitized to them. Interestingly, pollen-derived LTP allergens do not seem to cross-react with LTPs from plant foods [78].

Another group of pollen allergens is represented by the major olive pollen allergen, Ole e 1, which shares high sequence identity and cross-reactive epitopes with allergens from the closely related trees of the Oleaceae family, ash (Fra e 1) [79]; privet (Lig v 1) [48]; and lilac (Syr v 1) [80]. However, Ole e 1 does not cross-react with homologous allergens from other plants. The Ole e 1 pollen allergens are glycosylated proteins, and their glycan moieties seem to be involved in the antigenic and allergenic properties of these allergens. However, to date no functional role has been assigned to these allergens [49].

In the division of Gymnospermae, two separate groups of pollen allergens have been identified [10], the pectate lyases and the polymethylgalacturonases. The major Japanese cedar pollen allergen, Cry j 1, the most thoroughly studied member of the pectate lyases [81], displays high sequence homology and IgE cross-reactivity with major allergens of other trees from the order Pinales (e.g., Japanese cypress, Arizona cypress, Italian cypress, and mountain cedar). Interestingly, sequence identities of nearly 50% were also found with the major ragweed allergens, the pectate lyases, Amb a 1 and Amb a 2 [10,82]. The second major allergen from Japanese cedar pollen, Cry j 2, has been classified as a polymethylgalacturonase, with cross-reactivity to homologous pollen allergens from other members of the order Pinales [83]. Database searches further revealed significant sequence homologies (~40%) of Cry j 2 with polygalacturonases from a grass pollen allergen (Phl p 13) [84] and with polygalacturonases associated with fruit ripening in tomato [10], but no relevant IgE cross-reactivity seems to exist between Cry j 2 and these enzymes. The third member of Japanese cedar pollen, Cry j 3, an allergen homologous to isoflavone reductase shows a significant sequence similarity to those of plant isoflavone reductase-like proteins, which include a birch pollen allergen, Bet v 5 [85]. The first plant aspartic protease allergen from Japanese cedar pollen has been identified and might be helpful to further elucidate the role of protease activity in the pathogenesis of cedar pollinosis [86].

Table 10.1 describes the characterized tree pollen allergens to date and provides information about their sources, biological functions, and molecular weights (kDa). The main features that tree pollen allergens have in common are that they represent low molecular weight proteins or glycoproteins, which rapidly elute from pollen after contact with aqueous solutions [87]. This observation should be extrapolated to the release of pollen allergens on contact with mammal mucosal membranes (including human). The use of immunogold electron microscopy reveals that these allergens are mainly intracellular proteins that either elute from pollen or, under certain conditions, are expelled from pollen by rupture or abortive pollen germination [88]. Analyses of the three-dimensional structures of relevant pollen allergens do not identify the structural motifs common among all allergens. However, these studies show that cross-reactivity among allergens is based on structural similarities [89].

10.2.5 Cross-reactivity among tree pollen allergens

During the last decades, the most common allergens from different sources, including those derived from tree pollen, have been identified by molecular cloning and produced as recombinant allergens in Europe but not in other areas of the world [12]. In this context, IgE inhibition studies performed with purified recombinant allergens have greatly enhanced our understanding of cross-reactivity at the molecular level [12].

Figure 10.5a illustrates an example of the cross-reactivity within the group of Bet v 1–related allergens. Allergens containing cross-reactive IgE epitopes have been described in pollen, fruits (e.g., apple and pear), vegetables (e.g., carrot and celery), and tree nuts (e.g., hazelnut) [65]. Accordingly, Bet v 1–sensitized patients frequently experience oral allergy syndrome after the ingestion of foods containing cross-reactive allergens. Due to the extensive level of cross-reactivity among Bet v 1–related allergens, it is not surprising that immunotherapy with birch pollen vaccine alone also improves allergy to other pollen species of related trees and certain foods [90].

It appears that cross-reactivity has in principle two facets that can be applied to diagnosis and therapy. Certain allergens/epitopes are restricted to allergen sources, and thus they can be used as marker molecules to confirm sensitization to them [91]. For example, Bet v 1 cross-reacts mainly with pollen allergens of trees belonging to the Fagales order. The major olive pollen allergen, Ole e 1, cross-reacts with pollen allergens of trees belonging to the Oleaceae order, including ash [19,92]. The major pollen allergens from timothy grass (e.g., Phl p 1, Phl p 2, Phl p 5) also cross-react with allergens from other grasses, but certain weed allergens (e.g., Par j 2 from *Parietaria judaica*) cross-react with allergens only present in weeds [27]. Based on this observation, it has been proposed to use such species-specific marker allergens to confirm sensitization to certain allergen sources. These marker allergens could be used, at least theoretically, to confirm the suitability of patients for immunotherapy with a given allergen extract [19,92]. Another argument for using major species-specific marker allergens as an inclusion criterium for immunotherapy is that the currently used allergen extracts are mainly standardized regarding these major allergens. However, a consideration is that these extracts are standardized only in Europe but not in other areas of the world.

However, many allergens identified to date exhibit broad cross-reactivity and thus indicate polysensitization. These allergens include, for example, the group of profilins (Figure 10.5b) and two EF-hand calcium-binding allergens (Figure 10.5c). Patients sensitized to profilins (e.g., Bet v 2 or Phl p 12) show cross-reactivity in most cases with profilins from various unrelated plants and suffer from both pollen and plant food polysensitization (Figure 10.5b) [91].

Patients sensitized to calcium-binding allergens (e.g., Bet v 4, Phl p 7, the two EF-hand calcium-binding allergen from timothy grass) suffer in most cases from multiple pollen sensitization to trees, grasses, and weeds (Figure 10.5c) [44]. Such patients may benefit less from allergen vaccine-based immunotherapy because the currently used therapeutic vaccines are not standardized regarding these molecules, and polysensitized patients seem to benefit less from allergen-specific immunotherapy [93].

In vitro diagnostic tests equipped with recombinant marker allergens to facilitate the selection of patients for immunotherapy with tree and grass pollen extracts are available from a few diagnostic companies in Europe and can be used by clinicians [94]. However, these strategies are not available in many other areas of the world.

10.2.6 Diagnosis and therapy: Transition from allergen extract-based to recombinant

The rapid progress of allergen characterization through the application of molecular cloning techniques in Europe has provided recombinant allergens covering most allergen sources, including trees. Recombinant allergens allow for the determination of individual sensitization profiles of allergic patients, a process that has been designated as component-resolved diagnosis (CRD) [35]. The diagnostic information obtained by CRD is more precise than diagnosis based on extract-based methodology. To utilize the full spectrum of recombinant allergens for allergy diagnosis, novel forms of multiallergen tests have been developed [95]. Some of the new tests combine chip and microarray technology, whereas others simply utilize nitrocellulose-based test systems for the elucidation of a patient's reactivity profile in a single test [95,96]. In addition, recombinant allergens have been incorporated into established quantitative and automated *in vitro* allergy test systems, where they allow a more precise quantitative measurement of specific-IgE and other allergen-specific immunoglobulins. Many of these assay platforms have been developed in Sweden and have not yet received approval from the U.S. Food and Drug Administration to be used in the American market.

Using these recombinant allergen-based tests, it has been possible to dissect the sensitization profiles of patients from various populations in Europe [26,27], to detect fetal allergen-specific IgE in cord blood [96] to (1) monitor the development of allergies from early childhood to adulthood [97,98], (2) investigate the development of IgE profiles during the natural course of allergic disease [99], and (3) study the effects of allergen-specific immunotherapy [99]

Recombinant allergen-based tests and CRD have resulted in several interesting observations regarding the pathogenesis of allergic diseases and the potential mechanisms for allergen-specific immunotherapy. The monitoring of specific IgE, IgG, and IgG subclass responses during allergen-specific immunotherapy has reemphasized the importance of specific blocking antibodies for the success of this therapeutic option [99].

The finding that allergen vaccines induce a highly heterogeneous immune response against the individual components in the vaccine has underlined the need for improvement of therapeutic allergen preparations in Europe [100]. Moreover, it appears that injection of allergen vaccines may induce specific IgE reactivity to new allergens in treated patients [101]. Although the clinical relevance of these findings has not been confirmed in large population studies around the world, these data support the idea that patients perhaps would benefit from treatment according to their individual sensitization profiles. Furthermore, the results of molecular allergy diagnosis could change the prescription of allergen-specific immunotherapy in Europe but not in other areas of the world. Theoretically, specialists would perhaps prescribe a different allergen-specific immunotherapy in a percent of allergic patients after performing CRD [102].

The concept of treating allergic patients according to their sensitization profile with purified or recombinant allergens, termed component-resolved immunotherapy (CRIT), has been proposed [35]. During the last few years, several candidate molecules have been developed by recombinant DNA technology [12,103]. These molecules have reduced allergenic activity while T-cell epitopes and immunogenicity (i.e., capacity to induce protective IgG responses) are maintained [103]. The recombinant, hypoallergenic allergen derivatives have been evaluated *in vitro*, in experimental animal models and in *in vivo* provocation testing in humans [12,103]. The first immunotherapy study with recombinant allergen derivatives was performed with hypoallergenic molecules of the major birch pollen allergen, Bet v 1 [90,92], and subsequently, several other successful immunotherapy studies have been performed with recombinant allergens [103].

SALIENT POINTS

1. The most relevant tree pollen allergens are derived from wind-pollinated trees belonging to the orders Fagales (e.g., birch and oak), Scrophulariales (e.g., olive), and Pinales (e.g., cedar and cypress).
2. Whole allergen extracts for diagnosis and treatment of allergic diseases have been used for years and likely will continue to be used in many areas of the world for the time coming.
3. The most common and clinically relevant tree pollen allergens have been produced as recombinant allergens. Panels of recombinant allergens resembling the epitope complexity of natural allergen extracts are becoming available, particularly in Europe.
4. The molecular characterization of tree pollen allergens reveals that there are families of cross-reactive allergens that are characterized by high-sequence homology and immunologic cross-reactivity.
5. Recombinant allergen-based diagnostic tests to determine the sensitization profiles of patients and to improve the selection of the most accurate treatment forms are available for clinical use in Europe.
6. Recombinant allergen derivatives with reduced allergenic activity have been developed and evaluated experimentally.

REFERENCES

1. Brozek JL, Bousquet J, Baena-Cagnani CE et al. Allergic Rhinitis and its Impact on Asthma (ARIA) guidelines: 2010 revision. *J Allergy Clin Immunol* 2010; 126: 466–476.
2. D'Amato G, Bonini S, Bousquet J, Durham SR, Platts-Mills TAE. *Pollinosis 2000 Global Approach.* Naples, Italy: JGC Editions, 2001.
3. Niederberger V, Ring J, Rakoski J et al. Antigens drive memory IgE responses in human allergy via the nasal mucosa. *Int Arch Allergy Immunol* 2007; 142: 133–144.
4. Florido JF, Delgado PG, de San Pedro BS et al. High levels of *Olea europaea* pollen and relation with clinical findings. *Int Arch Allergy Immunol* 1999; 119: 133–137.
5. Ridolo E, Albertini R, Giordano D, Soliani L, Usberti I, Dall'Aglio PP. Airborne pollen concentrations and the incidence of allergic asthma and rhinoconjunctivitis in northern Italy from 1992 to 2003. *Int Arch Allergy Immunol* 2007; 142: 151–157.
6. Dvorin DJ, Lee JJ, Belecanech GA, Goldstein MF, Dunsky EH. A comparative, volumetric survey of airborne pollen in Philadelphia, Pennsylvania (1991–1997) and Cherry Hill, New Jersey (1995–1997). *Ann Allergy Asthma Immunol* 2001; 87: 394–404.
7. D'Amato G, Mullins J, Nolard N, Spieksma FT, Wachter R. City spore concentrations in the European Economic Community (EEC). VII. Oleaceae (Fraxinus, Ligustrum, Olea). *Clin Allergy* 1988; 18: 541–547.
8. Charpin D, Pichot C, Belmonte J et al. Cypress pollinosis: From tree to clinic. *Clin Rev Allergy Immunol* 2019; 56(2): 174–195.
9. Kaneko Y, Motohashi Y, Nakamura H, Endo T, Eboshida A. Increasing prevalence of Japanese cedar pollinosis: A meta-regression analysis. *Int Arch Allergy Immunol* 2005; 136: 365–371.
10. Elonard M, Lo E, Levetin E. Increasing *Juniperus virginiana* L. pollen in the Tulsa atmosphere: Long-term trends, variability, and influence of meteorological conditions. *Int J Biometeorol* 2016; 62: 229–241.

11. Jelks M. *Allergy Plants that Cause Sneezing and Wheezing.* Tampa, FL: World-Wide Publications.

12. Valenta, R. Biochemistry of allergens, recombinant allergens. In: Kay AB, Kaplan A, Bousquet J, Holt B, editors. *Allergy and Allergic Diseases*, 2nd ed. Oxford, England: Blackwell Publishing, 2008.

13. Linhart B, Valenta R. Vaccines for allergy. *Curr Opin Immunol* 2012; 24: 354–360.

14. Valenta R, Linhart B, Swoboda I, Niederberger V. Recombinant allergens for allergen-specific immunotherapy: 10 years anniversary of immunotherapy with recombinant allergens. *Allergy* 2011; 66: 775–783.

15. Grote M, Valenta R, Reichelt R. Abortive pollen germination: A mechanism of allergen release in birch, alder, and hazel revealed by immunogold electron microscopy. *J Allergy Clin Immunol* 2003; 111: 1017–1023.

16. van Ree R. Carbohydrate epitopes and their relevance for the diagnosis and treatment of allergic diseases. *Int Arch Allergy Immunol* 2002; 129: 189–197.

17. Altmann F. The role of protein glycosylation in allergy. *Int Arch Allergy Immunol* 2007; 142: 99–115.

18. Ferreira F, Hawranek T, Gruber P, Wopfner N, Mari A. Allergic cross-reactivity: From gene to the clinic. *Allergy* 2004; 59: 243–267.

19. Valenta R, Twaroch T, Swoboda I. Component-resolved diagnosis to optimize allergen-specific immunotherapy in the Mediterranean area. *J Investig Allergol Clin Immunol* 2007; 17(Suppl 1): 36–40.

20. D'Amato G, Spieksma FThM, Liccardi G et al. Pollen related allergy in Europe. Position Paper of the European Academy of Allergology and Clinical Immunology. *Allergy* 1998; 53: 567–578.

21. Lauer I, Miguel-Moncin MS, Abel T et al. Identification of a plane pollen lipid transfer protein (Pla a 3) and its immunological relation to the peach lipid-transfer protein, Pru p 3. *Clin Exp Allergy* 2007; 37: 261–269.

22. Pazouki N, Sankian M, Nejadsattari T, Khavari-Nejad RA, Varasteh AR. Oriental plane pollen allergy: Identification of allergens and cross-reactivity between relevant species. *Allergy Asthma Proc* 2008; 29: 622–628.

23. Phillips JF, Jelks ML, Lockey RF. Important Florida botanical aeroallergens. *Allergy Asthma Proc* 2010; 31: 337–340.

24. Liang KL, Su MC, Shiao JY, Wu SH, Li YH, Jiang RS. Role of pollen allergy in Taiwanese patients with allergic rhinitis. *J Formos Med Assoc* 2010; 109: 879–885.

25. Stablein JJ, Buchholtz GA, Lockey RF. Melaleuca tree and respiratory disease. *Ann Allergy Asthma Immunol* 2002; 89: 523–530.

26. Moverare R, Westritschnig K, Svensson M et al. Different IgE reactivity profiles in birch pollen-sensitive patients from six European populations revealed by recombinant allergens: An imprint of local sensitization. *Int Arch Allergy Immunol* 2002; 128: 325–335.

27. Stumvoll S, Westritschnig K, Lidholm J et al. Identification of cross-reactive and genuine *Parietaria judaica* pollen allergens. *J Allergy Clin Immunol* 2003; 111: 974–979.

28. Accorsi CA, Bandini-Mazzanti M, Romano B et al. Allergenic pollen: Morphology and microscopic photographs. In: D'Amato G, Spieksma FThM, Bonini S, editors. *Allergenic Pollen and Pollenosis in Europe.* Oxford: Blackwell, 1991: 24–44.

29. Smith G. 2000. *Sampling and Identifying Allergenic Pollens and Molds.* San Antonio, TX: Blewstone Press.

30. Jäger S, Emberlin J, Gallop R et al. The European pollen information service center in the internet. *Allergy Suppl* 1997; 52: 32.

31. Buters JT, Kasche A, Weichenmeier I et al. Year-to-Year Variation in Release of Bet v 1 Allergen from Birch Pollen: Evidence for Geographical Differences between West and South Germany. *Int Arch Allergy Immunol* 2007; 145: 122–130.

32. Aalberse RC, Nieuwenhuys EJ, Hey M, Stapel SO. "Horoscope effect" not only for seasonal but also for non-seasonal allergens. *Clin Exp Allergy* 1992; 22: 1003–1006.

33. Graf N, Johansen P, Schindler C et al. Analysis of the relationship between pollinosis and date of birth in Switzerland. *Int Arch Allergy Immunol* 2007; 143: 269–275.

34. Kihlstrom A, Lilja G, Pershagen G, Hedlin G. Exposure to birch pollen in infancy and development of atopic disease in childhood. *J Allergy Clin Immunol* 2002; 110: 78–84.

35. Valenta R, Lidholm J, Niederberger V, Hayek B, Kraft D, Gronlund H. The recombinant allergen-based concept of component-resolved diagnostics and immunotherapy (CRD and CRIT). *Clin Exp Allergy* 1999; 29: 896–904.

36. Focke M, Marth K, Flicker S, Valenta R. Heterogeneity of commercial grass-pollen extracts. *Clin Exp Allergy* 2008; 38: 1400–1408.

37. Valenta R, Vrtala S, Laffer S, Spitzauer S, Kraft D. Recombinant allergens. *Allergy* 1998; 53: 552–561.

38. Breiteneder H, Pettenburger K, Bito A et al. The gene coding for the major birch pollen allergen, Bet v 1, is highly homologous to a pea disease resistance response gene. *EMBO J* 1989; 8: 1935–1938.

39. Valenta R, Duchene M, Pettenburger K et al. Identification of profilin as a novel pollen allergen: IgE autoreactivity in sensitized individuals. *Science* 1991; 253: 557–560.

40. Seiberler S, Scheiner O, Kraft D, Lonsdale D, Valenta R. Characterization of a birch pollen allergen, Bet v 3, representing a novel class of Ca^{2+} binding proteins; specific expression in mature pollen and dependence of patients' IgE binding on protein-bound Ca^{2+}. *EMBO J* 1994; 13: 3481–3486.

41. Twardosz A, Hayek B, Seiberler S et al. Molecular characterization, expression in *Escherichia coli* and epitope analysis of a two EF-hand calcium-binding birch pollen allergen, Bet v 4. *Biochem Biophys Res Commun* 1997; 239: 197–204.

42. Hayek B, Vangelista L, Pastore A et al. Molecular and immunological characterization of a highly cross-reactive two EF-hand calcium-binding alder pollen allergens, Aln g 4. Structural basis for calcium-modulated IgE recognition. *J Immunol* 1998; 161: 7031–7039.

43. Breiteneder H, Ferreira F, Reikerstorfer A et al. cDNA cloning and expression in *Escherichia coli* of Aln g I, the major allergen in pollen of alder (*Alnus glutinosa*). *J Allergy Clin Immunol* 1992; 90: 909–917.

44. Larson JN, Stroman P, Ipsen H. PCR based cloning and sequencing of isogenes encoding the tree pollen major allergen Car b I from *Carpinus betulus*, hornbeam. *Mol Immunol* 1992; 1992; 29: 703–711.

45. Breiteneder H, Ferreira F, Hoffmann-Sommergruber K et al. Four recombinant isoforms of Cor a I, the major allergen of hazel pollen, show different IgE-binding properties. *Eur J Biochem* 1993; 212: 355–362.

46. Villalba M, Batanero E, Monsalve RI, Delapena MAG, Lahoz C, Rodriguez R. Cloning and expression of Ole e 1, the major allergen from olive tree pollen. Polymorphism analysis and tissue specificity. *J Biol Chem* 1994; 269: 15217–15222.

47. Asturias JA, Arilla MC, Gomez-Bayon N, Martinez J, Martinez A, Palacios R. Cloning and expression of the panallergen profilin and the major allergen (Ole e 1) from olive tree pollen. *J Allergy Clin Immunol* 1997; 100: 365–372.

48. Batanero E, Gonzalez de la Pena MA, Villalba M, Monsalve RI, Martin-Esteban M, Rodriguez R. Isolation, cDNA cloning and expression of Lig v 1, the major allergen from privet pollen. *Clin Exp Allergy* 1996; 26: 1401–1410.

49. Rodriguez R, Villalba M, Monsalve RI, Batanero E. The spectrum of olive pollen allergens. *Int Arch Allergy Immunol* 2001; 125: 185–195.

50. Sone T, Komiyama N, Shimizu K, Kusakabe T, Morikubo K, Kino K. Cloning and sequencing of cDNA coding for Cry j I, a major allergen of Japanese cedar pollen. *Biochem Biophys Res Commun* 1994; 199: 619–628.

51. Komiyama N, Sone T, Shimizu K, Morikubo K, Kino K. cDNA cloning and expression of Cry j II the second major allergen of Japanese cedar pollen. *Biochem Biophys Res Commun* 1994; 201: 1021–1028.

52. Vanek-Krebitz M, Hoffmann-Sommergruber K, Laimer da Camara Machado M et al. Cloning and sequencing of Mal d 1, the major allergen from apple (*Malus domestica*), and its immunological relationship to Bet v 1, the major birch pollen allergen. *Biochem Biophys Res Commun* 1995; 214: 538–551.

53. Breiteneder H, Hoffmann-Sommergruber K, O'Riordain G et al. Molecular characterization of Api g 1, the major allergen of celery (*Apium graveolens*), and its immunological and structural relationships to a group of 17 kDa tree pollen allergens. *Eur J Biochem* 1995; 233: 484–489.

54. Scheurer S, Pastorello EA, Wangorsch A, Kastner M, Haustein D, Vieths S. Recombinant allergens Pru av 1 and Pru av 4 and a newly identified lipid transfer protein in the *in vitro* diagnosis of cherry allergy. *J Allergy Clin Immunol* 2001; 107: 724–731.

55. Mittermann I, Zidarn M, Silar M et al. Recombinant allergen-based IgE testing to distinguish bee and wasp allergy. *J Allergy Clin Immunol* 2010; 125: 1300–1307.

56. Mothes N, Horak F, Valenta R. Transition from a botanical to a molecular classification in tree pollen allergy: Implications for diagnosis and therapy. *Int Arch Allergy Immunol* 2004; 135: 357–373.

57. Mari A. Importance of databases in experimental and clinical allergology. *Int Arch Allergy Immunol* 2005; 138: 88–96.

58. Valenta R, Kraft D. From allergen structure to new forms of allergen-specific immunotherapy. *Curr Opin Immunol* 2002; 14: 718–727.

59. Fernandes H, Michalska K, Sikorski M, Jaskolski M. Structural and functional aspects of PR-10 proteins. *FEBS J* 2013; 280: 1169–1199.

60. Hoffmann-Sommergruber K. Plant allergens and pathogenesis-related proteins. What do they have in common? *Int Arch Allergy Immunol* 2000; 122: 155–166.

61. Bufe A, Spangfort MD, Kahlert H, Schlaak M, Becker WM. The major birch pollen allergen, Bet v 1, shows ribonuclease activity. *Planta* 1996; 199: 413–415.

62. Ferreira F, Hirtenlehner K, Jilek A et al. Dissection of immunoglobulin E and T lymphocyte reactivity of isoforms of the major birch pollen allergen Bet v 1: Potential use of hypoallergenic isoforms for immunotherapy. *J Exp Med* 1996; 183: 599–609.

63. Laffer S, Hamdi S, Lupinek C et al. Molecular characterization of recombinant T1, a non-allergenic periwinkle (*Catharanthus roseus*) protein, with sequence similarity to the Bet v 1 plant allergen family. *Biochem J* 2003; 373: 261–269.

64. Spök A, Gaugitsch H, Laffer S et al. Suggestions for the assessment of the allergenic potential of genetically modified organisms. *Int Arch Allergy Immunol* 2005; 137: 167–180.

65. Hoffmann-Sommergruber K, O'Riordain G, Ahorn H et al. Molecular characterization of Dau c 1, the Bet v 1 homologous protein from carrot and its cross-reactivity with Bet v 1 and Api g 1. *Clin Exp Allergy* 1999; 840–847.

66. Valenta R, Ferreira F, Grote M et al. Identification of profilin as an actin-binding protein in higher plants. *J Biol Chem* 1993; 268: 22777–22781.

67. Batanero E, Villalba M, Ledesma A, Puente XSM, Rodriguez R. Ole e 3, an olive-tree allergen, belongs to a widespread family of pollen proteins. *Eur J Biochem* 1996; 241: 772–778.

68. Ledesma A, Villalba M, Rodriguez R. Cloning, expression and characterization of a novel four EF-hand Ca (2+)-binding protein from olive pollen with allergenic activity. *FEBS Lett* 2000; 466: 192–196.

69. van Ree R, Voitenko V, van Leeuwen WA, Aalberse RC. Profilin is a cross-reactive allergen in pollen and vegetable foods. *Int Arch Allergy Immunol* 1992; 98: 97–104.

70. Valenta R, Hayek B, Seiberler S et al. Calcium-binding allergens: From plants to man. *Int Arch Allergy Immunol* 1998; 117: 160–166.

71. Tinghino R, Barletta B, Palumbo S et al. Molecular characterization of a cross-reactive *Juniperus oxycedrus* pollen allergen, Jun o 2: A novel calcium-binding allergen. *J Allergy Clin Immunol* 1998; 101: 772–777.

72. Engel E, Richter K, Obermeyer G et al. Immunological and biological properties of Bet v 4, a novel birch pollen allergen with two EF-hand calcium-binding domains. *J Biol Chem* 1997; 272: 8630–8637.

73. Tinghino R, Twardosz A, Barletta B et al. Molecular, structural, and immunologic relationships between different families of recombinant calcium-binding pollen allergens. *J Allergy Clin Immunol* 2002; 109: 314–320.

74. Verdino P, Westritschnig K, Valenta R, Keller W. The cross-reactive calcium-binding pollen allergen, Phl p 7, reveals a novel dimer assembly. *EMBO J* 2002; 21: 5007–5016.

75. Rodriguez R, Villalba M, Batanero E et al. Olive pollen recombinant allergens: Value in diagnosis and immunotherapy. *J Investig Allergol Clin Immunol* 2007; 17(Suppl 1): 4–10.

76. Pascal M, Munoz-Cano R, Reina Z et al. Lipid transfer protein syndrome: Clinical pattern, cofactor effect and profile of molecular sensitization to plant-foods and pollens. *Clin Exp Allergy* 2012; 42: 1529–1539.

77. Salcedo G, Sanchez-Monge R, Diaz-Perales A, Garcia-Casado G, Barber D. Plant non-specific lipid transfer proteins as food and pollen allergens. *Clin Exp Allergy* 2004; 34: 1336–1341.

78. Tordesillas L, Sirvent S, Diaz-Perales A et al. Plant lipid transfer protein allergens: No cross-reactivity between those from foods and olive and Parietaria pollen. *Int Arch Allergy Immunol* 2011; 156: 291–296.

79. Hemmer W, Focke M, Wantke F, Götz M, Jarisch R, Jäger S. Ash (*Fraxinus excelsior*) pollen allergy in Central Europe: Specific role of pollen pan allergens and the major allergen of ash pollen, Fra e 1. *Allergy* 2000; 55: 923–930.

80. Batanero E, Villalba M, Lopez-Otin C, Rodriguez R. Isolation and characterization of an olive allergen-like protein from lilac pollen. Sequence analysis of three cDNA encoding protein isoforms. *Eur J Biochem* 1994; 221: 187–193.

81. Griffith IJ, Lussier A, Garman R, Koury R, Yeung H, Pollock J. The cDNA cloning of Cry j I, the major allergen of *Cryptomeria japonica* (Japanese cedar). *J Allergy Clin Immunol* 1993; 91: 339.

82. Rafnar T, Friffith IJ, Kuo M, Bond JF, Rogers BL, Klapper DG. Cloning of Amb a I (antigen E), the major allergen family of short ragweed pollen. *J Biol Chem* 1995; 95: 970–978.

83. Sakaguchi M, Inouye S, Taniai M, Ando S, Usui M, Matuhasi T. Identification of the second major allergen of Japanese cedar pollen. *Allergy* 1990; 45: 309–312.

84. Swoboda I, Grote M, Verdino P et al. Molecular characterization of polygalacturonases as grass pollen-specific marker allergens: Expulsion from pollen via submicronic respirable particles. *J Immunol* 2004; 172: 6490–6500.

85. Kawamoto S, Fujimura T, Nishida M et al. Molecular cloning and characterization of a new Japanese cedar pollen allergen homologous to plant isoflavone reductase family. *Clin Exp Allergy* 2002; 32: 1064–1070.

86. Ibrahim AR, Kawamoto S, Aki T et al. Molecular cloning and immunochemical characterization of a novel major Japanese cedar pollen allergen belonging to the aspartic protease family. *Int Arch Allergy Immunol* 2010; 152: 207–218.

87. Vrtala S, Grote M, Duchene M et al. Properties of tree and grass pollen allergens; reinvestigation of the linkage between solubility and allergenicity. *Int Arch Allergy Immunol* 1993; 102: 160–169.

88. Grote M, Vrtala S, Valenta R. Monitoring of two allergens, Bet v 1 and profilin, in dry and rehydrated birch pollen by immunogold electron microscopy and immunoblotting. *J Histochem Cytochem* 1993; 41: 745–750.

89. Valenta R, Kraft D. Recombinant allergen molecules: Tools to study effector cell activation. *Immunol Rev* 2001; 179: 119–127.

90. Niederberger V, Horak F, Vrtala S et al. Vaccination with genetically engineered allergens prevents progression of allergic disease. *Proc Natl Acad Sci USA* 2004; 101: 14677–14682.

91. Kazemi-Shirazi L, Niederberger V, Linhart B, Lidholm J, Kraft D, Valenta R. Recombinant marker allergens: Diagnostic gatekeepers for the treatment of allergy. *Int Arch Allergy Immunol* 2002; 127: 259–268.

92. Palomares O, Swoboda I, Villalba M et al. The major allergen of olive pollen Ole e 1 is a diagnostic marker for sensitization to Oleaceae. *Int Arch Allergy Immunol* 2006; 141: 110–118.

93. Bousquet J, Becker WM, Hejjaoui A et al. Differences in clinical and immunologic reactivity of patients allergic to grass pollens and to multiple-pollen species. II. Efficacy of a double-blind, placebo-controlled, specific immunotherapy with standardized extracts. *J Allergy Clin Immunol* 1991; 88: 43–53.

94. King EM, Filep S, Smith B et al. A multi-center ring trial of allergen analysis using fluorescent multiplex array technology. *J Immunol Methods* 2013; 387: 89–95.

95. Hiller R, Laffer S, Harwanegg C et al. Microarrayed allergen molecules: Diagnostic gatekeepers for allergy treatment. *FASEB J* 2002; 16: 414–416.

96. Kamemura N, Tada H, Shimojo N et al. Intrauterine sensitization of allergen-specific IgE analyzed by a highly sensitive new allergen microarray. *J Allergy Clin Immunol* 2012; 130: 113–121.e2.

97. Niederberger V, Niggemann B, Kraft D, Spitzauer S, Valenta R. Evolution of IgM, IgE and IgG (1–4) antibody responses in early childhood monitored with recombinant allergen components: Implications for class switch mechanisms. *Eur J Immunol* 2002; 32: 576–584.

98. Melioli G, Marcomini L, Agazzi A et al. The IgE repertoire in children and adolescents resolved at component level: A cross-sectional study. *Pediatr Allergy Immunol* 2012; 23: 433–440.

99. Lupinek C, Marth K, Niederberger V, Valenta R. Analysis of serum IgE reactivity profiles with microarrayed allergens indicates absence of *de novo* IgE sensitizations in adults. *J Allergy Clin Immunol* 2012; 130: 1418–1420.e4.

100. Mothes N, Heinzkill M, Drachenberg KJ et al. Allergen-specific immunotherapy with a monophosphoryl lipid A-adjuvanted vaccine: Reduced seasonally boosted IgE production and inhibition of basophil histamine release by therapy-induced blocking antibodies. *Clin Exp Allergy* 2003; 33: 1–11.

101. van Hage-Hamsten M, Valenta R. Specific immunotherapy—The induction of new IgE-specificities? *Allergy* 2002; 57: 375–378.

102. Sastre J, Landivar ME, Ruiz-Garcia M, Andregnette-Rosigno MV, Mahillo I. How molecular diagnosis can change allergen-specific immunotherapy prescription in a complex pollen area. *Allergy* 2012; 67: 709–711.

103. Valenta R, Niederberger V. Recombinant allergens for immunotherapy. *J Allergy Clin Immunol* 2007; 119: 826–830.

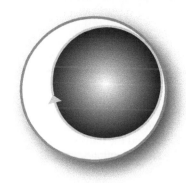

11 Grass pollen allergens

Robert E. Esch
Lenoir-Rhyne University

CONTENTS

11.1 INTRODUCTION

Grass pollen represents a major component of the airborne allergen load during the spring and summer months in most parts of the world. They are responsible for the symptoms in the majority of allergic rhinitis patients and can also trigger asthma. The diagnosis and treatment of grass pollen allergy with grass pollen allergen extracts/vaccines are nearly a hundred years old, and their use for immunotherapy is unequaled by any other allergen vaccine. Since Charles Blackley's initial investigations [1] during the 1870s that led to the identification of grass pollen as the cause of his own illness, the study of grass pollen allergens has continued to fascinate

botanists, allergists/immunologists, and more recently, molecular biologists. In this chapter, the grass family (Poaceae), their ecology, and pollen allergens are described. Special attention is given to the molecular characteristics of grass pollen allergens with regard to their cross-reactivities.

11.2 CLASSIFICATION AND TAXONOMY

The grasses belong to the family Poaceae (Gramineae) and are grouped with the sedges, rushes, and other monocots belonging to the order Poales. The family Poaceae is the fourth largest family of flowering plants, with more than 700 genera and 10,000 species. The family has historically been divided into two major groups, the pooids and the panicoids, based on the structure of the spikelet, the basic unit of inflorescence [2]. The pollen antigens of the pooids and panicoids are immunochemically distinct, as are other characteristics including leaf anatomy, embryo anatomy, and karyotype. These and additional morphologic, physiologic, biochemical, and cytologic comparisons have led to the recognition of up to nine subfamilies and as many as 60 tribes. Most agrostologists today have adopted a phylogenetic classification of grasses using DNA studies that is improving the understanding of the relationship among the grasses. A 2015 classification based on available molecular and morphologic evidence included 12,074 species and 771 genera placed into 12 subfamilies [3]. A taxonomic relationship of common allergenic grass genera is presented in Table 11.1. The classification system is based on that of Watson and Dallwitz [4] with modifications based on molecular studies [3]. Over 95% of the allergenically important grass species belong to the three subfamilies: Pooideae, Chloridoideae, and Panicoideae.

11.3 GRASS FLOWER AND POLLEN

Flowers of the allergenic grasses have obvious characteristics for wind pollination: reduced perianth, small and smooth pollen grains, a high pollen-ovule ratio, and feathery stigmas. The flower head, known as the inflorescence (Figure 11.1), is made up of spikelets that are highly modified branches consisting of a pair of bracts called glumes. They protect the immature spikelet and a rachilla, upon which are borne one to several florets. There is a wide variation in spikelet structure, size, and shape, and this is of great value in the identification and classification of grasses.

Pollination in grasses is of short duration, and it regularly occurs at a certain time of day or night. The breeding systems of the grasses are extremely varied. Some grasses are cleistogamous (self-fertile) or entomophilous (insect-pollinated) and therefore are not allergenically important. Polyploidy is common among the grasses, and hybridization is known to contribute to the adaptation and evolution of many grass groups, especially among the tribe Triticeae, the cereal grasses.

The pollen structure is unique to the family, but they are too uniform to be useful taxonomically (Figure 11.2). The pollen is more or less spheroidal to ovoid, 20–55 μm in diameter. The pollen grain wall consists of two layers, the exine (outer wall) and the intine (inner wall), and a single germination aperture or pore. Pollen antigens are stored in both the exine and intine walls, most being localized in the intine. A wide range of pollen antigens, including those that are allergenic, undoubtedly have a major role in the recognition of a suitable reproductive partner and thus may be expected to be species specific. Many grass pollen antigens also have wide taxonomic spans. Upon moistening, exine- and intine-associated components are released into the medium (Figure 11.3). The kinetics of antigen release from grass pollen suggest minimal structural compartmentalization as compared to pollen derived from other plant families [5].

Variations in a patient's allergic symptoms during the year depend, in part, on the pattern of seasonal pollen exposure. The expected seasonal levels of grass pollen for a given geographic locality in the United States can be obtained from various sources including the American Academy of Allergy, Asthma and Immunology's (AAAAI) Aerobiology Committee's Annual Pollen and Spore Reports [6]. Grass pollen are most abundant during the spring and summer months and account for a significant portion of the total pollen count during this time. Because whole pollen grains are too large to be respirable, it has been difficult to explain how grass pollen provoke asthmatic symptoms. Several possibilities, including the presence of submicronic particles possessing allergenic activity, are suggested as the trigger of asthma attacks. The existence of such particles is confirmed by specialized airborne sampling and immunochemical detection methods [7,8] and correlates to weather (e.g., thunderstorms) and epidemics of asthma [9]. A primary source of such particles is starch granules (0.6–2.5 μm in diameter) that are released from grass pollen upon contact with moisture. Other sources, including pollen fragments [10,11], orbicules [12], and allergen-adsorbed aerosols, remain to be investigated.

11.4 ECOLOGY AND HABITAT

Grasses occur on all continents, from desert to polar regions and in freshwater to marine habitats, and they account for about 25%–35% of the earth's vegetation. The steppes of Eurasia, the prairies and plains of central and western North America, and the pampa of Argentina represent the most extensive grassland areas of the temperate zone. Less extensive grasslands are found in the velds of South Africa and in Australia and New Zealand. Tropical and subtropical grasslands are located in central Africa and in central South America. In the grasslands, drought, fire, and grazing by animals are the major ecological challenges for a plant's survival. The growth tissue in most plants is located at the tip of the leaf or shoot; once clipped, it will not grow back. In contrast, the growth tissue in the grasses is located near the base of the leaf or the shoot, and growth continues even after the grass plant is cropped, burned, or grazed. This and other distinctive features including basal tillering, protection of the flower and fruit within the spikelet, a great diversity of habitats, alternative photosynthetic pathways, breeding systems, and dispersal mechanisms allow them to survive and dominate in areas where other plants cannot.

The distribution of grass species is delimited by conditions of soil, moisture, temperature, exposure, and altitude. Some species are restricted in habitat, being found only in salt marshes or alpine summits. Their geographic range, however, may be extensive. A species found on one mountain range also may be found at the same altitude on another mountain range. Other more tolerant species, such as *Festuca rubra,* can be found in meadows, bogs, marshes, and hills of North America, Eurasia, and North Africa.

Seventy percent of the world's farmland is planted in crop grasses with sugarcane (*Saccharum officinarum*), wheat (*Triticum aestivum*), rice (*Oryza sativa*), and maize (*Zea mays*) being the most widely cultivated. Bamboos are a critical part of the economy of many tropical areas because they contribute young shoots for food, fiber for paper, and stems for construction. Grasses are cultivated for livestock feed, erosion control, and as ornamentals. Many grasses introduced into cultivation escape and become established over wide areas. Their seeds may be carried long distances in cattle cars as impurities in the seed of crop plants and by birds and insects. Often, they may become troublesome weeds. The turfgrasses are planted to cover lawns, parks, roadsides, cemeteries, golf courses, and sporting fields. Considerable energy is spent maintaining turfgrasses in areas where they would normally not survive. The lawn industry, which accounts for more than a billion dollars of sales of seed, fertilizers, chemicals, paraphernalia, and services, supports the maintenance of grasses in regions that would otherwise be deciduous forests and deserts. Of

Table 11.1 Taxonomic relationships between common grasses

Subfamily	Tribe	Genus and species	Common name
Oryzoideae	Oryzeae	*Oryza sativa*	Cultivated rice
		Zizania aquatica	Wild rice
		Ehrharta erecta	Panic, veldt grass
Arundinoideae	Molinieae	*Phragmites communis*	Common reed
		Cortaderia	Pampas grass
Aristidoideae	Aristideae	*Aristida* spp.	Three-awns
Panicoideae	Paniceae	*Digitaria sanguinalis*	Crab grass
		Paspalum notatum	Bahia grass
		Panicum miliaceum	Common millet
		Panicum virgatum	Switch grass
		Stenotaphrum secundatum	Buffalo grass, Saint Augustine
	Andropogoneae	*Eremochloa ophiuroides*	Centipede grass
		Saccharum officinarum	Sugarcane
		Sorghum halepense	Johnson grass
		Sorghum sudanense	Sudan grass
		Zea mays	Corn, maize
Chloridoideae	Cynodonteae	*Bouteloua* spp.	Grama grass
		Buchloë dactyloides	Buffalo grass
		Chloris spp.	Finger grass
		Cynodon dactylon	Bermuda, couch grass
	Aeluropodeae	*Distichlis spicata*	Salt grass
		Eleusine indica	Goose grass
	Eragrostideae	*Eragrostis* spp.	Love grass
		Tridens flavus	Purpletop
Pooideae	Poeae	*Dactylis glomerata*	Orchard grass, cocksfoot
		Festuca elatior	Meadow fescue
		Lolium multiforme	Italian rye
		Lolium perenne	Perennial rye
		Poa compressa	Canada bluegrass
		Poa pratensis	Kentucky bluegrass (June grass)
		Agrostis alba	Redtop, bent grass
		Anthoxanthum odoratum	Sweet vernal
		Phalaris arundinacea	Reed canary
		Phalaris canariensis	Canary
		Koeleria cristata	June grass
		Avena sativa	Cultivated oat
		Holcus lanatus	Velvet grass
	Stipeae	*Stipa* spp.	Needle grass
	Bromeae	*Bromus* spp.	Brome grass, cheat grass
	Triticeae	*Agropyron repens*	Quack, wheat grass
		Elymus spp.	Wild rye
		Hordeum vulgare	Barley
		Secale cereale	Cultivated rye
		Triticum aestivum	Wheat

(a)

(b)

(c)

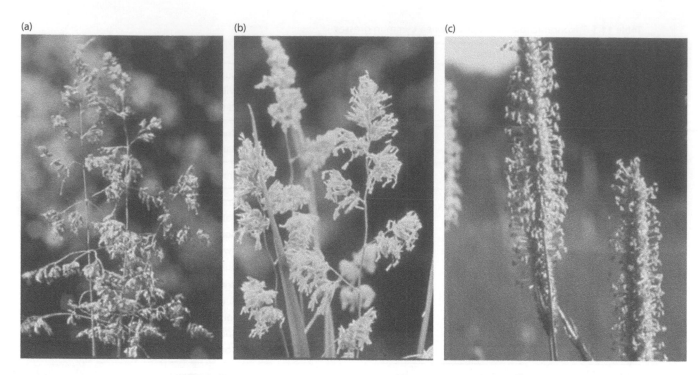

Figure 11.1 Grass inflorescence, the arrangement of the flowers on the stem, is illustrated by the three pooids: (a) Kentucky bluegrass with panicles, a compound inflorescence, bearing flowers along slender, spreading branches; (b) orchard grass with panicles bearing clusters of flowers near the ends of stout branches; and (c) timothy grass with spikes, or cylindrical clusters of flowers with no stalks.

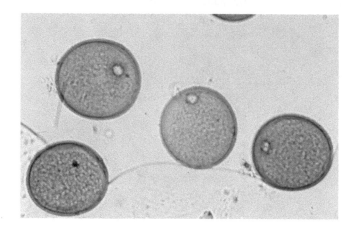

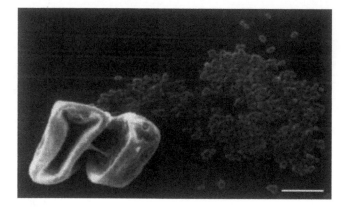

Figure 11.2 The pollen grains of the grasses are remarkably uniform. They are spheroidal, and in most allergenic species, they range from about 20 mm to less than 50 mm in diameter. The exine is thin and has a characteristically granular texture without adornments of any kind. The most distinctive characteristic is the single germ pore, consisting of a small aperture surrounded by a thickened rim of the exine and covered by a transparent membrane.

the hundreds of genera of grasses recognized, only a few are known to cause allergic disease. The major grass species responsible for inducing allergic symptoms are usually those that are cultivated and, therefore, prevalent where people live (Table 11.1).

11.4.1 Oryzoideae

The Oryzoideae belong to the BOP clade, one of two major lineages within the Poaceae. The group is represented by approximately 120

Figure 11.3 Ryegrass pollen ruptures after slight wetting with sedimenting mist droplets. The cytoplasmic debris from the ruptured pollen forms an aerosol of respirable particles that are loaded with allergens. (From Taylor PE et al. *J Allergy Clin Immunol* 2002; 109: 51–56.)

species in 20 genera. The Asian species *Oryza sativa* and the wild rice of North America, *Zizania aquatica,* are the best-known species. *O. sativa* is thought to have been first cultivated in Southeast Asia, India, and China between 8000 and 15,000 years ago [13] and today is grown worldwide, including in Asia, North America, South America, Europe, the Middle East, Africa, and Australia. Wild and cultivated species of rice are wind pollinated, but rice pollen is not considered to be highly allergenic.

11.4.2 Arundinoideae

The Arundinoideae are thought to represent the direct descendants of the earliest grasses that moved into the open savanna ecosystem.

This subfamily previously included a heterogeneous group of unrelated genera and tribes that did not fit into the other relatively well-defined subfamilies. Most of them are now moved to other subfamilies, e.g., Micrairoideae, Danthonioideae, and Aristidoideae. As a group, they are distributed mainly in the tropical and temperate regions of the southern hemisphere. Of the approximately 75 genera represented in the subfamilies, only about five are native in North America. This group includes the giant reed (*Arundo*) and the common reed (*Phragmites communis*), which are frequently planted to control erosion. The female plants of the South American pampas grass (*Cortaderia*), with their large, plumose panicles, are commonly grown as ornamentals in warmer regions of the world. The more than 250 species of *Aristida* (three-awns), having adapted to the semiarid habitats of South Africa and northern Mexico, are one of the more successful genera of this group.

11.4.3 Pooideae

The temperate zones are dominated by grasses belonging to the subfamily Pooideae, the largest subfamily of the Poaceae. The 14 major tribes, consisting of about 200 genera and 4200 species, are distributed across the world in relatively well-defined latitudinal belts, with the majority of genera found in the northern hemisphere. The center of pooid distribution is the Mediterranean area, and they have adapted to the cool and cold climates of the open steppe or meadows. They are virtually absent at low elevations in both humid and dry tropical areas. Species of *Bromus*, *Poa*, *Festuca*, and *Agropyron* can be found only at high altitudes in mountainous regions of tropical latitudes. The pooids account for approximately 70%–85% of the grasses in Canada and the northwestern United States, 40%–50% in the middle latitudes, and less 15%–25% in the southern United States. The cool-season turfgrasses representing this subfamily include the genera *Poa* (bluegrasses), *Agrostis* (bent grasses), *Festuca* (fescues), and *Lolium* (ryegrasses). These represent the major allergenic grass genera along with *Dactylis* (orchard grass), *Phleum* (timothy grass), and *Anthoxanthum odoratum* (vernal grass), which are common in meadows, pastures, and waste places. The subfamily also includes the important cultivated cereals *Triticum aestivum* (wheat), *Secale cereale* (rye), and *Hordeum vulgare* (barley).

11.4.4 Chloridoideae

The members of the subfamily Chloridoideae, represented by about 130 genera, are distributed throughout North American, African, and Australian continents. The chloridoids have adapted to a wide range of ecotypes, especially the warm and arid habitats, with high winter temperatures and summer or nonseasonal rainfall. Over 50% of the grass species in the southwestern United States are chloridoid, compared with less than 10% of the total in the northwestern United States. The centers of distribution are in the savannas of southern Africa and the open grasslands of Queensland. Their success in the warm, arid environments is due to the distinct physiologic and anatomical features of their C_4 dicarboxylic acid pathway of photosynthesis, referred to as the Kranz syndrome. The popular southern turfgrass *Cynodon dactylon* (Bermuda grass) is widespread throughout the warmer regions of the world and is a major allergenic species. Several species of *Bouteloua* (grama grass) and *Buchloë* (buffalo grass) are the outstanding range forage grasses and occur widely in the central and western United States.

11.4.5 Panicoideae

The subfamily Panicoideae dominates the humid, tropical to subtropical environments of the savannas of Indochina and Africa and the moist New World tropics, especially northeastern South America. Over 75% of the grasses in the Panama Canal Zone are panicoid, and 50% in the southern United States, but only about 5% of the species belong to this subfamily in the northwestern United States. The subfamily is the second largest subfamily of the Poaceae with 12 major tribes, 200 genera, and 3600 species. It includes the largest of the grass genera, *Panicum,* with about 600 species distributed throughout the warmer parts of the world and the cultivated species *Saccharum officinarum* (sugarcane) and *Sorghum vulgare* (sorghum). Allergenically important species include *Paspalum notatum* (Bahia grass), an important forage and erosion control grass in the Gulf Coast states of the United States, and *Sorghum halepense* (Johnson grass), a forage grass and frequently troublesome weed in the warmer and tropical regions of both hemispheres.

11.5 MOLECULAR CHARACTERISTICS AND CROSS-REACTIVITIES OF GRASS POLLEN ALLERGENS

Since the pioneering work of David Marsh and coworkers [14–16] with the perennial ryegrass group 1, 2, and 3 allergens during the 1960s and 1970s, a number of new allergens have been identified, isolated, and characterized. The International Union of Immunological Societies (IUIS) Allergen Nomenclature Sub-Committee's current official list identifies 13 grass pollen allergen groups (see Table 11.2). The techniques of molecular biology and protein chemistry have contributed to increased knowledge regarding the structure and possible function of grass pollen allergens. Murine monoclonal antibodies raised against specific allergens are used to define allergenically important and cross-reactive B-cell epitopes as well as to develop specific assays for their detection and quantitation in allergen extracts. Cloning of cDNA and nucleic acid sequencing accelerated the availability of primary structure data. Recombinant allergen fragments, mutated recombinant proteins, and synthetic peptides are useful to delineate determinants involved in B- and T-cell recognition. High-resolution protein separation and immunoblotting techniques and the application of proteomic approaches led to the identification of new allergen groups and the detection of microheterogeneity (isoallergens or isoforms) within the grass allergen groups.

11.5.1 Group 1 antigens

The grass group 1 allergens are acidic or basic glycoproteins with molecular weights (MW) in the 27–35 kDa range and exist in multiple isoallergenic forms or isoforms distinguished by their respective pIs and amino acid sequences. Histochemical examination localized this glycoprotein in the exine and cytoplasm of the pollen grain [17]. The protein can account for 6%–8% of the total extractable pollen protein and is detected in every grass species examined to date. The complete group 1 amino acid sequences from perennial ryegrass (Lol p 1), timothy grass (Phl p 1), velvet grass (Hol l 1), corn (Zea m 1), Johnson grass (Sor h 1), and Bermuda grass (Cyn d 1) are determined,

Table 11.2 Grass pollen allergen groups

Allergen group	Biochemical name/characteristics	IgE reactivity
1	β-Expansins; 27–35 kDa major grass pollen allergen produced by every grass species examined so far	>90%
2	Acidic protein (11 kDa); highly homologous to group 3 and C-terminal portion of group 1 allergens	35%–50%
3	Basic protein (11–14 kDa); highly homologous to group 2 and C-terminal portion of group 1 allergens	35%–70%
4	High-molecular-weight (50–60 kDa) basic glycoprotein; member of the berberine bridge enzyme family, plant pathogen response system	50%–75%
5/9	Heterogeneous proteins (27–35 kDa) found in pooid grass species; ribonuclease activity; associated with submicronic cytoplasmic starch particles	65%–85%
6	Phl p 6 (12–13 kDa), associated with submicronic cytoplasmic P-particles; homologous to internal Phl p 5 sequences	60%–70%
7	Calcium-binding protein (8–12 kDa) with novel dimer assembly; cross-reactive with birch (Bet v 4), olive (Ole e 3), and rape (Bra r 1) pollen allergens	10%–35%
10	Cytochrome c (11 kDa)	<20%
11	Glycoprotein (16–20 kDa); trypsin inhibitor; structurally similar to pollen allergens from olive tree (Ole e 1) and lamb's quarter (Che a 1)	35%
12	Profilin (13–14 kDa); possible association with pollen-plant food cross-sensitization	20%–50%
13	High-molecular-weight glycoprotein (45–60 kDa); polygalacturonase; highly susceptible to protease degradation; associated with submicronic cytoplasmic P-particles	30%–40%
22	Cyn d 22; Enolase (42 kDa)	Not determined
24	Cyn d 24; Pathogenesis-related protein (21 kDa)	65%

and the sequences of internal peptide fragments or N-terminal sequences from other several other grass species are reported [18–22]. The degree of glycosylation varies between 2% and 7%, and the monosaccharides fucose, arabinose, xylose, mannose, and N-acetylglucosamine detected. Up to eight glycoforms have been detected as part of glycoproteomic analyses of grass group 1 allergens [23,24]. The carbohydrate moiety does not appear to play an important role in the allergenicity of the group 1 allergens although IgE antibodies toward the carbohydrate structures have been detected in a select group of subjects [25–26].

The group 1 allergens belong to a subfamily of structurally related proteins called β-expansins, which are cell-wall-loosening proteins. Their activity shows specificity to grass cell walls, suggesting that they act on the matrix polymers specific to grasses, e.g., glucuronoarabinoxylan or mixed-linked 1,3: 1:4-β-glucan [27]. The expansin activity of grass group 1 allergens is attributed to a papain-like proteinase activity [28–30], but this proposed mechanism of action has been challenged [31]. Subsequently, the proteinase activity detected in the recombinant Phl p 1 has been attributed to contaminating proteinases derived from the *Pichia pastoris* expression system [32]; and the proteinase activity associated with native Phl p 1 preparations to a typsin-like protease that coelutes with Phl p 1 during conventional chromatographic purification [33]. The characteristics of Zea m 1 suggest a specialized role of β-expansins in pollen function [34–35]. A function of group 1 allergens is to facilitate growth of the pollen tube and penetration of the ovule to achieve fertilization and, thus, breeding success under conditions of pollen competition [36]. Evidence supports a nonenzymatic mechanism of wall loosening by weakening the middle lamella and thereby promoting the penetration of the pollen tube through the stigma and style [37]. Structural modeling of the presumed cellulose-binding domain of Lol p 1 suggests a close structural relationship between its cellulose-binding and allergenic properties [38].

Allergens homologous to Lol p 1 are detected in pollen extracts from all grass species examined to date; in each case, more than 90% of allergic subjects are highly reactive to the respective group 1 allergens. Patient sensitivity to the group 1 allergens correlates with their sensitivity to the whole pollen extract as measured by both skin test and histamine release assays. Extensive immunologic cross-reactivity among the group 1 allergens from taxonomically related grasses is also firmly established. For these reasons, a potency assay based on the group 1 content of grass pollen extracts has been proposed as an approach to grass pollen allergen extract standardization [39].

Two important cross-reactive allergenic determinants or sites are localized on the pooid grass group 1 allergen molecule with the aid of murine monoclonal antibodies selected for their ability to inhibit human IgE binding to grass group 1 allergens. One site is localized on a 28-mer located at the C-terminus [40] (amino acid residues 213–240) of the molecule and the second site within amino acid residues 23–35 [41]. Continuous B-cell epitopes on Phl p 1 that represent five major IgE-reactive regions of the allergen molecule have been identified by a gene fragmentation approach. The IgE-binding fragments, generated from a random fragment expression library of Phl p 1 [42] and Hol l 1 [21] cDNA, represent regions localized at C-terminus, N-terminus, and in the center of the allergen sequence. The C-terminal portion of the molecule accounts for the majority of the IgE-binding sites of Phl p 1, and they cluster in a sterically oriented manner that may facilitate the cross-linking of effector cell-bound IgE antibodies [43]. The importance of correct folding and a stable secondary structure for its allergenic activity is demonstrated by the difficulty to express active, soluble grass group 1 allergens as recombinant molecules. This is not unexpected considering that group 1 proteins possess seven cysteine residues and three disulfide bridges. The replacement of a single cysteine residue at position 77 of Lol p 1 with a serine residue using site-directed mutagenesis is sufficient to reduce the IgE-binding activity by more than 60% [44]. Insect-cell expressed Phl p 1 [45] and purified natural Dac g 1 [46] possess superior allergenic activity as compared to recombinant molecules expressed in bacteria. A recombinant variant of Phl p 1, introducing a cysteine residue to promote the formation of an additional disulfide bridge, yields a product that is stable, soluble, and comparable in activity to native Phl p 1 [47]. A conformational epitope on the N-terminal region of the Phl p 1, located at the interface region of the homodimeric protein, was elucidated using naturally occurring anti-idiotypic antibodies that mimic the Phl p 1 epitope [48]. One of the complementarity-determining regions (CDRs) from each of the four clones selected matches the highly conserved N-terminal epitope defined by monoclonal antibodies in the earlier studies. Other CDRs are mapped to more central regions of the molecule.

The allergenic epitopes of the group 1 allergen of Bermuda grass (Cyn d 1) and of Bahia grass (Pas n 1) appear to be different from those defined for the pooid grasses [49,50] in spite of a 65%–75% sequence homology. Nonconservative amino acid substitutions in allergenically important regions may explain the lack of cross-reactivity between Cyn d 1 and the other grass group 1 allergens [20,51]. Four major linear IgE-binding epitopes were mapped using synthetic peptides spanning the length of the Cyn d 1 molecule. These epitopes correspond to amino acid residues 70–79, 101–110, 159–167, and 172–181 and are all located on the surface of the simulated Cyn d 1 molecule. Three of them are also major epitopes for both IgE and IgG [52].

A major human T-cell determinant is localized within amino acid residues 191–210 utilizing overlapping peptides spanning the entire Lol p 1 molecule [18]. Subsequent studies revealed multiple T-cell determinants distributed throughout the molecule including cross-reactive T-cell epitopes shared with grass group 2, group 3, and group 5 allergens [53–57]. An immunodominant epitope within residues 126–134 was identified in a study employing class II MHC tetramers in grass pollen-allergic individuals [58]. DR*0401 tetramers loaded with this peptide consistently detect CD4+ T cells expressing a Th2 cytokine profile in allergic but not nonallergic subjects. Nonallergic subjects exhibit very low frequency of such tetramer-specific cells even after allergen stimulation and cell expansion, suggesting a fundamental difference in T-cell responses to group 1 allergens in allergic and nonallergic individuals. Unique and cross-reactive T-cell determinants were mapped using Bahia grass Pas n 1 peptide-specific T-cell clones isolated from allergic donors [59]. A majority (15 of 18) of the donors responded to one of more of three immunodominant epitopes.

11.5.2 Group 2 antigens

The grass group 2 allergens are acidic proteins (MW = 11,000) toward which 35%–50% of grass-allergic subjects are sensitive. The perennial ryegrass group 2 antigens exist in at least two immunochemically indistinguishable isoforms, Lol p 2A (pI = 5.0) and Lol P 2B (pI = 5.1–5.3). The complete primary structure of Lol p 2A was determined by peptide sequencing of the purified protein and found to contain 97 amino acids without evidence of glycosylation sites [57]. The complete primary structures of Lol p 2,

Dac g 2, and Phl p 2 were deduced from the nucleotide sequence of the cDNA encoding the protein and found to be homologous to the Lol p 2 sequence [60–62].

Mapping of IgE-reactive epitopes was attempted using a model based on the solution structure of Phl p 2 and recombinant Phl p 2 fragments spanning the entire molecule [63]. Only relatively long fragments representing the N-terminal and C-terminal regions of the molecule show strong IgE reactivity. No reactivity can be detected when synthetic dodecapeptides spanning the complete Ph1 p 2 sequence are evaluated. These results indicate that grass group 2 IgE epitopes are highly conformation dependent. The three-dimensional structure of a complex between Phl p 2 and a Phl p 2-specific Fab derived from an IgE antibody was determined by x-ray crystallography [64]. The IgE-binding epitope is composed of nine residues grouped in four sequentially distant segments of the allergen molecule.

The amino acid sequences of group 2 and 3 allergens are also highly homologous.

Lol p 2A and Lol p 3 possess 59% identical amino acids, and this percentage increases to 67% when similar amino acids are equated. A similar homology exists for Dac g 2 and Dac g 3 with 66% sequence identity and 79% sequence similarity. This sequence homology translates to a high degree of cross-reactivity at the B- and T-cell levels [53,65]. The grass group 2 and group 3 allergens also show sequence similarity with the C-terminal portion of the group 1 allergens. Only three residues are conserved based on the alignment of the Phl p 2 epitope sequence with the nine homologous sequences of the C-terminal portion of the group 1 allergens. This explains the lack of any significant cross-reactivity between groups 2 and 3 with group 1. The three allergen groups may share a common origin, with groups 2 and 3 being generated by partial gene duplication of the C-terminal portion of group 1 [66,67].

11.5.3 Group 3 antigens

The grass group 3 allergens are basic proteins (MW = 11–14 kDa, pI = 8.9–9.4) with a reported frequency of sensitization of 35%–70% among grass pollen allergic subjects. The group 3 allergens from perennial ryegrass, orchard grass, and timothy grass pollen have been isolated and characterized at the molecular level [67–69]. The complete primary structures of Lol p 3 and Dac g 3 reveal a 92.6% similarity and 84.2% identity, and the mature proteins lack cysteine and show no evidence of glycosylation. In spite of this high degree of homology, computer analyses detected differences in their predicted secondary structure and antigenic sites.

The three-dimensional structure of Phl p 3 was solved by x-ray crystallography and compared to the corresponding structures of group 1 and 2 grass pollen allergens [70]. Phl p 3 is a globular β-sandwich protein with structural similarity to Phl p 2 and the C-terminal domain of Phl p 1, consistent with the amino acid sequence data available for the three allergens. Epitope predictions using protein modeling software (SPADE) and immunologic cross-reactivity data help explain the structural basis of the observed cross-reactivity between group 3 and 2 allergens and not with group 1 allergens.

11.5.4 Group 4 antigens

The grass group 4 allergens are high-molecular-weight basic glycoproteins (MW = 50–60 kDa, pI = 8.6–10.4) with sequence similarity to the berberine bridge enzymes (BBEs), a member of a flavoprotein oxidoreductase superfamily. The initial report by Marsh found only a 20% sensitization rate toward Lol p 4 among grass allergic subjects, but other studies suggest that group 4 allergens from timothygrass, orchard grass, and Bermuda grass may be responsible for sensitization rates of 50%–75%. The complete primary structure of group 4 allergens was elucidated in 2005–2006 [71,72]. Based on the reported mass determination of native Phl p 4 and that deduced from the sequence, approximately 10% of its total mass appears to be made up of carbohydrate. Two potential N-glycosylation sites can be identified from the Phl p 4 sequence. A flavin-binding domain, first identified in BG60, the basic 60 kD allergen from Bermuda grass pollen, is consistent with other proteins of the BBE family thought to be involved in the plant pathogen response system [73]. Using monoclonal antibodies against Dac g 4, related proteins from various pooid and chlorodoid grass species can be detected on sodium dodecyl sulfate polyacrylamide gel electrophoresis (SDS-PAGE) immunoblots. Enzyme-linked immunosorbent assay (ELISA) inhibition experiments, however, reveal cross-reactivity only among the pooid grasses [74]. Allergenic determinants are localized on two Lol p 4 peptide fragments (MW = 17.4 and 11.0 kDa) by CNBr cleavage of the purified protein. Fragmentation of these Lol p 4 fragments with trypsin or chymotrypsin destroys their IgE-binding capacity, hampering further resolution and delineation of the allergenic sites [75]. A decapeptide sequence of Ph1 p 4 shows significant sequence similarity to peptides from the major allergen family of ragweed pollen, Amb a 1 and Amb a 2 [76]. Ph1 p 4 specific monoclonal antibody and human IgE-antibody binding can be inhibited by preadsorption with Amb a 1. Rabbit and human antibodies directed toward Ph1 p 4 react with allergens present in various tree and weed pollen as well as vegetables and fruits [77,78]. Together, these findings suggest the possibility of common IgE-binding epitopes on grass group 4 allergens and various unrelated pollen and plant foods. The three-dimensional structure of Phl p 4 was determined by x-ray crystallography [79]. The general structure is consistent with oxireductases with bicovalently attached FAD cofactor. Phl p 4 reacts as a dehydrogenase when 2,6-dichlorophenolindophenol is added as the electron acceptor, catalyzing dehydrogenation of glucose.

Studies with the group 4 allergen from Bermuda grass [80] suggest that the carbohydrate moiety, accounting for about 7.5% of the mass, may be important allergenic determinants of the molecule. Periodate oxidation reduces the IgE-binding activity of the allergen by approximately 50%. The predominant N-linked oligosaccharides of the molecule are unique among plant glycoproteins in that they possess a-(1,3)-linked fucose without any xylose [81]. Nine decapeptides corresponding to about 90% of the primary structure of Cyn d 4 were synthesized and tested negative for IgE reactivity with allergic sera positive to the whole molecule. This suggests that the IgE epitopes of Cyn d 4 are predominantly conformational in nature [82]. Huang et al. analyzed the crystal structure of Cyn d 4 in parallel with the modeled group 4 allergen structures from pooid grasses to predict possible cross-reactive and species-specific conformation epitopes. Five conserved clusters (Aps12-Lys19-Arg76-His77, Arg24-Lys110-Lys112, Arg195-Lys196-Glu200, Lys321-Lys335-Phe405, and Lys460-Glu464-Glu472-Arg473) were identified as putative cross-reactive epitopes. Of interest is a unique loop containing three consecutive acidic residues (Glu323-Asp324-Asp325) that could be an epitope specific to the pooid group 4 allergens.

11.5.5 Group 5 antigens (includes group 9 antigens)

The group 5 allergens are a heterogeneous group of proteins with multiple isoforms varying in pIs and primary sequences [83–86]. Comparison of the deduced amino acid sequences of the three group 5 allergens shows a high degree of homology (80%–90%), consistent with the high degree of cross-reactivity observed. Their having similar molecular weights to the group 1 allergens (27–35 kDa for the group 1 and 27–38 kDa for group 5) probably explains why traditional protein fractionation methods based on molecular size failed to establish the identity of the group 5 allergens. The group 5 allergens, together with the group 1 allergens, account for the majority of the IgE-binding reactivity of most grass-allergic sera. In contrast to the group 1 allergens, group 5 allergens have been identified only among the subfamily Pooideae, and polyclonal antibodies raised against group 5 allergens fail to detect cross-reactive antigens outside of the subfamily. Furthermore, Northern analysis with Poa p V probes could only identify homologous transcripts among the pooids [87]. Thus, it appears that group 5 allergens are restricted to a single subfamily of grasses, and if similar proteins are produced by the panicoid, chloridoid, and arundinoid grasses, they are immunochemically and genetically unique.

By using recombinant and synthetic allergen fragments, or site-directed mutagenesis, investigators have localized IgE-binding determinants in the central and C-terminal regions of the Lol p 5 molecule [88,89] to both the N-terminal and C-terminal ends of Ph1 p 5 [90–93) and predominantly on a C-terminal fragment of Poa p 5 (Poa p 9) [94]. At least four continuous and five discontinuous IgE-binding sites are localized on the group 5 allergen from velvet grass pollen (Hol l 5), and each are differentially recognized by individual patient IgE antibodies [95]. Conformational IgE epitopes of Phl p 5 were mapped using grass allergic patient sera and a random peptide-phage display library [96]. Peptide alignment with the solvent-accessible amino acids reveals at least three sequence sections on Phl p 5a. Taken together, these studies suggest either an extremely heterogeneous human B-cell response to group 5 allergens or a marked difference in the epitope structures of group 5 proteins derived from the different grass species. Nevertheless, a few point mutations in the group 5 sequence can yield mutants with significantly reduced allergenic activity [97,98]. In one study, a single deletion (amino acid residues 175–198) in the Phl p 5 sequence causes a large reduction in IgE reactivity in a subset of allergic sera, and a double deletion (amino acid residues 175–198 and 94–113) further reduces IgE reactivity in all sera tested. The hypoallergenic double mutant retains its T-cell reactivity, an important attribute for immunotherapy. A similar approach studied the effect of single and multiple mutations in the eight proline residues of the molecule. One of the mutated Phl p 5 molecules with five proline deletions and a substitution of proline 211 to leucine yielded a monomeric, soluble protein with diminished IgE reactivity and strong T-cell reactivity [99].

A characteristic of the group 5 allergens is their association with intracellular starch granules within the pollen grain. The cDNA sequence of Lol p 5 revealed the flanking transit peptide sequences typical of chloroplast-targeted proteins; thus, it was proposed that the Lol p 5 is synthesized as a preallergen in the cytosol and transported to the amyloplast for posttranslational modification [100]. This model may explain the existence of the multiple isoforms and the molecular weight heterogeneity of group

5 allergens isolated from pollen extracts. The size of the starch granules (0.6–2.5 μm in diameter) and their sudden appearance in air samples following rainfall are suggestive of a role in triggering asthmatic reactions. Phl p 5 possesses ribonuclease activity, and the homologous group 5 allergens from the other grass species may be expected to possess this activity as well [101]. It is interesting to speculate on the role of ribonuclease activity at the level of pollen-stigma interaction: Its release during hydration and stigma contact might facilitate the reproductive responses of the stigma.

T-cell determinants are localized on Lol p 5 and Phl p 5 allergens by generating specific T-cell lines or clones and measuring proliferative responses to a series of overlapping group 5 synthetic peptides spanning the entire sequence of the molecule [55,56,102,103]. T-cell determinates are spread throughout the allergen molecule. Regions of high reactivity are found in specific patients but differ among them. Isoform-specific T-cell epitopes also are detected with Phl p 5a and Phl p 5b fragments. Histocompatibility leukocyte antigen (HLA)-DR ligand prediction software (TEPITOPE) identified DR ligands within the Lol p 5a sequence that proved to be novel T-cell epitopes [104]. Most of these ligands are clustered at the C-terminal part of a repeated 32-amino acid sequence motif, which occupies about 50% of the Lol p 5 sequence, A similar structural organization is shared by other group 5 allergens, suggesting that this repeated motif may be a molecular signature of group 5 allergens. The observed diversity of the human T-cell response and specificity shown by individual patient responses suggest that immunotherapy with allergen peptides is not feasible.

The recognition of IgE and T-cell epitopes of Phl p5 was dissected using seven peptides (31–38 amino acids in length) that spanned the entire molecule [105]. The peptides were used to generate peptide-specific IgG antibodies for IgE-blocking studies as well as to evaluate lymphocyte proliferation and cytokine responses in peripheral blood mononuclear cells from grass pollen-allergic subjects. Although none of the peptides examined show detectable IgE-reactivity in sera from 51 patients with grass pollen allergy, antibodies directed toward those peptides defining the N-terminal and C-terminal domains of Phl p 5 show significant IgE-blocking activity. In contrast, the peptides inducing the IgE-blocking antibodies are relatively ineffective in inducing lymphocyte proliferation and cytokine responses. The apparent spatial dissociation of IgE and T-cell epitopes of Phl p 5 may allow for immunotherapeutic strategies based on selective targeting of IgE and/or T-cell responses.

11.5.6 Group 6 antigens

The group 6 allergens from timothy grass pollen, Phl p 6, are polypeptides (MW = 12–13 kDa, pI = 5.2–5.5) toward which a majority of timothy grass pollen-sensitive subjects react [106,107]. The group 6 allergens thus far have been detected only in timothy pollen extracts. Phl p 6 is a pollen-specific protein localized on the polysaccharide-containing wall-precursor bodies or P-particles [88]. The amino acid sequence deduced from the cDNA sequence revealed no cysteines and one potential glycosylation site, although no carbohydrate structures were detected [107]. The N-terminal sequence of Phl p 6 is highly homologous to internal Phl p 5 sequences, and epitope mapping studies with rPhl p 6 fragments indicate that the N-terminus of the molecule is required for IgE recognition. Sequence analysis of a cDNA encoding the complete Phl p 6 allergen provides evidence for an independent gene family

arising from gene duplication. Comparison of the complete Phl p 6 and Phl p 5 sequences shows only a 55%–60% match, even though the N- and C- termini of Phl p 6 demonstrate about a 95% similarity to the internal Phl p 5 protein sequence. Both unique and shared epitopes have been identified on Phl p 5 and 6 allergens using antibodies raised against Phl p 5 and Phl p 6, and allergenic cross-reactivity has been detected by immunoadsorption studies [108]. Epitope mapping studies with rPhl p 6 fragments indicate that the N-terminus of the molecule is required for IgE recognition.

11.5.7 Group 7 antigens

The group 7 allergens (MW = 8–12 kDa) from Bermuda (Cyn d 7) and timothy grass pollen (Phl p 7) were identified and isolated from a cDNA expression library using serum IgE from grass-allergic individuals [109,110]. The group 7 allergens belong to a family of Ca^{2+}-binding proteins, characterized by the presence of two potential EF-hand calcium-binding domains [111]. Approximately 35% of grass pollen-allergic subjects possess IgE antibodies toward the recombinant Cyn d 7. In addition, approximately 10% of pollen-allergic patients possess IgE antibodies toward group 7 homologous allergens present in pollen of monocotyledonic and dicotyledonic plants. The deduced amino acid sequence of this protein shows significant sequence similarity with a variety of Ca^{2+}-binding proteins, including the pollen allergens Bet v 4 from birch, Aln g 4 from alder, Ole e 3 from olive, Bra r 1 from oilseed rape, and calmodulin from the fungus *Fusarium oxysporum*. A three-dimensional model of Phl p 7 with two calcium-binding domains (FF-hands) shows a novel dimer assembly adopting a barrel-like structure with an extended hydrophobic cavity providing a ligand-binding site [112]. Structural similarities with other pollen allergens with two EF-hands (Che a 3, Bet v 4, Aln g 4, Ole e 3, Cyn d 7, and Bra r 1), three EF-hands (Bet v 3), and four EF-hands (Jun o 4 and Ole e 8) are also suggested by molecular modeling studies [113]. Cross-reactivity with Bet v 4 is established, and a cross-reactive allergenic epitope was localized to the region representing the Ca^{2+}-binding domain II of the molecule, which shows an 83.3% amino acid sequence identity between Bet v 4 and Cyn d 7. The Cyn d 7 clone hybridizes to transcripts in 13 other grass pollen using RNA gel blot analysis, suggesting that homologous proteins with similar allergenic activity may be present in other grass pollen. In addition, pollen extracts derived from 16 unrelated genera exhibited cross-reactivity with Aln g 4 and Jun o 4, suggesting that calcium-binding allergens are widely distributed in pollen from various plants. Disruption of the structure essential for calcium binding reduces the allergenic activity of Phl p 7 without affecting its ability to induce blocking antibodies [114]. Phl p 7, unlike Bet v 4 and all the other EF-hand proteins, appears to occur exclusively as a domain-swapped dimer [115]. A comparison of the three-dimensional structures of Phl p 7, Che a 3, and Bet v 4 shows essentially identical structural folds despite the observation that Che a 3 and Phl p 7 exist as a dimer and Bet v 4 a monomer [116]. Sequence alignments identified highly conserved amino acids at four clusters of putative cross-reactive epitopes on the surface of the molecules explaining the IgE cross-reactivities between weed, grass, and tree pollen allergens.

11.5.8 Group 10 antigens (cytochrome c)

Cytochrome c (MW = 11 kDa, pI = 10) from timothy grass, perennial ryegrass, and Bermuda grass pollen are allergenic in humans.

Their importance as allergens based on sensitization rates is not thoroughly documented. This allergen group has been proposed as a model system for studying the molecular basis of cross-reactivity because a vast knowledge base exists for cytochrome structure and function [117].

11.5.9 Group 11 antigens

The group 11 allergens are a group of glycoproteins (MW = 16–20 kDa, pI = 5.0–6.0) structurally similar to the Kunitz soybean trypsin inhibitor but lack the active site and appear not to possess inhibitory activity. Proteins that are homologous to Lol p 11 occur in other grass and nongrass pollen, most notably Ole e 1, the major allergen of olive tree pollen [118–120]. This allergen may have eluded detection in conventional immunoblotting techniques using SDS-PAGE under reducing conditions because there are three potential disulfide bridges present that may be required for maintaining the IgE-binding peptide epitopes.

Among individuals with IgE antibodies against grass pollen, approximately 65% possess IgE antibodies toward Lol p 11, and of these, about 35% possess IgE antibodies against the carbohydrate moiety. Monosaccharide analysis suggests that N-glycan (mannose-type) or arabinoxylan substitutions may represent the IgE-binding carbohydrate group(s). The N-glycan structures appear to be involved in IgE binding, as is bee venom phospholipase A_2, an allergen with known N-glycan IgE-binding epitopes, and a potential inhibitor of IgE binding to Lol p 11. The recombinant form of Ph1 p 11, expressed as a soluble fusion protein in *Escherichia coli*, induces histamine release from basophils and skin reactivity in grass pollen–sensitized subjects. The unglycosylated rPhl p 11 shows a reduced prevalence of IgE reactivity among grass pollen–positive sera and little or no cross-reactivity with other members of this allergen family, suggesting its diagnostic utility in identifying the primary sensitizer in allergic individuals.

11.5.10 Group 12 antigens (profilin)

Profilin, purified from grass pollen, is probably an important allergen because antiprofilin IgE antibodies can be detected in 20%–50% of grass-sensitive subjects [121]. Because profilin is a highly conserved protein present in all organisms, the potential role of this allergen as a "panallergen" has been proposed [122]. The cDNA sequences of timothy grass, Bermuda grass, and birch *(Betula verrucosa)* pollen encoding for the respective profilins are 80% homologous, but profilins from unrelated sources are much more variable and typically are less than 50% homologous [123,124]. Allergic patients with multiple pollen and plant-derived food sensitizations frequently possess IgE antibodies toward profilin. Evidence for both cross-reactive and unique IgE-binding epitopes exists, and potential conformational epitopes have been predicted by structural analyses [125]. However, the clinical relevance of the cross-reacting or species-specific IgE antibodies cannot be established [126]. Alvarado et al. investigated the potential role of profilin as a major respiratory allergen leading to clinically significant profilin-induced food allergies in patients from a geographic area with prolonged grass pollen seasons and relatively high grass pollen counts [127]. A patient's sensitivity in provocation tests to foods standardized on the basis of profilin content is associated not only with multiple grass pollen allergen sensitivities and increased antiprofilin IgE, but

with decreased sIgG4/sIgE ratios to Phl p 2 and Phl p 5. Additional studies in populations with severe profilin-mediated food reactions with concomitant grass pollen allergies may shed light on the clinical importance of cross-reactivity with this panallergen. T-cell responses to Phl p 12 were studied in grass-allergic subjects sensitized to profilin, and three immunodominant epitopes are identified within amino acid residues 22–51, 62–81, and 92–121 [128]. The T-cell epitopes include regions that are highly conserved (amino acid residues 92–121) among profilins from other allergen sources as well as those that are not highly conserved (amino acid residues 22–51; 62–81). The T-cell responses to profilins from olive, birch, apple, and date palm correspond to levels of sequence homology.

11.5.11 Group 13 antigens

The group 13 allergens (MW = 50–60 kDa, pI = 6.0–7.5) have similar molecular weights to the grass group 4 allergens and are difficult to distinguish by one-dimensional SDS-PAGE. This and the finding that group 13 allergens are highly susceptible to proteolytic degradation may explain why they were not identified until about 2000. Approximately 42%–75% of grass-sensitive subjects possess IgE antibodies to the group 13 allergens, and allergenic proteins homologous to the Ph1 p 13 are detected in all grass pollen extracts examined to date. The deduced amino acid sequence from the cloned cDNA of Ph1 p 13, consisting of 394 residues, indicates homology with pollen-specific polygalacturonases [129,130] and Pas n 13 from Bahia grass pollen [131]. IgE-binding epitopes are mapped to the less-conserved regions of the C-terminus of the molecule and cross-reactivity restricted to polygalacturonases from grass pollen. The carbohydrate moiety of Phl p 13 cross-links IgE receptors on basophils and induces mediator release [25]. This is attributed to the presence of multiple N-glycan epitopes on the molecule. In contrast, Phl p 1, which has at most a single N-glycosylation site, bound IgE antibodies but did not cause mediator release. Phl p 13 is localized on submicronic particles released from hydrated timothy pollen grains and, like Phl p 5, may be considered as environmental markers for grass pollen exposure [132,133].

11.5.12 Group 22 and 24 antigens

The group 22 (enolase) and group 24 (PR-1) antigens were identified in Bermuda grass pollen extract using a proteomic approach combining two-dimensional electrophoretic separations, immunoblotting, matrix-assisted laser desorption/ionization-mass spectrometry (MALDI-MS), liquid chromatography-mass spectrometry/mass spectrometry (LC-MS/MS), and bioinformatics to identify these novel pollen allergens [134]. Both proteins are purified from whole Bermuda grass pollen extracts and possess allergenic activity based on histamine release or skin test responses in allergic patients. Enolase is an IgE-binding protein in a variety of environmental sources including pollen, fungi, cockroach, and seafoods. Cyn d 24 is a glycoprotein (MW = 19–21 kDa, pI = 5.9) structurally similar to the plant pathogenesis-related proteins (PR-1). Sequence identity ranges from 45% to 50% with PR-1 s from barley, wheat, maize, and rice [135]. The carbohydrate moiety, which makes up about 6% of the total weight of the glycoprotein, resembles the structure possessed by Cyn d 4 (BG60): An L-fucose a-(1,3)-linked to an N-acetyl glucosamine without xylose linked to the branching mannose. As with Cyn d 4, there is evidence that the carbohydrate moiety is involved with IgE binding.

11.5.13 Novel IgE-binding antigens

Increasingly more sensitive analyses of complex allergen sources are being employed for standardizing allergen extracts [136,23]. Proteomic studies incorporating combinations of two-dimensional immunoelectrophoresis, mass spectrometry, and sophisticated computer software not only allow for the quantitation of specific isoforms of known allergens but also permit identification of the presence of additional IgE-reactive components in grass pollen. For example, a shotgun proteomic analysis of ryegrass pollen extract and immunoblotting pollen proteins separated by two-dimensional electrophoresis revealed the presence of novel IgE-reactive proteins that might be involved in polysensitization [137]. Cyclophilin (peptidyl-prolyl *cis-trans* isomerase), fructosyltransferase, an enzyme with invertase activity and multiple putative N-glycosylation sites, and legumin-like protein belonging to the Cupin superfamily were identified as potential allergens. Another proteomic study of timothy grass pollen allergens isolated from pollen and pollen cytoplasmic granules (PCGs) identified up to six novel IgE-binding proteins including ascorbate reductase and triosephosphate isomerase in pollen and PCGs; a ß-glucosidase in pollen only; and cinnamyl alcohol dehydrogenase, legumin-like protein, and UDP-glucose pyrophosphorylase in PCGs only [138]. The clinical significance of these IgE-reactive proteins is yet to be established.

Campbell et al. [139] performed a comprehensive transcriptome, proteome, and allergome analysis of Johnson grass pollen to reveal qualitative differences between the homologous allergenic components derived from other grass species. They established Sor h 1 and 13 as clinically important allergens and identified multiple cDNA transcripts, peptide spectra, belonging to groups 1, 2, 4, 7, 11, 12, 13, 22, 23, 24, and 25. Although IgE reactivity is not established for all of the identified putative allergens, the information generated will be crucial in elucidating the molecular differences between homologous allergens derived from different grass taxa.

Novel IgE-binding proteins localized to the pollen extracellular coat matrix are present in Bermuda grass pollen using an immunoproteomics approach. A cysteine protease (23 kDa) and an endoxylanase (30 kDa) were recovered from pollen grains by cyclohexane extraction, separated electrophoretically, and analyzed by IgE immunoblotting and proteomics [140]. A significant percentage (25%–57%) of grass pollen allergic subjects possess IgE reactivity toward these two proteins, suggesting that they may be clinically important Bermuda grass pollen allergens. Peptide sequencing of IgE-reactive bands from pollen coat fractions derived from timothy grass and Johnson grass pollen confirm the presence of homologous cysteine proteases. Additionally, the purified cysteine protease induces epithelial cell detachment and disruption of the integrity of airway epithelial cells.

PCGs released by the grass pollen grain are recognized as a source of specific allergens playing a role in triggering asthma symptoms [100,106,132,133]. A comprehensive proteomic analysis was conducted to characterize allergens intrinsic to the PCGs [141]. Among those already known grass pollen allergens, seven are associated with PCGs: Phl p 1, 3, 4, 5, 6, 11, and 12. Three novel IgE-reactive proteins were identified: an alcohol dehydrogenase unique to the PCGs, an ascorbic reductase detected in both the whole pollen grain as well as the PCGs, and a ß-glucosidase detected

only in pollen extracts. Five additional proteins were identified in PCGs which might be potential allergens: enolase, triosephosphate isomerase, legumin-like protein, UDP-glucose pyrophosphorylase, and a phosphomutase.

11.6 GRASS POLLEN ALLERGEN CROSS-REACTIVITY

Grass-allergic subjects almost always display multiple grass pollen sensitivities.

Because many grass species coexist in the same geographical area, simultaneous sensitization to pollen from multiple grass species is expected. Various approaches are used to investigate grass pollen allergen cross-reactivities, and most of these studies support the hypothesis that sensitization to one grass pollen species leads to multiple pollen sensitivities. Radioallergosorbent test (RAST) and ELISA inhibition assays reveal extensive allergenic cross-reactivity among taxonomically related grasses [142]. Data have been generated using whole pollen extracts, but more precise information about cross-reactivity, i.e., relative affinity, can only be obtained using individual specific allergens. Structural details of homologous grass pollen allergens also may reveal potential cross-reactive epitopes [143,144]. These studies may be based on the primary amino acid sequence data or on more sophisticated three-dimensional structural data of surface exposed residues.

The pattern of allergenic cross-reactivity among the pollen species closely follows taxonomic relationships (Figure 11.4). All studies find the highest degree of allergenic cross-reactivity among pollen extracts derived from grasses of the same subfamily. Martin et al. [145], using a human serum pool from allergic North American subjects with pollen extracts from the three subfamilies Pooideae (brome, meadow fescue, perennial ryegrass, timothy, sweet vernal, redtop, Kentucky bluegrass, and Western wheatgrass), Chloridoideae (salt grass, Bermuda grass, and grama grass), and Panicoideae (Bahia grass and Johnson grass), detected little or no cross-reactivity between pooid and chloridoid pollen, while the panicoid grasses showed moderate cross-reactivity with both the

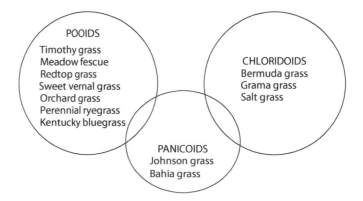

Figure 11.4 A Venn diagram representing the cross-relativity grouping of major allergenic grasses based on their taxonomic and immunologic relationship. The grass species within each subfamily group are highly cross-reactive and are difficult to differentiate immunologically. The two groups pooids and chloridoids are allergenically distinct and require separate diagnoses and immunotherapies. The panicoids, Johnson and Bahia grass, are allergenically cross-reactive with both pooids and chloridoids.

pooids and chloridoids. Little or no cross-reactivity occurs between ryegrass and Bahia or Bermuda grass pollen allergens as revealed by a study using IgE antibodies from Australian subjects and selected for reactivity to Lol p 1 and Lol p 5. However, in reciprocal experiments using antibodies selected for reactivity to Bahia pollen allergens, grass pollen from ryegrass, timothy, Johnson, and Bermuda are cross-reactive [146]. Gonzales et al. [147], employing sera from European subjects selected for reactivity toward each pollen group, detected little or no allergenic cross-reactivity between the pooids (perennial ryegrass, timothy, and cultivated rye) and Bermuda grass. *P. communis* (common reed), an arundinoid, shows moderate cross-reactivity with both the pooids and chloridoids. Extensive cross-reactivity was detected among 14 different species of pooids, with the highest responses directed toward *P. pratensis, F. rubra, P. pratense,* and *D. glomerata.* Excluding *P. communis,* an arundinoid; *C. dactylon,* a chloridoid; and *Z. mays,* a panicoid, any one grass species is sufficient for *in vitro* diagnosis of grass pollen allergy [148] in a study with 209 individual sera with reactivity toward grass pollen. No studies have examined possible allergenic cross-reactivities between arundinoid and panicoid pollen.

The availability of purified grass pollen allergens, allergen fragments, and recombinant allergens allowed for more refined studies that detect cross-reactivity among allergens derived from the same species as well as among homologous allergens from different species. Of particular interest is the strong homology between the C-terminal end of the group 1 molecule (amino acid residues 145–240) and the entire 97-amino acid sequence of the grass group 2 and group 3 allergens. The human immune response to the three ryegrass allergens is associated with HLA DR3, and concordant reactivity to all three allergens is common. These observations may be explained by cross-reactivity among Lol p 1, Lol p 2, and Lol p 3, detected at both the B-cell and T-cell levels [53,65]. Some human T-cell clones are reactive to the purified protein of the three allergen groups and the group 5 allergens. Stretches of homologous segments with an amphipathic nature suggest the presence of structural similarities that may account for this cross-reactivity.

The cross-reactive nature of the ubiquitous protein profilin is illustrated by the serological cross-reactivity between grass pollen profilins and profilins from other pollen and vegetable foods [128,149]. Human anti-profilin IgE antibodies cross-react with almost all plant profilins. The presence of highly conserved structures among plant profilins may explain the reports of coincident oral allergies to fruits and vegetables consumed by grass-allergic subjects [26,121,150] as well as allergenic cross-reactivities occasionally detected between unrelated pollen. The group 4 and group 7 allergens also may be useful diagnostic markers to identify patients with multiple sensitizations caused by cross-reactivity. For example, grass group 4–related proteins are present in unrelated plant foods including peanut, apple, celery, and carrot root as well as mugwort and birch pollen. Approximately 20% of polysensitized individuals possess IgE antibodies toward calcium-binding pollen proteins. Among the calcium-binding proteins, Ph1 p 7 contains most of the relevant IgE epitopes in the population studied and may be a useful molecule to detect sensitization to this group of cross-reactive pollen allergens.

Cross-reactive carbohydrate determinants (CCDs) of grass pollen allergens also are implicated in serological cross-reactions among a variety of pollen and vegetable foods [151–154]. The β (1–2)-xylose- and α-(1–3)-fucose-containing glycans on glycoproteins from several plants, molluscs, and insects are highly cross-reactive. The clinical significance of anticarbohydrate IgE antibodies is not established, and the role of CCD in allergic sensitization remains to be explored. In this regard, the grass group 11 allergens, Cyn d 4 (BG60), and Cyn d 24 may present a unique opportunity to investigate the role of both carbohydrate and peptide epitopes in allergenic cross-reactivity among glycoproteins from related and unrelated sources. The presence of conserved amino acids and cysteine positions in the primary structure of Lol p 11 suggests homology with pollen glycoproteins from maize, rice, tomato, olive tree, and privet.

Since grass pollen immunotherapy was pioneered by Freeman and Noon [155] almost a century ago, the specificity of grass immunotherapy has been questioned. Freeman advocated the use of only extracts/vaccines from timothy grass pollen for the diagnosis and treatment of grass allergy in Great Britain as did Cooke and Vander Veer [156] in the United States. Leavengood et al. [157] selected a group of patients showing multiple sensitivities to pooid, panicoid, and chloridoid grasses and treated them with vaccines prepared only from timothy and Bermuda grass pollen. The treatment significantly reduced the skin test responses to all of the grass pollen, suggesting that treatment with the two grass pollen vaccines may be sufficient for effective treatment in these grass-allergic patients. The current practice parameters for allergen immunotherapy, established by both the American Academy of Allergy, Asthma and Immunology and the American College of Allergy, Asthma, and Immunology, specifically state that information regarding allergen cross-reactivity should be used in the selection of relevant allergens for immunotherapy because limiting the number of allergens in a treatment vial may be necessary to attain optimal therapeutic doses for the individual patient [158]. The molecular and clinical evidence for cross-reactivity among grass pollen allergens supports the premise that effective diagnosis and immunotherapy can be accomplished with a limited number of grass pollen extracts [159]. The use of representative extracts/vaccines or mixtures of individual species from the major grass subfamilies appears to be a reliable strategy, and the selection of the species should be based on their prevalence [160,161]. For example, timothy grass (or a combination of relevant pooid species), Bermuda grass, and Johnson grass, which represent the three major allergenic grass subfamilies, should be sufficient for clinical practice.

11.7 CONCLUSION

Grasses are ubiquitous, and their pollen are important aeroallergens in most parts of the world. Only a few grass species are positively identified as important sources of allergens, but less conspicuous grass species may add to the aeroallergen load due to their cross-reactivity. The degree of allergenic cross-reactivity tends to correlate with their taxonomic grouping, and the treatment of grass allergy with vaccines derived from representative species is efficacious. Cross-reactivities between homologous proteins from different grass species and their clinical relevance are established. There is evidence of cross-reactivities between grass pollen allergens and proteins derived from diverse plant sources including other pollen, fruits, and vegetables. Clinical investigations to establish the relevance of such cross-reactivities are still needed.

New immunochemical and molecular biological approaches to the study of grass pollen allergens have greatly increased the knowledge about this important group of pollen allergens. Due to their worldwide importance, grass allergens are a subject of great interest among researchers from virtually every continent, and more than 100 grass pollen allergen structures were identified, purified, and sequenced between 2005 and 2017. The genomes of a variety of grasses were sequenced and analyzed [162–165]. Because the members of the grass family are closely related, and their genomes share extensive synteny, this genetic information undoubtedly will have a great impact on grass pollen allergen research. Only a few minor grass pollen allergen groups are yet to be identified, and it is expected that in the next few years the molecular structure of all of the major grass allergen groups will be established. The human immune responses at both the B-cell and T-cell levels are being studied to define relevant structures on the grass allergen molecules, and novel diagnostic and therapeutic approaches based on their immunologic activities are in progress. Together with advances being made with allergens from other environmental sources, the study of grass pollen will contribute to a better understanding of allergic responses to these ubiquitous allergens.

SALIENT POINTS

1. Grasses are ubiquitous, and grass pollen allergens are of worldwide importance.

2. Of the hundreds of grass genera and thousands of species, only a small number are allergenically important. Most of these species are cultivated.

3. The pooids account for most grass species in Canada and the northwestern United States and are prevalent in the cooler regions of the world; the chloridoids are well established especially in the warm and arid habitats with high winter temperatures such as the southwestern United States; and the panicoids dominate the humid tropical environments including the southern United States and northeastern South America.

4. Allergic symptoms depend on pollen exposure. Particles that are significantly smaller than the size of grass pollen grains and capable of entering the lower airway are implicated as major causes of allergic reactions.

5. At least 11 groups of structurally related allergens are identified and characterized across multiple grass subfamilies.

6. Grass-allergic patients often display multiple sensitivities. Simultaneous sensitizations to multiple species are expected based on the numerous grass species pollinating at a given time and place and on the high degree of cross-reactivity among them.

7. Allergenic cross-reactivities are documented among homologous allergens produced by taxonomically related grasses and between allergens produced in a single grass species.

8. The presence of conserved structures among the proteins and various carbohydrate determinants of pollen and vegetable foods is consistent with coincident allergic reactions to fruits and vegetables as well as unrelated pollen in grass pollen–allergic patients.

9. Diagnosis and immunotherapy with a limited number of grass allergen vaccines representing the subfamilies Pooideae, Chloridoideae, and Panicoideae may be effective in most grass-allergic patients.

10. Advances made with the grass genome projects should be leveraged to increase the understanding of the structure, expression, and function of grass pollen allergens.

REFERENCES

1. Waite KJ. Blackley and the development of hay fever as a disease of civilization in the nineteenth century. *Med Hist* 1995; 39: 186–196.

2. Hitchcock AS. *Manual of the Grasses of the United States*, 2nd ed., revised by A. Chase. Washington, DC: USDA Misc Publ 200, 1951.

3. Soreng RJ, Peterson PM, Romaschenko K et al. A worldwide phylogenetic classification of the Poaceae (Gramineae). *J Syst Evol* 2015; 53: 117–137.

4. Watson L, Dallwitz MJ. *The Grass Genera of the World*, 2nd ed. Wallingford, UK: CAB International, 1994.

5. Barunuik JN, Bolick M, Esch R., Buckley CE III. Quantification of pollen solute release using pollen grain column chromatography. *Allergy* 1992; 47: 411–417.

6. Aeroallergen Monitoring Network. *1996 Pollen and Spore Report*. Milwaukee, WI: AAAA&I, 1997.

7. Habenicht HA, Burge HA, Muilenburg ML, Solomon WR. Allergen carriage by atmospheric aerosol II. Ragweed-pollen determinants in submicronic atmospheric fractions. *J Allergy Clin Immunol* 1984; 74: 64–67.

8. Schumacher MJ, Griffith RD, O'Rourke MK. Recognition of pollen and other particulate aeroantigens by immunoblot microscopy. *J Allergy Clin Immunol* 1988; 82: 608–616.

9. Knox RB. Grass pollen, thunderstorms and asthma. *Clin Exp Allergy* 1993; 23: 354–359.

10. Taylor PE, Flagan RC, Valenta R, Glovsky MM. Release of allergens as respirable aerosols: A link between grass pollen and asthma. *J Allergy Clin Immunol* 2002; 109: 51–56.

11. Taylor PE, Jacobson KW, House JM, Glovsky MM. Links between pollen, atopy and the asthma epidemic. *Int Arch Allergy Immunol* 2007; 144: 162–170.

12. Vinckier S, Smets E. The potential role of orbicules as a vector of allergens. *Allergy* 2001; 56: 1129–1136.

13. Normile, D. Yangtze seen as earliest rice site. *Science* 2004; 275: 309.

14. Johnson P, Marsh DG. Allergens from common rye grass pollen (Lolium perenne): I. Chemical composition and structure. *Immunochemistry* 1966; 3: 91–100.

15. Johnson P, Marsh DG. Isoallergens from rye grass pollen. *Nature* 1965; 206: 935–937.

16. Marsh DG, Haddad ZH, Campbell DH. A new method for determining the distribution of allergenic fractions in biological materials: Its application to grass pollen extracts. *J Allergy* 1970; 46: 107–121.

17. Howlett BJ, Vithanage HIMV, Knox RB. Immunofluorescence localization of two water soluble glycoproteins, including the major allergen of rye-grass, Lolium perenne. *Histochem J* 1981; 13: 461–480.

18. Perez M, Ishioka GY, Walker LE, Chesnut RW. cDNA cloning and immunological characterization of the rye grass allergen Lol p I. *J Biol Chem* 1990; 265: 16210–16215.

19. Laffer S, Valenta R, Vrtala S et al. Complementary DNA cloning of the major allergen Phl p 1 from timothy grass (Phleum pratense); recombinant Phl p 1 inhibits IgE binding to group 1 allergens from eight different grass species. *J Allergy Clin Immunol* 1994; 94: 689–698.

20. Smith PM, Suphioglu C, Griffith IJ, Theriault K, Knox B, Singh MB. Cloning and expression in yeast *Pichia pastoris* of a biologically active form of Cyn d 1, the major allergen of Bermuda grass pollen. *J Allergy Clin Immunol* 1996; 98: 331–343.

21. Schramm G, Bufe A, Petersen A, Haas H, Schlaak M, Becker WM. Mapping of IgE-binding epitopes on the recombinant major group I allergen of velvet grass pollen, rHol l 1. *J Allergy Clin Immunol* 1997; 99: 781–789.

22. Broadwater AH, Rubinstein AL, Chay CH, Klapper DG, Bedinger PA. Zea ml, the maize homolog of the allergen-encoding Lol p I gene of rye grass. *Gene* 1993; 131: 227–230.

23. Fenaille F, Nony E, Chabre H et al. Mass spectrometric investigation of molecular variability of grass pollen group 1 allergens. *J Proteome Res* 2009; 8: 4014–4027.

24. Halim A, Carlsson MC, Madsen CB et al. Glycoproteomic analysis of seven major allergenic proteins reveals novel post-translational modifications. *Mol Cell Proteomics* 2015; 14: 191–204.

25. Petersen A, Becker W-M, Moll H, Blumke M, Schlaak M. Studies on the carbohydrate moieties of the timothy grass pollen allergen Phl p 1. *Electrophoresis* 1995; 16: 869–875.

26. Wicklein D, Lindner B, Moll H et al. Carbohydrate moieties can induce mediator release: A detailed characterization of two major timothy grass pollen allergens. *Biol Chem* 2004; 385: 397–407.

27. Cosgrove DJ. Loosening of plant cell walls by expansins. *Nature* 2000; 407: 321–326.

28. Grobe K, Becker WM, Schlaak M, Petersen A. Grass group 1 allergens (β-expansins) are novel, papain-related proteinases. *Eur J Biochem* 1999; 263: 33–40.

29. Grobe K, Poppelmann M, Becker WM, Petersen A. Properties of group 1 allergens from grass pollen and their relation to cathepsin B, a member of the C1 family of cysteine proteinases. *Eur J Biochem* 2002; 269: 2083–2092.

30. Raftery MJ, Saldanha RG, Geczy CL, Kumar RK. Mass spectrometric analysis of electrophoretically separated allergens and proteases in grass pollen diffusates. *Respir Res* 2003; 4: 10.

31. Li LC, Cosgrove DJ. Grass group 1 pollen allergens (β-expansins) lack proteinase activity and do not cause wall loosening via proteolysis. *Eur J Biochem* 2001; 268: 4217–4226.

32. Poppelmann M, Becker W-M, Petersen A. Combination of zymography and immunodetection to analyze proteins in complex culture supernatants. *Electrophoresis*. 2002; 23: 993–997.

33. Baeyens-Volant D, M'Rabet N, El Mahyaoui R et al. A contaminant trypsin-like activity from the timothy grass pollen is responsible for the conflicting enzymatic behavior of the major allergen Phl p 1. *Biochim Biophys Acta* 2013; 1834: 272–283.

34. Crosgrove DJ, Bedinger P, Durachko DM. Group 1 allergens of grass pollen as cell wall-loosening agents. *Proc Natl Acad Sci USA* 1997; 94: 6559–6564.

35. Li LC, Bedinger PA, Volk C, Jones AD, Cosgrove DJ. Purification and characterization of four β-expansins (Zea m 1 isoforms) from maize pollen. *Plant Physiol* 2003; 132: 2073–2085.

36. Valdivia ER, Wu Y, Li LC, Cosgrove DJ, Stephenson AG. A group 1 grass pollen allergen influences the outcome of pollen competition in maize. *PLOS ONE* 2007; 2: e154.

37. Tabuchi A, Li L-C, Cosgrove DJ. Matrix solubilization and cell wall weakening by β-expansin (group-1 allergen) from maize pollen. *Plant J* 2011; 68: 546–559.

38. Barre A, Rouge P. Homology modeling of the cellulose-binding domain of a pollen allergen from rye grass: Structural basis for the cellulose recognition and associated allergenic properties. *Biochem Biophys Res Commun* 2002; 296: 1346–1351.

39. Baer H, Maloney CJ, Norman P, Marsh DG. The potency and group I antigen content of six commercially prepared grass pollen extracts. *J Allergy Clin Immunol* 1974; 54: 157–164.

40. Esch RE, Klapper DG. Isolation and characterization of a major cross-reactive grass group I allergenic determinant. *Mol Immunol* 1989; 26: 557–561.

41. Hiller KM, Esch RE, Klapper DG. Mapping of an allergenically important determinant of grass group 1 allergens. *J Allergy Clin Immunol* 1997; 100: 335–340.

42. Ball T, Fuchs T, Sperr R et al. B cell epitopes of the major timothy grass pollen allergen, Phl p 1, revealed by gene fragmentation as candidates for immunotherapy. *FASEB J* 1999; 13: 1277–1290.

43. Flicker S, Steinberger P, Ball T et al. Spatial clustering of the IgE epitopes on the major timothy grass pollen allergen Phl p 1: Importance for allergenic activity. *J Allergy Clin Immunol* 2006; 117: 1336–1343.

44. de Weerd N, Bhalla PL, Singh MB. Effect of cysteine mutagenesis on human IgE reactivity of recombinant forms of the major rye grass pollen allergen Lol p 1. *Allergol Int* 2003; 52: 183–190.

45. Ball T, Ekstrom W, Mauch L et al. Gain of structure and IgE epitopes by eukaryotic expression of the major timothy grass pollen allergen, Phl p 1. *FEBS J* 2005; 272: 217–227.

46. van Oort E, de Heer PG, Dieker M, Van Leeuwen AW, Aalberse RC, van Ree R. Characterization of natural Dac g 1 variants: An alternative to recombinant group 1 allergens. *J Allergy Clin Immunol* 2004; 114: 1124–1130.

47. Suck R, Kamionka T, Schaffer B et al. Bacterially expressed and optimized recombinant Phl p 1 is immunobiochemically equivalent to natural Phl p 1. *Biochim Biophys Acta* 2006; 1764: 1701–1709.

48. Lukschal A, Fuhrmann J, Sobanov J et al. Anti-idiotypic Fab fragments image a conserved N-terminal epitope patch of grass pollen allergen Phl p 1. *Open Allergy J* 2011; 4: 16–23.

49. Han S, Chang Z, Chang H, Chi C, Wang J, Lin C. Identification and characterization of epitopes on Cyn d 1, the major allergen of Bermuda grass pollen. *J Allergy Clin Immunol* 1993; 91: 1035–1041.

50. Davies JM, Dang TD, Voskamp A et al. Functional immunoglobulin E cross-reactivity between Pas n 1 of Bahia grass pollen and other group 1 grass pollen allergens. *Clin Exp Allergy* 2011; 41: 281–291.

51. Davies JM, Mittag D, Dang TD et al. Molecular cloning, expression and immunological characterization of Pas n 1, the major allergen of Bahia grass *Paspalum notatum* pollen. *Mol Immunol* 2008; 46: 186–293.

52. Yuan HC, Wu KG, Chen CJ et al. Mapping of IgE and IgG4 antibody-binding epitopes in Cyn d 1, the major allergen of Bermuda grass pollen. *Int Arch Allergy Immunol* 2012; 157: 125–135.

53. Baskar S, Parronchi P, Mohapatra S, Romagnani S, Ansari AA. Human T cell responses to purified pollen allergens of the grass, *Lolium perenne*. Analysis of relationship between structural homology and T cell recognition. *J Immunol* 1992; 148: 2378–2383.

54. Mohapatra SS, Mohapatra S, Yang M et al. Molecular basis of cross-reactivity among allergen-specific human T cells: T-cell receptor Vα gene usage and epitope structure. *Immunology* 1994; 81: 15–20.

55. Mulller WD, Karamfilov T, Bufe A, Fahlbush B, Wolf I, Juger L. Group 5 allergens of timothy grass (Ph1 p 5] bear cross-reacting T cell epitopes with group 1 allergens of ryegrass (Lol p 1]. *Int Arch Allergy Immuno1* 1996; 109: 352–355.

56. Burton MD, Papalia L, Eusebius NP, Q'Hehir RE, Rolland JM. Characterization of the human T cell response to rye grass pollen allergens Lol p 1 and Lol p 5. *Allergy* 2002; 57: 1136–1144.

57. Ansari AA, Shenbagamurthi P, Marsh DG. Complete primary structure of a *Lolium perenne* (perennial rye grass) pollen allergen, Lol p II. *J Biol Chem* 1989; 265: 11181–11185.

58. Macaubas C, Wahlstrom J, Galvao da Silva AP et al. Allergen-specific MHC class II tetramer+ cells are detectable in allergic, but not in nonallergic individuals. *J Immunol* 2006; 176: 5069–5077.

59. Etto T, de Boer C, Prickett S et al. Unique and cross-reactive T cell epitope peptides of the major Bahia grass pollen allergen, Pas n 1. *Int Arch Allergy Immunol* 2012; 159: 355–366.

60. Roberts AM, Bevan LJ, Flora PS, Jepson I, Walker MR. Nucleotide sequence of cDNA encoding the group II allergen cocksfoot/orchard grass *(Dactylis glomerata)*, Dac g II. *Allergy* 1993; 48: 615–623.

61. Tomborini E, Brandazza A, De Lalla C et al. Recombinant allergen Lol p II: Expression, purification and characterization. *Mol Immunol* 1995; 32: 505–513.

62. Dolecek C, Vrtala S, Laffer S et al. Molecular characterization of Phl p II, a major timothy grass *(Phleum pratense)* pollen allergen. *FEBS Lett* 1993; 335: 299–304.

63. De Marino S, Castiglione Morelli MA, Fratemali F et al. An immunoglobulin-like fold in a major plant allergen: The solution structure of Phl p 2 from timothy grass pollen. *Structure Fold Des* 1999; 7: 943–952.

64. Padavattan S, Flicker S, Schirmer T et al. High-affinity IgE recognition of a conformational epitope of the major respiratory allergen Phl p 2 as revealed by x-ray crystallography. *J Immunol* 2009; 182: 2141–2151.

65. Ansari AA, Kihara TK, Marsh DG. Immunochemical studies of *Lolium perenne* (rye grass) pollen allergens Lol p I, II, and III. *J Immuno1* 1987; 139: 4034–4041.

66. Petersen A, Suck R, Lindner B et al. Phl p 3: Structural and immunological characterization of a major allergen of timothy grass pollen. *Clin Exp Allergy* 2006; 36: 840–849.

67. Ansari AA, Shenbagamurthi P, Marsh DG. Complete primary structure of a *Lolium perenne* (perennial rye grass) pollen allergen, Lol p III: Comparison with known Lol p I and II sequences. *Biochemistry* 1989; 28: 8665–8670.

68. Guerin-Marchand C, Senechal H, Bouin A-P et al. Cloning, sequencing and immunological characterization of Dac g 3, a major allergen from *Dactylis glomerata* pollen. *Mol Immunol* 1996; 33: 797–806.

69. Schweimer K, Petersen A, Suck R et al. Solution structure of Phl p 3, a major allergen from timothy grass pollen. *Biol Chem* 2008; 389: 919–923.

70. Devanaboyina SC, Cornelius C, Lupinek C et al. High-resolution crystal structure and IgE recognition of the major grass pollen allergen Phl p 3. *Allergy.* 2014; 69: 1617–1628.

71. Nandy A, Petersen A, Wald M et al. Primary structure, recombinant expression, and molecular characterization of Phl p 4, a major allergen of timothy grass *(Phleum pratense)*. *Biochem Biophys Res Comm* 2005; 305: 563–570.

72. DeWitt AM, Andersson K, Peltre G, Lidholm J. Cloning, expression and immunological characterization of full-length timothy grass pollen allergen Phl p 4, a berberine bridge enzyme-like protein with homology to celery allergen Api g 5. *Clin Exp Allergy* 2006; 36: 77–86.

73. Dittrich H, Kutchan TM. Molecular cloning, expression and induction of berberine bridge enzyme, an enzyme essential to the formation of benzophenanthridine alkaloids in the response of plants to pathogenic attack. *Proc Natl Acad Sci USA* 1991; 88: 9969–9973.

74. Leduc-Brodard V, Inacio F, Jaquinod M, Forest E, David B, Peltre G. Characterization of Dac g 4, a major basic allergen from *Dactylis glomerata* pollen. *J Allergy Clin Immunol* 1996; 98: 1065–1072.

75. Jaggi KS, Ekramoddoullah AKM, Kisil FT. Allergenic fragments of rye grass *(Lolium perenne)* pollen allergen Lol p IV. *Int Arch Allergy Appl Immunol* 1989; 89: 342–348.

76. Fischer S, Grote M, Fahlbusch B, Muller WD, Kraft D, Valenta R. Characterization of Ph1 p 4, a major timothy grass *(Phleum pratense)* pollen allergen. *J Allergy Clin Immunol* 1996; 98: 189–198.

77. Grote M, Stumvoll S, Reichelt R, Lidholm J, Rudolf V. Identification of an allergen related to Ph1 p 4, a major timothy grass pollen allergen, in pollen, vegetables, and fruits by immunogold electron microscopy. *Biol Chem* 2002; 383: 1441–1445.

78. Stumvoll S, Lidholm J, Thunberg R et al. Purification, structural and immunological characterization of a timothy grass *(Phleum pratense)* pollen allergen, Ph1 p 4, with cross-reactive potential. *Biol Chem* 2002; 383: 1383–1396.

79. Zafred D, Nandy A, Pump L et al. Crystal structure and immunologic characterization of the major grass pollen allergen Phl p 4. *J Allergy Clin Immunol.* 2013; 132: 696–703.

80. Su S-N, Shu P, Gai-Xuong L, Yang S-Y, Huang S-W, Lee, Y-C. Immunologic and physicochemical studies of Bermuda grass pollen antigen BG60. *J Allergy Clin Immunol* 1996; 98: 486–494.

81. Ohsuga H, Su S-N, Takahashi N et al. The carbohydrate moiety of the Bermuda grass antigen BG60: New oligosaccharides of plant origin. *J Biol Chem* 1996; 273: 26653–26658.

82. Huang T-H, Peng H-J, Su S-N, Liaw S-H. Various cross-reactivity of the grass pollen group 4 allergens: Crystallographic study of the Bermuda grass isoallergen Cyn d 4. *Acta Cryst.* 2012; D68: 1303–1310.

83. Matthiesen F, Lowenstein H. Group V allergens in grass pollen. 1. Purification and characterization of group V allergen from *Phleum pratense* pollen, Ph1 p V. *Clin Exp Allergy* 1991; 21: 297–307.

84. Silvanovich A, Astwood J, Zhang L et al. Nucleotide sequence analysis of three cDNAs coding for Poa p IX isoallergens of Kentucky bluegrass pollen. *J Biol Chem* 1991; 266: 1204–1210.

85. Ong EK, Griffith IJ, Knox RB, Singh MB. Cloning of a cDNA encoding a group V (group IX) allergen isoform from rye-grass pollen that demonstrates specific antigenic immunoreactivity. *Gene* 1993; 134: 235–240.

86. Suphioglu C, Mawdsley D, Schappi G et al. Molecular cloning, expression and immunological characterization of Lol p 5C, a novel allergen isoform of rye grass pollen demonstrating high IgE reactivity. *FEBS Lett* 1999; 462: 435–441.

87. Smith PM, Ong EK, Knox RB, Singh MB. Immunological relationships among group I and group V allergens from grass pollen. *Mol Immunol* 1994; 31: 491–498.

88. Ong EK, Knox RB, Singh MB. Mapping of the antigenic and allergenic epitopes of Lol p VB using gene fragmentation. *Mol Immunol* 1995; 32: 295–302.

89. Suphioglu C, Blaher B, Rolland JM et al. Molecular basis of IgE-recognition of Lol p 5, a major allergen of ryegrass pollen. *Mol Immunol* 1998; 35: 293–305.

90. Bufe A, Becker W-M, Schramm G et al. Major allergen Phl p Va (timothy grass) bears at least two different IgE-reactive epitopes. *J Allergy Clin Immunol* 1994; 94: 173–181.

91. Flicker S, Vrtala S, Steinberger P et al. A human monoclonal IgE antibody defines a highly allergenic fragment of the major timothy grass pollen allergen, Phl p 5: Molecular, immunological, and structural characterization of the epitope-containing domain. *J Immunol* 2000; 165: 3849–3859.

92. Gehlhar K, Rajashankar KR, Hofmann E et al. Lysine as a critical amino acid for IgE binding in Phl p 5b C terminus. *Int Arch Allergy Immunol* 2006; 140: 285–294.

93. Levin M, Rotthus S, Wendel S et al. Multiple independent IgE epitopes on the highly allergenic grass pollen allergen Phl p 5. *Clin Exp Allergy* 2014; 44: 1409–1419.

94. Zhang L, Olsen E, Kisil FT, Hill RD, Sehon AH, Mohapatra SS. Mapping of antibody binding epitopes of a recombinant Poa p IX allergen. *Mol Immunol* 1992; 29: 1383–1389.

95. Schramm G, Bufe A, Petersen A et al. Discontinuous IgE-binding epitopes contain multiple continuous epitope regions: Results of an epitope mapping on recombinant Hol l 5, a major allergen from velvet grass pollen. *Clin Exp Allergy* 2001; 31: 331–341.

96. Hantusch B, Krieger S, Untersmayr E et al. Mapping of conformational IgE epitopes on Phl p 5a by using mimotopes from a phage display library. *J Allergy Clin Immunol* 2004; 114: 1294–1300.

97. Wald M, Kahlert H, Weber B et al. Generation of a low immunoglobulin E-binding mutant of the timothy grass pollen major allergen Phl p 5a. *Clin Exp Allergy* 2007; 37: 441–450.

98. Swoboda I, De Weerd N, Bhalla PL et al. Mutants of the major ryegrass pollen allergen, Lol p 5, with reduced IgE-binding capacity: Candidates for grass pollen-specific immunotherapy. *Eur J Immunol* 2002; 32: 270–280.

99. Wald M, Kahlert H, Reese G et al. Hypoallergenic mutants of the timothy grass pollen allergen Phl p 5 generated by proline mutations. *Int Arch Allergy Immunol* 2012; 159: 130–142.

100. Singh MB, Hough T, Theerakulpisut P et al. Isolation of cDNA encoding a newly identified major allergenic protein of rye-grass pollen: Intracellular targeting to the amyloplast. *Proc Natl Acad Sci USA* 1991; 88: 1384–1388.

101. Bufe A, Uhlig U, Scholzen T, Matousek J, Schlaak M, Weber W. A nonspecific, single-stranded nuclease activity with characteristics of a topoisomerase found in a major grass pollen allergen: Possible biological significance. *Biol Chem* 1999; 380: 1009–1016.

102. Blaher B, Suphioglu C, Knox RB, Singh MB, McCluskey J, Rolland JM. Identification of T-cell epitopes of Lol p 9, a major allergen of rye grass *(Latium perenne)* pollen. *J Allergy Clin Immunol* 1996; 98: 124–132.

103. Wurtzen P, Wissenbach M, Ipsen H, Bufe A, Arnved J, van Neerven RJ. Highly heterogeneous Phl p 5-specific T cells from patients with allergic rhinitis differentially recognize recombinant Phl p 5 isoallergens. *J Allergy Clin Immunol* 1999; 104: 115–122.

104. de Lalla C, Sturniolo T, Abbruzzese L et al. Identification of novel T cell epitopes in Lol p 5a by computational prediction. *J Immunol* 1999; 163: 1725–1729.

105. Focke-Tejkl M, Campana R, Reininger R et al. Dissection of the IgE and T-cell recognition of the major group 5 grass pollen allergen Phl p 5. *J Allergy Clin Immunol* 2014; 133: 836–845.

106. Vrtala S, Fischer S, Grote M et al. Molecular, immunological and structural characterization of Phl p 6, a major allergen and P-particle-associated protein from Timothy grass *(Phleum pratense)* pollen. *J Immunol* 1999; 163: 5489–5496.

107. Petersen A, Bufe A, Schramm G, Schlaak M, Becker W-M. Characterization of the allergen group VI in timothy grass pollen (Phl p 6] II. cDNA cloning of Phl p 6 and structural comparison to group V. *Int Arch Allergy Immunol* 1995; 108: 55–59.

108. Petersen A, Bufe A, Schlaak M, Becker W-H. Characterization of the allergen group VI in timothy grass pollen (Phl p 6) I. Immunological and biochemical studies. *Int Arch Allergy Immunol* 1995; 108: 49–54.

109. Suphioglu C, Ferreira F, Knox RB. Molecular cloning and immunological characterisation of Cyn d 7, a novel calcium-binding allergen from Bermuda grass pollen. *FEBS Lett* 1997; 402: 167–172.

110. Niederberger V, Hayek B, Vrtala S et al. Calcium-dependent immunoglobulin E recognition of the apo- and calcium-bound form of a cross-reactive two EF-hand timothy grass pollen allergen, Phl p 7. *F ASEB J* 1999; 13: 843–856.

111. Wopfner N, Dissertori O, Ferreira F, Lackner P. Calcium-binding proteins and their role in allergic disease. *Immunol Allergy Clin North Am* 2007; 27: 29–44.

112. Verdino P, Westritschnig K, Valenta R, Keller W. The cross-reactive calcium-binding pollen allergen Phl p 7, reveals a novel dimer assembly. *EMBO J* 2002; 21: 5007–5016.

113. Tinghino R, Twardosz A, Barletta B et al. Molecular, structural and immunological relationships between different families of recombinant calcium-binding pollen allergens. *J Allergy Clin Immunol* 2002; 109: 314–320.

114. Westritschnig K, Focke M, Verdino P et al. Generation of an allergy vaccine by disruption of the three-dimensional structure of the cross-reactive calcium-binding allergen, Phl p 7. *J Immunol* 2004; 172: 5684–5692.

115. Neukecker P, Nerkamp J, Eisenmann A et al. Solution structure, dynamics, and hydrodynamics of the calcium-bound cross-reactive birch pollen allergen Bet v 4 reveal a canonical monomeric two EF-hand assembly with a regulatory function. *J Mol Biol* 2004; 336: 1141–1157.

116. Verdino P, Barderas R, Villalba M et al. Three-dimensional structure of the cross-reactive pollen allergen Che a 3: Visualizing cross-reactivity on the molecular surfaces of weed, grass, and tree pollen allergens. *J Immunol* 2008; 180: 2313–2321.

117. Ekramoddoullah AKM, Kisil FT, Sehon AH. Allergenic cross-reactivity of cytochromes c of Kentucky bluegrass and perennial ryegrass pollen. *Mol Immunol* 1982; 19: 1527–1534.

118. van Ree R, Hoffman DR, Vandijk W et al. Lol p XI, a new major grass pollen allergen, is a member of a family of soybean trypsin inhibitor-related proteins. *J Allergy Clin Immunol* 1995; 95: 970–978.

119. Marknell DeWitt A, Niederberger V, Lehtonen P et al. Molecular and immunological characterization of a novel timothy grass *(Phleum pratense)* pollen allergen, Phl p 11. *Clin Exp Allergy* 2002; 32: 1329–1340.

120. Barderas R, Villalba M, Lombardero M, Rodriguez R. Identification and characterization of Che a 1 allergen from *Chenopodium album* pollen. *Int Arch Allergy Immunol* 2002; 127: 47–54.

121. van Ree R, Voitenko V, van Leeuwen WA, Aalberse RC. Profilin is a cross-reactive allergen in pollen and vegetable foods. *Int Arch Allergy Immunol* 1992; 98: 97–104.

122. Valenta R, Duchene M, Vrtala S et al. Profilin, a novel plant pan-allergen. *Int Arch Allergy Immunol* 1992; 99: 271–273.

123. Valenta R, Ball T, Vrtala S, Duchene M, Kraft D, Scheiner O. cDNA cloning and expression of timothy grass *(Phleum pratense)* pollen profilin in *Escherichia coli:* Comparison with birch pollen profilin. *Biochem Biophys Res Commun* 1994; 199: 106–118.

124. Asturias JA, Arilla MC, Gomez-Bayon N, Martinez J, Martinez A, Palacios R. Cloning and high level expression of *Cynodon dactylon* (Bermuda grass) pollen profilin (Cyn d 12) in *Escherichia coli*: Purification and characterization of the allergen. *Clin Exp Allergy* 1997; 27: 1307–1313.

125. Asturias JA, Arilla MC, Gomez-Bayon N, Martinez A, Martinez J, Palacios R. Recombinant DNA technology in allergology: Cloning and expression of plant profilins. *Allergol Immunopathol (Madr)* 1997; 25: 127–134.

126. Wensing M, Akkerdaas JH, van Leeuwen WA et al. IgE to Bet v 1 and profilin: Crossreactivity patterns and clinical relevance. *J Allergy Clin Immunol* 2002; 11: 435–442.

127. Alvarado MI, Jimeno L, De La Torre F et al. Profilin as a severe food allergen in allergic patients overexposed to grass pollen. *Exp Allergy Immunol* 2014; 69: 1610–1616.

128. Lund G, Brand S, Ramos T et al. Strong and frequent T-cell responses to the minor allergen Phl p 12 in Spanish patients IgE-sensitized to profilins. *Allergy* 2018; 73: 1013–1021.

129. Suck R, Petersen A, Hagen S, Cromwell O, Becker WM, Fiebig H. Complementary DNA cloning and expression of a newly recognized high molecular mass allergen Ph1 p 13 from timothy grass (*Phleum pratense*). *Clin Exp Allergy* 2000; 30: 324–332.

130. Petersen A, Suck R, Hagen S, Cromwell O, Fiebig H, Becker WM. Group 13 grass allergens: Structural variability between different grass species and analysis of proteolytic stability. *J Allergy Clin Immunol* 2001; 107: 856–862.

131. Davies JM, Voskamp A, Dang TD et al. The dominant 55 kDa allergen of the subtropical Bahia grass (*Paspalum notatum*) pollen is a group 13 pollen allergen, Pas n 13. *Mol Immunol.* 2011; 48: 931–940.

132. Swoboda I, Grote M, Verdino P et al. Molecular characterization of polygalacturonases as grass pollen-specific marker allergens: Expulsion from pollen via submicronic respirable particles. *J Immunol* 2004; 172: 6490–6500.

133. Grote M, Swoboda I, Valenta R, Reichelt R. Group 13 allergens as environmental and immunological markers for grass pollen allergy: Studies by immunogold field emission scanning and transmission electron microscopy. *Int Arch Allergy Immunol* 2005; 136: 303–310.

134. Kao SH, Su SN, Huang SW, Tsai JJ, Chow LP. Sub-proteome analysis of novel IgE-binding proteins from Bermuda grass pollen. *Proteomics* 2005; 5: 3805–3813.

135. Chow LP, Chiu LL, Khoo KH et al. Purification and structural analysis of the novel glycoprotein allergen Cyn d 24, a pathogenesis-related protein PR-1, from Bermuda grass pollen. *FEBS J* 2005; 272: 6218–6227.

136. Sepplala U, Dauly C, Robinson S et al. Absolute quantification of allergen from complex mixtures: A new sensitive tool for standardization of allergen extracts for specific immunotherapy. *J Proteome Res* 2011; 10: 2113–2122.

137. De Canio M, D'Aguanno S, Sacchetti C et al. Novel IgE recognized components of *Lolium perenne* pollen extract: Comparative proteomics evaluation of allergic patients' sensitization profiles. *J Proteome Res* 2009; 8: 4383–4391.

138. Chakra ORA, Sutra J-P, Thomas ED et al. Proteomic analysis of major and minor allergens from isolated pollen cytoplasmic granules. *J Proteome Res* 2012; 11: 1208–1216.

139. Campbell BC, Gilding EK, Timbrell V et al. Total transcriptome, proteome, and allergome of Johnson grass pollen, which is important for allergic rhinitis in subtropical regions. *J Allergy Clin Immunol* 2015; 135: 133–142.

140. Bashir MEH, Ward JM, Cummings M et al. Dual function of novel pollen coat (surface) proteins: IgE-binding capacity and proteolytic activity disrupting the airway epithelial barrier. *PLOS ONE* 2013; 8: e53337.

141. Chakra ORA, Sutra J-P, Demey Thomas E et al. Proteomic analysis of major and minor allergens from isolated pollen cytoplasmic granules. *J Proteome Res* 2012; 11: 1208–1216.

142. Weber RW. Cross-reactivity of plant and animal allergens. *Clin Rev Allergy Immunol* 2001; 21: 153–202.

143. Aalberse RC, Akkerdaas JH, van Ree R. Cross-reactivity of IgE antibodies to allergens. *Allergy* 2001; 56: 478–490.

144. Aalberse RC. Structural biology of allergens. *J Allergy Clin Immunol* 2000; 106: 228–238.

145. Martin BG, Mansfield LE, Nelson HS. Cross-allergenicity among the grasses. *Ann Allergy* 1985; 54: 99–104.

146. Davies JM, Bright ML, Rolland JM, O'Hehir RE. Bahia grass pollen specific IgE is common in seasonal rhinitis patients but has limited cross-reactivity with ryegrass. *Allergy* 2005; 60: 251–255.

147. Gonzales RM, Cortes C, Conde J et al. Cross-reactivity among five major pollen allergens. *Ann Allergy* 1987; 59: 149–154.

148. van Ree R, van Leeuwen WA, Aalberse RC. How far can we simplify *in vitro* diagnostics for grass pollen allergy? A study with 17 whole pollen extracts and purified natural and recombinant major allergens. *J Allergy Clin Immunol* 1998; 102: 184–190.

149. Radauer C, Willerroider M, Fuchs H et al. Cross-reactive and species-specific immunoglobulin E epitopes of plant profilins: An experimental and structure-based analysis. *Clin Exp Allergy* 2006; 36: 920–929.

150. De Martino M, Novembre E, Cozza G, De Marco A, Bonazza P, Vierucci A. Sensitivity to tomato and peanut allergens in children monosensitized to grass pollen. *Allergy* 1988; 43: 206–213.

151. Petersen A, Vieths S, Aulepp H, Schlaak M, Becker W-H. Ubiquitous structures responsible for IgE cross-reactivity between tomato fruit and grass pollen allergens. *J Allergy Clin Immunol* 1996; 98: 805–813.

152. Calkhoven PG, Aalbers M, Koshte VL, Pos O, Oie HD, Aalberse RC. Crossreactivity among birch pollen, vegetables and fruits as detected by IgE antibodies is due to at least three distinct cross-reactive structures. *Allergy* 1987; 42: 382–390.

153. Mari A. Multiple pollen sensitization: A molecular approach to the diagnosis. *Int Arch Allergy Immunol* 2001; 125: 57–65.

154. Aalberse RC, van Ree R. Cross-reactive carbohydrate determinants. *Clin Rev Allergy Immunol* 1997; 15: 375–387.

155. Freeman J, Noon L. Further observations on the treatment of hay fever by hypodermic inoculations of pollen vaccine. *Lancet* 1911; 2: 814–817.

156. Cooke RA, Vander Veer A. Human sensitization. *J Immunol* 1916; 1: 201–237.

157. Leavengood DC, Renard RL, Martin BG, Nelson HS. Cross allergenicity among grasses determined by tissue threshold changes. *J Allergy Clin Immunol* 1985; 76: 789–794.

158. Joint Task Force on Practice Parameters (AAAAI, ACAAI, JCAAI). Allergen immunotherapy: A practice parameter, second update. *J Allergy Clin Immunol* 2007; 120: S25–S85.

159. Gangl K, Niederberger V, Valenta R. Multiple grass mixes as opposed to single grasses for allergen immunotherapy in allergic rhinitis. *Clin Exp Allergy* 2013; 43: 1202–1216.

160. Davies JM. Grass pollen allergens globally: The contribution of subtropical grasses to burden of allergic respiratory diseases. *Clin Exp Allergy* 2014; 44: 790–801.

161. Chabre H, Gouyon B, Huet A et al. Molecular variability of group 1 and 5 grass pollen allergens between Pooideae species: Implications for immunotherapy. *Clin Exp Allergy* 2009; 40: 505–519.

162. Paterson AH, Bowers JE, Bruggmann R et al. The Sorghum bicolor genome and the diversification of grasses. *Nature* 2009; 457: 551–556.

163. International Rice Genome Sequencing Project. The map-based sequence of the rice genome. *Nature* 2005; 436: 793–800.

164. Schnable PS, Ware D, Fulton RS et al. The B73 maize genome: Complexity, diversity, and dynamics. *Science* 2009; 326: 1112–1115.

165. The International Brachypodium Initiative. Genome sequencing and analysis of the model grass *Brachypodium distachyon*. *Nature* 2010; 463: 763–768.

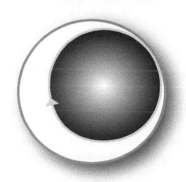

12 Weed pollen allergens

Michael Hauser, Gabriele Gadermaier, Sabrina Wildner,
Lisa Pointner, Michael Wallner, and Fatima Ferreira
University of Salzburg

CONTENTS

12.1 INTRODUCTION

Worldwide, pollen originating from weeds represents one of the most important sources of allergenic proteins. Although pollination seasons vary according to species and geographical locations of the weeds, typically, sensitized patients will experience allergic reactions from midsummer until late autumn. Among allergenic weeds, *Ambrosia* (ragweed), *Artemisia* (mugwort), *Parietaria* (pellitory), *Chenopodium* (chenopod), *Salsola* (Russian thistle), *Plantago* (plantain), and *Mercurialis* (annual mercury) are the most clinically relevant species. Taxonomy as well as biological aspects of these species are briefly discussed in this chapter. Presently, 47 weed pollen allergens are listed in the official International Union of Immunological Societies (IUIS) allergen nomenclature database (http:// www.allergen.org). In this review, special attention is given to the description of major weed pollen allergens as well as cross-reactive pan-allergens, including their biological function and allergenic relevance.

12.2 TAXONOMY OF WEEDS

The term *weed* does not refer to any particular botanical group of plants. It describes a group of plants mostly lacking appreciable economic or aesthetic value, in contrast to trees and grasses. The Oxford English Dictionary defines a weed as a "herbaceous plant not valued for use or beauty, growing wild and rank, and regarded as cumbering the ground or hindering the growth of superior vegetation." Consequently, the classification and taxonomy of plants into "weeds" is rather complex and challenging.

Given the absence of an all-encompassing classification system of weeds, this chapter focuses on the prominent and most clinically relevant weeds. Figure 12.1 and Table 12.1 show the most clinically relevant sources of weed pollen with corresponding allergenic molecules and their geographical distribution.

Besides some exceptions (e.g., Poales and Lamiales orders within the Monocots), weeds are found predominantly in the Eudicots, from which they divide into several subclasses. Within the Eudicots, the most prominent groups are the Rosids and the Asterids, containing 10–20 orders, respectively, depending on classification. The Asterids can be further subdivided into several orders and families. The family of Asteraceae comprises a large number of flowering plants of approximately 20,000 species. Prominent allergenic members in this family are ragweed (*Ambrosia*), mugwort (*Artemisia*), feverfew (*Parthenium*), and sunflower (*Helianthus*). To date, about 40 different species are known within the genus *Ambrosia*. The most widespread *Ambrosia* species and major elicitors of allergic reactions are common and short ragweed (*Ambrosia artemisiifolia, A. elatior*) and giant ragweed (*A. trifida*). Sensitization rates toward ragweed increased in the United States from 10% in the 1970s, toward 26.2% in the 1990s, and reached 32.8% in the 2000s, as assessed by the National Health and Nutrition Examination Survey (NHANES) [1–3]. A larger number of species (around 350) can be found in the genus *Artemisia*, with *Artemisia vulgaris* representing the best-studied allergenic species. In Europe, *Artemisia* pollen causes allergic reactions in 10%–14% of pollinosis patients [4]. Within the family of Plantaginaceae, the genus *Plantago* causes allergic reactions in 20%–40% of pollinosis patients [5,6].

In addition to the Asteraceae and Plantaginaceae, the Amaranthaceae family within the Asterids contains a number of clinically important allergenic weeds (e.g., *Chenopodium*, *Salsola*, *Amaranthus*). The best-studied members are (1) *Chenopodium album*, the main sensitizer in the desert areas of Saudi Arabia, Iran, and Kuwait; (2) *Salsola kali*; and (3) *Amaranthus retroflexus* [5,7].

Important sources of allergenic pollen within the Rosids are found in the Urticaceae family, with *Parietaria* (pellitory) being the most important weed within this family. The sensitization frequencies of *Parietaria* in some coastal areas in Southern Europe

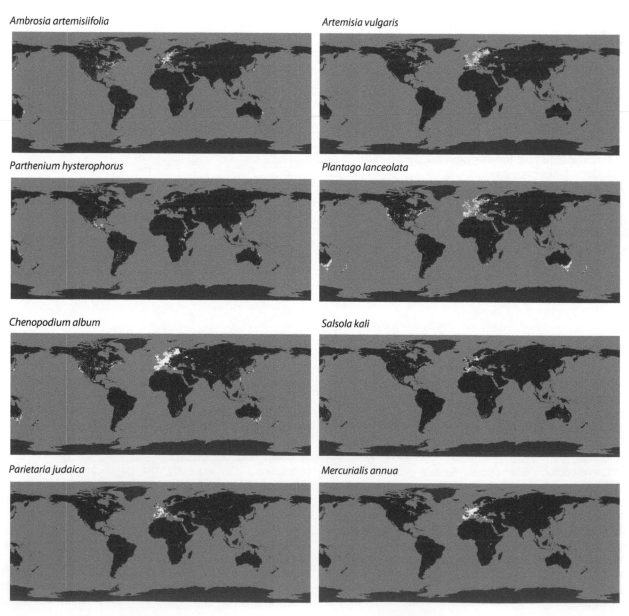

Ambrosia artemisiifolia

Artemisia vulgaris

Parthenium hysterophorus

Plantago lanceolata

Chenopodium album

Salsola kali

Parietaria judaica

Mercurialis annua

Figure 12.1 Geographical distribution of major allergenic weeds. (From Biodiversity database: https:// www.gbif.org.)

Table 12.1 Weed pollen allergens listed by the International Union of Immunological Societies Allergen Nomenclature Sub-Committee

	Allergen	SF in pollen (%)	Allergenicity assayed	Protein function/family	MW (kDa)	PDB code
Asteraceae						
Short ragweed (*Ambrosia artemisiifolia*)	Amb a 1	>95	IVR, MR, SPT	Pectate lyase family	38	
	Amb a 3	30–50	IVR	Plastocyanin protein family, *N*-terminal sequence	11	
	Amb a 4	20–40	IVR	Defensin-like protein linked to proline-rich glycosylated *C*-terminal domain, PR-12 protein family	13–15	
	Amb a 5	10–15	IVR, MR	Secreted disulfide-stabilized basic protein	5	
	Amb a 6	21	IVR	Nonspecific lipid transfer protein 1, PR-14 protein family	10	
	Amb a 7	15–20	IVR	Plastocyanin protein family, *N*-terminal sequence	12	
	Amb a 8	35–50	IVR, MR	Profilin	14	5EM1
	Amb a 9	10–15	IVR, MR	Polcalcin, 2 EF-hand calcium-binding protein	9	
	Amb a 10	10–15	IVR, MR	Polcalcin, 3 EF-hand calcium-binding protein	17	
	Amb a 11	60	IVR	Cysteine protease	37	5EF4
	Amb a 12	66	IVR	Enolase	48	
Giant ragweed (*Ambrosia trifida*)	Amb t 5	5	IVR	Secreted basic protein	5	1BBG
Cuman ragweed (*Ambrosia psilostachya*)	Amb p 5	10–15	IVR, MR	Secreted basic protein	5	
Mugwort (*Artemisia vulgaris*)	Art v 1	95	IVR, MR, SPT	Defensin-like protein linked to proline-rich glycosylated *C*-terminal domain, PR-12 protein family, NMR structure	13–16	2KPY
	Art v 2	58	IVR, SPT	Secreted basic glycoprotein, PR-1 protein family	16	
	Art v 3	22–70	IVR, MR, SPT	Nonspecific lipid transfer protein 1, PR-14 protein family	10	6FRR
	Art v 4	35	IVR, MR	Profilin	14	5EM0
	Art v 5	10–28	IVR, MR	Polcalcir, 2 EF-hand calcium-binding protein	10	
	Art v 6	26	IVR	Pectate lyase family, Amb a 1 homologue	38	
Annual mugwort (*Artemisia annua*)	Art an 7	>95	IVR, SPT	Putative galactose oxidase	62	
Chinese mugwort (*Artemisia argyi*)	Art ar 2	41	IVR	Pathogenesis-related protein PR-1	18	
Sunflower (*Helianthus annuus*)	Hel a 1	65	IVR	Sequence not available	34	
	Hel a 2	31	IVR	Profilin	14	
	Hel a 6	36	IVR	Pectate lyase	42	
Feverfew (*Parthenium hysterophorus*)	Par h 1	40–60	IVR, MR	Defensin-like protein linked to proline-rich glycosylated *C*-terminal domain, PR-12 protein family	12	

(Continued)

Table 12.1 (Continued) Weed pollen allergens listed by the International Union of Immunological Societies Allergen Nomenclature Sub-Committee

	Allergen	SF in pollen (%)	Allergenicity assayed	Protein function/family	MW (kDa)	PDB code
Amaranthaceae						
Chenopod (*Chenopodium album*)	Che a 1	70	IVR, SPT[a]	Ole e 1-like protein, glycosylated	18	
	Che a 2	55	IVR, SPT[a]	Profilin	14	
	Che a 3	46	IVR, SPT[a]	Polcalcin, 2 EF-hand calcium-binding protein, crystal structure	10	2OPO
Russian thistle (*Salsola kali*)	Sal k 1	65	IVR, SPT	Pectin methylesterase family	38	
	Sal k 2	n.d.	IVR	Protein kinase homologue	36	
	Sal k 3	63	IVR	Cobalamin-independent methionine synthase	85 (35 + 45)	
	Sal k 4	46	IVR	Profilin	14	
	Sal k 5	30–60	IVR	Ole e 1-like protein	18	
	Sal k 6	30	IVR	Polygalacturonase	47 (28)	
	Sal k 7	40	IVR	Polcalcin	9	
Redroot pigweed (*Amaranthus retroflexus*)	Ama r 1	38	IVR	Ole e 1-like protein	18	
	Ama r 2	33	IVR, SPT	Profilin	14	
Burning bush (*Kochia/Bassia scoparia*)	Koc s 1	35	IVR, SPT	Ole e 1-like protein	18	
	Koc s 2	50–60	IVR, SPT	Profilin	14	
Plantaginaceae						
English plantain (*Plantago lanceolata*)	Pla l 1	86	IVR	Ole e 1-like protein, glycoprotein	17–20	4Z8W
	Pla l 2	70	IVR	Profilin	15	
Urticaceae						
Pellitory of the wall (*Parietaria judaica*)	Par j 1	95	IVR, MR, SPT	Nonspecific lipid transfer protein 1	15	
	Par j 2	80	IVR, MR, SPT	Nonspecific lipid transfer protein 1	11	
	Par j 3	n.d.	IVR	Profilin, 3 isoallergen	14	
	Par j 4	6	IVR	Polcalcin, 2 EF-hand calcium-binding protein	9	
Pellitory (*Parietaria officinalis*)	Par o 1	100	IVR	Nonspecific lipid transfer protein 1, N-terminal sequence available	15	
Euphorbiaceae						
Mercury (*Mercurialis annua*)	Mer a 1	50–60	IVR	Profilin	14	

Abbreviations: IVR, *in vitro* reactivity (e.g., immunoblot, enzyme-linked immunosorbent assay, radioallergosorbent assay); MR, mediator release; MW, molecular weight; n.d., not determined; SF, sensitization frequency; SPT, skin prick test.

[a] Tested as mixture of Che a 1, Che a 2, and Che a.

can reach 60%–90%. Furthermore, a high prevalence of asthma and bronchial hyperresponsiveness has been observed in *Parietaria*-sensitized patients [5,8].

12.3 BIOLOGY OF WEEDS

According to their life cycle, weeds can be classified into annual weeds (summer and winter), biennial weeds, and perennial weeds (warm-season and cool-season perennials). Summer annual weeds germinate in spring or early summer, produce seeds during the summer, and die with cold weather or frost. *Amaranthus* is a good example of a summer annual weed. Winter annual weeds (e.g., pepperweed, *Lepidium*) germinate in fall or winter, overwinter during the coolest months, grow and produce seeds in spring, and die in summer. In contrast, biennial weeds germinate in spring and survive the first year in rosette stage. The production of seeds follows in the second growing season. Some *Brassica* species are biennial weeds.

Perennial weeds can be further classified into (1) warm-season perennial weeds that germinate in spring or summer and produce seeds in the first summer (e.g., *Artemisia* sp., *Rumex* sp., *Mentha* sp.) and (2) cool-season perennial weeds that germinate in fall or winter and produce their seeds in the first spring. In general, perennial weeds reproduce vegetatively and can survive for many years due to remaining underground structures.

During evolution, weeds acquired some special and advantageous characteristics: (1) a high reproductive output, (2) a bimodal reproduction with biennial and perennial members, (3) a discontinuous germination, (4) a high degree of adaptability and resistance to many given environmental extremes, and (5) fast growth and development.

Weeds are presently found worldwide and are often considered as an unwanted type of vegetation due to their aforementioned characteristics, their widespread distribution, and continuous spreading beyond their natural geographical locations. In man-made monocultures, weeds will normally fill in niches where the former vegetation, such as trees and forests, was eradicated. They can be collected and transported along with crops during harvesting processes because they are commonly found in agricultural environments. For example, ragweed was imported as ballast weed from North America to Europe at the beginning of the last century. Although initially confined to Hungary, ragweed is highly abundant in a number of European countries and spreading steadily. Another example is *Plantago*, originally native to Europe, but now growing abundantly worldwide [9].

Finally, pollen of weeds may cause allergic reactions. However, weeds can also have some beneficial effects. Some weeds are edible, their leaves and/or roots are used for herbal medicines, and some can be used in organic farming to attract insects that are beneficial for the crop.

12.4 WEED POLLEN ALLERGENS AND IgE CROSS-REACTIVITY

Ragweed, mugwort, pellitory, chenopod, Russian thistle, plantain, and annual mercury represent the most clinically relevant sources of pollen capable of eliciting allergic symptoms. Major weed pollen allergens can be found in the family of pectate lyases, defensin-like, Ole e 1–like, and nonspecific lipid transfer proteins (nsLTPs).

In addition, profilin and polcalcin are cross-reactive pan-allergens. At present, 47 weed pollen allergens are listed in the IUIS allergen nomenclature database (http:// www.allergen.org). An overview of identified molecules, biological function, and allergenic relevance is provided in Table 12.1. The geographical distribution of clinically important allergenic pollen sources is shown in Figure 12.1. Representative three-dimensional (3D) structures or models of weed pollen allergens are depicted in Figure 12.2.

12.4.1 Polysaccharide lyases

Pectate lyases are enzymes catalyzing the eliminative cleavage of pectin, a major component of the cell wall of many higher plants. They loosen the cell wall to facilitate pollen tube growth and breakdown of the cell wall. Amb a 1 represents the most important allergenic member of this protein family with a sensitization frequency of greater than 95% among ragweed-allergic individuals [5,10]. So far, five isoallergens with sequence homologies from 59% to 86% were identified. Amb a 1 is an acidic, nonglycosylated single-chain protein with a molecular weight of 38 kDa. In the past, it was reported that the protein undergoes proteolytic cleavage during extract preparation as well as purification of the natural protein, resulting in two fragments designated as α- (26kDa) and β- (12kDa) chains showing distinct immunologic properties [5,11]. Both chains of Amb a 1 isoform 1.0301 were produced as recombinant molecules after determination of the exact cleavage site. The α-chain, located at the C-terminus of the protein, displays limited IgE-binding capacity in contrast to the β-chain, which shows comparable allergenic potential as the natural molecule. Thus, the Amb a 1 α-chain was considered as a potential candidate to treat ragweed pollen allergy, since dominant T-cell epitopes of Amb a 1 are located in this C-terminal domain [12]. To further investigate the immunologic properties of the Amb a 1 isoallergens and due to the lack of high-quality recombinant molecules, the purification and characterization of natural allergens were pursued. Recently, a study was published describing a method for purification of natural Amb a 1 isoallergens without the appearance of proteolytic cleavage products. Detailed characterization of the purified Amb a 1 isoforms showed that these molecules exhibit distinct patterns in IgE binding and immunogenicity, with Amb a 1.0101 showing the highest IgE-binding activity [13]. Further, it was revealed that isoform 1.0101 is capable of inducing a strong TH2 immune response in mice in the absence of (extrinsic) adjuvants [14].

In contrast to the dominant IgE-binding activity of Amb a 1, only 26% sensitization prevalence was found for Art v 6, the homologous pectate lyase in mugwort pollen [15]. A study demonstrated that Art v 6 elicits less diverse IgE and T-cell responses than Amb a 1, even though Art v 6 shares 65% sequence identity with Amb a 1 [16]. In a further study, a hybrid molecule consisting of the α-chains of Amb a 1 and Art v 6 was designed, expressed in *Escherichia coli*, and purified to homogeneity. This accumulation of T-cell epitopes and deletion of IgE-reactive areas of the two allergens modulated the immunologic properties of the hybrid, leading to a promising novel candidate for therapeutic approaches [17]. Nevertheless, primary sensitization to Art v 6, which is commonly observed in areas with high mugwort pollen exposure, may also play a role in the development of cross-sensitization to Amb a 1. This was further investigated in enzyme-linked immunosorbent assay (ELISA) and ELISA inhibition experiments with clinically relevant pectate lyase

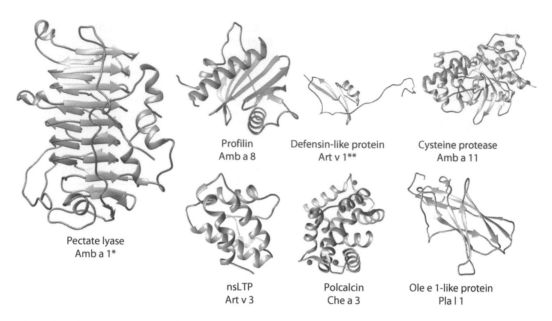

Figure 12.2 Three-dimensional structures of weed pollen allergens. PDB codes are given in Table 12.1. (*Amb a 1 model generated by Swiss Modeller [template 1PXZ]. **Defensin-like domain of Art v 1. Bound calcium depicted in red.)

allergens Amb a 1 and Art v 6, as well as tree pollen pectate lyase allergens from cypress and Japanese cedar (Cup a 1, Jun a 1, and Cry j 1) using serum samples from various cohorts. Results showed specific sensitization patterns for each geographic region, which reflected the natural allergen exposure of the patients. Significant cross-reactivity was found between the plant orders (Asteraceae and Cupressaceae); however, cross-reactivity was limited between the orders [18].

Sal k 1, the major allergen from Russian thistle, is a member of the pectin methylesterase family and thus part of the polysaccharide family. The polymorphic and slightly basic allergen has a molecular weight of 37 kDa and may be a marker allergen for genuine sensitization to *Salsola* [19]. About 67% of patients sensitized to *Salsola kali* recognized Sal k 1 when using a natural preparation [20]. Recently, the production of recombinant Sal k 1 was also shown as a further potential candidate for clinical diagnosis [21]. Additionally, an IgE-reactive polygalacturonase was identified and termed Sal k 6. The molecule shares IgE epitopes with Oleaceae members with IgE-inhibition values ranging from 20% to 60% [22]. A study was published using Sal k 1 expressed in *Lactococcus lactis* in a sublingual immunotherapy approach showing downregulation of the TH2 immune response in allergic mice [23]. In general, allergic reactions to Russian thistle can be frequent among individuals living in dry areas.

A further pectate lyase allergen was identified in sunflower and termed Hel a 6. A natural preparation of the allergenic molecule was used in skin prick test as well as basophil activation test, resulting in about 30% recognition and activation, respectively (data obtained from the World Health Organization [WHO]/IUIS Allergen Nomenclature Sub-Committee database).

12.4.2 Defensin-like proteins

Plant defensins are small, basic proteins stabilized by four disulfide bonds and were included in the pathogenesis-related (PR)-12 family. Art v 1, the major allergen of mugwort pollen, is a two-domain

protein consisting of an *N*-terminal defensin-like fold linked to a hydroxyproline-rich *C*-terminal region carrying plant-specific *O*-glycans. Among *Artemisia vulgaris*–allergic patients, up to 95% demonstrated IgE binding to Art v 1 [24,25]. Although patients' IgE are mainly reactive to the defensin-like domain [26], glycan moieties were also shown to be involved in antibody binding while their biological relevance in mediator release assays was negligible. The defensin-like fold is highly conserved and crucial for epitope formation since upon disruption of disulfide bonds, a loss in IgE reactivity was observed [27,28]. Nuclear magnetic resonance (NMR) studies identified two discontinuous human IgE epitopes located in the defensin-like and transitional domain [29]. Art v 1 presents a single immune-dominant T-cell epitope that is recognized by 96% of mugwort-allergic patients and presented by HLA-DRB*01 in a restricted manner [30]. Mugwort has been shown to trigger allergic reactions in 10%–14% of pollinosis patients in Europe and up to 11.3% of asthma and/or rhinitis patients in China [24,31,32]. Highly cross-reactive Art v 1 homologous molecules were shown to be present in other *Artemisia* species as well as sunflower pollen [33, unpublished data].

In contrast to Art v 1, the homologous allergen Amb a 4 does not represent a dominant IgE-binding protein in ragweed pollen. Using recombinant Amb a 4, a sensitization prevalence of 39%–42% could be demonstrated in different cohorts of weed pollen–allergic patients [28,34]. IgE reactivity of the recently cloned homologue Par h 1 from feverfew showed diverse sensitization profiles, and further studies in larger cohorts including patients with high feverfew pollen exposure are required to elucidate its primary sensitization capacity [6,28,35].

Art v 1, Amb a 4, and Par h 1 show high sequence homology within the defensin-like domain and overall similar structural features [28]. However, the *C*-terminus of Art v 1 is different regarding amino acid sequence as well as in *O*-glycosylation pattern [28,34–36]. Extensive, but patient-specific IgE cross-reactivity was observed in different patients' cohorts, and inhibition results suggest that mostly mugwort pollen Art v 1 is involved in primary sensitization. However, for a group of patients, primary sensitization to ragweed pollen Amb a 4 was also noted, which seems to be attributed to linear epitopes not depending on the cysteine-stabilized structure [28]. Simulated endolysosomal degradation revealed a distinct cleavage pattern, while the peptide region harboring the immunodominant T-cell epitope was preserved in all three allergens [37]. Interestingly, limited T-cell cross-reactivity was revealed between the three allergens when using T-cell lines or a cell line with the T-cell receptor specific for the immunodominant Art v 1 T-cell epitope [38].

12.4.3 Nonspecific lipid transfer proteins

Type I nonspecific lipid transfer proteins (nsLTPs) are small (9 kDa) basic proteins with a disulfide bond-stabilized α-helical structure, and binding of lipids was shown to impact the allergic sensitization [39]. They are members of the prolamin superfamily and were classified as PR-14 proteins due to their involvement in responses to abiotic and biotic stress. Allergenic nsLTPs are important food allergens, predominantly in the Mediterranean area, but are also present in pollen and latex. The 3D structure of Art v 3 (PDB: 6FRR) was recently solved presenting a high flexibility of the hydrophobic cavity (Wildner et al., manuscript in preparation). Art v 3 demonstrates a broad range of sensitization prevalence (22%–89%), which is particularly high in the Mediterranean areas but can also be observed in other geographic regions [40–42]. Four mugwort isoallergens were identified, and the recombinant proteins were suggested to be used as replacement for purified natural Art v 3, which is difficult to obtain in sufficient quantity and purity [43]. It was initially suggested that Art v 3 reactivity is merely observed as a consequence of sensitization to Pru p 3, a dominant allergen from peach, while later studies also showed its clinical relevance as a trigger of pollen allergies [44,45]. In mugwort highly exposed patients, primary sensitization to Art v 3 was also able to trigger pollen-food related syndromes with peaches [46].

In contrast to Art v 3, Amb a 6 is considered a minor allergen in ragweed pollen with a sensitization prevalence of 14% [24]. The allergen demonstrates less than 35% sequence identity to other allergenic nsLTPs and does not cross-react with Art v 3 [47]. Recent studies also revealed the presence of an Art v 3 cross-reactive molecule in pollen of feverfew [6]. While mass spectrometry–based analysis of IgE-reactive proteins in sunflower using Indian patients' sera did not identify a homolog in pollen, Hel a 3 was suggested to represent a food allergen in sunflower seeds [48,49].

The nsLTPs Par j 1 and Par j 2 were both identified as major allergens in the pollen from pellitory with a sensitization prevalence of 80%–95% [24]. The molecules show very low sequence identity to other allergenic members of the nsLTP family and display an elongated C-terminal region. The N-terminal region of both molecules constitutes a major target for IgE antibodies, and due to lacking IgE cross-reactivity with other nsLTPs, Par j 2 was suggested as the marker allergen for diagnosis of *Parietaria* pollen allergy [50–52].

12.4.4 Ole e 1–like proteins

The common feature of proteins within this family is the presence of six conserved cysteine residues and the Ole e 1 consensus pattern sequence [EQT]-G-x-V-Y-C-D-[TNP]-C-R. Otherwise, Ole e 1–like glycoproteins can show a high degree of heterogeneity in the amino acid sequence. Allergenic members of this protein family in weeds can be found in pollen from plantain (Pla l 1), chenopod (Che a 1), Russian thistle (Sal k 5), and redroot pigweed (Ama r 1).

Among plantain-sensitized patients, up to 92% react to the major allergen Pla l 1 [53,54]. Recently, the 3D structure of Pla l 1 was solved by x-ray crystallography, revealing for the first time the Ole e 1–like structure consistent of a seven-stranded β-barrel with four pronounced loop regions (PDB: 4Z8W) [55]. The highest structural similarity was found with cell-wall surface anchor proteins, while the previously suggested trypsin inhibitor function was experimentally ruled out. Inhibition studies using various Ole e 1–like allergens showed lack of IgE cross-reactivity with other allergenic Ole e 1–like family members. Thus, the primary sensitization capacity of Pla l 1 was unequivocally proven, also rendering the molecule an excellent diagnostic tool for English plantain pollen allergy [54,55].

Other Ole e 1–like weed pollen allergens were found in the Amaranthaceae family [7]. Che a 1 is an important allergen of chenopod displaying a sensitization frequency up to 77% [56]. Sal k 5 from Russian thistle represents a minor allergen in the source with a sensitization prevalence between 30% and 40% [57]. While high IgE cross-reactivity between Che a 1 and Sal k 5 was observed, limited cross-inhibition with Ole e 1 was detected, presumably due to low sequence homology [56,57]. Recombinant Pla l 1, Che a 1, and Sal k 5 were produced in *E. coli* or *Pichia pastoris*, resulting in nonglycosylated and yeast-specific glycosylated molecules. Since antibody reactivity was comparable to the purified natural allergens, it was concluded that respective glycan moieties do not constitute relevant epitopes, which is in contrast to results reported for Ole e 1 [55,57–60]. A similar sensitization prevalence of 38% was found for the recently identified Ama r 1 from amaranth [61] and based on high sequence similarity with Che a 1, IgE cross-reactivity is anticipated. Another new member is Koc s 1 from pollen of *Kochia scoparia*, a plant abundant in tropical and subtropical areas [62]. In an *in vitro* assay simulating endolysosomal processing upon antigen uptake, similar kinetics and peptide pattern of the investigated weed pollen allergens were found for Che a 1 and Sal k 5, while Pla l 1 showed divergent results [63].

12.4.5 Profilins

The members of the profilin family are small proteins (14 kDa) expressed in all eukaryotic cells and some viruses, sharing greater than 75% sequence identities [64,65]. Their conformation displays a central antiparallel β-sheet core surrounded by α helices representative of α/β proteins. Profilins are actin-monomer-binding proteins promoting the polymerization of actin filaments for the cytoskeleton's turnover and are, therefore, involved in cell motility, cytokinesis, and outgrowth of the pollen tube [66–69]. Additional binding partners have been identified, including phosphatidylinositols and L-proline-rich proteins, suggesting the contribution of profilins in other essential cellular processes, such as exocytosis-endocytosis and in signaling pathways [70].

The prevalence of sensitization to profilin allergens is about 5%–40% worldwide [64,65,71]. This variability results from various influencing factors including geographical factors. For example, sensitization rates to mugwort and ragweed profilins among weed pollen–allergic patients was found to be lower in Italian individuals (20%) compared to Austrians (45%–50%) [71].

To date, 43 profilin allergens have officially been acknowledged by the WHO/IUIS Allergen Nomenclature Sub-Committee. The first allergenic profilin identified was Bet v 2 from birch pollen

(*Betula pendula*) in 1991 [72]. Since, more have been identified in tree, grass, and weed pollens, in various plant-derived food (fruits, vegetables, legumes, nuts) and in latex [64].

Due to their ubiquitous distribution and their highly conserved 3D structure, profilins are classified as pan-allergens that are responsible for many IgE reactions [65,73]. For example, profilins from ragweed (Amb a 8), mugwort (Art v 4), and sunflower pollen (Hel a 2), which are considered minor allergens with sensitization frequencies ranging from 30% to 35%, demonstrate a high level of identity at the amino acid level leading to extensive IgE cross-reactivity among the Asteraceae family [71,74,75]. Interestingly, some profilins from other weed pollen sources seem to play an even more significant role in weed pollen allergy. Che a 2, for instance, the chenopod profilin, showed IgE reactivity with 55% of tested sera suggesting a relevant role in chenopod allergy [76]. Par j 3 from pellitory also showed limited IgE cross-reactivity among profilin-sensitized patients although it shares high sequence homology with other profilins [77]. In contrast, considerable IgE cross-reactivity has been observed between Sal k 4 and Ama r 2, the profilins from Russian thistle and pigweed, respectively [78,79].

Profilin pan-allergens are both found in pollen and in food sources and have been associated with the pollen-food allergy syndrome. Symptoms are usually limited to reactions in the oral cavity because these allergens are labile to heat and gastric digestion. Therefore, it is assumed that they cannot cause sensitization through the gastrointestinal tract [80].

12.4.6 Polcalcins

Polcalcins are α-helical proteins that belong to the calcium-binding protein family and contain the characteristic EF-hand motifs (helix-loop-helix structure) enabling the binding of calcium. According to the number of EF-hand motifs, polcalcins are classified into three groups: those with two (Art v 5, Amb a 9), three (Amb a 10), or four calcium-binding domains [71]. Depending on this and the formation of dimers for some polcalcins, their molecular weight varies between 9 and 28 kDa.

The biological function of polcalcin proteins is still uncertain, but their ability to bind calcium contributing to the regulation of intracellular calcium levels suggests a role in pollen tube growth [81]. The binding of calcium induces a conformational change that influences the IgE reactivity and the thermal stability of the polcalcin protein. In fact, unlike the closed, Ca-free apo-form, which is less thermostable, the open, Ca-bound holo-form is more stable and results in stronger interaction with IgE antibodies [82].

So far, 15 polcalcin allergens have been identified and officially acknowledged by the WHO/IUIS Allergen Nomenclature Sub-Committee. As polcalcins are pan-allergens restrictively expressed in pollen, these proteins are highly cross-reactive but are not implicated in pollen-food allergy syndromes. They cause respiratory reactions upon inhalation with a sensitization frequency of 5%–10% among pollen-allergic patients [64,65].

Concerning weed pollen allergens, Amb a 9 and Amb a 10 from ragweed and Art v 5 from mugwort pollen represent minor allergens, displaying around 10% and 25% IgE reactivity for patients from central and southern Europe, respectively [71]. Pellitory polcalcin, Par j 4, displays a much lower level of IgE reactivity, which seems to be due to cross-reactivity to other polcalcins that can act as primary sensitizers [83]. In contrast, 46% of chenopod-sensitized patients recognized the polcalcin, Che a 3 [76].

12.4.7 Cysteine proteases

A new protein family has been added to the classification of weed pollen allergens since the identification of a further major allergen from ragweed pollen, namely, Amb a 11 [84]. Amb a 11 is a 28 kDa glycosylated protein belonging to the peptidase family C1 (papain family, clan CA) [85]. This family includes other major allergens from different sources, such as Der p 1 and Der f 1 from house dust mites, Act d 1 from kiwi, and papain Car p 1 from papaya, that share sequence similarities with Amb a 11. Its 3D structure has been determined by x-ray crystallography showing two distinct globular domains representative of the folding of cysteine proteases [84,86]. The enzymatic activity of cysteine proteases can cause epithelial barrier disruption and modulate immune cell regulation, thus contributing to the severity of allergic inflammations.

Besides Amb a 1 showing a sensitization rate of greater than 90% [87], Amb a 11 is also considered as an important major allergen from ragweed with a sensitization prevalence of around 66% among ragweed-allergic individuals from Europe and North America [85]. Therefore, both Amb a 1 and Amb a 11 should be considered as marker allergens for diagnostics and immunotherapeutic approaches.

12.5 POLLEN–FOOD SYNDROMES ASSOCIATED WITH WEED SENSITIZATION

Pollen–food syndromes with association to weed pollen allergy were mainly described for allergens found in the Asteraceae family [88]. For *Artemisia*, the most prominent examples are the mugwort-celery-spice syndrome and the mugwort-peach association. Ragweed sensitization seems to be involved in the ragweed-melon-banana association. At the molecular level, identified causative IgE cross-reactive allergens are suggested to be nsLTPs, profilins, high-molecular-weight components, and/or glycoallergens [46,89–92].

12.6 DIAGNOSIS OF WEED POLLEN ALLERGY

Skin prick testing with allergen extracts allows clinicians to identify sensitivity to a given pollen. But extract-based allergy diagnosis of weed pollen is often difficult due to multisensitization of patients, overlapping flowering seasons, and similar allergen profiles [87]. However, component-resolved diagnosis offers the possibility to study IgE reactivity to individual allergens. Correctly confirming the diagnosis of ragweed and mugwort pollen allergy represents a major clinical problem in areas where both plants are endemic. Discrimination between cosensitization and cross-reactivity is essential for decision-making regarding allergen immunotherapy. Sensitization to both commonly occurs; however, ragweed Amb a 1 belongs to the pectate lyase family, whereas mugwort Art v 1 represents a defensin-like glycoprotein belonging to the pathogenesis-related protein family 12 (PR-12) [4,47]. Although ragweed Amb a 4 and mugwort Art v 6 are minor allergens, they are homologous to the major allergens, Art v 1 and Amb a 1, respectively. In addition, the cross-reactive pan-allergens, profilins, and nsLTPs, as well as polcalcins present in both pollens hamper the accurate diagnosis when using pollen extracts. However, the pan-allergens are only to a minor extent accountable for the cross-reactivity of IgE antibodies [4,15].

A study performed by Asero et al. addressed the question of cosensitization versus cross-reactivity of ragweed and mugwort pollen allergy in Italy. Analyses of the sensitization profiles of a cohort of 372 Asteraceae-allergic individuals show that 31% reacted with extracts of plants, 32% with ragweed, and 7% with mugwort only; 46% of selected double-positive patients reacted with Art v 1 and showed limited cross-reactivity with Amb a 4, whereas 92% recognized Amb a 1 but only 25% cross-reacted with mugwort Art v 6. Thus, ragweed- and mugwort-allergic patients seem to be cosensitized to both weed species, and cross-reactivity seems to be mainly due to pan-allergens [15].

Another study by Jahn-Schmid et al. further investigated the IgE cross-reactivity between Amb a 1 and Art v 6, showing that the IgE cross-reactivity highly depends on the exposure to mugwort pollen. Ragweed-allergic patients from Italy showed no or only low cross-reactivity, whereas mugwort-allergic patients from Austria displayed distinct cross-reactivity patterns. However, inhibition experiments demonstrated that Art v 6 contains additional, non-cross-reactive IgE epitopes; thus, Art v 6 can also act as the primary sensitizing allergen. The primary sensitizing capacity of Art v 6 could play a role in the development of cross-sensitization to ragweed pollen [16].

Helianthus, as well as *Parthenium,* also belong to the family of Asteraceae, and although both plants have been reported as allergenic sources, knowledge on allergens is limited. Currently, three allergenic molecules from sunflower pollen (the 34 kDa protein Hel a 1, the profilin Hel a 2, and Hel a 6, a pectate lyase) and one from sunflower seed (Hel a 3, a nsLTP) have been identified, and IgE cross-reactivity with other Asteraceae pollen has been reported [48,93]. In *Parthenium,* Par h 1, a hydroxyproline-rich protein has been identified and purified, which is a member of the PR-12 protein family. A study by Pablos et al. showed that sensitization to Par h 1 in weed pollen-allergic patients from Austria, Canada, and Korea is mainly due to cross-reactivity with Art v 1 and Amb a 4. However, some patients reacted exclusively to Amb a 4 and Pa h 1, indicating a common epitope that is not shared with Art v 1. Therefore, Amb a 4 should be included in molecule-based diagnosis of weed pollen allergies [6,28].

Cross-reactivity versus cosensitization is not an exclusive problem associated with ragweed and mugwort allergies. This question also needs to be addressed at the molecular level for Amaranthaceae allergies. Three purified recombinant allergens from *Chenopodium* (Che a 1–3) versus white goosefoot pollen extracts have been tested for efficacy to diagnose clinical allergy [94]. Only one out of 30 *Chenopodium*-allergic individuals could not be successfully diagnosed with the selected panel of allergens. Besides *Chenopodium, Salsola kali* pollen is frequently associated with clinical Amaranthaceae allergy. A certain degree of cross-reactivity between the two species is reported mainly due to the Ole e 1-homologues Sal k 5 and Che a 1 as well as the profilins Sal k 4 and Che a 2. However, Sal k 1 seems to be the main sensitizer of *Salsola* pollen, whereas Che a 1, Che a 2, and Che a 3 seem to be responsible for sensitization to *Chenopodium.* Thus, cross-reactivity and clinical allergy caused by related species belonging to the Amaranthaceae family should be investigated in more detail resulting in improved diagnosis and management of allergic patients [95].

English plantain represents the most important allergen source from the Plantaginaceae family. Although English plantain pollen is

an important cause of allergic reactions, it is usually not included in routine diagnosis [24]. However, extract-based diagnosis is often difficult due to the multisensitization of plantain pollen-sensitized patients. Pla l 1, the major allergen of English plantain, is a member of the Ole e 1–like family sharing only around 40% sequence identity with other homologous allergens. Recent studies showed that Pla l 1 represents the most reliable diagnostic marker for genuine plantain sensitization due to the lacking IgE cross-reactivity with homologous allergens [55,96].

Concomitant exposure to several weeds makes a correct diagnosis difficult. In a study by Moverare et al., the sensitization patterns of mugwort-allergic individuals from different geographic areas (North America, northern and southern Europe) were compared [97]. IgE reactivity to mugwort Art v 1 was common in patients from northern and southern Europe but quite rare among individuals from North America. In contrast, only a minority of the European serum samples contained antibodies against ragweed Amb a 1, whereas among the American weed pollen-allergic population, the prevalence of sensitization to Amb a 1 was around 68%. Of note, sensitization to botanically unrelated allergenic weed species, such as *Parietaria,* was also common in regions where the plants were endemic. These differences in sensitization pattern most likely reflect the geographic distribution of different weeds.

In parts of Asia, allergic reactions to *Artemisia* seem to play an even more intriguing role, since they demonstrate an 11.3% sensitization rate among pollinosis patients [32,98]. Although mugwort is considered one of the most important pollen sources to trigger respiratory allergy symptoms, detailed information regarding the sensitization profile toward single mugwort pollen allergens in an Asian cohort is limited [99]. The relevance of Art v 1 and Art v 3 for *Artemisia*-sensitized patients living in Asia has been demonstrated. Since ragweed is also endemic in Asia, component-resolved diagnosis is particularly useful to help discriminate between cross-reactivity and cosensitization. Sensitization to ragweed pollen in China is reported to range between 6.5% and 7.4% among patients suffering from pollinosis, making ragweed an important elicitor of pollen allergy in this country [32,98].

To conclude, the correct diagnosis of weed pollen allergy is a challenging task. Skin and *in vitro* testing are still performed using difficult-to-standardize allergen extracts; however, determining specific IgE to individual allergens would be advantageous. Great progress in allergen identification and characterization has been achieved within the past several years. Molecule-based allergy diagnosis will not only help to identify specific disease-eliciting allergens but also to understand sensitization patterns and IgE cross-reactivity, enabling the physician to make a more accurate characterization of an allergic condition.

Currently, molecule-based allergy diagnostic tests are available for clinical use in a single or multiplex format. The ImmunoCAP platform (Phadia) quantifies IgE binding to six distinct weed pollen allergens: Amb a 1, Art v 1, Art v 3, Par j 2, Pla l 1, and Sal k 1. The Immuno Solid-phase Allergen Chip (ImmunoCAP ISAC, ThermoFisher Scientific) multiplex microarray system or the Mechanisms of the Development of ALLergy (MeDALL) chip will identify two additional weed pollen allergens, Che a 1 and Mer a 1 [100]. Another type of macroarray is based on the nanobead technology in which allergen molecules or allergen extracts are coupled to chemically activated nanoparticles and are then arrayed to a solid-phase matrix. Examples based on this technology are the FABER chip with 122 purified allergens (4 weed allergens) and 122 protein extracts (3 weed extracts) or the Allergy Explorer kit called ALEX with 282 allergen extracts and molecular allergens (15 weed extracts and 7 weed allergens) [101]. ALEX is the first *in vitro* multiplex allergy test allowing the simultaneous measurement of total and specific IgE (sIgE). Nevertheless, additional research on allergenic molecules will facilitate their accessibility and broaden the panel of allergens commercially available for component-resolved diagnosis.

12.7 SPECIFIC IMMUNOTHERAPY: PAST AND NOVEL DEVELOPMENTS

The first successful weed pollen allergen immunotherapy (AIT) trial was reported by George Clowes in 1913. The author used aqueous ragweed pollen extracts injected subcutaneously to ameliorate allergic symptoms of eight ragweed-allergic subjects [102]. More than 100 years have passed, but weed pollen allergies are still routinely treated with pollen extracts. The major disadvantages of extract-based subcutaneous immunotherapy (SCIT) are related to the risk of treatment-induced systemic reactions including anaphylaxis, and the frequent and long-lasting dosing schedule, which usually lasts for several years.

The first modifications that successfully attenuated adverse side effects caused by injections of pollen extracts were formulations of allergen extracts with aluminum hydroxide, which is currently the most widely used adjuvant in AIT. In general, the effectiveness of ragweed pollen IT has been demonstrated to be highly dose dependent, with high doses being required for effectiveness, but at the same time increasing the risk of IgE-mediated side effects. Thus, the optimal treatment dose of ragweed pollen extract for immunotherapy was determined to be between 0.6 μg and 12.4 μg per injection in terms of Amb a 1 equivalents [103]. The next development in ragweed IT aimed to introduce modifications causing structural changes of proteins in the allergenic extracts and leading to reduced IgE-binding activity. However, due to difficulties in reproducibility, only chemical cross-linking of allergen preparations yielding allergoids had a sustainable effect [104].

The anti-IgE therapy (Omalizumab) has been developed as a general, allergen-independent approach and shown to reduce circulating levels of IgE, to inhibit early and late-phase responses to allergen, and to clinically protect against disease exacerbation [105]. The use of anti-IgE therapy in combination with allergen-specific immunotherapy has been explored for ragweed allergy. Omalizumab was administered during a 9-week pretreatment phase and during the 12-week period of rush immunotherapy with ragweed extracts. The results demonstrated that the combination of anti-IgE with ragweed immunotherapy reduced seasonal severity scores and had fewer adverse events compared to extract immunotherapy alone [106]. Further studies demonstrated that the benefit of the combined anti-IgE and ragweed immunotherapy is due to prolonged and complete inhibition of allergen-IgE interactions by immunotherapy-induced "blocking" IgG4 antibodies and direct blocking of IgE binding to its low-affinity receptor CD23 [107].

The cross talk of antigen with receptors of the innate immune system is crucial for the subsequent development of immune responses. In this regard, several approaches are being developed to improve allergen IT. The nonpyrogenic component of *Salmonella minnesota* LPS monophosphoryl lipid (MPL) A was combined with chemically cross-linked ragweed pollen extracts adsorbed to L-tyrosine in order to boost immunogenicity while modifying the immunologic properties of ragweed allergens [108]. MPL acts as a toll-like receptor 4 (TLR4) agonist and is capable of potentiating ragweed-specific immune responses. In this way, the use of MPL allowed a shorter treatment schedule of four injections in a 3-week interval. This represents a great improvement over the standard IT regimen, which uses approximately 50 injections over a period of 3–5 years.

A very interesting approach was the chemical coupling of purified ragweed Amb a 1 to a TLR9 agonist for allergy vaccination. This strategy addressed two common problems associated with IT: (1) safety and standardization problems (total allergen content, composition) of allergenic extracts by using the purified allergen and (2) poor immunogenic activity and TH2 bias by using a TLR agonist as adjuvant. In a randomized placebo-controlled study, purified Amb a 1 conjugated to immune-modulatory oligodeoxynucleotide (AIC) (mean conjugation efficacy 1:4) was administered in six injections with increasing concentrations in weekly intervals prior to the start of the pollen season. In the first posttreatment season, no differences in the patients' symptom and medication scores were observed. However, in the second year of the follow-up phase, the chest symptoms were significantly decreased [109]. Using the same treatment schedule described earlier, Creticos et al. performed a randomized, double-blind, placebo-controlled phase II trial with AIC [110]. The actively treated group showed a reduction in rhinitis symptoms during the ragweed season when compared to the placebo group, and this effect was maintained through the following year. Of note, AIC treatment induced only a transient increase in allergen-specific IgG but suppressed the seasonal increase in Amb a 1–specific IgE antibodies. Based on these promising results, a large AIC clinical study including 738 ragweed-allergic patients in 30 centers was initiated. However, no significant improvements in the treatment groups could be detected when evaluating the total nasal symptom scores. Consequently, the AIC program was discontinued (http://www.drugs.com).

The advent of the recombinant DNA technology opened exciting new possibilities to replace allergen extracts with purified recombinant allergens [111]. Moreover, genetic engineering approaches were introduced allowing the design of low-IgE binding, highly immunogenic molecules able to selectively target and modify the allergic immune response. In this regard, the knowledge of the structures of the major allergens of *Parietaria* Par j 1 and *Artemisia* Art v 1, which were shown to be stabilized by disulfide bonds, was successfully used to generate cysteine variants showing reduced IgE binding but conserved T-cell activating properties [5,27]. Moreover, two studies reported on the generation of hybrid molecules of *Parietaria* Par j 1 and 2 as candidates for IT. The hybrids were engineered as head-to-tail fusion proteins. In one approach, both nsLTP allergens were additionally mutated at distinct cysteine residues to disrupt IgE epitopes on the hybrid [112], whereas in another approach the amino acid residues shown to be crucial for IgE binding to the nsLTPs were mutated in the hybrid molecule [113]. Both hybrids showed patients had reduced IgE-binding activity and retained T-cell reactivity, and both were able to induce protective IgG antibodies against wild-type allergens in preclinical animal models. More recently, a novel vaccine candidate for mugwort allergy has been developed consisting of a fusion of the TLR5-ligand Flagellin A from *Listeria* and wild-type or hypoallergenic versions of Art v 1. In animal models, the Flagellin-Art v 1 fusion proteins induced a strong mTOR-dependent secretion of IL-10 in dendritic cells and suppressed the secretion of allergen-specific TH2 cytokines, both *in vitro* and *in vivo* [114]. The fusion technology was also used to engineer a hybrid molecule containing the T-cell epitope-rich and low IgE-binding C-terminal domains of Amb a 1 and Art v 6, respectively. The hybrid hypoallergenic molecule induced T-cell proliferative responses in human PBMC comparable to those of the natural allergens and induced a mixed TH1-TH2 response in a mouse immunization model [17].

Besides subcutaneous injections, the oral/sublingual route has been suggested as an alternative for allergy vaccine application. Oral delivery of allergens has in general the problem that the proteins are destroyed during digestion. As a possible solution to this problem, Litwin et al. performed a double-blind placebo-controlled study with encapsulated ragweed pollen extracts, which allowed delivery of immunologically intact antigen to the small intestine. Active therapy induced the induction of ragweed-specific IgG antibodies, had a suppressive effect on the rise of IgE titers during the pollen season, and could decrease the medication scores in the active group compared to the placebo [115]. Another clinical study tested the safety and efficacy profiles of ragweed pollen extracts formulated as tablets and drops for sublingual administration. In a cohort of 110 outpatients, 50% received active treatment and 50% placebo. Mild to moderate adverse reactions in the oral cavity as well as in the gastrointestinal tract were reported in the actively treated group. The treatment group that received the highest dose of IT showed significant improvement of rhinitis and conjunctivitis scores compared to lower doses as well as to placebo. Thus, this study demonstrated the potential of pollen sublingual immunotherapy but also showed high dose dependence for treatment efficacy and the risk of side effects associated with the use of pollen extracts [116]. Such dose dependence was confirmed in a clinical trial by Skoner et al. in which 48 μg Amb a 1 per day (high maintenance dose) formulated as glycerinated pollen extract and applied in a sublingual swallow regimen was shown to be effective in reducing symptoms of weed pollen allergy [117]. Of note, a 10-fold lower dose was almost as effective as the high-dose treatment regime. More recently, a phase 3, randomized, placebo-controlled trial was conducted in North America using a standardized glycerinated short ragweed sublingual extract solution (RW-SAIL) in subjects with ragweed-related allergic rhinoconjunctivitis [118]. The study successfully demonstrated the tolerability and efficacy of the RW-SAIL sublingual liquid preparation. Another study investigated the clinical efficacy of ragweed sublingual tablets. Canadian patients treated once daily with MK-3641 immunotherapy tablet with 12 Amb a 1 units showed significant reduction of ragweed-induced allergic rhinoconjunctivitis during the entire ragweed pollen season [119].

It should be mentioned that in addition to the previously mentioned ragweed studies, other clinical trials with *Parietaria* showed that sublingual IT is effective not only in adults but also in children with allergic rhinoconjunctivitis [120]. In summary, the future perspectives for IT look very promising: novel treatment forms with higher efficacy and safety profiles are being evaluated in clinical trials, which will help to improve the outlook for weed pollen-allergic patients [24,121–124].

SALIENT POINTS

- The term *weed* is not a botanical classification but is used to describe a highly heterogeneous group of plants mostly lacking appreciable economic or esthetic value.
- *Ambrosia* (ragweed), *Artemisia* (mugwort), *Parietaria* (pellitory), *Chenopodium* (chenopod), *Salsola* (Russian thistle), *Plantago* (plantain), and *Mercurialis* (annual mercury) represent the most clinically relevant sources of pollen capable of eliciting allergenic symptoms.
- Forty-seven weed pollen allergens are listed in the WHO/IUIS Allergen Nomenclature Sub-Committee database. Major weed pollen allergens belong to the family of pectate lyases, defensin-like, Ole e 1–like, and nonspecific lipid transfer proteins. Profilin and polcalcin are cross-reactive weed pollen pan-allergens.
- Commercially available molecule-based diagnostic tests make it possible to quantify IgE binding to nine distinct weed pollen allergens: ragweed Amb a 1 and Amb a 4, mugwort Art v 1 and Art v 3, pellitory Par j 2, Russian thistle Sal k 1, chenopod Che a 1, annual mercury Mer a 1, and plantain Pla l 1.
- Clinical trials with allergenic extracts utilized both subcutaneous and sublingual immunotherapy routes. Different adjuvants such as alum, TLR agonists (monophosphoryl lipid A for TLR4, CpG for TLR9), and optimal doses have been tested. In addition, a combination of anti-IgE and ragweed immunotherapy delivered promising results.
- Novel allergen derivatives based on ragweed Amb a 1, mugwort Art v 1, and pellitory Par j 1 and Par j 2 are being developed for safer and more effective forms of specific immunotherapy.

REFERENCES

1. Gergen PJ, Turkeltaub PC, Kovar MG. The prevalence of allergic skin test reactivity to eight common aeroallergens in the U.S. population: Results from the second National Health and Nutrition Examination Survey. *J Allergy Clin Immunol* 1987; 80(5): 669–679.
2. Arbes SJ, Jr., Gergen PJ, Elliott L, Zeldin DC. Prevalences of positive skin test responses to 10 common allergens in the US population: Results from the third National Health and Nutrition Examination Survey. *J Allergy Clin Immunol* 2005; 116(2): 377–383.
3. Salo PM, Arbes SJ Jr., Jaramillo R et al. Prevalence of allergic sensitization in the United States: Results from the National Health and Nutrition Examination Survey (NHANES) 2005–2006. *J Allergy Clin Immunol* 2014; 134(2): 350–359.
4. Wopfner N, Gadermaier G, Egger M et al. The spectrum of allergens in ragweed and mugwort pollen. *Int Arch Allergy Immunol* 2005; 138(4): 337–346.
5. Gadermaier G, Dedic A, Obermeyer G, Frank S, Himly M, Ferreira F. Biology of weed pollen allergens. *Curr Allergy Asthma Rep* 2004; 4(5): 391–400.
6. Pablos I, Eichhorn S, Briza P et al. Proteomic profiling of the weed feverfew, a neglected pollen allergen source. *Sci Rep* 2017; 7(1): 6049.
7. Villalba M, Barderas R, Mas S, Colas C, Batanero E, Rodriguez R. Amaranthaceae pollens: Review of an emerging allergy in the Mediterranean area. *J Investig Allergol Clin Immunol* 2014; 24(6): 371–381; quiz 2 p preceding 82.
8. Bonura A, Di Blasi D, Barletta B et al. Modulating allergic response by engineering the major Parietaria allergens. *J Allergy Clin Immunol* 2018; 141(3): 1142–1144.e3.
9. D'Amato G, Cecchi L, Bonini S et al. Allergenic pollen and pollen allergy in Europe. *Allergy* 2007; 62(9): 976–990.
10. Bordas-Le Floch V, Le Mignon M, Bouley J et al. Identification of novel short ragweed pollen allergens using combined transcriptomic and immunoproteomic approaches. *PLOS ONE* 2015; 10(8): e0136258.

11. Wopfner N, Jahn-Schmid B, Schmidt G et al. The α and β subchain of Amb a 1, the major ragweed-pollen allergen show divergent reactivity at the IgE and T-cell level. *Mol Immunol* 2009; 46(10): 2090–2097.

12. Jahn-Schmid B, Wopfner N, Hubinger G et al. The T-cell response to Amb a 1 is characterized by 3 dominant epitopes and multiple MHC restriction elements. *J Allergy Clin Immunol* 2010; 126(5): 1068–1071, 1071.e1–2.

13. Wolf M, Twaroch TE, Huber S et al. Amb a 1 isoforms: Unequal siblings with distinct immunological features. *Allergy* 2017; 72(12): 1874–1882.

14. Wolf M, Aglas L, Twaroch TE et al. Endolysosomal protease susceptibility of Amb a 1 as a determinant of allergenicity. *J Allergy Clin Immunol* 2018; 141(4): 1488–1491.e5.

15. Asero R, Wopfner N, Gruber P, Gadermaier G, Ferreira F. *Artemisia* and *Ambrosia* hypersensitivity: Co-sensitization or co-recognition? *Clin Exp Allergy* 2006; 36(5): 658–665.

16. Jahn-Schmid B, Hauser M, Wopfner N et al. Humoral and cellular cross-reactivity between Amb a 1, the major ragweed pollen allergen, and its mugwort homolog Art v 6. *J Immunol* 2012; 188(3): 1559–1567.

17. Sancho AI, Wallner M, Hauser M et al. T cell epitope-containing domains of ragweed Amb a 1 and Mugwort Art v 6 modulate immunologic responses in humans and mice. *PLOS ONE* 2017; 12(1): e0169784.

18. Pichler U, Hauser M, Wolf M et al. Pectate lyase pollen allergens: Sensitization profiles and cross-reactivity pattern. *PLOS ONE* 2015; 10(5): e0120038.

19. Barderas R, Garcia-Selles J, Salamanca G et al. A pectin methylesterase as an allergenic marker for the sensitization to Russian thistle (*Salsola kali*) pollen. *Clin Exp Allergy* 2007; 37(7): 1111–1119.

20. Carnes J, Fernandez-Caldas E, Marina A et al. Immunochemical characterization of Russian thistle (*Salsola kali*) pollen extracts. Purification of the allergen Sal k 1. *Allergy* 2003; 58(11): 1152–1156.

21. Mas S, Boissy P, Monsalve RI et al. A recombinant Sal k 1 isoform as an alternative to the polymorphic allergen from *Salsola kali* pollen for allergy diagnosis. *Int Arch Allergy Immunol* 2015; 167(2): 83–93.

22. Mas S, Oeo-Santos C, Cuesta-Herranz J et al. A relevant IgE-reactive 28kDa protein identified from *Salsola kali* pollen extract by proteomics is a natural degradation product of an integral 47kDa polygalacturonase. *Biochim Biophys Acta Proteins Proteom* 2017; 1865(8): 1067–1076.

23. Ghasemi Z, Varasteh AR, Moghadam M, Jalali SA, Anissian A, Sankian M. Sublingual immunotherapy with Sal k1 expressing *Lactococcus Lactis* down-regulates Th2 immune responses in Balb/c mice. *Iran J Allergy Asthma Immunol* 2018; 17(3): 281–290.

24. Gadermaier G, Hauser M, Ferreira F. Allergens of weed pollen: An overview on recombinant and natural molecules. *Methods* 2014; 66(1): 55–66.

25. Himly M, Jahn-Schmid B, Dedic A et al. Art v 1, the major allergen of mugwort pollen, is a modular glycoprotein with a defensin-like and a hydroxyproline-rich domain. *FASEB J* 2003; 17(1): 106–108.

26. Dedic A, Gadermaier G, Vogel L et al. Immune recognition of novel isoforms and domains of the mugwort pollen major allergen Art v 1. *Mol Immunol* 2009; 46(3): 416–421.

27. Gadermaier G, Jahn-Schmid B, Vogel L et al. Targeting the cysteine-stabilized fold of Art v 1 for immunotherapy of *Artemisia* pollen allergy. *Mol Immunol* 2010; 47(6): 1292–1298.

28. Pablos I, Eichhorn S, Machado Y et al. Distinct epitope structures of defensin-like proteins linked to proline-rich regions give rise to differences in their allergenic activity. *Allergy* 2018; 73(2): 431–441.

29. Razzera G, Gadermaier G, de Paula V et al. Mapping the interactions between a major pollen allergen and human IgE antibodies. *Structure* 2010; 18(8): 1011–1021.

30. Jahn-Schmid B, Fischer GF, Bohle B et al. Antigen presentation of the immunodominant T-cell epitope of the major mugwort pollen allergen, Art v 1, is associated with the expression of HLA-DRB1 *01. *J Allergy Clin Immunol* 2005; 115(2): 399–404.

31. Hao GD, Zheng YW, Gjesing B et al. Prevalence of sensitization to weed pollens of *Humulus scandens*, *Artemisia vulgaris*, and *Ambrosia artemisiifolia* in northern China. *J Zhejiang Univ Sci B* 2013; 14(3): 240–246.

32. Li J, Sun B, Huang Y et al. A multicentre study assessing the prevalence of sensitizations in patients with asthma and/or rhinitis in China. *Allergy* 2009; 64(7): 1083–1092.

33. Gruber P, Gadermaier G, Bauer R et al. Role of the polypeptide backbone and post-translational modifications in cross-reactivity of Art v 1, the major mugwort pollen allergen. *Biol Chem* 2009; 390(5–6): 445–451.

34. Leonard R, Wopfner N, Pabst M et al. A new allergen from ragweed (*Ambrosia artemisiifolia*) with homology to Art v 1 from mugwort. *J Biol Chem* 2010; 285(35): 27192–27200.

35. Gupta N, Martin BM, Metcalfe DD, Rao PV. Identification of a novel hydroxyproline-rich glycoprotein as the major allergen in Parthenium pollen. *J Allergy Clin Immunol* 1996; 98(5 Pt 1): 903–912.

36. Leonard R, Petersen BO, Himly M et al. Two novel types of O-glycans on the mugwort pollen allergen Art v 1 and their role in antibody binding. *J Biol Chem* 2005; 280(9): 7932–7940.

37. Jahn-Schmid B, Kelemen P, Himly M et al. The T cell response to Art v 1, the major mugwort pollen allergen, is dominated by one epitope. *J Immunol* 2002; 169(10): 6005–6011.

38. Leb VM, Jahn-Schmid B, Schmetterer KG et al. Molecular and functional analysis of the antigen receptor of Art v 1-specific helper T lymphocytes. *J Allergy Clin Immunol* 2008; 121(1): 64–71.

39. Scheurer S, Schulke S. Interaction of non-specific lipid-transfer proteins with plant-derived lipids and its impact on allergic sensitization. *Front Immunol* 2018; 9: 1389.

40. Egger M, Hauser M, Mari A, Ferreira F, Gadermaier G. The role of lipid transfer proteins in allergic diseases. *Curr Allergy Asthma Rep* 2010; 10(5): 326–335.

41. Azofra J, Berroa F, Gastaminza G et al. Lipid transfer protein syndrome in a non-Mediterranean area. *Int Arch Allergy Immunol* 2016; 169(3): 181–188.

42. Scala E, Till SJ, Asero R et al. Lipid transfer protein sensitization: Reactivity profiles and clinical risk assessment in an Italian cohort. *Allergy* 2015; 70(8): 933–943.

43. Gadermaier G, Harrer A, Girbl T et al. Isoform identification and characterization of Art v 3, the lipid-transfer protein of mugwort pollen. *Mol Immunol* 2009; 46(10): 1919–1924.

44. Sanchez-Lopez J, Tordesillas L, Pascal M et al. Role of Art v 3 in pollinosis of patients allergic to Pru p 3. *J Allergy Clin Immunol* 2014; 133(4): 1018–1025.

45. Mota I, Gaspar A, Benito-Garcia F et al. Anaphylaxis caused by lipid transfer proteins: An unpredictable clinical syndrome. *Allergol Immunopathol (Madr)* 2018; 46.

46. Gao ZS, Yang ZW, Wu SD et al. Peach allergy in China: A dominant role for mugwort pollen lipid transfer protein as a primary sensitizer. *J Allergy Clin Immunol* 2013; 131(1): 224–226.e1-3.

47. Gadermaier G, Wopfner N, Wallner M et al. Array-based profiling of ragweed and mugwort pollen allergens. *Allergy* 2008; 63(11): 1543–1549.

48. Ghosh N, Sircar G, Saha B, Pandey N, Gupta Bhattacharya S. Search for allergens from the pollen proteome of sunflower (*Helianthus annuus* L.): A major sensitizer for respiratory allergy patients. *PLOS ONE* 2015; 10(9): e0138992.

49. Berecz B, Clare Mills EN, Paradi I et al. Stability of sunflower 2S albumins and LTP to physiologically relevant *in vitro* gastrointestinal digestion. *Food Chem* 2013; 138(4): 2374–2381.

50. Asturias JA, Gomez-Bayon N, Eseverri JL, Martinez A. Par j 1 and Par j 2, the major allergens from *Parietaria judaica* pollen, have similar immunoglobulin E epitopes. *Clin Exp Allergy* 2003; 33(4): 518–524.

51. Tordesillas L, Sirvent S, Diaz-Perales A et al. Plant lipid transfer protein allergens: No cross-reactivity between those from foods and olive and *Parietaria* pollen. *Int Arch Allergy Immunol* 2011; 156(3): 291–296.

52. Comite P, Ferrero F, Mussap M, Ciprandi G. Par j 2 IgE measurement for distinguishing between sensitization and allergy. *Allergol Int* 2015; 64(4): 384–385.

53. Calabozo B, Barber D, Polo F. Purification and characterization of the main allergen of *Plantago lanceolata* pollen, Pla l 1. *Clin Exp Allergy* 2001; 31(2): 322–330.

54. Gadermaier G, Eichhorn S, Vejvar E et al. *Plantago lanceolata*: An important trigger of summer pollinosis with limited IgE cross-reactivity. *J Allergy Clin Immunol* 2014; 134(2): 472–475.

55. Stemeseder T, Freier R, Wildner S et al. Crystal structure of Pla l 1 reveals both structural similarity and allergenic divergence within the Ole e 1-like protein family. *J Allergy Clin Immunol* 2017; 140(1): 277–280.

56. Barderas R, Villalba M, Lombardero M, Rodriguez R. Identification and characterization of Che a 1 allergen from *Chenopodium album* pollen. *Int Arch Allergy Immunol* 2002; 127(1): 47–54.

57. Castro L, Mas S, Barderas R et al. Sal k 5, a member of the widespread Ole e 1-like protein family, is a new allergen of Russian thistle (*Salsola kali*) pollen. *Int Arch Allergy Immunol* 2014; 163(2): 142–153.

58. Calabozo B, Diaz-Perales A, Salcedo G, Barber D, Polo F. Cloning and expression of biologically active *Plantago lanceolata* pollen allergen Pla l 1 in the yeast *Pichia pastoris*. *Biochem J* 2003; 372(Pt 3): 889–896.

59. Barderas R, Villalba M, Rodriguez R. Che a 1: Recombinant expression, purification and correspondence to the natural form. *Int Arch Allergy Immunol* 2004; 135(4): 284–292.

60. Vahedi F, Sankian M, Moghadam M, Mohaddesfar M, Ghobadi S, Varasteh AR. Cloning and expression of Che a 1, the major allergen of *Chenopodium album* in *Escherichia coli*. *Appl Biochem Biotechnol* 2010; 163(7): 895–905.

61. Morakabati P, Assarehzadegan MA, Khosravi GR, Akbari B, Dousti F. Cloning and expression of Ama r 1, as a novel allergen of *Amaranthus retroflexus* pollen. *J Allergy (Cairo)* 2016; 2016: 4092817.

62. Akbari B, Assarehzadegan MA, Morakabati P, Khosravi GR, Dousti F. Molecular characterization of a new allergen from *Kochia scoparia* pollen, Koc s 1. *Int J Biosci* 2015; 7(4): 128–138.

63. Wildner S, Elsasser B, Stemeseder T et al. Endolysosomal degradation of allergenic Ole e 1-like proteins: Analysis of proteolytic cleavage sites revealing T cell epitope-containing peptides. *Int J Mol Sci* 2017; 18(8).

64. Hauser M, Roulias A, Ferreira F, Egger M. Panallergens and their impact on the allergic patient. *Allergy Asthma Clin Immunol* 2010; 6(1): 1.

65. McKenna OE, Asam C, Araujo GR, Roulias A, Goulart LR, Ferreira F. How relevant is panallergen sensitization in the development of allergies? *Pediatr Allergy Immunol* 2016; 27(6): 560–568.

66. Valenta R, Duchene M, Ebner C et al. Profilins constitute a novel family of functional plant pan-allergens. *J Exp Med* 1992; 175(2): 377–385.

67. Ramachandran S, Christensen HE, Ishimaru Y et al. Profilin plays a role in cell elongation, cell shape maintenance, and flowering in Arabidopsis. *Plant Physiol* 2000; 124(4): 1637–1647.

68. Valster AH, Pierson ES, Valenta R, Hepler PK, Emons A. Probing the plant actin cytoskeleton during cytokinesis and interphase by profilin microinjection. *Plant Cell* 1997; 9(10): 1815–1824.

69. Witke W. The role of profilin complexes in cell motility and other cellular processes. *Trends Cell Biol* 2004; 14(8): 461–469.

70. Gibbon BC, Zonia LE, Kovar DR, Hussey PJ, Staiger CJ. Pollen profilin function depends on interaction with proline-rich motifs. *Plant Cell* 1998; 10(6): 981–993.

71. Wopfner N, Gruber P, Wallner M et al. Molecular and immunological characterization of novel weed pollen pan-allergens. *Allergy* 2008; 63(7): 872–881.

72. Valenta R, Duchene M, Pettenburger K et al. Identification of profilin as a novel pollen allergen; IgE autoreactivity in sensitized individuals. *Science* 1991; 253(5019): 557–560.

73. Hauser M, Egger M, Wallner M, Wopfner N, Schmidt G, Ferreira F. Molecular properties of plant food allergens: A current classification into protein families. *Open Immunol J* 2008; 1: 1–12.

74. Oberhuber C, Ma Y, Wopfner N et al. Prevalence of IgE-binding to Art v 1, Art v 4 and Amb a 1 in mugwort-allergic patients. *Int Arch Allergy Immunol* 2008; 145(2): 94–101.

75. Asturias JA, Arilla MC, Gomez-Bayon N et al. Cloning and immunological characterization of the allergen Hel a 2 (profilin) from sunflower pollen. *Mol Immunol* 1998; 35(8): 469–478.

76. Barderas R, Villalba M, Pascual CY, Batanero E, Rodriguez R. Profilin (Che a 2) and polcalcin (Che a 3) are relevant allergens of *Chenopodium album* pollen: Isolation, amino acid sequences, and immunologic properties. *J Allergy Clin Immunol* 2004; 113(6): 1192–1198.

77. Asero R, Mistrello G, Roncarolo D, Amato S. *Parietaria* profilin shows only limited cross-reactivity with birch and grass profilins. *Int Arch Allergy Immunol* 2004; 133(2): 121–124.

78. Assarehzadegan MA, Amini A, Sankian M, Tehrani M, Jabbari F, Varasteh A. Sal k 4, a new allergen of *Salsola kali*, is profilin: A predictive value of conserved conformational regions in cross-reactivity with other plant-derived profilins. *Biosci Biotechnol Biochem* 2010; 74(7): 1441–1446.

79. Tehrani M, Sankian M, Assarehzadegan MA et al. Identification of a new allergen from *Amaranthus retroflexus* pollen, Ama r 2. *Allergol Int* 2011; 60(3): 309–316.

80. Popescu FD. Cross-reactivity between aeroallergens and food allergens. *World J Methodol* 2015; 5(2): 31–50.

81. Wopfner N, Dissertori O, Ferreira F, Lackner P. Calcium-binding proteins and their role in allergic diseases. *Immunol Allergy Clin North Am* 2007; 27(1): 29–44.

82. Ledesma A, Gonzalez E, Pascual CY, Quiralte J, Villalba M, Rodriguez R. Are Ca^{2+}-binding motifs involved in the immunoglobin E-binding of allergens? Olive pollen allergens as model of study. *Clin Exp Allergy* 2002; 32(10): 1476–1483.

83. Bonura A, Gulino L, Trapani A et al. Isolation, expression and immunological characterization of a calcium-binding protein from *Parietaria* pollen. *Mol Immunol* 2008; 45(9): 2465–2473.

84. Bouley J, Groeme R, Le Mignon M et al. Identification of the cysteine protease Amb a 11 as a novel major allergen from short ragweed. *J Allergy Clin Immunol* 2015; 136(4): 1055–1064.

85. Bordas-Le Floch V, Groeme R, Chabre H et al. New insights into ragweed pollen allergens. *Curr Allergy Asthma Rep* 2015; 15(11): 63.

86. Groeme R, Airouche S, Kopecny D et al. Structural and functional characterization of the major allergen Amb a 11 from short ragweed pollen. *J Biol Chem* 2016; 291(25): 13076–13087.

87. Stemeseder T, Hemmer W, Hawranek T, Gadermaier G. Marker allergens of weed pollen—Basic considerations and diagnostic benefits in the clinical routine: Part 16 of the series molecular allergology. *Allergo J Int* 2014; 23(8): 274–280.

88. Egger M, Mutschlechner S, Wopfner N, Gadermaier G, Briza P, Ferreira F. Pollen-food syndromes associated with weed pollinosis: An update from the molecular point of view. *Allergy* 2006; 61(4): 461–476.

89. Gadermaier G, Hauser M, Egger M et al. Sensitization prevalence, antibody cross-reactivity and immunogenic peptide profile of Api g 2, the non-specific lipid transfer protein 1 of celery. *PLOS ONE* 2011; 6(8): e24150.

90. Ukleja-Sokolowska N, Gawronska-Ukleja E, Zbikowska-Gotz M, Bartuzi Z, Sokolowski L. Sunflower seed allergy. *Int J Immunopathol Pharmacol* 2016; 29(3): 498–503.

91. Lukschal A, Wallmann J, Bublin M et al. Mimotopes for Api g 5, a relevant cross-reactive allergen, in the Celery-Mugwort-Birch-Spice syndrome. *Allergy Asthma Immunol Res* 2016; 8(2): 124–131.

92. Borghesan F, Mistrello G, Amato S, Giuffrida MG, Villalta D, Asero R. Mugwort-fennel-allergy-syndrome associated with sensitization to an allergen homologous to Api g 5. *Eur Ann Allergy Clin Immunol* 2013; 45(4): 130–137.

93. Fernandez C, Martin-Esteban M, Fiandor A et al. Analysis of cross-reactivity between sunflower pollen and other pollens of the Compositae family. *J Allergy Clin Immunol* 1993; 92(5): 660–667.

94. Nouri HR, Sankian M, Vahedi F et al. Diagnosis of *Chenopodium album* allergy with a cocktail of recombinant allergens as a tool for component-resolved diagnosis. *Mol Biol Rep* 2012; 39(3): 3169–3178.

95. Ferrer L, Carnes J, Rojas-Hijazo B, Lopez-Matas MA, Sobrevia MT, Colas C. Assessing degree of flowering implicates multiple Chenopodiaceae/Amaranthaceae species in allergy. *Int Arch Allergy Immunol* 2012; 158(1): 54–62.

96. Stemeseder T, Metz-Favre C, de Blay F, Pauli G, Gadermaier G. Do *Plantago lanceolata* skin prick test-positive patients display IgE to genuine plantain pollen allergens? Investigation of pollen allergic patients from the North-East of France. *Int Arch Allergy Immunol* 2018; 177(2): 97–106.

97. Moverare R, Larsson H, Carlsson R, Holmquist I. Mugwort-sensitized individuals from North Europe, South Europe and North America show different IgE reactivity patterns. *Int Arch Allergy Immunol* 2011; 154(2): 164–172.

98. Huang F, Zhao Y, He J et al. [Analyzing of the inhaled allergens profiles of allergic rhinitis patients in district of Jingmen]. *Lin Chung Er Bi Yan Hou Tou Jing Wai Ke Za Zhi* 2010; 24(8): 341–343.

99. Han D, Lai X, Gjesing B, Zhong N, Zhang L, Spangfort MD. The specific IgE reactivity pattern of weed pollen-induced allergic rhinitis patients. *Acta oto-laryngologica* 2011; 131(5): 533–538.

100. Lupinek C, Wollmann E, Baar A et al. Advances in allergen-microarray technology for diagnosis and monitoring of allergy: The MeDALL allergen-chip. *Methods* 2014; 66(1): 106–119.

101. Heffler E, Puggioni F, Peveri S, Montagni M, Canonica GW, Melioli G. Extended IgE profile based on an allergen macroarray: A novel tool for precision medicine in allergy diagnosis. *World Allergy Organ J* 2018; 11(1): 7.

102. Clowes GHR. A preliminary communication on the treatment of autumnal hay fever by vaccination with an aqueous extract of the pollen of ragweed. *Proc Soc Exp Biol Med* 1913; 10(3): 70–72.

103. Creticos PS, Marsh DG, Proud D et al. Responses to ragweed-pollen nasal challenge before and after immunotherapy. *J Allergy Clin Immunol* 1989; 84(2): 197–205.

104. Niederberger V. Allergen-specific immunotherapy. *Immunol Lett* 2009; 122(2): 131–133.

105. Milgrom H, Fick RB, Jr., Su JQ et al. Treatment of allergic asthma with monoclonal anti-IgE antibody. rhuMAb-E25 Study Group. *N Engl J Med* 1999; 341(26): 1966–1973.

106. Casale TB, Busse WW, Kline JN et al. Omalizumab pretreatment decreases acute reactions after rush immunotherapy for ragweed-induced seasonal allergic rhinitis. *J Allergy Clin Immunol* 2006; 117(1): 134–140.

107. Klunker S, Saggar LR, Seyfert-Margolis V et al. Combination treatment with omalizumab and rush immunotherapy for ragweed-induced allergic rhinitis: Inhibition of IgE-facilitated allergen binding. *J Allergy Clin Immunol* 2007; 120(3): 688–695.

108. Baldrick P, Richardson D, Woroniecki SR, Lees B. Pollinex Quattro Ragweed: Safety evaluation of a new allergy vaccine adjuvanted with monophosphoryl lipid A (MPL) for the treatment of ragweed pollen allergy. *J Appl Toxicol* 2007; 27(4): 399–409.

109. Tulic MK, Fiset PO, Christodoulopoulos P et al. Amb a 1-immunostimulatory oligodeoxynucleotide conjugate immunotherapy decreases the nasal inflammatory response. *J Allergy Clin Immunol* 2004; 113(2): 235–241.

110. Creticos PS, Schroeder JT, Hamilton RG et al. Immunotherapy with a ragweed-toll-like receptor 9 agonist vaccine for allergic rhinitis. *N Engl J Med* 2006; 355(14): 1445–1455.

111. Valenta R, Ferreira F, Focke-Tejkl M et al. From allergen genes to allergy vaccines. *Annu Rev Immunol* 2010; 28: 211–241.

112. Bonura A, Corinti S, Artale A et al. A hybrid expressing genetically engineered major allergens of the *Parietaria* pollen as a tool for specific allergy vaccination. *Int Arch Allergy Immunol* 2007; 142(4): 274–284.

113. Bonura A, Passantino R, Costa MA et al. Characterization of a Par j 1/Par j 2 mutant hybrid with reduced allergenicity for immunotherapy of *Parietaria* allergy. *Clin Exp Allergy* 2012; 42(3): 471–480.

114. Schulke S, Kuttich K, Wolfheimer S et al. Conjugation of wildtype and hypoallergenic mugwort allergen art v 1 to flagellin induces IL-10-DC and suppresses allergen-specific TH2-responses *in vivo. Sci Rep* 2017; 7(1): 11782.

115. Litwin A, Flanagan M, Entis G et al. Oral immunotherapy with short ragweed extract in a novel encapsulated preparation: A double-blind study. *J Allergy Clin Immunol* 1997; 100(1): 30–38.

116. Andre C, Perrin-Fayolle M, Grosclaude M et al. A double-blind placebo-controlled evaluation of sublingual immunotherapy with a standardized ragweed extract in patients with seasonal rhinitis. Evidence for a dose-response relationship. *Int Arch Allergy Immunol* 2003; 131(2): 111–118.

117. Skoner D, Gentile D, Bush R, Fasano MB, McLaughlin A, Esch RE. Sublingual immunotherapy in patients with allergic rhinoconjunctivitis caused by ragweed pollen. *J Allergy Clin Immunol* 2010; 125(3): 660–666, 6.e1–6.e4.

118. Creticos PS, Esch RE, Couroux P et al. Randomized, double-blind, placebo-controlled trial of standardized ragweed sublingual-liquid immunotherapy for allergic rhinoconjunctivitis. *J Allergy Clin Immunol* 2014; 133(3): 751–758.

119. Kim H, Waserman S, Hebert J et al. Efficacy and safety of ragweed sublingual immunotherapy in Canadian patients with allergic rhinoconjunctivitis. *Allergy Asthma Clin Immunol* 2014; 10(1): 55.

120. Wilson DR, Lima MT, Durham SR. Sublingual immunotherapy for allergic rhinitis: Systematic review and meta-analysis. *Allergy* 2005; 60(1): 4–12.

121. Chen KW, Marusciac L, Tamas PT, Valenta R, Panaitescu C. Ragweed pollen allergy: Burden, characteristics, and management of an imported allergen source in Europe. *Int Arch Allergy Immunol* 2018; 176(3-4): 163–180.

122. Ferreira F, Briza P, Infuhr D et al. Modified recombinant allergens for safer immunotherapy. *Inflamm Allergy Drug Targets* 2006; 5(1): 5–14.

123. Wallner M, Briza P, Thalhamer J, Ferreira F. Specific immunotherapy in pollen allergy. *Curr Opin Mol Ther* 2007; 9(2): 160–167.

124. Wallner M, Pichler U, Ferreira F. Recombinant allergens for pollen immunotherapy. *Immunotherapy* 2013; 5(12): 1323–1338.

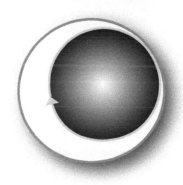

13 Fungal allergens

Robert E. Esch
Lenoir-Rhyne University

Jonathan A. Bernstein
University of Cincinnati College of Medicine

Hari M. Vijay
VLN Biotech, Inc.

CONTENTS

13.1 INTRODUCTION

Fungi are eukaryotic, nonchlorophyllic, mostly spore-bearing organisms that exist as saprophytes or as parasites of animals and plants [1–3]. Fungi constitute unicellular to multicellular organisms, and their presence in the environment depends on the climate, vegetation, and other ecological factors. The presence and prevalence of fungi indoors depend on the moisture content, ventilation, and presence or absence of carpets, pets, and houseplants [4–6]. Spores of *Aspergillus fumigatus, Alternaria alternata, Cladosporium herbarum, Penicillium,* and *Fusarium* are universally present in the indoor and outdoor environments (Figure 13.1). The development of allergies to fungi follows the same biological phenomena as allergies to other environmental agents.

Fungi are associated with several allergic diseases in humans. The prevalence of respiratory allergy to fungi is estimated to be 20%–30% of atopic individuals and up to 6% in the general population [7–10]. The major allergic manifestations induced by these agents are allergic asthma, rhinoconjunctivitis, bronchopulmonary mycoses, and hypersensitivity pneumonitis [3–6,11–13]. These diseases result from exposure to spores, vegetative cells, or metabolites of the fungi. Spores from some fungi are shown in Figure 13.1. Fungal spores vary in size and can be associated with both upper and lower respiratory symptoms. Spores and hyphal fragments less than 5 μM can penetrate the lower airways, where allergic reactions may manifest as asthma. The site of deposition of spores also depends on whether spores enter the respiratory tract

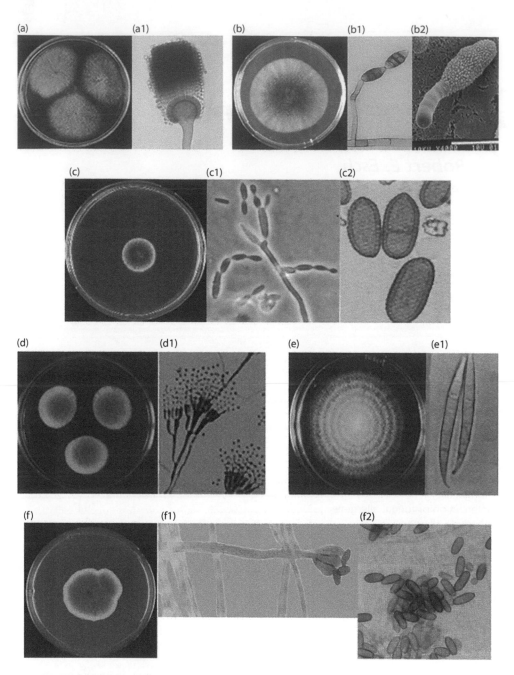

Figure 13.1 Some common allergenic molds. Colonies of *Aspergillus fumigatus* (a); *Alternaria alternata* (b); *Cladosporium herbarum* (c); *Penicillium chrysogenum* (d); *Fusarium solani* (e); and *Stachybotrys chartarum* (f). Conidiospores of *A. fumigatus* (a1); *A. alternata* showing vertical and horizontal septa (b1). Scanning electron micrograph of *A. alternata* (b2); conidiophores and conidia of *C. herbarum* (c1 and c2); broom-shaped sporophores of *Penicillium* sp. (d1); spores (macroconidia) of *Fusarium* sp. (e1); and conidiophores and conidia of *S. chartarum* (f1 and f2).

as individual spores or as aggregates. For example, the clusters of small conidia of *Aspergillus* and *Penicillium* are usually deposited in the upper respiratory tract, while the smaller individual spores and possibly fungal fragments (<1 um) reach the lower airways [14,15]. Spore and fungal extracts both cause early- and late-phase allergic asthmatic reactions in allergic subjects. More than 80 genera of the major fungal groups have been associated with symptoms of respiratory tract allergy [3]; however, only a few genera such as *Alternaria, Cladosporium, Aspergillus*, and *Penicillium*, have been systematically investigated for causing allergic diseases [3,16,17]. Exposure to toxin-producing fungi such as *Aspergillus, Alternaria,* and *Stachybotrys* often contaminating foods, agricultural products,

and water-damaged buildings, has also been reported to cause symptoms [18–20].

Fungal allergenic extracts are highly heterogeneous and complex. They can contain partly or completely shared antigenic components from a number of fungal species and identically labeled products produced by different manufacturers may not be interchangeable Therefore, accurate interpretation of skin tests and serological test results requires understanding the cross-reactivity between fungal allergens and how they are manufactured [21–23]. Even though a number of fungal allergens have been isolated and characterized, standardized extracts (vaccines) are still not available to more reliably diagnose and treat allergic diseases.

13.2 CLASSIFICATION OF FUNGI

Fungi belong to the botanical kingdom that includes molds, yeasts, mildews, bracket fungi, rusts, smuts, and mushrooms. They constitute a very large and diverse group of organisms with a complex taxonomy. The hyphae are the basic structural unit for most fungi and typically are branched with tubular filaments possessing a defined cell wall composed of chitin, a polymer of N-acetylglucosamine and other complex carbohydrates. These hyphae may be divided into individual cells by cross-walls, called "septa" [1]. Some fungi exist exclusively as single-cell yeast forms, while others demonstrate extensive hyphae. Mushrooms belong to the phylum Basidiomycota, where clumping of mycelium results in the development of large macroscopic structures of diverse color and shape. The pleomorphism of fungi further complicates the classification and antigenicity and poses problems for accurate identification.

Fungi, like animals, are heterotrophs, which means they must obtain their energy for growth by digesting organic molecules from their environment. The various modes of fungal reproduction include fragmentation, fission, budding, and spore production, and most produce both sexual and asexual spores. Fungal spores can be thick-walled, dry, pigmented, hydrophobic, or colorless and slimy. Fungal cell walls are composed of chitin and also may contain mannans, glucans, and cellulose. The fungal cell membrane is composed of ergosterol; DNA content is very low, whereas RNA in the form of ribosomal RNA may comprise up to 10% of the dry weight of a fungus. Glycogen is the main storage carbohydrate of fungi, which allows them to metabolize glucose by aerobic respiration into CO_2 and water or by fermentation into CO_2 and alcohol or lactic acid. Fungi produce many unique protease enzymes that are important for the degradation of resistant materials like cellulose and polyethylene.

Until recently, the taxonomy of fungi was based primarily on morphology of their sexual stage. True fungi are categorized based on patterns of sexual reproduction into two divisions: the Zygomycota (characterized by the cytoplasms and nuclei of two hyphal cells fusing to make one cell) and Dikarya (cytoplasmic fusion occurs first, followed later by nuclear fusion). The Dikarya are further subdivided into Ascomycota (sexual spores in the ascus, a membranous, club-shaped structure typically composed of eight ascospores) and Basidiomycota (sexual spores on a basidium which is a small, club-shaped structure composed of four basidiospores at the tips of tiny projections). Fungi without an identifiable sexual stage were classified as fungi imperfecti or Deuteromycetes. This system led to the creation of different names for the sexual (teleomorph) and asexual (anamorph) forms of the same species. Today, fungal molecular systematics based on DNA sequencing have become the established standard, and mycologists have launched a "One fungus, one name" campaign aimed at ending the system of dual nomenclature [24]. Choosing the correct name for the thousands of pleomorphic fungi will take time and will undoubtedly cause confusion among nonmycologists. Maintaining consistency between the revised code, allergen nomenclature, and labeling of commercially available allergenic extracts will also require attention. Under the current classification system, the known allergenic fungi belong to one of three phyla, Zygomycota, Ascomycota, or Basidiomycota. Allergenic fungi previously belonging to the Deuteromycetes now belong to the Ascomycota (see Table 13.1). Fungi are divided into standard taxonomic categories including phylum, class, order, family, genus, and species, and each of these categories may contain further subphyla, subclasses, and suborders. The Ascomycota is the largest phylum with over 65,000 species, the Basidiomycota with over 30,000 species and the Zygomycota with about 1000 species known [1,2].

13.3 IDENTIFICATION OF FUNGI

The most important group of air-disseminated fungi that causes respiratory allergic diseases in humans is the conidial fungi, which produce asexual, nonmotile spores on specialized structures called conidiophores. The spores are genetically identical and serve in biological dispersal. Fungal spores vary in shape, size, texture, color, number of cells, thickness of the cell wall, and methods by which they are attached to each other and to their conidiophores. These morphologic characteristics are often distinctive and are used in identification of the species. The identification of the common fungi can be difficult as their fungal colony characteristics and even microscopic characteristics vary according to the medium on which they are grown, the incubation temperature, and the strain variation and pleomorphic nature of the spores [25,26].

13.4 FUNGAL ALLERGENS

Fungi are ubiquitous in nature, and at least one million fungal species occur on earth [27,28]. *Alternaria*, *Cladosporium*, *Aspergillus*, and *Penicillium* are found throughout the world. The airborne spores of these fungi are important causes of allergic diseases (allergic rhinitis, asthma, bronchopulmonary mycoses, and hypersensitivity pneumonitis) [29,30].

The accurate *in vivo* and *in vitro* diagnosis of fungal allergies depends on the availability of well-characterized allergen preparations. Aerobiological identification and assessment of fungi in outdoor and indoor environments are necessary to determine their role in causing allergic diseases. Such surveys conducted in different parts of the world in conjunction with skin and *in vitro* tests for IgE specific to mold have identified relevant fungal allergens for type 1 hypersensitivity. Based on such data, extracts from *Alternaria alternata*, *Cladosporium herbarum*, *Aspergillus fumigatus*, *Epicoccum nigrum* synonym (*E. purpurascens*), *Fusarium roseum*, and *Penicillium chrysogenum* (formerly *P. notatum*) and others are commercially available. Selection of species and strains of fungi is crucial for utilizing representative allergens. As the prevalence of fungi and their allergenicity varies, relevant fungi need to be identified for consistent and reproducible results, both for diagnosis and treatment of allergic diseases [3,4,31–33].

Because of the variability among strains and species in morphology, biochemistry, and allergenicity, it is difficult to obtain relevant antigens with consistent allergenic activity. In addition, there is considerable immunologic cross-reactivity among various taxonomically and antigenically related strains, species, and even genera. It is almost impossible with some fungi to grow two consecutive cultures with identical antigenic profiles [34]. Factors contributing to the differences among commercial and laboratory extracts are (1) variability in the proper identification of stock cultures used to prepare allergenic extracts; (2) the use of mycelial-rich material as the source of allergens; (3) variable conditions in which fungi are grown and extracts prepared; (4) the differing stability

Table 13.1 Taxonomy of allergenic fungi

Phylum	Subphylum	Class	Order	Family	Genus
Zygomycota	Zygomycotina	Incertae sedis	Mucorales	Mucoraceae	*Mucor*
					Rhizopus
Ascomycota	Saccharomycetina	Saccharomycetes	Saccharomycetales	Saccharomycetaceae	*Candida*
					Saccharomyces
				Dipodascaceae	*Geotrichum*
	Pezizomycotina	Dothideomycetes	Capnodiales	Davidiellaceae	*Cladosporium*
			Pleosporales	Pleosporaceae	*Alternaria*
					Curvularia
					Drechslera
					Bipolaris
					Helminthosporium
					Stemphylium
					Ulocladium
					Epicoccum
				Didymellaceae	*Phoma*
			Dothideales	Dothioraceae	*Aureobasidium*
		Eurotiomycetes	Eurotiales	Trichocomaceae	*Aspergillus*
					Penicillium
					Paecilomyces
			Onygenales	Arthrodermataceae	*Trichophyton*
					Epidermophyton
		Sordariomycetes	Hypocreales	Nectriaceae	*Fusarium*
				Hypocreaceae	*Trichoderma*
					Acremonium
				Stachybotryaceae	*Stachybotrys*
				Incertae sedis	*Trichothecium*
			Sordariales	Sordariaceae	*Neurospora*
				Chaetomiaceae	*Chaetomium*
			Trichosphaeriales	Trichosphaeriaceae	*Nigrospora*
		Leotiomycetes	Helotiales	Sclerotiniaceae	*Botrytis*
Basidiomycota	Pucciniomycotina	Microbotryomycetes	Sporidiobolales	Sporidiobolaceae	*Rhodotorula*
	Ustilaginomycotina	Ustilaginomycotina	Ustilaginales	Ustilaginaceae	*Ustilago*
		Malasseziomycetes	Malasseziales	Malasseziaceae	*Malassezia*
	Agaricomycotina	Agaricomycetes	Agaricales	Agaricaceae	*Coprinus*
				Strophariaceae	*Psilocybe*
				Schizophyllaceae	*Schizophyllum*

of the extracts; and (5) the type of quality control measures used. Allergenic fungi may be cultured in synthetic, simplified media rather than in complex media containing macromolecules. These allergenic extracts show less variability and demonstrate more specific reactivity in allergic patients [35,36]. However, for the production of certain relevant allergens, complex media components are essential.

The extraction procedure should be optimized for consistent results by the use of a suitable extraction buffer, optimal duration of extraction, appropriate cell disruption, and select use of protease inhibitors and preservatives [22,33,37]. The allergenic activity of an extract, or fraction, can be evaluated either by prick or intradermal skin testing. The intradermal method, however, is more quantitative and sensitive than prick testing [38,39]. The most common *in vitro* tests that correlate with allergen-specific IgE in the serum are radioallergosorbent test (RAST) and enzyme-linked immunosorbent assay (ELISA). Semiautomated specific IgE assays, such as Immuno-CAP, are preferred due to their simplicity and reliability for a spectrum of aeroallergens, including fungi [40–43].

Antibody response to allergens and their specificity can also be studied by competitive inhibition assays. Patients' sera are incubated with varying dilutions of the allergens before adding the sera to the solid-phase bound reference allergens. ELISA is performed, and the percent inhibition of binding of the preadsorbed sera to the reference allergen is determined. A 50% inhibition in binding of the patient's IgE to the reference allergen is interpreted as a measure of potency of the test allergen [44]. Direct challenge of allergic patients by inhalation of small doses of various fungal extracts has been used in patient evaluation studies; however, the use of mold allergens for inhalation studies is controversial because of possible late-phase reactions and other adverse effects including the development of new sensitizations [45,46].

The stability of allergenic extracts depends on the type and quality of the allergen, the storage temperature, and the presence of preservatives and other nonallergic materials in the mixture. For most extracts, lyophilization is the best method to maintain the allergenic potency, but some allergens may be permanently altered and inactivated by this process. The loss of potency of any extract may be due to degradation of a specific allergen by proteases rather than a general reduction in activity of all allergens. Moreover, the reconstituted extract must contain a stabilizer such as human serum albumin, glycerol, phenol, or aminocaproic acid to preserve the integrity of allergenic extracts [47].

13.5 DISTRIBUTION OF INDOOR AND OUTDOOR FUNGAL ALLERGENS

Fungi grow on almost any material if sufficient moisture is available. Large numbers of airborne spores are usually present in outdoor air throughout the year, frequently exceeding the pollen population by 100- to 1000-fold, depending on environmental factors, such as water, nutrients, temperature, and wind [48–50]. Most fungi commonly considered allergenic, such as *Alternaria*, *Cladosporium*, *Epicoccum*, or *Ganoderma*, have a seasonal spore-releasing pattern [51,52].

Indoor fungi are a mixture of those that have entered from outdoors and those that grow and multiply indoors [53]. *Aspergillus* and *Penicillium* usually are less common outdoors and are primarily considered to be indoor fungi [54]. *Alternaria* can be found in house dust samples in the absence of environmental mold spores [55]. Some investigators find good correlation between outdoor spore counts and allergic symptoms; however, little information is available on the effects of indoor spore concentrations and allergic symptoms [56]. Dampness, excess moisture, and mold growth in buildings are associated with an increased prevalence of asthma and bronchitis. The indoor versus the outdoor air fungal flora may differ, both quantitatively and qualitatively; and most of the time, outdoor concentrations of fungal spores outnumber those of indoor environments. The indoor sources of fungi result in a different composition of indoor airborne fungi compared to the outdoor air [57]. The health effects caused by fungal propagules are primarily allergic but can be infectious [58]. Finally, health effects may result

from irritation of mucosa secondary to fungal spores and hyphal particles and the release of volatile organic compounds. Therefore, the overall concentration of both viable and nonviable spores may give a more accurate estimate of the actual exposure [59].

Most studies of indoor fungal spores in the air have been performed with a discontinuous sampler to collect viable fungi. Surveys on outdoor mold spores are mostly done with continuous techniques to collect nonviable samples [60]. The spectrum of airborne mold spores in homes, offices, and other workplaces differs due to the influx of spores from outdoor air through ventilations and air exchangers. Hence, it is important to have a standardized approach for sampling if one hopes to arrive at any significant conclusion regarding the effect of indoor mold spore exposure on the allergic response [61,62]. Distribution of indoor and outdoor mold spore counts varies regionally in the United States and around the world [20,63,65]. Most experts believe that a spore count as low as $500/m^3$ has a sufficient antigen load to be harmful for exposed susceptible individuals [66]. Garrett and colleagues found that most common fungal genera/groups were *Cladosporium*, *Penicillium*, and yeast, both indoor and outdoor in winter and late spring, in their studies of airborne fungal spores in southeastern Australian homes [67]. Outdoor versus indoor levels were higher throughout the year, and significant seasonal variation in spore levels occurred indoors and outdoors with maximum levels usually found during the summer. On the contrary, the levels of *Aspergillus*, *Cephalosporium*, *Gliocladium*, and yeasts were higher in winter. *Penicillium* was detected more commonly indoors than outdoors. However, outdoor mold spore levels can have a significant influence on indoor spore levels [67].

13.6 CROSS-REACTIVITY OF FUNGAL ALLERGENS

The term *cross-reactivity* refers to the antigenic determinants shared by different molecules from different fungi [68,69]. Studies with techniques such as immunoprecipitation, immunoblotting, and ELISA or RAST inhibition have contributed to the understanding of this phenomenon [6,21,32]. Cross-reactivity should be distinguished from parallel, independent sensitization to multiple fungal allergens. The degree of cross-reactivity among different species and strains of fungi depends on the number of antigenic components that cross-react, the immunogenicity of epitopes, and the method used to detect the reactivity. The presence of cross-reactive epitopes among allergens is advantageous to diagnose allergic diseases because it reduces the number of antigens required in the panel of extracts for testing [21,32]. However, the results may lack specificity and necessitate secondary testing to determine the specific sensitizing mold. Cross-reactive antigens are advantageous for allergen immunotherapy due to their broad-spectrum effect.

There are shared allergenic and antigenic components from cytoplasmic and cell-wall antigens of fungi. The cell-wall antigens usually contain carbohydrates, which may contribute to the cross-reactivity. In addition, several of the related genera of fungi share similar proteins. For example, *Aspergillus* and *Penicillium* species share a number of proteases, and these proteins cross-react [70]. A recent cluster analysis of fungal sensitization patterns from 668 individuals revealed a close relationship between their sensitization to 17 different fungal species and fungal phylogenetic relationships [71].

Allergens from unrelated sources can also cross-react. Mold-latex allergy is such an example. A number of minor and major allergens from *Hevea brasiliensis* (the source of latex) share partial homology with fungal allergens [72,73]. These cross-reactive allergens belong to families of highly conserved proteins involved in vital cellular processes called pan-allergens [74]. The concept was first described among cross-reacting pollen and plant-food allergens but has now expanded to include fungal allergens as their molecular identities are resolved [21,75–77].

Monoclonal antibodies and antibodies raised to defined epitopes or peptides can be used to more precisely define fungal allergen cross-reactivity as compared to using antibodies raised against extracts [69,78]. The increased availability of allergen sequence and fungal genome data has allowed comparative genomic analysis and searches for potential cross-reactive allergens. Bowyer et al. [79] used a database of 82 allergen sequences to search 22 fungal genomes for homologous allergen orthologue classes. One highly conserved set of allergen orthologues including enolase, heat shock proteins, cyclophilins, proteases, redoxins, and disulfide isomerases was present across the entire fungal kingdom. Other sets of allergens were less well conserved and appeared to be restricted to a limited number of species, e.g., Asp f 1 and Alt a 1. It should be pointed out that although allergenic cross-reactivity can be associated with sequence homology, a single amino acid change within an epitope can have a significant impact on IgE reactivity. A better understanding of cross-reactivity between different fungi is important as it may be relevant for diagnosis, treatment, and development of more effective disease prevention control measures.

13.7 ISOLATION AND CHARACTERIZATION OF FUNGAL ALLERGENS

Over 100 genera of fungi are thought to cause allergic diseases, but the understanding of fungal allergens is limited to less than about 20. In the present discussion, only the predominant fungi associated with IgE mediated-allergy are discussed. These include those allergens that have been sufficiently characterized to be approved by the World Health Organization and International Union of Immunological Societies (WHO/IUIS) Allergen Nomenclature Sub-Committee (see Tables 13.2 through 13.9).

13.7.1 *Alternaria alternata* allergens

Alternaria is the most widely studied allergenic fungus belonging to the order Pleosporales in the class Dothideomycetes. Other members of the order include *Curvularia*, *Drechslera*, *Biopolaris*, *Helminthosporium*, *Stemphylium*, *Ulocladium*, *Epicoccum*, and *Phoma*. *Alternaria alternata* is one of the most important allergenic fungi. This species is an important cause of bronchospasm and is clinically associated with asthma [80,81]. Hypersensitivity pneumonitis, a condition associated with IgG precipitating antibodies, may also be caused by *Alternaria* [82]. Most fungi, including *A. alternata* and *C. herbarum*, have a seasonal spore-releasing pattern. Although other *Alternaria* species are probably clinically relevant, most research has been performed on *A alternata*. Twelve allergenic proteins have been accepted by the WHO/IUIS Allergen Nomenclature Sub-Committee (see Table 13.2).

The first allergenic fraction of *A. alternata* reported was a glycoprotein fraction of a mycelial extract partially purified by gel chromatography. This allergenic fraction was referred to as Alt-I with a molecular weight ranging between 25 and 50 kDa [83,84]. The major allergen, Alt a 1 was purified to homogeneity and identified as a 29–31 kDa acidic glycoprotein that dissociated into two subunits (approximately 15 kDa) under reducing conditions [85–87]. More than 80% of *Alternaria*-allergic patients are sensitized to Alt a 1. The localization of Alt a 1 to the spore wall [88] might explain its particular importance as an aeroallergen and its ability to sensitize susceptible individuals. The allergen was subsequently cloned [89,90] and the three-dimensional crystal structure elucidated [91].

Table 13.2 *Alternaria* allergens

Fungus	MW (kDa)	Biological activity	Sequence accession number
Alternaria alternata			
Alt a 1	30	Unknown	U82633
Alt a 3	70	Heat shock protein 70	U87807
Alt a 4	57	Protein disulfide-isomerase	CAA58999
Alt a 5	11	Ribosomal protein P2	CAA55066, AAB48041
Alt a 6	45	Enolase	AAG42022
Alt a 7	22	YCP4 protein, Flavodoxin	CAA55069
Alt a 8	29	Mannitol dehydrogenase	AAO91800
Alt a 10	53	Aldehyde dehydrogenase	CAA55071
Alt a 12	11	Acid ribosomal protein P1	CAA58998
Alt a 13	26	Glutathione-*S*-transferase	AAR98813
Alt a 14	24	Manganese superoxide dismutase	AGS80276
Alt a 15	58	Serine protease	AHZ97469

Table 13.3 *Cladosporium* allergens

Fungus	MW (kDa)	Biological activity	Sequence accession number
C. herbarum			
Cla h 1	13	Unknown	
Cla h 2	45	Unknown	
Cla h 5	11	Acid ribosomal protein P2	CAA55067
Cla h 6	46	Enolase	CAA55070
Cla h 7	22	YCP4 protein	CAA55068
Cla h 8	28	Mannitol dehydrogenase	AAO91801
Cla h 9		Vacuolar serine protease	AAX14379
Cla h 10	53	Aldehyde dehydrogenase	CAA55072
Cla h 12	11	Acid ribosomal protein P1	CAA59463
C. cladosporioides			
Cla c 14	36.5	Transaldolase	ADK47394
Cla c 9	36	Vacuolar serine protease	ABQ59329

Alt a 1 was shown to be a dimer with a unique β-barrel comprising 11 β-strands held together by a disulfide bridge. There were no equivalent structures identified after bioinformatic analyses comparing the Alt a 1 sequence and structure with proteins derived from other sources. Homologues of Alt a 1 have been identified within members of the Pleosporaceae family by DNA sequencing with phylogenetic analyses [92] as well by immunochemical methods [93,94]. The presence of Alt a 1 homologues could not be detected in *Cladosporium*, *Aspergillus*, and *Penicillium* extracts or culture filtrates. Together, these studies suggest that Alt a 1 homologues are restricted to *Alternaria* and closely related taxa within the family Pleosporaceae, e.g., *Ulocladium*, *Curvularia*, and *Stemphylium*.

IgE-binding epitopes were identified by screening overlapping peptides spanning the complete Alt a 1 sequence. Four peptides (amino acid residues 41–50, 54–63, 87–96, and 119–128) bound IgE antibodies from *Alternaria*-allergic subjects, and two of them (amino acid residues 41–50 and 54–63) showed consistent reactivity across all subjects [95]. The two major epitopes were mapped on the surface on the three-dimensional structure of Alt a 1 [91]. Another peptide representing the *N*-terminus (amino acid residues 4–23) showed weak binding to human IgE antibodies [96].

Highly sensitive and specific immunoassays for Alt a 1 have been developed for the detection and measurement of Alt a 1 in environmental samples as well as in diagnostic and therapeutic extracts [97–100]. Airborne Alt a 1 levels correlated with clinical symptoms recorded through the year by patients with allergic asthma and/or rhinitis monosensitized to *Alternaria* [101]; and the Alt a 1 content of commercial *Alternaria* extracts correlated with their biological activity as assessed by quantitative skin testing [98]. Although the performance characteristics for these assays have been well documented, their regulatory acceptance as a suitable potency test for commercial extracts still awaits validation.

Several investigators [90,102,103] have cloned and sequenced seven allergens derived from *Alternaria* cDNA libraries: Alt a 3 (hsp-70), Alt a 4 (disulfide isomerase), Alt a 5 (ribosomal protein P2, formerly Alt a 6), Alt a 8 (mannitol dehydrogenase), Alt a 10 (aldehyde dehydrogenase), and Alt a 7 (YCP4 protein). All are minor allergens because less than 50% of *Alternaria*-allergic patients are sensitized to these allergens. Most are potentially cross-reactive, and some are highly conserved proteins that have been identified as cross-reactive across fungal classes and even phyla. These proteins bound IgE antibodies from 2% to 42% of *Alternaria*-sensitized subjects and represent "housekeeping" proteins involved in maintaining basic cellular function.

Alt a 6 (enolase) is a highly conserved, ubiquitous enzyme with allergenic cross-reactivity with *Cladosporium*, *Aspergillus*, *Candida*, and *Saccharomyces* [104,105]. The potential clinical and diagnostic importance of this allergen in addition to Alt a 1 has been proposed [106]. The amino acid sequences of Alt a 6 and Cla h 6 are 89% identical and 73% identical compared to the *S. cerevisiae* and *C. albicans* enolase [105]. Epitope mapping of *Cladosporium* enolase Cla h 6 using 10 fusion peptides produced by polymerase chain reaction (PCR) cloning localized a major IgE-binding epitope on a peptide (amino acid residues 120–189) [105]. Competitive immunoassays using this peptide to deplete IgE antibodies from allergic serum cosensitized to Cla h 6 and Alt a 6 suggest that the corresponding region on Alt a 6 also constitutes a major IgE-binding epitope. Enolase from *Curvularia lunata* (Cur l 2) was described as a major allergen based on the presence of specific IgE toward rCur l 2 in sera from 15 patients with skin test sensitivity to *C. lunata* extract [107]. *C. lunata* is phylogenetically related to *Alternaria* and *Cladosporium* (see Table 13.1), and the protein sequence of Cur l 2 is 83% and 88% similar to Cla h 6 and Alt a 6, respectively. In contrast, enolase allergens from phylogenetically more distant fungi show less similarity: *Candida albicans* (71%) and *Penicillium citrinum* (79%). One of the 10 computationally predicted epitopes of Cur l 2 (amino acid residues 138–162) was within the peptide sequence identified as a major IgE-binding epitope for Cla h 6.

Alt a 13 (glutathione-*S*-transferase) was characterized as a major allergen from *Alternaria* based on positive intradermal skin test

Table 13.4 *Aspergillus* allergens

Fungus	MW (kDa)	Biological activity	Sequence accession number
A. fumigatus			
Asp f 1	18	Mitogillin family, Ribotoxin	AAB07779
Asp f 2	37	Fibrinogen-binding protein	AAC69357
Asp f 3	18.5	Peroxysmal protein	AAB95638
Asp f 4	30	Unknown	CAA04959
Asp f 5	40	Metalloprotease	CAA83015
Asp f 6	26.5	Mn superoxide dismutase	AAB60779
Asp f 7	12	Unknown	CAA11255
Asp f 8	11	Ribosomal protein P2	CAB64688
Asp f 9	34	Glycosyl hydrolase	CAA11266
Asp f 10	34	Aspartic protease	CAA59419
Asp f 11	24	Cyclophilin, Rotamase	CAB44442
Asp f 12	90	Heat shock protein P90	AAB51544
Asp f 13	34	Serine protease	CAA77666
Asp f 14		Transaldolase	AFUA-5G09230
Asp f 15	16	Unknown	CAA05149
Asp f 16	43	Glycosyl hydrolase	AAC61261
Asp f 17		Galactomannoprotein	CAA12162
Asp f 18	34	Vacuolar serine protease	CAA73782
Asp f 22	46	Enolase	AAK49451
Asp f 23	44	Ribosomal protein L3	AAM43909
Asp f 26		Acidic ribosomal protein P1	AFUB_007210
Asp f 27	18	Cyclophilin, Rotamase	CAI78448
Asp f 28	13	Thioredoxin	CAI78449
Asp f 29	13	Thioredoxin	CAI78450
Asp f 34	20	PhiA cell wall protein	CAM54066
A. flavus			
Asp fl 13	34	Alkaline serine protease	
A. niger			
Asp n 14	105	β-Xylosidase	AAD13106
Asp n 18	34	Vacuolar serine protease	
Asp n 25	66–100	3-Phytase B	AAA02934
A. oryzae			
Asp o 13	34	Alkaline serine protease	CAA35594
Asp o 21	53	TAKA-amylase A	AAA32708, BAA00336
A. versicolor			
Asp v 13	43	Alkaline serine protease	ADE74975

Table 13.5 *Penicillium* allergens

Fungus	MW (kDa)	Biological activity	Sequence accession number
P. brevicompactum			
Pen b 13	33	Alkaline serine protease	
Pen b 26	11	Acidic ribosomal protein P1	AAX11194
P. citrinum			
Pen c 3	18	Peroxisomal membrane protein	AAD42074
Pen c 13	33	Alkaline serine protease	Q9URH1
Pen c 19	70	Heat shock protein P70	AAB06397
Pen c 22	46	Enolase	AAK51201
Pen c 24		Elongation factor 1-β	AAR17475
Pen c 30	97	Catalase	ABB89950
Pen c 32	40	Pectate lyase	ABM60783
P. chrysogenum			
Pen ch 13	34	Alkaline serine protease	AAF23726
Pen ch 18	32	Vacuolar serine protease	AAF71379
Pen ch 20	68	*N*-acetyl-glucosaminidase	AAB34785
Pen ch 31		Calreticulin	AAX45072
Pen ch 33	16	Unknown	ABP04053
Pen ch 35	36.5	Transaldolase	ADK27483
P. crustosum			
Pen cr 26	11	Acidic ribosomal protein P1	AEX34122
P. oxalicum			
Pen o 18	34	Vacuolar serine protease	AAG44478

responses to native and recombinant forms of the allergen in 14 of 17 (82%) *Alternaria*-sensitized patients [108]. The IgE-binding epitopes were mapped to an *N*-terminal fragment (aa residues 1–50) using a combination of skin testing, IgE-ELISA inhibition, and histamine release assays [109]. Cross-reactivity with glutathione-*S*-transferases from other fungal genera (*Cladosporium, Curvularia, Aspergillus,* and *Epicoccum*) was shown by immunoblot and ELISA inhibition experiments using antibodies raised against recombinant Alt a 13 [110].

Alt a 14 (manganese-dependent superoxide dismutase) was first identified as a potentially important *Alternaria* allergen in a study evaluating the utility of component-resolved diagnostic testing to fungal allergens [106]. Although Alt a 14 is a minor *Alternaria* allergen (7 of 61 *Alternaria*-sensitized subjects are reactive to Alt a 14), it accounted for approximately 7% of allergy to *Alternaria* after excluding patients with Alt a 1 sensitization. Cross-reactivity with a homologous allergen, Asp f 6, has been established [111]. The importance of Asp f 6 as a marker for allergic bronchopulmonary aspergillosis (ABPA) suggests that the cross-reactive Alt a 14 may be related to the pathogenesis of ABPA [112].

Alt a 15 (vacuolar serine protease) is a minor allergen with about a 10% prevalence among *Alternaria*-sensitized patients.

The allergen was cloned and expressed as a recombinant protein in *Escherichia coli* [113]. The deduced amino acid sequence revealed a high similarity to the subtilisin-like serine proteases from a variety of filamentous fungi. Significant homologies with vacuolar serine proteases across multiple fungal taxonomic groups identified in *Curvularia* (90%), *Cladosporium* (70%–76%), *Penicillium* (68%–71%), *Aspergillus* (71%), and *Rhodotorula* (64%) were confirmed. Two critical amino acid residues (His157, Phe160) for IgE binding mapped on Pen ch 13 [114] were conserved on all fungal serine protease allergens including Alt a 15. Specific IgE analyses suggested that sensitization to Alt a 15 (or the homologous Cur l 4) may be a marker for *Curvularia* sensitization in the absence of Alt a 1 sensitization among patients sensitized to multiple fungi [113].

13.7.2 *Cladosporium* allergens

Cladosporium species is the predominant member belonging to the order Capnodiales in the class Dothideomycetes. Spores of *Cladosporium* species (previously referred to as *Hormodendrum*)

Table 13.6 Basidiomycetes allergens

Fungus	MW (kDa)	Biological activity	Sequence accession number
Psilocybe cubensis			
Psi c 1	48	Unknown	
Psi c 2	16	Cyclophilin, Rotamase	
Coprinus comatus			
Cop c 1	11	Leucine zipper protein	CAB39376
Cop c 2	11.7	Thioredoxin	CAB52130
Cop c 3		Nucleotide-binding protein	CAB52131
Cop c 5	15.6	Unknown	CAB52132
Cop c 7		Unknown	CAB52133
Schizophyllum commune			
Sch c 1	61	Glucoamylase	XP003030591
Malassezia furfur			
Mala f 2	21	Peroxisomal membrane protein	BAA32435
Mala f 3	20	Peroxisomal membrane protein	BAA32436
Mala f 4	35	Malate dehydrogenase	AAD25927
Malassezia sympodialis			
Mala s 1		Peroxisomal protein MF1	CAA65341
Mala s 4		Malate dehydrogenase	UniProt-M5E482
Mala s 5	18	Oxidoreductase	CAA09883
Mala s 6	17	Cyclophilin, Rotamase	CAA09884
Mala s 7		Unknown	CAA09885
Mala s 8	19	Unknown	CAA09886
Mala s 9	37	Unknown	CAA09887
Mala s 10	86	Heat shock protein 70	CAD20981
Mala s 11	23	Mn-superoxide dismutase	CAD68071
Mala s 12	67	G-M-C Oxidoreductase	CAI43283
Mala s 13	13	Thioredoxin	CAI78451
Rhodotorula mucilaginosa			
Rho m 1	47	Enolase	AAP30720
Rho m 2	31	Serine protease	AAT37679

probably occur more abundantly worldwide than any other spore type and are the dominant airborne spores, especially in temperate climates [115]. The recent classification of the genus *Cladosporium* identifies 169 species within three species complexes represented by *C. herbarum*, *C. cladosporioides*, and *C. sphaerospermum* [116]. Although *Cladosporium cladosporioides* in some areas is the most prevalent airborne species, *Cladosporium herbarum* may be the predominant fungal allergen in other locations. *Cladosporium sphaerospermum* can contribute to a significant proportion of indoor fungal allergen load due to its growth at lower water activity (≥0.82) as compared to *C. herbarum* and *C. cladosporioides* (≥0.85) [117]. All three species complexes have been implicated in causing fungal allergies with *C. herbarum* being the most studied. Currently, nine allergens from *C. herbarum* and two from *C. cladosporiodes* have been accepted by the WHO/IUIS Allergen Nomenclature Sub-Committee (see Table 13.3).

Table 13.7 *Candida* allergens

Fungus	MW (kDa)	Biological activity	Sequence accession number
C. albicans			
Cand a 1	40	Alcohol dehydrogenase	CAA57342
Cand a 3	20	Peroxisomal protein	AAN11300
C. boidinii			
Cand b 2	20	Peroxisomal protein	AAA34357

Table 13.8 *Trichophyton* allergens

Fungus	MW (kDa)	Biological activity	Sequence accession number
T. rubrum			
Tri r 2		Serine protease	AAD52013
Tri r 4	83	Serine protease	AAD52012
T. tonsurans			
Tri t 1	30	Unknown	
Tri t 4	83	Serine protease	P80814

The classic crossed-immunoelectrophoretic characterization of *C. herbarum* allergens by Aukrust and colleagues was the first comprehensive analysis of fungal allergenic extracts [118–120]. Over 60 antigenic components were identified using hyperimmunized rabbit antisera raised against *C. herbarum*. Four important and 10–20 less important allergens were demonstrated by crossed radioimmunoelectrophoresis using sera from 35 individuals with allergy to *C. herbarum*. Two of these allergens, Ag-54 (Cla h 1) and Ag-32 (Cla h 2), were partially purified. Ag-32 was reported as a small (13 kDa) acidic allergen existing in multiple isoallergenic forms (pI 3.4–4.4), and Ag-54 (25 kDa) was reported as an acidic glycoprotein (pI 5.0) containing 80% carbohydrate. The carbohydrate moiety of Ag-54 was extensively studied [120,121] and found not to contribute to the IgE-binding properties of the allergen. The application of recombinant technology to fungal allergen identification in the 1990s led to the cloning and sequencing of additional *C. herbarum* allergens [90,122,123]: aldehyde dehydrogenase (Cla h 10, formerly Cla h 3), acid ribosomal proteins P2 (Cla h 5, formerly Cla h 4) and P1 (Cla h 12), YCP4 protein (Cla h 7, formerly Cla h 5), and enolase (Cla h 6). The nomenclature assigned to these allergens was initially based on the order of discovery; now, their names are revised to reflect their assignment to homologous groups (see Table 13.1). The utility of this revised nomenclature is especially relevant when one considers the growing number of orthologous allergens identified among the fungi.

The only *Cladosporium* allergen to be currently recognized as a major allergen is Cla h 8 (mannitol dehydrogenase). The allergen is recognized by 12 of 21 (57%) of *Cladosporium*-allergic patients as determined by IgE immunoblotting [124]. The native allergen exists as a 28 kDa protein with a pI of 5.8. Enzymatic analysis established that Cla h 8 is a nicotinamide adenine dinucleotide phosphate (NADP[H])-dependent mannitol dehydrogenase that is likely induced in response to environmental stress. The crystal structure of Cla h 8 was determined [125] and showed that the protein can exist as a monomer, dimer, or tetramer in solution. Metal cations were shown to stabilize oligomer formation by bridging the C-terminal carboxy termini of the individual subunits. It would be of interest to study how these varying structures might influence their allergenic properties.

The vacuolar serine protease from *C. cladosporioides* (Cla c 9) was isolated as a 36 kDa protein showing extensive cross-reactivity with fungal serine proteases derived from *Aspergillus fumigatus* and *Penicillium chrysogenum*. Chou et al. [126] found 41 of 74 (55%) prevalence of IgE binding toward Cla c 9 in *C. cladosporioides*–sensitized patients and designated the allergen as a major allergen. Subsequently, the homologue from *C. herbarum*, Cla h 9, was cloned and expressed for immunologic studies [127]. High sequence homologies were confirmed between the vacuolar serine proteases from *A. fumigatus* (A fum 18), *P. oxalicum* (Pen o 18), *P. chrysogenum* (Pen ch 18) (64%–78%), as well as with Cla c 9 (97%). The Cla h 9 allergen bound IgE antibodies from 17 of 110 *C. herbarum*–sensitized patients (15.5%) and was shown to be highly allergenically cross-reactive to Asp f 18, Pen ch 18, and Pen ch 13, an alkaline serine protease. Epitope mapping using IgE antibodies from *Cladosporium*-sensitized subjects and peptide fragments distributed along the entire protein sequence revealed a potential cross-reactive epitope localized on one of the peptides corresponding to amino acid residues 244–298 on Cla h 9.

A novel family of cross-reacting fungal transaldolases is represented by Cla c 14. About 38% of *C. cladosporioides*–sensitized patients showed IgE binding against Cla c 14. Chou et al. [128] cloned the full-length cDNAs encoding the transaldolase from *C. cladosporioides* and *P. chrysogenum* (Pen ch 35). Sequence alignment revealed that the Cla c 14 sequence has 65%, 75%, and 76% amino acids identical to that of *S. cerevisiae*, *A. fumigatus*, and *P. chrysogenum* transaldolases. Human transaldolase revealed 61% amino acid sequence identity. IgE cross-reactivity was detected by immunoblot inhibition testing using human allergic sera, and a linear IgE-reactive fragment (aa residues 257–278) was localized on Cla c 14. Interestingly, residues 271–285 on human transaldolase, recognized by autoantibodies from multiple sclerosis patients [129], correspond to residues 261–275 on Cla c 14.

13.7.3 *Aspergillus* allergens

The genus *Aspergillus*, with about 250 species, belongs to the order Eurotiales in the class Eurotiomycetes. *Aspergillus fumigatus* is one of the predominant fungi implicated in the pathogenesis of allergic diseases in humans and the principal etiological agent of ABPA [130]. Clinical diagnosis of ABPA includes asthma, proximal bronchiectasis, immediate skin reactivity to *A. fumigatus* antigenic extracts, elevated total serum IgE (>417 kU/L), and elevated sIgE and/or IgG to *A. fumigatus*. Other species, such as *A. nidulans*, *A. oryzae*, *A. terreus*, *A. flavus*, and *A. niger*, also cause allergic diseases in humans [131–135]. All of these organisms are freely distributed in most environments, although in certain conditions they grow much faster and liberate numerous spores. The ability to diagnose and differentiate ABPA would be greatly improved using standardized antigen preparations.

Early studies with *A. fumigatus* extracts showed that they were diverse in their physiochemical and immunologic characteristics [136–140]. Depending on the source materials used to prepare the

Table 13.9 Other fungal allergens

Fungus	MW (kDa)	Biological activity	Sequence accession number
Curvularia lunata			
Cur l 1	31	Serine protease	
Cur l 2	48	Enolase	AAK67491
Cur l 3	12	Cytochrome c	AAK67492
Cur l 4	54	Serine protease	ACF19589
Cur l 6		Mn superoxide dismutase	UniProt-Q1EHH3
Epicoccum purpurascens			
Epi p 1	30	Serine protease	P83340
Epi p 13		Glutathione-*S*-transferase	UniProt-Q45X97
Fusarium culmorum			
Fus c 1	11	Ribosomal protein P2	AAL79930
Fus c 2	13	Thioredoxin	AAL79931
Fus c 3		Unknown	UniProt-5516
Fusarium proliferatum			
Fus p 4	37.5	Transaldolase	AHY02994
Fus p 9	36.5	Serine protease	AJA79001
Fusarium solani			
Fus s 1		Unknown	UniProt P81010
Stachybotrys chartarum			
Sta c 3	21	Exodeoxyribonuclease	ACT37324
Rhizopus oryzae			
Rhi o 1	44	Aspartyl endopeptidase	AIS82656, AIS82657
Rhi o 2	18	Cyclophilin, Rotamase	ALM24136

extracts and the detection systems employed, about 100 different antigenic components could be detected. Varying numbers of antigens were found to bind IgE antibodies using sera from patients with ABPA. Thus, the use of antigenic preparations derived from *A. fumigatus* cultured and processed under different conditions led to confusion and discord regarding their identity, purity, and specificity. The application of molecular approaches based on the use of purified or recombinant allergens has not only provided powerful diagnostic tools but also allowed for the standardization of antigen preparations [75]. Currently, no fewer than 23 different allergens have been identified in *A. fumigatus* (see Table 13.4), and they represent a wide range of proteins and glycoproteins ranging in molecular weight from 11 kDa to about 100 kDa.

Asp f 1 is an 18 kDa allergen to which about 85% of ABPA patients possess IgE antibodies. Amino acid sequencing of Asp f 1 shows extensive homology to mitogillin, a cytotoxin produced by *A. restrictus* [142,143]. Asp f 1 is a secreted antigen and is rarely detected in environmental samples [144,145]. The linear B-cell epitopes of Asp f 1 were localized using synthetic decapeptides spanning the entire molecule and analyzed for their IgE-binding

properties using sera from ABPA patients [146]. Six peptides representing the C-terminal end of the molecule demonstrated strong IgE binding. Two of them representing amino acid residues 116–130 showed 80%–91% inhibition of IgE binding to the whole molecule, while the extreme end (aa residues 140–149) achieved 100% inhibition of IgE binding. Nine peptides bound IgE antibodies.

Another major allergen, a 37 kDa protein of *A. fumigatus* (Asp f 2), has been cloned, expressed, and characterized [147]. Recombinant Asp f 2 exhibits specific IgE binding with sera of ABPA patients and discriminates ABPA without evidence of central bronchiectasis (ABPA-S) from ABPA with definitive central bronchiectasis (ABPA-CB). Banerjee et al. [148] identified both conformational and linear IgE-binding on Asp f 2 using synthetic decamer peptides spanning the entire molecule and testing them for reactivity using sera from patients with ABPA. Reduction and alkylation of the molecule significantly diminished its IgE binding suggesting the importance of conformational-dependent epitopes. Point mutations responsible for the loss of IgE binding indicated that intrachain disulfide loops between cysteine residues residing near the C-terminus are involved in forming IgE-binding epitopes of Asp f 2 [242].

Asp f 3 has been identified as a major allergen based on immediate skin test reactivity, peripheral blood mononuclear cell proliferation, and strong IgE binding in up to 94% of patients with ABPA. The primary structure reveals sequence homology among identified IgE epitopes of peroxisomal membrane proteins from *Candida boidinii* [149], *Malassezia furfur* [150], and *Pencillium citrinum* [151]. Linear IgE-binding regions were demonstrated using synthetic peptides spanning the entire molecule using sera from patients with ABPA in IgE-ELISA and Western blotting. Conformational determinants were identified at the *N*-terminal and *C*-terminal ends using mutant recombinant Asp f 3 proteins deleted off the specific IgE-binding regions. The IgE-binding patterns of the respective mutant Asp f 3 molecules suggested that together the *N*-terminal residues 1–12 and the *C*-terminal residues 143–150 were necessary for maintaining the IgE-binding conformational structure [152].

Asp f 4 is one of several recombinant allergens derived by screening a cDNA library from *A. fumigatus* displayed on the surface of the filamentous phage M13 with sera from patients with ABPA [153]. Asp f 4 along with Asp f 2, and Asp f 6 showed differential binding to IgE antibodies in sera of ABPA patients when compared to *A. fumigatus*–sensitized asthmatic patients without ABPA [112,155]. In contrast, Asp f 1 and Asp f 3 showed significant binding in both patient groups and lacked diagnostic specificity. The biological function of Asp f 4 is not known. Ramachandran et al. [156] evaluated the role of the four cysteine residues present in Asp f 4 in the immune responses in ABPA. They selectively deleted the cysteine residues and tested the mutant Asp f 4 molecules for IgE binding using serum from ABPA patients. Based on the IgE-binding patterns toward the respective mutant Asp f 4 proteins, the authors determined that the *N*-terminal IgE epitope regions are critical in maintaining the IgE-binding conformational structure.

Asp f 3 (peroxisomal membrane protein), Asp f 6 (manganese superoxide dismutase), Asp f 8 (P2 acidic ribosomal protein), Asp f 11 (peptidyl-prolyl isomerase), Asp f 12 (heat shock protein 90), Asp f 22 (enolase), and Asp f 27 (cyclophilin) belong to a group of highly conserved proteins with structural similarities and cross-reactivity with homologous proteins across phyla. Some of these proteins share more than 50% sequence identity with their corresponding human homologues. The allergens Asp f 6 and Asp f 8, as well as the human homologues, stimulated peripheral blood lymphocytes and induced positive skin reactions in patients with ABPA, suggesting a role for IgE-mediated and cell-mediated autoreactivity in patients suffering from chronic inflammatory responses to *A. fumigatus* [157,158]. The *A. fumigatus* gene encoding a polypeptide fragment of a heat shock protein 90 family, Asp f 12, has been expressed and its allergenicity confirmed [159]. Asp f 12 has homologous counterparts in *Candida albicans*, *Saccharomyces*, *Trypanosoma*, housefly, mouse, and humans. Asp f 22 or enolase has been shown to be cross-reactive with other fungal enolases. Enolase was first identified as an allergen in *S. cerevisiae* [160] and *C. albicans* [161,162]. Subsequently, enolase has been identified as an allergen in *C. herbarum*, *A. alternata*, *A. fumigatus*, *C. lunata*, and *P. citrinum* [105]. Asp f 27 and Asp f 11 are members of the cyclophilin family of cytosolic proteins, which play a role in protein folding and is highly conserved among different phyla. As an allergen, cyclophilins have been found to be cross-reactive across other fungi, including the basidiomycete *Psilocybe cubensis* [163], the yeast *Malassezia furfur* [150], as well as the phylogenetically more distant birch pollen [164] and human cyclophilin [165].

Asp f 16 is a 43 kDa protein with unknown biological function that strongly binds to IgE from ABPA patients. Seventy-five percent of ABPA patients demonstrated high levels of IgE to the recombinant allergen, but no detectable IgE was found in patient sera from *Aspergillus* skin-test-positive asthmatics without ABPA [166]. Thus, Asp f 16 showed specificity toward ABPA as found with Asp f 2, Asp f 4, and Asp f 6. Asp f 16 failed to show any significant sequence homology with known structural proteins except for a 36% identity and 46% similarity within the region of amino acid residues 99–214 with a probable membrane protein from the yeast *Saccharomyces cerevisiae*. In addition, Asp f 14 exhibited an overall sequence homology of 53% with the 31 kDa Asp f 9, another *Aspergillus fumigatus* allergen with unknown biological function.

The alkaline and vacuolar serine proteases have been identified as pan-fungal allergens in prevalent airborne fungal species including *Aspergillus*, *Penicillium*, *Cladosporium*, *Curvularia*, *Rhodotorula*, and *Trichophyton* [70,167–174]. These fungal proteases exhibit high sequence homologies with the known enzymes of other fungi and have been identified as important cross-reacting aeroallergens in *A. fumigatus* (Asp f 13 and Asp f 18), *A. flavus* (Asp fl 13 and Asp fl 18), *A. oryzae* (Asp o 13), *A. niger* (Asp n 18), as well as in *Pencillium citrinum* (Pen c 13 and Pen c 18), *P. oxalicum* (Pen o 18), and *P. chrysogenum* (Pen ch 13 and Pen ch 18). Serine proteases from *Cladosporium* (Cla c 9), *Curvularia* (Cur l 1), and *Rhodotorula* (Rho m 2) have also been identified as cross-reacting allergens [167]. Chow et al. [167] localized IgE-binding epitopes on Asp f 13 (alkaline serine protease) peptides generated by cyanogen bromide (CNBr) cleavage or proteolysis. Three peptides corresponding to amino acid residues 165–202, 188–259, and 243–282 showed strong reactivity to a serum pool from *Aspergillus*-sensitized patients. These epitopes were mapped at the *C*-terminal end of the Asp f 13 molecule.

The biological function of the *Aspergillus* allergens Asp f 2, Asp f 4, Asp f 7, Asp f 9, Asp f 11, Asp f 15, Asp f 16, and Asp f 17 is still not known, and homologous proteins have not yet been identified among other taxa. For this reason, these allergens could be regarded as species-specific allergens. In contrast, Asp f 3, Asp f 6, Asp f 8, Asp f 12, Asp f 13, Asp f 18, Asp f 22, and Asp f 27 are highly conserved proteins with homologous, cross-reacting proteins from other taxa that might be considered important as environmental fungal respiratory allergens.

Aspergillus allergen groups not identified in *A. fumigatus* include Asp n 14 (β-xylosidase) and Asp n 25 (3-phytase B) from *A. niger*; and Asp o 21 (TAKA α-amylase A) from *A. oryzae*. All of these are enzymatic proteins causing occupational respiratory allergies in the food industry [175–177].

13.7.4 *Penicillium* species allergens

The genus *Penicillium* belongs to the order Eurotiales in the class Eurotiomycetes and to the same family Trichocomaceae as the genus *Aspergillus* and *Paecilomyces*. They are ubiquitous soil fungi commonly found in both indoor and outdoor environments [6]. Inhalation of *Penicillium* spores in quantities comparable with those encountered by natural exposure can induce both immediate and late asthma in sensitive persons [53]. Among more than 300 different *Penicillium* species, *P. citrinum*, *P. chrysogenum* (*P. notatum*), *P. oxalicum*, *P. brevicompactum*, and *P. spinulosum* are the five most frequently recovered species of *Penicillium* in the United States, while *P. citrinum* is the most prevalent *Penicillium* species reported from Taiwan [178]. Seventeen allergens representing 13 allergen groups from five *Penicillium* species have been identified and accepted by the WHO/IUIS Allergen Nomenclature Sub-Committee (see Table 13.5).

The group 13 (alkaline serine proteases) and group 18 (vacuolar serine proteases) allergens have been identified as major allergens of *P. citrinum*, *P. brevicompactum*, *P. chrysogenum*, and *P. oxalicum* [70]. Immunoblotting showed that IgE antibodies against components of these prevalent *Penicillium* species are detected in the sera of 16%–26% of asthmatic patients [172]. The majority of the positive serum samples tested showed IgE-binding to the group 13 allergens, with a frequency greater than 80% in different fungal species tested. Vijay et al. studied 14 *Penicillium* species and found that *P. viridicatum*, *P. janthinellium*, *P. oxalicum*, *P. brevicompactum*, and *P. italicum* are highly immunogenic as well as allergenic and possibly good candidates for allergen cloning studies [179].

The cDNAs of the alkaline serine protease allergens from *P. citrinum* (Pen c 13) and *P. chrysogenum* (Pen ch 13), and the vacuolar serine proteases from *P. citrinum* (Pen c 18), *P. oxalicum* (Pen o 18), and *P. chrysogenum* (Pen ch 18) have been cloned and characterized [114,168,169,171,173,174,180–182]. IgE cross-reactivity occurs among the group 13 and 18 allergens of *Penicillium* and *Aspergillus* species, and results suggest that patients primarily sensitized to serine protease allergens from one of these genera may develop allergic symptoms after exposure to the other due to cross-reactivity [70]. Allergen-specific IgE epitopes have been identified between group 13 and 18 allergens. Shen et al. [181] used immunoblot cross-inhibition experiments using allergic sera positive to Asp o 13 and Asp o 18 to evaluate the cross-reactivity between group 13 and 18 allergens. The extent of cross-inhibition varied significantly depending on the individual patient serum used, suggesting the presence of both cross-reactive and allergen-specific IgE-binding epitopes on these molecules. Moreover, Chou et al. [171] evaluated the cross-reactivity between the homologous group 13 allergens from *P. chrysogenum* (Pen ch13) and *A. fumigatus* (Asp f 13) using ELISA inhibition with Pen ch 13 as the allergosorbent and serum from patients sensitized to both species. Both homologues completely inhibited IgE binding to Pen ch 13, but the relative inhibitory potency varied from 4 to 16 times in favor of Pen ch 13. Further insight into the structural features of the IgE epitopes of Pen ch 13 and its homologues was pursued by Lai et al. [114]. They tested for linear IgE-binding epitopes using 11 overlapping phage-displayed peptide fragments spanning the entire molecule, and the results were used to further localize the putative epitopes on the surface of a three-dimensional model of Pen ch 13. Site-directed mutagenesis of the Pen ch 13 molecule at one location (His49 and Phe52), which corresponded to one of the highest IgE-binding regions, significantly reduced the overall IgE reactivity of the molecule. Interestingly, these residues represented a highly conserved region located on the surface of fungal serine proteases. Yu et al. [183] mapped IgE-binding epitopes on the Pen ch 18 molecule to nine different peptide fragments generated by proteolytic digestion. The corresponding residues of the reactive peptides were distributed along the entire length of the molecule. One of the peptides (aa residues 44–62) was recognized by six of eight (75%) of the patients tested and was classified as a dominant epitope. Using a molecular model, this immunodominant IgE-binding epitope was localized on a structurally conserved solvent-exposed surface region at the *N*-terminal end of the molecule.

Several minor *Penicillium* allergens have been identified. They include the fungal pan-allergens peroxisomal membrane protein, Pen c 3 [151]; heat shock protein P70, Pen c 19 [184]; *N*-acetylglucosaminase, Pen ch 20 [185]; enolase, Pen c 22 [186]; elongation factor 1-β, Pen c 24 [187]; acidic ribosomal protein P1, Pen b 26 [75,189] and Pen cr 26 [190]; catalase, Pen c 30

[188]; calreticulin, Pen ch 31; pectate lyase, Pen c 32 [188]; and transaldolase, Pen ch 35 [128]. No biological function has been attributed to Pen ch 33. The relative clinical importance of these allergens with respect to the alkaline and vacuolar serine proteases has not yet been critically evaluated.

13.7.5 Basidiomycetes allergens

There are over 20,000 Basidiomycetes species, including the familiar mushrooms and puffballs belonging to the fungal order Agaricales; the pathogenic fungi belonging to orders Pucciniales and Ustilaginales that cause plant diseases called rusts and smuts; and the yeast-like *Malessezia* and *Rhodotorula*. Reports indicate that basidiospores occur in the air in high concentrations throughout the world [3,191]. Respiratory allergy and asthma have been correlated to outdoor basidiospore levels, and occupational exposure can result in hypersensitivity pneumonitis. About 50 species have tested for allergenicity, and about 25 have been determined to be allergenic. Positive skin tests, sIgE measurements, and provocation tests to their extracts occur in sensitized subjects [192–194].

Calvatia species are seasonally occurring puffballs that are prolific producers of basidiospores. Two major allergens, one with a pI of 9.3 and the other with a pI of 6.6, were identified from IgE immunoprints using crude and fractionated extracts of *Calvatia cyathiformis* [195]. The pI 9.3 allergen, to which 68% of *C. cyathiformis*–sensitized patients possessed IgE antibodies, was purified using preparative isoelectric focusing and was found to have a molecular weight of 16 kDa [196].

Pleurotus ostreatus (oyster mushroom) is cultivated for food and has been identified as a cause of hypersensitivity pneumonitis among mushroom workers [197]. Their spores contain at least five allergens that have been identified by crossed-radioimmunoelectrophoresis analyses [198].

Psilocybe cubensis (magic mushroom) mycelial and spore extracts have been characterized by immunoblotting and RAST inhibition [198]. The major allergen Psi c 2 was cloned and found to be 78% identical to the homologous cyclophilin from the fission yeast *Schizosaccharomyces pombe* [163].

The allergenicity of *Coprinus* (inky cap) spores and mycelium extracts has been demonstrated by skin tests and RAST [192,199,200]. Several allergens from *C. comatus* have been identified and cloned (see Table 13.6). Sequence analysis of the 11 kDa Cop c 1 reveals the periodic repetition of leucine residues, a characteristic of leucine zipper structural domains that are common among plant transcription factors. Thirty-four percent of individuals sensitized to *C. comatus* and 25% from basidiomycete-sensitized subjects showed serum IgE binding to rCop c 1 [201]. The sequence for a second recombinant allergen, Cop c 2, codes for *C. comatus* thioredoxin, which is a highly conserved protein involved in a variety of cellular processes including DNA synthesis, protein folding, and stress responses. No information other than the sequences of the remaining cloned Cop c allergens has been published.

Schizophyllum commune is a causative agent for allergic bronchopulmonary mycosis (ABPM) and allergic fungal sinusitis. A major allergen, designated Sch c 1, was identified from Western blots of concentrated *S. commune* culture filtrates and subsequently cloned [202]. The cloned and sequenced rSch c 1 was identified as a glucoamylase. The majority of patients with *S. commune*–induced ABPM had both Sch c 1–specific IgG and IgE antibody. Two of 10 sera from patients with ABPA had positive IgG titers against Sch c 1, and none were positive for IgE against Sch c 1, suggesting the diagnostic utility of this allergen in immunoassays for differentiating ABPM caused by different fungal species, especially A. fumigatus.

Ganoderma belongs to the fungal class Agaricomycetes, order Polyporales, which includes many of the common bracket fungi found on decaying trees. *Ganoderma* is used in traditional Asian medicines, and their lignin- and cellulose-degrading enzymes have industrial applications, especially in biopulping and bioremediation. Spores of *Ganoderma* occur widely in air-sampling surveys [203–205]. The allergenicity of G. meredithae spore and cap extracts was investigated using Western blots with serum from sensitized individuals. Ten allergens ranging in size from 14 kDa to greater than 66 kDa with pls ranging from less than 3.5 to 6.6 were identified [206]. A similar range of IgE-binding proteins was also detected in G. applanatum spores and fruiting body extracts. In another study of G. applanatum spores, 14 allergens were detected by crossed radioimmunoelectrophoresis (CRIE) and immunoblotting [207]. This study also revealed that IgE-binding bands are mostly between 18 and 82 kDa. Even though several *Ganoderma* extracts are reasonably well-characterized, no allergens have been purified, sequenced, or cloned.

Malassezia (*Pityrosporum*) belongs to fungal class Malasseziomycetes, order Malasseziales, and includes 11 species of *Malassezia*, the most clinically important being M. globosa, M. sympodialis, M. furfur, M. restricta, and M. obtusa. They are yeast-like, lipophilic fungi that are normal flora on human skin but can cause opportunistic infections, tinea versicolor, folliculitis, and seborrheic dermatitis. They can also be an exacerbating factor in atopic dermatitis, psoriasis, and neonatal cephalic pustulosis [208].

Malassezia produces a complex array of species-specific as well as cross-reacting allergenic proteins [209,210], and 13 of them have been cloned, sequenced, and accepted by the WHO/IUIS Allergen Nomenclature Sub-Committee (see Table 13.6). They include the highly cross-reactive fungal pan-allergens peroxisomal proteins, Mala f 2 and Mala f 3 [211]; cyclophilin, Mala s 6 [150,165,212]; heat shock protein 70, Mala s 10 [213]; manganese superoxide dismutase, Mala s 11 [213]; and thioredoxin, Mala s 13 [214]. Several allergens have no homology with known fungal proteins and are prospective genus- or species-specific allergens: Mala s 1 [215], Mala s 5 [150], Mala s 7, Mal f 8, and Mala s 9 [216]. Mala s 12 is a major allergen based on its IgE reactivity with 62% of sera from atopic eczema (AE) patients sensitized to M. sympodialis. The sequence of the 67 kDa protein showed similarity to the glucose-methanol-choline (GMC) oxidoreductase enzyme superfamily [217]. Laboratory cultures of M. sympodialis grown at pH 6.1 to 5.0 were analyzed for the presence of IgE-binding components by immunoblotting and quantitative PCR [218]. The biosynthesis of allergens, especially Mala s 12, was greatly enhanced under the higher pH conditions associated with skin of AE patients, suggesting a host-microbe interaction where *Malassezia* on the skin of patients with increased pH will produce more allergen into the skin environment, leading to increased inflammation in AE patients.

The availability of a panel of individual recombinant *Malassezia* allergenic proteins has allowed for enhanced diagnostic resolution not achieved by whole cell extracts. Casagrande et al. investigated the differential reactivity to M. sympodialis allergens in various atopic patients including those with urticaria, asthma, contact dermatitis, and AE. In addition, AE patients were further evaluated by skin prick tests, atopic patch tests, IgE-ELISA, and peripheral blood mononuclear cell (PBMC) proliferation assays with six recombinant M. sympodialis allergens, rMala s 1 and rMala s 5–9 [219]. Sensitization to M. sympodialis and its individual allergens was specific for AE patients. Frequencies of positive IgE antibodies among the AE patients were 39%, 47%, 55%, 10%, 31%, and 61% for rMala s 1, 5, 6, 7, 8, and 9, respectively. Response rates were similar when the allergens were applied by atopic patch tests. Frequencies of positive PBMC proliferation assay were 46%, 0, 38%, 8%, 31%, and 54%, respectively. The results indicated that Mala s 9 was the dominant allergen among those evaluated in terms of IgE and T-cell responses in AE patients.

Rhodotorula belong to the fungal class Microbotryomycetes, order Sporidiobolales, and are among the most common environmental yeasts found in air, soil, water, milk, and fruits [220]. They can colonize human skin, and R. mucilaginosa (R. rubra), R. glutinis, and R. minuta are known opportunistic pathogens. In a study evaluating antibody responses to common yeasts in atopic patients, Savolainen et al. [221] identified five IgE-binding components using Western blotting and sera from eight patients sensitized to R. mucilaginosa. Two allergens have been cloned and sequenced: Enolase, Rho m 1 [222]; and vacuolar serine protease, Rho m 2 [223]. Among R. mucilaginosa–sensitized bronchial asthmatic patients, 21% demonstrated IgE antibodies to Rho m 1, while 57% demonstrated IgE to the 31 kDa Rho m 2. Both allergens are highly cross-reactive with their respective homologues from other prevalent fungal species. Enolase allergens from C. albicans, S. cerevisiae, P. citrinum, A. fumigatus, C. herbarum, and A. alternata have 74%–85% sequence identity with Rho m 1 and serine protease allergens from three different *Penicillium* species share 67%–68% sequence identity with Rho m 2.

13.7.6 *Candida albicans* allergens

Candida albicans belongs to the fungal class Saccharomycetes, order Saccharomycetales, and family Saccharomycetaceae, which include yeasts that reproduce by budding. Another member of the same family, *Saccharomyces cerevisiae*, is perhaps the most economically important fungus and has served as a model eukaryotic organism for molecular and cell biologists. S. cerevisiae enolase has been identified as an important inhalant allergen associated with baker's asthma in occupational settings, with cross-reactivity to C. albicans enolase [160–162].

C. albicans is one of the most prevalent fungal species of the normal human microbiota, colonizing much of the mucosa including the skin, oral cavity, and gastrointestinal and genitourinary tracts. It can cause life-threatening opportunistic infections supported by a wide range of virulence factors and the ability to adapt to changing environmental conditions [224]. Sensitization to C. albicans is associated with a variety of atopic diseases including atopic dermatitis, eosinophilic esophagitis, chronic urticaria, and allergic asthma [225–229]. Although several allergenic proteins have been identified [161,162,229,230], only two allergens from C. albicans and one from C. boidinii have been accepted by the WHO/IUIS Allergen Nomenclature Sub-Committee (see Table 13.7). Cand a 1, a 40 kDa C. albicans alcohol dehydrogenase, was cloned and its sequence identity revealed 70% homology with S. cerevisiae alcohol dehydrogenase [231]. Cand a 3 is a 20 kDa peroxisomal protein that has 62% sequence identity with the homologous protein from S. cerevisiae [232]. Cand b 2 is the C. boidinii peroxisomal membrane protein showing 58% sequence similarity with the homologous protein from A. fumigatus [149].

13.7.7 *Trichophyton* species

Trichophyton belongs to the fungal order Onygenales in the class Eurotiomycetes. They are members of the family Arthrodermataceae, which includes three dermatophytes, *Epidermophyton* and *Microsporum*. Humans and other animals are natural reservoirs for these fungi. *T. rubrum*, *T. mentagrophytes*, and *T. tonsurans* are the three anthropophilic species most often associated with dermatophytosis. Both immediate hypersensitivity (IH) and delayed-type hypersensitivity (DTH) to *Trichophyton* are common in humans, with the latter considered as protective against infection [232]. The role of *Trichophyton* spp. in IgE-mediated urticaria, asthma, and rhinitis has been supported in clinical studies [232–235], and four allergens have been identified and studied (see Table 13.8).

Tri t 1 is a 30 kDa major allergen of *T. tonsurans* to which 54% of *Trichophyton*-sensitized, skin test-positive and 73% of RAST-positive patients possess IgE antibodies [236]. The allergen has a sequence similarity to *S. cerevisiae* exo 1,3-β-glucanase [237] The *Trichophyton* group 4 allergens have been identified in *T. tonsurans* (Tri t 4) and *T. rubrum* (Tri r 4) as an 83 kDa protein associated with DTH skin test reactions. The cloned and sequenced rTri r 4 [238] showed limited sequence identity to the prolyl oligopeptidase family of serine proteinases. Tri r 2 was also cloned and sequenced [238], and the 29 kDa protein has a high degree of sequence identity to the subtilase enzyme family.

Slunt et al. [239] examined *in vitro* T-cell cytokine production in patients with either IH or DTH skin test reactions to *Trichophyton* extract. T-cell clones from subjects with immediate hypersensitivity to *Trichophyton* produced a Th2/Th0 cytokine profile in response to stimulation with *T. tonsurans* extract, Tri t 1, or Tri t 4, while those from subjects with DTH had a Th 1 profile after stimulation. These results demonstrated that *T. tonsurans* can elicit distinct T-cell profiles that correspond to *in vivo* hypersensitivity skin test responses in sensitized subjects. In another study, Woodfolk et al. [240] further delineated differences in T-cell repertoires between subjects with IH and DTH reactions to *Trichophyton*. T-cell epitopes were mapped using PBMC proliferation assays with Tri r 2, an allergen capable of eliciting both IH and DTH skin responses in sensitized individuals. A set of 27 synthetic, overlapping peptides spanning the entire Tri r 2 molecule was used to stimulate PBMCs from each test subject. The results showed that differential responsiveness to a single peptide (P5) in the amino-terminal end of the molecule gave a 95% predictive accuracy for classifying subjects into the IH or DTH group. It would be of interest to evaluate whether T-cell hyporesponsiveness to this epitope predisposes individuals to develop IH to *Trichophyton*.

13.7.8 Other fungi

Aerobiological studies performed in various geographical locations and different countries demonstrate the prevalence of other fungi including *Mucor*, *Rhizopus*, *Geotrichum*, *Curvularia*, *Drechslera*, *Bipolaris*, *Helminthosporium*, *Stemphylium*, *Ulocladium*, *Epicoccum*, *Phoma*, *Aureobasidium*, *Paecilomyces*, *Fusarium*, *Trichoderma*, *Acremonium* (*Cephalosporium*), *Stachybotrys*, *Trichothecium*, *Neurospora*, *Chaetomium*, *Nigrospora*, *Botrytis*, *Ustilago*, and *Puccinia*, and these genera have been implicated in allergic disorders in humans [2–6,22,48–51,54,65]. In cases where allergens from these fungi have been identified, they have been orthologous allergenic proteins previously identified in related fungi [17,21,79,94, 107,108,110,141,154,241].

13.8 CONCLUSION AND FUTURE DIRECTIONS

Significant progress in fungal allergen identification and characterization has been made, particularly since the 1990s, because of the availability of purified and recombinant allergens. The increase in sequence data of fungal allergens has allowed for comparative genomic analyses and the identification of species-specific and potentially cross-reactive allergens. This knowledge base should serve to better define sensitization toward fungal species and improve diagnostic testing.

Progress in the standardization of fungal extracts used clinically has been nonexistent. Enough information is now available to begin characterizing the allergenic composition of commercially available *Alternaria*, *Cladosporium*, *Aspergillus*, and *Penicillium* extracts to evaluate their quality, potency, and consistency. This would be the first step toward standardization.

The use of fungal extracts in skin testing does not generate the information needed to differentiate the primary sensitizing fungi from those that are cross-reactive. The knowledge of individual species-specific and cross-reacting allergens is needed to improve diagnostic testing with respect to their positive and negative predictive value, especially in polysensitized patients. Component-resolved diagnostics (CRDs) have been used with increasing utility especially in food, pollen, and insect venom allergy patients [64]. A promising application in fungal allergy patients would be in differentiating ABPA from fungal sensitization [155,156]. The feasibility of CRD in fungal allergy is made possible with the increased availability of purified, recombinant fungal allergens, and there is no shortage of patients who could benefit from improved diagnostics and immunotherapy outcomes.

SALIENT POINTS

1. Fungi are ubiquitous, and of the more than 80 genera of major fungal groups that have been associated with symptoms of respiratory allergy, only a few genera have been systematically investigated for causing allergic diseases.
2. Many common fungi still await clinical evaluation and testing to determine their relevance in allergic disease.
3. Although the fungal spores in the outdoor air are seasonal, in cold climates some fungal-sensitive patients have perennial symptoms, possibly because of growth and sporulation of fungi in the indoor environment.
4. Fungal spores are structurally very different from pollens since inhaled particles consist of entire living cells, capable of growing and secreting allergens *in vivo*.
5. Progress in standardization of fungal extracts (vaccines) has been impeded by the variations in the inclusion of mycelia, spore, and culture filtrate-derived allergens in extracts; conditions in which the fungi are cultivated and extracts prepared; and types of quality control measured employed.
6. Recombinant allergens including engineered allergens and synthetic peptides have facilitated epitope identification and production of allergens that may provide safer and more effective diagnosis and treatment of fungal allergy.
7. Allergenic cross-reactivity has been observed among homologous allergens across fungal taxonomic groups and at times with nonfungal species. The ability to differentiate the

primary sensitizing fungi from those that are cross-reactive is needed to improve diagnostic testing, especially in polysensitized patients.

REFERENCES

1. Axelopoulos CJ, Mims CW, Blackwell M. *Introductory Mycology*, 4th ed. New York, NY: John Wiley & Sons, 1996.
2. Levetin E, Horner WE, Scott JA; Environmental Allergens Workgroup. Taxonomy of allergenic fungi. *J Allergy Clin Immunol Pract* 2016; 4: 375–385.
3. Horner WE, Helbling A, Salvaggio JE, Lehrer SB. Fungal allergens. *Clin Microbiol Rev* 1995; 8(2): 161–179.
4. Kurup VP, Shen HD, Banerjee B. Respiratory fungal allergy. *Microbes Infect* 2000; 2: 1101–1110.
5. Twaroch TE, Curin M, Valenta R, Swoboda I. Mold allergens in respiratory allergy: From structure to therapy. *Allergy Asthma Immunol Res* 2015; 7: 205–220.
6. Vijay HM, Kurup VP. Fungal allergens. *Clin Allergy Immunol* 2008; 21: 141–160.
7. Rick EM, Woolnough K, Pashley CH, Wardlaw AJ. Allergic fungal airway disease. *J Investig Allergol Clin Immunol* 2016; 26: 344–354.
8. Baxi SN, Portnoy JM, Larenas-Linnemann D, Phippatanuakul W. Exposure and health effects of fungi on humans. *J Allergy Clin Immunol Pract* 2016; 4(3): 396–404.
9. Heinzerling L, Frew AJ, Bindslev-Jensen C et al. Standard skin prick testing and sensitization to inhalant allergens across Europe—A survey from the GALEN network. *Allergy* 2005; 60: 1287–1300.
10. Salo PM, Arbes SJ, Jr., Sever M et al. Exposure to *Alternaria alternata* in US homes is associated with asthma symptoms. *J Allergy Clin Immunol* 2006; 118: 892–898.
11. Selman M, Pardo A, King TE. Hypersensitivity pneumonitis. *Am J Resp Crit Care Med* 2012; 186: 314–324.
12. Greenberger PA. Allergic bronchopulmonary aspergillosis, allergic fungal sinusitis, and hypersensitivity pneumonitis. *Clin Allergy Immunol* 2002; 16: 449–468.
13. Adhikari A, Reponen T, Rylander R. Airborne fungal cell fragments in homes in relation to total fungal biomass. *Indoor Air* 2013; 23(2): 142–147.
14. Gorny RL, Reponen T, Willeke K et al. Fungal fragments as indoor air biocontaminants. *Appl Environ Microbiol* 2002; 68: 3522–3531.
15. Fukutomi Y, Taniguchi M. Sensitization to fungal allergens: Resolved and unresolved issues. *Allergol Int* 2015; 64: 321–331.
16. Crameri R, Garbani M, Rhyner C, Huitema C. Fungi: The neglected allergenic sources. *Allergy* 2014; 69: 176–185.
17. Simon-Nobbe B, Denk U, Poll V et al. The spectrum of fungal allergy. *Int Arch Allergy Immunol* 2008; 145: 58–86.
18. Pinto VE, Patriarca A. *Alternaria* species and their associated mycotoxins. *Methods Mol Biol* 2017; 1542: 13–32.
19. Woloshuk CP, Shim WB. Aflatoxins, fumonisins, and trichothecenes: A convergence of knowledge. *FEMS Microbiol Rev* 2013; 37(1): 94–109.
20. Gravesen S, Nielsen PA, Iversen R, Nielsen KF. Microfungal contamination of damp buildings—Examples of risk constructions and risk materials. *Environ Health Perspect* 1999; 107(Suppl 3): 505–508.
21. Crameri R, Zeller S, Glaser AG et al. Cross-reactivity among fungal allergens: A clinically relevant phenomenon? *Mycoses* 2008; 52: 99–106.
22. Esch RE, Codina R. Fungal raw materials used to produce allergen extracts. *Ann Allergy Asthma Immunol* 2017; 118: 399–405.
23. Larsen JN, Houghton CG, Vega ML, Lowenstein H. Manufacturing and standardizing allergen extracts in Europe. *Clin Allergy Immunol* 2008; 21: 283–301.
24. Hawksworth DL, Crous PW, Redhead SA et al. The Amsterdam Declaration on Fungal Nomenclature. *IMA Fungus* 2011; 2: 105–112.
25. St-Germain G, Summerbell R. *Identifying Fungi*. 2nd ed. Belmont, CA: Star Publishing, 2011.
26. Kendrick B, Nag Raj TR. Morphological terms in fungi imperfecti. In: Kendrick B, editor. *The Whole Fungus: The Sexual-Asexual Synthesis*. Ottawa: National Museums of Canada, 1979.
27. Wicklow TT, Carrol, GC. *The Fungal Community: Its Organization and Role in the Ecosystem*. New York, NY: Marcell Dekker, 1981.
28. Bold HC, Alexopoulos CJ, Delevoryas T. *Morphology of Plants and Fungi*. New York, NY: Harper and Row, 1973.
29. Kurup VP, Fink JN. Fungal allergy. In: Murphy JW, editor. *Fungal Infections and Immune Responses*. New York, NY: Plenum Press, 1993.
30. Latge JP, Paris S. The fungal spore: Reservoir of allergens. In: Cole GT, Moch HC, editors. *The Fungal Spores and Disease Initiation in Plants and Animals*. New York, NY: Plenum Press, 1991.
31. Heederik D, von Mutius E. Does diversity of environmental microbial exposure matter for the occurrence of allergy and asthma? *J Allergy Clin Immunol* 2012; 130: 44–50.
32. Kurup VP, Banerjee B. Fungal allergens and peptide epitopes. *Peptides* 2000; 21: 589–599.
33. Lehrer SB, Salvaggio JE. Allergens: Standardization and impact of biotechnology: A review. *Allergy Proc* 1990; 11: 197–208.
34. Aukrust L. Crossed radioimmunoelectrophoretic studies of distinct allergens in two extracts of *Cladosporium herbarum*. *Int Arch Allergy Appl Immunol* 1979; 58: 375–390.
35. Kim SJ, Chaparas SD. Characterization of antigens from *Aspergillus fumigatus*. I. Preparation of antigens from organisms grown in completely synthetic medium. *Am Rev Respir Dis* 1978; 118: 547–551.
36. Kurup VP, Barboriak JJ, Fink JN. Indirect immunofluorescent detection of antibodies against thermophilic actinomycetes in patients with hypersensitivity pneumonitis. *J Lab Clin Med* 1977; 89: 533–539.
37. Hauck PR, Williamson S. The manufacture of allergenic extracts in North America. *Clin Rev Allergy Immunol* 2001; 21: 93–110.
38. Aas K, Backman A, Belin L, Weeke B. Standardization of allergen extracts with appropriate methods. The combined use of skin prick testing and radio-allergosorbent tests. *Allergy* 1978; 33: 130–137.
39. Dreborg S, Agrell B, Foucard T, Kjellman NI, Koivikko A, Nilsson S. A double-blind, multicenter immunotherapy trial in children, using a purified and standardized *Cladosporium herbarum* preparation. I. Clinical results. *Allergy* 1986; 41: 131–140.
40. Larenas-Linnemann D, Baxi S, Phipatanakul W, Portnoy JM. Clinical evaluation and management of patients with suspected fungus sensitivity. *J Allergy Clin Immunol Pract* 2016; 4: 405–414.

41. Hamilton RG. Proficiency survey-based evaluation of clinical total and allergen-specific IgE assay performance. *Arch Pathol Lab Med* 2010; 134: 975–982.

42. Hamilton RG. Clinical laboratory assessment of immediate-type hypersensitivity. *J Allergy Clin Immunol* 2010; 125: S284–S296.

43. Kurup VP, Banerjee B, Hemmann S, Greenberger PA, Blaser K, Crameri R. Selected recombinant *Aspergillus fumigatus* allergens bind specifically to IgE in ABPA. *Clin Exp Allergy* 2000; 30: 988–993.

44. Becker WM, Vogel L, Vieths S. Standardization of allergen extracts for immunotherapy: Where do we stand? *Curr Opin Allergy Clin Immunol* 2006; 6: 470–475.

45. Kabe J. Late asthmatic reactions to inhalation of fractions from extracts of *Candida albicans* and *Aspergillus fumigatus*. *Allergie und Immunologie* 1974; 20–21: 393–401.

46. Stevens EA, Hilvering C, Orie NG. Inhalation experiments with extracts of *Aspergillus fumigatus* on patients with allergic aspergillosis and aspergilloma. *Thorax* 1970; 25: 11–18.

47. Weber RW. Allergen immunotherapy and standardization and stability of allergen extracts. *J Allergy Clin Immunol* 1989; 84: 1093–1096.

48. Lehrer SB, Aukrust L, Salvaggio JE. Respiratory allergy induced by fungi. *Clin Chest Med* 1983; 4: 23–41.

49. Burge HA. Airborne-allergenic fungi. *Immunol Allergy Clin North Am* 1989; 9: 307–319.

50. Hoppe KA, Metwali N, Perry SS, Hart T, Kostle PA, Thorne PS. Assessment of airborne exposures and health in flooded homes undergoing renovation. *Indoor Air* 2012; 22: 446–456.

51. Beaumont F, Kauffman HF, Sluiter HJ, De Vries K. Sequential sampling of fungal air spores inside and outside the homes of mould-sensitive, asthmatic patients: A search for a relationship to obstructive reactions. *Ann Allergy* 1985; 55: 740–746.

52. de Ana SG, Torres-Rodriguez JM, Ramirez EA, Garcia SM, Belmonte-Soler J. Seasonal distribution of *Alternaria, Aspergillus, Cladosporium* and *Penicillium* species isolated in homes of fungal allergic patients. *J Investig Allergol Clin Immunol* 2006; 16: 357–363.

53. Dassonville C, Demattei C, Detaint B, Barral S, Bex-Capelle V, Momas I. Assessment and predictors determination of indoor airborne fungal concentrations in Paris newborn babies' homes. *Environ Res* 2008; 108: 80–85.

54. Lee T, Grinshpun SA, Martuzevicius D, Adhikari A, Crawford CM, Reponen T. Culturability and concentration of indoor and outdoor airborne fungi in six single-family homes. *Atmos Enivron* 2006; 40: 2902–2910.

55. Cho SH, Reponen T, Bernstein DI et al. The effect of home characteristics on dust antigen concentrations and loads in homes. *Sci Total Environ* 2006; 371: 31–43.

56. Malling HJ. Diagnosis and immunotherapy of mould allergy. IV. Relation between asthma symptoms, spore counts and diagnostic tests. *Allergy* 1986; 41: 342–350.

57. Lechtonen M, Reponen T, Nevalainen A. Everyday activities and variation of fungal spore concentrations in indoor air. *Int Biodeterior Biodegradation* 1993; 31: 25–39.

58. Bobbitt RC, Jr., Crandall MS, Venkataraman A, Bernstein JA. Characterization of a population presenting with suspected mold-related health effects. *Ann Allergy Asthma Immunol* 2005; 94: 39–44.

59. Portnoy JM, Kwak K, Dowling P, VanOsdol T, Barnes C. Health effects of indoor fungi. *Ann Allergy Asthma Immunol* 2005; 94: 313–319.

60. Portnoy JM, Kennedy K, Barnes C. Sampling for indoor fungi: What the clinician needs to know. *Curr Opin Otolaryngol Head Neck Surg* 2005; 13: 165–170.

61. Barnes CS, Horner WE, Kennedy K et al. Home assessment and remediation. *J Allergy Clin Immunol Pract* 2016; 4: 423–431.

62. Horner WE, Barnes C, Codina R, Levetin E. Guide for interpreting reports from inspections/investigations of indoor mold. *J Allergy Clin Immunol* 2008; 121: 592–597.

63. D'Amato G, Spieksma FT. Aerobiologic and clinical aspects of mould allergy in Europe. *Allergy* 1995; 50: 870–877.

64. Kozak PP, Gallup J, Cummins LH, Gillman SA. Factors of importance in determining the prevalence of indoor molds. *Ann Allergy* 1979; 43: 88–94.

65. Solomon WR. A volumetric study of winter fungus prevalence in the air of midwestern homes. *J Allergy Clin Immunol* 1976; 57: 46–55.

66. Jacob B, Ritz B, Gehring U et al. Indoor exposure to molds and allergic sensitization. *Environ Health Perspect* 2002; 110: 647–653.

67. Garrett MH, Rayment PR, Hooper MA et al. Indoor airborne fungal spores, house dampness and associations with environmental factors and respiratory health in children. *Clin Exp Allergy* 1998; 28: 459–467.

68. Aukrust L, Borch SM. Cross reactivity of moulds. *Allergy* 1985; 40: 57–60.

69. Twaroch TE, Curin M, Sterflinger K et al. Specific antibodies for the detection of *Alternaria* allergens and the identification of cross-reactive antigens in other fungi. *Int Arch Allergy Immunol* 2016; 170: 269–278.

70. Shen HD, Ming FT, Tang RBm, Chou H. *Aspergillus* and *Penicillium* allergens: Focus on proteases. *Curr Allergy Asthma Rep* 2007; 7: 351–356.

71. Soeria-Atmadja D, Onell A, Borga A. IgE sensitization to fungi mirrors fungal phylogenetic systematics. *J Allergy Clin Immunol* 2010; 125: 1379–1386.

72. Wagner S, Sowka S, Mayer C et al. Identification of a *Hevea brasiliensis* latex manganese superoxide dismutase (Hev b 10) as a cross-reactive allergen. *Int Arch Allergy Immunol* 2001; 125: 120–127.

73. Wagner S, Breiteneder H, Simon-Nobbe B et al. Hev b 9, an enolase and a new cross-reactive allergen from Hevea latex and molds: Purification, characterization, cloning and expression. *Eur J Biochem* 2000; 267: 7006–7014.

74. Hauser M, Roulias A, Ferreira F, Egger M. Panallergens and their impact on the allergic patient. *Allergy Asthma Clin Immunol* 2010; 6: 1–14.

75. Crameri R. Structural aspects of fungal allergens. *Semin Immunopathol* 2015; 37: 117–121.

76. Rid R, Onder K, Hawranek T et al. Isolation and immunological characterization of a novel *Cladosporium herbarum* allergen structurally homologous to the α/β hydrolase fold superfamily. *Mol Immunol* 2010; 47(6): 1366–1377.

77. Sharma V, Singh BP, Gaur SN, Arora N. Molecular and immunological characterization of cytochrome c: A potential cross-reactive allergen in fungi and grasses. *Allergy* 2008; 63: 189–197.

78. Shen HD, Choo KB, Yu KW, Ling WL, Chang FC, Han SH. Characterization of a monoclonal antibody (RJ5) against the immunodominant 41-kD antigen of *Candida albicans*. *Int Arch Allergy Immunol* 1991; 96: 142–148.

79. Bowyer P, Fraczek M, Denning DW. Comparative genomics of fungal allergens and epitopes shows widespread distribution of closely related allergen and epitope orthologues. *BMC Genomics* 2006; 7: 51.

80. Bush RK, Prochnau JJ. *Alternaria*-induced asthma. *J Allergy Clin Immunol* 2002; 113: 227–234.

81. Nelson HS, Szefler SJ, Jacobs J et al. The relationships among environmental exposure, pulmonary function, and bronchial hyperresponsiveness in the Childhood Asthma Management Program. *J Allergy Clin Immunol* 1999; 104: 775–785.

82. Schlueter DP, Fink JN, Hensley GT. Wood-pulp workers' disease: A hypersensitivity pneumonitis caused by *Alternaria*. *Ann Intern Med* 1972; 77: 907–914.

83. Yunginger JW, Jones RT, Nesheim ME, Geller M. Studies on *Alternaria* allergens. III. Isolation of a major allergenic fraction (ALT-I). *J Allergy Clin Immunol* 1980; 66: 138–147.

84. Nyholm L, Lowenstein H, Yunginger JW. Immunochemical partial identity between two independently identified and isolated major allergens from *Alternaria alternata* (Alt-I and Ag 1). *J Allergy Clin Immunol* 1983; 71: 461–467.

85. Portnoy J, Olson I, Pacheco F, Barnes C. Affinity purification of a major *Alternaria* allergen using a monoclonal antibody. *Ann Allergy* 1990; 65: 109–114.

86. Deards MJ, Montague AE. Purification and characterisation of a major allergen of *Alternaria alternata*. *Mol Immunol* 1991; 28: 409–415.

87. Paris S, Debeaupuis JP, Prevost MC, Casotto M, Latge JP. The 31 kd major allergen, Alt a I1563, of *Alternaria alternata*. *J Allergy Clin Immunol* 1991; 88: 902–908.

88. Twaroch TE, Arcalis E, Sterflinger K et al. Predominant localization of the major *Alternaria* allergen Alt a 1 in the cell wall of airborne spores. *J Allergy Clin Immunol* 2012; 129: 1148–1149.

89. De Vouge MW, Thaker AJ, Curran IH et al. Isolation and expression of a cDNA clone encoding an *Alternaria alternata* Alt a 1 subunit. *Int Arch Allergy Immunol* 1996; 111: 385–395.

90. Achatz G, Oberkofler H, Lechenauer E et al. Molecular cloning of major and minor allergens of *Alternaria alternata* and *Cladosporium herbarum*. *Mol Immunol* 1995; 32: 213–227.

91. Chruszcz M, Chapman M, Osinski T et al. *Alternaria alternata* allergen Alt a 1: A unique β-barrel protein dimer found exclusively in fungi. *J Allergy Clin Immunol* 2012; 130: 241–247.

92. Hong SG, Cramer RA, Lawrence CB et al. Alt a 1 homologs from *Alternaria* and related taxa: Analysis of phylogenetic content and secondary structure. *Fungal Genet Biol* 2005; 42: 119–129.

93. Saenz-de-Santamaria M, Postigo I, Gutierrez-Rodriguez A et al. The major allergen *Alternaria alternata* (Alt a 1) is expressed in other members of the Pleosporaceae family. *Mycoses* 2006; 49: 91–95.

94. Moreno A, Pineda F, Alcover J et al. Orthologous allergens and diagnostic utility of major allergen Alt a 1. *Allergy Asthma Immunol Res* 2016; 8: 428–437.

95. Kurup VP, Vijay HM, Kumar V, Castillo L, Elms N. IgE binding synthetic peptides of Alt a 1, a major allergen of *Alternaria alternata*. *Peptides* 2003; 24(2): 179–185.

96. Zhang L, Curran IH, Muradia G et al. N-terminus of a major allergen Alt a I, of *Alternaria alternata* defined to be an epitope. *Int Arch Allergy Immunol* 1995; 108: 254–259.

97. Barnes C, Portnoy J, Sever M, Arbes S Jr., Vaughn B, Zeldin DC. Comparison of enzyme immunoassay-based assays for environmental *Alternaria alternata*. *Ann Allergy Asthma Immunol* 2006; 97(3): 350–356.

98. Aden E, Weber B, Bossert J et al. Standardization of *Alternaria alternata*: Extraction and quantification of Alt a 1 by using an mAb-based 2-site binding assay. *J Allergy Clin Immunol* 1999; 104: 128–135.

99. Asturias JA, Arilla MC, Ibarrola I et al. A sensitive two-site enzyme-linked immunosorbent assay for measurement of the major *Alternaria alternata* allergen Alt a 1. *Ann Allergy Asthma Immunol* 2003; 90: 529–535.

100. Abebe M, Kumar V, Rajan S, Thaker A, Sevinc S, Vijay HM. Detection of recombinant Alt a1 in a two-site, IgM based, sandwich ELISA opens up possibilities of developing alternative assays for the allergen. *J Immunol Methods* 2006; 312: 111–117.

101. Feo Brito F, Alonso AM, Carnes J et al. Correlation between Alt a 1 levels and clinical symptoms in *Alternaria alternata*-monosensitized patients. *J Investig Allergol Clin Immunol* 2012; 22: 154–159.

102. De Vouge MW, Thaker AJ, Zhang L, Muradia G, Rode H, Vijay HM. Molecular cloning of IgE-binding fragments of *Alternaria alternata* allergens. *Int Arch Allergy Immunol* 1998; 116(4): 261–268.

103. Schneider PB, Denk U, Breitenbach M et al. *Alternaria alternata* NADP-dependent mannitol dehydrogenase is an important fungal allergen. *Clin Exp Allergy* 2006; 36(12): 1513–1524.

104. Breitenbach M, Simon B, Probst G et al. Enolases are highly conserved fungal allergens. *Int Arch Allergy Immunol* 1997; 113: 114–117.

105. Simon-Nobbe B, Probst G, Kajava AV et al. IgE-binding epitopes of enolases, a class of highly conserved fungal allergens. *J Allergy Clin Immunol* 2000; 106: 887–895.

106. Postigo I, Gutierrez-Rodriguez A, Fernandez J et al. Diagnostic value of Alt a 1, fungal enolase and manganese-dependent superoxide dismutase in the component-resolved diagnosis of allergy to Pleosporaceae. *Clin Exp Allergy* 2011; 41: 443 451.

107. Sharma V, Gupta R, Jhingran A et al. Cloning, recombinant expression and activity studies of a major allergen "enolase" from the fungus *Curvularia lunata*. *J Clin Immunol* 2006; 26: 360–369.

108. Shankar J, Singh BP, Gaur SN, Arora N. Recombinant glutathione-S-transferase a major allergen from *Alternaria alternata* for clinical use in allergy patients. *Mol Immunol* 2006; 43: 1927–1932.

109. Shankar J, Singh BP, Gaur SN, Arora N. Engineered Alt a 13 fragment of *Alternaria alternata* abrogated IgE binding without affecting T-cell stimulation. *J Clin Immunol* 2009; 29: 63–70.

110. Shankar J, Gupta PD, Sridhara S et al. Immunobiochemical analysis of cross-reactive glutathione-S-transferease allergen from different fungal sources. *Immunol Invest* 2005; 34: 37–51.

111. Gabriel MF, Postigo I, Gutierrez-Rodriguez A et al. Characterization of *Alternaria alternata* manganese-dependent superoxide dismutase, a cross-reactive allergen homologue to Asp f 6. *Immunobioogy* 2015; 220: 851–858.

112. Hemmann S, Menz G, Ismail C et al. Skin test reactivity to 2 recombinant *Aspergillus fumigatus* allergens in *A. fumigatus*-sensitized asthmatic subjects allows diagnostic separation of allergic bronchopulmonary aspergillosis from fungal sensitization. *J Allergy Clin Immunol* 1999; 104: 601–607.

113. Gabriel MF, Postigo I, Gutierrez-Rodriguez A et al. Alt a 15 is a new cross-reactive minor allergen of *Alternaria alternata*. *Immunobiology* 2016; 221: 153–160.

114. Lai HY, Tam MF, Chou H et al. Molecular and structural characterization of immunoglobulin E-binding epitopes of Pen ch 13, and alkaline serine protease major allergen from *Penicillium chrysogenum*. *Clin Exp Allergy* 2004; 34: 1926–1933.

115. Esch RE, Bush RK. Aerobiology of outdoor allergens. In: Adkinson Jr NR, Bochner BS, Busse WW et al. editors. *Middleton's Allergy: Principles and Practice*, 7th ed. St. Louis, MO: Mosby-Elsevier, 2009.

116. Bensch K, Braun U, Groenewald JZ, Crous PW. The genus *Cladosporium. Stud Mycol* 2012; 72: 1–401.

117. Segers FJJ, Meijer M, Houbraken J et al. Xerotolerant *Cladosporium sphaerospermum* are predominant on indoor surfaces compared to other *Cladosporium* species. *PLOS ONE* 2015; 10: e0145415.

118. Aukrust L, Borch SM. Partial purification and characterization of two *Cladosporium herbarum* allergens. *Int Arch Allergy Immunol* 1979; 60: 68–79.

119. Sward-Nordmo M, Wold JK, Paulsen BS, Aukrust L. Purification and partial characterization of the allergen Ag-54 from *Cladosporium herbarum. Int Arch Allergy Appl Immunol* 1985; 78: 249–255.

120. Sward-Nordmo M, Smestad Paulsen B, Wold JK. Immunological studies of the glycoprotein allergen Ag-54 (Cla h II) in *Cladosporium herbarum* with special attention to the carbohydrate and protein moieties. *Int Arch Allergy Appl Immunol* 1989; 90: 155–161.

121. Sward-Nordmo M, Paulsen BS, Wold JK et al. Further structural studies of the carbohydrate moeity of the allergen Ag-54 (Cla h II) from the mould *Cladosporium herbarum. Carbohydr Res* 1991; 214: 267–279.

122. Zhang L, Muradia G, Curran IH et al. A cDNA clone coding for a novel allergen, Cla h III, of *Cladosporium herbarum* identified as a ribosomal P2 protein. *J Immunol* 1995; 154: 710–717.

123. Breitenbach M, Achatz G, Oberkofler H et al. Molecular characterization of allergen of *Cladosporium herbarum* and *Alternaria alternaria. Int Arch Allergy Immunol* 1995; 107: 458–459.

124. Simon-Nobbe B, Denk U, Schneider PB et al. NADP-dependent mannitol dehydrogenase, a major allergen of *Cladosporium herbarum. J Biol Chem* 2006; 281(24): 16354–16360.

125. Nuss D, Goettig P, Magler I et al. Crystal structure of the NADP-dependent mannitol dehydrogenase from *Cladosporium herbarum*: Implications for oligomerisation and catalysis. *Biochimie* 2010; 92: 985–993.

126. Chou H, Tam MF, Lee LH et al. Vacuolar serine protease is a major allergen of *Cladosporium cladosporioides. Int Arch Allergy Immunol* 2008; 146: 277–286.

127. Poll V, Denk U, Shen HD et al. The vacuolar serine protease, a cross-reactive allergen from *Cladosporium herbarum. Mol Immunol* 2009; 46: 1360–1373.

128. Chou H, Tam MF, Chiang CH et al. Transaldolases are novel and immunoglobulin-E cross-reacting fungal allergens. *Clin Exp Allergy* 2011; 41: 739–749.

129. Esposito M, Venkatesh V, Otvos L et al. Human transaldolase and cross-reactive viral epitopes identified by autoantibodies of multiple sclerosis patients. *J Immunol* 1999; 163: 4027–4032.

130. Greenberger PA, Bush RK, Demain JG et al. Allergic bronchopulmonary aspergillosis. *J Allergy Clin Immunol Pract* 2014; 2: 703–708.

131. Laham MN, Allen RC, Greene JC. Allergic bronchopulmonary aspergillosis (ABPA) caused by *Aspergillus terreus*: Specific lymphocyte sensitization and antigen-directed serum opsonic activity. *Ann Allergy* 1981; 46: 74–80.

132. Quirce S, Cuevas M, Diez-Gomez M et al. Respiratory allergy to *Aspergillus*-derived enzymes in baker's asthma. *J Allergy Clin Immunol* 1992; 90: 970–978.

133. Yoshida K, Ando M, Ito K et al. Hypersensitivity of a mushroom worker due to *Aspergillus glaucus. Arch Environ Health* 1990; 45: 245–247.

134. Itabashi T, Hosoe T, Toyasaki N et al. Allergen activity of xerophilic fungus, *Aspergillus restrictus. Arerugi* 2007; 56: 101–108.

135. Aggarwal S, Chhabra SK, Saxena RK, Agarwal MK. Heterogeneity of immune responses to various *Aspergillus* species in patients with allergic respiratory diseases. *Indian J Chest Dis Allied Sci* 2000; 42: 249–258.

136. Hearn VM, Wilson EV, Latge JP, Mackenzie DW. Immunochemical studies of *Aspergillus fumigatus* mycelial antigens by polyacrylamide gel electrophoresis and western blotting techniques. *J Gen Microbiol* 1990; 136(8): 1525–1535.

137. Kurup VP. Production and characterization of a murine monoclonal antibody to *Aspergillus fumigatus* antigen having IgG- and IgE-binding activity. *Int Arch Allergy Appl Immunol* 1988; 86(4): 400–406.

138. Longbottom JL, Austwick PKC. Antigens and allergens of *Aspergillus fumigatus* I. Characterization by quantitative immunoelectric techniques. *J Allergy Clin Immunol* 1986; 78: 9–17.

139. Longbottom JL, Harvey C, Taylor ML et al. Characterization of immunologically important antigens and allergens of *Aspergillus fumigatus. Int Arch Allergy Appl Immunol* 1989; 88: 185–186.

140. Latge JP. *Aspergillus fumigatus* and aspergillosis. *Clin Microbiol Rev* 1999; 12: 310–350.

141. Tripathi P, Nair S, Singh BP, Arora N. Molecular and immunological characterization of subtilisin like serine protease, a major allergen of *Curvularia lunata. Immunobiology* 2011; 216: 402–408.

142. Arruda LK, Platts-Mills TA, Fox JW, Chapman MD. *Aspergillus fumigatus* allergen I, a major IgE-binding protein, is a member of the mitogillin family of cytotoxins. *J Exp Med* 1990; 172: 1529–1532.

143. Moser M, Crameri R, Menz G et al. Cloning and expression of recombinant *Aspergillus fumigatus* allergen I/a (rAsp f I/a) with IgE binding and type I skin test activity. *J Immunol* 1992; 149: 454–460.

144. Arruda LK, Platts-Mills TA, Longbottom JL, el-Dahr JM, Chapman MD. *Aspergillus fumigatus*: Identification of 16, 18, and 45 kd antigens recognized by human IgG and IgE antibodies and murine monoclonal antibodies. *J Allergy Clin Immunol* 1992; 89(6): 1166–1176.

145. Sporik RB, Arruda LK, Woodfolk J et al. Environmental exposure to *Aspergillus fumigatus* allergen (Asp f I). *Clin Exp Allergy* 1993; 23: 326–331.

146. Kurup VP, Banerjee B, Murali PS et al. Immunodominant peptide epitopes of allergen, Asp f 1 from the fungus *Aspergillus fumigatus. Peptides* 1998; 19: 1469–1477.

147. Banerjee B, Kurup VP, Phadnis S, Greenberger PA, Fink JN. Molecular cloning and expression of a recombinant *Aspergillus fumigatus* protein Asp f II with significant immunoglobulin E reactivity in allergic bronchopulmonary aspergillosis. *J Lab Clin Med* 1996; 127: 253–262.

148. Banerjee B, Greenberger PA, Fink JN, Kurup VP. Conformational and linear B-cell epitopes of Asp f 2, a major allergen of *Aspergillus fumigatus*, bind differently to immunoglobulin E antibody in the sera of allergic bronchopulmonary aspergillosis patients. *Infect Immun* 1999; 67: 2284–2291.

149. Hemmann S, Blaser K, Crameri R. Allergens of *Aspergillus fumigatus* and *Candida boidinii* share IgE-binding epitopes. *Am J Respir Crit Care Med* 1997; 156: 1956–1962.

150. Linborg M, Magnusson CG, Zargari A et al. Selective cloning of allergens from the skin colonizing yeast *Malassezia furfur* by phase surface display technology. *J Invest Dermatol* 1999; 113: 156–161.

151. Shen HD, Wang CW, Chou H et al. Complementary DNA cloning and immunologic characterization of a new *Penicillium citrinum* allergen (Pen c 3). *J Allergy Clin Immunol* 2000; 105: 827–833.

152. Ramachandran H, Jayaraman V, Banerjee B et al. IgE binding conformational epitopes of Asp f 3, a major allergen of *Aspergillus fumigatus*. *Clin Immunol* 2002; 103: 324–333.

153. Crameri R, Jaussi R, Menz G, Blaser K. Display of expression products of cDNA libraries on phage surfaces. A versatile screening system for selective isolation of genes by specific gene-product/ligand interaction. *Eur J Biochem* 1994; 226: 53–58.

154. Bisht V, Arora N, Singh BP et al. Epi p 1, an allergenic glycoprotein of *Epicoccum purpurascens* is a serine protease. *FEMS Immunol Med Microbiol* 2004; 42: 205–211.

155. Kurup VP, Banerjee B, Hemmann S et al. Selected recombinant *Aspergillus fumigatus* allergens bind specifically to IgE in ABPA. *Clin Exp Allergy* 2000; 30: 988–993.

156. Ramachandran H, Banerjee B, Greenberger PA et al. Role of C-terminal cysteine residues of *Aspergillus fumigatus* allergen Asp f 4 in immunoglobulin E binding. *Clin Diagn Lab Immunol* 2004; 11: 261–265.

157. Crameri R, Faith A, Hemmann S et al. Humoral and cell-mediated autoimmunity in allergy to *Aspergillus fumigatus*. *J Exp Med* 1996; 184: 265–270.

158. Mayer C, Appenzeller U. Seelbach H et al. Humoral and cell-mediated autoimmune reactions to human acidic ribosomal protein P2 protein in individuals sensitized to *Aspergillus fumigatus* P2 protein. *J Exp Med* 1999; 189: 1507–1512.

159. Kumar A, Reddy LV, Sochanik A, Kurup VP. Isolation and characterization of a recombinant heat shock protein of *Aspergillus fumigatus*. *J Allergy Clin Immunol* 1993; 91: 1024–1030.

160. Baldo BA, Baker RS. Inhalant allergies to fungi: Reactions to bakers' yeast (*Saccharomyces cerevisiae*) and identification of bakers' yeast enolase as an important allergen. *Int Arch Allergy Appl Immunol* 1988; 86: 201–208.

161. Kortekangas-Savolainen O, Kalimo K, Lammintausta K, Savolainen J. IgE-binding components of baker's yeast (*Saccharomyces cerevisiae*) recognized by immunoblotting analysis. Simultaneous IgE binding to mannan and 46–48 kD allergens to *Saccharomyces cerevisiae* and *Candida albicans*. *Clin Exp Allergy* 1993; 23: 179–184.

162. Ito K, Ishiguro A, Kanbe T et al. Detection of IgE antibody against *Candida albicans* enolase and its crossreactivity to *Saccharomyces cerevisiae* enolase. *Clin Exp Allergy* 1995; 25: 522–528.

163. Horner WE, Reese G, Lehrer SB. Identification of the allergen Psi c 2 from the basidiomycete *Psilocybe cubensis* as a fungal cyclophilin. *Int Arch Allergy Immunol* 1995; 107: 298–300.

164. Cadot P, Diaz JF, Proost P et al. Purification and characterization of an 18-kd allergen of birch (*Betula verrucosa*) pollen: Identification as cyclophilin. *J Allergy Clin Immunol* 2000; 105: 286–291.

165. Fluckiger S, Fijten H, Whitley P et al. Cyclophilins, a new family of cross-reactive allergens. *Eur J Immunol* 2002; 32: 10–17.

166. Banerjee B, Kurup VP, Greenberger PA, Johnson BD, Fink JN. Cloning and expression of *Aspergillus fumigatus* allergen Asp f 16 mediating both humoral and cell-mediated immunity in allergic bronchopulmonary aspergillosis (ABPA). *Clin Exp Allergy* 2001; 31: 761–770.

167. Chow LP, Liu SL, Yu CJ et al. Identification and expression of an allergen Asp f 13 from *Aspergillus fumigatus* and epitope mapping using human IgE antibodies and rabbit polyclonal antibodies. *Biochem J* 2000; 346: 423–431.

168. Su NY, Yu CJ, Shen HD, Pan FM, Chow LP. Pen c 1, a novel enzymic allergen protein from *Penicillium citrinum*. Purification, characterization, cloning and expression. *Eur J Biochem* 1999; 261: 115–123.

169. Shen HD, Lin WL, Liaw SF, Tam MF, Han SH. Characterization of the 33-kilodalton major allergen of *Penicillium citrinum* by using MoAbs and N-terminal amino acid sequencing. *Clin Exp Allergy* 1997; 27: 79–86.

170. Shen HD, Lin WL, Tam MF et al. Alkaline serine proteinase: A major allergen of *Aspergillus oryzae* and its cross-reactivity with *Penicillium citrinum*. *Int Arch Allergy Immunol* 1998; 116: 29–35.

171. Chou H, Lai HY, Tam MF et al. cDNA cloning, biological and immunological characterization of the alkaline serine protease major allergen from *Penicillium chrysogenum*. *Int Arch Allergy Immunol* 2002; 127: 15–26.

172. Shen HD, Tam MF, Chou H, Han SH. The importance of serine proteinases as aeroallergens associated with asthma. *Int Arch Allergy Immunol* 1999; 119: 259–264.

173. Shen HD, Lin WL, Tam MF et al. Identification of vacuolar serine proteinase as a major allergen of *Aspergillus fumigatus* by immunoblotting and N-terminal amino acid sequence analysis. *Clin Exp Allergy* 2001; 31: 295–302.

174. Shen HD, Lin WL, Tsai JJ, Liaw SF, Han SH. Allergenic components in three different species of *Penicillium*: Cross-reactivity among major allergens. *Clin Exp Allergy* 1996; 26: 444–451.

175. Sander I, Raulf-Heimsoth M, Slethoff C et al. Allergy to *Aspergillus*-derived enzymes in the baking industry: Identification of β-xylosidase from *Aspergillus niger* as a new allergen (Asp n 14). *J Allergy Clin Immunol* 1998; 102: 256–264.

176. Baur X, Chen Z, Sander I. Isolation and denomination of an important allergen in baking additives: α-Amylase from *Aspergillus oryzae* (Asp o II). *Clin Exp Allergy* 1994; 24: 465–470.

177. van Heemst RC, Sander I, Rooyackers J et al. Hypersensitivity pneumonitis caused by occupational exposure to phytase. *Eur Resp J* 2009; 33: 1507–1509.

178. Wei DL, Chen JH, Jong SC, Shen HD. Indoor airborne *Penicillium* species in Taiwan. *Curr Microbiol* 1993; 26: 485–490.

179. Vijay HM, Abebe M, Kumar V et al. Allergenic and mutagenic characterization of 14 Penicillium species. *Aerobiologia* 2005; 21: 95–103.

180. Shen HD, Wang C, Lin WL et al. cDNA cloning and immunologic characterization of Pen o 18, the vacuolar serine protease major allergen of *Penicillium oxalicum*. *J Lab Clin Med* 2001; 137: 115–124.

181. Shen HD, Chou H, Tam MF et al. Molecular and immunological characterization of Pen ch 18, the vacuolar serine protease major allergen of *Penicillium chrysogenum*. *Allergy* 2003; 58: 993–1002.

182. Lin WL, Chou H, Tam MF et al. Production and characterization of monoclonal antibodies to serine proteinase allergens in *Penicillium* and *Aspergillus* species. *Clin Exp Allergy* 2000; 30: 1653–1662.

183. Yu CJ, Chen YM, Su SN et al. Molecular and immunological characterization and IgE epitope mapping of Pen n 18, a major allergen of *Penicillium notatum*. *Biochem J* 2002; 363: 707–183.

184. Shen HD, Au LC, Lin WL et al. Molecular cloning and expression of a *Penicillium citrinum* allergen with sequence

homology and antigenic crossreactivity to a hsp 70 human heat shock protein. *Clin Exp Allergy* 1997; 27: 682–690.

185. Shen HD, Liaw SF, Lin WL et al. Molecular cloning of cDNA coding for the 68kDa allergen of *Penicillium notatum* using MoAbs. *Clin Exp Allergy* 1995; 25: 350–356.

186. Lai HY, Tam MF, Tang RB et al. cDNA cloning and immunological characterization of a newly identified enolase allergen from *Penicillium citrinum* and *Aspergillus fumigatus*. *Int Arch Allergy Immunol* 2002; 127: 181–190.

187. Tang RB, Chen YS, Chou H et al. cDNA cloning and immunologic characterization of a novel EF-1β allergen from *Pencillium citrinum*. *Allergy* 2005; 60: 366–371.

188. Chiu LL, Lee KL, Lin YF et al. Secretome analysis of novel IgE-binding proteins from *Penicillium citrinum*. *Proteomics Clin Appl* 2008; 2: 33–45.

189. Sevinc MS, Kumar V, Abebe M et al. Expression and characterization of Pen b 26 allergen of *Pencillium brevicompactum* in *Escherichia coli*. *Prot Expr Purif.* 2009; 65: 8–14.

190. Sevinc MS, Kumar V, Abebe M et al. Isolation, expression and characterization of a minor allergen from *Penicillium crustosum*. *Med Mycol* 2014; 52: 81–89.

191. Levetin E. Studies on airborne basidiospores. *Aerobiologia* 1990; 6: 177–180.

192. Lehrer SB, Lopez M, Butcher BT et al. Basidiomycete mycelia and spore-allergen extracts: Skin test reactivity in adults with symptoms of respiratory allergy. *J Allergy Clin Immunol* 1986; 78: 478–485.

193. Helbling A, Gayer F, Pichler WJ, Brander KA. Mushroom (Basidiomycete) allergy: Diagnosis established by skin test and nasal challenge. *J Allergy Clin Immunol* 1998; 102: 853–858.

194. Lopez M, Voigtlander JR, Lehrer SB, Salvaggio JE. Bronchoprovocation studies in basidiospore-sensitive allergic subjects with asthma. *J Allergy Clin Immunol* 1989; 84: 242–246.

195. Horner WE, Ibanez MD, Lehrer SB. Immunoprint analysis of *Calvatia cyathiformis* allergens. I. Reactivity with individual sera. *J Allergy Clin Immunol* 1989; 87: 784–792.

196. Horner WE, Lopez M, Salvaggio JE, Lehrer SB. Basidiomycete allergy: Identification and characterization of an important allergen from *Calvatia cyathiformis*. *Int Arch Allergy Appl Immunol* 1991; 94: 359–361.

197. Lockey SD. Mushroom workers' pneumonitis. *Ann Allergy* 1974; 33: 282–288.

198. Weissman DN, Halmepura L, Salvaggio JE, Lehrer SB. Antigenic/allergenic analysis of basidiomycete cap, mycelia and spore extracts. *Int Arch Allergy Appl Immunol* 1987; 84: 56–61.

199. Butcher BT, O'Neil CE, Reed MA et al. Basidiomycete allergy: Measurement of spore-specific IgE antibodies. *J Allergy Clin Immunol* 1987; 80: 803–809.

200. Davis WE, Horner WE, Salvaggio JE, Lehrer SB. Basidiospore allergens: Analysis of *Coprinus quadrifidus* spore, cap, and stalk extracts. *Clin Allergy* 1988; 18: 261–267.

201. Brander KA, Brbely P, Crameri R et al. IgE-binding proliferative responses and skin test reactivity to Cop c 1, the first recombinant allergen from the basidiomycete *Corpinus comatus*. *J Allergy Clin Immunol* 1999; 104: 630–636.

202. Toyotome T, Satoh M, Yahiro M et al. Glucoamylase is a major allergen of *Schizophyllum commune*. *Clin Exp Allergy* 2014; 44: 450–457.

203. Tarlo SM, Bell B, Srinivasan J et al. Human sensitization to *Ganoderma* antigen. *J Allergy Clin Immunol* 1979; 64: 43–49.

204. Cutten AE, Hasnain SM, Segedin BP, Bai TR, McKay EJ. The basidiomycete *Ganoderma* and asthma: Collection, quantitation and immunogenicity of the spores. *NZ Med J* 1988; 101: 361–363.

205. Singh AB, Kumar P. Common environmental allergens causing respiratory allergy in India. *Indian J Pediatr* 2002; 69(3): 245–250.

206. Horner WE, Helbling A, Lehrer SB. Basidiomycete allergens: Comparison of three *Ganoderma* species. *Allergy* 1993; 48: 110–116.

207. Vijay HM, Helbling A, Lehrer SB. Allergenic components of *Gandoderma applanatum*. *Grana* 1991; 30: 167–170.

208. Ashbee HR. Recent developments in the immunology and biology of *Malassezia* species. *FEMS Immunol Med Microbiol* 2006; 47: 14–23.

209. Zargari A, Midgley G, Back O et al. IgE-reactivity to seven *Malassezia* species. *Allergy* 2003; 58: 306–311.

210. Nissen D, Petersen LJ, Esch R et al. IgE-sensitization to cellular and culture filtrate of fungal extracts in patients with atopic dermatitis. *Ann Allergy Asthma Immunol* 1998; 81: 247–255.

211. Yasueda H, Hashida-Okado T, Saito A et al. Identification and cloning of two novel allergens from the lipophilic yeast, *Malassezia furfur*. *Biochem Biophys Res Comm* 1998; 248: 240–244.

212. Glaser AG, Limacher A, Fluckiger S et al. Analysis of the cross-reactivity and of the 1.5 A crystal structure of the *Malassezia sympodialis* Mala s 6 allergen, a member of the cyclophilin pan-allergen family. *Biochem J* 2006; 396: 41–49.

213. Andersson A, Rasool O, Schmidt M et al. Cloning, expression and characterization of two new IgE-binding proteins from the yeast *Malassezia sympodialis* with sequence similarities to heat shock proteins and manganese superoxide dismutase. *Eur J Biochem* 2004; 271: 1885–1894.

214. Limacher A, Glasesr AG, Meier C et al. Cross-reactivity and 1.4-A crystal structure of *Malassezia sympodialis* thioredoxin (Mala s 13), a member of a new pan-allergen family. *J Immunol* 2007; 178: 389–396.

215. Schmidt M, Zargari A, Holt P et al. The complete cDNA sequence and expression of the first major allergenic protein of *Malassezia furfur*, Mal f 1. *Eur J Biochem* 1997; 246: 181–185.

216. Rasool O, Zargari A, Almqvist J et al. Cloning, characterization and expression of complete coding sequences of three IgE binding *Malassezia furfur* allergens, Mal f 7, Mal f 8 and Mal f 9. *Eur J Biochem* 2000; 267: 282–287.

217. Zargaru A, Selander C, Rasool O et al. Mala s 12 is a major allergen in patients with atopic eczema and has sequence similarities to the GMC oxidoreductase family. *Allergy* 2007; 62: 695–703.

218. Selander C, Zargari A, Mollby R et al. Higher pH level, corresponding to that on the skin of patients with atopic eczema, stimulates the release of *Malassezia sympodialis* allergens. *Allergy* 2006; 61: 1002–1008.

219. Casagrande BF, Fluckiger S, Linder MT et al. Sensitization to the yeast *Malassezia sympodialis* is specific for extrinsic and intrinsic atopic eczema. *J Invest Dermatol.* 2006; 126: 2414–2421.

220. Wirth F, Goldani LZ. Epidemiology of *Rhodotorula*: An emerging pathogen. *Interdiscip Perspect Infect Dis* 2012; 2012: 465717.

221. Savolainen J, Kortekangas-Savolainen O, Nermes M et al. IgE, IgA, and IgG responses to common yeasts in atopic patients. *Allergy* 1998; 53: 506–512.

222. Chang CY, Chou H, Tam M et al. Characterization of enolase allergen from *Rhodotorula mucilaginosa*. *J Biomed Sci* 2002; 9: 645–655.

223. Chou H, Tam MF, Lee SS et al. A vacuolar serine protease (Rho m 2) is a major allergen of *Rhodotorula mucilaginosa* and belongs to a class of highly conserved pan-fungal allergens. *Int Arch Allergy Immunol* 2005; 138: 134–141.

224. Mayer FL, Wilson D, Hube B. *Candida albicans* pathogenicity mechanisms. *Virulence* 2013; 4: 119–128.

225. Simon D, Straumann A, Dahinden C, Simon HU. Frequent sensitization to *Candida albicans* and profilins in adult eosinophilic esophagitis. *Allergy* 2013; 68: 945–948.

226. Khosravi AR, Bandghorai AN, Moazzeni N et al. Evaluation of *Candida albicans* allergens reactive with specific IgE in asthma and atopic eczema patients. *Mycoses* 2009; 52: 326–333.

227. Savolainen J, Lammintausta K, Kalimo K, Viander M. *Candida albicans* and atopic dermatitis. *Clin Exp Allergy* 1993; 23: 332–339.

228. Staubach P, Vonend A, Burow G et al. Patients with chronic urticaria exhibit increased rates of sensitisation to *Candida albicans*, but not to common moulds. *Mycoses* 2009; 52: 334–338.

229. Ishiguro A, Homma M, Torii S, Tanaka K. Identification of *Candida albicans* antigens reactive with immunoglobulin E antibody of human sera. *Infect Immun* 1992; 60: 1550–1557.

230. Akiyama K, Shida I, Yasueda H et al. Allergenicity of acid protease secreted by *Candida albicans*. *Allergy* 1996; 51: 887–892.

231. Shen HD, Choo KB, Lee HH et al. The 40-kilodalton allergen of *Candida albicans* is an alcohol dehydrogenase: Molecular cloning and immunological analysis using monoclonal antibodies. *Clin Exp Allergy* 1991; 21: 675–681.

232. Woodfolk JA. Allergy and dermatophytes. *Clin Microbiol Rev* 2005; 18: 30–43.

233. Mungan D, Bavbek S, Peksari V et al. *Trichophyton* sensitivity in allergic and nonallergic asthma. *Allergy* 2001; 56: 558–562.

234. Ward GW Jr, Karlsson G, Rose G, Platts-Mills TA. Trichophyton asthma: Sensitization of bronchi and upper airways to dermatophyte antigen. *Lancet* 1989; 1(8643): 859–862.

235. Platts-Mills TAE, Fiocco GP, Hayden ML et al. Serum IgE antibodies to *Trichophyton* in patients with urticaria, angioedema, asthma, and rhinitis: Development of a radioallergosorbent test. *J Allergy Clin Immunol* 1987; 79: 40–45.

236. Deuell B, Arruda LK, Hayden ML et al. *Trichophyton tonsurans* allergen. I. Characterization of a protein that causes immediate but not delayed hypersensitivity. *J Immunol* 1991; 147: 96–101.

237. Stewart GA. Sequence similarity between a major allergen from the dermatophyte *Trichophyton tonsurans* and exo 1,3-β-glucanase. *Clin Exp Allergy* 1993; 23: 154–155.

238. Woodfolk JA, Wheatley LM, Piyasena RV et al. *Trichophyton* antigens associated with IgE antibodies and delayed type hypersensitivity: Sequence homology to two families of serine proteinases. *J Biol Chem* 1998; 273: 29489–29496.

239. Slunt JB, Taketomi EA, Woodfold JA et al. The immune response to *Trichophyton tonsurans*: Distinct T cell cytokine profiles to a single protein among subjects with immediate and delayed hypersensitivity. *J Immunol* 1996; 157: 5192–5197.

240. Woodfolk JA, Sung S-SJ, Benjamin DC et al. Distinct human T cell repertoires mediate immediate and delayed-type hypersensitivity to *Trichophyton* antigen, Tri t 2. *J Immunol* 2000; 165: 4379–4387.

241. Hoff M, Ballmer-Weber BK, Niggemann B et al. Molecular cloning and immunological characterisation of potential allergens from the mould *Fusarium culmorum*. *Mol Immunol* 2003; 39: 965–975.

242. Banerjee B, Kurup VP, Greenberger PA et al. C-terminal cysteine residues determine the IgE binding of Aspergillus fumigatus allergen Asp f 2. *J Immunol* 2002; 169: 5137–5144.

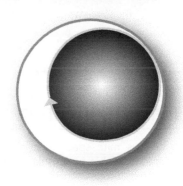

14 Mite allergens

Enrique Fernández-Caldas
Inmunotek S.L.
University of South Florida Morsani College of Medicine

Leonardo Puerta and Luis Caraballo
University of Cartagena

Victor Iraola
Inmunotek S.L.

Richard F. Lockey
University of South Florida Morsani College of Medicine

CONTENTS

14.1 INTRODUCTION

Numerous mite species have been described as the source of allergens capable of sensitizing and inducing allergic symptoms in sensitized and genetically predisposed individuals. Allergic diseases triggered by mite allergens include allergic rhinoconjunctivitis, asthma, atopic dermatitis, and other skin diseases. The most studied house dust mite (HDM) species belong to the family Pyroglyphidae and include *Dermatophagoides pteronyssinus*, *Dermatophagoides farinae*, and *Euroglyphus maynei*. HDMs are commonly present in human dwellings and are especially abundant in mattresses, sofas, carpets, and blankets. Other species, such as *Dermatophagoides microceras*, *Dermatophagoides siboney*, *Gymnoglyphus longior*, and other genera, such as *Hirstia* and *Malayoglyphus*, are also allergenic, although their study is limited [1].

Another important group of mites, referred to as "storage mites," comprises members of the Acaridae and Glycyphagidae families that live in stored food and grains. All mite species present in the home environment capable of inducing IgE-mediated sensitization are called "domestic mites" [2]. Approximately 150 storage mite species are known [3], of which perhaps 20 can be considered important from an economic and sanitary perspective. The most studied species are *B. tropicalis*, due to its abundance in tropical and subtropical regions of the world [4], and *L. destructor*, because of its frequent presence in barns. Storage mite species can be present in kitchen floor dust, cupboards, and pantries. They can be an important plague with economic consequences and cause occupational respiratory allergies in farmers and other occupationally exposed individuals. The most important genera are *Blomia* (family Echimyopodidae), *Lepidoglyphus* and *Glycyphagus* (family Glycyphagidae), *Acarus*, *Tyrophagus* and *Aleuroglyphus* (family Acaridae), *Suidasia* (family Suidasidae), *Chortoglyphus* (family Chortoglyphidae), and *Cheyletus* (family Cheyletidae). Since *B. tropicalis* is present in large quantities in house dust in tropical and subtropical regions, it could also be considered an HDM species.

14.2 ALLERGENS FROM HOUSE DUST MITES

The main sources of allergens in house dust are the mite species *D. pteronyssinus*, *D. farinae*, *E. maynei*, and the storage mite *B. tropicalis* [5]. Most studies in temperate climates demonstrate that *D. pteronyssinus*, originally known as the European HDM, and *D. farinae*, American HDM, are the predominant HDM species worldwide. In tropical and subtropical areas of the world, *B. tropicalis* occurs with a very high frequency and in some regions is present to the same degree as is *D. pteronyssinus* [6,7].

Mite allergens can be extracted and isolated by conventional biochemical methods, by a proteomic approach or by molecular cloning. Mite allergens are present in mite bodies, secreta, and excreta [8]. Mite allergens can be detected in many areas of the home, including beds, carpets, upholstered furniture, and clothing. Leather-covered couches, wood furniture, and bare floors contain fewer mites. Beds are the ideal habitat for mites, since they provide the ideal temperature, food (skin scales, molds, etc.), and moisture for their proliferation. The allergens they produce may accumulate inside mattresses, pillows, and carpets, especially when they are old. They also can be detected in the air using volumetric samplers equipped with sizing devices. Mite allergens remain airborne for a short period of time. Allergenic activity can be detected in particles smaller than 1 μm and in particles larger than 10 μm. Mite fecal pellets may occasionally enter the lung and cause inflammation and bronchoconstriction. Fergusson and Broide [9] demonstrated the presence of Der p 1 in bronchial alveolar lavage fluids of asthmatic children after an overnight exposure to Der p 1 and Der p 2.

Mite allergens display polymorphism in their sequences due to the existence of multigene families or gene duplication. Therefore, some allergens may exist as several variants, or isoforms, including hypoallergenic isoforms, which may have different impacts on the sensitization profile of mite-allergic individuals [10,11].

14.3 CHARACTERIZED HOUSE DUST MITE ALLERGENS

Most of the isolated allergens are placed in groups based on their chronological characterization and/or homology with previously described allergens (Table 14.1).

14.3.1 Group 1

Der p 1 and Der f 1 are considered major allergens based on frequency of recognition by specific IgE of sensitized patients, amount of specific IgE directed to them, and relative content in mite extract. Der p 1 is a glycoprotein with sequence homology and thiol protease functions similar to the enzymes papain, actinidin, bromelain, and human cathepsins B and H [12]. Several isoforms of Der p 1 and Der f 1 have been reported for Der p 1 [10,13].

Several mechanisms are proposed to be involved in the hyperresponsiveness and airway inflammation caused by these allergens. Der p 1 upregulates IgE synthesis by cleaving the low-affinity IgE receptor (CD23) from the surface of human B-cell lymphocytes [14]. Der p 1 cleaves the α subunit of the IL-2 receptor (IL-2R or CD25) from the surface of human peripheral blood T cells, and as a result, these cells show markedly diminished proliferation and interferon γ (IFN-γ) secretion, which consequently causes an immune response toward Th2 cells. The cysteine protease activity of Der p 1 seems to selectively enhance the IgE response and conditions T cells to produce more IL-4 and less IFN-γ [15,16].

The enzymatic activity for Der p 1, and other mite allergens, may also contribute to their immunogenicity by increasing mucosal permeability. The peptidase activity creates specific conditions that favor delivery of any allergen to antigen-presenting cells by a process that involves cleavage of tight junctions that regulate paracellular permeability [17]. Studies using A549 epithelial cells demonstrate that Der p 1 produces both damage and activation of airway epithelial cells. It activates the release of cytokines from this cell line in a protease-activated receptor (PAR) independent manner [18,19]. However, studies in mouse fibroblasts expressing the human PAR1, PAR2, or PAR4 show that Der p 1 and Der p 5 do not affect intracellular calcium mobilization in these cells, providing considerable evidence against a PAR-mediated mechanism. Der p 1 and Der f 1 cleave surfactant protein-A (SP-A) and SP-D lung collectins, which have protective roles in allergy, in a time- and concentration-dependent manner at multiple sites. The cleavage and consequent inactivation of SP-A and SP-D may be a novel mechanism that could explain the potent allergenicity of Der p 1 and Der f 1 [20]. Studies in animal models suggest that the cysteine protease activity of Der p 1 contributes to the *in vivo* immune

Table 14.1 Biological function, molecular weight, and prevalence of specific IgE binding of several mite allergens

Group	Biological function	MW (kDa)	Mite species	IgE binding frequency (%)
1	Cysteine protease	25	Dp, Df, Dm, Ds, Em, Bt, As, Ao, Sm, Tp	70–100
2	Niemann-Pick type C2 (NPC2) protein Recognition and binding of lipids; similar to MD-2	14	Dp, Df, Dm, Ds, Em, Ld, Gd, Bt, As, Ao, Sm, Tp	80–100
3	Trypsin	28–30	Dp, Df, Dm, Ds, Em, Gd, Bt, As, Ao, Sm, Tp	16–100
4	α-Amylase	57	Dp, Df, Em, Bt, As, Sm, Tp	25–46
5	Unknown	15	Dp, Df, Ds, Ld, Gd, Bt, Ao, Sm, Tp	50–70
6	Chymotrypsin	25	Dp, Df, Ds, Bt, Ao, Sm	40
7	Lipid-binding protein Similar to proteins in the TLR pathway	22–31	Dp, Df, Ld, Gd, Bt, As, Ao, Sm, Tp	50
8	Glutatthione-S-transferase	26	Dp, Df, Ld, Gd, Bt, As, Ao, Sm	40
9	Collagenolytic serine protease	30	Dp, Df, Dm, Bt, Ao, Sm	90
10	Tropomyosin	33–37	Dp, Df, Ld, Gd, Bt, As, Ao, Sm, Tp, Ca	50–95
11	Paramyosin	92–110	Dp, Df, Dm, Bt	80
12	Unknown	14	Bt	50
13	Fatty acid-binding proteins	14–15	Dp, Df, Ld, Gd, Bt, As, Ao, Sm, Tp	10–23
14	Lipid-binding apolipophorin	177	Dp, Df, Dm, Em, Bt	90
15	Chitinase	98–109	Dp, Df, Dm, Bt	70
16	Gelsolin-like protein/villin	53	Df	35
17	EF-hand calcium-binding protein	53	Df	35
18	Chitinase	60	Dp, Df	50–60
19	Antimicrobial peptide	7.2	Bt	
20	Arginine kinase	40	Dp, Df, Ao	67
21	Unknown	13.2	Dp, Bt	29–42
22	MD-2-related lipid recognition	14	Dp, Df, Ao, As, Tp	40–42
23	Chitin-binding domain type 2	14	Dp	74
24	ubiquinol-cytochrome c reductase-binding protein/Troponin C	18	Df, Tp	11

(Continued)

Table 14.1 (*Continued*) Biological function, molecular weight, and prevalence of specific IgE binding of several mite allergens

Group	Biological function	MW (kDa)	Mite species	IgE binding frequency (%)
25	Triose-phosphate isomerase	34	Dp, Df	42
26	Myosin light-chain/translation elongation factor 2	43	Dp, Df	
27	Serpin		Df, Dp	42
28	Heat shock protein	70	Dp, Df, Tp	47.5
29	Cyclophilin	29	Dp, Df	24
30	Ferritin	16	Dp, Df	63–100
31	Cofilin		Dp, Df	32
32	Inorganic pyrophosphatase		Dp, Df	
33	Alpha tubulin	52	Dp, Df, Tp	23–29
34	Endoribonuclease		Dp, Df	68–68
35	Aldehyde dehydrogenase		Dp, Tp	77–80
36	Unknown		Dp	42

Sources: Adapted from Ong ST, Chew FT. Reconstructing the Repertoire of Mite Allergens by Recombinant DNA Technology. In: R. Pawankar et al., editors, *Allergy Frontiers: Future Perspectives*, © Springer, 2010; www.allergen.org; and unpublished data with sequence data available in World Health Organization/International Union of Immunological Societies Allergen Nomenclature, or GenBank.

Abbreviations: Ao, *Aleuroglyphus ovatus*; As, *Acarus siro*; Bt, *B. Tropicalis*; Ca, *Chortoglyphus arcuatus*; Df, *Dermatophagoides farinae*; Dm, *Dermatophagoides microceras*; Dp, *Dermatophagoides pteronyssinus*; Ds, *Dermatophagoides siboney*; Em, *Euroglyphus maynei*; Gd, *Glycyphagus domesticus*; Ld, *L. Destructor*; Sm, *Suidasia medanensis*; Tp, *T. Putrescentiae*.

responses, including the production, not only of IgE, but also IgG. Intranasal administration of proteolytically active Der p 1 to sensitized mice leads to an enhanced inflammatory cellular infiltration of the lungs and systemic production of IgE in comparison to inactive Der p 1, which has no effect [15].

Blo t 1, homologous to Der p 1, is a cysteine protease. Blo t 1, with an estimated molecular weight of 26 kDa, is an important allergen. Recombinant Blo t 1 reacted positively with IgE in 90% and 65% of sera from asthmatic children and adults from Singapore, respectively. Furthermore, there is a low correlation between IgE reactivity to Blo t 1 and Der p 1 [21]. Recently, the crystal structure of recombinant Blo t 1 was determined and indicated a fold characteristic for the pro-form of cysteine proteases from the C1A class. Structural comparison of experimentally mapped Der f 1/Der p1 IgG epitopes to the same surface patch on Blo t 1, and the sequence identity of surface-exposed residues, suggests limited cross-reactivity between these allergens and Blo t 1 [22].

Eur m 1 is an allergen of *E. maynei* and has amino acid (aa) sequence similarities of approximately 85% with Der p 1 and Der f 1 [23]. Der s 1, a major allergen of *D. siboney*, has an 89% frequency of specific IgE binding [24]. Due to its high prevalence in house dust and worldwide distribution, the group 1 allergen is used as a standard to estimate environmental exposure to *Dermatophagoides* spp. in the indoor environment and is an important reagent in the component-resolved diagnosis of mite allergy.

14.3.2 Group 2

Der p 2 and Der f 2 are heat- and pH-stable, lipid-binding proteins [25]. These allergens have 88% sequence similarity. In their native stage and as recombinant allergens, both have more than 80% frequency of specific IgE recognition [26]. Der p 2 and Der f 2 show a significant degree of sequence polymorphism. The polymorphic residues are also found in regions containing T-cell epitopes [27]. Eur m 2 from *E. maynei* is characterized by having 84%–86% sequence identity with the corresponding allergens from *Dermatophagoides* spp. [28,29]. Suzuki et al. demonstrated that the conformation of Der f 2 is critical in the determination of the Th1/Th2 shift [30].

Group 2 allergens bind lipopolysaccharides (LPS) with a nanomolar affinity and in a manner similar to the binding by myeloid differentiation protein-2 (MD-2). The hydrophobic LPS-binding residues are similar in all group 2 allergen sequences [31]. Considering that MD-2 loads LPS onto toll-like receptor 4 (TLR4), the allergenicity of group 2 mite allergens might be enhanced by a similar interaction. Der p 2 complexed with LPS induces Th2 responses in MD-2- but not TLR4-deficient animals [32]. Tsai et al. demonstrated that Der p2 is capable of triggering human B-cell activation and TLR4 induction. Der p 2 specifically upregulates mitogen-activated protein kinase phosphatase-1 (MKP-1) expression and activity in human B cells, which in turn, results in p38 mitogen-activated protein kinase (p38/MAPK) dephosphorylation, triggering TLR4 induction [33]. *In vitro* and animal model studies suggest that Der p 2 induces airway inflammation and elevated nerve growth factor (NGF) release through increasing reactive oxygen species (ROS) production and the mitogen-activated protein kinases (MAPK)-dependent pathway [34]. Furthermore, rDer p2 could act directly on airway smooth muscle cells activating the TLR2 signaling pathway. rDer p2 seems to be essential for the promotion of the myeloid differentiation primary response gene/interleukin-1 receptor-associated kinase 1/nuclear factor κ-light-chain-enhancer

of activated B cells (MyD88/IRAK1/NF-kB) pathway to induce an inflammatory response and bronchial hyperresponsiveness [35].

In Central Europe, more than 95% of mite-allergic patients are primarily sensitized to Der p 1 or Der p 2. Diagnostic tests containing these allergens plus the highly cross-reactive allergen Der p 10 may improve the diagnostic selection of patients for immunotherapy with *D. pteronyssinus* vaccines [36]. In China, among 100 selected patients, 95% had specific IgE directed against Der f 1, Der f 2, and Der p 2 and 94% against Der p 1; 60% of sera contained IgE reacting against the allergen Eur m 2 [37]. In the tropical city of Cartagena, Colombia, the prevalence of specific IgE to Der p 1 was 64% and to Der p 2, 69%. However, when Der p 10 reactivity was incorporated in the serological test, 93.5% of the mite-allergic subjects were positively diagnosed [38]. In France, the prevalence of serum-specific IgE to Der p 1 was 93%, to Der p 2 77% (Der p 1 or Der p 2 94%), and to Der p 10, 28%. Levels of specific IgE against *D. pteronyssinus* strongly correlated with levels against Der p 1 and Der p 2 ($r = .89$ and 0.85, respectively), but not to Der p 10 [39], suggesting that this allergen is a minor contributor to the overall allergenicity of *D. pteronyssinus*. The serum IgE reactivity of 95% against Der p 1 and 93% for Der p 2 was found in Chinese patients, with HDM allergy being the Der p 2 sensitization predominant in adults [40]. The development of hybrid proteins containing mite group 1 and group 2 allergens could be adequate to treat mite-allergic patients [41,42].

Sera from subjects in Bangkok and Perth, where different variants of Der p 2 are found, were compared by the affinity (IC_{50}) of IgE cross-reactivity to different variants and by direct IgE binding. The secondary structures of the recombinant variants resembled the natural allergen but with differences in 1-anilinonaphthalene 8-sulfonic acid binding. The IC_{50} of Der p 2.0101 required sevenfold higher concentrations to inhibit IgE binding to the high-IgE-binding Der p 2.0104 than for homologous inhibition in sera from Bangkok where it is absent, while in sera from Perth that have both variants, the IC_{50} was the same and low. Direct binding revealed that Der p 2.0104 was best for detecting IgE in both regions, Bangkok and Perth, followed by Der p 2.0101 with binding to other variants showing larger differences [43].

The major allergen Lep d 2 is a protein of 14–18 kDa by sodium dodecyl sulfate polyacrylamide gel electrophoresis (SDS-PAGE) [44]. It is present in the digestive tract of the mite [45]. Lep d 2 is cloned, sequenced, and expressed as a recombinant protein (rLep d 2) [46]. This allergen possesses high IgE reactivity *in vitro* [47] and *in vivo* [48]. Lep d 2 presents a high degree of polymorphism, with two distinct isoforms, Lep d 2.01 and Lep d 2.02, differing in 13 aa. Lep d 2.02 has two variants, and Lep d 2.01 has three variants. The frequency of these variants may differ between wild and cultured mites [49].

G. domesticus is a phylogenetically closely related species to *L. destructor*. A 15 kDa allergen belonging to group 2, and termed Gly d 2, is cloned and expressed as a recombinant protein. Gly d 2 shows a high degree of homology with Lep d 2. Three isoforms of Gly d 2 are isolated; 16 out of 17 sera of sensitized patients recognized this recombinant protein [50].

Tyr p 2 is a 16 kDa protein [51]. The recombinant protein demonstrated high IgE reactivity *in vitro* [47] and *in vivo* [48]. This major allergen is recognized by 80% of sera from sensitized patients [52].

14.3.3 Groups 3 and 4

Group 3 has a trypsin-like serine protease activity and 50% sequence similarity with other serine proteases, including chymotrypsin [53].

The sequence of Der p 3 has 81% sequence identity with Der f 3 and both have a 41% sequence identity with bovine trypsin. A frequency of IgE binding between 51% and 90% for Der p 3 and between 42% and 70% for Der f 3 is described [54]. Immature Der p 3 obtained in *Pichia pastoris* displayed a very weak IgE reactivity by sandwich enzyme-linked immunosorbent assay (ELISA) and competitive inhibition. In a model of mouse allergy, Der p 3 induced a TH1-biased immune response that prevented allergic response but retained Der p 3-specific T-cell reactivity [55].

Der p 4 is an enzyme similar to carbonic anhydrases, which shows significant homology with mammalian α-amylase. It is recognized as an allergen by 25% to 46% of mite-allergic individuals [56].

Similar allergens have been found in *B. tropicalis*. Blo t 4 is an allergen homologous to amylase, with 68% aa sequence identity with group 4 allergen of *Dermatophagoides* [57] and *A. siro*. Aca s 4 has a high level of α-amylase activity and 74%, 70%, 64%, and 66% sequence similarity with Tyr p 4, Blo t 4, Eur m 4, and Der p 4, respectively [58].

14.3.4 Group 5

Der p 5 is a 15 kDa allergen, which has an estimated IgE-binding prevalence of 50% [59]. Studies with epithelial cells demonstrate that Der p 5 also induces the secretion of IL-6 and IL-8, even to a higher extent than Der p 1. This effect of Der p 5 is dose-dependent and -specific and could not be blocked by protease inhibitors.

rDer p 5 is a heat-stable protein with predominantly α-helical secondary structure. IgE reactivity was tested with sera from 117 mite-allergic patients and in a basophil histamine release experiment. It reacted with IgE from 31% of mite-allergic patients' sera and showed no relevant cross-reactivity to group 5 allergens from storage mites and tropical mites. rDer p 5-specific rabbit IgG antibodies and immunogold electron microscopy localize the allergen to secretory granules of midgut epithelial cells of HDMs [60]. Biophysical analysis showed that rDer p 5 was monomeric and adopted a similar α-helix-rich fold at both physiological and acidic pH. Spectrofluorimetry experiments showed that rDer p 5 is able to selectively bind lipid ligands but only under mild acidic pH conditions. Computer-based docking simulations identified potential binding sites for these ligands. This allergen, with putatively associated lipid(s), triggered the production of IL-8 in respiratory epithelial cells through a TLR2-, NF-kB- and MAPK-dependent signaling pathway [61]. A similar localization of conformational IgE-binding epitopes on Der p 5 and Der p 21, despite limited IgE cross-reactivity, has been described [62].

Five polymorphic variants of Blo t 5 were identified with 26 DNA base and 12 amino acid substitutions, thus implying a high degree of sequence diversity. Of the 115 cases, 68.70% and 59.13% showed reactivity to *B. tropicalis* extract and rBlo t 5, respectively. Blo t 5 gene exhibits polymorphic variants with predicted amino acid sequences resulting in changes in its IgE epitopes. These polymorphisms may suggest variability of allergenic properties of Blo t 5 [63].

Several studies focused on the *in vitro* cross-reactivity of purified Blo t 5 and Der p 5 [6,64,65]. Most group 5 studies demonstrate low to moderate cross-reactivity at the molecular level. Blo t 5 is recognized by 40% to 70% of *B. tropicalis*-sensitive patients, especially those residing in tropical areas [66,67,126]. Unlike in *D. pteronyssinus*, where group 1 and 2 allergens are the major

allergens, Blo t 5 is the dominant major allergen in *B. tropicalis* [68]. The recombinant Blo t 5 shows up to 70% of IgE reactivity in sensitized asthmatic patients, whereas the homologous Der p 5 reacts with 40%–50% of sera from mite-allergic asthmatic individuals [69]. Despite the high-sequence homology between group 5 allergens, IgE cross-reactivity of the major allergen Blo t 5 and the minor allergen Der p 5 is surprisingly low. The solution structure of Blo t 5 shows a monomeric three-helical structure tightly packed into an antiparallel bundle [70,71].

The structure of Der p 5 is a three-helical bundle with a kinked *N*-terminal helix that assembles in an entangled dimer with a large hydrophobic cavity that could be involved in the binding of ligands, like LPS, and thus shifting the immune response from tolerance to allergic inflammation [72]. Der p 5 and Der f 5 have the propensity to form dimeric structures, unlike Blo t 5. This may have important consequences in the allergenicity of these molecules [73].

Lep d 5 is cloned and expressed as a partial molecule. This partial clone of 110 aa and a molecular mass of 12.5 kDa is recognized by 9% of 45 sera from patients sensitized to *L. destructor* [74]. Two isoforms are sequenced, Lep d 5.02 with 171 aa and 19.5 kDa and Lep d 5.04 with 169 aa and 19.3 kDa.

14.3.5 Groups 6 and 7

Der p 6 is a chymotrypsin-like serine protease, which shows a 40%–60% frequency of IgE binding [75]. Der p 7 and Der f 7 have 86% similarity in aa sequences. Frequency of sensitization of approximately 50% is reported with these *D. pteronyssinus* allergens in mite-allergic children and adults [76]. The structure of Der p 7 reveals a distant homology to a family of proteins involved in the human innate immune recognition of bacterial lipid products. It does not bind LPS but binds with weak affinity to the bacterial lipopeptide polymyxin B. Therefore, it has the potential to interact with the innate immune system [77]. Der p 7 is homologous to Der f 7 in terms of its aa sequence and overall three-dimensional (3D) structure but with significant differences in the region proximal to the IgE epitope and in thermal stability [78].

The allergen Lep d 7 is sequenced and cloned, and the calculated molecular mass is 22 kDa, without *N*-glycosylation sites. The recombinant protein rLep d 7 is recognized by the 62% of the sera of *L. destructor*-positive subjects. The biochemical function of the group 7 mite allergens is unknown, and Lep d 7 does not show significant homologies to proteins other than to the group 7 mite allergens [74].

14.3.6 Groups 8 and 9

Der p 8 is a 26 kDa allergen with strong homology with rat and mouse glutathione-*S*-transferase (GST). Approximately 40% of mite-allergic subjects tested with recombinant Der p 8 had detectable levels of specific IgE to this allergen [79]. At least eight isoforms of native Der p 8 were detected by two-dimensional gel and immunoblot analyses. Sera from Taiwanese asthmatics show 96% and 84% IgE reactivity to native Der p 8 and recombinant Der p 8, respectively. Native Der p 8 showed 75% and 65% IgE reactivity with sera from Malaysia and Singapore, respectively. In Australia, the prevalence was reported between 25% and 40%. Der p 8 and Blo t 8 are similar to mammalian GST. A distinctive difference of the mite GST appears to be the rare occurrence of a large aromatic moiety at position 14 in the active site loop instead of the usual leucine. This indicates that these enzymes may have different substrate specificities from other mu-class GST. The cross-reactivity between Der p 8 and GST in *Periplaneta americana* suggests that the GST in mites and cockroaches may be considered a pan-allergen [80].

The allergenicity of Tyr p 8 was demonstrated by antibody recognition, IgE inhibition, and the triggering of basophil-sensitized release of histamine [81]. Tyr p 8 contains 218 aa with the MW of 26 kDa and exhibits 83% sequence homology with Der p8. Specific IgE-binding assays showed that 45.3% of the subjects had specific IgE against rTyr p8. However, only 17.9% had specific IgE against rTyr p 8 after Der p 8 absorption, suggesting cross-reactivity between these two allergens.

Der p 9 is a 24 kDa protein, as indicated by mass spectroscopy, with collagenolytic serine protease activity and a frequency of IgE reactivity higher than 80% [82].

14.3.7 Groups 10 and 11

These groups are composed of tropomyosin and paramyosin, respectively. They are involved in muscle contraction in invertebrates and are present in low concentrations in mite extracts. The invertebrate tropomyosins are allergenic in man with high IgE cross-reactivity and, therefore, are referred to as pan-allergens. Der f 10 and Der p 10 are allergens with significant homology with tropomyosins from different species [83] and are involved in the cross-reactivity process between mites, shrimp, and insects in seafood-allergic patients [84]. Although Blo t 10 and Der p 10 are highly conserved and significantly cross-react, unique IgE epitopes exists [85]. Der p 10 is recognized by 10%–20% of HDM-allergic patients. The allergenic activity of Der p 10 is generally low, but some patients can be identified as suffering from clinically relevant HDM allergy due to Der p 10 sensitization [86].

Lep d 10 is an allergenic protein homologous to tropomyosin. It was identified as an allergen from a phage display cDNA library. The molecule of 284 aa is formed by two polypeptide chains. The IgE-binding frequencies of the recombinant Lep d 10 are estimated at 13% among subjects with IgE reactivity to mites and/or crustaceans [87]. Recombinant Tyr p 10 has 64%–94% of amino acid identity with other allergenic tropomyosins and was recognized by 12.5% of sera from sensitized patients [88,137].

The tropomyosin allergen, Cho a 10, was cloned and sequenced from a *C. arcuatus* expression library. The homology between Cho a 10 and Der p 10 is 94% and between Cho a 10 and Lep d 10, 95% [89].

Der f 11 is a paramyosin [90]. Skin test and IgE-binding studies showed that 62% and 50% of mite-sensitive asthmatic patients reacted with recombinant Der f 11 [91], respectively. rDer p 11 has a frequency of specific IgE binding in the sera of allergic patients of 60%, slightly higher than to Der f 11 (52.5%), suggesting that Der p 11 is also an important allergen [92]. The aa sequence of Der p 11 shares over 89% identity with the aa sequence of Der f 11 and Blo t 11 [93].

14.3.8 Group 12

Blo t 12 has a mature sequence of 14 kDa, binds specific IgE with a 50% frequency, and does not show homology with other known proteins [94]. Genome and transcriptome analysis of *D. pteronyssinus* and *D. farinae* fail to identify group 12 in these mite species [95]. Two isoforms of Blo t 12 have been described; one isoform, with 14.4% prevalence of specific IgE reactivity, was isolated in Singapore. The IgE reactivity of this isoform was tested in Colombia using sera of mite-allergic patients and showed 23.4% and 17% reactivity by ELISA and skin prick test (SPT), respectively [11]. The two isoforms bound chitin, but Blo t 12.0101 showed a stronger binding capacity. In sensitized mice, the chitin reinforces the effects of Blo t 12 on total IgE production [96].

14.3.9 Group 13

Group 13 allergens belong to the fatty acid-binding protein (FABP) family and have been cloned and characterized from several mite species [97–99]. Der p 13 has 7% of IgE-binding frequency in Thai HDM-allergic patients as well as limited propensity to activate basophil degranulation. Nevertheless, the protein with its presumptively associated lipid(s) triggered the production of IL-8 and granulocyte-macrophage colony-stimulating factor (GM-CSF) in respiratory epithelial cells through a TLR2, MyD88, NF-κB, and MAPK-dependent signaling pathway. Der p 13 may, through its lipid-binding capacity, play a role in the initiation of the HDM-allergic response through TLR2 activation [100].

Der f 13 shares a medium- to high-sequence homology with human FABPs, with the closest one being human brain FABP, having a 39.1% amino acid identity and 58.6% similarity. A solution structure study reveals that Der f 13 adopts the typical β barrel fold of an FABP, similar to that of other human FABPs [101]. ELISA inhibition assays with monoclonal antibody specific for Blo t 13 suggest that the homologous allergen Der s 13 is also present in *D. siboney* [102,103]. Tyr p 13 was isolated from a cDNA library of the mite *T. putrescentiae*, showing 62.3% of identity in the amino acid sequence with Blo t 13. The recombinant allergen shows 6.4% of reactivity in allergic individuals from Korea [98]. In the sheep scab mite, *Psoroptes ovis*, a genomic sequence encoding for a FABP with 55% similarity with Blo t 13 was identified [97].

The recombinant protein rLep d 13 is recognized by approximately 13% of the sera of *L. destructor*-sensitized patients [74]. The recombinant allergen Aca s 13 from *Acarus siro* is recognized by 23% of the sera of patients sensitized to this mite species [106]. The genomic sequence data from *Euroglyphus maynei* predicted two homologs of the group 13 allergens: one was most closely related to a version of Blo t 13, and one was most closely related to Der p 13 [23].

14.3.10 Groups 14 and 15

Group 14 is an apolipophorin-like lipid transport protein, isolated by molecular cloning from *Dermatophagoides* spp. [107]. This allergen, along with Der p 15 and Der 18, appeared as the last allergen in the evolution of IgE response in a German population [108]. Group 15 is homologous to insect chitinases. Der f 15 is a major allergen for dogs and cats. McCall et al. isolated a pair of natural Der f 15 proteins with apparent molecular weight masses of 98 and 109 kDa, which reflect different degrees of glycosylation [109]. Der p 15–specific IgE was detected in 70% of a panel of 27 human allergic sera [110]. Chitin-binding proteins are of interest because they are the dominant allergens for HDM-allergic dogs and might interact with chitin, which is a TH2 adjuvant [111,112].

14.3.11 Groups 16, 17, and 18

The allergen Der f 16 has sequence similarity to gelsolin, a Ca^{2+} and phosphatidylinositol 4,5-bisphosphate (PIP2)-regulated actin filament severing and capping protein. In allergic individuals, IgE reactivity by skin and serological tests has been reported between 62% and 50%, respectively [113]. Der f 17 is a calcium-binding protein that binds IgE in 35% of the sera from mite-allergic patients.

Der p 18 encodes a mature protein of 49.2 kDa with 88% sequence identity with Der f 18. Specific IgE to this allergen is reported in 63% of human allergic sera [110,114]. Using the basophil activation test with samples from allergic patients, rDer p 18 induced basophil activation in an IgE-dependent manner, albeit to a lower extent than Derp 2. Der p 18 is localized in the peritrophic matrix of *D. pteronyssinus* but is almost absent in feces. Der p 18 and another chitinase-like HDM allergen, Der p 15, bound weakly to chitin, which could only be detected with the purified, recombinant allergens but not with the natural allergens in a HDM extract in which natural chitin-binding proteins may already be bound to chitin [116].

14.3.12 Groups 19 and 20

Blo t 19 is a 7 kDa allergen showing homology to an antimicrobial peptide. The structure of a 68-amino-acid peptide has been elucidated by nuclear magnetic resonance (NMR) spectroscopy and registered in the Protein Data Bank database (code 2MFJ). It has a 10% frequency of IgE reactivity in mite-allergic subjects [117]. The Der f 20 is an arginine kinase [118]. It has similarities with arginine kinase from *D. pteronyssinus* and *Aleuroglyphus ovatus*. Western-blot and ELISA studies showed IgE-binding capacity of 66.7% in the sera from dust mite-allergic patients from Guangzhou, China [119,120].

14.3.13 Group 21

Der p 21 has been identified and isolated by molecular cloning from the gut of the dust mite *D. pteronyssinus*. It has sequence homology with Der p 5. rDer p 21 binds high levels of patients' IgE antibodies and shows high allergenic activity in basophil activation experiments. Rabbit anti-Der p 21 IgG antibodies allowed the ultrastructural localization of the allergen in the midgut (epithelium, lumen, and feces) of *D. pteronyssinus* by immunogold electron microscopy [121]. The recombinant Der f 21 protein was characterized by Western-blot, ELISA, and SPT. It showed 28.9% of serum IgE reactivity in 38 dust mite-allergic children, and 42% in 98 dust mite-allergic patients displaying positive responses to skin prick testing. Immune inhibition assays showed an important degree of IgE cross-reactivity between rDer f 21 and rDer f 5 [122,123].

Blo t 21 is a 129 amino acid protein with an α-helical secondary structure and localizes in the midgut and hindgut of *B. tropicalis* as well as fecal particles. Positive specific IgE responses to Blo t 21

were shown in 93% of allergic individuals by ELISA and in 95% by skin prick testing in 43 adult patients with allergic rhinitis [124]. Blo t 21 shares 41% and 39% aa identity with Der p 21 and Blo t 5, respectively [125]. In a study, 253 children were tested with Der p 21 and Blo t 21. A 64% and 56% frequency of IgE reactivity was reported, respectively [126]. Blo t 21 has a low to moderate cross-reactivity with Blo t 5 and Der p 5. The Blo t 21 3D structure determined by NMR mapped its IgE-binding epitopes almost to the same region as Blo t 5 but with an additional conformational epitope [127].

14.3.14 Groups 22 and 23

The full-length sequence of Der f 22 coded for mature proteins of 135 amino acids containing six cysteine residues. Phylogenetic analysis shows that Der f 22 is a paralogue of Der f 2. Both allergens showed specific IgE binding to over 40% of the atopic patients, with limited cross-reactivity. Der f 22 contains the Der-p2–like domain, which is a member of the MD-2-related lipid-recognition domain family. The ML domain is predicted to be involved in lipid binding, and its structure is characterized by two antiparallel β-pleated sheets and an accessible central hydrophobic cavity. By immunostaining of *D. farinae* sections, Der f 22 was strongly localized at the anterior midgut region. It was able to bind sera IgE in about 42% of allergic individuals and has limited cross-reactivity with Der f 2 [128].

Der p 23 has sequence homology to peritrophins, which contain chitin-binding domains and is part of the peritrophic matrix lining the gut of arthropods. Recombinant Der p 23 reacted with IgE antibodies from 74% of *D. pteronyssinus*-allergic patients ($n = 347$) at levels comparable to the two major HDM allergens, Der p 1 and Der p 2, and exhibits high allergenic activity as demonstrated by upregulation of CD203c expression on basophils from *D. pteronyssinus*-allergic patients. Immunogold electron microscopy localized the allergen in the peritrophic matrix lining the midgut of *D. pteronyssinus* as well as on the surface of the fecal pellets. The high allergenic activity of Der p 23 and its frequent recognition as a respiratory allergen may be explained by the fact that it becomes airborne and respirable through its association with mite feces [129]. Fifty-four percent of Thai HDM-allergic patients displayed Der p 23–specific IgE responses, and rDer p 23 was able to induce basophil degranulation of rat basophil leukemia cells [130].

14.3.15 Group 24

A cDNA encoding a 17.7 kDa troponin C, with homology to cockroach allergen Bla g 6, was identified from *T. putrescentiae*–expressed sequence tags and termed Tyr p 24. The recombinant *T. putrescentiae* troponin C shares 62.7%–85.5% homology with troponin C from various arthropods. Sera from 5 of 47 subjects in the study group (10.6%) show IgE binding to the recombinant protein [131].

Der f 24 was identified as an ubiquinol-cytochrome c reductase binding protein (UQCRB)–like protein homologue. *D. farinae* UQCRB-like protein clustered with proteins of other arthropods but branched away from the cluster, underscoring its uniqueness. Serum IgE reactivity was demonstrated in 22 sera from mite-allergic patients to the recombinant UQCRB by ELISA and positive SPT in five of ten subjects tested [132].

14.3.16 Groups 25, 26, and 27

By a proteomic approach, several D. farinae allergens, including Der f 25, Der f 26, and Der f 27, were identified by coupling two-dimensional electrophoresis with two-dimensional immunoblotting and IgE from allergic sera. The allergenicity was further examined by ELISA using the recombinant allergens and mouse models of asthma. Der f 25 was purified and characterized as homologous to triose-phosphate from the mite extract of D. farinae. Competitive SPT with recombinant rDer f 25 showed that 16 of 42 (38%) dust mite-allergic patients were positive to this allergen. The IgE binding to D. farinae extract can be inhibited by recombinant Der f 25 in a dose-dependent manner [133].

Der f 26 was identified as a translational factor elongation 2, with capacity to bind IgE. Several isoforms of Der p 26 have been identified [134].

Der f 27 is a serpin, which shares significant similarity with serpin allergens (Tri a 33 and Gal d 2) from *Triticum aestivum* and *Gallus domesticus*. Using the SPT, 8 out of 19 mite allergic patients (42%) showed a positive SPT reaction to r-Der f 27, The specific immune reactivity of IgE against purified Der f 27 was also confirmed by ELISA. In a mouse model of asthma, airways disease was induced by administration of r-Der f 27 [135].

14.3.17 Group 28

Der f 28, homologous to heat shock protein, was confirmed as allergen by proteomics and two-dimensional immunoblotting of D. farinae extracts in an induced allergic pulmonary inflammation in a mouse model of allergic asthma [136]. Tyr p 28 from *Tyrophagus putrescentiae* has 64% amino acid sequence similar to Der f 28. Frequency of IgE reactivity of 47.1% in allergic patients from China was demonstrated by Western blotting using the recombinant allergen [137].

14.3.18 Groups 29 and 30

The gene of Der f 29b consists of 495 bases and encodes 164 amino acids. Positive responses to r-Der f 29b were shown in 24.3% of 37 HDM-allergic patients by SPT [138]. Der f 30 has been identified by a proteomic approach in D. farinae. It has the structure of the ferritin heavy chain. Ferritin was reported as an allergen in *Procambarus clarkii* (freshwater crayfish). No other ferritin allergens have been identified. Native ferritin was purified from D. farinae allergen extracts. Sixty-three percent of the sera reacted by immunoblotting of electrophoresed natural allergen, 100% by specific IgE binding to partially purified natural by ELISA, and 60% by skin testing [139].

14.3.19 Groups 31, 32, 33, 34, 35, and 36

r-Der f 31 is capable of modulating dendritic cells (DCs) and facilitates Th2 cell differentiation. It is suggested that Der f 31 can activate lung-resident ILC2s. Hui et al. found that the levels of TSLP and IL-33 were increased by r-Der f 31 in a concentration-dependent manner, an effect that was abolished in the presence of an anti-TLR2 antibody but not a TLR4 inhibitor [140,141].

Der f 32 has the biological function of an inorganic secreted pyrophosphatase. It produced skin test reactivity and specific IgE binding in subjects by immunoblot and ELISA [142,143].

Der f 33 was identified and characterized as having a molecular weight of 52 kDa and belonging to the α-tubulin protein family. The positive rate of SPT to Der f 33 was 23.5% (4/17 patients). It can modulate the functions of DCs and induce airway hyperreactivity [144,145].

An α-tubulin is a putative allergen from a phage display cDNA library of T. putrescentiae. The IgE-binding frequency of the recombinant allergen was 29.3% among subjects with IgE reactivity to mites and/or crustaceans [146].

Der f 34 has imine deaminase activity that preferentially acts on leucine and methionine. Native Der f 34 showed a high IgE-binding frequency as revealed by two-dimensional immunoblotting (62.5%) or ELISA (68%), which was comparable with those of a major HDM allergen Der f 2 (77.5% and 79%, respectively) [147].

Der f 35 shows a similar amino acid sequence to group 2 allergens from sheep scab mite and storage mites. Native Der f 35 showed 77.5% IgE-binding frequency in HDM-allergic patients, comparable to nDer f 2 (77.5% and 65%) [148]. Similarly, Tyr p 35, homologous to aldehyde dehydrogenase (ALDH), also showed an IgE-binding frequency higher than 80% [137].

A recent study has established that a group of 23 kDa proteins represents a novel mite allergen group, namely, group 36. They are present in D. farinae and D. pteronyssinus. Der f 36 and Der p 36 have amino acid sequence identity of 79% and a 46% identity with the KPM0996 putative protein from the scabies mite *Sarcoptes scabiei*. Der f 36 and Der p 36 react with serum-specific IgE from 42% (8/19) of HDM-allergic individuals [150].

Tyr p 36 represents the first mite profilin allergen to be officially named. rTyr p 36 reacted with greater than 60% of sera from patients allergic to T. putrescentiae [137].

14.4 ALLERGENICITY OF THE STORAGE MITES

The allergenicity of B. tropicalis, Lepidoglyphus destructor, Glycyphagus domesticus, Tyrophagus putrescentiae, Acarus siro, Aleuroglyphus ovatus, Suidasia medanensis, and Thyreophagus entomophagus has been demonstrated in different populations, and for most of them several allergens are characterized [151]. Some of these allergens can be considered as pan-allergens, while some have sequence homology and biological functions like those previously described in the Dermatophagoides spp. As we presented before, the main allergens described in storage mites include FABPs, tropomysin and paramyosin homologues, apolipophorine-like proteins, α-tubulines, and others, such as groups 2, 5, and 7 allergens. The allergenicity of other species such as *Acarus farris, Austroglycyphagus malaysiensis, B. kulagini, B. tjibodas, Cheyletus eruditus, Chortoglyphus arcuatus, Gohieria fusca, Thyreophagus entomophagus,* and *Tyrophagus longior* also has been investigated. Table 14.2 shows a list of the main families and species of storage mites described as allergenic [152].

In vivo studies using provocation tests to investigate the clinical significance of sensitivity to B. tropicalis and its cross-reactivity with D. pteronyssinus are scarce. Stanaland et al. [153] demonstrated that 83% of B. tropicalis-sensitive patients in Florida had a positive nasal challenge with a *B. tropicalis* extract. Therefore, a positive skin test to *B. tropicalis* is a good indicator of possible allergic symptoms after inhalation of *B. tropicalis* allergens. Other studies in Brazil and Singapore demonstrate the allergenicity of *B. tropicalis* using nasal challenges [154,155]. In Brazil, a group of *D. pteronyssinus*- and *B. tropicalis*-sensitive patients was evaluated; 90% of the patients had a positive nasal challenge to *D. pteronyssinus* and 60% to *B. tropicalis*. The study conducted in Singapore included 20 adults with persistent allergic rhinitis, 5 of whom had a history of asthma. Significant increases in subjective and objective nasal symptoms, together with a significant increase of tryptase and LTC4 concentrations in nasal secretion, were found in all patients after each challenge with *B. tropicalis*. Furthermore, a study conducted by García Robaina et al. [156] demonstrates that patients sensitized to two mite species, *D. pteronyssinus* and *B. tropicalis*, may only react to one of them upon allergen-specific challenges. This was previously suggested for even more closely related species, such as *D. pteronyssinus* and *D. farinae* [157]. The study confirms previous *in vivo* and *in vitro* cross-reactivity observations using whole extracts as well as purified allergens. It suggests that although there is some *in vitro* and *in vivo* allergenic cross-reactivity between *B. tropicalis* and *D. pteronyssinus*, clinical symptoms induced by the inhalation of *B. tropicalis* and *D. pteronyssinus* allergens seem to be species specific, although some patients may react to common allergens. Standardized extracts of *B. tropicalis* are only available in some European and Asian countries, in Cuba, and in some African and South American countries. *B. tropicalis* extracts are only available

Table 14.2 Main families and species of storage mites that have been described as allergenic

Family	Species
Glycyphagidae	*Glycyphagus domesticus*
	G. privatus
	Gohieria fusca
	L. destructor
Echimyopodidae	*B. tropicalis*
	B. kulagini
	B. tjibodas
Chortoglyphidae	*Chortoglyphus arcuatus*
Ebertiidae	*Suidasia medanensis*
Acaridae	*T. putrescentiae*
	T. longior
	Acarus siro
	A. farris
	Thyreophagus entomophagus
	Aleuroglyphus ovatus
Cheyletidae	*Cheyletus eruditus*
	Ch. tenuipilis
	Ch. malaccensis

under experimental conditions in the United States and other countries throughout the world. There is a definitive need to use standardized extracts of *B. tropicalis* in countries with tropical, subtropical, and temperate climates of the world where *Blomia* species are endemic. For example, in the subtropical Canary Islands, Spain, a strong association between sensitization to *B. tropicalis* and bronchial hyperreactivity and asthma, before and after the age of 15 years, was found [158]. Table 14.3 contains the most important allergens of *B. tropicalis*. It is firmly established that *B. tropicalis* is the source of numerous clinically relevant allergens [159].

T. putrescentiae is one of the most important pest mite species on stored products. At least 14 allergens are demonstrated for this mite species [98,131,160]. Recombinant Tyr p 10 has 64%–94% shared aa identity with other allergenic tropomyosins and was recognized by 12.5% of sera from sensitized patients [88].

S. medanensis exhibits minimal to moderate cross-reactivity with HDMs [162,163]. The most frequently detected allergens in the tropical mite, *S. medanensis* have molecular weights of 30–31, 24.5, 21, 47, and 58 kDa. Sui m 2, with a molecular weight of 15 kDa (Q2TUH5), is considered an important major allergen in this species. There is a high degree of cross-reactivity between *S. medanensis* and *B. tropicalis*, and *D. farinae* [164]. Anaphylaxis after the ingestion of flour contaminated with *S. medanensis* has also been reported [165]. The mite species *Th. entomophagus* also is implicated in cases of anaphylaxis after the ingestion of contaminated flour [166].

Chortoglyphus arcuatus is also frequently found in house dust in storage food in Spain and elsewhere [167]. The tropomyosin allergen, Cho a 10, is cloned and sequenced from a *C. arcuatus* expression library. The homology between Cho a 10 and Der p 10 is 94% and between Cho a 10 and Lep d 10 is 95% [89]. *Cheyletus eruditus* is a predator mite species frequently identified in house dust, especially in rural environments, where it feeds on storage mites. Numerous allergens have been demonstrated by immunoblotting [168] with a prominent band at approximately 16 kDa. There is a variable degree of cross-reactivity of this mite with the other domestic mites. Allergenicity to this predatory mite has been demonstrated by SPT and nasal provocation [169].

14.5 ALLERGENS OF MITES PRESENT IN AGRICULTURAL SETTINGS AND OF PARASITIC IMPORTANCE

The spider mites are main pests of fruit and horticultural crops and are common sensitizing allergens that are related to the prevalence of allergic diseases [170]. Epidemiologic studies demonstrate high rates of sensitization in the surrounding population, not occupationally exposed to orchard trees [171]. Major allergens with 10, 14, 19, 29, 67, and 75 kDa are described by immunoblotting in extracts of the two-spotted spider mite, *Tetranychus urticae* [172] and three in *Panonychus ulmi*, the apple spider mite, with molecular weights of 33, 41, and 51 kDa. Specific IgE binding against *T. urticae* and *P. ulmi* is partially inhibited by crude extracts of *D. pteronyssinus* and *T. putrescentiae* [173]. In the case of the citrus spider mite, *P. citri*, two allergens of 24 and 35 kDa are identified. The N-terminal aa sequences of these major allergens of the spider mites are not homologous with any characterized allergens [174].

Allergens of mites, used as biological control agents against spider mites and other pests, such as the Phytoseiidae, *Phytoseiulus*

Table 14.3 Described allergens in *Blomia tropicalis*

Allergens	Dp/Df allergens	Identity (identical residues/total residues)	MW (kDa)	Molecular function	IgE Reactivity Bt	IgE Reactivity Dp/Df
Blo t 1	Der p 1	32% (108/333)	26	Cysteine protease	62%–90%	80%
Blo t 2	Der p 2	39% (57/146)	14	Unknown	ND	80%
Blo t 3	Der p 3	49% (131/266)	25	Trypsin	50%–57%	16%–100%
Blo t 4	Der p 4	65% (335/515)	56	α-Amylase	<15%	40%
Blo t 5	Der p 5	42% (56/134)	14	Unknown	43%–92%	50%–70%
Blo t 6	Der p 6	58% (164/281)	25	Chymotrypsin	<10%	40%
Blo t 10	Der p 10	95% (270/284)	33	Tropomyosin	29%	50%–95%
Blo t 11	Der f 11	89% (781/875)	110	Paramyosin	12%–52%	80%
Blo t 12	ND	ND	14	Unknown	50%	ND
Blo t 13	Der f 13	80% (105/131)	15	Fatty acid-binding protein	11%	ND
Blo t 19	ND	ND	7.2	Antimicrobial peptide	3%	ND
Blo t 21						

Abbreviations: Bt, *B.* tropicalis; Df, *Dermatophagoides farinae*; Dp, *Dermatophagoides pteronyssinus*; MW, molecular weight.

persimilis and *Amblyseius cucumeris,* or the Dermanyssidae, *Hypoaspis miles,* are described [175,176]. These predator mites have species-specific as well as common antigens that are cross-reactive with *D. pteronyssinus* [177].

Several parasitic mite species are in frequent contact with humans and domestic animals. The itch mite, *Sarcoptes scabiei,* causes skin lesions and IgE-mediated sensitization in parasitized individuals [178–180]. Allergens homologous to serine proteases (group 3) [181], GST (group 8) [182], paramyosin (group 11) [183], tropomyosin [184], and apolipoprotein [185] have been identified. Tropomyosin (Sar s 10) of scabies has a high sequence similarity with the tropomyosin of other invertebrate species. Results of a study suggest that *S. scabiei* paramyosin is primarily recognized by individuals infested with ordinary scabies and not HDM-allergic subjects, and that serum IgE reactivity to *S. scabei* paramyosin is a sensitive method to diagnose scabies infestation in clinical practice [186].

Ticks (Ixodida), belonging to the families Ixodidae and Argasidae, have several proteins in their saliva that can induce IgE-mediated reactions after a bite. Several cases of anaphylaxis after tick bites are reported [187]. The allergenic composition of these mites has been analyzed [188], and an important allergen of *Argas reflexus,* the European pigeon tick, is cloned. Arg r 1 is a protein belonging to the lipocalin family [189]. In the case of the paralysis tick, *Ixodes holocyclus,* an allergen of 28 kDa from the salivary gland, has been identified [190]. Other allergenic proteins, with molecular masses of 51, 38, and 35 kDa from *I. pacificus, I. ricinus, Haemaphysalis punctata,* and *Rhipicephalus* sp. are described [191–194].

Other parasitic mites that are involved in allergic reactions in humans are the bee parasite, *Varroa jacobsoni,* with an allergenic protein of 13 kDa [195], and the feather mite of domestic birds, *Diplaegidia columbae,* with 20 IgE-binding components ranging from 22 to 200 kDa [196]. Two allergens from *Hemisarcoptes cooremani,* a predator of scale insects, of 16 kDa and 19 kDa

are described [197]. Other mite families and species of allergenic mites, excluding house dust and storage mites, are shown in Table 14.4 [152].

14.6 CROSS-REACTIVITY OF MITE AND OTHER ALLERGEN SOURCES

Cross-reactivity is a common feature among mite allergens, especially in those from taxonomically related species. This phenomenon may be the cause of polysensitization occurring in some mite-allergic individuals, although species-specific reactions do occur and should not be neglected. Originally, cross-reactivity was studied using whole extracts and radioallergosorbent test (RAST) inhibition techniques. In recent years, new tools, such as purified native or recombinant allergens, epitope mapping, T-cell proliferation techniques, and bioinformatics prediction have been applied [198]. When serum pools are used in cross-reactivity studies, the result depends to a great extent on the characteristics of the individual sera in the serum pool.

The allergenic cross-reactivity between *L. destructor* and *B. tropicalis* was initially demonstrated by specific IgE inhibition studies using whole allergen extracts. Puerta et al. [199] demonstrated a greater degree of cross-reactivity between *B. tropicalis* and *L. destructor* than between *B. tropicalis* and *Dermatophagoides* spp. The sequence identity of Lep d 2 with Gly d 2 is high (79%), but only 40% between Tyr p 2 and Der p 2 [50]. However, the cross-reactivity among group 2 allergens from storage mites, *L. destructor, T. putrescentiae,* and *G. domesticus,* is significant, whereas there is only limited cross-inhibition between Der p 2 and the nonpyroglyphid mite allergens [50]. This lack of cross-reactivity between Der p 2 and the group 2 storage mites is a result

Table 14.4 Other mite families and species of allergenic mites, excluding house dust and storage mites

Family	Parasite of plants
Tetranychidae	Tetranychus urticae
	Panonychus ulmi
	Panonychus citri
Tydeidae	Pronematus davisi
	Predator mites
Phytoseiidae	Amblyseius cucumeris
	Phytoseiulus persimilis
Hypoaspidae	Hypoaspis miles
Hemisarcoptidae	Hemisarcoptes cooremani
	Parasites of animals
Varroaidae	Varroa sp.
Sarcoptidae	Sarcoptes scabiei
Analgidae	Diplaegidia columbae
Ixodidae	Ixodes pacificus
	I. holocyclus
	I. ricinus
	Rhipicephalus sp.
Argasidae	Argas reflexus

of the multiple aa substitutions across the surface [200]. Studies have shown limited cross-reactivity between D. pteronyssinus, L. destructor, and T. putrescentiae [201,202], but others reported a greater cross-reactivity between Dermatophagoides and T. putrescentiae [203]. A low degree of cross-reactivity between D. pteronyssinus, A. siro and T. putrescentiae was described in one study, whereas cross-reactivity between L. destructor and A. siro is high [52].

The degree of allergenic cross-reactivity in group 1 allergens, although variable, is high. Analysis of their structures reveals that the sequence differences between Der f 1 and Der p 1 are not distributed evenly in relation to their molecular surfaces. The uneven spatial arrangement of conserved versus altered residues could explain both the specificity and cross-reactivity of antibodies against Der f 1 and Der p 1 [204,205]. ELISA inhibition studies between Der p 1 and Blo t 1 show that although cross-reactive human IgE epitopes exist, there are unique IgE epitopes for both Blo t 1 and Der p 1 [22].

Der p 5 and Der p 21 contain a major conformational IgE epitope-containing area located on similar portions of their structure, but they lack relevant IgE cross-reactivity [62].

Individuals allergic to the Dermatophagoides ssp. may experience allergic symptoms after the consumption of crustaceans and mollusks. Der f 10 and Der p 10 proteins with homology to tropomyosin from various animals are involved in the cross-reactivity among Dermatophagoides spp., mollusks, and crustaceans. The cross-reactive tropomyosin present in mites, various insects (chironomids, mosquito, and cockroach), and shrimp [207,208]

is responsible for cross-reactivity among different arthropods. Immunochemical studies demonstrate that allergens from snails, crustaceans, cockroaches, and chironomids cross-react with HDM allergens. However, HDMs are usually the primary source of sensitizing allergens. The nematode, Anisakis simplex, a common fish parasite, can be a hidden food allergen, inducing IgE-mediated reactions. Allergic cross-reactivity between this nematode and the domestic mites, A. siro, L. destructor, T. putrescentiae, and D. pteronyssinus, is reported, in which tropomyosin seems to be involved. The clinical relevance of this cross-reactivity needs further investigation [209].

Tropomyosin is also involved in the cross-reactivity between mites and parasites. A high degree of IgE cross-reactivity between allergenic extracts from HDMs and Ascaris has been demonstrated with the participation of several allergens such as tropomyosin and GST [210]. The allergenic cross-reactivity between Blo t 10 and Ascaris tropomyosin was demonstrated by ELISA inhibition and immunoblotting using sera from asthmatic mite-allergic patients. The tropomyosin of A. lumbricoides (Asc l 3) is an allergen that cross-reacts with mite tropomyosins. IgE reactivity to this allergen is very frequent in both asthmatic and normal subjects sensitized to an Ascaris extract [211]. Evidence suggests that cross-reactivity between mites and Ascaris tropomyosins could be important.

Filarial and mite tropomyosins are similar, with 72% identity at the aa level. Filarial infection induces strong cross-reactive antitropomyosin antibody responses that may affect sensitization and regulation of the allergic reactivity, especially in the tropics. The prevalence of IgE and IgG to Der p 10 was increased in filaria-infected individuals compared with uninfected subjects. There was a strong correlation between the serum levels of Onchocerca volvulus- and Der p 10-tropomyosin-specific IgE, IgG, and IgG4 ($P <$ .0001; $r >$ .79). Antifilarial tropomyosin IgE is entirely cross-reactive with Der p 10 using sera from experimentally filaria-infected nonhuman primates [212].

Several excretory/secretory (ES) and somatic Anisakis allergens have been cloned and characterized [213]. Among these, Ani s 1 (21 kDa) and Ani s 7 (139 kDa) are probably the most important ES major allergens described, as they are recognized by 85% and 100% of infected patients, respectively. Ani s 2 (paramyosin) [214] and Ani s 3 (tropomyosin) are somatic A. simplex allergens that cross-react with other common allergens. Ani s 7 is the most important ES Anisakis simplex allergen, as it is the only one recognized by 100% of infected patients. A fragment of recombinant Ani s 7 is a useful target for differentiating immunoglobulin E antibodies induced by true Anisakis infections from those induced by other antigens that may cross-react with Anisakis allergens [215,216].

The feather mite, Diplaegidia columbae, is a major source of clinically relevant allergens for pigeon breeders. The results of RAST inhibition experiments suggest that this feather mite cross-reacts with D. pteronyssinus [196]. Arlian et al. [217] demonstrated that antigens of the parasitic mite, S. scabiei, cross-react with antigens of D. pteronyssinus. Proteins with homology to different groups of mite allergens have been identified by genomic and molecular cloning approaches as the parasitic mites S. scabiei [183,218] and Psoroptes ovis [219].

GST seems to be an important cross-reactive allergen between mites and parasites in some populations. Inhibition studies with cockroach extract and native purified GST show that Der p 8 is cross-reactive with cockroach GST [80]. Different classes of GST have been described as allergens, which seem to influence the profile of IgE reactivity against GST from different allergen sources.

Mueller et al. [221] found lack of cross-reactivity among GST from cockroach, HDM, and helminths in North American populations, which is especially relevant for the development of more accurate molecular diagnostic techniques. This suggests that the use of species-specific GST should be included in diagnostic panels for evaluating allergies, especially to cockroach, for the identification of sources of IgE cross-reactivity.

Cross-reactivity among GSTs in tropical environments, where a simultaneous exposure to cockroach, mosquitoes, and mites occurs, could generate a stronger and more diverse immune response. Evidence of cross-reactivity of the GSTs allergens using extracts from *Ascaris* and *B. tropicalis* has been observed [222,223].

Group 13 mite allergens, the FABPs homologues, are involved in cross-reactivity among different taxonomic groups, which include different mite species, shrimp, and humans. The clinical importance of these findings is under evaluation. In the case of IgE autoreactivity, exposure to mites seems to induce specific IgE antibodies that recognize, by cross-reactivity, the human homologous protein, due to a high structural homology, sharing IgE-binding epitopes.

In general, patients sensitized to HDMs can be subdivided, based on their component-resolved responses, into two main groups: those sensitized only to the HDM major allergens (group 1 and group 2 in the *Pyroglyphid* mites) and those with a broader pattern of sensitization, including highly cross-reactive epitopes (e.g., the group 10 tropomyosins). In geographic areas with dual or multiple mite species exposure, component-resolved diagnosis of allergic diseases in children enables a better definition of clinical reactivity, challenge-associated severity, and prognostic accuracy than the commonly available quantitative, allergen-specific tests. These data are important for the future formulation of a component-based immunomodulatory vaccine as well as to tailor immunotherapy for individual patients.

14.7 ENZYMATIC ACTIVITY IN MITE EXTRACTS

Important airborne allergens may possess hydrolytic enzymatic activities, such as proteases, glycosidases, and ribonucleases. Several of these enzymes are important allergens, including cysteine and serine proteases and glycosidases (amylase) in mites and molds and ribonucleases in grass and tree pollens and molds. Mite extracts have enzymes capable of degrading a wide range of substances, including other proteins and allergens, and could have negative effects on the efficacy and stability of therapeutic extracts. Allergens with enzymatic activity are in groups 1, 3, 4, 6, 8, 9, 15, 18, and 20 [224,225]. Other mite species, such as *Glycyphagus domesticus* [226], *Acarus farris* [227], *T. putrescentiae* [228], *B. tropicalis* [229,230], *Psoroptes cuniculi* [231], and *Aleuroglyphus ovatus* [232] also contain allergens with enzymatic activity. Serine proteases (trypsin and chymotrypsin) seem to be more abundant in fecal than in whole-body extracts [233,234].

The presence of proteolytic activity in feces extracts is of great clinical importance since fecal pellets are more susceptible to become airborne and inhaled, thus reaching the respiratory mucosa. This enzymatic activity seems to play an important role in the allergenicity of certain mites, since it can facilitate the access of the allergen to the immune system and has an adjuvant proallergic role influencing its immunogenicity [15]. The enzymatic activity is present in body and mainly in fecal extracts, suggesting a role in the

protein digestion of the mites. The presence or absence of certain digestive enzymes reflects the trophic specialization, showing different "enzyme patterns" among house dust and storage mites. This may have important consequences when standardizing mite allergen extracts [235].

The protease activity of allergens may induce a range of inflammatory effects modulating the adaptive immune response by cleavage of CD23 and CD25, including induction of vascular permeability, edema, activation of neural reflex leading to bronchoconstriction, and stimulation of gland secretion and cough [236]. Der p 1 has additional effects on the innate defense mechanisms of the lung by inactivating *in vitro* and *ex vivo* the elastase inhibitors in humans. Der p 1 may also increase the susceptibility to infection of patients with allergic inflammation [237]. Der p 1 can damage bronchial epithelium and thereby increase permeability and detaching of cells *in vitro*. The resulting breach of the epithelial barrier may increase exposure to antigen-presenting cells and the likelihood that IgE will be formed against proteins in mite fecal pellets. Allergens, such as Der p 3 and Der p 9, with serine protease activity may also induce a nonallergic inflammatory response in the airways through the release of proinflammatory cytokines from the bronchial epithelium [238].

An influence on the innate mechanism of defense also has been described. The proteolytic activity of mite feces interacts with pulmonary elastase, inactivating a human elastase inhibitor *in vivo* and *ex vivo*. Because these elastase inhibitors have antimicrobial as well as antielastase activity, the inactivation of these innate components of the lung defense system by proteolytic enzymes present in mite feces may increase the susceptibility of patients with allergic inflammation to infection and thereby exacerbate allergic respiratory diseases [237]. Following exposure of the bronchial mucosa to HDM fecal pellets, the mite proteases can access the lung interstitium and promote Th2 responses [236].

14.8 GENETICS OF IgE RESPONSES TO MITE ALLERGENS

Molecular genetic studies about the influence of specific genes and genetic variants on the control of the IgE response began with the discovery of the major histocompatibility complex (MHC, also known as human leukocyte antigen [HLA]), under the hypothesis of the existence of immune response genes. Following the pioneering research developed by McDevitt and Benacerraf in the field of immunogenetics of immune-related diseases, specialists worked together in several international histocompatibility workshops and individual projects trying to find associations between MHC genes and the IgE response to allergens derived from many different sources, including dust mites. Marsh was the first to demonstrate strong associations between class II MHC molecules and the IgE response to allergens, particularly ragweed, and promoted the search for more genes in other chromosomal regions. After a long period of exploration of the entire genome, where many associations were found (not all confirmed) between variants (usually single-nucleotide polymorphisms [SNPs]) and IgE response to allergens, the genetic reasons for the predisposition to overreact against the apparently innocuous natural molecules remain an enigma. One of the important aspects of these investigations is their relation to the question of why a molecule is an allergen, since it seems that the IgE response of the genetically predisposed host (and not any particular intrinsic property of the molecules) is the main determinant of whether or not a molecule is an allergen. In regard to mite allergens, there are associations between different genetic variants and the specific IgE response.

Most data showing genetic influence (linkage or association) with mite-specific IgE responses in humans are related to HLA. In 1990, Caraballo and Hernandez, using affected sib pair analysis, showed that IgE hyperresponsiveness to *D. farinae* in patients with allergic asthma was linked to HL [239].

Years later, a genome-wide search found strong evidence of linkage between the specific IgE responsiveness to *D. pteronyssinus* and chromosomes 6p21 (HLA-D region), 2q21-q23, 8p23-p21, 13q32-q34, and 5q23-q33 in Caucasian families [240]. The role of HLA on the IgE response to this mite was further analyzed by the same authors, evaluating the IgE responses to several allergen components of *D. pteronyssinus* extract [241]. Linkage studies involving HLA loci and mite IgE responses have been replicated in other populations [242–244].

Associations between HLA class II genes and IgE hyperresponsiveness to mite allergens are both positive and negative, involving different alleles and loci and often showing no replication among different studies. This could be explained by the large number of mite allergenic epitopes, the variable level of exposure to each epitope, the ability of each HLA class II allele to present more than one peptide, and the participation of genes from other chromosome regions. In a case-control study, the frequency of allele HLA-DPB1*0401 was remarkably decreased in patients with IgE hyperresponsiveness to mite allergens, suggesting that it could be suppressing this phenotype in the nonallergic population [245]. Also, the protective role of other DPB1 allele (*0201) in controlling IgE response to mites has been reported [246]. Furthermore, a genome-wide association study (GWAS) in Asian populations confirmed the important role of the HLA-DPB locus in asthma [247]. Besides, the protective role of DRB1 locus against mite sensitization, as detected by skin test, also has been reported in a recent study in Brazil [248,249].

Other associations include IgE hyperresponsiveness to *B. tropicalis* and *D. pteronyssinus* purified allergens with HLA-DRB1*03 in nonrelated subjects [250] and family studies [251], although the role of other HLA alleles has also been documented [252–255]. The 6p21 region contains additional genes (e.g., butyrophilin-like 2, BTNL2) that have been associated with the risk of mite sensitization [256], but it is unclear whether those associations are due to linkage disequilibrium with HLA alleles or other yet unclear mechanisms.

As the complex nature of IgE synthesis became more evident, the discovery of "beyond MHC" immune response genes influencing IgE was more frequent. Polymorphisms in Th2 genes, for instance, those in the gene encoding interleukin 4 at the 5q31 locus [257,258] and the signal transducer and activator of transcription 6 (STAT6) [259], have been replicated in different populations. Associations with mite sensitization also have been reported with polymorphisms in the genes encoding interleukin-18 (IL-18) [260,261], leukotriene C4 synthase (LTC4S) [262], nitric oxide synthase 1 (NOS1) [263], interleukin-4 receptor alpha (ILR4A) [257], dendritic cell associated nuclear protein 1 (DCNP1) [264], interferon regulatory factor 1 (IRF-1) [265], CD14 [266,267], Janus kinase 2 (JAK2), GATA binding protein 3 (GATA3), CD40, and interleukin-5 receptor alpha (IL5RA) [268], all of them participating in any of the multiple steps of IgE synthesis. The significant associations with polymorphisms in innate immune genes suggest that genetic effects exert their influences at very early phases of the response. These loci include

the complement component 3 (C3) associated with the specific IgE levels to *D. pteronyssinus* [269], the myeloid differentiation factor 2 (MD2) associated with the specific IgE levels to *D. pteronyssinus* and Der p 2 [270], and the nucleotide-binding oligomerization domain containing 1 (NOD1) associated with mite sensitization [268].

At the beginning, the search for IgE-modulating genes was based mainly on candidate gene approaches, but in the last decade GWASs and gene expression analyses revealed associations with mite sensitization in new chromosomal regions [271–274] and confirmed the role of previously described HLA alleles [259,275]. The associations detected by GWAS include the kinase domain-containing protein (PKDCC) with allergen sensitization in Europeans [271]; thymic stromal lymphopoietin (TSLP) and leucine-rich repeat containing 32 (LRRC32) with sensitization to *D. pteronyssinus* and *B. tropicalis* in Singapore (ethnic Chinese) [273]. There are still regions to be fine-mapped because the underlying genes in the associated loci are unknown. That is the case of rs10142119, associated with the sensitization to *D. farinae* in Koreans [274] and rs10174949, associated with mite sensitization in Lithuanians [276] (2p25.1).

Since allergen exposure varies according to the geographic region, it can be anticipated that genetic epidemiology studies on the same genes but in distinct locations can obtain different results. For example, IL-4 is an important candidate gene for asthma and atopy susceptibility. In Caucasians the effect of IL-4 C-590T on mite sensitization was dependent of Der p 1 levels. The rare allele T confers a high risk of sensitization only in children exposed to excessive levels of Der p 1, while the reference allele C was not associated with mite sensitization, independent of the level of allergen exposure [277]. Similar findings have been obtained with the polymorphisms in the gene encoding interleukin 10 (IL-10), which were significantly associated with specific IgE levels to Der p 1 only if effect modification by allergen exposure levels was considered in the model [278].

The search for genes controlling the specificity and intensity of specific IgE responses continues, with genome sequencing approaches and the investigation on epigenetic influences on the forefront. For example, by resequencing several genomic regions harboring genes related to the IgE immune responses in a Colombian population, it was found that the SNP rs12584136 of the Insulin Receptor Substrate 2 (*IRS2*) gene was associated with high IgE response to *D. pteronyssinus*, and the rs3783118 of AB hydrolase domain containing protein 13 (*ABHD13*) was associated with low IgE response to this mite [279].

Studies reveal that the epigenome might influence the susceptibility to mite sensitization by modifying DNA methylation in B cells [280], and the hypomethylation of the interleukin 13 gene [281]. More interesting, HDM can induce epigenetic modifications in mice experimental airways inflammation, changing the methylation pattern of important genes such as *Phosphodiesterase 4 D* [282] and *tgfb1* [283]. In addition, using an *ex vivo* model of inflammation in human bronchial epithelial cells, HDM induces the same epigenetic modifications as does diesel exhaust [284]. These studies suggest that HDMs, in addition to inducing IgE-mediated bronchial inflammation, can alter the epigenetic patterns of cells involved in bronchial homeostasis, inducing inflammation. In contrast, allergen-specific immunotherapy is able to change DNA methylation levels at the forkhead box P3 gene (FOXP3) and, by improving the function of T-regulatory cells, can modify the IgE response to mites [285]. Hence, environmental exposures affecting the epigenome or polymorphisms influencing the interaction between the genome and the epigenetic machinery may play a role in modulating the gene-environment signals that lead to mite sensitization.

Defining the genetic variants underlying complex traits has intrinsic scientific relevance; in addition, when associated with diseases, polymorphisms are expected to be useful for evaluating the relative importance of the genetic component in multifactorial diseases such as asthma. However, although mite sensitization is one of the most confirmed risk factors for asthma, the impact of the involved polymorphisms in relation to other heritable traits also influencing the pathogenesis of the disease remains to be established, which makes it difficult to detect the real effect and heritability of the whole genetic component. Therefore, the usefulness of the variants described in this chapter as early predictors of mite-induced asthma, as expected in terms of precision medicine, is still limited. However, the knowledge of so many variants potentially influencing the IgE response to mite allergens could help to answer fundamental questions of immunology such as the origin of allergenicity and allergenic activity.

SALIENT POINTS

1. The main sources of allergens in house dust worldwide are the HDM species *D. pteronyssinus*, *D. farinae*, *E. maynei*, and *B. tropicalis*, and the storage mites *L. destructor* and *T. putrescentiae*. Other species can also be locally important.
2. Several storage mite allergens are purified, cloned, and sequenced. Some of these allergens can be considered as pan-allergens.
3. The main allergens described in storage mites include FABPs, tropomyosin and paramyosin homologues, apolipophorine-like proteins, alpha-tubulines, and others, such as group 2, 5, and 7 allergens.
4. The spider mites are main pests of fruit and horticultural crops and are common sensitizing allergens in occupationally exposed patients.
5. Cross-reactivity has been traditionally studied using whole extracts and RAST inhibition techniques. Purified native or recombinant allergens, epitope mapping, and T-cell proliferation techniques are now being used. Due to cross-reactivity, individuals allergic to the *Dermatophagoides* ssp. may experience allergic symptoms after the consumption of crustaceans and mollusks.
6. It is becoming increasingly evident that most mite species contain similar allergens. These allergens may have the same biological functions, and only small changes in aa sequences and allergen exposure may condition their recognition by specific IgE of mite allergic patients.
7. Mite allergen extracts contain enzymes capable of degrading a wide range of substances, including other proteins and allergens, and could have negative effects on the efficacy and stability of therapeutic extracts. Most mite allergens are potent enzymes.
8. Patients sensitized to HDMs can be subdivided on the basis of their component-resolved responses into two main groups: those sensitized only to the HDM major allergens (groups 1 and 2 in the Pyroglyphid mites) and those with a broader pattern of sensitization, including highly cross-reactive epitopes (e.g., the group 10 tropomyosins).
9. In geographic areas with dual or multiple mite species exposure, component-resolved diagnosis of allergic diseases in children enables better definition of clinical reactivity, challenge-associated severity, and prognostic accuracy than the commonly available quantitative, allergen-specific tests.
10. Advances in genomics and molecular biology of mite allergens will improve the ability to dissect the genetics of specific IgE response, especially because this can now be investigated at the epitope level. Genome-wide scans for association studies are available.
11. Environmental control and mite immunotherapy remain the two allergen-specific treatments for mite-allergic patients.

REFERENCES

1. Colloff MJ. *Dust Mites*. Collingwood, Australia: CSIRO Publishing, 2009: 268–271.
2. Platts-Mills TA, Vervloet D, Thomas WR et al. Indoor allergens and asthma: Report of the Third International Workshop. *J Allergy Clin Immunol* 1997; 100: S2–S24.
3. Smiley RL. The ordinal and subordinal names of mites with a list of mite pests of stored food products. *Proc Int Working Conf on Stored Product Entomology* 1983; 3: 37–43.
4. Fernández-Caldas E, Lockey RF. *Blomia tropicalis*, a mite whose time has come. *Allergy* 2004; 59(11): 1161–1164.
5. Arlian L, Bernstein D, Bernstein L et al. Prevalence of dust mites in the homes of people with asthma living in eight different geographic areas of the United States. *J Allergy Clin Immunol* 1992; 90: 292–300.
6. Fernández-Caldas E, Fox R, Bucholtz G, Truedeau W, Ledford, Lockey R. House dust mite allergy In Florida. Mite survey in households of mite sensitive individuals in Tampa, Florida. *Allergy Clin Immunol* 1990; 11: 263–267.
7. Caraballo L, Zakzuk J, Lee BW et al. Particularities of allergy in the Tropics. *World Allergy Organ J* 2016; 9: 20.
8. Tovey ER, Chapman MD, Platts-Mills TAE. Mite feces are a major source of house dust allergens. *Nature* 1982; 289: 592–593.
9. Fergusson P, Broide DH. Environmental and bronchoalveolar lavage *Dermatophagoides pteronyssinus* antigen levels in tropic asthmatics. *Am J Respir Crit Care Med* 1995; 151: 71–74.
10. Piboonpocanun S, Malainual N, Jirapongsananuruk O, Vichyanond P, Thomas WR. Genetic polymorphisms of major house dust mite allergens. *Clin Exp Allergy*. 2006; 36(4): 510–516.
11. Zakzuk J, Jimenez S, Cheong N et al. Immunological characterization of a Blo t 12 isoallergen: Identification of immunoglobulin E epitopes. *Clin. Exp. Allergy* 2009; 39: 608–616.
12. Chua KY, Stewart GA, Thomas WR et al. Sequence analysis of cDNA coding for a major house dust mite allergen, Der p I homology with cysteine proteases. *J Exp Med* 1988; 167: 175–182.
13. Shafique RH, Klimov PB, Inam M, Chaudhary FR, OConnor BM. Group 1 allergen genes in two species of house dust mites, *Dermatophagoides farinae* and *D. pteronyssinus* (Acari: Pyroglyphidae): Direct sequencing, characterization and polymorphism. *PLOS ONE* 2014; 9(12): e114636.
14. Hewitt CRA, Brown AP, Hart BJ et al. A major house dust mite allergen disrupts the immunoglobulin E network by selectively clearing CD23: Innate protection by antiproteases. *J Exp Med* 1995; 182: 1537–1544.

15. Kikuchi Y, Takai T, Kuhara T et al. Crucial commitment of proteolytic activity of a purified recombinant major house dust mite allergen Der p 1 to sensitization toward IgE and IgG responses. *J. Immunol* 2006; 177: 1609–1617.

16. Ghaemmaghami AM, Robins A, Gough L, Sewell HF, Shakib F. Human T cell subset commitment determined by the intrinsic property of antigen: The proteolytic activity of the major mite allergen Der p 1 conditions T cells to produce more IL-4 and less IFN-γ. *Eur J Immunol* 2001; 31: 1211–1216.

17. Wan H, Winton HL, Soeller C et al. The transmembrane protein occluding of epithelial tight junctions is a functional target for serine peptidases from faecal pellets of *Dermatophagoides pteronyssinus*. *Clin Exp Allergy* 2001; 31: 279–294.

18. Kauffman HF, Tamm M, Timmerman JA, Borger P. House dust mite major allergens Der p 1 and Der p 5 activate human airway-derived epithelial cells by protease-dependent and protease-independent mechanisms. *Clin Mol Allergy* 2006; 4: 5.

19. Adam E, Hansen KK, Astudillo Fernandez O et al. The house dust mite allergen DER P 1, unlike DER P 3, stimulates the expression of IL-8 in human airway epithelial cells via a proteinase-activated receptor -2 (PAR2) independent mechanisms. *J Biol Chem* 2006; 281: 6910–6923.

20. Deb R, Shakib F, Reid K, Clark H. Major house dust mite allergens Der p 1 and Der f 1 degrade and inactivate lung surfactant proteins –A and –D. *J Biol Chem* 2007; 282: 36808–36819.

21. Cheong N, Soon SC, Ramos JD et al. Lack of human IgE cross-reactivity between mite allergens Blo t 1 and Der p 1. *Allergy* 2003; 58(9): 912–920.

22. Meno KH, Kastrup JS, Kuo IC, Chua KY, Gajhede M. The structure of the mite allergen Blo t 1 explains the limited antibody cross-reactivity to Der p 1. *Allergy* 2017; 72(4): 665–670.

23. Rider SD Jr, Morgan MS, Arlian LG. Allergen homologs in the *Euroglyphus maynei* draft genome. *PLOS ONE* 2017; 12(8): 22.

24. Ferrándiz R, Casas R, Dreborg S, Einarsson R, Bonachea I, Chapman M. Characterization of allergenic components from house dust mite *Dermatophagoides siboney*. Purification of Der s I and Der s 2 allergens. *Clin Exp Allergy* 1995; 25: 922–928.

25. Derewenda U, Li J, Derewenda Z et al. The crystal structure of a major dust mite allergen Der p 2, and its biological implications. *J Mol Biol* 2002; 318: 189–197.

26. Weghofer M, Thomas WR, Kronqvist M et al. Variability of IgE reactivity profiles among European mite allergic patients. *Eur J Clin Invest* 2008; 38(12): 959–965.

27. Chua KY, Huang CH, Shen HD, Thomas WR. Analysis of sequence polymorphism of a major mite allergen, Der p 2. *Clin Exp Allergy* 1996; 26: 829–837.

28. Morgan MS, Arlian LG, Barnes KC, Fernández-Caldas E. Characterization of the allergens of the house dust mite *Euroglyphus maynei*. *J Allergy Clin Immunol* 1997; 100: 222–228.

29. Gruber A, Mancek M, Wagner H et al. Structural model of MD-2 and functional role of its basic amino acid clusters involved in cellular lipopolysaccharide recognition. *J Biol Chem* 2004; 279: 28475–28482.

30. Suzuki M, Tanaka Y, Korematsu S, Mikami B, Minato N. Crystal structure and some properties of a major house dust mite allergen, Der f 2. *Biochem Biophys Res Commun* 2006; 339: 679–686.

31. Ichikawa S, Takai T, Yashiki T et al. Lipopolysaccharide binding of the mite allergen Der f 2. *Genes Cells* 2009; 14(9): 1055–1065.

32. Trompette A, Divanovic S, Visintin A et al. Allergenicity resulting from functional mimicry of a Toll-like receptor complex protein. *Nature* 2009; 457(7229): 585–588.

33. Tsai JJ, Liu SH, Yin SC et al. Mite allergen Der-p2 triggers human B lymphocyte activation and Toll-like receptor-4 induction. *PLOS ONE* 2011; 6(9): e23249.

34. Ye Y, Wu H, Lin C et al. *Dermatophagoides pteronyssinus* 2 regulates nerve growth factor release to induce airway inflammation via a reactive oxygen species-dependent pathway. *Am J Physiol Lung Cell Mol Physiol* 2011; 300: L216–L224.

35. Chiou YL, Lin CY. Der p2 activates airway smooth muscle cells in a TLR2/MyD88-dependent manner to induce an inflammatory response. *J Cell Physiol* 2009; 220: 311–318.

36. Pittner G, Vrtala S, Thomas WR et al. Component-resolved diagnosis of house dust mite allergy with purified natural and recombinant purified allergens. *Clin Exp Allergy* 2004; 34: 597–603.

37. Zheng YW, Li J, Lai XX et al. Allergen micro-array detection of specific IgE-reactivity in Chinese allergy patients. *Chin Med J (Engl)* 2011; 124(24): 4350–4354.

38. Jiménez S, Puerta L, Mendoza D, Chua KY, Mercado D, Caraballo L. IgE antibody responses to recombinant allergens of *Blomia tropicalis* and *Dermatophagoides pteronyssinus* in a tropical environment. *Allergy Clin Immun Int* 2007; 19: 233–238.

39. Bronnert M, Mancini J, Birnbaum J et al. Component-resolved diagnosis with commercially available *D. pteronyssinus* Der p 1, Der p 2 and Der p 10: Relevant markers for house dust mite allergy. *Clin Exp Allergy* 2012; 42(9): 1406–1415.

40. Wang HY, Gao ZS, Zhou X et al. Evaluation of the role of IgE responses to Der p 1 and Der p 2 in Chinese house dust mite-allergic patients. *Int Arch Allergy Immunol* 2015; 167: 203–210.

41. Chen KW, Blatt K, Thomas WR et al. Hypoallergenic Der p 1/Der p 2 combination vaccines for immunotherapy of house dust mite allergy. *J Allergy Clin Immunol* 2012; 130(2): 435–443.

42. Martínez D, Cantillo JF, Herazo H et al. Characterization of a hybrid protein designed with segments of allergens from *Blomia tropicalis* and *Dermatophagoides pteronyssinus*. *Immunol Lett* 2018; 196: 103–112.

43. Tanyaratsrisakul S, Jirapongsananuruk O, Kulwanich B, Hales BJ, Thomas W, Piboonpocanun S. Effect of amino acid polymorphisms of house dust mite Der p 2 variants on allergic sensitization 1. *Allergy Asthma Immunol Res* 2016; 8: 55–62.

44. Ventas P, Carreira J, Polo F. Purification and characterization of Lep d I, a major allergen from the mite *Lepidoglyphus destructor*. *Clin Exp Allergy* 1992; 22(4): 454–460.

45. Van Hage-Hamsten M, Olsson S, Emilson A, Harfast B, Svensson A, Scheynius A. Localization of major allergens in the dust mite *Lepidoglyphus destructor* with confocal laser scanning microscopy. *Clin Exp Allergy* 1995; 25: 536–542.

46. Olsson S, van Hage-Hamsten M, Whitley P et al. Expression of two isoforms of Lep d 2, the major allergen of *Lepidoglyphus destructor*, in both prokaryotic and eukaryotic systems. *Clin Exp Allergy* 1998; 28: 984–991.

47. Johansson E, Eriksson TL, Olsson S et al. Evaluation of specific IgE to the recombinant group 2 mite allergens Lep d 2 and Tyr p 2 in the Pharmacia CAP system. *Int Arch Allergy Immunol* 1999; 120: 43–49.

48. Kronqvist M, Johansson E, Magnusson CG et al. Skin prick test and serological analysis with recombinant group 2 allergens of the dust mites *L. destructor* and *T. putrescentiae*. *Clin Exp Allergy* 2000; 30: 670–676.

49. Kaiser L, Gafvelin G, Johansson E, van Hage-Hamsten M, Rasool O. Lep d 2 polymorphisms in wild and cultured *Lepidoglyphus destructor* mites. *Eur J Biochem* 2003; 270(4): 646–653.

50. Gafvelin G, Johansson E, Lundin A et al. Crossreactivity studies of a new group 2 allergen from the dust mite *Glycyphagus domesticus*, Gly d 2, and group 2 allergens from *Dermatophagoides pteronyssinus*, *Lepidoglyphus destructor*, and *Tyrophagus putrescentiae* with recombinant allergens. *J Allergy Clin Immunol* 2001; 107: 511–518.

51. Eriksson TL, Johansson E, Whitley P, Schmidt M, Elsayed S, van Hage-Hamsten M. Cloning and characterisation of a group II allergen from the dust mite *Tyrophagus putrescentiae*. *Eur J Biochem* 1998; 251(1-2): 443–447.

52. Johansson E, Johansson SG, Van Hage-Hamsten M. Allergenic characterization of *Acarus siro* and *Tyrophagus putrescentiae* and their crossreactivity with *Lepidoglyphus destructor* and *Dermatophagoides pteronyssinus*. *Clin Exp Allergy* 1994; 24: 743–751.

53. Stewart GA, Ward LD, Simpson RJ, Thompson PJ. The group III allergen from the house dust mite *Dermatophagoides pteronyssinus* is a trypsin-like enzyme. *J Immunol* 1992; 75: 29–35.

54. Stewart GA, Thompson PJ. The biochemistry of common aeroallergens. *Clin Exp Allergy* 1996; 26: 1020–1044.

55. Bouaziz A, Walgraffe D, Bouillot C et al. Development of recombinant stable house dust mite allergen Der p 3 molecules for component-resolved diagnosis and specific immunotherapy. *Clin Exp Allergy* 2015; 45: 823–834.

56. Lake FR, Ward LD, Simpson RJ, Thompson PJ, Stewart GA. House dust mite derived amylase: Allergenicity and physicochemical characterization. *J Allergy Clin Immunol* 1991; 87: 1035–1042.

57. Cheon N, Ramos JD, Tang CY et al. Mite amylase from *Blomia tropicalis* (Blo t 4): Differential allergenicity linked to geographical regions. *Int Arch Allergy Immunol* 2009; 149: 25–32.

58. Pytelkova J, Lepsik M, Sandra M, Talacko P, Mares M. Enzymatic activity and immunoreactivity of Aca s4, an α-amylase allergen from the storage mite *Acarus siro*. *BMC Biochem* 2012; 13(3): 1–1.

59. Lin KL, Hsieh KH, Thomas WR, Chiang BL, Chua KY. Characterization of Der p 5 allergen, cDNA analysis and IgE-mediated reactivity of the recombinant protein. *J Allergy Clin Immunol* 1995; 94: 989–996.

60. Weghofer M, Grote M, Dall'Antonia Y et al. Characterization of folded recombinant Der p 5, a potential diagnostic marker allergen for house dust mite allergy. *Int Arch Allergy Immunol* 2008; 147: 101–109.

61. Pulsawat P, Soongrung T, Satitsuksanoa P et al. The house dust mite allergen Der p 5 binds lipid ligands and stimulates airway epithelial cells through a TLR2-dependent pathway. *Clin Exp Allergy* 2019; 49(3): 378–390.

62. Curin M, Garmatiuk T, Resch-Marat Y et al. Similar localization of conformational IgE epitopes on the house dust mite allergens Der p 5 and Der p 21 despite limited IgE cross-reactivity. *Allergy* 2018; 73(8): 1653–1661.

63. Medina LR, Malainual N, Ramos JD. Genetic polymorphisms and allergenicity of Blo t 5 in a house dust mite allergic Filipino population. *Asian Pac J Allergy Immunol* 2017; 35(4): 203–211.

64. Simpson A, Green R, Custovic A, Woodcock A, Arruda LK, Chapman MD. Skin test reactivity to natural and recombinant *Blomia* and *Dermatophagoides* spp. allergens among mite allergic patients in the UK. *Allergy* 2003; 58(1): 53–56.

65. Kuo IC, Cheong N, Trakultivakorn M, Lee BW, Chua KY. An extensive study of human IgE cross-reactivity of Blo t 5 and Der p 5. *J Allergy Clin Immunol* 2003; 111(3): 603–609.

66. Arruda K, Vailes LD, Platts-Mills AE et al. Sensitization to *Blomia tropicalis* in patients with asthma and identification of allergen Blo t 5. *Am J Respir Crit Care Med* 1997; 155: 343–350.

67. Caraballo L, Mercado D, Jiménez S, Moreno L, Puerta L, Chua KY. Analysis of the cross-reactivity between BtM and Der p 5, two group 5 recombinant allergens from *Blomia tropicalis* and *Dermatophagoides pteronyssinus*. *Int Arch Allergy Immunol* 1998; 117: 38–45.

68. Yi FC, Shek LP, Cheong N, Chua KY, Lee BW. Molecular cloning of *Blomia tropicalis* allergens—A major source of dust mite allergens in the tropics and subtropics. *Inflamm Allergy Drug Targets* 2006; 5(4): 261–266.

69. Chua KY, Cheong N, Kuo IC et al. The *Blomia tropicalis* allergens. *Protein Pept Lett* 2007; 14(4): 325–333.

70. Naik MT, Chang CF, Kuo IC et al. Roles of structure and structural dynamics in the antibody recognition of the allergen proteins: An NMR study on *Blomia tropicalis* major allergen. *Structure* 2008; 16(1): 125–136.

71. Chan SL, Ong TC, Gao YF et al. Nuclear magnetic resonance structure and IgE epitopes of Blo t 5, a major dust mite allergen. *J Immunol* 2008; 181(4): 2586–2596.

72. Mueller GA, Gosavi RA, Krahn JM et al. Der p 5 crystal structure provides insight into the group 5 dust mite allergens. *J Biol Chem* 2010; 285(33): 25394–25401.

73. Khemili S, Kwasigroch JM, Hamadouche T, Gilis D. Modelling and bioinformatics analysis of the dimeric structure of house dust mite allergens from families 5 and 21: Der f 5 could dimerize as Der p 5. *J Biomol Struct Dyn* 2012; 29(4): 663–675.

74. Eriksson TL, Rasool O, Huecas S et al. Cloning of three new allergens from the dust mite *Lepidoglyphus destructor* using phage surface display technology. *Eur J Biochem* 2001; 268: 287–294.

75. Bennett BJ Thomas WR. Cloning and sequencing of the group 6 allergen of *Dermatophagoides pteronyssinus*. *Clin Exp Allergy* 1996; 26: 1150–1154.

76. Shen HD, Chua KY, Lin WL, Hsieh KH, Thomas WR. Molecular cloning and immunological characterization of the house dust mite allergen Der f 7. *Clin Exp Allergy* 1995; 25: 1000–1006.

77. Mueller GA, Edwards LL, Aloor JJ et al. The structure of the dust mite allergen Der p 7 reveals similarities to innate immune proteins. *J Allergy Clin Immunol* 2010; 125(4): 909–917.

78. Tan KW, Jobichen C, Ong TC et al. Crystal structure of Der f 7, a dust mite allergen from *Dermatophagoides farinae*. *PLOS ONE* 2012; 7(9): e44850.

79. O'Neill GM, Donavan GR, Baldo BA. Cloning and characterization of a major allergen of the house dust mite, *Dermatophagoides pteronyssinus*, homologous with glutathione-S-transferase. *Biochim Biophys Acta* 1994; 1219: 521–528.

80. Huang CH, Liew LM, Mah KW, Kuo IC, Lee BW, Chua KY. Characterization of glutathione S-transferase from dust mite, Der p 8 and its immunoglobulin E cross-reactivity with cockroaches glutathione S-transferase. *Clin Exp Allergy* 2006; 36: 369–376.

81. Liao EC, Lin YH, Chiu CL, Lin TC, Tsai JJ. Identification of allergenic component Tyr p 8 from *Tyrophagus putrescentiae* and cross-reactivity with Der p 8. *Clin Vaccine Immunol* 2013; 20(4): 506–512.

82. King C, Simpson RJ, Moritz RL, Reed GL, Thompson PJ, Stewart GA. The isolation and characterization of a novel

collagenolitic serine protease allergen (Der p 9) from the dust mite *Dermatophagoides pteronyssinus. J Allergy Clin Immunol* 1996; 98: 739–747.

83. Aki T, Kodama T, Fujikawa A et al. Immunochemical characterization of recombinant and native tropomyosin as a new allergen from the house dust mite, *Dermatophagoides farinae. J Allergy Clin Immunol* 1995; 96: 74–83.

84. Cantillo JF, Puerta L, Lafosse-Marin S, Subiza JL, Caraballo L, Fernandez-Caldas E. Allergens involved in the cross-reactivity of *Aedes aegypti* with other arthropods. *Ann Allergy Asthma Immunol* 2017; 118(6): 710–718.

85. Yi FC, Cheong N, Shek PC, Wang DY, Chua KY, Lee BW. Identification of shared and unique immunoglobulin E epitopes of the highly conserved tropomyosins in *Blomia tropicalis* and *Dermatophagoides pteronyssinus. Clin Exp Allergy* 2002; 32: 1203–1210.

86. Resch Y, Weghofer M, Seiberler S et al. Molecular characterization of Der p 10: A diagnostic marker for broad sensitization in house dust mite allergy. *Clin Exp Allergy* 2011; 41(10): 1468–1477.

87. Saarne T, Kaiser L, Rasool O, Huecas S, van Hage-Hamsten M, Gafvelin G. Cloning and characterisation of two IgE-binding proteins, homologous to tropomyosin and alpha-tubulin, from the mite *Lepidoglyphus destructor. Int Arch Allergy Immunol* 2003; 130: 258–265.

88. Jeong KY, Lee H, Lee JS et al. Molecular cloning and the allergenic characterization of tropomyosin from *Tyrophagus putrescentiae. Protein Pept Lett* 2007; 14: 431–436.

89. López-Matas MA, Iraola V, Moya R et al. Cloning and characterization of tropomyosin from the mite *Chortoglyphus arcuatus. Mol Immunol* 2015; 68: 634–640.

90. Tsai LC, Chao P, Hung MW et al. Protein sequence analysis and mapping of IgE and IgG epitopes of an allergenic 98-kDa *Dermatophagoides farinae* paramyosin, Der f 11. *Allergy* 2000; 55: 141–147.

91. Tsai LC, Sun YC, Chao PL et al. Sequence analysis and expression of a cDNA clone encoding a 98-KDa allergen in *Dermatophagoides farinae. Clin Exp Allergy* 1999; 29: 1606–1613.

92. Lee CS, Tsaiw LC, Chaow PL et al. Protein sequence analysis of a novel 103-kDa *Dermatophagoides pteronyssinus* mite allergen and prevalence of serum immunoglobulin E reactivity to rDer p 11 in allergic adult patients. *Clin Exp Allergy* 2004; 34: 354–362.

93. Tsai LC, Peng HJ, Lee CS et al. Molecular cloning and characterization of full-length cDNAs encoding a novel high-molecular-weight *Dermatophagoides pteronyssinus* mite allergen, Der p 11. *Allergy* 2005; 60: 927–937.

94. Puerta L, Caraballo L, Fernández-Caldas E et al. Nucleotide sequence analysis of a complementary DNA coding for a *Blomia tropicalis* allergen. *J Allergy Clin Immunol* 1996; 98: 932–937.

95. Randall TA, Mullikin JC, Geoffrey A, Mueller G. The draft genome assembly of *Dermatophagoides pteronyssinus* supports identification of novel allergen isoforms in *Dermatophagoides* species. *Int Arch Allergy Immunol* 2018; 175(3): 136–146.

96. Zakzuk J, Benedetti I, Fernández-Caldas E, Caraballo L. The influence of chitin on the immune response to the house dust mite allergen Blo t 12. *Int Arch Allergy Immunol* 2014; 163(2): 119–129.

97. Kenyon F, Welsh M, Parkinson J, Whitton C, Blaxter ML, Knox DP. Expressed sequence tag survey of gene expression in the scab mite *Psoroptes ovis* allergens, proteases and free-radical scavengers. *Parasitology* 2003; 126: 451–460.

98. Jeong KY, Kim WK, Lee JS et al. Immunoglobulin E reactivity of recombinant allergen Tyr p 13 from *Tyrophagus putrescentiae* homologous to fatty acid binding protein. *Clin Diag Lab Immunol* 2005; 12(5): 581–585.

99. Angus AC, Ong ST, Chew FT. Sequence tag catalogs of dust mite-expressed genomes: Utility in allergen and acarologic studies. *Am J Pharmacogenomics* 2004; 4:357–369.

100. Satitsuksanoa P, Kennedy M, Gilis D et al. The minor house dust mite allergen Der p 13 is a fatty acid-binding protein and an activator of a TLR2-mediated innate immune response. *Allergy* 2016; 71(10): 1425–1434.

101. Siew LC, Seow TO, Su YO, Fook TC, Yu KM. Nuclear magnetic resonance structure-based epitope mapping and modulation of dust mite group 13 allergen as a hypoallergen. *J Immunol* 2006; 176: 4852–4860.

102. Labrada M, Uyema K, Sewer M et al. Monoclonal antibodies against Blo t 13, a recombinant allergen from *Blomia tropicalis. Int Arch Allergy Immunol* 2002; 129: 212–218.

103. Caraballo L, Puerta L, Jiménez S et al. Cloning and IgE binding of a recombinant allergen from the mite *Blomia tropicalis*, homologous with fatty acid-binding proteins. *Int Arch Allergy Immunol* 1997; 112: 341–347.

104. Cheng RY, Shang Y, Limjunyawong N et al. Alterations of the lung methylome in allergic airway hyper-responsiveness. *Environ Mol Mutagen* 2014; 55(3): 244–255.

105. Zhang X, Chen X, Weirauch MT et al. Diesel exhaust and house dust mite allergen lead to common changes in the airway methylome and hydroxymethylome. *Environ Epigenet* 2018; 4(3): dvy020.

106. Eriksson TL, Whitley P, Johansson E, van Hage-Hamsten M, Gafvelin G. Identification and characterisation of two allergens from the dust mite *Acarus siro*, homologous with fatty acid-binding proteins. *Int Arch Allergy Immunol* 1999; 119: 275–281.

107. Epton MJ, Dilworth RJ, Smith W, Hart BJ, Thomas WR. High-molecular-weight allergens of the house dust mite: An apolipophorin-like cDNA has sequence identity with the major M-177 allergen and the IgE-binding peptide fragments Mag1 and Mag3. *Int Arch Allergy Immunol* 1999; 120: 185–191.

108. Posa D, Perna S, Resch Y et al. Evolution and predictive value of IgE responses toward a comprehensive panel of house dust mite allergens during the first 2 decades of life. *J Allergy Clin Immunol* 2017; 139: 541–549.

109. McCall C, Hunter S, Stedman K et al. Characterization and cloning of a major high molecular weight house dust mite allergen (Der f 15) for dogs. *Vet Immunol Immunopathol* 2001; 78(3–4): 231–247.

110. O'Neil SE, Heinrich TK, Hales BJ et al. The chitinase allergens Der p 15 and Der p 18 from *Dermatophagoides pteronyssinus. Clin Exp Allergy* 2006; 36: 831–839.

111. Sutherland TE, Maizels RM, Allen JE. Chitinases and chitinase-like proteins: Potential therapeutic targets for the treatment of T-helper type 2 allergies. *Clin Exp Allergy* 2009; 39(7): 943–955.

112. Fernández-Caldas E. On mite allergy in dogs and humans. *Int Arch Allergy Immunol* 2012; 160(4): 329–330.

113. Kawamoto S, Suzuki T, Aki T et al. Der f 16: A novel gelsolin-related molecule identified as an allergen from the house dust mite, *Dermatophagoides farinae. FEBS Lett* 2002; 516: 234–238.

114. Weber E, Hunter S, Stedman K et al. Identification, characterization, and cloning of a complementary DNA encoding a 60-kd house dust mite allergen (Der f 18) for human beings and dogs. *J Allergy Clin Immunol* 2003; 112: 79–86.

115. Li JY, Zhang Y, Lin XP et al. Association between DNA hypomethylation at IL13 gene and allergic rhinitis in house dust mite-sensitized subjects. *Clin Exp Allergy* 2016; 46(2): 298–307.

116. Resch Y, Blatt K, Malkus U et al. Molecular, structural and immunological characterization of Der p18, a chitinase-like house dust mite allergen. *PLOS ONE* 2016; 11(8): e0160641.

117. Stewart GA. Studies of house dust mites can now fully embrace the "-omics" era. *J Allergy Clin Immunol* 2015; 135(2): 549–550.

118. Teng F, Yu L, Sun J, Wang N, Cui Y. Homology modeling and prediction of B-cell and T-cell epitopes of the house dust mite allergen Der f 20. *Mol Med Rep* 2018; 17: 1807–1812.

119. Xing P, Yu H, Li M et al. Characterization of arginine kinase, a novel allergen of *Dermatophagoides farinae* (Der f 20). *Am J Transl Res* 2015; 7(12): 2815–2823.

120. Teng F, Yu L, Sun J, Wang N, Cui Y. Homology modeling and prediction of B-cell and T-cell epitopes of the house dust mite allergen Der f 20. *Mol Med Rep* 2018; 17(1): 1807–1812.

121. Weghofer M, Dall'Antonia Y, Grote M et al. Characterization of Der p 21, a new important allergen derived from the gut of house dust mites. *Allergy* 2008;63(6): 758–767.

122. Wu Y, Jiang C, Li M et al. Der f 21, a novel allergen from *Dermatophagoides farinae*. *Am J Transl Res* 2016; 8(1): 49–59.

123. Pang SL, Ho KL, Waterman J, Teh AH, Chew FT, Ng CL. Cloning, expression, purification, characterization, crystallization and X-ray crystallographic analysis of recombinant Der f 21 (rDer f 21) from *Dermatophagoides farinae*. *Acta Crystallogr F Struct Biol Commun* 2015; 71(Pt 11): 1396–1400.

124. Gao YF, Wang de Y, Ong TC, Tay SL, Yap KH, Chew FT. Identification and characterization of a novel allergen from *Blomia tropicalis*: Blo t 21. *J Allergy Clin Immunol* 2007; 120: 105–112.

125. Yun G, De YW, Tan CO, Su LT, Kwong HY, Chew FT. Identification and characterization of a novel allergen from *Blomia tropicalis*: Blo t 21. *J Allergy Clin Immunol* 2007; 120: 105–112.

126. Kidon MI, Chin CW, Kang LW et al. Mite component–specific IgE repertoire and phenotypes of allergic disease in childhood: The tropical perspective. *Pediatr Allergy and Immunol* 2011; 22: 202–210.

127. Tan KW, Ong TC, Gao YF et al. NMR structure and IgE epitopes of Blo t 21, a major dust mite allergen from *Blomia tropicalis*. *J Biol Chem* 2012; 287(41): 34776–34785.

128. Reginald K, Tan CL, Chen S, Yuen L, Goh SY, Chew FT. Characterization of Der f 22—A paralogue of the major allergen Der f 2. *Sci Rep* 2018; 8(1): 11743.

129. Weghofer M, Grote M, Casset A et al. Identification of Der p 23, a peritrophin-like protein, as a new major *Dermatophagoides pteronyssinus* allergen associated with the peritrophic matrix of mite fecal pellets. *J Immunol* 2013; 190(7): 3059–3067.

130. Soh WT, Le Mignon M, Suratannon N et al. The house dust mite major allergen Der p 23 displays O-glycan-independent IgE reactivities but no chitin-binding activity. *Int Arch Allergy Immunol* 2015; 168(3): 150–160.

131. Jeong KY, Kim CR, Un S et al. Allergenicity of recombinant troponin C from *Tyrophagus putrescentiae*. *Int Arch Allergy Immunol* 2010; 151: 207–213.

132. Chan T-F, Ji K-M, Yim AK-Y et al. The draft genome, transcriptome, and microbiome of *Dermatophagoides farinae* reveal a broad spectrum of dust mite allergens. *J Allergy Clin Immunol* 2015; 135: 539–548.

133. Lin J, Wan Q, Gao A et al. Characterization of a novel allergen Der f 25 homologous to triose-phosphate isomerase, from *Dermatophagoides farinae*. *Int J Clin Exp Med* 2016; 9:10829–10837.

134. World Health Organization/International Union of Immunological Societies Allergen Nomenclature Sub-Committee. Allergen Nomenclature. http://www.allergen.org/viewallergen.php?aid=815

135. Lin J, Li M, Liu Y et al. Expression, purification and characterization of Der f 27, a new allergen from *Dermatophagoides farinae*. *Am J Transl Res* 2015; 15(7): 1260–1270.

136. Lin JL, Wang YY, Xiao XJ et al. Characterization of a new subtype of allergen in *Dermatophagoides farinae*-Der f 28. *J Thorac Dis* 2015; 7:1842–1849.

137. Cui Y, Yu L, Teng F et al. Transcriptomic/proteomic identification of allergens in the mite *Tyrophagus putrescentiae*. *Allergy* 2016; 71: 1635–1639.

138. Lin J, Wang H, Li M et al. Characterization and analysis of a cDNA coding for the group 29b (Der f 29b) allergen of *Dermatophagoides farinae*. *Am J Transl Res* 2016; 15(8): 568–577.

139. An S, Chen L, Long C et al. *Dermatophagoides farinae* allergens diversity identification by proteomics. *Mol Cell Proteomics* 2013; 12: 1818–1828.

140. Wang H, Lin J, Zeng L et al. Der f 31, a novel allergen from *Dermatophagoides farinae*, activates epithelial cells and enhances lung-resident group 2 innate lymphoid cells. *Sci Rep* 2017; 7(1): 8519.

141. Lin J, Huang N, Wang H et al. Identification of a novel cofilin-related molecule (Der f 31) as an allergen from *Dermatophagoides farinae*. *Immunobiology* 2018; 223(2): 246–251.

142. WHO/IUIS Allergen Nomenclature Sub-Committee, www.allergen.org; http://allergen.org/viewallergen.php?aid=817

143. Thomas WR. House dust mite allergens: New discoveries and relevance to the allergic patient. *Curr Allergy Asthma Rep* 2016; 16(9): 69.

144. Wang H, Lin J, Liu X et al. Identification of a-tubulin, Der f 33, as a novel allergen from *Dermatophagoides farinae*. *Immunobiology* 2016; 221: 911–917.

145. Teng F, Sun J, Yu L, Li Q, Cui Y. Homology modeling and epitope prediction of Der f 33. *Braz J Med Biol Res* 2018; 51(5): e6213.

146. Jeong KY, Lee H, Lee JS et al. Immunoglobulin E binding reactivity of a recombinant allergen homologous to α-tubulin from *Tyrophagus putrescentiae*. *Clin Diagn Lab Immunol* 2005; 12(12): 1451–1454.

147. El Ramlawy KG, Fujimura T, Baba K et al. Der f 34, a novel major house dust mite allergen belonging to a highly conserved Rid/YjgF/YER057c/UK114 family of imine deaminases. *J Biol Chem* 2016; 291(41): 21607–21615.

148. Fujimura T, Aki T, Isobe T et al. Der f 35: An MD-2-like house dust mite allergen that cross-reacts with Der f 2 and Pso o 2. *Allergy* 2017; 72(11): 1728–1736.

149. Pascual M, Suzuki M, Isidoro-Garcia M et al. Epigenetic changes in B lymphocytes associated with house dust mite allergic asthma. *Epigenetics* 2011; 6(9): 1131–1137.

150. Bordas-Le Floch V, Le Mignon M, Bussières L et al. A combined transcriptome and proteome analysis extends the allergome of house dust mite *Dermatophagoides* species. *PLOS ONE* 2017; 12(10).

151. Fernández-Caldas E, Iraola V, Carnés J. Molecular and biochemical properties of storage mites (except *Blomia* species). *Protein Pept Lett* 2007; 14(10): 954–959.

152. Fernández-Caldas E, Iraola Calvo V. Mite allergens. *Curr Allergy Asthma Rep* 2005; 5(5): 402–410.

153. Stanaland BE, Fernández-Caldas E, Jacinto CM, Trudeau WL, Lockey RF. Positive nasal challenge response to *Blomia tropicalis*. *J Allergy Clin Immunol* 1996; 97: 1045–1049.

154. Barreto BA, Daher S, Naspitz CK, Sole D. Specific and non-specific nasal provocation tests in children with perennial allergic rhinitis. *Allergol Immunopathol* 2001; 29(6): 255–263.

155. Wang DY, Goh DY, Ho AK, Chew FT, Yeoh KH, Lee BW. The upper and lower airway responses to nasal challenge with house-dust mite *Blomia tropicalis*. *Allergy* 2003; 58(1): 78–82.

156. Garcia Robaina JC, Sanchez Machin I, Fernandez-Caldas E et al. Skin tests and conjunctival and bronchial challenges with extracts of *Blomia tropicalis* and *Dermatophagoides pteronyssinus* in patients with allergic asthma and/or rhinoconjunctivitis. *Int Arch Allergy Immunol* 2003; 131(3): 182–188.

157. Niggemann B, Kleinau I, Schou C, Hansen GN, Wahn U. Discrepancies between *in vitro* and *in vivo* tests for house dust mite allergy: Is domestic exposure a better predictor than sensitization? *Clin Exp Allergy* 1994; 24(10): 946–948.

158. Juliá-Serdá G, Cabrera-Navarro P, Acosta-Fernández O, Martín-Pérez P, García-Bello MA, Antó-Boqué J. Prevalence of sensitization to *Blomia tropicalis* among young adults in a temperate climate. *J Asthma* 2012; 49(4): 349–354.

159. Santos da Silva E, Asam C, Lackner P et al. Allergens of *Blomia tropicalis*: An overview of recombinant molecules. *Int Arch Allergy Immunol* 2017; 172(4): 203–214.

160. Arlian LG, Vyszenski-Moher DL, Johansson SG, van Hage-Hamsten M. Allergenic characterization of *Tyrophagus putrescentiae* using sera from occupationally exposed farmers. *Ann Allergy Asthma Immunol* 1997; 79: 525–529.

161. Shang Y, Das S, Rabold R, Sham JS, Mitzner W, Tang WY. Epigenetic alterations by DNA methylation in house dust mite-induced airway hyperresponsiveness. *Am J Respir Cell Mol Biol* 2013; 49(2): 279–287.

162. Silton RP, Fernández-Caldas E, Trudeau WL, Swanson MC, Lockey RF. Prevalence of specific IgE to the storage mite, *Aleuroglyphus ovatus*. *J Allergy Clin Immunol* 1991; 88: 595–603.

163. Puerta L, Fernández Caldas E, Lockey R, Caraballo L. Sensitization to *Chortoglyphus arcuatus* and *Aleuroglyphus ovatus* in *Dermatophagoides* spp. allergic individuals. *Clin Exp Allergy* 1993; 23: 117–123.

164. Puerta L, Lagares A, Mercado D, Fernández-Caldas E, Caraballo L. Allergenic composition of the mite *Suidasia medanensis* and cross-reactivity with *Blomia tropicalis*. *Allergy* 2005; 60: 41–47.

165. Sánchez-Borges M, Capriles-Hulett A, Fernández-Caldas E et al. Mite-contaminated foods as a cause of anaphylaxis. *J Allergy Clin Immunol* 1997; 99(6 Pt 1): 738–743.

166. Blanco C, Quiralte J, Castillo R et al. Anaphylaxis after ingestion of wheat flour contaminated with mites. *J Allergy Clin Immunol* 1997; 99(3): 308–313.

167. Boquete M, Carballas C, Carballada F, Iraola V, Carnes J, Fernández-Caldas E. *In vivo* and *in vitro* allergenicity of the domestic mite *Chortoglyphus arcuatus*. *Ann Allergy Asthma Immunol* 2006; 97: 203–208.

168. Fernández-Caldas E, Lafosse Marin S, Ochoa C et al. Allergenicity of the predator mite *Cheyletus eruditus*. *XXIII EAACI Congress (abstract book)*, June 12–18, 2004: 183.

169. Poza Guedes P, Sánchez Machín I, Matheu V, Iraola V, González Pérez R. Role of predatory mites in persistent nonoccupational allergic rhinitis. *Can Respir J* 2016; 2016: 5782317.

170. Kim YK, Lee MH, Jee YK et al. Spider mite allergy in apple-cultivating farmers: European red mite (*Panonychus ulmi*) and two-spotted spider mite (*Tetranychus urticae*) may be important allergens in the development of work-related asthma and rhinitis symptoms. *J Allergy Clin Immunol* 1999; 104: 1285–1292.

171. Lee MH, Cho SH, Park HS et al. Citrus red mite (*Panonychus citri*) is a common sensitizing allergen among children living around citrus orchards. *Ann Allergy Asthma Immunol* 2000; 85: 200–204.

172. Park HS, Jee YK, Kim YK, Lee SK, Lee MH, Kim YY. Identification of immunoglobulin E binding components of the two-spotted spider mite *Tetranychus urticae*: Allergenic relationships with the citrus red mite and house-dust mite. *Allergy Asthma Proc* 2002; 23(3): 199–204.

173. Kim YK, Oh SY, Jung JW, Min KU, Kim YY, Cho SH. IgE binding components in *Tetranychus urticae* and *Panonychus ulmi*-derived crude extracts and their crossreactivity with domestic mites. *Clin Exp Allergy* 2001; 31: 1457–1463.

174. Kim HY, Park HS, Kim YK et al. Identification of IgE-binding components of citrus red mite in sera of patients with citrus red mite-induced asthma. *J Allergy Clin Immunol* 2001; 107: 244–248.

175. van Hage-Hamsten M, Kolmodin-Hedman B, Johansson E. Predatory mites, *Phytoseiulus persimilis* and *Amblyseius cucumeris*, used for biological crop protection, cause sensitization among greenhouse workers. *Allergy* 2000; 55: 30.

176. Kronqvist M, Johansson E, Kolmodin-Hedman B, Oman H, Svartengren M, van Hage-Hamsten M. IgE-sensitization to predatory mites and respiratory symptoms in Swedish greenhouse workers. *Allergy* 2005; 60: 521–526.

177. de Jong NW, Groenewoud GC, van Ree R et al. Immunoblot and radioallergosorbent test inhibition studies of allergenic cross-reactivity of the predatory mite *Amblyseius cucumeris* with the house dust mite *Dermatophagoides pteronyssinus*. *Ann Allergy Asthma Immunol* 2004; 93: 281–287.

178. Falk ES, Bolle R. IgE antibodies to house dust mites in patients with scabies. *Br J Dermatol* 1980; 103: 283–288.

179. Morgan MS, Arlian LG, Estes SA. Skin test and radioallergosorbent test characteristics of scabietic patients. *Am J Trop Med Hyg* 1997; 57: 190–196.

180. Arlian LG, Morgan MS, Estes SA et al. Circulating IgE in patients with ordinary and crusted scabies. *J Med Entomol* 2004; 41: 74–77.

181. Holt DC, Fischer K, Allen GE et al. Mechanisms for a novel immune evasion strategy in the scabies mite *Sarcoptes scabiei*: A multigene family of inactivated serine proteases. *J Invest Dermatol* 2003; 121(6): 1419–1424.

182. Dougall A, Holt DC, Fischer K, Currie BJ, Kemp DJ, Walton SF. Identification and characterization of *Sarcoptes scabiei* and *Dermatophagoides pteronyssinus* glutathione-S-transferases: Implication as a potential major allergen in crusted scabies. *Am J Trop Med Hyg* 2005; 73: 977–984.

183. Fischer K, Holt DC, Harumal P, Currie BJ, Walton SF, Kemp DJ. Generation and characterization of cDNA clones from *Sarcoptes scabiei* var. *hominis* for an expressed sequence tag library: Identification of homologues of house dust mite allergens. *Am J Trop Med Hyg* 2003; 68: 61–64.

184. Zhang R, Jise Q, Zheng W et al. Characterization and evaluation of a *Sarcoptes scabiei* allergen as a candidate vaccine. *Parasit Vectors* 2012; 5:176.

185. Harumal P, Morgan M, Walton SF et al. Identification of a homologue of a house dust mite allergen in a cDNA library from *Sarcoptes scabiei* var. hominis and evaluation of its vaccine potential in a rabbit/*S. scabiei* var. canis model. *Am J Trop Med Hyg* 2003; 68(1): 54–60.

186. Naz S, Desclozeaux M, Mounsey KE, Chaudhry FR, Walton SF. Characterization of *Sarcoptes scabiei* tropomyosin and paramyosin: Immunoreactive allergens in scabies. *Am J Trop Med Hyg* 2017;97(3): 851–860.

187. Kleine-Tebbe J, Heinatz A, Graser I et al. Bites of the European pigeon tick (*Argas reflexus*): Risk of IgE-mediated sensitizations and anaphylactic reactions. *J Allergy Clin Immunol* 2006; 117: 190–195.

188. Rolla G, Nebiolo F, Marsico P et al. Allergy to pigeon tick (*Argas reflexus*): Demonstration of specific IgE-binding components. *Int Arch Allergy Immunol* 2004; 135: 293–295.

189. Hilger C, Bessot JC, Hutt N et al. IgE-mediated anaphylaxis caused by bites of the pigeon tick *Argas reflexus*: Cloning and expression of the major allergen Arg r 1. *J Allergy Clin Immunol* 2005; 115: 617–622.

190. Gauci M, Loh RK, Stone BF, Thong YH. Evaluation of partially purified salivary gland allergens from the Australian paralysis tick *Ixodes holocyclus* in diagnosis of allergy by RIA and skin prick test. *Ann Allergy* 1990; 64(3): 297–299.

191. Van Wye JE, Hsu YP, Terr AI, Moss RB, Lane RS. Anaphylaxis from a tick bite. *N Engl J Med* 1991; 324: 777–778.

192. Fernández-Soto P, Dávila I, Laffond E, Lorente F, Encinas-Grandes A, Pérez-Sánchez R. Tick-bite-induced anaphylaxis in Spain. *Ann Trop Med Parasitol* 2001; 95: 97–103.

193. Acero S, Blanco R, Bartolomé B. Anaphylaxis due to a tick bite. *Allergy* 2003; 58: 824–825.

194. Miadonna A, Tedeschi A, Leggieri E et al. Anaphylactic shock caused by allergy to the venom of *Argas reflexus*. *Ann Allergy* 1982; 49: 293–294.

195. Rudeschko O, Machnik A, Dorfelt H et al. A novel inhalation allergen present in the working environment of beekeepers. *Allergy* 2004; 59: 332–337.

196. Colloff MJ, Merrett TG, Merret J et al. Feather mites are potentially an important source of allergens for pigeon and budgerigar keepers. *Clin Exp Allergy* 1998; 27: 60–67.

197. Arlian LG, Morgan MS, Houck MA. Allergenicity of the mite *Hemisarcoptes cooremani*. *Ann Allergy Asthma Immunol* 1999; 83: 401–409.

198. Ivanciuc O, Midoro-Horiuti T, Schein CH et al. The property distance index PD predicts peptides that cross-react with IgE antibodies. *Mol Immunol* 2009; 46(5): 873–883.

199. Puerta L, Fernández-Caldas E, Caraballo Gracia LR, Lockey RF. Sensitization of *Blomia tropicalis* and *Lepidoglyphus destructor* in *Dermatophagoides* spp. Allergic individuals. *J Allergy Clin Immunol* 1991; 88: 943–950.

200. Smith AM, Benjamin DC, Hozic N et al. The molecular basis of antigenic cross-reactivity between the group 2 mite allergens. *J Allergy Clin Immunol* 2001; 107(6): 977–984.

201. Luczynska CM, Griffin P, Davies RJ, Topping MD. Prevalence of specific IgE to storage mites (*A. siro, L. destructor* and *T. longior*) in an urban population and cross-reactivity with the house dust mite (*D. pteronyssinus*). *Clin Exp Allergy* 1990; 20(4): 403–406.

202. van Hage-Hamsten M, Johansson SG, Johansson E, Wiren A. Lack of allergenic cross-reactivity between storage mites and *Dermatophagoides pteronyssinus*. *Clin Allergy* 1987; 17: 23–31.

203. Park JW, Ko SH, Yong TS, Ree HI, Jeoung BJ, Hong CS. Cross-reactivity of *Tyrophagus putrescentiae* with *Dermatophagoides farinae* and *Dermatophagoides pteronyssinus* in urban areas. *Ann Allergy Asthma Immunol* 1999; 83: 533–539.

204. Chruszcz M, Chapman MD, Vailes LD et al. Crystal structures of mite allergens Der f 1 and Der p 1 reveal differences in surface-exposed residues that may influence antibody binding. *J Mol Biol* 2009; 386(2): 520–530.

205. Chruszcz M, Pomés A, Glesner J et al. Molecular determinants for antibody binding on group 1 house dust mite allergens. *J Biol Chem* 2012; 287(10): 7388–7398.

206. Ong ST, Chew FT. Reconstructing the repertoire of mite allergens by recombinant DNA technology. In: Pawankar R et al. editors. *Allergy Frontiers: Future Perspectives.* New York, NY: Springer, 2010.

207. Witteman AM, Akkerdaas JH, van Leeuwen J, van der Zee JS, Aalberse RC. Identification of a cross-reactive allergen (presumably tropomyosin) in shrimp, mite and insects. *Int Arch Allergy Immunol* 1994; 105(1): 56–61.

208. Cantillo JF, Puerta L, Fernandez-Caldas E et al. Tropomyosins in mosquito and house dust mite cross-react at the humoral and cellular level. *Clin Exp Allergy* 2018; 48(10): 1354–1363.

209. Johansson E, Aponno M, Lundberg M, van Hage-Hamsten M. Allergenic cross-reactivity between the nematode Anisakis simplex and the dust mites *Acarus siro, Lepidoglyphus destructor, Tyrophagus putrescentiae,* and *Dermatophagoides pteronyssinus. Allergy* 2001; 56: 660–666.

210. Acevedo N, Sánchez J, Erler A et al. IgE cross-reactivity between Ascaris and domestic mite allergens: The role of tropomyosin and the nematode polyprotein ABA-1. *Allergy* 2009; 64(11): 1635–1643.

211. Acevedo N, Erler A, Briza P, Puccio F, Ferreira F, Caraballo L. Allergenicity of *Ascaris lumbricoides* tropomyosin and IgE sensitization among asthmatic patients in a tropical environment. *Int Arch Allergy Immunol* 2011; 154(3): 195–206.

212. Santiago HC, Bennuru S, Boyd A, Eberhard M, Nutman TB. Structural and immunologic cross reactivity among filarial and mite tropomyosin: Implications for the hygiene hypothesis. *J Allergy Clin Immunol* 2010; 127: 479–486.

213. Arlian LG, Morgan MS, Quirce S, Marañón F, Fernández-Caldas E. Characterization of allergens of Anisakis simplex. *Allergy* 2003; 58(12): 1299–1303.

214. Pérez-Pérez J, Fernández-Caldas E, Marañón F et al. Molecular cloning of paramyosin, a new allergen of Anisakis simplex. *Int Arch Allergy Immunol* 2000; 123(2): 120–129.

215. Anadón AM, Rodríguez E, Gárate MT et al. Diagnosing human anisakiasis: Recombinant Ani s 1 and Ani s 7 allergens versus the UniCAP 100 fluorescence enzyme immunoassay. *Clin Vaccine Immunol* 2010; 17(4): 496–502.

216. Sastre J, Lluch-Bernal M, Quirce S et al. A double-blind, placebo-controlled oral challenge study with lyophilized larvae and antigen of the fish parasite, Anisakis simplex. *Allergy* 2000; 55(6): 560–564.

217. Arlian LG, Vyszenski-Moher DL, Ahmed SG, Estes SA. Cross-antigenicity between the scabies mite, *Sarcoptes scabiei*, and the house dust mite, *Dermatophagoides pteronyssinus*. *J Invest Dermatol* 1991; 96: 349–354.

218. Dean Rider Jr. S, Morgan MS, Arlian LG. Draft genome of the scabies mite. *Parasites Vectors* 2015; 8: 585.

219. Temeyer KB, Soileau LC, Pruett JH. Cloning and sequence analysis of a cDNA encoding Pso II, a group II mite allergen of the sheep scab mite (Acari: Psoroptidae). *J Med Entomol* 2002; 39: 384–391.

220. Swamy RS, Reshamwala N, Hunter T et al. Epigenetic modifications and improved regulatory T-cell function in subjects undergoing dual sublingual immunotherapy. *J Allergy Clin Immunol* 2012; 130(1): 215–24e7.

221. Mueller GA, Pedersen LC, Glesner J et al. Analysis of glutathione S-transferase allergen cross-reactivity in a North American population: Relevance for molecular diagnosis. *J Allergy Clin Immunol* 2015; 136: 1369–1377.

222. Acevedo N, Caraballo L. IgE cross-reactivity between *Ascaris lumbricoides* and mite allergens: Possible influences on allergic sensitization and asthma. *Parasite Immunol* 2011; 33: 309–321.

223. Acevedo N, Mohr J, Zakzuk J et al. Proteomic and immunochemical characterization of glutathione transferase as a new allergen of the nematode *Ascaris lumbricoides*. *PLOS ONE* 2013; 8: e78353.

224. Fernández-Caldas E, Puerta L, Caraballo L, Lockey RF. Mite allergens. *Clin Allergy Immunol* 2004; 18: 251–270.

225. Stewart GA, Kollinger MR, King CM, Thompson PJ. A comparative study of three serine proteases from *Dermatophagoides pteronyssinus* and *D. farinae*. *Allergy* 1994; 49: 553–560.

226. Bowman CE. Comparative enzymology of economically important astigmatid mites. In: Griffiths DA, Bowman CE, editors. *Acarology VI*. Chichester: Ellis Horwood 1984; 2: 993.

227. Sánchez-Ramos I, Hernández CA, Castanera P, Ortego F. Proteolytic activities in body and faecal extracts of the storage mite, *Acarus farris*. *Med Vet Entomol* 2004; 18: 378–386.

228. Ortego F, Sánchez-Ramos I, Ruiz M, Castanera P. Characterization of proteases from a stored product mite, *Tyrophagus putrescentiae*. *Arch Insect Biochem Physiol* 2000; 43: 116–124.

229. Montealegre F, Quinones C, Torres N, Goth K. Detection of serine proteases in extracts of the domestic mite *Blomia tropicalis*. *Exp Appl Acarol* 2002; 26: 87–100.

230. Flores I, Mora C, Rivera E, Donnelly R, Montealegre F. Cloning and molecular characterization of a cDNA from *Blomia tropicalis* homologous to dust mite group 3 allergens (trypsin-like proteases). *Int Arch Allergy Immunol* 2003; 130: 12–16.

231. Nisbet AJ, Billingsley PF. Hydrolytic enzymes of *Psoroptes cuniculi* (Delafond). *Insect Biochem Mol Biol* 1999; 29: 25–32.

232. Edwards TB, Trudeau WL, Fernández-Caldas E, Lee DK, Seleznick MJ, Lockey RF. Proteinases in extracts of the storage mite, *Aleuroglyphus ovatus*. *J Allergy Clin Immunol* 1992; 90: 129–131.

233. Ando T, Homma R, Ino Y et al. Trypsin-like protease of mites: purification and characterization of trypsin-like protease from mite faecal extract *Dermatophagoides farinae*. Relationship between trypsin-like protease and Der f III. *Clin Exp Allergy* 1993; 23: 777–784.

234. Stewart GA, Lake FR, Thompson PJ. Faecally derived hydrolytic enzymes from *Dermatophagoides pteronyssinus*: Physicochemical characterisation of potential allergens. *Int Arch Allergy Appl Immunol* 1991; 95: 248–256.

235. Fernández-Caldas E. Towards a more complete standardization of mite allergen extracts. *Int Arch Allergy Immunol* 2013; 160(1): 1–3.

236. Reithofer M, Jahn-Schid B. Allergens with protease activity from house dust mites. *Int J Mol Sci* 2017; 18: 1368.

237. Brown A, Farmer K, MacDonald L et al. House dust mite Der p 1 downregulates defenses of the lung by inactivating elastase inhibitors. *Am J Respir Cell Mol Biol* 2003; 29: 381–389.

238. Sun G, Stacey MA, Schmidt M, Mori L, Mattoli S. Interaction of mite allergens Der p 3 and Der p 9 with protease-activated receptor-2 expressed by lung epithelial cells. *J Immunol* 2001; 167: 1014–1021.

239. Caraballo LR, Hernandez M. HLA haplotype segregation in families with allergic asthma. *Tissue Antigens* 1990; 35(4): 182–186.

240. Hizawa N, Freidhoff LR, Chiu YF et al. Genetic regulation of *Dermatophagoides pteronyssinus*-specific IgE responsiveness: A genome-wide multipoint linkage analysis in families recruited through 2 asthmatic sibs. Collaborative Study on the Genetics of Asthma (CSGA). *J Allergy Clin Immunol* 1998; 102(3): 436–442.

241. Hizawa N, Collins G, Rafnar T et al. Linkage analysis of *Dermatophagoides pteronyssinus*-specific IgE responsiveness with polymorphic markers on chromosome 6p21 (HLA-D region) in Caucasian families by the transmission/disequilibrium test. Collaborative Study on the Genetics of Asthma (CSGA). *J Allergy Clin Immunol* 1998; 102(3): 443–448.

242. Stephan V, Kuehr J, Seibt A et al. Genetic linkage of HLA-class II locus to mite-specific IgE immune responsiveness. *Clin Exp Allergy* 1999; 29(8): 1049–1054.

243. Torres-Galván MJ, Quiralte J, Blanco C et al. Linkage of house dust mite allergy with the HLA region. *Ann Allergy Asthma Immunol* 1999; 82(2): 198–203.

244. Blumenthal MN, Ober C, Beaty TH et al. Genome scan for loci linked to mite sensitivity: The Collaborative Study on the Genetics of Asthma (CSGA). *Genes Immun* 2004; 5(3): 226–231.

245. Caraballo L, Marrugo J, Jimenez S, Angelini G, Ferrara GB. Frequency of DPB1*0401 is significantly decreased in patients with allergic asthma in a mulatto population. *Hum Immunol* 1991; 32(3): 157–161.

246. Hu C, Hsu PN, Lin RH, Hsieh KH, Chua KY. HLA DPB1*0201 allele is negatively associated with immunoglobulin E responsiveness specific for house dust mite allergens in Taiwan. *Clin Exp Allergy* 2000; 30(4): 538–545.

247. Noguchi E, Sakamoto H, Hirota T et al. Genome-wide association study identifies HLA-DP as a susceptibility gene for pediatric asthma in Asian populations. *PLOS Genet* 2011; 7(7): e1002170.

248. da Costa Lima Caniatti MC, Borelli SD, Guilherme AL, Tsuneto LT. Association between HLA genes and dust mite sensitivity in a Brazilian population. *Hum Immunol* 2017; 78(2): 88–94.

249. Caniatti MCDCL, Borelli SD, Guilherme ALF, Franzener SB, Tsuneto LT. Association between KIR genes and dust mite sensitization in a Brazilian population. *Hum Immunol* 2018; 79(1): 51–56.

250. Caraballo L, Martínez B, Jiménez S, Puerta L. HLA-DR3 is associated with the IgE immune responsiveness to a recombinant allergen from *Blomia tropicalis* (BT). *Adv Exp Med Biol* 1996; 409: 81–83.

251. Young RP, Dekker JW, Wordsworth BP et al. HLA-DR and HLA-DP genotypes and immunoglobulin E responses to common major allergens. *Clin Exp Allergy* 1994; 24(5): 431–439.

252. Lara-Marquez ML, Yunis JJ, Layrisse Z et al. Immunogenetics of atopic asthma: Association of DRB1*1101 DQA1*0501 DQB1*0301 haplotype with *Dermatophagoides* spp.-sensitive asthma in a sample of the Venezuelan population. *Clin Exp Allergy* 1999; 29(1): 60–71.

253. Blumenthal MN. Positive association between HLA-DRB1*07 and specific IgE responses to purified major allergens of *D. pteronyssinus* (Der p 1 and Der p 2). *Ann Allergy Asthma Immunol* 2002; 88(2): 147–149.

254. Kim YK, Oh HB, Oh SY, Cho SH, Kim YY, Min KU. HLA-DRB1*07 may have a susceptibility and DRB1*04 a protective effect upon the development of a sensitization to house dust mite *Dermatophagoides pteronyssinus*. *Clin Exp Allergy* 2001; 31(1): 110–115.

255. Pino-Yanes M, Corrales A, Acosta-Herrera M et al. HLA-DRB1*15:01 allele protects from asthma susceptibility. *J Allergy Clin Immunol* 2014; 134(5): 1201–1203.

256. Konno S, Takahashi D, Hizawa N et al. Genetic impact of a butyrophilin-like 2 (BTNL2) gene variation on specific IgE responsiveness to *Dermatophagoides farinae* (Der f) in Japanese. *Allergol Int* 2009; 58(1): 29–35.

257. Caniatti MC, Marchioro AA, Guilherme AL, Tsuneto LT. Association of cytokines in individuals sensitive and insensitive to dust mites in a Brazilian population. *PLOS ONE* 2014; 9(9): e107921.

258. Lu MP, Chen RX, Wang ML et al. Association study on IL4, IL13 and IL4RA polymorphisms in mite-sensitized persistent allergic rhinitis in a Chinese population. *PLOS ONE* 2011; 6(11): e27363.

259. Hinds DA, McMahon G, Kiefer AK et al. A genome-wide association meta-analysis of self-reported allergy identifies shared and allergy-specific susceptibility loci. *Nat Genet* 2013; 45(8): 907–911.

260. Shin HD, Kim LH, Park BL et al. Association of interleukin 18 (IL18) polymorphisms with specific IgE levels to mite allergens among asthmatic patients. *Allergy* 2005; 60(7): 900–906.

261. Kruse S, Kuehr J, Moseler M et al. Polymorphisms in the IL 18 gene are associated with specific sensitization to common allergens and allergic rhinitis. *J Allergy Clin Immunol* 2003; 111(1): 117–122.

262. Acevedo N, Vergara C, Mercado D, Jiménez S, Caraballo L. The A-444C polymorphism of leukotriene C4 synthase gene is associated with IgE antibodies to *Dermatophagoides pteronyssinus* in a Colombian population. *J Allergy Clin Immunol* 2007; 119(2): 505–507.

263. Martínez B, Barrios K, Vergara C et al. A NOS1 gene polymorphism associated with asthma and specific immunoglobulin E response to mite allergens in a Colombian population. *Int Arch Allergy Immunol* 2007; 144(2): 105–113.

264. Kim Y, Park CS, Shin HD et al. A promoter nucleotide variant of the dendritic cell-specific DCNP1 associates with serum IgE levels specific for dust mite allergens among the Korean asthmatics. *Genes Immun* 2007; 8(5): 369–378.

265. Schedel M, Pinto LA, Schaub B et al. IRF-1 gene variations influence IgE regulation and atopy. *Am J Respir Crit Care Med* 2008; 177(6): 613–621.

266. Tan CY, Chen YL, Wu LS, Liu CF, Chang WT, Wang JY. Association of CD14 promoter polymorphisms and soluble CD14 levels in mite allergen sensitization of children in Taiwan. *J Hum Genet* 2006; 51(1): 59–67.

267. Jackola DR et al. CD14 promoter polymorphisms in atopic families: Implications for modulated allergen-specific immunoglobulin E and G1 responses. *Int Arch Allergy Immunol* 2006; 139(3): 217–224.

268. Tripathi P, Hong X, Caruso D, Gao P, Wang X. Genetic determinants in the development of sensitization to environmental allergens in early childhood. *Immun Inflamm Dis* 2014; 2(3): 193–204.

269. Purwar R, Langer K, Werfel T. Polymorphisms within the C3 gene are associated with specific IgE levels to common allergens and super-antigens among atopic dermatitis patients. *Exp Dermatol* 2009; 18(1): 30–34.

270. Liao EC, Chang CY, Wu CC, Wang GJ, Tsai JJ. Association of single nucleotide polymorphisms in the MD-2 gene promoter region with Der p 2 allergy. *Allergy Asthma Immunol Res* 2015; 7(3): 249–255.

271. Castro-Giner F, Bustamante M, Ramon González J et al. A pooling-based genome-wide analysis identifies new potential candidate genes for atopy in the European Community Respiratory Health Survey (ECRHS). *BMC Med Genet* 2009; 10: 128.

272. Wan YI, Strachan DP, Evans DM et al. A genome-wide association study to identify genetic determinants of atopy in subjects from the United Kingdom. *J Allergy Clin Immunol* 2011; 127(1): 223–231, 231.e1–3.

273. Andiappan AK, Wang de Y, Anantharaman R et al. Replication of genome-wide association study loci for allergic rhinitis and house dust mite sensitization in an Asian population of ethnic Chinese in Singapore. *J Allergy Clin Immunol* 2013; 131(5): 1431–1433.e8.

274. Kim JH, Cheong HS, Park JS et al. A genome-wide association study of total serum and mite specific IgEs in asthma patients. *PLOS ONE* 2013; 8(8): e71958.

275. Bønnelykke K, Matheson MC, Pers TH et al. Meta-analysis of genome-wide association studies identifies ten loci influencing allergic sensitization. *Nat Genet* 2013; 45(8): 902–906.

276. Šauliené I, Grečiuvlené I, Šukiené L et al. Genetic loci associated with allergic sensitization in Lithuanians. *PLOS ONE* 2015; 10(7): e0134188.

277. Liu X, Beaty TH, Deindl P et al. Associations between specific serum IgE response and 6 variants within the genes IL4, IL13, and IL4RA in German children: The German Multicenter Atopy Study. *J Allergy Clin Immunol* 2004; 113(3): 489–495.

278. Hunninghake GM, Soto-Quirós ME, Lasky-Su J et al. Dust mite exposure modifies the effect of functional IL10 polymorphisms on allergy and asthma exacerbations. *J Allergy Clin Immunol* 2008; 122(1): 93–98, 98e1–5.

279. Acevedo N, Bornacelly A, Mercado D et al. Genetic Variants in CHIA and CHI3L1 are associated with the IgE response to the Ascaris resistance marker ABA-1 and the birch pollen allergen Bet v 1. *PLOS ONE* 2016; 11(12): e0167453.

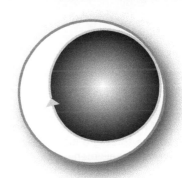

15 Cockroach and other inhalant insect allergens

Anna Pomés
INDOOR Biotechnologies, Inc.

Coby Schal
North Carolina State University

CONTENTS

15.1 INTRODUCTION

Insect inhalant allergy is a health problem worldwide due to the cosmopolitan distribution of these arthropods. The great diversity of insects, their presence in all terrestrial and aquatic environments, and the accumulation of debris associated with large populations vary significantly with season and geography. Insect inhalant allergens are found indoors, outdoors, in homes, and at the workplace. Sensitization can be due to airborne insect emanations in house dust or to occupational exposures, encountered by professionals such as research entomologists [1]. The concept of inhalant insect allergies was developed by the early observations of Figley (1929), Parlato (1930 and 1932), and Kern (1938) of asthma associated with sensitization to the mayfly, sand fly, mushroom fly, moths, and butterflies [2,3]. In the animal kingdom, the phylum Arthropoda constitutes 75% of known animal species that can contribute significant organic material for airborne dispersal. Three arthropod taxonomic groups, Insecta, Crustacea, and Arachnida, are of major concern as allergen producers. Some of the allergens from the three groups share amino acid sequence homology that manifests in allergenic cross-reactivity [2].

This chapter focuses on the class Insecta, which includes more than 80% of the total number of species from the three groups combined. Insects have three pairs of legs; their body is divided into head, thorax, and abdomen; and adults are either wingless or have one or two pairs of wings. All insects molt through several immature stages, representing different instars, before they reach the adult reproductive stage. The cuticle that is shed at each molt consists of chitin and cuticular proteins, and the latter can be highly allergenic. Cockroaches, mayflies, caddisflies, moths, butterflies, flies, fleas, midges, ants, bees, and wasps are representative members of this class (Table 15.1). Insect allergy (i.e., IgE-mediated sensitivity) may be induced by a wide variety of insect-derived allergens in the environment either on a seasonal (vast emergences of aquatic insects, such as caddisflies, mayflies, and midges) or perennial basis (terrestrial pests, such as cockroaches). In certain places, inhalant insect "dust" is clearly visible and associated with the mass emergence of caddisflies in the summer months. In Japan, sensitization to moths and butterflies is common. Chironomidae (nonbiting midges) larvae and adults cause allergic reactions in approximately 20% of exposed subjects (Table 15.1). These are predominantly aquarists using insect larvae as fish food and environmentally exposed subjects living in areas abounding streams and lakes. Exposure to large numbers of the "green nimitti" midge in Sudanese communities is associated with an increased incidence of both asthma and allergic rhinitis. Honeybees produce "bee dust," which causes inhalant allergy in beekeepers, and subjects extracting bee venom can develop inhalant allergy to phospholipase C. Wherever allergenic exposure (onset, intensity, and frequency) and adjuvants (ozone, NO_2, tobacco smoke, viruses, etc.) are present in the environment, allergic symptoms are more likely to develop, particularly in those with a genetic atopic predisposition.

Cockroach allergy is especially important for the development of asthma in inner cities among lower socioeconomic groups [4–9]. Over 4000 species of cockroaches (Order Blattodea) have been described and named worldwide, the majority of which are not directly associated with humans in their home and work environments. Infestations of cockroaches in primary dwellings and workplaces represent one of the most intimate and chronic associations of pests with humans. All cockroach species are adept crawlers. Species differ in capacity of flight, morphology (size, color), response to light, geographic distribution, and domestic habitat. The two most common species associated with allergic disease are the American (*Periplaneta americana*) and German (*Blattella germanica*) cockroaches, although other species might be involved (e.g., *Blatta orientalis*), as well as closely related species within the genera *Periplaneta* and *Blattella* (Table 15.2, Figure 15.1). The American cockroach is 34–53 mm long, reddish brown, and capable of flight, whereas the German cockroach is 16 mm long, brown, nocturnal, incapable of flight, and strictly domestic. Taxonomy and details of species identification are available in the literature [3,10].

15.2 PUBLIC HEALTH IMPORTANCE OF COCKROACHES

Cockroaches may adversely affect human health in several ways, including causing psychological stress, contaminating food (with excrement resulting in vomiting and diarrhea), causing exposure to associated pathogens, and inducing inhalant allergy. In addition, cockroaches affect human health indirectly, as large amounts of insecticides are used in efforts to control cockroaches, exposing residents to pesticide residues. Bernton and Brown reported cockroach sensitization for the first time in the 1960s [4]. Kang and colleagues showed that 60% of patients with asthma in the Chicago area had positive skin tests, serum IgE antibodies, or positive bronchial challenge tests to *B. germanica* allergens [11]. Sensitization and exposure to cockroach allergens are risk factors for emergency room admissions with asthma [12]. The National Cooperative Inner City Asthma Study found that exposure and sensitization to cockroach allergens were associated with asthma morbidity in children from eight major inner-city areas in the United States. Of 476 children with asthma (age 4–7 years), 36.8% were allergic to cockroach allergens, followed by those of the dust mite (34.9%) and cat (22.7%) allergens [6]. The same association was found in children for cockroaches, but not for mite, cat, and dog, in another inner city asthma study, reporting a 69% prevalence of sensitization to cockroach allergens in 937 children and reaching the highest value of 81% in the Bronx, New York [9]. Women from Boston sensitized and exposed to cockroach allergens were at least three times more likely to have used steroids and to have attended a hospital emergency room with asthma [13]. Other exposures may affect sensitization to cockroach. Repeatedly high levels of urinary polycyclic aromatic hydrocarbon metabolites during childhood may increase likelihood of sensitization to cockroach allergen in urban inner-city children at age 9 years [14]. Association between exposure to cockroach allergens and asthma has been confirmed by studies outside the United States. However, an association of exposure to cockroach protein with asthma has been documented also without evidence of allergy in other studies, suggesting that this association can be independent of specific IgE [15,16]. Thus, asthma prevalence or severity may be due to cofactors related to cockroach exposure other than allergy, potentially including urban environmental influences such as pollutant exposure and lack of sun exposure.

Importantly, in heavy cockroach infestations, their fecal deposits, their shed cuticles, and dead cockroaches constitute an appreciable mass of organic matter that can serve as substrate for bacteria and fungi. A recent study has shown that the microbiome of cockroach-infested apartments is significantly different from that of uninfested apartments [17]. Moreover, the bacterial communities associated with household dust in infested apartments overlap more with those in cockroach gut than in uninfested homes. In some cases, potentially pathogenic microbes can also be associated with cockroaches [18]. Finally, a study in Hong Kong demonstrated that cockroach feces contains massive amounts of endotoxin [19], suggesting that cockroaches likely contribute to endotoxin levels in infested homes both directly through their feces and indirectly by adding organic substrate to the home.

Cockroach allergy can result from initial sensitization to allergens mostly through inhalation but also by ingestion or transdermal exposure due to abrasion or injection. Americans now spend more than 95% of their time indoors in homes that are better insulated and temperature controlled, while outdoor air exchange has been drastically reduced, creating conditions that support both pest growth and associated dust accumulation in the home. Infestations by domiciliary cockroaches are largely dependent upon housing conditions, and high-rise apartments have higher levels of cockroach allergens [9,20,21]. Potential sources of relevant cockroach allergens in the environment include whole bodies, cast cuticle,

Table 15.1 Inhalant insect allergies

Species	Common name	Order	Place of exposure	Studies by
Apis mellifera	Honey bee	Hymenoptera	Environment of beekeepers (O)	Rudeschko (2004), Bousquet (1982), Abdullah (2016)
Attagenus unicolor	Black carpet beetle	Coleoptera	House dust, museum (O)	Cuesta-Herranz (1997)
Bombyx mori	Silk moth	Lepidoptera	Bedding, clothes; silk workers (O)	Kino (1987), Wen (1990), Uragoda (1991), Suzuki (1995), Komase (1997), Hirabayashi (1997), Zhao (2015), Zuo (2015), Jeong (2016), Wang (2016), Jeong (2017)
Chironomus sp.	Midges, chironomids	Diptera	Hypereutrophic lake in Japan; outdoors	Kino (1987), Eriksson (1989), Baur (1992), Liebers (1993), Witteman (1995), Teranishi (1995), Ree (1996), Komase (1997), Hirabayashi (1997), Yong (1999), Morsy (2000), Jeong (2004), Ballesteros (2006), Selden (2013), Arce (2013), Nandi (2014)
Cimex lectularius	Bedbug[a]	Hemiptera	Infested homes; bedding	Reinhardt (2009), Leverkus (2006), Gries [76], DeVries [77]
Coptotermes formosanus	Formosan subterranean termite	Blattodea	Infested homes	Mattison [79], Vargas (2018)
Ctenocephalides felis	Cat flea	Siphonaptera	House dust	Trudeau (1993), Bond (2006), Werr (2009)
Drosophila melanogaster	Fruit fly	Diptera	Laboratories (O)	Jones (2017)
Ephestia kuehniella	Flour moth	Lepidoptera	Bakers (O)	Makinen-Kiljunen (2001), Armentia (2004)
Halyomorpha halys	Brown marmorated stink bug	Hemiptera	Infested homes	Mertz (2012)
Harmonia axyridis	Asian lady beetle	Coleoptera	Infested homes	Yarbrough (1999), Albright (2006), Goetz (2007), Nakazawa (2007), Knuffman (2007), Goetz (2009), Clark (2009), Girodet (2016)
Lepisma saccharina	Silverfish	Zygentoma	Infested homes	Witteman (1995), (1996), Barletta (2002, 2005, 2007), Boquete (2008)
Liposcelis bostrychophila	Booklouse	Psocoptera	House dust	Fukutomi (2012), Ishibashi (2017)

(Continued)

Table 15.1 (*Continued*) Inhalant insect allergies

Species	Common name	Order	Place of exposure	Studies by
Liposcelis decolor	Booklouse	Psocoptera	House dust	Marco (2016)
Locusta migratoria	Grasshopper	Orthoptera	Research laboratories (O)	Soparkar (1993), Lopata (2005)
Lucilia cuprina	Blowfly	Diptera	Entomological research laboratory (O)	Kaufman (1986)
Monomorium pharaonis	Pharaoh ant	Hymenoptera	Indoor infested environments	Kim (2005), Kim (2007)
Musca domestica	Common house fly	Diptera	Closed breeding rooms; livestock stables, barns; pharmaceutical industry workers (O)	Baldo (1988), Wahl (1997), Tas (2007), Focke (2003), Barletta (2003), Smith (2005)
Plodia interpunctella	Indianmeal moth	Lepidoptera	Household and dry stored food	Binder (2001), Hoflehner (2012)
Sitophilus oryzae	Rice weevil	Coleoptera	Infested homes; food storage (O)	Kleine-Tebbe (1992), Jeebhay (2005), Hubert (2018)
Sitophilus granarius	Granary weevil	Coleoptera	Infested homes; food storage (O)	Jeebhay (2005), Jakubas-Zawalska (2016), Hubert (2018)
Tenebrio molitor	Yellow mealworm	Coleoptera	Warehouse fishing bait handling (O)	Bernstein (1983), Siracusa (1994), Lamberti (2018)
Thaumetopoea pityocampa	Pine processionary caterpillar[b]	Lepidoptera	Airborne urticating hairs	Werno (1993), Rebollo (2002), Moneo (2003), Fuentes (2006), Rodriguez-Mahillo (2012), Vega (2014), Berardi (2015)
Triatoma infestans	Kissing bug	Hemiptera	Indoor and outdoor environments	Alonso (1996), Walter (2012)
Trogoderma variabile	Warehouse beetle	Coleoptera	Warehouse (O)	Bernstein (2009)
Several species	Caddisflies	Trichoptera	Outdoor environments; hydroelectric plant workers (O)	Kino (1987), Koshte (1989), Warrington (2003), Smith (2005), McNutty (2017)
Several species	**Mayflies**	Ephemeroptera	Outdoor rural environment	Smith (2005)

Notes: Occupational exposures are indicated by (O). Usually the terms *caddisfly* and *mayfly* imply multiple species. Studies are cited by first author and year of publication.
[a] Although allergic hypersensitivity to bedbug has been described for bites, this insect excretes histamine and might produce potential inhalant allergens.
[b] Sensitization may occur by urticating hairs (setae), not necessarily inhalation, that induce cutaneous reactions in animals and humans.

Table 15.2 Taxonomy of cockroaches[a]

Phylum: Arthropoda

Class: Insecta

Order: Blattodea

Family	Genus/species	Common name
Blaberidae	*Leucophaea (=Rhyparobia) maderae*	Madeira
Ectobiidae	*Blattella germanica*	German
	Blattella asahinai	Asian
	Supella longipalpa	Brown-banded
Blattidae	*Periplaneta americana*	American
	Periplaneta australasiae	Australian
	Periplaneta brunnea	Brown
	Periplaneta fuliginosa	Smokybrown
	Blatta orientalis	Oriental
	Blatta (= Shelfordella) lateralis[b]	Turkestan

[a] Some taxonomic group names have changed since previous versions of this chapter.
[b] New invasive species that has spread throughout the United States.

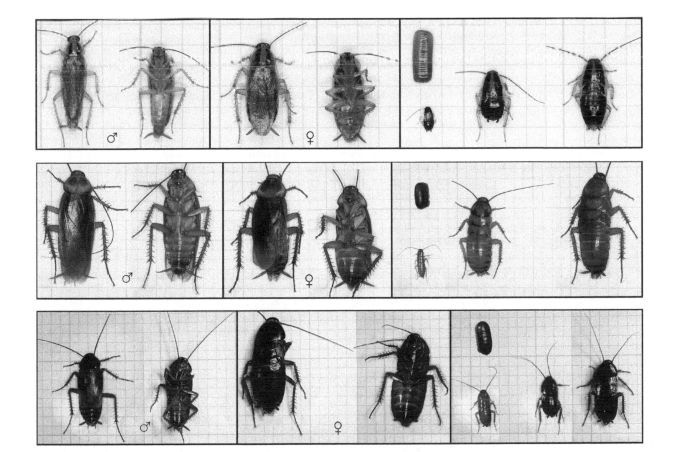

Figure 15.1 Images of three cockroach species: Top to bottom, German cockroach (*Blattella germanica*), American cockroach (*Periplaneta americana*), and Oriental cockroach (*Blatta orientalis*). For each of the three panels, from left to right: Adult male dorsal and ventral views; adult female dorsal and ventral views; small, medium, and large nymph; and an egg case. Scale: Each square is 1/8 inch (3.12 mm). (Photo credit: Benoit Guenard.)

secretions, egg cases, and/or fecal material. Airborne cockroach allergens are associated primarily with amorphous and larger particles (10 μm) (which settle after disturbance) than are particles from animals like cat and dog [22]. The threshold levels of allergen exposure, above which susceptible individuals are at increased risk for sensitization or asthma symptoms, have been considered for a long time to be 2 and 8 U/g of dust, respectively, for either Bla g 1 or Bla g 2 (1 U of Bla g 1 is equivalent to 0.1 μg [23] and 1 U of Bla g 2 is equivalent to 0.04 μg) [6,7,24–26]. However, rather than the existence of specific thresholds, there is evidence of the existence of a dose-response relationship between exposure and sensitization or disease. In a nationally representative sample, cockroach allergen (Bla g 1) concentrations exceeded 2 U/g in 11% of U.S. living room floors and 13% of kitchen floors and exceeded 8 U/g in 3% of living room floors and 10% of kitchen floors. Detectable concentrations of greater than 0.4 U/g were found in 27.4% of U.S. homes [21]. Mild-to-moderate symptoms induced by cockroach allergen inhalation include sneezing and rhinorrhea, skin reactions (mild dermatitis), and eye irritation, with difficulty in breathing and possible anaphylactic episodes occurring in more severely allergic individuals. Children aged 2–3 years who have anti-cockroach IgE are at increased risk of wheeze, rhinitis, or atopic dermatitis [26]. Two studies of the Inner-City Asthma Consortium (ICAC) report on the complex relationships between cockroach allergen exposure, sensitization, and asthma. Cumulative exposure to cockroaches over the first 3 years of life correlated with allergen sensitization at 3 years of age that was positively associated with recurrent wheezing. However, contrary to expectations, exposure to high levels of cockroaches in the first year of life showed a strong inverse correlation with recurrent wheeze at age 3 years. The authors subsequently found that exposure to high levels of allergens in combination with an environment rich in specific bacteria in early childhood might be beneficial, leading to a protective effect against wheeze and atopy [27]. Similarly, higher indoor levels of cockroach allergen exposure in the first 3 years of life were associated with lower risk of asthma at 7 years of age [28].

Only few studies report associations between sensitization to specific allergens and disease. In Taiwan, sensitization to Per a 2 (81% of patients) correlated with more severe airway allergy and elevated proinflammatory cytokines, but more patients with rhinitis only were sensitized to Per a 9 (80%) [29]. In New York, Bla g 2 levels greater than 1 U/g in children's bedroom and kitchen dust samples were independently associated with cockroach-specific IgE among children with asthma [30]. A recent analysis of IgE reactivity to eight recombinant cockroach allergens (allergen components) reports the emergence of additional major cockroach allergens (e.g., from groups 6, 9, and 11 among highly cockroach sensitized subjects) in addition to the originally identified major allergens Bla g 2 and Bla g 5 [31]. The role of these cockroach allergens in disease is currently being investigated.

15.3 MOLECULAR BIOLOGY OF COCKROACH ALLERGENS

Initial identification of cockroach allergens was performed by several groups using conventional physicochemical techniques reviewed in Pomés [3]. Allergenic proteins with molecular weights ranging from 6 to 120 kD were recognized in cockroach extracts by serum IgE from cockroach-sensitive individuals. In the last two

decades, 13 groups (group 13 is not yet published) of cockroach allergens have been identified by molecular cloning or proteomic approaches, and their biochemical activities and biological roles have been investigated. Molecular cloning involved the construction of American and German cockroach cDNA expression libraries that were screened with human IgE or murine monoclonal antibodies to identify clones expressing allergens. The official list of cockroach allergens listed in the World Health Organization/ International Union of Immunological Societies (WHO/IUIS) Allergen Nomenclature Database (http:// www.allergen.org) is shown in Table 15.3. It is also noteworthy that the recent sequencing and annotation of the genomes of the German and American cockroaches, and broader availability of transcriptomes, will likely facilitate the identification of new cockroach allergens [32,33].

15.3.1 Group 1

Bla g 1 is an acidic allergen that cross-reacts with homologous proteins from other cockroach species, such as Per a 1. It was first identified by Twarog et al. and subsequently purified [34–36]. Molecular cloning revealed that group 1 cockroach allergens consist of tandem nucleotide repeats, each encoding two consecutive ~100 amino acid repeats [37–40]. DNA sequence analysis showed that group 1 cockroach allergens originated from gene duplication and subsequent mutagenesis of an original DNA domain [38]. The origin of the duplex has been confirmed and only found in other species of insects [41]. Group 1 cockroach allergens are a mixture of allergenic proteins of different sizes (6, 21, 32, 43 kD up to 90 kD), containing different numbers of repeats [38,42]. Bla g 1 is most prevalent in the midgut, the only tissue where the Bla g 1 gene is expressed [38,43]. Adult females produce and excrete significantly more Bla g 1 in their feces than males and nymphs, most likely because females process more food, and production is related to food intake [44]. The x-ray crystal structure of Bla g 1 has been determined, revealing a capsule-like fold made of two consecutive repeats with an internal lipid-binding cavity [23] (Figure 15.2). Evidence supports a digestive function for Bla g 1, associated with nonspecific transport of lipids.

15.3.2 Group 2

Bla g 2 has long been considered one of the most important cockroach allergens, with the highest (approximately twofold higher) prevalence of IgE antibody binding (54.4%; $n = 118$) compared to rBla g 1, rBla g 4, rBla g 5, and rPer a 7 [45]. Among sera with high IgE antibody levels to cockroach extract (3.5–100 IU/mL), the prevalence of IgE antibodies to Bla g 2 and Bla g 5 was 71% and 58%, respectively [45]. These results confirm previous findings that Bla g 2 elicits IgE responses in 58%–70% of cockroach-allergic patients ($n = 106$) (compared to 30%–40% for Bla g 1) [46].

Bla g 2 is homologous to aspartic proteases, which are a widely distributed group of digestive enzymes (Figure 15.2). Several studies support the idea that allergens with proteolytic activity (e.g., Der p 1, Der p 3, Der p 6) may achieve access to antigen-presenting cells in the absence of inflammation by damaging the epithelium and facilitating their own access and penetration into the mucosa (reviewed in Chapman et al. [47]). The proteolytic activity of allergens may contribute to allergenicity. However, Bla g 2 is proteolytically inactive and yet is a potent allergen, inducing sensitization at exposure

Table 15.3 Nomenclature and function of cockroach allergens (World Health Organization/International Union of Immunological Societies)

Allergen	MW[a] (kD)	Function/homology	GenBank accession number
Blattella germanica			
Bla g 1 [37,38]			
Bla g 1.0101	46, 21	Midgut microvilli protein-homolog	AF072219, AF072221
Bla g 1.0102	90	Midgut microvilli protein-homolog	L47595
Bla g 1.0201	56	Midgut microvilli protein-homolog	AF072220
Bla g 2 [46,48,49]	36	Inactive aspartic protease[b]	U28863
Bla g 3 [57]	78.9	Arylphorin/hemocyanin	GU086323
Bla g 4 [58,59]	21	Lipocalin[c]	U40767
Bla g 5 [64]	23	Glutathione *S*-transferase	U92412
Bla g 6 [65]			
Bla g 6.0101	17	Troponin C	DQ279092
Bla g 6.0201	17	Troponin C	DQ279093
Bla g 6.0301	17	Troponin C	DQ279094
Bla g 7 [68]	33	Tropomyosin	AF260897
Bla g 8 [65]	21	Myosin light chain	DQ389157
Bla g 9 [72]	40	Arginine kinase	DQ358231
Bla g 11 [74]	57	α-Amylase	KC207403
Periplaneta americana			
Per a 1 [39,40]			
Per a 1.0101	26	Midgut microvilli protein-homolog	AF072222
Per a 1.0102	26	Midgut microvilli protein-homolog	U78970
Per a 1.0103	45	Midgut microvilli protein-homolog	U69957
Per a 1.0104	31	Midgut microvilli protein-homolog	U69261
Per a 1.0201	51	Midgut microvilli protein-homolog	U69260
Per a 2 [29]	42	Inactive aspartic protease	GU188391
Per a 3 [56]			
Per a 3.0101	79	Arylphorin/hemocyanin	L40818
Per a 3.0201	75	Arylphorin/hemocyanin	L40820
Per a 3.0202	56	Arylphorin/hemocyanin	L40819
Per a 3.0203	46	Arylphorin/hemocyanin	L40821
Per a 5 [120,121]	23		
Per a 5.0101	25	Glutathione *S*-transferase	MG255130
Per a 5.0102	25	Glutathione *S*-transferase	FJ855485
Per a 6 [65]	17	Troponin C	AY792950

(Continued)

Table 15.3 (*Continued*) Nomenclature and function of cockroach allergens (World Health Organization/International Union of Immunological Societies)

Allergen	MWᵃ (kD)	Function/homology	GenBank accession number
Per a 7 [66,67]			
Per a 7.0101	33	Tropomyosin	Y14854
Per a 7.0102	33	Tropomyosin	AF106961
Per a 9 [70]	43	Arginine kinase	EU429466
Per a 10 [71]	28	Serine protease	AY792954
Per a 11 [73]	55	α-Amylase	KR019685
Per a 12 [73]	45	Chitinase	KR019686

ᵃ Molecular weight calculated from amino acid sequence, except for Bla g 3 (mass spectrometry).

ᵇ The x-ray crystal structures of Bla g 2 alone and in combination with monoclonal antibodies that inhibit IgE antibody binding are accessible in the Protein Data Bank under the accession numbers 1YG9, 2NRS, and 3LIZ.

ᶜ The x-ray crystal structures of Bla g 4 and a *P. americana* homolog are accessible under the accession numbers 3EBK and 3EBW, respectively.

levels that are one or two orders of magnitude lower than other allergens such as Der p 1 [24,48,49]. The x-ray crystallographic structure of Bla g 2 reveals interesting features that explain why Bla g 2 is not an active aspartic protease [48]. Aspartic proteases have a bilobal molecular structure, and the catalytic activity depends on a couple of amino acid triads (aspartate-threonine-glycine or DTG) at the bottom of a cleft between the two lobes. However, Bla g 2 has important amino acid substitutions in the catalytic site, especially at the level of the triads (aspartate-serine-threonine [DST] and aspartate-threonine-serine [DTS] instead of DTG) that make this molecule enzymatically inactive [48–50]. Distortions in the catalytic site, due to these substitutions, lead to a bigger distance of the catalytic aspartates, which is expected to impair enzymatic activity. In addition, there is an insertion (F75a) that interferes with the typical substrate-binding site, providing an autoinhibitory mechanism of enzymatic activity [3]. These structural studies indicate that proteolytic activity is not necessary for allergenicity [49–51]. Two unique structural characteristics of Bla g 2 may contribute to allergenicity

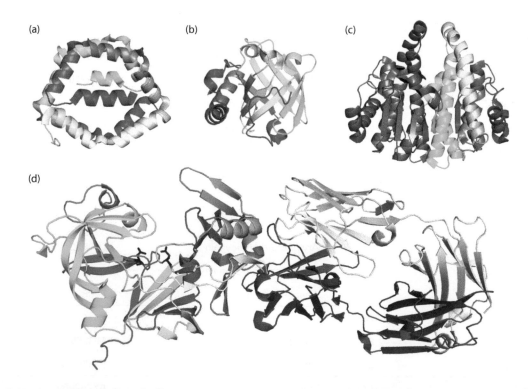

Figure 15.2 Crystal structures of the cockroach allergens Bla g 1 (a), Bla g 4 (b), Bla g 5 (c), and Bla g 2 in combination with the Fab of the monoclonal antibody 4C3 (d) (Protein Data Bank accession numbers are 4jrb, 3ebk, 4q5r, and 3liz, respectively). The allergen molecules are shown from the *N*- (blue) to the *C*-termini (red). One of the two molecules in the Bla g 5 dimer is shown in gray. In Bla g 2, the two aspartates in positions 32 and 215 are indicated as black sticks. The heavy and light chains of the mAb 4C3 Fab are shown in dark and light grays, respectively.

by conferring stability to the molecule: (1) the allergen has five disulfide bonds in contrast to only two or three in active aspartic proteases, and (2) Bla g 2 binds one atom of zinc [48]. Chronic exposure to low doses (1–10 μg/year) of this stable cockroach allergen may explain why sensitization and exposure to Bla g 2 are associated with asthma. Recent analysis of the antigenic surface of Bla g 2 was performed by solving the x-ray crystal structure of the allergen in combination with monoclonal antibodies that inhibit IgE antibody binding [52–55] (Figure 15.2). These studies revealed IgE antibody binding sites and the contribution of carbohydrates in IgE antibody recognition and led to the production of recombinant allergens with reduced IgE antibody binding capacity (see Section 15.7.2) [54,55].

15.3.3 Group 3

Cockroach allergens from group 3 show high homology to insect hemolymph proteins [56]. Although Per a 3 isoallergenic variants display significant differences in skin reactivity, suggesting a high degree of polymorphism among these allergens, they are considered minor allergens in cockroach. A minor allergen from the German cockroach, Bla g 3, has also been identified [57]. Hemoglobins of the Diptera (insect) family Chironomidae are causative agents of asthma in patients living in regions where large swarms of nonbiting midges occur. Chi t 1, the hemoglobin from the European midge species (*Chironomus thummi*), represents the major allergenic component causing rhinitis, conjunctivitis, and bronchial asthma in exposed populations. There is considerable immunologic cross-reactivity between hemoglobins of the same and closely related Chironomidae species, suggesting that hemoglobins and hemocyanins of insects may also represent an important source of arthropod allergens (Table 15.1).

15.3.4 Group 4

Bla g 4 belongs to the family of proteins called lipocalins or calycins [58]. Apart from another insect lipocalin allergen in the biting reduviid *Triatoma protracta*, most of the known lipocalin allergens are of mammalian origin: Bos d 2 (cow); Can f 1 (2, 4, and 6) (dog); Cav p 1 (2, 3, and 6) (guinea pig); Equ c 1 (2) (horse); Fel d 4 (cat); Mes a 1 (Golden or Syrian hamster); Mus m 1 (mouse); Ory c 1 (4) (rabbit); Phod s 1 (Siberian hamster); and Rat n 1 (rat). The milk allergen β-lactoglobulin (Bos d 5) is also a lipocalin. The molecular structures of Bla g 4 and the *P. americana* homologue have been determined [59]. Lipocalins are very stable, and their structure consists of a C-terminal α-helix and a β-barrel enclosing an internal hydrophobic cavity that binds small ligands such as retinoids, glucocorticosteroids, and pheromones (Figure 15.2) [60]. In fact, a structural analysis of native Bla g 4 revealed tyramine and octopamine as ligands that might control pheromone production [61]. The homology of Bla g 4 with rodent urinary proteins raises the possibility of pheromone or lipid transport proteins being potential families of inhalant arthropod allergens. Immunohistochemical localization studies show that Bla g 4 is only expressed in the accessory glands of the male cockroach reproductive system (conglobate gland and utricles) and is transferred to the female during copulation. The study suggests that Bla g 4 has a reproductive function, and the allergen could be released from dried seminal secretions, spermatophores, or dead males into the environment [62].

15.3.5 Group 5

Bla g 5 is a major cockroach allergen that shares homology and three-dimensional structure with glutathione S-transferases (GSTs) (Figure 15.2) [63]. This enzymatic activity is associated to a detoxifying function, which has been speculated for Bla g 5. IgE antibody was bound to natural and recombinant Bla g 5 in 68% and 73% of subjects' sera, respectively [64]. A comparative study of the relative importance of five cockroach allergens revealed that Bla g 2 and Bla g 5 dominated the IgE antibody response to cockroach (54% and 37%, respectively, and up to 71% and 58% among sera with high IgE to cockroach extract [3.5–100 IU/mL]) [45].

15.3.6 Groups 6–8

These three allergen groups comprise proteins involved in muscle contraction: troponin C (group 6), tropomyosin (group 7), and myosin light chain (group 8) [65–68]. Bla g 6 and Bla g 8 have a calcium-dependent regulatory function based on the presence of EF-hand motifs, which are helix-loop-helix structural domains. Calcium binding to Bla g 6 induces changes in the molecular structure that affect IgE antibody binding [65]. A low IgE prevalence to both allergens was reported in the original cloning studies (~14%) [65]. However, higher prevalences to Bla g 6 were found among cockroach-allergic patients in the United States (44% for $n = 23$ and 66% in a subgroup of 15 subjects with CAP class ≥3) and in Korea (33%–46%) [31,69]. Troponins and tropomyosins include a diverse group of proteins with distinct isoforms found in muscle, brain, and nonmuscle tissue. Structurally, tropomyosins are elongated two-stranded proteins wound around each other with dimeric α-helical coiled structures along their length. The IgE prevalence to cockroach tropomyosins varies from 13% to 54% depending on the technique used to detect IgE antibody binding and the population studied [31,45,66–68]. The high degree of amino acid sequence identity of tropomyosins from different species explains part of the allergenic cross-reactivity among arthropods and mollusks (see Section 15.5.2).

15.3.7 Groups 9 and 10

Groups 9 and 10 comprise the enzymes arginine kinases and serine proteases, respectively [70,71]. Arginine kinases are involved in the metabolism of ATP, and serine proteases are proteolytic enzymes. Originally identified in *P. americana* [70], an arginine kinase allergen has also been reported from German cockroach in a Taiwanese population, using a combination of proteomic techniques and bioinformatic allergen database analysis, and in a U.S. population [31,72]. Additional IgE-binding proteins were also identified in the Taiwanese study, including the high molecular weight protein vitellogenin (which breaks down into fragments of up to 97 kDa), aldolase, enolase, and heat shock protein 70 (Hsp70) [72]. The relevance of these additional allergens in cockroach allergy needs to be further investigated.

15.3.8 Groups 11 and 12

These two groups of allergens comprise the enzymes α-amylases and chitinases, respectively. In the gastrointestinal tract, α-amylases hydrolyze polysaccharides to yield glucose and maltose, and chitinases hydrolyze chitin polymers [73]. An α-amylase was first reported as an allergen from *B. germanica* in Korea, with an IgE prevalence of 41% [74]. This allergen, Bla g 11, was found to be major in a group of 23 cockroach-allergic patients from the United States (57% IgE prevalence), which included a subgroup of highly allergic patients (CAP class $\geq$3) highly sensitized to Bla g 11 (73%) [31]. Both allergen groups were first reported as major allergens from *P. americana* in China, with IgE prevalences of 83% and 64% on immunoblots, respectively [73]. Bla g 11, together with Bla g 5 and Bla g 9, were found to be immunodominant regarding T-cell responses in cockroach-sensitized asthmatic individuals [75].

15.4 OTHER SOURCES OF INSECT ALLERGENS

The role of insects as producers of inhalant allergens has widely been reported and supported by data showing positive bronchial or nasal challenge. Table 15.1 shows a summary of insect species and their association to inhalant allergies. Airborne insect-derived particles include shed hairs, scales, excreta, and disintegrated body parts that contribute to amorphous dust. The composition of dust is influenced by geographical location, diligence and thoroughness of cleaning, and use of insecticides.

Dogs and cats contribute dander, hair, and body secretions to allergenic loads in household dust. Not widely known is the contribution of the common flea. When dogs and cats are present in the house, populations of the dog flea, *Ctenocephalides canis*, and cat flea, *C. felis*, can reach high levels. Most flea allergenicity has been attributed to bites from these insects. However, IgE antibodies to cat flea allergens were detected in 33.3% (16 of 48) of cat flea skin test positive sera of individuals in the Tampa Bay area of Florida, and the allergens were different from the antigenic components of the salivary secretions of the cat flea (Table 15.1). These results suggest a mode of sensitization other than by bite. Furthermore, using an in-house flea extract, flea allergens were quantified in eight house dust samples using RAST inhibition assays. Such evidence indicates that insects are a significant source of both indoor and outdoor inhalant allergens.

Additional inhalant allergens released by insects to the environment, not injected as venoms, have been described (Table 15.1). The Indianmeal moth *Plodia interpunctella* is a stored food pest in human dwellings and produces an arginine kinase (Plo i 1), and the first thioredoxin identified as an animal allergen, Plo i 2 (25% and 8% IgE prevalences, respectively) (Table 15.1). A major allergen from processionary caterpillar *Thaumetopoea pityocampa* has been identified that is recognized by 82% of patients clinically sensitive to caterpillar (Table 15.1). A relatively new inhalant allergy is associated with the multicolored Asian lady beetle or ladybug (*Harmonia axyridis*) (Table 15.1). This insect was repeatedly introduced into the United States between 1916 and 1990, as a biological control for aphids. The first report of allergy to Asian lady beetle was published in 1999 and describes two cases of allergic rhinoconjunctivitis (Table 15.1). *Harmonia axyridis* seeks refuge in homes during fall and winter, leading to patient sensitization and allergic symptoms including rhinitis, wheezing, urticaria, conjunctivitis, chronic cough, and asthma. Reports on lady beetle allergy come from St. Louis (Missouri), Appleton (Wisconsin), Louisville (Kentucky), West

Virginia, and Georgia, and a survey reveals positive responses in North Central, Mid-Atlantic, and New England states (Table 15.1). Five lady beetle proteins, with molecular weights of approximately 8.6, 21, 28, 31, and 75 kD, bind IgE antibody in Western blots. Partial protein sequences of purified Har a 1 (10 kD) and Har a 2 (55 kD), as well as the complete cDNA sequence encoding two additional lady beetle allergens (16.6 and a 30 kD), have been reported (Table 15.1). Further analysis of the allergens involved in Asian lady beetle allergy will help to better understand this novel inhalant allergy.

The presence in insects of highly expressed homologous proteins, such as microvillar components, arginine kinases, α-amylases, chitinases, serine proteases, GSTs, and muscle proteins, suggests that many insects have the potential to serve as sources of allergens if their populations reach high numbers, particularly in confined residential and occupational settings. The bedbug (*Cimex lectularius*) has become a major global indoor pest in the last two decades. Without adequate intervention, bedbug populations can reach very high levels. Its intimate association with humans and propensity to shelter in the bed would suggest that dead bedbugs, feces, and shed cuticles might sensitize people. Bedbug bites can cause severe local and systemic reactions, and IgE-mediated allergy to bedbug bites has been reported (Table 15.1). It is likely that bedbugs produce yet-to-be-identified inhalant allergens. Interestingly, bedbugs defecate histamine that also serves as an aggregation pheromone [76]. A recent study found large amounts of histamine in household dust in bedbug-infested homes but not in uninfested homes [77]. It remains to be determined whether house dust-associated bedbug histamine is involved in inhalant allergies.

15.5 COCKROACH ALLERGEN CROSS-REACTIVITY

15.5.1 Interspecific cross-reactivity among cockroaches

Allergen cross-reactivity refers to the concordance of IgE reactivity between two or more crude extracts or allergens from different species due to the presence of homologous proteins that share antibody binding epitopes. Skin test or *in vitro* test panels are unlikely to identify primary sources of sensitization without adequate histories and evidence of exposure. In the attempt to control allergic disease by reducing allergen exposure, it is necessary to minimize exposure to all sources of the sensitizing and the cross-reacting allergens.

Early clinical studies provided evidence that cross-reactivity occurs among homologous allergens from American, German, Madagascar (*Gromphadorhina portentosa*), Asian (*Blattella asahinai*), and Oriental cockroaches (reviewed in *Allergens and Allergen Immunotherapy*, Chapter 11, 4th edition [3]). An analysis of 45 antigens in *P. americana* and 29 antigens in *B. germanica* by crossed immunoelectrophoresis and immunoblots identified Per a 1 and Bla g 1 as cross-reactive homologous allergens [35]. A 70%–72% amino acid identity between these two allergens reveals the molecular basis of the allergenic cross-reactivity [37–40]. Similarly, homologous allergens among cockroach species (e.g., group 7) are known to be cross-reactive (Table 15.3). Other cockroach proteins have been cloned that share homology to German and American cockroach allergens and most likely also contribute to intercockroach species' cross-reactivity. For example, a *P. americana* protein homologous to Bla g 4 has been cloned (AY792948). However, these proteins are not yet present in the official WHO/IUIS Allergen Nomenclature Database. The Sub-Committee encourages submission of new allergens to the database (http:// www.allergen.org). Given the cross-reactivity between the German and American cockroaches, which share a relatively distant evolutionary relationship, it is expected that more closely related species to *B. germanica* (e.g., *B. asahinai*, *Supella longipalpa*) and *P. americana* (several *Periplaneta* and *Blatta* species) will also share homologous and cross-reactive allergens with their respective relatives (Table 15.2).

15.5.2 Cross-reactivity among cockroaches and other insects

Indoor, outdoor, and workplace exposure to large numbers of insect species in different geographic regions makes it extremely difficult to determine whether multiple sensitivities are explained by multiple exposures or by insect allergen cross-reactivity. From clinical and immunologic observations, allergy to a single arthropod is uncommon, and cross-reactivity can extend to foods and other arthropods. Arthropods that have been most studied as sources of allergens include crustaceans (shrimp, crayfish, crabs, lobsters), insects (caddisflies or "sedges," mayflies, moths and butterflies, fleas, chironomid midges, and cockroaches), and arachnids (mites). Several other arthropods, including houseflies, ants, spiders, locusts and grasshoppers, bees, and silverfish, cause sensitization either in the home or in occupational settings (Table 15.1). The term *pan-allergy*, sensitization to one or a few insects with allergenic similarities that may extend to other noninsect members of the phylum Arthropoda, defines this phenomenon [2].

Several reports in the literature prove cross-reactivity between allergens from cockroach and other species. IgE antibodies in patients' sera were shown to react with silverfish, cockroach, and/ or chironomid extracts in 30% of house dust mite-allergic patients in the Netherlands (Table 15.1). Tropomyosin, a protein involved in muscle contraction, is a cross-reactive allergen among members of the phyla Arthropoda and Mollusca. The arthropods producing allergenic tropomyosin include species from Crustacea (shrimp, crab, lobster, crawfish), Arachnida (dust mites), and Insecta (cockroaches, chironomids, silverfish). The Mollusca include Bivalvia (oysters, mussels, scallops, clams, pen shells), Gastropoda (snails, abalones, whelks), and Cephalopoda (squids, octopus, and cuttlefish). An insect tropomyosin from the silverfish *Lepisma saccharina*, Lep s 1, has been immunologically characterized and shows cross-reactivity with rPer a 7, the dust mite rDer p 10, and natural shrimp tropomyosin (Table 15.1). These invertebrate tropomyosins share approximately 80% amino acid sequence identity, whereas they are only ~45% homologous to human and edible meat (chicken, beef, pork, lamb, etc.) tropomyosins. This difference in homology may explain why humans do not develop allergies to edible meat tropomyosin. Interesting observations illustrate the clinical relevance of tropomyosin cross-reactivity. Exposure and sensitization to a particular food tropomyosin (dietary source) may lead to reactivity to aeroallergen exposure, and vice versa (e.g., due to immunotherapy) [3]. It is worth noting that as insects become more accepted as human food [78], cross-reactivities are expected to increase.

Termites produce proteins that could cross-react with cockroach allergens, due to the evolutionary relationship between both groups of insects [79]. In particular, the termite hemocyanin and tropomyosin orthologs of Bla g 3 and Bla g 7 were found to cross-react with cockroach allergens (Table 15.1). The tropomyosin allergen, Copt f 7, from the Formosan subterranean termite (*Coptotermes formosanus*) is listed in the WHO/IUIS Allergen Nomenclature Database with an IgE prevalence of 31%.

An interesting cross-reactivity has been described between GSTs from German cockroach (Bla g 5) and the helminth *Wuchereria bancrofti*, a major lymphatic filarial pathogen of humans, despite a low level of amino acid identity (30%) [80]. The GST from dust mite, Der p 8, also shows cross-reactivity with a cockroach homolog [81]. However, a lack of significant IgE cross-reactivity among four GSTs from cockroach (Bla g 5), mite (Der p 8 and Blo t 8), and *Ascaris* (Asc s 13) was observed in a study that also analyzed the three-dimensional structure of these allergens, in agreement with the low shared amino acid identity at the molecular surface [63].

Other cockroach allergens show cross-reactivity with arthropod homologs. The arginine kinases (group 9) share homology with Pen m 2 from giant tiger shrimp (*Penaeus monodon*), Bomb m 1 from silk moth (*Bombyx mori*), Der p 20 from house dust mite, and Plo i 1 from the Indianmeal moth, *P. interpunctella*. The arginine kinases from silk moth and American cockroach cross-react [82]. Inhibition experiments, using dust mite, cockroach, king prawn, lobster, and mussel extracts, suggest that arginine kinase is an invertebrate pan-allergen (Table 15.1). A myosin light chain from white pacific shrimp, Lit v 3, was identified as a major allergen that could potentially cross-react with the cockroach homolog [83]. Mealworms produce larval cuticle proteins that might be the dominant allergens in primary mealworm allergy, and cross-reactive allergens such as tropomyosin, arginine kinase, and myosin heavy chain [84]. α-Amylases from cockroach share approximately 50% amino acid identity with the group 4 mite homologs [74]. Other proteins from *P. americana* are homologous to the mite allergens from groups 2, 3 (trypsin), and 13 (fatty acid binding protein) (GenBank accession numbers AY792953, AY792954, and AY792955). Additional cross-reactivities among some of these proteins, not yet characterized as allergens, would be expected.

15.6 MECHANISMS ASSOCIATED WITH COCKROACH ALLERGEN SENSITIZATION

Several groups have investigated the underlying mechanisms of cockroach sensitization, including genetic factors, and innate and adaptive immunity. Anthony et al. observed that American cockroach extracts (lacking serine and aspartic proteinase activity) induced the release of a vascular permeability factor (VEGF) in bronchial airway epithelial cells causing endothelial barrier abnormalities and increased microvascular permeability [85]. The authors proposed a mechanism for increased sensitization to cockroach allergens by suggesting that this barrier breakdown facilitates allergen entry into the bronchial airways causing both sensitization and the allergic response. In contrast, Bhat et al. demonstrated that German cockroach extracts contain serine protease activity, presumably a homolog of Per a 10, which has a direct inflammatory effect upon airway epithelial cells [86]. Per a 10 biases dendritic cells toward type 2 by upregulating CD86 and reducing IL-12 secretions [87]. Cockroach proteases increase IL-8 expression in human bronchial epithelial cells via extracellular-signal-regulated kinase and activation of protease-activated receptors-2 (PAR-2), which are upregulated in respiratory epithelium from asthmatic patients [86,88]. Moreover, the IL-8 expression, dependent upon a serine protease activity, was not induced by endotoxin at levels present in cockroach extracts, even though endotoxin is capable of inducing airway inflammation and worsening asthma [86].

The involvement of a mannose receptor in mediating uptake of glycosylated allergens, such as Bla g 2, by dendritic cells has been reported [89]. The mannose receptor (MRC1/CD206) recognizes cockroach allergens and leads to macrophage polarization [90]. Cockroach extracts induced oxidative stress in human bronchial epithelial cells, and cyclooxygenase-2 (COX-2) was the most significantly upregulated gene related to this effect [91]. This study also reports that in a mouse model of asthma, COX-2 was regulated by microRNA (miR-155–3p), which could serve as a marker for diagnosis or therapeutic target of asthma. Activation of other receptors (e.g., toll-like receptor 2, aryl hydrocarbon receptor) and induction of release of cytokines and chemokines have been reported as mechanisms leading to cockroach allergy (reviewed in [92]). In addition, chitin is part of the exoskeleton of cockroaches and has an effect in adaptive and innate immune responses associated with allergy [93]. Thus, environmental control of allergen, chitin, and endotoxin levels may modify sensitization and allergic response.

At the molecular level, analysis of the antigenic surface of Bla g 2 has revealed new insights on IgE binding sites and interpatient variability of the allergic response [52–55] (Figure 15.2). T-cell epitopes from six *B. germanica* allergens have been identified among cockroach-allergic subjects, with a dominant response for Bla g 5 [94]. T-cell responses to Bla g allergens appeared uncorrelated with IgE responses. In another study, asthmatic and nonasthmatic cockroach-sensitized individuals exhibited similar Th2-polarized responses. However, asthmatic individuals had T-cell responses of higher magnitude and different allergen specificity [75]. The characterization of B- and T-cell epitopes in cockroach allergens will permit a better understanding of the immunopathogenic mechanisms involved in insect hypersensitivity.

15.7 DIAGNOSIS AND IMMUNOTHERAPY

15.7.1 Diagnosis

Skin testing using crude whole-body extracts is the gold standard to diagnose cockroach allergies. At present, cockroach extracts used for skin testing are not standardized, and those commercially marketed are prepared from whole-body extracts of the three most common species: American, German, and Oriental (Figure 15.1). Assays, using allergen-specific monoclonal antibodies, showed up to 200-fold differences in Bla g 1 levels in six commercial extracts, ranging from 4.7 to 1085 U/mL, whereas only two extracts contained detectable Bla g 2 (248 and 324 U/mL) [36]. Variability in content of Bla g 1, Bla g 2, and Bla g 5 has recently been reported as a determinant of *in vitro* IgE potency of cockroach extracts [31]. The lack of an immunodominant cockroach allergen hampers standardization of cockroach extracts. Serologic studies suggest that a cocktail of *B. germanica* allergens, Bla g 1, Bla g 2, Bla g 4, and Bla g 5, would diagnose 95% of U.S. patients with a cockroach allergy

[95]. The use of recombinant allergens that can be produced as pure proteins, using *in vitro* expression systems, should allow diagnosis of IgE sensitization to specific allergens in the future.

15.7.2 Immunotherapy

Allergen immunotherapy is effective for patients with insect sting hypersensitivity. However, at present, efficacy of cockroach immunotherapy is not well established (reviewed in [92,95]). In 1988, Kang et al. showed that allergen immunotherapy, using cockroach extracts in sensitive individuals, decreased symptom scores and medication requirements. It also increased specific IgG levels and decreased basophil histamine release in response to cockroach antigen [96]. A double-blind, placebo-controlled cockroach immunotherapy trial from India showed significant clinical improvement after 1 year and an increase of cockroach-specific IgG4 [97]. Wood et al. performed four pilot clinical trials of sublingual (SLIT) and subcutaneous (SCIT) immunotherapy with German cockroach extracts [98]. SCIT was immunologically more active than SLIT. Based on these results, the ICAC is currently conducting a subcutaneous cockroach immunotherapy trial in the United States. However, a lack of standardization of cockroach extracts is presently a strong limitation for assessing efficacy of immunotherapy. The U.S. Food and Drug Administration (FDA) has reported variability of commercially available cockroach allergen extracts in protein content, electrophoretic banding patterns, relative potency, and Bla g 2 levels [99]. Mindaye et al. quantified the levels of *B. germanica* allergens in cockroach commercial extracts by liquid chromatography coupled to multiple reactions monitoring mass spectrometry (LC-MRM MS) and found Bla g 1 and Bla g 3 in all extracts, but Bla g 5 and Bla g 8 were found in some extracts but not others [100]. Standards to measure allergens in settled dust samples and for standardization of allergy diagnostics have been developed by the FDA and the WHO [101]. Similarly, efforts to standardize cockroach extracts have been reported and will be necessary to properly develop effective immunotherapy for cockroach allergies [102,103]. A recent study showed that the content of three cockroach allergens in the extract and the subject's sensitization profile to eight recombinant cockroach allergens determine the *in vitro* IgE potency of the cockroach extract [31]. These two factors should be considered for the design and interpretation of cockroach clinical trials. The ongoing ICAC clinical trial has been designed to shed light onto the influence of these factors on the effectiveness of cockroach immunotherapy.

As with any other allergy, cockroach allergy therapy should be based on three approaches: (1) environmental control (avoidance) (see Section 15.8); (2) pharmacotherapy; and (3) immunotherapy with the appropriate allergens. The use of recombinant cockroach allergens is envisioned as a way to improve therapy for cockroach hypersensitivity. Benefits include better control of batch-to-batch variability and the assurance of representation of minor allergens in standard amounts. Additionally, immunotherapy with specific hypoallergenic recombinant allergens or peptides lacking IgE binding epitopes rather than crude allergen vaccine mixtures could prove to be a more effective regimen to avoid anaphylactic reactions. A recombinant Bla g 2 mutant, with reduced IgE antibody binding capacity and potential to modulate cytokines differently than the wild-type allergen, has been developed as a result of crystallographic studies mentioned in Section 15.3.2 and has potential therapeutic use [54,55]. However, specific immunotherapy with recombinant cockroach allergens has yet to be performed.

15.8 ENVIRONMENTAL CONTROL

Integrated pest management (IPM) is an effective way to control and reduce exposure to potentially harmful substances released by cockroaches (allergens, endotoxin, chitin) [10,104–107]. This strategy involves a combination of source reduction, abatement, and mitigation with the goal of reducing the ability of the environment to support pest infestations. The Joint Council of Allergy, Asthma and Immunology (a joint group of the American Academy of Allergy, Asthma and Immunology and the American College of Allergy, Asthma and Immunology) published a comprehensive document on "Environmental Assessment and Exposure Reduction of Cockroaches: A practice parameter" covering this topic [108]. This document acknowledges that a cutoff of 0.04 µg/g dust for Bla g 2 has been proposed as a threshold for sensitization, and 0.08 µg/g are levels associated with development of disease and symptoms. In New York City, Bla g 2 levels higher than 0.04 µg/g in the beds and kitchens of 4-year-old children were independently associated with cockroach-specific IgE [30], and 2 to 3 year olds with anticockroach and antimouse IgE were at increased risk of wheeze and atopy [26].

The specific tactics and expenses associated with multicomponent IPM programs are highly variable. While source elimination, the process of eradicating cockroach populations, is central to all programs, its implementation relative to mitigation and abatement efforts varies dramatically, as do the resources committed to suppressing cockroach infestations. For example, practical recommendations often consider mitigation, which involves the removal of facilitating factors (food, water, shelter, warmth, means of ingress, etc.), as the first step in an integrated intervention. Abatement then follows, which includes removing, treating, or isolating reservoirs of contaminants (air filtration, vacuuming or removal of carpeting, use of denaturing chemicals, removal of contaminated building materials), followed by pest control. There are several compelling reasons for reversing this order and starting all interventions with intensive pest control efforts, as also recognized in the Practice Parameter by Portnoy et al. [108]. First, as long as live cockroaches are present, they deposit fresh allergens as they defecate (e.g., Bla g 1, Bla g 2, endotoxin), molt (chitin), mate (Bla g 4), and die (all allergens). Second, although early studies with insecticide sprays highlighted the importance of mitigation (e.g., remedial sanitation) for effective pest control, recent studies using much more effective baits (see later in this section) conclude that baits can be highly effective as a stand-alone pest control intervention. For example, Arbes et al. conducted an IPM intervention that included providing professional cleaning, educating residents, instructing residents on how to use a HEPA vacuum cleaner, and controlling cockroach populations with baits [109]. While this intervention significantly reduced, and in many cases eliminated, cockroach infestations (and significantly reduced cockroach allergens in infested homes), it did not produce better results than intensive cockroach control alone without the mitigation and abatement components [110]. Finally, cockroach control is generally much less expensive and less time-consuming than mitigation and abatement, because the latter often include extensive cleaning, repairs, and even renovations. Therefore, limited resources should be directed to source control first, because ineffective pest control will compromise all the other more expensive interventions.

The first step in cockroach control is determining if cockroaches are present and where aggregations are located. This is best implemented with a combined thorough visual inspection for live cockroaches and signs of infestation and the overnight use of multiple sticky traps throughout the home. Some studies use only two or three traps in the kitchen, and this approach can easily miss substantial aggregations of cockroaches elsewhere in the home. The presence of live cockroaches is a clear indication of allergen exposure. However, allergen levels may still be significant without obvious presence of live cockroaches, and measurement of allergen levels provides an estimate of exposure and the need for abatement. Specific enzyme-linked immunoassays for Bla g 1 and Bla g 2 are used to monitor environmental cockroach exposure [36,95]. The goal is to keep contaminant exposure below threshold levels for adverse health effects (see Section 15.2).

Cockroaches can be controlled using a variety of insecticides formulated as baits, dusts, sprays, and aerosols. Organochlorine, organophosphate, and carbamate insecticides, which were extensively used in sprays against cockroaches, are no longer registered with the U.S. Environmental Protection Agency (EPA) for cockroach control indoors. Other classes of insecticides (namely pyrethroids and neonicotinoids), which disrupt the insect's nervous system, are used as residual insecticides in spray formulations. However, their use is not recommended in most residential settings because they deposit residues that may be contacted by children and pets. Moreover, most populations of the German cockroach are highly resistant to pyrethroid insecticides, significantly compromising their effectiveness. Many do-it-yourself aerosols and total release foggers (TRFs, "bug bombs") contain pyrethroids; they have marginal or no efficacy but cause the evolution of resistance and contaminate surfaces in the indoor environment [111]. Effective dusts include boric acid and diatomaceous earth (silica), but their use requires some skill, and they are often applied excessively and in improper locations. Biological approaches to environmental control are being researched but are still far from being commercially developed.

The effectiveness of pest control in reducing cockroaches and allergens is significantly influenced by the tactics used in the intervention. Gel baits are without a doubt the most effective and safest chemical approach in cockroach control. Their effectiveness stems from several biological, ecological, and toxicological characteristics: (1) Insecticides, like pharmaceuticals, are generally more bioavailable and effective by ingestion than by dermal contact. (2) More classes of insecticides with unique modes of action can be formulated in baits than in sprays, including novel approaches such as biopesticides and RNAi technology. (3) While resistance to insecticides in baits has been documented, it is generally lower than to insecticides in sprays, aerosols, and TRFs, and it can be managed through rotation of bait products with different modes of action. (4) Baits are applied near cockroach aggregation sites without disrupting and dispersing the cockroaches, as other formulations often do. (5) Baits contain attractants and feeding stimulants, whereas many spray formulations repel cockroaches so they have less contact with the insecticide. (6) Baits also can be placed in protected areas, away from children and pets. (7) Baits can be used in cluttered environments and even in relatively unsanitary conditions, whereas spray applications require some preparation by residents. (8) Overall, homes can be effectively treated with much less insecticide in bait form than in spray form. (9) All mobile stages of cockroaches must feed to grow and reproduce. Finally, (10) cockroaches engage in coprophagy (ingestion of feces within an aggregation) and other social feeding behaviors, so unmetabolized insecticide in their feces can kill other cockroaches within the resting aggregation.

Common insecticides in bait products include, among others, abamectin, boric acid, clothianidin, dinotefuran, emamectin benzoate, fipronil, hydramethylnon, indoxacarb, and pyriproxyfen. The availability of effective baits has revolutionized cockroach control and dramatically increased the effectiveness of interventions and allergen reduction. Cockroach population reductions of 95%–100% are common when baits are properly deployed and multiple sticky traps are used during the intervention to guide bait placement, determine amount, assess efficacy, and steer further actions [10,110,112]. Although baits have been shown to be highly effective, and cockroach control alone can significantly reduce cockroach allergens in infested homes [110,113], an integrated intervention should include cleaning, vacuuming, making repairs to eliminate water and hiding places, and improving sanitation (Table 15.4). The extent of cockroach allergen stability and allergen persistence in the environment following cockroach eradication measures is unknown, so thorough cleaning and vacuuming are especially recommended after cockroaches have been eliminated to remove cockroach allergen found in feces, cast cuticles, and body parts from the environment.

An ongoing debate in the environmental intervention community is the relative effectiveness of single interventions, designed to reduce a major pest (e.g., cockroaches) and the indoor allergens it produces, and multicomponent interventions (that integrate cleaning, remedial sanitation, air filtration, repairs, pest control, education, etc., and often target multiple indoor allergens). A recent review of single and multicomponent interventions concluded that results of both approaches are variable, and we know little about the contribution of specific approaches to multicomponent interventions [114]. A central concern, not addressed in this report, is how the effectiveness of environmental interventions is assessed, whether cockroach populations were monitored, and the durability and sustainability of the home-based intervention. Most interventions either subcontract the cockroach control to a pest control company or provide residents the tools to implement their own pest control; in both cases, little detail is disclosed on how the intervention was conducted and which and how much insecticide used. Personal experience, as well as a blinded study [112], demonstrate that these approaches frequently fail to reduce cockroach infestations in low-income communities. Moreover, most reports neither objectively assess nor report the effectiveness of cockroach control, often relying on resident or pest control technician testimonials instead of the standard unbiased use of multiple sticky traps. Because extensive allergen reduction can be accomplished only after cockroaches are substantially reduced or eradicated, the relative effectiveness of single and multicomponent interventions can

Table 15.4 Cockroach control measures

I. Chemical measures—Direct cockroach eradication

Note: All sprays and aerosols of organochlorine (chlordane), organophosphate (chlorpyrifos, diazinon, propetamphos), and carbamate (bendiocarb, propoxur) insecticides were banned by the U.S. Environmental Protection Agency from indoor use.

1. Sprays and aerosols: Pyrethrins, pyrethroids, neonicotinoids, and insect growth regulators (IGRs). High levels of resistance to pyrethroids. All except IGRs are not recommended for use in typical residential settings.

2. Total release foggers ("bug bombs"): Pyrethroids and synergists (e.g., piperonyl butoxide, PBO). High levels of resistance in cockroach populations. Should not be used in residential environments.

3. Dusts: Boric acid, diatomaceous earth. Effective, but difficult to use.

4. Repellents: Many essential oils available in do-it-yourself products. Limited data on their effectiveness at reducing cockroach populations.

5. Baits (gels, pastes, granules, stations): abamectin, boric acid, clothianidin, dinotefuran, emamectin benzoate, fipronil, hydramethylon, indoxacarb, and pyriproxifen. Most gel baits are highly effective if properly placed in many small dots near cockroach hiding places. There is some evidence of physiologic and behavioral resistance to baits, but both can be minimized and mitigated with rotations among baits with different modes of action.

II. Physical mitigation measures

A. Reduce access to food
   1. Store food in sealed containers
   2. Eliminate sources of organic debris
   3. Do not leave food exposed overnight

B. Reduce access to water
   1. Repair leaking faucets and pipes
   2. Wrap pipes to prevent condensation
   3. Eliminate damp areas beneath sinks
   4. Repair damp, damaged wood
   5. Service and clean water tray under the refrigerator

C. Improve ventilation by eliminating clutter beneath sinks

D. Eliminate hiding places and access points
   1. Caulk and seal cracks and crevices in foundations, walls, and cabinets
   2. Caulk around water pipes' entry into house and beneath sinks
   3. Eliminate clutter within household (e.g., remove all newspaper and magazine storage areas)
   4. Isolate and seal the refuse/garbage bin

be adequately assessed only when cockroach control has been shown to be highly effective using objective and unbiased assessment tools. Most early reports of cockroach interventions neglected to do so. For example, Sarpong et al., using several rooms in a college dormitory as a model for cockroach control studies, showed that Bla g 2 allergen levels of dust of 5.2 U/g could be reduced to 0.95 U/g following insecticide spray applications and regular vacuuming [115]. However, sustained decrease of cockroach allergens was difficult to achieve, and the levels, in this and other studies, remained above those reported to be clinically significant (reviewed in [95]). As pointed out by Gore and Schal, because the effectiveness of the cockroach intervention was not assessed, it is possible that live cockroaches continued to disseminate allergens in the dormitory rooms. Moreover, the relative contribution of the two interventions (pest control, cleaning) could not be discerned in this and many other multicomponent interventions. This early example of a cockroach intervention that is not sufficiently characterized is typical of many subsequent interventions. Some recent studies aiming to document that reduction in exposure can be associated with improvement in disease have begun to monitor cockroach populations to assess the effectiveness of the intervention, but two important shortcomings remain. First, some studies report extremely low baseline cockroach populations and low allergen levels, so the quantification of further pest reduction would require greater sensitivity (lower limit of detection) that can only be achieved with more traps placed in critical locations. Second, some recent pest interventions have adopted "integrated pest management" but with no further details on the specific tactics and intensity of each intervention. This oversight constitutes a significant barrier for transparent and unbiased critical assessment of the intervention.

The availability of effective baits (discussed earlier in this section) has dramatically changed cockroach interventions. Several single-component interventions have been reported, using only baits, coupled with cockroach population monitoring with sticky traps, and allergen quantification by ELISA [110,112,113]. The results, reviewed by Krieger et al. [116], are compelling and show that effective single pest control interventions can be effective in reducing cockroaches, allergens, and allergy symptoms, in stark contrast to the findings of the 2018 review [114]. Of particular significance are the recent findings by Rabito et al. that an intensive intervention with baits not only reduced cockroaches and allergens but also significantly improved clinical health outcomes for asthmatic children, including significant reductions in emergency department or unscheduled clinic visits, significantly improved FEV1 (forced expiratory volume in 1 second), and significantly fewer school days missed [113].

Given the high efficacy of properly implemented bait treatments, it is important to note several inadequacies in how they are treated in some reviews, meta-analyses, and even policy decisions [114,117]. First, pest control interventions that target different pests are often grouped as "multicomponent interventions," with the tacit expectation of equivalent outcomes with all pests. In fact, acaricides targeting house dust mites are not nearly as effective as baits targeting cockroaches, and it is nearly impossible to eradicate mite populations with pesticides alone. It is not surprising therefore that acaricide-based interventions have contributed little to allergen reductions and clinical outcomes. Second, the requirements in randomized controlled trials of blinding participants and study personnel, and of placebo controls, severely limit the number of studies included in reviews and meta-analyses. The requirement for randomized controlled trials, in itself, disqualifies many excellent entomological interventions on the effectiveness of innovative tactics for cockroach

control. Blinding participants is clearly required when they are the target of the intervention. But the target of cockroach interventions is the pest population, not participants, and blinding, while useful, is neither practical nor useful if unbiased assessment tools (e.g., sticky traps) are used to quantify effectiveness. Finally, placebo treatments with baits lacking insecticide are ill-advised, because they supplement the home environment with highly palatable cockroach food that can unintentionally increase the pest population.

Despite limited evidence, cockroach eradication and reduced exposure to cockroach allergens in infested structures could lead to improvements in asthma morbidity among cockroach-sensitized patients [108,116], reviewed by Gore et al. and Morgan et al. [118,119]. Nevertheless, as mentioned in Section 15.2, the relationships between cockroach allergen exposure, sensitization, and asthma are complex, as also highlighted in recent studies showing that higher indoor levels of pests and pest allergens, including from cockroaches, in early childhood may lower the risk of asthma in high-risk inner-city children [28].

SALIENT POINTS

1. Sensitization to indoor inhalant allergens is strongly associated with the development of asthma. In urban and inner-city areas, up to 80% of children with asthma may have IgE antibody to cockroach allergens.
2. Infestations of domiciliary cockroaches are largely dependent on housing conditions. The average American spends approximately 95% of time indoors in controlled environments that lead to continued low-dose allergen exposure, which may lead to sensitization in predisposed individuals.
3. Amorphous cockroach particles containing allergens are recognized as an important source of indoor allergens, together with dust mite particles.
4. Cross-reactivity of arthropod allergens can be identified among members of the taxonomic groups Crustacea, Arachnida, and Insecta, described as "pan-allergy."
5. Molecular cloning of cockroach and other insect allergens has provided the basis for investigating the relationship between allergen function/structure and allergenicity.
6. Currently, cockroach immunotherapy is based on the use of nonstandardized allergens with variable allergen content. Recombinant cockroach allergens are potential new tools for the future diagnosis and treatment of cockroach hypersensitivity.
7. The x-ray crystal structures of Bla g 2 alone and in combination with fragments of antibodies that interfere with IgE antibody binding revealed molecular features that contribute to allergenicity and antigenic determinants for design of hypoallergens.
8. Eradication of cockroaches and other insect infestations is essential to control inhalant insect allergic diseases.
9. The composition of environmental dust includes a wide range of components from the biosystem, and given the widespread distribution of insects in the world, their involvement in allergic reactions will continue to be of major social, economic, and medical importance.
10. Future directions for research should include the study of cockroach reduction strategies, development of specific assays to detect clinically relevant insect inhalant allergens, and measures to reduce exposure to environmental allergens (including patient education for pest management and the safe use of insecticides and nontoxic traps). The analysis of B- and

T-cell allergen epitopes involved in disease and the mechanisms of cockroach allergy will provide new insights for allergy treatment.

ACKNOWLEDGMENTS

Thanks to Dr. Ricki M. Helm for his contributions to cockroach allergy research and to previous versions of the chapter that evolved into the present one. Part of the research described in this chapter was supported by Indoor Biotechnologies, Inc., and by the National Institute of Allergy and Infectious Diseases of the National Institutes of Health under award number R01AI077653 (PI: AP), and by the Housing and Urban Development Healthy Homes program (award NCHHU0017-13 to CS). The content is solely the responsibility of the authors and does not necessarily represent the official views of the National Institutes of Health or the Department of Housing and Urban Development.

REFERENCES

1. Barletta B, Pini C. Does occupational exposure to insects lead to species-specific sensitization? *Allergy* 2003; 58: 868–870.
2. Panzani RC, Ariano R. Arthropods and invertebrates allergy (with the exclusion of mites): The concept of panallergy. *Allergy* 2001; 56(Suppl 69): 1–22.
3. Pomés A. Cockroach and other inhalant insect allergens. *Clin Allergy Immunol* 2008; 21: 183–200.
4. Bernton HS, Brown H. Insect allergy—Preliminary studies of the cockroach. *J Allergy Clin Immunol* 1964; 35: 506–513.
5. Pollart SM, Chapman MD, Fiocco GP, Rose G, Platts-Mills TA. Epidemiology of acute asthma: IgE antibodies to common inhalant allergens as a risk factor for emergency room visits. *J Allergy Clin Immunol* 1989; 83: 875–882.
6. Rosenstreich DL, Eggleston P, Kattan M et al. The role of cockroach allergy and exposure to cockroach allergen in causing morbidity among inner-city children with asthma. *N Engl J Med* 1997; 336: 1356–1363.
7. Arruda LK, Vailes LD, Ferriani VP, Santos AB, Pomés A, Chapman MD. Cockroach allergens and asthma. *J Allergy Clin Immunol* 2001; 107: 419–428.
8. Huss K, Adkinson NF, Jr., Eggleston PA, Dawson C, Van Natta ML, Hamilton RG. House dust mite and cockroach exposure are strong risk factors for positive allergy skin test responses in the Childhood Asthma Management Program. *J Allergy Clin Immunol* 2001; 107: 48–54.
9. Gruchalla RS, Pongracic J, Plaut M et al. Inner city asthma study: Relationships among sensitivity, allergen exposure, and asthma morbidity. *J Allergy Clin Immunol* 2005; 115: 478–485.
10. Schal C. Cockroaches. In: Hedges S, Moreland D, editors. *Handbook of Pest Control*. GIE Media, 2011: 150–291.
11. Kang B, Sulit N. A comparative study of prevalence of skin hypersensitivity to cockroach and house dust antigens. *Ann Allergy* 1978; 41: 333–336.
12. Gelber LE, Seltzer LH, Bouzoukis JK, Pollart SM, Chapman MD, Platts-Mills TA. Sensitization and exposure to indoor allergens as risk factors for asthma among patients presenting to hospital. *Am Rev Respir Dis* 1993; 147: 573–578.
13. Lewis SA, Weiss ST, Platts-Mills TA, Burge H, Gold DR. The role of indoor allergen sensitization and exposure in causing morbidity in women with asthma. *Am J Respir Crit Care Med* 2002; 165: 961–966.
14. Jung KH, Lovinsky-Desir S, Perzanowski M et al. Repeatedly high polycyclic aromatic hydrocarbon exposure and cockroach sensitization among inner-city children. *Environ Res* 2015; 140: 649–656.
15. Rabito FA, Carlson J, Holt EW, Iqbal S, James MA. Cockroach exposure independent of sensitization status and association with hospitalizations for asthma in inner-city children. *Ann Allergy Asthma Immunol* 2011; 106: 103–109.
16. Wisnivesky JP, Sampson H, Berns S, Kattan M, Halm EA. Lack of association between indoor allergen sensitization and asthma morbidity in inner-city adults. *J Allergy Clin Immunol* 2007; 120: 113–120.
17. Kakumanu ML, Maritz JM, Carlton JM, Schal C. Overlapping community compositions of gut and fecal microbiomes in lab-reared and field-collected German cockroaches. *Appl Environ Microbiol* 2018; 84(17): e01037–18.
18. Ahmad A, Ghosh A, Schal C, Zurek L. Insects in confined swine operations carry a large antibiotic resistant and potentially virulent enterococcal community. *BMC Microbiol* 2011; 11: 23.
19. Lai KM. Are cockroaches an important source of indoor endotoxins? *Int J Environ Res Public Health* 2017; 14(1): E91.
20. Chew GL, Higgins KM, Gold DR, Muilenberg ML, Burge HA. Monthly measurements of indoor allergens and the influence of housing type in a northeastern US city. *Allergy* 1999; 54: 1058–1066.
21. Cohn RD, Arbes SJ, Jr., Jaramillo R, Reid LH, Zeldin DC. National prevalence and exposure risk for cockroach allergen in U.S. households. *Environ Health Perspect* 2006; 114: 522–526.
22. de Blay F, Sanchez J, Hedelin G et al. Dust and airborne exposure to allergens derived from cockroach (*Blattella germanica*) in low-cost public housing in Strasbourg (France). *J Allergy Clin Immunol* 1997; 99: 107–112.
23. Mueller GA, Pedersen LC, Lih FB et al. The novel structure of the cockroach allergen Bla g 1 has implications for allergenicity and exposure assessment. *J Allergy Clin Immunol* 2013; 132: 1420–1426.
24. Sporik R, Squillace SP, Ingram JM, Rakes G, Honsinger RW, Platts-Mills TA. Mite, cat, and cockroach exposure, allergen sensitisation, and asthma in children: A case-control study of three schools. *Thorax* 1999; 54: 675–680.
25. Eggleston PA, Rosenstreich D, Lynn H et al. Relationship of indoor allergen exposure to skin test sensitivity in inner-city children with asthma. *J Allergy Clin Immunol* 1998; 102: 563–570.
26. Donohue KM, Al-alem U, Perzanowski MS et al. Anti-cockroach and anti-mouse IgE are associated with early wheeze and atopy in an inner-city birth cohort. *J Allergy Clin Immunol* 2008; 122: 914–920.
27. Lynch SV, Wood RA, Boushey H et al. Effects of early-life exposure to allergens and bacteria on recurrent wheeze and atopy in urban children. *J Allergy Clin Immunol* 2014; 134: 593–601.
28. O'Connor GT, Lynch SV, Bloomberg GR et al. Early-life home environment and risk of asthma among inner-city children. *J Allergy Clin Immunol* 2018; 141: 1468–1475.
29. Lee MF, Song PP, Hwang GY, Lin SJ, Chen YH. Sensitization to Per a 2 of the American cockroach correlates with more clinical severity among airway allergic patients in Taiwan. *Ann Allergy Asthma Immunol* 2012; 108: 243–248.
30. Chew GL, Perzanowski MS, Canfield SM et al. Cockroach allergen levels and associations with cockroach-specific IgE. *J Allergy Clin Immunol* 2008; 121: 240–245.

31. Glesner J, Filep S, Vailes LD et al. Allergen content in German cockroach extracts and sensitization profiles to a new expanded set of cockroach allergens determine *in vitro* extract potency for IgE reactivity. *J Allergy Clin Immunol* 2019 Apr; 143(4): 1474–1481.

32. Harrison MC, Jongepier E, Robertson HM et al. Hemimetabolous genomes reveal molecular basis of termite eusociality. *Nat Ecol Evol* 2018; 2: 557–566.

33. Li S, Zhu S, Jia Q et al. The genomic and functional landscapes of developmental plasticity in the American cockroach. *Nat Commun* 2018; 9: 1008.

34. Twarog FJ, Picone FJ, Strunk RS, So J, Colten HR. Immediate hypersensitivity to cockroach. Isolation and purification of the major antigens. *J Allergy Clin Immunol* 1977; 59: 154–160.

35. Schou C, Lind P, Fernández-Caldas E, Lockey RF, Lowenstein H. Identification and purification of an important cross-reactive allergen from American (*Periplaneta americana*) and German (*Blattella germanica*) cockroach. *J Allergy Clin Immunol* 1990; 86: 935–946.

36. Pollart SM, Mullins DE, Vailes LD et al. Identification, quantitation, and purification of cockroach allergens using monoclonal antibodies. *J Allergy Clin Immunol* 1991; 87: 511–521.

37. Helm R, Cockrell G, Stanley JS, Brenner RJ, Burks W, Bannon GA. Isolation and characterization of a clone encoding a major allergen (Bla g Bd90K) involved in IgE-mediated cockroach hypersensitivity. *J Allergy Clin Immunol* 1996; 98: 172–180.

38. Pomés A, Melén E, Vailes LD, Retief JD, Arruda LK, Chapman MD. Novel allergen structures with tandem amino acid repeats derived from German and American cockroach. *J Biol Chem* 1998; 273: 30801–30807.

39. Melén E, Pomés A, Vailes LD, Arruda LK, Chapman MD. Molecular cloning of Per a 1 and definition of the cross-reactive Group 1 cockroach allergens. *J Allergy Clin Immunol* 1999; 103: 859–864.

40. Wu CH, Wang NM, Lee MF, Kao CY, Luo SF. Cloning of the American cockroach Cr-PII allergens: Evidence for the existence of cross-reactive allergens between species. *J Allergy Clin Immunol* 1998; 101: 832–840.

41. Randall TA, Perera L, London RE, Mueller GA. Genomic, RNAseq, and molecular modeling evidence suggests that the major allergen domain in insects evolved from a homodimeric origin. *Genome Biol Evol* 2013; 5: 2344–2358.

42. Pomés A, Vailes LD, Helm RM, Chapman MD. IgE reactivity of tandem repeats derived from cockroach allergen, Bla g 1. *Eur J Biochem* 2002; 269: 3086–3092.

43. Gore JC, Schal C. Gene expression and tissue distribution of the major human allergen Bla g 1 in the German cockroach, *Blattella germanica* L. (Dictyoptera: Blattellidae). *J Med Entomol* 2004; 41: 953–960.

44. Gore JC, Schal C. Expression, production and excretion of Bla g 1, a major human allergen, in relation to food intake in the German cockroach, *Blattella germanica*. *Med Vet Entomol* 2005; 19: 127–134.

45. Satinover SM, Reefer AJ, Pomés A, Chapman MD, Platts-Mills TA, Woodfolk JA. Specific IgE and IgG antibody-binding patterns to recombinant cockroach allergens. *J Allergy Clin Immunol* 2005; 115: 803–809.

46. Arruda LK, Vailes LD, Mann BJ et al. Molecular cloning of a major cockroach (*Blattella germanica*) allergen, Bla g 2. Sequence homology to the aspartic proteases. *J Biol Chem* 1995; 270: 19563–19568.

47. Chapman MD, Wunschmann S, Pomés A. Proteases as Th2 adjuvants. *Curr Allergy Asthma Rep* 2007; 7: 363–367.

48. Gustchina A, Li M, Wünschmann S, Chapman MD, Pomés A, Wlodawer A. Crystal structure of cockroach allergen Bla g 2, an unusual zinc binding aspartic protease with a novel mode of self-inhibition. *J Mol Biol* 2005; 348: 433–444.

49. Wünschmann S, Gustchina A, Chapman MD, Pomés A. Cockroach allergen Bla g 2: An unusual aspartic proteinase. *J Allergy Clin Immunol* 2005; 116: 140–145.

50. Pomés A, Chapman MD, Vailes LD, Blundell TL, Dhanaraj V. Cockroach allergen Bla g 2: Structure, function, and implications for allergic sensitization. *Am J Respir Crit Care Med* 2002; 165: 391–397.

51. Pomés A. Intrinsic properties of allergens and environmental exposure as determinants of allergenicity. *Allergy* 2002; 57: 673–679.

52. Li M, Gustchina A, Alexandratos J et al. Crystal structure of a dimerized cockroach allergen Bla g 2 complexed with a monoclonal antibody. *J Biol Chem* 2008; 283: 22806–22814.

53. Li M, Gustchina A, Glesner J et al. Carbohydrates contribute to the interactions between cockroach allergen Bla g 2 and a monoclonal antibody. *J Immunol* 2011; 186: 333–340.

54. Glesner J, Wunschmann S, Li M et al. Mechanisms of allergen-antibody interaction of cockroach allergen Bla g 2 with monoclonal antibodies that inhibit IgE antibody binding. *PLOS ONE* 2011; 6: e22223.

55. Woodfolk JA, Glesner J, Wright PW et al. Antigenic determinants of the bilobal cockroach allergen Bla g 2. *J Biol Chem* 2016; 291: 2288–2301.

56. Wu CH, Lee MF, Liao SC, Luo SF. Sequencing analysis of cDNA clones encoding the American cockroach Cr-PI allergens. Homology with insect hemolymph proteins. *J Biol Chem* 1996; 271: 17937–17943.

57. Khurana T, Collison M, Chew FT, Slater JE. Bla g 3: A novel allergen of German cockroach identified using cockroach-specific avian single-chain variable fragment antibody. *Ann Allergy Asthma Immunol* 2014; 112: 140–145.

58. Arruda LK, Vailes LD, Hayden ML, Benjamin DC, Chapman MD. Cloning of cockroach allergen, Bla g 4, identifies ligand binding proteins (or calycins) as a cause of IgE antibody responses. *J Biol Chem* 1995; 270: 31196–31201.

59. Tan YW, Chan SL, Ong TC et al. Structures of two major allergens, Bla g 4 and Per a 4, from cockroaches and their IgE binding epitopes. *J Biol Chem* 2009; 284: 3148–3157.

60. Flower DR. The lipocalin protein family: Structure and function. *Biochem J* 1996; 318: 1–14.

61. Offermann LR, Chan SL, Osinski T et al. The major cockroach allergen Bla g 4 binds tyramine and octopamine. *Mol Immunol* 2014; 60: 86–94.

62. Fan Y, Gore JC, Redding KO, Vailes LD, Chapman MD, Schal C. Tissue localization and regulation by juvenile hormone of human allergen Bla g 4 from the German cockroach, *Blattella germanica* (L.). *Insect Mol Biol* 2005; 14: 45–53.

63. Mueller GA, Pedersen LC, Glesner J et al. Analysis of glutathione S-transferase allergen cross-reactivity in a North American population: Relevance for molecular diagnosis. *J Allergy Clin Immunol* 2015; 136: 1369–1377.

64. Arruda LK, Vailes LD, Platts-Mills TA, Hayden ML, Chapman MD. Induction of IgE antibody responses by glutathione S-transferase from the German cockroach (*Blattella germanica*). *J Biol Chem* 1997; 272: 20907–20912.

65. Hindley J, Wünschmann S, Satinover SM et al. Bla g 6: A troponin C allergen from *Blattella germanica* with IgE binding calcium dependence. *J Allergy Clin Immunol* 2006; 117: 1389–1395.

66. Asturias JA, Gomez-Bayon N, Arilla MC et al. Molecular characterization of American cockroach tropomyosin (*Periplaneta americana* allergen 7), a cross-reactive allergen. *J Immunol* 1999; 162: 4342–4348.

67. Santos AB, Chapman MD, Aalberse RC et al. Cockroach allergens and asthma in Brazil: Identification of tropomyosin as a major allergen with potential cross-reactivity with mite and shrimp allergens. *J Allergy Clin Immunol* 1999; 104: 329–337.

68. Jeong KY, Lee J, Lee IY, Ree HI, Hong CS, Yong TS. Allergenicity of recombinant Bla g 7, German cockroach tropomyosin. *Allergy* 2003; 58: 1059–1063.

69. Un S, Jeong KY, Yi MH, Kim CR, Yong TS. IgE binding epitopes of Bla g 6 from German cockroach. *Protein Pept Lett* 2010; 17: 1170–1176.

70. Sookrung N, Chaicumpa W, Tungtrongchitr A et al. *Periplaneta americana* arginine kinase as a major cockroach allergen among Thai patients with major cockroach allergies. *Environ Health Perspect* 2006; 114: 875–880.

71. Sudha VT, Arora N, Gaur SN, Pasha S, Singh BP. Identification of a serine protease as a major allergen (Per a 10) of *Periplaneta americana*. *Allergy* 2008; 63: 768–776.

72. Chuang JG, Su SN, Chiang BL, Lee HJ, Chow LP. Proteome mining for novel IgE-binding proteins from the German cockroach (*Blattella germanica*) and allergen profiling of patients. *Proteomics* 2010; 10: 3854–3867.

73. Fang Y, Long C, Bai X et al. Two new types of allergens from the cockroach, *Periplaneta americana*. *Allergy* 2015; 70: 1674–1678.

74. Jeong KY, Kim CR, Park J, Han IS, Park JW, Yong TS. Identification of novel allergenic components from German cockroach fecal extract by a proteomic approach. *Int Arch Allergy Immunol* 2013; 161: 315–324.

75. Dillon MB, Schulten V, Oseroff C et al. Different Bla-g T cell antigens dominate responses in asthma versus rhinitis subjects. *Clin Exp Allergy* 2015; 45: 1856–1867.

76. Gries R, Britton R, Holmes M, Zhai H, Draper J, Gries G. Bed bug aggregation pheromone finally identified. *Angew Chem Int Ed Engl* 2015; 54: 1135–1138.

77. DeVries ZC, Santangelo RG, Barbarin AM, Schal C. Histamine as an emergent indoor contaminant: Accumulation and persistence in bed bug infested homes. *PLOS ONE* 2018; 13: e0192462.

78. Fischer ARH, Steenbekkers LPAB. All insects are equal, but some insects are more equal than others. *Br Food J* 2018; 120: 852–863.

79. Mattison CP, Khurana T, Tarver MR et al. Cross-reaction between Formosan termite (*Coptotermes formosanus*) proteins and cockroach allergens. *PLOS ONE* 2017; 12: e0182260.

80. Santiago HC, Leevan E, Bennuru S et al. Molecular mimicry between cockroach and helminth glutathione S-transferases promotes cross-reactivity and cross-sensitization. *J Allergy Clin Immunol* 2012; 130: 248–256.

81. Huang CH, Liew LM, Mah KW, Kuo IC, Lee BW, Chua KY. Characterization of glutathione S-transferase from dust mite, Der p 8 and its immunoglobulin E cross-reactivity with cockroach glutathione S-transferase. *Clin Exp Allergy* 2006; 36: 369–376.

82. Liu Z, Xia L, Wu Y, Xia Q, Chen J, Roux KH. Identification and characterization of an arginine kinase as a major allergen from silkworm (*Bombyx mori*) larvae. *Int Arch Allergy Immunol* 2009; 150: 8–14.

83. Ayuso R, Grishina G, Bardina L et al. Myosin light chain is a novel shrimp allergen, Lit v 3. *J Allergy Clin Immunol* 2008; 122: 795–802.

84. Broekman HCHP, Knulst AC, den Hartog Jager CF et al. Primary respiratory and food allergy to mealworm. *J Allergy Clin Immunol* 2017; 140: 600–603.

85. Antony AB, Tepper RS, Mohammed KA. Cockroach extract antigen increases bronchial airway epithelial permeability. *J Allergy Clin Immunol* 2002; 110: 589–595.

86. Bhat RK, Page K, Tan A, Hershenson MB. German cockroach extract increases bronchial epithelial cell interleukin-8 expression. *Clin Exp Allergy* 2003; 33: 35–42.

87. Goel C, Govindaraj D, Singh BP, Farooque A, Kalra N, Arora N. Serine protease Per a 10 from *Periplaneta americana* bias dendritic cells towards type 2 by upregulating CD86 and low IL-12 secretions. *Clin Exp Allergy* 2012; 42: 412–422.

88. Page K, Strunk VS, Hershenson MB. Cockroach proteases increase IL-8 expression in human bronchial epithelial cells via activation of protease-activated receptor (PAR)-2 and extra-cellular-signal-regulated kinase. *J Allergy Clin Immunol* 2003; 112: 1112–1118.

89. Royer PJ, Emara M, Yang C et al. The mannose receptor mediates the uptake of diverse native allergens by dendritic cells and determines allergen-induced T cell polarization through modulation of IDO activity. *J Immunol* 2010; 185: 1522–1531.

90. Zhou Y, Do DC, Ishmael FT et al. Mannose receptor modulates macrophage polarization and allergic inflammation through miR-511–3p. *J Allergy Clin Immunol* 2018; 141: 350–364.

91. Qiu L, Zhang Y, Do DC et al. miR-155 modulates cockroach allergen- and oxidative stress-induced cyclooxygenase-2 in asthma. *J Immunol* 2018; 201: 916–929.

92. Pomés A, Mueller GA, Randall TA, Chapman MD, Arruda LK. New insights into cockroach allergens. *Curr Allergy Asthma Rep* 2017; 17: 25.

93. Reese TA, Liang HE, Tager AM et al. Chitin induces accumulation in tissue of innate immune cells associated with allergy. *Nature* 2007; 447: 92–96.

94. Oseroff C, Sidney J, Tripple V et al. Analysis of T cell responses to the major allergens from German cockroach: Epitope specificity and relationship to IgE production. *J Immunol* 2012; 189: 679–688.

95. Arruda LK, Ferriani VP, Vailes LD, Pomés A, Chapman MD. Cockroach allergens: Environmental distribution and relationship to disease. *Curr Allergy Asthma Rep* 2001; 1: 466–473.

96. Kang BC, Johnson J, Morgan C, Chang JL. The role of immunotherapy in cockroach asthma. *J Asthma* 1988; 25: 205–218.

97. Srivastava D, Gaur SN, Arora N, Singh BP. Clinico-immunological changes post-immunotherapy with *Periplaneta americana*. *Eur J Clin Invest* 2011; 41: 879–888.

98. Wood RA, Togias A, Wildfire J et al. Development of cockroach immunotherapy by the Inner-City Asthma Consortium. *J Allergy Clin Immunol* 2014; 133: 846–852.

99. Patterson ML, Slater JE. Characterization and comparison of commercially available German and American cockroach allergen extracts. *Clin Exp Allergy* 2002; 32: 721–727.

100. Mindaye ST, Spiric J, David NA, Rabin RL, Slater JE. Accurate quantification of 5 German cockroach (GCr) allergens in complex extracts using multiple reaction monitoring mass spectrometry (MRM MS). *Clin Exp Allergy* 2017; 47: 1661–1670.

101. Filep S, Tsay A, Vailes LD et al. Specific allergen concentration of WHO and FDA reference preparations measured using a multiple allergen standard. *J Allergy Clin Immunol* 2012; 129: 1408–1410.

102. Slater JE, James R, Pongracic JA et al. Biological potency of German cockroach allergen extracts determined in an inner city population. *Clin Exp Allergy* 2007; 37: 1033–1039.

103. Khurana T, Dobrovolskaia E, Shartouny JR, Slater JE. Multiplex assay for protein profiling and potency measurement of German cockroach allergen extracts. *PLOS ONE* 2015; 10: e0140225.

104. Schal C, Hamilton RL. Integrated suppression of synanthropic cockroaches. *Annu Rev Entomol* 1990; 35: 521–551.

105. Nalyanya G, Gore JC, Linker HM, Schal C. German cockroach allergen levels in North Carolina schools: Comparison of integrated pest management and conventional cockroach control. *J Med Entomol* 2009; 46: 420–427.

106. Kass D, McKelvey W, Carlton E et al. Effectiveness of an integrated pest management intervention in controlling cockroaches, mice, and allergens in New York City public housing. *Environ Health Perspect* 2009; 117: 1219–1225.

107. Wang C, Bennett GW. Cost and effectiveness of community-wide integrated pest management for German cockroach, cockroach allergen, and insecticide use reduction in low-income housing. *J Econ Entomol* 2009; 102: 1614–1623.

108. Portnoy J, Chew GL, Phipatanakul W et al. Environmental assessment and exposure reduction of cockroaches: A practice parameter. *J Allergy Clin Immunol* 2013; 132: 802–808.

109. Arbes SJ, Jr., Sever M, Archer J et al. Abatement of cockroach allergen (Bla g 1) in low-income, urban housing: A randomized controlled trial. *J Allergy Clin Immunol* 2003; 112: 339–345.

110. Arbes SJ, Jr., Sever M, Mehta J et al. Abatement of cockroach allergens (Bla g 1 and Bla g 2) in low-income, urban housing: Month 12 continuation results. *J Allergy Clin Immunol* 2004; 113: 109–114.

111. DeVries ZC, Santangelo RG, Crissman J, Mick R, Schal C. Exposure risks and ineffectiveness of total release foggers (TRFs) used for cockroach control in residential settings. *BMC Public Health* 2019; 19: 96.

112. Sever ML, Arbes SJ, Jr., Gore JC et al. Cockroach allergen reduction by cockroach control alone in low-income urban homes: A randomized control trial. *J Allergy Clin Immunol* 2007; 120: 849–855.

113. Rabito FA, Carlson JC, He H, Werthmann D, Schal C. A single intervention for cockroach control reduces cockroach exposure and asthma morbidity in children. *J Allergy Clin Immunol* 2017; 140: 565–570.

114. Leas BF, D'Anci KE, Apter AJ, Bryant-Stephens T, Schoelles K, Umscheid CA. *Effectiveness of indoor allergen reduction in management of asthma. Comparative effectiveness review No. 201. (Prepared by the ECRI Institute-Penn Medicine Evidence-based Practice Center under Contract No. 290-2015-0005-I).* Report of the Effective Health Care Program.

115. Sarpong SB, Wood RA, Eggleston PA. Short-term effects of extermination and cleaning on cockroach allergen Bla g 2 in settled dust. *Ann Allergy Asthma Immunol* 1996; 76: 257–260.

116. Krieger J, Jacobs DE, Ashley PJ et al. Housing interventions and control of asthma-related indoor biologic agents: A review of the evidence. *J Public Health Manag Pract* 2010; 16: S11–S20.

117. Gold DR, Adamkiewicz G, Arshad SH et al. NIAID, NIEHS, NHLBI, and MCAN Workshop Report: The indoor environment and childhood asthma-implications for home environmental intervention in asthma prevention and management. *J Allergy Clin Immunol* 2017; 140: 933–949.

118. Gore JC, Schal C. Cockroach allergen biology and mitigation in the indoor environment. *Annu Rev Entomol* 2007; 52: 439–463.

119. Morgan WJ, Crain EF, Gruchalla RS et al. Results of a home-based environmental intervention among urban children with asthma. *N Engl J Med* 2004; 351: 1068–1080.

120. Wei JF, Yang H, Li D, Gao P, He S. Preparation and identification of Per a 5 as a novel American cockroach allergen. *Mediators Inflamm* 2014, 2014: 591468.

121. Sookrung N, Reamtong O, Poolphol R et al. Glutathione S-transferase (GST) of American cockroach, *Periplaneta americana*: Classes, isoforms, and allergenicity. *Sci Rep* 2018; 8: 484.

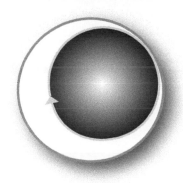

16 Mammalian allergens

Tuomas Virtanen and Marja Rytkönen-Nissinen
University of Eastern Finland

CONTENTS

16.1 INTRODUCTION

People come into contact with animals in many different occupations and activities. Household animals are significant sources of allergens in the indoor environment. Exposure to these allergens is usually perennial and not limited to immediate contact with the animals.

Mammalian inhalant allergens are especially associated with severe allergic disorders, including asthma [1,2]. If children are cosensitized to both cat and dog allergens, the condition is associated with increased cat Fel d 1– and dog Can f 1–specific IgE levels and more frequent symptoms than sensitization to the allergens of one animal only [3]. The likelihood of having allergic symptoms to cat or dog at age 16 years increases depending on the level of polysensitization, i.e., the number of IgE-recognized cat or dog allergens in early childhood [3].

Almost all important mammalian respiratory allergens belong to the lipocalin family of proteins, the major exception being cat Fel d 1 [4]. Despite all accumulated data on the characteristics of lipocalin allergens, causes for their allergenic capacity remain enigmatic [4,5]. In asthmatic children sensitized to mammals, sensitization to three or more lipocalin allergens is associated with severe asthma [6]. In dog allergy, sensitization to lipocalin allergens is a characteristic feature [7].

16.2 TAXONOMY OF MAMMALS

Figure 16.1 shows the condensed taxonomy of 10 mammals that are sources of allergens. Sensitization also occurs to other members of

the order Cetartiodactyla (e.g., reindeer, *Rangifer tarandus*, family Cervidae, and pig, *Sus scrofa domestica*, family Suidae). Several members of the family Felidae, in addition to the house cat, are also possible sources of allergens. Hair extracts from animal members of Felidae other than cat contain allergens that are similar to and IgE cross-react with the house cat allergen, Fel d 1. Although mouse, rat, hamster, and guinea pig are the only rodents included in the current Allergen Nomenclature database (ANDB) by the World Health Organization/International Union of Immunological Societies (WHO/IUIS) Allergen Nomenclature Sub-Committee (http://www.allergen.org), other members of the order, such as gerbils (family Muridae), cause allergy.

16.3 HUMAN CONTACT WITH OTHER MAMMALS

People come into direct contact with mammalian animals in multiple ways. Household pets, especially cats and dogs, are found in many (30%–40%) homes in industrialized countries. Consequently, high levels of Can f 1 or Fel d 1 allergens occur in the homes of dog and cat owners. The levels are substantially lower in the homes without pets [8].

The effects of exposure to inhalant animal allergens depend on a complex array of host-related factors, such as epithelial barriers, innate and adaptive immunity, and genetics, as well as environmental factors. Therefore, high levels of exposure may lead to allergen-specific tolerance: the highest rate of sensitization in children exposed to Fel d 1 was observed with "intermediate"

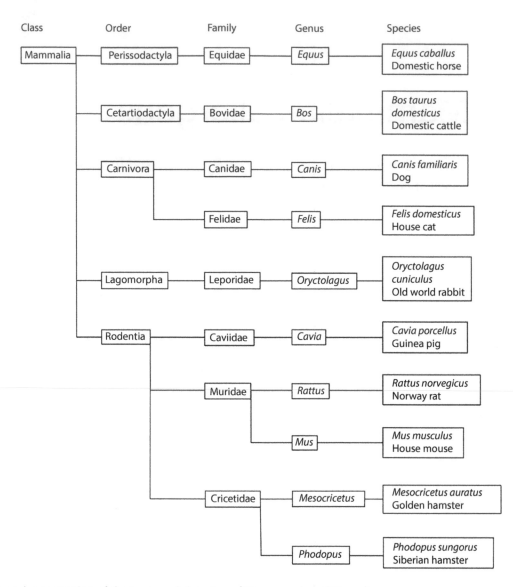

Figure 16.1 Condensed presentation of the taxonomic location of 10 mammals emitting allergens.

levels of the allergen [9]. This suggests that the dose-response relationship between exposure to cat and sensitization is bell-shaped. The protective effect is hypothetically due to a modified T-helper type 2 (Th2) response ("healthy immune response") involving the synthesis of specific IgG4. Accordingly, a recent study found that cat-allergic adult cat owners (chronic allergen exposure) had significantly higher levels of serum Fel d 1– and Fel d 4–specific IgG4 and lower sensitization than cat-allergic adults without a pet cat [10]. However, nonallergic adults with or without a cat also had low levels of specific IgG4. In an experimental human study of nasal neoantigen exposure, specific IgE demonstrated a bell-shaped dose-response, while the specific IgG response increased with increasing exposure [11]. There are also studies that provide no evidence for the protective effect of high exposure to mammalian allergens. This may reflect the multifaceted nature of the nonallergic state, such as immunity, age, genetics, and several exposure-related factors. Discussion on the development of the allergen-specific antibody response is continuing [12–14].

Exposure to pet allergens is not only limited to direct contact. Dog and cat allergens adhere to clothing, and they are consistently found in homes without pets as well as in public buildings, including schools and day care centers, and public transport vehicles. The concentrations are low but may be sufficient to cause sensitization and symptoms in sensitized persons.

Mice, hamsters, guinea pigs, and gerbils are also popular household pets, and handling the pets and cleaning their cages expose their owners to allergens. The presence of rodent allergens in the home depends not only on the presence of pets but also on the living conditions: mouse Mus m 1 and rat Rat n 1 are detectable in apartments infested with these animals. In U.S. studies, 20%–25% of inner-city children with asthma show sensitization to mouse and rat allergens. Keeping guinea pigs as pets is associated with a more than a threefold increased risk of atopic eczema, an effect not seen with other pets such as cats, dogs, or hamsters. Rodent bites have been reported to cause anaphylaxis, whereas it is not common with other mammals.

Sensitization associated with the handling of laboratory animals is a worldwide occupational problem. The exposure occurs through the respiratory tract, conjunctiva, and skin contact. One review of seven studies found that 15.6% of workers in laboratory animal facilities had work-related symptoms, and 22.5% were skin prick tests positive to animal allergens [15]. The common laboratory animals (mouse, rat, guinea pig, hamster, rabbit, and dog) appear to be equally potent sensitizers. The level of exposure varies according to the task. The highest concentrations of airborne allergens are encountered during the emptying and cleaning of the cages. However, several exposure factors are incompletely understood, for example, whether mean or peak exposures are the most relevant for sensitization [16]. One study suggests that both the level and variability of mouse allergen exposure are associated with specific immunophenotypes in the exposed workers [17].

An example of a work-related allergy caused by domestic animals is occupational asthma in Finnish dairy farmers. An interesting feature is the prolonged exposure time (median, 22 years) before cattle asthma becomes clinically evident. In contrast, symptoms of laboratory animal allergies appear within 2–3 years of exposure in 70%–80% of cases.

Horse allergy is a health problem because of horseback riding as a hobby or occupation. Sensitization to a variety of allergens associated with horses is also a concern. These allergens include those derived from the feeding of horses and allergens, in addition to horse, within barns and stables.

16.4 MOLECULAR CHARACTERISTICS OF MAMMALIAN ALLERGENS

16.4.1 Protein families of mammalian allergens

16.4.1.1 LIPOCALINS

Lipocalins are a large protein family (https://prosite.expasy.org/PS00213) comprising proteins from vertebrate and invertebrate animals, plants, and bacteria. In addition to mammalian respiratory allergens, the family contains a milk allergen, Bos d 5 (β-lactoglobulin), and arthropodan lipocalins, cockroach allergens Bla g 4 and Per a 4, a "kissing bug" (*Triatoma protracta)* allergen Tria p 1, and a pigeon tick (*Argas reflexus*) allergen Arg r 1. Lipocalins form, together with fatty acid–binding proteins, avidins, triabin, and a group of metalloproteinase inhibitors, the calycin superfamily [18]. A protein should fulfill the requirements for sequence homology, biological function, and structural similarity to be included in the family (https://prosite.expasy.org/PDOC00187).

The sequential length of lipocalins is 160–230 amino acids, the average predicted molecular mass being about 20 kDa (without posttranslational modifications) [18]. The overall amino acid identity between lipocalins is low, at the level of 20%–30%. In some cases, the sequential identity among animal species can be much higher (Table 16.1). For example, dog Can f 1 exhibits a 61% identity with human lipocalin-1 (von Ebner gland protein/tear lipocalin), and human epididymal-specific lipocalin-9 exhibits identities about 55% with several nonprimate mammalian proteins (analyzed in UniProt Knowledgebase (UniProtKB), a hub for information on proteins, with the Basic Local Alignment Search Tool (BLAST; https://www.uniprot.org/blast/).

Lipocalins contain large structurally conserved regions (SCRs; Figure 16.2) in defined positions of the molecule [18]. More than 90% of lipocalins have SCR1, which contains the motif glycine-x-tryptophan, and SCR3 which contains arginine/lysine. SCR2, which contains the motif threonine-aspartic acid-tyrosine-x-x-tyrosine, is found in more than 60% of lipocalins. Moreover, most lipocalins contain one or more intramolecular disulfide bonds. Lipocalins can be *N*- and/or *O*-glycosylated or nonglycosylated (Table 16.2).

Despite the low sequential identities between lipocalins, they share a common three-dimensional structure (Figure 16.3) [18]. The central β-barrel of lipocalins is composed of eight antiparallel β-strands, and it encloses an internal ligand-binding site (Figures 16.2 and 16.3). At the *N*-terminus, there is a 3_{10} helix, whereas at the *C*-terminus, there is an α-helix of variable length. The oligomerization (arrangement in multisubunit complexes) of lipocalins is variable (Table 16.2). The three-dimensional structures of several lipocalin allergens are known (Table 16.2).

These typically small, extracellular proteins have a capacity to bind small, principally hydrophobic molecules, to attach to specific cell-surface receptors, and to form covalent and noncovalent complexes with soluble macromolecules [18]. Most of the mammalian lipocalins are produced in the liver or secretory glands. Although they were originally characterized as transport proteins for diverse molecules, such as odorants, steroids, and pheromones, they are involved in a wide range of other biological functions.

Some lipocalins show immunomodulatory activity. One such protein, glycodelin (placental protein 14), exerts its anti-inflammatory activity by attenuating T-cell receptor (TCR) signaling and in this way favors the Th2 deviation of immune response [19]. Some lipocalins can be enzymes, such as β-lactoglobulin (Bos d 5) and human lipocalin-1 (tear lipocalin), which have nonspecific endonuclease activity [20]. The glutamic acid at position 128 in lipocalin-1, important for the enzyme activity, is present in several lipocalin allergens, such as Bos d 2, Mus m 1, Rat n 1, Equ c 1, and Can f 1. It is not known whether other lipocalin allergens exhibit enzyme activity and what would be the significance of such activity for the allergenicity of lipocalins. As the evolutionary conserved amino acid at position 128 in human lipocalin-1 is found at or adjacent to the cores of the immunodominant T-cell epitopes of Bos d 2 [21] and Can f 1 [22], it might be implicated in modifying human T-cell response against these allergens (see later discussion). Can f 1 is also proposed to act as a cysteine proteinase inhibitor because of its sequential homology with lipocalin-1. The motifs crucial for this potential function are only partially conserved in Can f 1.

Why Th2 responses specific for lipocalin proteins occur is unknown [4]. One requirement for the allergenicity of a protein, its effective dispersal in the environment, is fulfilled with lipocalin allergens, as they are found in animal dander and excretions. However, the crucial element for sensitization to occur is that the protein is recognized by the immune system. Therefore, it is noteworthy that endogenous lipocalins are recognized by specific receptors [4,23]. For example, food allergen β-lactoglobulin (Bos d 5) is taken up by the lipocalin-interacting membrane receptor (LIMR) [23]. This receptor mediates the uptake of another lipocalin allergen, horse Equ c 1 (B. Redl, personal communication). A glycosylated lipocalin allergen, dog Can f 1, is reported to be recognized by two distinct receptors, mannose receptor (MR) and dendritic cell-specific intracellular adhesion molecule (ICAM)-3-grabbing nonintegrin (DC-SIGN, CD209). Further results with another glycosylated (nonlipocalin) allergen, mite Der p 1, however, are conflicting in that the supposed outcome, Th2 immune deviation, is only favored by recognition with MR [24], whereas DC-SIGN recognition favors Th1 immune deviation [25]. Confusingly, several mammalian lipocalin allergens are reported to be quite inert, as they were not able to induce or inhibit the

Table 16.1 Amino acid identities (%) between lipocalin allergens

	LCN1	LCN9	Bos d 2	Can f 1	Can f 2	Can f 4	Can f 6	Cav p 2	Cav p 3	Cav p 6	Equ c 1	Fel d 4	Fel d 7	Mes a 1	Mus m 1	Ory c 4	Phod s 1
LCN9	28																
Bos d 2	27																
Can f 1	61	32															
Can f 2	26																
Can f 4	36	33															
Can f 6	37	28	26	25		28											
Cav p 2	26	40					33										
Cav p 3	40	33	28					44									
Cav p 6	35	25		29		27	54										
Equ c 1	36	33	28	26		30	57	33	27	48							
Fel d 4	35	31	27	25		27	67	32	29	53	67						
Fel d 7	58			63		33	33										
Mes a 1	28	33	33	34		37	42	27	31	31							
Mus m 1	37	29	27				47	28	25	46	47	49	25	26			
Ory c 4	36	29		30		34	60	30	26	51	54	64	27		53		
Phod s 1	31	34					31			39	43	26	26	41			
Rat n 1	39	27		30			52	31	25	51	49	55	29		65	56	25

Note: The UniProt Knowledgebase BLAST (https://www.uniprot.org/blast/) was used to analyze the amino acid identities of lipocalins without their signal peptides. Gray-shaded cells indicate lipocalin pairs with greater than 50% amino acid identities, while empty cells indicate those with identities less than 25%. Two endogenous human lipocalins included are LCN1 (human lipocalin-1/von Ebner gland protein/tear lipocalin) and LCN9 (human epididymal-specific lipocalin-9).

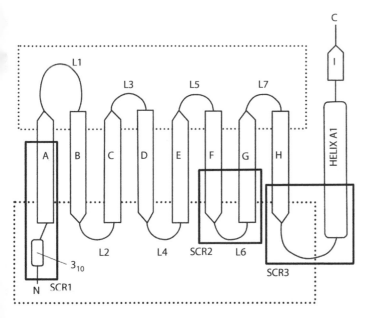

Figure 16.2 Schematic structure of the lipocalin fold. An unwound view of the lipocalin fold orthogonal to the axis of the barrel. The nine β-strands of the antiparallel β-sheet are shown as arrows. The C-terminal α-helix A1 and N-terminal 3_{10}-like helix are also marked. Loops are labeled L1–L7. A pair of dotted lines indicates the hydrogen-bonded connection of two strands. Those parts that form the three main conserved regions (SCRs) of the fold (SCR1, SCR2, and SCR3) are marked as heavy boxes. (Reproduced from Ganfornina M et al. *Lipocalins.* Georgetown, TX: Landes Bioscience, 2006: 17–27, with permission of Taylor & Francis Group, LLC, a division of Informa plc.)

maturation of human monocyte-derived dendritic cells (DCs) or to promote the proliferation or Th2 deviation of naive CD4+ T cells [26]. In another study, however, the human endogenous counterpart of Can f 1, lipocalin-1, was curiously found to be more stimulatory for human monocyte-derived DCs *in vitro* than the dog allergen [27]. Subsequently, lipocalin-1 induced a Th1-type response, whereas the response to Can f 1 was of Th2-type in an allogeneic coculture setting. In one additional study, a dog lipocalin allergen, Can f 6, enhanced lipopolysaccharide (LPS)-induced activation of toll-like receptor (TLR) 4 signaling in murine, bone marrow–derived macrophages [28]. The finding is reconcilable with the development of allergic sensitization in that low-level LPS stimulation promotes Th2 immunity [29]. All things considered, it is implausible that the recognition of LPS or other ligands by pattern recognition receptors provides an overall rationale accounting for allergen-specific sensitization [30]. However, the active uptake of an allergen, by binding to pattern recognition receptors, can facilitate its access to the immune system [23,31].

A peculiar characteristic of lipocalin allergens examined (cow Bos d 2 [21], dog Can f 1 [22,32], horse Equ c 1 [33], or rat Rat n 1 [34]) is their weak capacity to stimulate *in vitro* proliferation of peripheral blood mononuclear cells (PBMCs) of sensitized subjects. Moreover, Bos d 2 is a weak immunogen in a mouse model [35,36]. In line with these observations, T-cell epitope-containing Can f 1 peptides were only twofold more potent in inducing specific CD4+ T-cell lines from PBMCs than the peptides of human endogenous lipocalin-1, the human homolog of Can f 1 [37]. Unexpectedly, the Can f 1–specific T-cell lines exhibited as strong, but not stronger, proliferative responses upon stimulation with dog Can f 1 peptides

as the lipocalin-1-specific T-cell lines stimulated with human lipocalin-1 peptides in allergic or healthy subject groups. A weak stimulatory capacity is also a characteristic of another animal-derived (nonlipocalin) allergen, cat Fel d 1 [38,39]. With lipocalin allergens, this phenomenon may be attributed to the low number of T-cell epitopes detected: on average, an individual recognizes three epitopes in Bos d 2, Can f 1, Equ c 1, or Can f 4 [21,22,33,40]. Moreover, as the epitope regions in lipocalin allergens colocalize (Figure 16.4) [22,33,34,40], it is possible that thymic tolerance, due to sequential similarity of lipocalin allergens with endogenous lipocalins, limits the strength of T-cell response to the allergens. In particular, this hypothesis implies that due to thymic deletion, there is an absence of high-avidity lipocalin allergen-reactive T cells [4,5]. Findings compatible with this hypothesis suggest that the two T-cell epitopes examined from two distinct lipocalin allergens, Bos d 2 and Can f 1, are suboptimal: optimal (or heteroclitic, that is, more potent than the natural one) peptide analogs (altered peptide ligands [APLs]) of the natural epitopes stimulated human T-cell clones at 10- to 100-fold lower concentrations than the natural ligands [41,42]. Further experiments indicated that the strong stimulation by APLs was attributed to their more efficient recognition by TCR [41–43]. Accordingly, the frequency of Can f 1 and human endogenous lipocalin-1-specific CD4+ T-cell lines with high functional TCR avidity was at a similarly low level and was statistically significantly lower than that of the T-cell lines specific to the control, influenza hemagglutinin peptide [37]. As the suboptimal recognition of antigen through TCR favors the development of Th2-biased immunity [4,44], a characteristic accounting for the allergenic capacity of lipocalin allergens may indeed be their evolutionary relatedness with human endogenous lipocalins [4,5]. It is plausible, however, that CD4+ T cells need to recognize a lipocalin allergen in a certain avidity window: (1) a protein too close to immunologic self is probably tolerated and therefore not allergenic [4,45,46]; (2) an evolutionary distant, for example bacterial protein, is probably recognized as foreign and immunogenic, and therefore does not give rise to a Th2-type response [4,46,47]; (3) a protein that can cross the threshold for TCR activation, without being too stimulatory (the borderline of self and nonself), probably has potential to be allergenic [4,46]. One study suggests that 30%–40% identity with self proteins may be optimal for the allergenic capacity of a protein [46], it is of interest that mammalian lipocalin allergens often fulfill that requirement (BLAST).

It is possible that evolutionary relatedness of human endogenous lipocalins with lipocalin allergens is also reflected in the frequency of lipocalin allergen-specific CD4+ T cells, as Can f 1–allergic subjects have 10- to 20-fold lower frequency of Can f 1–specific cells than microbe antigen-specific cells in their peripheral blood [48] (S. Parviainen, unpublished results). Indeed, the frequencies of Bos d 2– [49], Can f 1– [37,48], Can f 4– [40], Equ c 1– [50], and Fel d 7–specific [10] CD4+ T cells of sensitized subjects are very low in peripheral blood, in the range of 10^{-5} and 10^{-6} circulating CD4+ T cells, and the frequencies with nonallergic subjects are even lower or nonexistent. The frequency of cat Fel d 4–specific CD4+ T cells in the peripheral blood of cat-allergic subjects appears to be somewhat higher than those found with other lipocalin allergens mentioned earlier [10]. Because the frequency of naive Bos d 2–specific [49] and cat Fel d 1/4/7/8–specific [10] CD4+ T cells in the peripheral blood of sensitized and healthy subjects is largely the same, the allergen-specific cells of healthy subjects inexplicably are not expanded *in vivo*. One factor with Bos d 2 could be the lower

Table 16.2 Physicochemical characteristics of mammalian lipocalin allergens causing respiratory sensitization

Allergen	Animal	MM[a], kDa	Amino acids	Isoelectric point	Glycosylation	Oligomeric state[b]	UniProtKB accession number[c]	Structure, PDB entry[d]	Key reference
Bos d 2	Cow	20	156	4.2	No	M/D	Q28133	1BJ7	[119]
Can f 1	Dog	22–25	156	5.2	Yes	D	O18873		[90]
Can f 2	Dog	22–27	162	4.9	Putative	M/D/T	O18874	3L4R	[90]
Can f 4	Dog	16–18	158	6.2	No	M/D	D7PBH4	4ODD	[101]
Can f 6	Dog	27, 29	175	4.9	Putative		H2B3G5		[110]
Cav p 1[e]	Guinea pig	20		4.3	No	M/D	P83507		[137]
Cav p 2	Guinea pig	17	154	4.3–4.5	No		F0UZ11		[138]
Cav p 3	Guinea pig	18	155	5.2	No		F0UZ12		[138]
Equ c 1	Horse	22	172	3.9	Yes	D	Q95182	1EW3	[113]
Equ c 2[e]	Horse	16		3.4–3.5	No		P81216 P81217		[117]
Fel d 4	Cat	20	171	4.6	Putative		Q5VFH6		[82]
Fel d 7	Cat	18	154	4.9	No	D	E5D2Z5		[86]
Mes a 1	Golden hamster	20.5, 24, 30	157		Both		Q9QXU1		[143]
Mus m 1	Mouse	18–21	162	4.6–5.3	No	M/D	P02762	1MUP	[131]
Ory c 1[e]	Rabbit	17–18			Yes				[140]
Ory c 4	Rabbit	24	172				U6C8D6		[142]
Phod s 1	Siberian hamster	18, 21, 23	151				S5ZYD3		[145]
Rat n 1	Rat	17–21	162	4.2–5.5	Yes	M/T	P02761	2A2U	[131]

[a] Molecular mass.
[b] D, dimer; M, monomer; T, tetramer.
[c] UniProtKB, https://www.uniprot.org.
[d] Protein Data Bank, https://www.rcsb.org.
[e] Only N-terminus known.

TCR avidity exhibited by the naive allergen-specific T cells of healthy subjects [49]. In summary, TCR-mediated recognition and signaling may be one of the factors governing the process of sensitization [51] to lipocalin allergens, due to evolutionary relatedness with human endogenous lipocalins [4] and/or among allergenic lipocalins from different species [52].

Finally, a property possibly contributing to the function of lipocalins as allergens can be their propensity for oligomerization, that is, the formation of complexes of a few monomeric molecules (Table 16.2). Mostly, lipocalin allergen oligomers are considered transient in nature [53]. It is conceivable that dimerization, for example, promotes IgE cross-linking on immune cells by offering two identical IgE epitopes [53,54].

16.4.1.2 SECRETOGLOBINS

The secretoglobin protein family (https://prosite.expasy.org/PS51311; https://prosite.expasy.org/PDOC00338) contains two allergens, the main allergen of cat, Fel d 1, and rabbit, Ory c 3. The features of secretoglobins and the two allergens are discussed later (Sections 16.4.2.1.1 and 16.4.2.8.2).

16.4.1.3 ALBUMINS

Albumins constitute another protein family (https://prosite.expasy.org/PDOC00186) containing respiratory allergens from several mammals. Albumin is produced in the liver, and it is a major constituent of plasma. It is involved in transporting various molecules and in maintaining the colloidal osmotic pressure of blood. The molecular mass of albumins is approximately 67 kDa [55]. Albumins share about 80% amino acid identity among mammals [55]. They are present in the dander and secretions of animals. Some studies suggest that IgE to mammalian albumins, minor allergens, is an indication of more severe airway disease [56,57], while other studies with children do not confirm this view [6,58]. For IgE cross-reactivity among albumins, see Section 16.5.

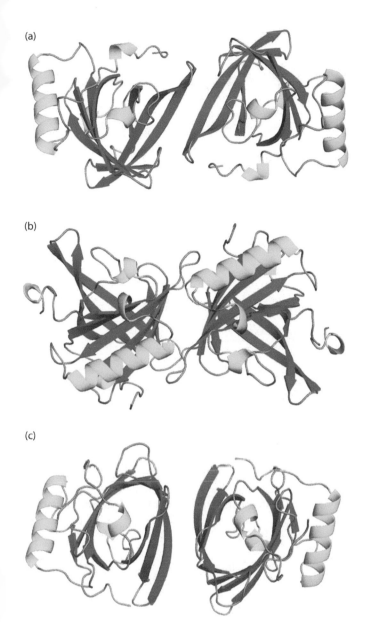

(a)

(b)

(c)

Figure 16.3 Ribbon representations of three lipocalin allergen dimers, bovine Bos d 2 (a), horse Equ c 1 (b), and mouse Mus m 1 (c), as observed in crystals. (Courtesy of Juha Rouvinen, Department of Chemistry, University of Eastern Finland, Joensuu, Finland.)

16.4.2 Allergenic proteins from mammals

16.4.2.1 CAT

16.4.2.1.1 Fel d 1

Cat dander contains several IgE-binding components, the most important being Fel d 1 (P30438 and P30440 at UniProtKB [https://www.uniprot.org]). Fel d 1, formerly cat-1, is a potent allergen sensitizing over 90% of cat-allergic individuals [59]. It is also responsible for 80%–90% of the IgE-binding capacity of cat allergen extracts [59]. A more recent study found that on average Fel d 1 bound 55% of cat allergen–specific IgE. The other cat allergens examined bound together more than 50% of cat allergen–specific IgE in 25% of the subjects [60]. The removal of

Fel d 1 from a dander extract decreases the histamine-releasing capacity of the preparation 200- to 300-fold. The presence of Fel d 1–specific IgE at 4 and 8 years of age is significantly associated with allergic symptoms to cat at age 16 years [3]. In two independent cohorts, Fel d 1 was found to be the only mammalian allergen among four to five risk allergens to which specific IgE (to three or more risk allergens) early in life identifies children with a high risk of asthma and/or allergic rhinitis in adolescence [61]. Fel d 1–specific IgE is considered a species-specific marker of sensitization to cat [62].

Fel d 1 is a glycoprotein with a molecular mass of 38 kDa [63]. It is a tetramer composed of two noncovalently linked heterodimers, each with a molecular mass of about 19 kDa. These dimers are composed of an 8-kDa chain 1 (α-chain) and 10-kDa chain 2 (β-chain), which are linked together covalently by three disulfide bonds. Chain 1 contains 70 amino acids, and the dominant forms of chain 2 contain 90 or 92 amino acids [64,65]. Chain 1 has a 29% amino acid identity with human uteroglobin, an anti-inflammatory protein (BLAST). Chain 2 has an amino acid identity of 39% with a putative human protein in a segment of 41 amino acids (BLAST). Both chains are classified as members of the secretoglobin (uteroglobin) family. Fel d 1 exists in several isoforms [63] and can be produced in a recombinant form. The three-dimensional structure of Fel d 1 is strikingly similar to that of uteroglobin and contains two cavities with potential for ligand binding [66].

Genes encoding Fel d 1 chains are expressed in the cat salivary glands and skin [65]. Fel d 1 is found in hair roots and sebaceous glands; in dander, saliva, and lacrimal fluid; and, in high concentrations, in anal glands. The production of Fel d 1 is hormonally controlled, and male cats produce more than females. The biological function of Fel d 1 is unknown, but it may be related to the protection of epithelia [64], to ligand transport [66], or to chemical communication [67]. It is speculated that Fel d 1 has an intrinsic capacity to promote allergy by sequestering calcium ions from phospholipase A$_2$ [66]. Fel d 1 does not have enzymatic activity [66]. Fel d 1 is also recognized by mannose receptor (MR), facilitating its internalization by antigen-presenting cells [31]. Further murine experiments suggest that the glycan component of Fel d 1 is involved in the Th2 immune deviation. A more recent study found that Fel d 1 enhanced LPS and lipoteichoic acid–induced TLR signaling (TLR4 and TLR2, respectively) in an experimental setting [28]. Interestingly, TLR4 signaling was independent of the glycosylation of Fel d 1 and thus MR activity. Moreover, Fel d 1 enhanced LPS-induced TNF-α production in primary human PBMCs.

Most of the IgE-binding epitopes on Fel d 1 are conformational, and glycosylation, present in chain 2 only, does not play a major role in IgE binding [68]. Analyses with overlapping synthetic peptides suggest that IgE-binding epitopes are localized at residues 25–38 and 46–59 in chain 1 and at residues 15–28 in chain 2 [69]. Among the sera tested, the highest percentage of positive reactions (46%) is against peptide 25–38. Another conformational B-cell epitope has been described on helices 1–4 of chain 1 [70].

The proliferative response of PBMCs induced by Fel d 1 is, in general, not strong [38,39,71]. In contrast, Fel d 1–specific T-cell clones and lines proliferate vigorously upon stimulation with Fel d 1 [72,73]. T-cell responses against Fel d 1 exhibit no correlation with human leukocyte antigen (HLA) phenotypes in two studies [38,72]. A third study found a possible excess of HLA-DR1 (odds ratio = 2, $p = .002$) among subjects with Fel d 1–specific IgE [74]. A fourth study found no association between specific IgE and the alleles of the HLA loci examined (including HLA-DRB1) [75].

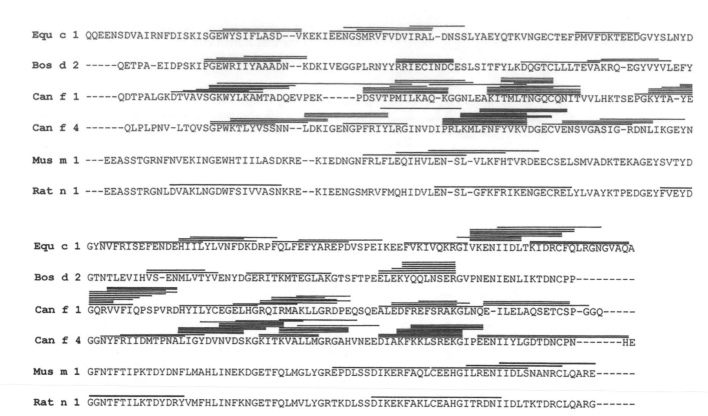

Figure 16.4 Alignment of the amino acid sequences of the lipocalin allergens of horse Equ c 1 [33], cow Bos d 2 [21], dog Can f 1 [22], dog Can f 4 [40], mouse Mus m 1 [52], and rat Rat n 1 [34]. For the first four allergens, lines above the sequences represent the cores of the epitopes recognized by individual T-cell lines and clones. The core sequence is defined as those amino acids that are shared by two to five consecutive peptides able to stimulate the T cells. The epitopes of Mus m 1 were defined by reactivity to immunodominant peptides in the ELISPOT analysis of allergen-specific T-cell lines [52] and those of Rat n 1 by peptide pools eliciting the highest number of positive responses upon stimulation of peripheral blood mononuclear cells of rat-allergic and nonallergic subjects [34]. (Modified from [33] with permission from John Wiley and Sons.)

Fel d 1 contains a few human T-cell epitope regions [71]. The recognition of Fel d 1 T-cell epitopes differs between allergic and nonallergic subjects in that the frequency of specific CD4+ T cells is substantially higher in the former group [10,76,77]. In allergic subjects, there is considerable variation in the frequency of specific cells, ranging from a few, to tens, and occasionally to 100 or more per 10^6 CD4+ T cells. Cat-allergic cat owners tend to have a higher frequency of Fel d 1– and Fel d 4–specific memory Th2 cells than cat-allergic subjects without cats [10]. The cytokine profiles of the specific Th2 cells did not differ between the two groups of allergic subjects. Distinct Fel d 1 epitopes may be able to induce qualitatively different T-cell responses [71,78]. For additional information, refer also to Section 16.3, and for IgE cross-reactivity, see Section 16.5.

16.4.2.1.2 Fel d 2

Fel d 2, cat serum albumin (P49064 at UniProtKB), is a minor allergen with IgE reactivity in about 20% of cat-allergic individuals [59], although higher figures are also reported. It has been cloned from cat liver and produced as a recombinant protein [79]. The role of Fel d 2 in respiratory allergy is uncertain, in that dominant IgE response against it occurs only in 2% of cat-allergic individuals [59]. Moreover, the significance of cat albumin as a primary sensitizer is difficult to assess [59], since albumins exhibit IgE cross-reactivity across animal species. (See Section 16.5, which also includes

pork-cat syndrome.) Component-resolved diagnostics, however, can be helpful in this context. IgE to Fel d 2 (and to Fel d 4) may be associated with atopic dermatitis in cat-allergic children [80]. IgE to this minor allergen may also be associated with more severe airway disease [56,57], although this was not confirmed in studies with children [6,58]. Consistent with IgE determinations, polyclonal T-cell lines, created with cat dander extract, proliferate weakly upon stimulation with cat albumin, whereas the response is stronger against Fel d 1 [72].

16.4.2.1.3 Fel d 3

Fel d 3, cystatin (Q8WNR9 at UniProtKB), was cloned from cat skin [81]. The prevalence of IgE reactivity among cat-allergic subjects is about 10% when measured using *Escherichia coli*–produced recombinant protein in a solid-phase enzyme-linked immunosorbent assay (ELISA) [81].

Fel d 3 is a 11-kDa protein containing 98 amino acids. There is one potential *N*-linked glycosylation site in the sequence. Fel d 3 exhibits approximately 80% amino acid identity with human cystatin A (BLAST). As endogenous protease inhibitors, cystatins control the function of cysteine proteases. Fel d 3 contains the signature motif conserved in cysteine protease inhibitors. Dog allergens, Can f 1 and Can f 2, which are lipocalins, show some homology with this sequence motif.

16.4.2.1.4 Fel d 4

One of the two cat allergens belonging to the lipocalin family of proteins is Fel d 4 (Q5VFH6 at UniProtKB). Up to 63% of cat-allergic subjects have IgE to it [57,82], based on measurements using recombinant Fel d 4. In general, the level of the antibody is low compared to that induced by Fel d 1, but about half of the Fel d 4–sensitized subjects have higher Fel d 4– than Fel d 1–specific IgE levels. IgE to Fel d 4 (and to Fel d 2) is associated with atopic dermatitis in cat-allergic children [80]. Sensitization to Fel d 4 is also linked with asthma [2,56,58,83]. In cat-allergic subjects, Fel d 4– and Fel d 1–specific Th2 cells are predominant in the T-cell response to cat allergens [10]. The responses to these allergens are independent, as they do not correlate. See also Sections 16.3, 16.4.1.1, and 16.4.2.1.1 for more information. The physicochemical characteristics of Fel d 4 are shown in Table 16.2. See Section 16.5 for IgE cross-reactivity.

Fel d 4 was cloned from submandibular salivary glands [82]. The expression of Fel d 4 is likely limited to this tissue, since Fel d 4 mRNA is not found in several other tissues examined. Isoallergens were not detected. Fel d 4 shows considerable amino acid identity, up to 67%, with horse Equ c 1, dog Can f 6, and rabbit Ory c 4, as well as with some other lipocalin allergens (Table 16.1).

16.4.2.1.5 Fel d 5w and Fel d 6w

Cat IgA (Fel d 5w) and IgM (Fel d 6w) may be respiratory allergens. Thirty-eight percent of cat-sensitized patients have IgE to cat IgA [84]. The IgE reactivity is mainly directed to the carbohydrate moiety of the IgA heavy chain. It potentially causes false IgE reactivity to cat dander (containing IgA) in the serological tests of subjects with IgE induced by carbohydrates from biting insects or other parasites [85]. Further studies are needed to clarify the clinical significance of cat immunoglobulins as aeroallergens. See Section 16.5 for IgE cross-reactivity.

16.4.2.1.6 Fel d 7

The other lipocalin allergen of cat is Fel d 7 (E5D2Z5 at UniProtKB). Thirty-eight to 47% of cat-allergic subjects have IgE to the recombinant form of the allergen [57,86,87]. The median concentration of Fel d 7–specific IgE is clearly lower than that of Fel d 1–specific IgE, but 10% of cat-allergic subjects have more IgE to Fel d 7 than to Fel d 1 [86]. In about 10% of cat-allergic subjects, a considerable Fel d 7–specific memory Th2 response is observed [10]. Additional information is available in Section 16.4.1.1. The physicochemical characteristics of Fel d 7 are shown in Table 16.2.

Fel d 7 is mainly found in cat saliva but is also present in hair. Estimates are that Fel d 7 constitutes 0.3% of proteins in the saliva. Fel d 7 was cloned from tongue tissue. Its gene is not expressed in skin, anal gland, parotid, or submandibular salivary glands. Fel d 7 is a homolog of dog Can f 1 and human lipocalin-1, the amino acid identity being about 60% with them (Table 16.1). See Section 16.5 for IgE cross-reactivity.

16.4.2.1.7 Fel d 8

Fel d 8 (F6K0R4 at UniProtKB), a latherin-like protein, is a 208-amino acid protein with a molecular mass of 24 kDa [86] and a predicted isoelectric point (pI) of 6.7. Latherins are surfactants that reduce water surface tension [88]. Nineteen percent of cat-allergic subjects have specific IgE to rFel d 8. The median concentration of Fel d 8–specific IgE is similar to that of Fel d 7–specific IgE. The memory CD4+ T-cell response to Fel d 8 is not strong [10].

Fel d 8 was cloned from the submandibular salivary gland. Several other tissues examined did not contain amplifiable cDNA for the allergen. Fel d 8 shows a 42% amino acid identity with horse allergen Equ c 4 (horse latherin, see Section 16.4.2.3.4). The amino acid identity with putative human latherin (Q86YQ2 at UniProtKB) is 39% (BLAST).

16.4.2.2 DOG

16.4.2.2.1 Can f 1

The major allergen of dog, Can f 1 (O18873 at UniProtKB), formerly called Ag 8, Ag 13, or Ag X, sensitizes 50%–75% of dog-allergic subjects [89–92]. It accounts for about 50% of the IgE-binding capacity of dog hair and dander extract [89] and for 60%–70% of the IgE-binding capacity of a dog saliva preparation [93]. Can f 1–specific IgE at 4 and 8 years of age is significantly associated with allergic symptoms to dog at age 16 years [3]. As Can f 1 shows IgE cross-reactivity with cat Fel d 7 (see Section 16.5), Can f 1–specific IgE together with IgE to Can f 2 and Can f 5 can be considered a species-specific marker of sensitization to dog [62]. Can f 1 belongs to the lipocalin family of proteins [90]. Its physicochemical characteristics are shown in Table 16.2.

Can f 1 is primarily found in dog saliva, but it is also present in dog dander [93]. It is absent or in very low concentrations in serum, urine, and feces. The allergen is detected in the hair extracts of all dog breeds examined, with variable amounts among individual dogs within a breed [93,94]. Male dogs may produce more Can f 1 than female dogs [94], although data are inconsistent [95]. Hypoallergenic dog breeds do not exist [96]. Can f 1 has been cloned from the parotid gland and produced in a recombinant form [90]. Its amino acid identity with human lipocalin-1 and cat Fel d 7 is about 60% (Table 16.1). Can f 1 mRNA is present in parotid and mandibular glands, tongue epithelial tissue, and skin but not in liver or kidney [90,97].

The IgE-binding capacity of Can f 1 is strongly dependent on the intact three-dimensional structure of the allergen [98]. Analyses suggest that the amino- and carboxy-terminal ends of Can f 1 come close to one another to form a major IgE-binding area on the surface of the molecule.

Human cellular immune responses to Can f 1 have been examined (see Section 16.4.1.1). One study found that the TCR Vβ5.1+ CD4+ T cells and the DR4-DQ8 haplotype may be protective against allergy to Can f 1 [32]. In two studies, no association between the Can f 1–specific IgE response and the HLA class II genotype was observed [74,75].

16.4.2.2.2 Can f 2

Can f 2 (O18874 at UniProtKB), formerly called dog allergen 2 or Dog 2, is a minor allergen sensitizing 25%–40% of dog-allergic subjects [90–92]. Sensitization to Can f 2 without sensitization to Can f 1 is rare. The average IgE response of dog-allergic subjects to Can f 2 is estimated to be 23% of that to dog dander extract [93]. Sensitization to this minor allergen is associated with asthma [2,6,56,58]. Can f 2 belongs to the lipocalin family of proteins [90,92]. Its physicochemical characteristics are illustrated in Table 16.2.

Can f 2 is found in dog dander and in saliva, whereas urine or feces contain very little of the allergen [93]. The amount of Can f 2 in the hair extracts of nine dog breeds varied widely. It has been cloned from the parotid gland and produced as a recombinant protein [90]. Can f 2 exhibits amino acid identities at the level of

30% with rodent urinary proteins [90] and other allergens (Table 16.1). A few human proteins show amino acid identities at the level of 25% with Can f 2 (BLAST). The mRNA of Can f 2 is predominantly expressed in parotid and mandibular glands and to a lesser extent in skin and tongue [90,97]. It is not found in kidney or liver. See Section 16.5 for IgE cross-reactivity.

16.4.2.2.3 Can f 3

Thirty-five percent of dog-allergic patients have IgE against Can f 3, dog serum albumin (P49822 at UniProtKB) [99], although both lower and higher figures are also reported. In individual patients, a major part of dog-specific IgE is directed to Can f 3 [99]. IgE to Can f 3 may be a marker of more severe airway disease [56] and/or multisensitization [7], although two pediatric studies did not confirm these findings [6,58]. Can f 3 is found, for example, in dog saliva [99,100]. The allergen has been cloned from dog liver and produced as a recombinant protein [55]. See Section 16.5 for IgE cross-reactivity of serum albumins.

16.4.2.2.4 Can f 4

Can f 4 (D7PBH4 at UniProtKB), a lipocalin, is a dog allergen sensitizing 35%–60% of dog-allergic subjects [91,101,102]. Sensitization to Can f 4 may serve as a marker of clinically relevant dog allergy [7]. The IgE-binding capacity of Can f 4 strongly depends on its intact three-dimensional structure [102]. The physicochemical characteristics of Can f 4 are shown in Table 16.2.

Can f 4 is found in dog saliva and dander. It was cloned from the lateral segment of the dog tongue for recombinant protein production [101]. The allergen is proposed to have isoforms. It shows an amino acid identity up to about 40% with odorant-binding and other proteins from mammals, as well as about a 30% identity with several lipocalin allergens (Table 16.1). In stretches of approximately 50 amino acids, Can f 4 exhibits identities up to 37% with human proteins (BLAST). The three-dimensional structure of Can f 4 has been determined [103]. See Section 16.5 for IgE cross-reactivity.

A study on human cellular immune response to Can f 4 (see Section 16.4.1.1) revealed, for example, that one sequential region (amino acids 43–67) is widely recognized, shows promiscuous HLA binding, and is therefore a potential target for developing allergen immunotherapy [40].

16.4.2.2.5 Can f 5

Can f 5 (P09582 at UniProtKB), a dog prostatic kallikrein (arginine esterase), is a 236-amino acid protein with a predicted pI of 8.0. In the natural glycosylated form, its molecular mass is approximately 33 kDa [104]. It is available as a recombinant protein. Can f 5 sensitizes up to 70% of dog-allergic subjects [104]. Approximately 50% of the Can f 5-sensitized subjects have no IgE to Can f 1-3. Although Can f 5 is associated with severe forms of allergic diseases in some studies [2,56,58], this does not appear to be true in Can f 5 monosensitized subjects [3,7].

Can f 5 is found in dog urine. A closely related or equivalent component is present in dog dander [104]. As Can f 5 is specifically expressed in prostate tissue, there may be subjects allergic specifically to male dogs [105,106]. The castration of male dogs strongly reduces the production of prostatic kallikrein.

Can f 5 shows amino acid identities of about 60% with kallikreins from different mammals, including human (BLAST). No other mammalian kallikrein is a known allergen, except human prostate-specific antigen (PSA), which is implicated in allergy to human semen [107]. In one case of human seminal plasma allergy, Can f 5 was considered the primary sensitizer [105]. Ten to 24% of dog-allergic subjects have IgE to PSA [104,107]. Allergy to Can f 5 may be involved in certain cases of infertility [104,107]. See Section 16.5 for IgE cross-reactivity.

Human CD4+ T-cell responses to Can f 5 and lipocalin allergens largely resemble one another [108]. For example, the frequency of Can f 5–specific cells in allergic subjects is low, as is the case with lipocalin allergen-specific T cells in sensitized subjects. Moreover, the frequency of Can f 5–specific cells in nonallergic subjects is about 10-fold lower compared to allergic ones.

16.4.2.2.6 Can f 6

Can f 6 (H2B3G5 at UniProtKB) is a lipocalin allergen sensitizing up to 61% of dog-allergic subjects based on IgE measurements using recombinant proteins [109,110]. Sensitization to Can f 6 may serve as a marker of clinically relevant dog allergy [7]. Its physicochemical characteristics are shown in Table 16.2.

Can f 6 is present in dog dander and saliva [100,109,110]. Although not systematically investigated, genes for the allergen appear to be expressed in dog submaxillary gland, skin, and bladder tissues [109,110]. Can f 6 exhibits considerable amino acid identities with several lipocalin allergens, up to 67%, including horse Equ c 1, rabbit Ory c 4, and cat Fel d 4, and others (Table 16.1). The amino acid identity with human epididymal-specific lipocalin-9 is 37% (Table 16.1). Can f 6 contains five linear B-cell epitopes [111]. See Section 16.5 for IgE cross-reactivity.

16.4.2.2.7 Can f 7

Can f 7 (Q28895 at UniProtKB), NPC intracellular cholesterol transporter 2 (NPC2) expressed in dog epididymis, is recognized as an allergen in dog epithelial extract [112]. The molecular mass of this 128-amino acid glycoprotein with pI of 8.5 is about 16 kDa. About 15% of dog-allergic subjects have specific IgE to Can f 7, measured using recombinant proteins [112].

Can f 7 has high amino acid identities with NPC2 proteins from other mammals. The amino acid identity with its human counterpart is over 80% (BLAST). Of interest, the NPC2 family also contains group 2 mite allergens with which the amino acid identity of Can f 7 is low, at the level of 20%–30% (BLAST). See Section 16.5 for IgE cross-reactivity.

16.4.2.2.8 Other dog allergens

Dog can be a source of up to 20 allergens. In an analysis of a hair and dander extract, 11 allergens in the molecular mass range of 14–68 kDa were detected. One of these is an immunoglobulin. Uncharacterized allergens in dog saliva may account for allergic symptoms in a proportion of subjects without IgE to dog dander [100].

16.4.2.3 HORSE

16.4.2.3.1 Equ c 1

IgE against Equ c 1 (Q95182 at UniProtKB), a lipocalin [113], probably previously named Ag 6, is found in up to 76% of horse-allergic subjects' sera [114]. Ag 6 accounts for 55% of skin prick test reactivity of a horse hair and dandruff extract according to one study. Sensitization to Equ c 1 may be associated with more severe forms of allergic disease [6,56]. Equ c 1 is not an ideal marker of species-specific sensitization because of its IgE cross-reactivity with lipocalin allergens from other mammals (see Section 16.5). The physicochemical characteristics of Equ c 1 are shown in Table 16.2.

In addition to horse dander [114], Equ c 1 is found in a high concentration in horse saliva. Equ c 1 mRNA expression is about 100-fold higher in sublingual salivary glands than in submaxillary salivary glands or liver [113]. The allergen has been cloned from sublingual salivary glands and produced in a recombinant form [113]. As mentioned previously, Equ c 1 belongs to the group of lipocalin allergens with considerable amino acid identities among one another (see Sections 16.4.2.1.4 and 16.4.2.2.6; Table 16.1). The amino acid identity with human epididymal-specific lipocalin-9 is 36% (BLAST). There are several isoforms of the allergen. Equ c 1 may bind histamine and has a surfactant-like property [115]. See Section 16.5 for IgE cross-reactivity.

An analysis of the IgE-binding epitopes of Equ c 1 suggests that the dominant epitopes are localized in a restricted region of the molecule [116]. Carbohydrates may affect IgE binding [115,116]. Human cellular immune response to Equ c 1 has been explored (see Section 16.4.1.1).

16.4.2.3.2 Equ c 2

Horse Equ c 2 has been preliminarily characterized. The N-terminal sequences of two horse dander allergens, with slightly different isoelectric points, were identical, and the allergens were named Equ c 2.0101 and Equ c 2.0102 (P81216 and P81217 at UniProtKB) [117]. A 29-amino acid fragment exhibits a 44% identity with bovine Bos d 2 and also contains the highly conserved G-X-W motif of lipocalins. Analyses of the amino acid compositions of the allergens also suggest that they are lipocalins (Table 16.2). Up to 50% of horse-allergic patients have IgE against Equ c 2 [117].

16.4.2.3.3 Equ c 3

As with albumins from other mammals, the significance of horse serum albumin, Equ c 3 (P35747 at UniProtKB), as an inhalant allergen is difficult to assess, but component-resolved diagnostics can be helpful. In one study, sensitization to Equ c 3 was associated with more severe forms of airway disease [56], while this was not observed in a pediatric study [6]. The prevalence of IgE reactivity against Equ c 3 is between 20% [118] and 50%.

16.4.2.3.4 Equ c 4

Equ c 4, the former Equ c 5, horse latherin (P82615 at UniProtKB), and surfactant protein, is a 208-amino acid, nonglycosylated protein with a molecular mass of 24.7 kDa and a pI of 4.1. Its transcripts are detectable only in skin and submaxillary salivary gland [88]. It is available as a recombinant protein [88]. As mentioned earlier, cat Fel d 8 and horse and human latherins exhibit homology at the level of 40%. Seventy-seven percent of horse-allergic patients have IgE to Equ c 4 [115].

16.4.2.3.5 Other horse allergens

Horse dander contains more than 10 IgE-binding proteins [117]. The designation Equ c 5 has been deleted from ANDB.

16.4.2.4 COW

16.4.2.4.1 Bos d 2

Bos d 2 (Q28133 at UniProtKB), a lipocalin allergen [119] also known as Ag 3 or BDA20, is the major respiratory allergen in cow dander (Table 16.2). About 90% of dairy farmers with asthma of bovine origin have Bos d 2–specific IgE on immunoblotting [120] or have positive bronchial challenge with Bos d 2. Both Ag 3 (Bos d 2) and an uncharacterized bovine allergen Ag 1 account for about 70% of the IgE-binding capacity of cow hair and dander extract. Together they bind about 80% of the IgE. While the Bos d 2 content in the hair samples of individual cows is highly variable, no significant differences are found among the breeds studied or between genders [121]. Bos d 2 can be considered a species-specific marker of sensitization to cow, as it has not been shown to be IgE-cross-reactive with other lipocalin allergens studied [102,122].

Bos d 2 is found in cow skin [123], although the same or an immunologically related allergen is present in urine [120]. In skin, Bos d 2 is localized in the secretory cells of the apocrine sweat glands and the basement membranes of the epithelium and hair follicles. It is probably a pheromone carrier [123]. There are several isoforms of Bos d 2. It has been cloned from cow skin [119] and produced as a recombinant protein [124]. Bos d 2 exhibits almost complete amino acid identity with a putative protein from another Bos species, wild yak (BLAST). The amino acid identity of Bos d 2 is at the level of 30%–40% with several lipocalin allergens (Table 16.1).

Bos d 2 has been produced in fragments and in mutated forms to reduce its IgE-binding capacity. IgE binding is highly dependent on an intact three-dimensional structure. The epitopes responsible for IgE binding are localized in the C-terminal part of Bos d 2. Many studies on cellular immune response to lipocalin allergens have been performed with Bos d 2 (see Section 16.4.1.1), including a study demonstrating that the HLA class II alleles DRB1*0101, DRB1*0404, DQB1*0302, and DQB1*0501 are associated with sensitization to Bos d 2, whereas HLA-DRB1*0301 and DQB1*0201 are protective [125].

16.4.2.4.2 Bos d 3

Bos d 3 (Q28050 at UniProtKB), known also as BDA11, is a minor bovine respiratory allergen [126]. According to the immunoblotting analysis with recombinant Bos d 3, about 40% of patients with cow dust-induced asthma have IgE against the allergen [126].

Bos d 3 is an 11-kDa protein with a predicted pI of 5.19 [126]. It is found in the bovine skin, mammary gland, and amniotic fluid. This 101-amino acid long allergen belongs to the S-100 family of proteins and is a homolog of horse and human psoriasins with amino acid identities of more than 60% (BLAST). Human psoriasin (S100-A7) is a calcium-binding keratinocyte protein found in normal skin, and it is highly upregulated in psoriatic skin. The protein has chemokine-like properties selective for CD4+ T cells and neutrophils as well as antimicrobial activity against E. coli. The latter property is shared with Bos d 3 [127].

16.4.2.4.3 Other bovine respiratory allergens

Using crossed radioimmunoelectrophoresis, serum proteins, including albumin (Bos d 6; P02769 at UniProtKB) and IgG (Bos d 7), are allergens in cow hair and dander [128]. By immunoblotting, up to 10 IgE-binding components are detected in the bovine epithelial extract and four in the urine preparation in the molecular mass range of 16 kDa to over 100 kDa [120]. Two of the allergens with the molecular masses of 20 kDa (Bos d 2) and 22 kDa are major allergens [120]. In another study, an 11-kDa protein showing almost complete homology with the bovine oligomycin sensitivity-conferral protein of the mitochondrial adenosine triphosphate synthase complex (P13621 at UniProtKB) was identified as a minor allergen in cow dander [129].

16.4.2.5 MOUSE

16.4.2.5.1 Mus m 1

There are multiple existing and potential murine proteins highly homologous with the major urinary protein MUP6 (P02762 at UniProtKB), which was originally designated as Mus m 1. It was previously known as Ag 1, prealbumin, or mouse allergen 1 (MA1) [130]. ANDB also contains another isoform for Mus m 1 (P11589 at UniProtKB). Mus m 1 accounts for the majority of the IgE-binding capacity of the crude male urine [130]. Sensitization rates to Mus m 1 vary considerably among studies; one study found it to be 66% among mouse-allergic subjects [122]. Mus m 1 belongs to the lipocalin family of proteins [131]. The physicochemical characteristics of Mus m 1 are shown in Table 16.2.

Mus m 1 is found in mouse urine, serum, pelt, and especially in liver [130], where it is primarily produced [131]. The production of major urinary proteins (MUPs) is under hormonal control and influenced by androgens [131]. Forms of MUPs are also expressed constitutively in the exocrine glands of mice and rats [131]. Mus m 1 is found in about fourfold higher concentrations in male compared to female mouse urine [130]. Mouse MUPs are encoded by approximately 35 genes, and 15 forms of MUPs are detected in male urine. Mouse MUP has been produced as a recombinant protein [132]. The amino acid identity between mouse and rat MUPs is about 65% [131]. The amino acid identity of Mus m 1 with rabbit Ory c 4 is 53%, approximately 50% with several other lipocalin allergens, and 37% with human epididymal-specific lipocalin-9 (Table 16.1). See Section 16.5 for IgE cross-reactivity.

In mouse-allergic subjects with asthma or rhinitis, T-cell response to Mus m 1 is dominant among murine antigens analyzed [52] (see also Section 16.4.1.1).

16.4.2.5.2 Other mouse allergens

The other major allergen of mouse, Ag 3, tentatively named Mus m 2, is a glycoprotein [133]. It is found in mouse dander and fur. It is localized in the hair follicles, coating the hairs, and on the skin [133]. Mouse albumin is also an allergen. It is not listed in ANDB.

16.4.2.6 RAT

16.4.2.6.1 Rat n 1

Rat n 1, also known as rat MUP (P02761 at UniProtKB), prealbumin, or α_2-globulin (α_2-euglobulin), is closely related to the major urinary proteins of mouse (see Section 16.4.2.5.1) and is a lipocalin [131]. Its physicochemical characteristics are shown in Table 16.2. Sixty-six percent of rat-exposed laboratory workers with asthma and rhinitis have Rat n 1–specific IgE [134]. Adult female rats excrete about one-sixth of the amount of MUPs in urine as male rats. Similar to Mus m 1, Rat n 1 exhibits considerable amino acid identities with rabbit Ory c 4 and other lipocalin allergens (Table 16.1).

Rat urinary prealbumin and α_2-globulin were considered distinct allergens in the 1980s. Subsequent analyses of these strongly cross-reactive proteins [134] showed that prealbumin is an isoform of α_2-globulin. Therefore, a more appropriate name for prealbumin is Rat n 1.01, and for α_2-globulin, Rat n 1.02 [135]. α_2-globulin has been cloned and produced as a recombinant protein. One study suggests that the IgE-binding epitopes of Rat n 1.02 tend to cluster toward the N- and C-terminal parts of the allergen.

Human cellular immune response to Rat n 1 has been examined (see Section 16.4.1.1). One study found that HLA-DR7 is positively associated and HLA-DR3 negatively associated with sensitization to rat urinary proteins [136].

16.4.2.6.2 Other rat allergens

Male rat urine contains a total of eight allergens in the molecular mass range of 17–75 kDa. About 20 allergens have been observed in rat fur and in saliva. Rat serum proteins, including albumin, transferrin, and IgG, are allergens.

16.4.2.7 GUINEA PIG

16.4.2.7.1 Cav p 1

Cav p 1 (P83507 at UniProtKB) is a major guinea pig allergen. Seventy percent of guinea pig allergic subjects have IgE to Cav p 1 in hair extract and 87% in urine preparation [137]. The allergen was purified from the hair extract. The physicochemical characteristics of Cav p 1 are shown in Table 16.2. The complete amino acid sequence of this allergen is unknown, but the analysis of the 15 aminoterminal residues shows that Cav p 1 is a lipocalin with a 57% amino acid identity with the major mouse allergen, Mus m 1 [137].

16.4.2.7.2 Cav p 2 and Cav p 3

Cav p 2 (F0UZ11 at UniProtKB) and Cav p 3 (F0UZ12) are major guinea pig allergens and both are lipocalins. According to a study with recombinant allergens, 65% of guinea pig allergic subjects have IgE against the former and 54% against the latter allergen [138]. The allergens were cloned from submaxillary gland. However, Cav p 2 appears to be mainly synthesized in the eye-associated Harderian gland. The physicochemical characteristics of the allergens are shown in Table 16.2. The amino acid identity of Cav p 2 and Cav p 3 is 43% [138]. Their amino acid identities are at the level of 30%–40% with several other lipocalin allergens (Table 16.1). The identities with human proteins are up to 29% (BLAST). See Section 16.5 for IgE cross-reactivity.

16.4.2.7.3 Other guinea pig allergens

Guinea pig hair extract and urine contain several IgE-binding components in addition to Cav p 1–3 with molecular mass range between 8 and 70 kDa [137]. Sixty-five percent of guinea pig allergic individuals have IgE against an 8-kDa allergen, whereas IgE reactivity to the other allergens is below 33%. Eight to 33% of guinea pig allergic patients exhibit IgE reactivity to Cav p 4 (Q6WDN9 at UniProtKB), guinea pig serum albumin [137,138]. An additional guinea pig allergen in ANDB is an 18 kDa lipocalin, Cav p 6 (S0BDX9 at UniProtKB).

16.4.2.8 RABBIT

16.4.2.8.1 Ory c 1

The major allergen Ory c 1, also known as Ag R1, is found in saliva and, to a slightly lesser extent, in fur [139]. It is present in dander in small amounts but not in urine. The physicochemical characteristics of Ory c 1 are shown in Table 16.2. The aminoterminal sequence of the allergen suggests that the allergen is a lipocalin with a 72% amino acid identity with rabbit odorant-binding protein 2 [140].

16.4.2.8.2 Ory c 3

The other allergen in the secretoglobin family of proteins, in addition to cat Fel d 1, is rabbit Ory c 3 [141]. Seventy-seven percent of rabbit-allergic subjects have IgE to Ory c 3 [141]. As Ory c 3 has not been found to be IgE cross-reactive with other allergens (see Section 16.5), it may be a species-specific marker of sensitization to rabbit.

Ory c 3 (Q9GK63 and Q9GK67 at UniprotKB) is a glycosylated heterodimer composed of lipophilins CL2 (75 amino acids) and AL (69 amino acids), with a total molecular mass of 18–19 kDa. The amino acid identities of the Ory c 3 chains with those of Fel d 1 are less than 25% [141]. The allergens nevertheless are structurally similar. Lipophilin CL2 exhibits a surprising 100% amino acid identity with a potential human secretoglobin (BLAST). The amino acid identities of both chains with other human secretoglobins are at the level of 45%–55%, whereas their identities with proteins from other mammals are somewhat lower.

Ory c 3 was isolated from rabbit hair extract [141]. Lipophilins are known to be present in various mammalian secretions. Glycosylation is not involved in IgE binding to Ory c 3 [141].

16.4.2.8.3 Ory c 4

The third rabbit allergen in ANDB is Ory c 4, a lipocalin (U6C8D6 at UniprotKB). It sensitizes 46% of rabbit-allergic subjects, measured using recombinant Ory c 4 in ELISA [142]. Ory c 4 exhibits amino acid identities of greater than 50% with dog Can f 6, guinea pig Cav p 6, horse Equ c 1, cat Fel d 4, mouse Mus m 1, and rat Rat n 1 (Table 16.1). The physicochemical characteristics of Ory c 4 are shown in Table 16.2.

16.4.2.8.4 Other rabbit allergens

Rabbit urine, fur, and saliva extracts contain several allergens with molecular masses from 8 to 80 kDa [140]. Saliva, which contains 12 allergens, is the most potent of the extracts according to radioallergosorbent test (RAST) inhibition experiments [140]. Rabbit serum albumin is of minor importance, although in individual cases sensitization can be strong [140]. The minor allergen Ag2, previously also referred to as Ory c 2, is not included in ANDB.

16.4.2.9 HAMSTER

16.4.2.9.1 Mes a 1

There are two allergens from two species of hamster in ANDB. Mes a 1 (Q9QXU1 at UniprotKB), also known as male-specific submandibular salivary gland protein (MSP), is a lipocalin allergen from the Golden (Syrian) hamster (Figure 16.1) [143]. The physicochemical characteristics of Mes a 1 are shown in Table 16.2.

Mes a 1 (MSP) is found in saliva, tears, urine, and fur. It is expressed in the male submandibular salivary gland and the female lacrimal glands [144]. It is under complicated sex-hormonal regulation in both sexes. Mes a 1 has been produced as a recombinant protein [143].

The amino acid identity of Mes a 1 with those of other characterized lipocalin allergens is relatively low (Table 16.1), the highest ones being with Cav p 3 of guinea pig (42%) and Phod s 1 of Siberian hamster (41%). The identity with female-specific lacrimal

gland protein from Golden hamster (Q99MG7) is 85% (BLAST). See Section 16.5 for IgE cross-reactivity.

16.4.2.9.2 Phod s 1

The characterized allergen from the Siberian hamster (Figure 16.1) is Phod s 1 (S5ZYD3 at UniprotKB), a lipocalin [145]. Its physicochemical characteristics are shown in Table 16.2. Phod s 1 is found in hair, urine, and saliva. The allergen was cloned from submaxillary glands and produced as a recombinant protein [145]. Phod s 1 exhibits the highest amino acid identities with guinea pig Cav p 3 (43%) and Golden hamster Mes a 1 (41%) among characterized allergens (Table 16.1). See Section 16.5 for IgE cross-reactivity.

16.4.2.10 HUMAN AUTOALLERGENS

IgE antibodies against human proteins occur in subjects with chronic inflammatory conditions. Some of these are evolutionary conserved proteins and homologous with recognized exogenous allergens (see later), and the IgE binding to these human proteins can be explained by molecular mimicry and shared B-cell epitopes.

However, screening of human cDNA libraries with sera from patients with atopic dermatitis reveals a large repertoire of IgE-binding self antigens that do not have homology to known allergens [146,147]. It is therefore possible that sensitization against these antigens is a direct result of autoimmunity, and these proteins can be considered as true autoallergens. Recombinant forms of several of these autoantigens induce basophil activation and a positive skin prick test in subjects with atopic dermatitis [146,147]. The clinical relevance of IgE autoantibodies in the pathogenesis of allergic conditions is unclear but is more likely in atopic dermatitis and chronic urticaria [148].

16.4.2.10.1 Hom s 1

Hom s 1 (O43290 at UniProtKB) is one of the five autoallergens listed in ANDB. Six out of 65 sera from atopic dermatitis patients had IgE antibodies against Hom s 1 [149]. Deduced from the cDNA sequence, it has a molecular mass of 73 kDa. However, a rabbit anti-serum against Hom s 1 detected proteins of variable size in extracts of human tissues [149]. Hom s 1 is a cytoplasmic protein, although SART-1, a protein with an almost complete sequence identity with Hom s 1, is localized to nuclei of normal and malignant cells.

16.4.2.10.2 Hom s 2-5

Hom s 2-5, like Hom s 1, are autoallergens that were found by screening a cDNA library from a human epithelial cell line using IgE antibodies from patients with atopic dermatitis [146]. The presence of IgE antibodies was restricted to a few individuals with atopic dermatitis. The cDNAs of Hom s 2–5 code for fragments of intracellular proteins. Hom s 2 shows sequence identity with a portion of the nascent polypeptide-associated complex subunit α (NAC-α) (Q13765 at UniProtKB). An isoform of Hom s 2, containing 21 amino acid exchanges compared with NAC-α, has been identified [150]. Hom s 3 has sequence identity with the oncoprotein BCL7B (Q9BQE9 at UniProtKB). Hom s 4 (Q9BPX6 at UniProtKB) is a 54-kDa basic protein with a pl of 8.7 [151]. It appears to belong to a subfamily of calcium-binding proteins and shows IgE cross-reactivity with exogenous calcium-binding allergens from plants (Phl p 7) and fish (Cyp c 1). Hom s 5 is identical to a portion of keratin, type II cytoskeletal 6A (P02538 at UniProtKB).

16.4.2.10.3 Human homologues of exogenous allergens

Several fungal allergens are phylogenetically highly conserved, and the corresponding human proteins react with IgE antibodies from patients with severe fungal allergies. Asp f 6 is a manganese superoxide dismutase (MnSOD) allergen of *A. fumigatus*. Recombinant human MnSOD, with a 48% amino acid identity with Asp f 6 (BLAST), reacts with IgE and stimulates T cells from patients with chronic *A. fumigatus* allergy [152]. Similarly, IgE cross-reactivity between several other fungal allergens, such as acidic ribosomal phosphoprotein type 2 (P2 protein) [153], thioredoxin [154], and cyclophilins [155], and their human homologues has been described. Profilins are another group of conserved proteins identified as allergens of several plants, e.g., Bet v 2 of birch. IgE from sera of subjects sensitized to plant profilins cross-react with human profilin [156].

16.5 ALLERGENIC CROSS-REACTIVITY AMONG MAMMALS

Evidence of the IgE cross-reactivity between pure mammalian, non-serum-derived inhalant allergens has accumulated mostly with the advent of recombinant allergens. The introduction of component-resolved diagnostics in allergy, exploiting recombinant allergens, can help to distinguish primary sensitizers from cross-sensitizers/IgE cross-reactive allergens. Ideally, a marker allergen indicating sensitization to a particular animal is widely IgE reactive in the sensitized population without IgE cross-reactivity with allergens from other animals.

rFel d 1 (100 µg/mL) inhibited the binding of IgE from Fel d 1–sensitized, cat-allergic patients to a dog allergen preparation by an average of 41% in one study [157]. An inhibition of more than 50% was detected with 25% of the sera. The probable IgE-cross-reactive dog allergen of 20 kDa was not characterized further. No IgE cross-reactivity exists between Fel d 1 and rabbit Ory c 3, two secretoglobin allergens [141].

The IgE cross-reactivity of another cat allergen, Fel d 4, a lipocalin, was initially characterized with allergen extracts from cow, horse, and dog [82]. Cow extract inhibited IgE binding to rFel d 4 by 66% on average, while horse and dog extracts were less potent. The bovine homologue remains unidentified. Fel d 4, Mus m 1, Rat n 1, Can f 6, Cav p 6, Ory c 4, and Equ c 1 form a group with considerable amino acid identities (47%–67%) (Table 16.1). In a study in which the IgE cross-reactivities between pure lipocalin allergens across species were examined for the first time, rEqu c 1 (200 µg/mL) almost completely prevented IgE binding to rMus m 1 [122]. As the opposite was not true, the IgE cross-reactivity being asymmetric, the allergens obviously contain both common and unique IgE epitopes. In this group, the rodent allergens Mus m 1 and Rat n 1 are also likely to be IgE cross-reactive, according to a study with rat and mouse urinary extracts [158]. In another study, rEqu c 1, rCan f 6, and rFel d 4 IgE cross-reacted variably between one another, the level of which could be strong with some serum-inhibitor combinations [109]. Another study with rCan f 6 and rFel d 4 obtained similar results, and in some cases, the IgE cross-reactivity was clearly asymmetric [110]. The IgE cross-reactivity between Equ c 1 and Can f 6 is also asymmetric [159]. Finally, a high amount of rFel d 4 (125 µg/mL) can serum-dependently inhibit up to 58% of IgE binding to dog rCan f 2, although the amino acid identity between the two lipocalins is only about 23% [92].

Although the amino acid identity of dog Can f 1 and 2 is also low (21%, BLAST), two studies, one with *E. coli*–produced [160] and the other *Pichia pastoris*–produced [122] allergens, found asymmetric IgE cross-reactivity between these two lipocalins. Can f 1 also exhibits IgE cross-reactivity with its human homolog, lipocalin-1 [122], and the cat homolog, Fel d 7 [87]. In the latter study, rFel d 7 (1 µg/mL) inhibited at least 70% of IgE binding to rCan f 1 in 30% of cat dander-sensitized patients who were IgE positive to both allergens, whereas rCan f 1 (1 µg/mL) inhibited more than 90% of IgE binding to rFel d 7 in about 50% of subjects [87]. The surface-exposed amino- and carboxyterminal ends coming close to one another in the allergens are assumed to account for the cross-reactivity [87,98]. A further dog allergen, Can f 4 (100 µg/mL), strongly inhibits IgE binding to a bovine odorant-binding protein with a 37% amino acid identity [101], whereas several lipocalins with amino acid identity of about 30%, including cow Bos d 2 and horse Equ c 1, do not show IgE cross-reactivity with Can f 4 [102].

A study with lipocalin allergens from guinea pig suggests that there is IgE cross-reactivity between Cav p 1 and Cav p 2 [161]. The 43% homologous Cav p 2 and 3 show asymmetric IgE cross-reactivity, as rCav p 3 (100 µg/mL) inhibits 16%–28% of IgE binding to rCav p 2 with four of the six sera tested [138].

Immunoblot inhibition studies suggest that the Golden hamster allergen Mes a 1 is not IgE cross-reactive with the allergens of the fur extracts from Siberian (presumable containing Phod s 1) and Roborovski hamsters (*Phodopus roborovskii*) [143]. While the Siberian hamster allergen Phod s 1 does not show IgE cross-reactivity with the proteins of submandibular salivary gland extracts (100 µg/mL) from Golden hamster (containing Mes a 1) and European hamster (*Cricetus cricetus*) in IgE ELISA inhibition with a serum pool, the extract from Roborovski hamster inhibited about 60% of IgE binding to Phod s 1, probably due to the phylogenetic proximity of the species [145].

A monoclonal antibody specific for Bos d 5 (β-lactoglobulin), a bovine food allergen of the lipocalin family, reacted against human serum retinol-binding protein, another lipocalin [162]. The core of the antibody-binding epitope, DTDY, is localized in the second structurally conserved region of lipocalins. The sequence is found, for example, in human glycodelin (BLAST).

Dog Can f 5 and human prostate-specific antigen (PSA) are about 60% homologous kallikrein proteins. Strong IgE cross-reactivity was detected in one study with two of the four PSA-reactive sera upon inhibition with rCan f 5 (100 µg/mL), whereas one serum showed partial and the other no IgE cross-reactivity [104].

Two proteins from the NPC2 family, dog Can f 7 and mite Der p 2, showed weak IgE cross-reactivity [112]. Their amino acid identity is low (see Section 16.4.2.2.7).

Although methodological and other differences interfere with the interpretation of these data, it seems that the IgE cross-reactivity between mammalian, non-serum-derived respiratory allergens is not very strong in general, as 100–200 µg/mL concentrations of the allergens are often needed to obtain significant inhibitions. One study shows that to obtain a 50% inhibition, the concentration of an inhibiting protein must be hundreds of times greater than that of the control protein [122]. In some cases, no IgE cross-reactivity is observed or it is asymmetric. Individual variation can be considerable. The IgE cross-reactivity mostly reflects the sequential similarity of the proteins, but structural similarity with low sequential similarity is sufficient in some cases [92,122]. Therefore, the clinical significance of IgE cross-reactivity between these allergens is largely unclear, with a possible exception of Can f 5 allergy (see Section 16.4.2.2.5) and allergy to certain lipocalin allergens. It has been suggested that sensitization to lipocalin allergens would promote sensitization to other IgE cross-reactive lipocalin allergens [1,109]. Alternatively, the apparent sensitization to more than one lipocalin allergen can be a reflection of cross-sensitization [7,159]—that is, one of the IgE cross-reacting allergens is the primary sensitizer. In this context, it is of interest that the IgE levels of asthmatic children to the homologous allergens Fel d 4, Equ c 1, and Mus m 1 correlate strongly, which is not the case with respect to IgE specific to the major birch pollen allergen, Bet v 1 [1]. Other studies show a considerable correlation in IgE reactivity between Fel d 4 and Equ c 1 [163] and a strong correlation between IgE levels to Fel d 4 and Can f 6 [110]. The latter finding was not confirmed in a study that also failed to show significant correlation between the IgE levels to Equ c 1 and Can f 6 [163]. Fel d 7 and Can f 1, which have somewhat higher level of homology than Equ c 1 and Can f 6, show a considerable correlation with specific IgE levels [60,87]. Cross-sensitization may explain why about half of dog-allergic subjects with Can f 1–specific IgE also have IgE to human lipocalin-1, whereas virtually no animal-allergic subject without IgE to Can f 1 has IgE to lipocalin-1 [122].

Animal-allergic patients may have IgE antibodies against a number of serum albumins, such as Fel d 2, Can f 3, and Equ c 3. Inhibition experiments show that albumin-specific IgE is often cross-reactive, although patients exhibit individual variation in this respect [118,164]. As pointed out for Fel d 2, the primary sensitizer can be difficult to identify [59], but component-resolved diagnostics can help in this respect. A study with three tryptic peptides from horse serum albumin identified regions involved in IgE cross-reactivity with dog albumin [165]. Inhibition of a monoclonal anti–human albumin antibody with cat or dog albumin suggests that cat, dog, and human albumins have similar epitopes [55]. In another study, monoclonal antibodies specific to cat or dog albumin recognize the albumin of both species [166]. The study also suggests that the monoclonal antibodies and human IgE recognize identical or closely related epitopes on cat and dog albumin. Moreover, the IgE responses of animal-allergic subjects to Fel d 2, Can f 3, and Equ c 3 correlate significantly [163]. Although the clinical significance of albumins in respiratory allergy still needs further clarification, albumin allergy, particularly in an occupational exposure, can be a significant cause of disease. Moreover, respiratory sensitization to cat epithelium containing Fel d 2 may lead to pork-cat syndrome in which IgE cross-reactivity between albumins leads to hypersensitivity symptoms upon ingestion of pork meat containing pork albumin [167].

Finally, galactose-α-1,3-galactose (α-gal), a cross-reactive carbohydrate determinant (CCD), expressed in the tissues of nonprimate mammals, is involved in certain allergy syndromes, typically associated with the consumption of red (mammalian) meat [168,169]. This IgE cross-reactive glycan, present in cat Fel d 5w (IgA), can also interfere with the cat dander-specific IgE measurements of parasite-infected individuals [85]. The IgE cross-reactivity of human autoallergens was discussed earlier.

16.6 ENVIRONMENTAL CONTROL

Exposure to indoor allergens can be reduced by control measures. It is conceivable that avoiding contact with pets would restrain sensitization and the clinical manifestations of allergy. However, several studies suggest a protective effect of a high-level exposure to cat and dog-derived dust early in childhood [170–173]. Thus, avoiding infants' and preschool children's exposure to pets does not appear justified at home [174].

The guidelines are straightforward for persons already sensitized to mammalian allergens. Avoidance, or reduction of exposure when total avoidance is not possible, is the primary strategy to prevent or to reduce allergic symptoms.

Mammalian pet allergen concentrations in homes with pets are 10 to 100 times higher than in homes without pets. Removing the pet from the household results in a gradual reduction of the allergen levels. In practice, families often wish to keep their pets for emotional reasons, and various measures have been proposed to reduce the exposure in these circumstances. These include keeping the pet out of a bedroom; using vacuum cleaners and air purifiers with HEPA filters; repetitive cleaning of flooring, household furnishings, and bedding; frequent washing of the pet's bedding and the pet; and utilizing allergen-proof mattresses and pillow covers [175]. Although a reduction in the allergen levels can be achieved, the beneficial effect on health is not straightforward. The measurement of allergen concentrations in dust samples may help to evaluate the efficacy of control measures [8].

As the first line of prevention against laboratory animal allergy, persons with an atopic background, especially if they are already allergic to animals, should be discouraged from engaging in these jobs [176]. Personal protection against occupational exposure should be used when appropriate. Planning of tasks to reduce stable intermediate-level exposure might help to reduce sensitization [17]. Preventive measures include the reduction of airborne allergen levels within laboratory animal facilities. Ideally, a comprehensive plan should be utilized, starting from the appropriate design of the facilities and ventilation system.

The use of curtains in front of cage racks or filter-topped animal cages reduce the dispersion of rodent allergens in the animal room. In one study, individually ventilated cage systems decreased ambient rodent allergen levels 250-fold or more under optimal conditions. Automated cage-handling machines reduce the exposure to persons emptying and cleaning soiled cages. Handling animals during experimental procedures in class II ventilated cabinets results in a greater than 10-fold protection factor. The most effective personal protection against airborne allergens is achieved with ventilated, motorized helmets in which inhaled air is pumped through type P2 or P3 filters. Although somewhat inconvenient to use, the helmet enables asthmatic persons to work safely with animals.

SALIENT POINTS

1. Mammalian respiratory allergens are primarily dispersed in dander, saliva, and urine.
2. Exposure to mammalian allergens is not limited to immediate contact with animals; these allergens are commonly present in indoor environments.
3. Almost all important mammalian aeroallergens belong to the lipocalin family of proteins. Factors accounting for the allergenicity of lipocalins remain to be identified.
4. Environmental control measures can help symptomatic individuals, although complete avoidance of exposure is preferable.
5. High exposure to pets in early childhood may be protective against sensitization.
6. Both mammalian serum albumins and lipocalin allergens exhibit IgE cross-reactivity. The clinical significance of the IgE cross-reactivities needs further study.

REFERENCES

1. Nordlund B, Konradsen JR, Kull I et al. IgE antibodies to animal-derived lipocalin, kallikrein and secretoglobin are markers of bronchial inflammation in severe childhood asthma. *Allergy* 2012; 67: 661–669.

2. Perzanowski MS, Ronmark E, James HR et al. Relevance of specific IgE antibody titer to the prevalence, severity, and persistence of asthma among 19-year-olds in northern Sweden. *J Allergy Clin Immunol* 2016; 138: 1582–1590.

3. Asarnoj A, Hamsten C, Waden K et al. Sensitization to cat and dog allergen molecules in childhood and prediction of symptoms of cat and dog allergy in adolescence: A BAMSE/MeDALL study. *J Allergy Clin Immunol* 2016; 137: 813–817.

4. Virtanen T, Kinnunen T, Rytkönen-Nissinen M. Mammalian lipocalin allergens—Insights into their enigmatic allergenicity. *Clin Exp Allergy* 2012; 42: 494–504.

5. Virtanen T, Zeiler T, Rautiainen J et al. Allergy to lipocalins: A consequence of misguided T-cell recognition of self and nonself? *Immunol Today* 1999; 20: 398–400.

6. Konradsen JR, Nordlund B, Onell A et al. Severe childhood asthma and allergy to furry animals: Refined assessment using molecular-based allergy diagnostics. *Pediatr Allergy Immunol* 2014; 25: 187–192.

7. Kack U, Asarnoj A, Grönlund H et al. Molecular allergy diagnostics refine characterization of children sensitized to dog dander. *J Allergy Clin Immunol* 2018; 142: 1113–1119.

8. Zahradnik E, Raulf M. Animal allergens and their presence in the environment. *Front Immunol* 2014; 5: 76.

9. Platts-Mills T, Vaughan J, Squillace S et al. Sensitisation, asthma, and a modified Th2 response in children exposed to cat allergen: A population-based cross-sectional study. *Lancet* 2001; 357: 752–756.

10. Renand A, Archila LD, McGinty J et al. Chronic cat allergen exposure induces a TH2 cell-dependent IgG4 response related to low sensitization. *J Allergy Clin Immunol* 2015; 136: 1627–1635.

11. Riedl M, Landaw E, Saxon A et al. Initial high-dose nasal allergen exposure prevents allergic sensitization to a neoantigen. *J Immunol* 2005; 174: 7440–7445.

12. Huang X, Tsilochristou O, Perna S et al. Evolution of the IgE and IgG repertoire to a comprehensive array of allergen molecules in the first decade of life. *Allergy* 2018; 73: 421–430.

13. Aalberse RC, Platts-Mills TA. Does a strong IgG response precede allergic sensitization? *Allergy* 2018; 73: 1924–1925.

14. Matricardi PM, Hofmaier S, Perna S et al. Reply to: "Allergen-specific IgG responses preceding allergic sensitization." *Allergy* 2018; 73: 1926–1928.

15. Bush Bus R, Wood R, Eggleston P. Laboratory animal allergy. *J Allergy Clin Immunol* 1998; 102: 99–112.

16. Pacheco KA. New insights into laboratory animal exposures and allergic responses. *Curr Opin Allergy Clin Immunol* 2007; 7: 156–161.

17. Peng RD, Paigen B, Eggleston PA et al. Both the variability and level of mouse allergen exposure influence the phenotype of the immune response in workers at a mouse facility. *J Allerg Clin Immunol* 2011; 128: 390–397.

18. Ganfornina M, Sanchez D, Greene L et al. The lipocalin protein family: Protein sequence, structure and relationship to the calycin superfamily. In: Åkerstrom B, Borregaard N, Flower D, Salier J-P, editors. *Lipocalins*. Georgetown, TX: Landes Bioscience, 2006: 17–27.

19. Mishan-Eisenberg G, Borovsky Z, Weber M et al. Differential regulation of TH1/TH2 cytokine responses by placental protein 14. *J Immunol* 2004; 173: 5524–5530.

20. Yusifov T, Abduragimov A, Gasymov O et al. Endonuclease activity in lipocalins. *Biochem J* 2000; 347: 815–819.

21. Zeiler T, Mäntyjärvi R, Rautiainen J et al. T cell epitopes of a lipocalin allergen colocalize with the conserved regions of the molecule. *J Immunol* 1999; 162: 1415–1422.

22. Immonen A, Farci S, Taivainen A et al. T cell epitope-containing peptides of the major dog allergen Can f 1 as candidates for allergen immunotherapy. *J Immunol* 2005; 175: 3614–3620.

23. Fluckinger M, Merschak P, Hermann M et al. Lipocalin-interacting-membrane-receptor (LIMR) mediates cellular internalization of β-lactoglobulin. *Biochim Biophys Acta* 2008; 1778: 342–347.

24. Royer P-J, Emara M, Yang C et al. The mannose receptor mediates the uptake of diverse native allergens by dendritic cells and determines allergen-induced T cell polarization through modulation of IDO activity. *J Immunol* 2010; 185: 1522–1531.

25. Emara M, Royer P-J, Mahdavi J et al. Retagging identifies dendritic cell-specific intercellular adhesion molecule-3 (ICAM3)-grabbing non-integrin (DC-SIGN) protein as a novel receptor for a major allergen from house dust mite. *J Biol Chem* 2012; 287: 5756–5763.

26. Parviainen S, Kinnunen T, Rytkönen-Nissinen M et al. Mammal-derived respiratory lipocalin allergens do not exhibit dendritic cell-activating capacity. *Scand J Immunol* 2013; 77: 171–176.

27. Posch B, Irsara C, Gamper FS et al. Allergenic Can f 1 and its human homologue Lcn-1 direct dendritic cells to induce divergent immune responses. *J Cell Mol Med* 2015; 19: 2375–2384.

28. Herre J, Grönlund H, Brooks H et al. Allergens as immunomodulatory proteins: The cat dander protein Fel d 1 enhances TLR activation by lipid ligands. *J Immunol* 2013; 191: 1529–1535.

29. Eisenbarth SC, Piggott DA, Huleatt JW et al. Lipopolysaccharide-enhanced, toll-like receptor 4-dependent T helper cell type 2 responses to inhaled antigen. *J Exp Med* 2002; 196: 1645–1651.

30. Zakeri A, Russo M. Dual role of Toll-like receptors in human and experimental asthma models. *Front Immunol* 2018; 9: 1027.

31. Emara M, Royer P-J, Abbas Z et al. Recognition of the major cat allergen Fel d 1 through the cysteine-rich domain of the mannose receptor determines its allergenicity. *J Biol Chem* 2011; 286: 13033–13040.

32. Kinnunen T, Taivainen A, Partanen J et al. The DR4-DQ8 haplotype and a specific T cell receptor Vbeta T cell subset are associated with absence of allergy to Can f 1. *Clin Exp Allergy* 2005; 35: 797–803.

33. Immonen A, Kinnunen T, Sirven P et al. The major horse allergen Equ c 1 contains one immunodominant region of T cell epitopes. *Clin Exp Allergy* 2007; 37: 939–947.

34. Jeal H, Draper A, Harris J et al. Determination of the T cell epitopes of the lipocalin allergen, Rat n 1. *Clin Exp Allergy* 2004; 34: 1919–1925.

35. Saarelainen S, Zeiler T, Rautiainen J et al. Lipocalin allergen Bos d 2 is a weak immunogen. *Int Immunol* 2002; 14: 401–409.

36. Immonen A, Saarelainen S, Rautiainen J et al. Probing the mechanisms of low immunogenicity of a lipocalin allergen, Bos d 2, in a mouse model. *Clin Exp Allergy* 2003; 33: 834–841.

37. Liukko ALK, Kinnunen TT, Rytkönen-Nissinen MA et al. Human CD4+ T cell responses to the dog major allergen Can f 1 and its human homologue tear lipocalin resemble each other. *PLOS ONE* 2014; 9: e98461.

38. Counsell C, Bond J, Ohman J et al. Definition of the human T-cell epitopes of Fel d 1, the major allergen of the domestic cat. *J Allergy Clin Immunol* 1996; 98: 884–894.

39. Marcotte G, Braun C, Norman P et al. Effects of peptide therapy on *ex vivo* T-cell responses. *J Allergy Clin Immunol* 1998; 101: 506–513.

40. Rönkä AL, Kinnunen TT, Goudet A et al. Characterization of human memory CD4+ T-cell responses to the dog allergen Can f 4. *J Allergy Clin Immunol* 2015; 136: 1047–1054.

41. Kinnunen T, Buhot C, Närvänen A et al. The immunodominant epitope of lipocalin allergen Bos d 2 is suboptimal for human T cells. *Eur J Immunol* 2003; 33: 1717–1726.

42. Juntunen R, Liukko A, Taivainen A et al. Suboptimal recognition of a T cell epitope of the major dog allergen Can f 1 by human T cells. *Mol Immunol* 2009; 46: 3320–3327.

43. Kinnunen T, Kwok WW, Närvänen A et al. Immunomodulatory potential of heteroclitic analogs of the dominant T-cell epitope of lipocalin allergen Bos d 2 on specific T cells. *Int Immunol* 2005; 17: 1573–1581.

44. Paul W, Zhu J. How are T(H)2-type immune responses initiated and amplified? *Nat Rev Immunol* 2010; 10: 225–235.

45. Jenkins J, Breiteneder H, Mills E. Evolutionary distance from human homologs reflects allergenicity of animal food proteins. *J Allergy Clin Immunol* 2007; 120: 1399–1405.

46. da Costa Santiago H, Bennuru S, Ribeiro JMC et al. Structural differences between human proteins and aero- and microbial allergens define allergenicity. *PLOS ONE* 2012; 7: e40552.

47. Emanuelsson C, Spangfort M. Allergens as eukaryotic proteins lacking bacterial homologues. *Mol Immunol* 2007; 44: 3256–3260.

48. Parviainen S, Taivainen A, Liukko A et al. Comparison of the allergic and nonallergic CD4+ T-cell responses to the major dog allergen Can f 1. *J Allergy Clin Immunol* 2010; 126: 406–408.

49. Kinnunen T, Nieminen A, Kwok WW et al. Allergen-specific naïve and memory CD4+ T cells exhibit functional and phenotypic differences between individuals with or without allergy. *Eur J Immunol* 2010; 40: 2460–2469.

50. Kailaanmäki A, Kinnunen T, Kwok WW et al. Differential CD4+ T-cell responses of allergic and non-allergic subjects to the immunodominant epitope region of the horse major allergen Equ c 1. *Immunology* 2014; 141: 52–60.

51. Datta S, Milner J. Altered T-cell receptor signaling in the pathogenesis of allergic disease. *J Allergy Clin Immunol* 2011; 127: 351–354.

52. Schulten V, Westernberg L, Birrueta G et al. Allergen and epitope targets of mouse-specific T cell responses in allergy and asthma. *Front Immunol* 2018; 9: 235.

53. Niemi MH, Rytkönen-Nissinen M, Miettinen I et al. Dimerization of lipocalin allergens. *Sci Rep* 2015; 5: 13841.

54. Rouvinen J, Jänis J, Laukkanen M-L et al. Transient dimers of allergens. *PLOS ONE* 2010; 5: e9037.

55. Pandjaitan B, Swoboda I, Brandejsky-Pichler F et al. *Escherichia coli* expression and purification of recombinant dog albumin, a cross-reactive animal allergen. *J Allerg Clin Immunol* 2000; 105: 279–285.

56. Uriarte SA, Sastre J. Clinical relevance of molecular diagnosis in pet allergy. *Allergy* 2016; 71: 1066–1068.

57. Tsolakis N, Malinovschi A, Nordvall L et al. Sensitization to minor cat allergen components is associated with type-2 biomarkers in young asthmatics. *Clin Exp Allergy* 2018; 48: 1186–1194.

58. Bjerg A, Winberg A, Berthold M et al. A population-based study of animal component sensitization, asthma, and rhinitis in schoolchildren. *Pediatr Allergy Immunol* 2015; 26: 557–563.

59. van Ree R, van Leeuwen W, Bulder I et al. Purified natural and recombinant Fel d 1 and cat albumin in *in vitro* diagnostics for cat allergy. *J Allergy Clin Immunol* 1999; 104: 1223–1230.

60. Hales BJ, Chai LY, Hazell L et al. IgE and IgG binding patterns and T-cell recognition of Fel d 1 and non-Fel d 1 cat allergens. *J Allergy Clin Immunol Pract* 2013; 1: 656–665.

61. Wickman M, Lupinek C, Andersson N et al. Detection of IgE reactivity to a handful of allergen molecules in early childhood predicts respiratory allergy in adolescence. *EBioMedicine* 2017; 26: 91–99.

62. Hilger C, van Hage M, Kuehn A. Diagnosis of allergy to mammals and fish: Cross-reactive vs. specific markers. *Curr Allergy Asthma Rep* 2017; 17: 64.

63. Kristensen AK, Schou C, Roepstorff P. Determination of isoforms, N-linked glycan structure and disulfide bond linkages of the major cat allergen Fel d1 by a mass spectrometric approach. *Biol Chem* 1997; 378: 899–908.

64. Morgenstern J, Griffith I, Brauer A et al. Amino acid sequence of Fel dI, the major allergen of the domestic cat: Protein sequence analysis and cDNA cloning. *Proc Natl Acad Sci USA* 1991; 88: 9690–9694.

65. Griffith IJ, Graig S, Pollock J et al. Expression and genomic structure of the genes encoding FdI, the major allergen from the domestic cat. *Gene* 1992; 113: 263–268.

66. Kaiser L, Velickovic TC, Badia-Martinez D et al. Structural characterization of the tetrameric form of the major cat allergen Fel d 1. *J Mol Biol* 2007; 370: 714–727.

67. Bienboire-Frosini C, Cozzi A, Lafont-Lecuelle C et al. Immunological differences in the global release of the major cat allergen Fel d 1 are influenced by sex and behaviour. *Vet J* 2012; 193: 162–167.

68. Duffort O, Carreira J, Nitti G et al. Studies on the biochemical structure of the major cat allergen *Felis domesticus* I. *Mol Immunol* 1991; 28: 301–309.

69. van Milligen FJ, van't Hof W, van den Berg M et al. IgE epitopes on the cat (*Felis domesticus*) major allergen Fel d I—A study with overlapping synthetic peptides. *J Allergy Clin Immunol* 1994; 93: 34–43.

70. Tasaniyananda N, Tungtrongchitr A, Seesuay W et al. A novel IgE-binding epitope of cat major allergen, Fel d 1. *Biochem Biophys Res Commun* 2016; 470: 593–598.

71. Worm M, Lee H, Kleine-Tebbe J et al. Development and preliminary clinical evaluation of a peptide immunotherapy vaccine for cat allergy. *J Allergy Clin Immunol* 2011; 127: 89–97.

72. van Neerven RJ, van de Pol MM, van Milligen FJ et al. Characterization of cat dander-specific T lymphocytes from atopic patients. *J Immunol* 1994; 152: 4203–4210.

73. Mark P, Segal D, Dallaire M et al. Human T and B cell immune responses to Fel d 1 in cat-allergic and non-cat-allergic subjects. *Clin Exp Allergy* 1996; 26: 1316–1328.

74. Young R, Dekker J, Wordsworth B et al. HLA-DR and HLA-DP genotypes and immunoglobulin E responses to common major allergens. *Clin Exp Allergy* 1994; 24: 431–439.

75. Howell W, Standring P, Warner J et al. HLA class II genotype, HLA-DR B cell surface expression and allergen specific IgE production in atopic and non-atopic members of asthmatic family pedigrees. *Clin Exp Allergy* 1999; 29: 35–38.

76. Bateman EAL, Ardern-Jones MR, Ogg GS. Persistent central memory phenotype of circulating Fel d 1 peptide/DRB1*0101 tetramer-binding CD4+ T cells. *J Allergy Clin Immunol* 2006; 118: 1350–1356.

77. Kwok W, Roti M, Delong J et al. Direct *ex vivo* analysis of allergen-specific CD4+ T cells. *J Allergy Clin Immunol* 2010; 125: 1407–1409.

78. Reefer A, Carneiro R, Custis N et al. A role for IL-10-mediated HLA-DR7-restricted T cell-dependent events in development of the modified Th2 response to cat allergen. *J Immunol* 2004; 172: 2763–2772.

79. Reininger R, Swoboda I, Bohle B et al. Characterization of recombinant cat albumin. *Clin Exp Allergy* 2003; 33: 1695–1702.

80. Wisniewski JA, Agrawal R, Minnicozzi S et al. Sensitization to food and inhalant allergens in relation to age and wheeze among children with atopic dermatitis. *Clin Exp Allergy* 2013; 43: 1160–1170.

81. Ichikawa K, Vailes L, Pomes A et al. Molecular cloning, expression and modelling of cat allergen, cystatin (Fel d 3), a cysteine protease inhibitor. *Clin Exp Allergy* 2001; 31: 1279–1286.

82. Smith W, Butler A, Hazell L et al. Fel d 4, a cat lipocalin allergen. *Clin Exp Allergy* 2004; 34: 1732–1738.

83. Patelis A, Gunnbjörnsdottir M, Malinovschi A et al. Population-based study of multiplexed IgE sensitization in relation to asthma, exhaled nitric oxide, and bronchial responsiveness. *J Allergy Clin Immunol* 2012; 130: 397–402.

84. Adedoyin J, Grönlund H, Öman H et al. Cat IgA, representative of new carbohydrate cross-reactive allergens. *J Allergy Clin Immunol* 2007; 119: 640–645.

85. Arkestål K, Sibanda E, Thors C et al. Impaired allergy diagnostics among parasite-infected patients caused by IgE antibodies to the carbohydrate epitope galactose-α1,3-galactose. *J Allergy Clin Immunol* 2011; 127: 1024–1028.

86. Smith W, O'Neil SE, Hales BJ et al. Two newly identified cat allergens: The von Ebner gland protein Fel d 7 and the latherin-like protein Fel d 8. *Int Arch Allergy Immunol* 2011; 156: 159–170.

87. Apostolovic D, Sanchez-Vidaurre S, Waden K et al. The cat lipocalin Fel d 7 and its cross-reactivity with the dog lipocalin Can f 1. *Allergy* 2016; 71: 1490–1495.

88. McDonald RE, Fleming RI, Beeley JG et al. Latherin: A surfactant protein of horse sweat and saliva. *PLOS ONE* 2009; 4: e5726.

89. Schou C, Svendsen U, Lowenstein H. Purification and characterization of the major dog allergen, Can f I. *Clin Exp Allergy* 1991; 21: 321–328.

90. Konieczny A, Morgenstern JP, Bizinkauskas CB et al. The major dog allergens, Can f 1 and Can f 2, are salivary lipocalin proteins: Cloning and immunological characterization of the recombinant forms. *Immunology* 1997; 92: 577–586.

91. Saarelainen S, Taivainen A, Rytkönen-Nissinen M et al. Assessment of recombinant dog allergens Can f 1 and Can f 2 for the diagnosis of dog allergy. *Clin Exp Allergy* 2004; 34: 1576–1582.

92. Madhurantakam C, Nilsson O, Uchtenhagen H et al. Crystal structure of the dog lipocalin allergen Can f 2: Implications for cross-reactivity to the cat allergen Fel d 4. *J Mol Biol* 2010; 401: 68–83.

93. de Groot H, Goei K, van Swieten P et al. Affinity purification of a major and a minor allergen from dog extract: Serologic activity of affinity-purified Can f I and of Can f I-depleted extract. *J Allergy Clin Immunol* 1991; 87: 1056–1065.

94. Ramadour M, Guetat M, Guetat J et al. Dog factor differences in Can f 1 allergen production. *Allergy* 2005; 60: 1060–1064.

95. Heutelbeck ARR, Schulz T, Bergmann K-C et al. Environmental exposure to allergens of different dog breeds and relevance in allergological diagnostics. *J Toxicol Environ Health Part A* 2008; 71: 751–758.

96. Vredegoor DW, Willemse T, Chapman MD et al. Can f 1 levels in hair and homes of different dog breeds: Lack of evidence to describe any dog breed as hypoallergenic. *J Allergy Clin Immunol* 2012; 130: 904–907.

97. Kamata Y, Miyanomae A, Nakayama E et al. Characterization of dog allergens Can f 1 and Can f 2. 1. Preparation of their recombinant proteins and antibodies. *Int Arch Allergy Immunol* 2007; 142: 291–300.

98. Curin M, Weber M, Hofer G et al. Clustering of conformational IgE epitopes on the major dog allergen Can f 1. *Sci Rep* 2017; 7: 616.

99. Spitzauer S, Schweiger C, Sperr W et al. Molecular characterization of dog albumin as a cross-reactive allergen. *J Allergy Clin Immunol* 1994; 93: 614–627.

100. Polovic N, Waden K, Binnmyr J et al. Dog saliva—An important source of dog allergens. *Allergy* 2013; 68: 585–592.

101. Mattsson L, Lundgren T, Olsson P et al. Molecular and immunological characterization of Can f 4: A dog dander allergen cross-reactive with a 23 kDa odorant-binding protein in cow dander. *Clin Exp Allergy* 2010; 40: 1276–1287.

102. Rytkönen-Nissinen M, Saarelainen S, Randell J et al. IgE reactivity of the dog lipocalin allergen Can f 4 and the development of a sandwich ELISA for its quantification. *Allergy Asthma Immunol Res* 2015; 7: 384–392.

103. Niemi MH, Rytkönen-Nissinen M, Jänis J et al. Structural aspects of dog allergies: The crystal structure of a dog dander allergen Can f 4. *Mol Immunol* 2014; 61: 7–15.

104. Mattsson L, Lundgren T, Everberg H et al. Prostatic kallikrein: A new major dog allergen. *J Allergy Clin Immunol* 2009; 123: 362–368.

105. Kofler L, Kofler H, Mattsson L et al. A case of dog-related human seminal plasma allergy. *Eur Ann Allergy Clin Immunol* 2012; 44: 89–92.

106. Schoos A-MM, Bonnelykke K, Chawes BL et al. Precision allergy: Separate allergies to male and female dogs. *J Allergy Clin Immunol Pract* 2017; 5: 1754–1756.

107. Basagaña M, Bartolomé B, Pastor C et al. Allergy to human seminal fluid: Cross-reactivity with dog dander. *J Allergy Clin Immunol* 2008; 121: 233–239.

108. Kailaanmäki A, Kinnunen T, Rönkä A et al. Human memory CD4+ T cell response to the major dog allergen Can f 5, prostatic kallikrein. *Clin Exp Allergy* 2016; 46: 720–729.

109. Nilsson OB, Binnmyr J, Zoltowska A et al. Characterization of the dog lipocalin allergen Can f 6: The role in cross-reactivity with cat and horse. *Allergy* 2012; 67: 751–757.

110. Hilger C, Swiontek K, Arumugam K et al. Identification of a new major dog allergen highly cross-reactive with Fel d 4 in a population of cat- and dog-sensitized patients. *J Allerg Clin Immunol* 2012; 129: 1149–1151.

111. Wang Y-J, Li L, Song W-J et al. *Canis familiaris* allergen Can f 6: Expression, purification and analysis of B-cell epitopes in Chinese dog allergic children. *Oncotarget* 2017; 8: 90796–90807.

112. Khurana T, Newman-Lindsay S, Young PR et al. The NPC2 protein: A novel dog allergen. *ANAI* 2016; 116: 440–442.

113. Gregoire C, Rosinski-Chupin I, Rabillon J et al. cDNA cloning and sequencing reveal the major horse allergen Equ c 1 to be a glycoprotein member of the lipocalin superfamily. *J Biol Chem* 1996; 271: 32951–32959.

114. Dandeu J-P, Rabillon J, Divanovic A et al. Hydrophobic interaction chromatography for isolation and purification of Equ.cl, the horse major allergen. *J Chromatogr* 1993; 621: 23–31.

115. Goubran Botros H, Poncet P, Rabillon J et al. Biochemical characterization and surfactant properties of horse allergens. *Eur J Biochem* 2001; 268: 3126–3136.

116. Lascombe M-B, Gregoire C, Poncet P et al. Crystal structure of the allergen Equ c 1—A dimeric lipocalin with restricted IgE-reactive epitopes. *J Biol Chem* 2000; 275: 21572–21577.

117. Bulone V, Krogstad-Johnsen T, Smestad-Paulsen B. Separation of horse dander allergen proteins by two-dimensional electrophoresis—Molecular characterisation and identification of Equ c 2.0101 and Equ c 2.0102 as lipocalin proteins. *Eur J Biochem* 1998; 253: 202–211.

118. Cabanas R, Lopez-Serrano M, Carreira J et al. Importance of albumin in cross-reactivity among cat, dog and horse allergens. *J Investig Allergol Clin Immunol* 2000; 10: 71–77.

119. Mäntyjärvi R, Parkkinen S, Rytkönen M et al. Complementary DNA cloning of the predominant allergen of bovine dander: A new member in the lipocalin family. *J Allergy Clin Immunol* 1996; 97: 1297–1303.

120. Ylönen J, Mäntyjärvi R, Taivainen A et al. IgG and IgE antibody responses to cow dander and urine in farmers with cow-induced asthma. *Clin Exp Allergy* 1992; 22: 83–90.

121. Zahradnik E, Sander I, Bruning T et al. Allergen levels in the hair of different cattle breeds. *Int Arch Allergy Immunol* 2015; 167: 9–15.

122. Saarelainen S, Rytkönen-Nissinen M, Rouvinen J et al. Animal-derived lipocalin allergens exhibit immunoglobulin E cross-reactivity. *Clin Exp Allergy* 2008; 38: 374–381.

123. Rautiainen J, Rytkönen M, Syrjänen K et al. Tissue localization of bovine dander allergen Bos d 2. *J Allergy Clin Immunol* 1998; 101: 349–353.

124. Rouvinen J, Rautiainen J, Virtanen T et al. Probing the molecular basis of allergy. Three-dimensional structure of the bovine lipocalin allergen Bos d 2. *J Biol Chem* 1999; 274: 2337–2343.

125. Kauppinen A, Peräsaari J, Taivainen A et al. Association of HLA class II alleles with sensitization to cow dander Bos d 2, an important occupational allergen. *Immunobiology* 2012; 217: 8–12.

126. Rautiainen J, Rytkönen M, Parkkinen S et al. cDNA cloning and protein analysis of a bovine dermal allergen with homology to psoriasin. *J Invest Dermatol* 1995; 105: 660–663.

127. Regenhard P, Leippe M, Schubert S et al. Antimicrobial activity of bovine psoriasin. *Vet. Microbiol.* 2009; 136: 335–340.

128. Prahl P, Weeke B, Lowenstein H. Quantitative immunoelectrophoretic analysis of extract from cow hair and dander. Characterization of the antigens and identification of the allergens. *Allergy* 1978; 33: 241–253.

129. Parkkinen S, Rytkönen M, Pentikäinen J et al. Homology of a bovine allergen and the oligomycin sensitivity-conferring protein of the mitochondrial adenosine triphosphate synthase complex. *J Allergy Clin Immunol* 1995; 95: 1255–1260.

130. Lorusso JR, Moffat S, Ohman JL. Immunologic and biochemical properties of the major mouse urinary allergen (Mus m 1). *J Allergy Clin Immunol* 1986; 78: 928–937.

131. Cavaggioni A, Mucignat-Caretta C. Major urinary proteins, α2U-globulins and aphrodisin. *Biochim Biophys Acta* 2000; 1482: 218–228.

132. Ferrari E, Lodi T, Sorbi RT et al. Expression of a lipocalin in *Pichia pastoris*: Secretion, purification and binding activity of a recombinant mouse major urinary protein. *FEBS Lett* 1997; 401: 73–77.

133. Price J, Longbottom J. Allergy to mice. II. Further characterization of two major mouse allergens (AG 1 and AG 3) and immunohistochemical investigations of their sources. *Clin Exp Allergy* 1990; 20: 71–77.

134. Platts-Mills T, Longbottom J, Edwards J et al. Occupational asthma and rhinitis related to laboratory rats: Serum IgG and IgE antibodies to the rat urinary allergen. *J Allergy Clin Immunol* 1987; 79: 505–515.

135. Virtanen T, Zeiler T, Mäntyjärvi R. Important animal allergens are lipocalin proteins: Why are they allergenic? *Int Arch Allergy Immunol* 1999; 120: 247–258.

136. Jeal H, Draper A, Jones M et al. HLA associations with occupational sensitization to rat lipocalin allergens: A model for other animal allergies? *J Allergy Clin Immunol* 2003; 111: 795–799.

137. Fahlbusch B, Rudeschko O, Szilagyi U et al. Purification and partial characterization of the major allergen, Cav p 1, from guinea pig *Cavia porcellus*. *Allergy* 2002; 57: 417–422.

138. Hilger C, Swiontek K, Kler S et al. Evaluation of two new recombinant guinea-pig lipocalins, Cav p 2 and Cav p 3, in the diagnosis of guinea-pig allergy. *Clin Exp Allergy* 2011; 41: 899–908.

139. Price J, Longbottom J. Allergy to rabbits. II. Identification and characterization of a major rabbit allergen. *Allergy* 1988;43: 39–48.

140. Baker J, Berry A, Boscato LM et al. Identification of some rabbit allergens as lipocalins. *Clin Exp Allergy* 2001; 31: 303–312.

141. Hilger C, Kler S, Arumugam K et al. Identification and isolation of a Fel d 1-like molecule as a major rabbit allergen. *J Allergy Clin Immunol* 2014; 133: 759–766.

142. Hilger C, Kler S, Hentges F. Reply: To PMID 24369805. *J Allergy Clin Immunol* 2014; 133: 284–285.

143. Hilger C, Dubey VP, Lentz D et al. Male-specific submaxillary gland protein, a lipocalin allergen of the golden hamster, differs from the lipocalin allergens of Siberian and Roborovski dwarf hamsters. *Int Arch Allergy Immunol* 2015; 166: 30–40.

144. Srikantan S, Parekh V, De PK. cDNA cloning and regulation of two sex-hormone-repressed hamster tear lipocalins having homology with odorant/pheromone-binding proteins. *Biochim Biophys Acta* 2005; 1729: 154–165.

145. Torres JA, Las Heras de M, Maroto AS et al. Molecular and immunological characterization of the first allergenic lipocalin in hamster: The major allergen from Siberian hamster (*Phodopus sungorus*). *J Biol Chem* 2014; 289: 23382–23388.

146. Natter S, Seiberler S, Hufnagl P et al. Isolation of cDNA clones coding for IgE autoantigens with serum IgE from atopic dermatitis patients. *FASEB J* 1998; 12: 1559–1569.

147. Zeller S, Rhyner C, Meyer N et al. Exploring the repertoire of IgE-binding self-antigens associated with atopic eczema. *J Allergy Clin Immunol* 2009; 124: 278–285.

148. Maurer M, Altrichter S, Schmetzer O et al. Immunoglobulin E-mediated autoimmunity. *Front Immunol* 2018; 9: 689.

149. Valenta R, Natter S, Seiberler S et al. Molecular characterization of an autoallergen, Hom s 1, identified by serum IgE from atopic dermatitis patients. *J Invest Dermatol* 1998; 111: 1178–1183.

150. Mossabeb R, Seiberler S, Mittermann I et al. Characterization of a novel isoform of α-nascent polypeptide-associated complex as IgE-defined autoantigen. *J Invest Dermatol* 2002; 119: 820–829.

151. Aichberger K, Mittermann I, Reininger R et al. Hom s 4, an IgE-reactive autoantigen belonging to a new subfamily of calcium-binding proteins, can induce Th cell type 1-mediated autoreactivity. *J Immunol* 2005; 175: 1286–1294.

152. Fluckiger S, Scapozza L, Mayer C et al. Immunological and structural analysis of IgE-mediated cross-reactivity between manganese superoxide dismutases. *Int Arch Allergy Immunol* 2002; 128: 292–303.

153. Mayer C, Appenzeller U, Seelbach H et al. Humoral and cell-mediated autoimmune reactions to human acidic ribosomal P2 protein in individuals sensitized to *Aspergillus fumigatus* P2 protein. *J Exp Med* 1999; 189: 1507–1512.

154. Limacher A, Glaser AG, Meier C et al. Cross-reactivity and 1.4-Å crystal structure of *Malassezia sympodialis* thioredoxin (Mala s 13), a member of a new pan-allergen family. *J Immunol* 2007; 178: 389–396.

155. Flückiger S, Fijten H, Whitley P et al. Cyclophilins, a new family of cross-reactive allergens. *Eur J Immunol* 2002; 32: 10–17.

156. Valenta R, Duchene M, Pettenburger K et al. Identification of profilin as a novel pollen allergen; IgE autoreactivity in sensitized individuals. *Science* 1991; 253: 557–560.

157. Reininger R, Varga E, Zach M et al. Detection of an allergen in dog dander that cross-reacts with the major cat allergen, Fel d 1. *Clin Exp Allergy* 2007; 37: 116–124.

158. Jeal H, Harris J, Draper A et al. Dual sensitization to rat and mouse urinary allergens reflects cross-reactive molecules rather than atopy. *Allergy* 2009; 64: 855–861.

159. Jakob T, Hilger C, Hentges F. Clinical relevance of sensitization to cross-reactive lipocalin Can f 6. *Allergy* 2013; 68: 690–691.

160. Kamata Y, Miyanomae A, Nakayama E et al. Characterization of dog allergens Can f 1 and Can f 2. 2. A comparison of Can f 1 with Can f 2 regarding their biochemical and immunological properties. *Int Arch Allergy Immunol* 2007; 142: 301–308.

161. Fahlbusch B, Rudeschko O, Schlott B et al. Further characterization of IgE-binding antigens from guinea pig hair as new members of the lipocalin family. *Allergy* 2003; 58: 629–634.

162. Reddy B, Karande A, Adiga P. A common epitope of β-lactoglobulin and serum retinol-binding proteins: Elucidation of its core sequence using synthetic peptides. *Mol Immunol* 1992; 29: 511–516.

163. Curin M, Swoboda I, Wollmann E et al. Microarrayed dog, cat, and horse allergens show weak correlation between allergen-specific IgE and IgG responses. *J Allergy Clin Immunol* 2014; 133: 918–921.

164. Spitzauer S, Pandjaitan B, Söregi G et al. IgE cross-reactivities against albumins in patients allergic to animals. *J Allerg Clin Immunol* 1995; 96: 951–959.

165. Goubran Botros H, Gregoire C, Rabillon J et al. Cross-antigenicity of horse serum albumin with dog and cat albumins: Study of three short peptides with significant inhibitory activity towards specific human IgE and IgG antibodies. *Immunology* 1996; 88: 340–347.

166. Boutin Y, Hebert J, Vrancken E et al. Mapping of cat albumin using monoclonal antibodies: Identification of determinants common to cat and dog. *Clin Exp Immunol* 1989; 77: 440–444.

167. Hilger C, Kohnen M, Grigioni F et al. Allergic cross-reactions between cat and pig serum albumin. Study at the protein and DNA levels. *Allergy* 1997; 52: 179–187.

168. Commins SP, Platts-Mills TAE. Anaphylaxis syndromes related to a new mammalian cross-reactive carbohydrate determinant. *J Allergy Clin Immunol* 2009; 124: 652–657.

169. Morisset M, Richard C, Astier C et al. Anaphylaxis to pork kidney is related to IgE antibodies specific for galactose-α-1,3-galactose. *Allergy* 2012; 67: 699–704.

170. Bufford JD, Reardon CL, Li Z et al. Effects of dog ownership in early childhood on immune development and atopic diseases. *Clin Exp Allergy* 2008; 38: 1635–1643.

171. Wegienka G, Johnson CC, Havstad S et al. Lifetime dog and cat exposure and dog- and cat-specific sensitization at age 18 years. *Clin Exp Allergy* 2011; 41: 979–986.

172. Lynch SV, Wood RA, Boushey H et al. Effects of early-life exposure to allergens and bacteria on recurrent wheeze and atopy in urban children. *J Allergy Clin Immunol* 2014; 134: 593–601.

173. Schoos A-MM, Chawes BL, Jelding-Dannemand E et al. Early indoor aeroallergen exposure is not associated with development of sensitization or allergic rhinitis in high-risk children. *Allergy* 2016; 71: 684–691.

174. Brozek JL, Bousquet J, Baena-Cagnani CE et al. Allergic Rhinitis and its Impact on Asthma (ARIA) guidelines: 2010 revision. *J Allergy Clin Immunol* 2010; 126: 466–476.

175. Matsui EC. Role of environmental control in the management of asthma and allergy. *J Allergy Clin Immunol* 2012; 129: 271–272.

176. Cullinan P, Cook A, Gordon S et al. Allergen exposure, atopy and smoking as determinants of allergy to rats in a cohort of laboratory employees. *Eur Respir J* 1999; 13: 1139–1143.

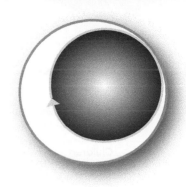

17 Food allergens

Anusha Penumarti and Mike Kulis
University of North Carolina at Chapel Hill

CONTENTS

17.1 INTRODUCTION

Food allergy is an immune system–mediated adverse reaction to food proteins that can affect multiple organs. Organ or systemic involvement includes cutaneous, gastrointestinal, respiratory, oral, and generalized reactions, including potentially lethal anaphylaxis [1]. Fatal anaphylactic reactions to foods have been reported from multiple locations throughout the world, including the United States and Europe. Accidental reactions occur approximately once per year per allergic person [2]. These data indicate that avoidance of food allergen triggers is not easy and can lead to anxiety and decreased quality of life in food-allergic patients [3]. Reactions to small quantities of food allergens have led to the Food Allergen Labeling and Consumer Protection Act (FALCPA) in the United States, which requires food manufacturers to list all ingredients and clearly identify the food source; i.e., *whey* would have to be labeled as derived from *milk*. Europe has a similar food allergen labeling law called Annex IIIa.

Food allergies affect an estimated 3%–6% of children in the United States, with similar prevalence estimates from Europe, Canada, Australia, and China [4]. These findings indicate an increase in prevalence over the past two decades. In young children, the most common food allergies are cow's milk, egg, peanut, wheat, soy, tree nuts, fish, and shellfish. Early childhood allergies to milk, egg, soy, and wheat often resolve by school age, whereas only approximately 20% of peanut allergies and 10% of tree nut allergies will resolve. Adult food allergies primarily include shellfish, peanut, tree nuts, and fish (see Table 17.1). Risk factors for developing food allergy include a family history of atopic disorders with environmental factors seemingly modulating the expression of food allergies. The mechanism of sensitization to foods is not clear, but epicutaneous sensitization is a possibility, as demonstrated in various mouse model studies [5,6]. Interestingly, a defect in skin barrier function caused by a loss-of-function mutation in the filaggrin gene was associated with peanut allergy in a European population [7].

The sensitizing ability of individual foods and severity of clinical reactivity to food allergens correlate with the following classification of food allergens [8]. Class 1 food allergens both sensitize and trigger allergic reactions via the oral route because they are quickly absorbed and distributed to the systemic immune system. However, class 2 food allergens do not sensitize orally because they are easily digested into small peptides and lose their sensitization potential. They elicit allergy indirectly when ingested by the fact that they cross-react with other allergens, typically inhalant allergens, often described

Table 17.1 Major allergenic foods in children and adults

Children	Adults
Milk	Peanut
Eggs	Tree nuts
Peanut	Fish
Soybean	Shellfish
Tree nuts	
Wheat	
Fish	
Shellfish	

as pollen–food allergy syndrome. Examples include apple, celery, and carrot, and their homologue in birch pollen, Bet v 1. Sequential epitopes of allergens consist of amino acids in the primary sequences, while conformational epitopes exist as a consequence of three-dimensional folding of the proteins. Allergen-specific IgE binding sites are routinely limited to short amino acid sequences, either sequential or conformational. Conformational determinants result from proximity of nonsequential amino acids following folding into a three-dimensional structure. Specific cross-reactivity with proteins sharing sufficient sequential and/or conformational homology occurs with similar food allergens as well as other proteins. Therefore, divergent patterns of cross-reactivity and clinically relevant allergic reactions to foods occur in individual patients.

Not all proteins in foods are allergenic. Major food allergens are generally water-soluble glycoproteins with molecular weights ranging from 10 to 60 kDa. However, structural characteristics are important for a protein's allergenicity, and many food allergens occur naturally as dimers or trimers with molecular weights of 150–200 kDa [9]. These oligomeric forms might have a higher allergenic potential than monomers because larger molecules have additional epitopes for IgE-mediated histamine release. There are no known unique biochemical or immunochemical characteristics for food allergens versus other allergens. Comparisons of primary structure (amino acid sequences) of allergenic proteins do not reveal patterns that could be related to allergenicity. Class 1 food allergens tend to be resistant to the usual food processing and preparation conditions and are comparatively resistant to heat and acid treatment, proteolysis, and digestion. For example, treatment of food allergens with acid concentrations simulating stomach acid typically has little effect on the specific IgE binding of the class 1 food allergens. In contrast, class 2 allergens, principally found in fresh fruits and select vegetables, are affected by these physical conditions, resulting in rapid digestion and dissociation into smaller peptides, bringing about the destruction of conformational epitopes and loss of allergenicity.

At least two different epitopes on the surface of the allergen must cross-link IgE on mast cells and basophils to result in a physiologic response causing an allergic reaction [10]. Evidence for conformational epitopes is provided by crystallographic resolution of antigen-antibody complex structures, by site-directed mutagenesis to alter the amino acid sequences, and by peptide mimics (individual peptides isolated from peptide libraries that frequently yield peptides mimicking the binding site of the cognate antigen for the specific antibody but do not correspond to the linear sequence) [11]. Using

peptides or mimotopes for allergen molecules, epitopes in a three-dimensional format can be studied by crystallographic comparisons. IgE epitopes identified in this manner were all conformational and responsible for high-affinity interactions with specific IgE preferentially forming di-, tri-, or multimers that display repetitive IgE epitopes. As B lymphocytes are pattern recognizers, the tendency for allergens to form multimers may be critical in initiation of the IgE response.

17.2 TAXONOMY OF FOOD ALLERGENS

Food allergens, found in plants and animals, are classified as to their biologic function or protein family group. Plant food allergens are contained in 31 of 8296 protein families [12], with the most important animal food allergens present in milk, egg, and various seafood. Examples of animal groups include birds (chicken and duck), crustaceans (crab and lobster), and red meats (beef and lamb). Examples of plant groups include the apple family (apple and pear), grass family (corn and wheat), legume family (lentil and peanut), and walnut family (black walnut and pecan). Allergy may result in a variable degree of clinical reactivity to other members of the same group because of cross-reacting allergens.

All allergens, including food allergens, are named using the first three letters of the genus, followed by a single letter for the species and a number indicating the chronologic order of allergen purification and immunologic characterization. For example, the first peanut (*Arachis hypogaea*) allergen reported in 1991 is designated as Ara h 1 [13], the second is Ara h 2, and so on. Allergens are named by the World Health Organization (WHO) and the International Union of Immunological Societies (IUIS) Allergen Nomenclature Sub-Committee [14,15]. The WHO/IUIS subcommittee began in 1984 and is composed of international experts in allergen characterization. Table 17.2 provides an overview of the key information needed before an allergen is officially recognized and named. An abbreviated listing of the families and examples of plant and animal protein allergens is presented in Table 17.3, along with the number of known allergens in several significant protein families [16].

Once an antigen meets the criteria in Table 17.2 and receives a name, it is customary to designate the allergen as either "major" or "minor." A major allergen typically designates an allergen that binds to IgE, or is otherwise immunologically active, in greater than 50% of patients studied. A minor allergen is defined as an allergen for which less than 50% of sensitive individuals have detectable IgE. The designation of major or minor is not always consistent from study to study. For example, Ara h 3, a peanut allergen, was found to be a "minor" allergen in a population in the United States [17] but qualified as "major" in an Italian study [18]. Various reasons could exist as to why an allergen would not behave the same way in different studies, including geographical location of subjects, age of subjects, or method used to determine the allergen's importance (i.e., IgE binding by Western blot or enzyme-linked immunosorbent assay [ELISA]; *in vitro* histamine release assays; skin prick testing). Although the designation of major and minor allergens in food is useful, it does not mean that minor allergens will not trigger severe reactions in some patients.

17.3 "BIG 8" FOOD ALLERGEN SOURCES

The WHO/IUIS Allergen Nomenclature Sub-Committee maintains a database of named allergens (http://www.allergen.org) [14]. The database contains links to key allergen information (see Table 17.2)

Table 17.2 Information requested for establishing and naming an allergen

Allergen source
Genus and species names
Common name
Taxonomic family and order
Biochemistry
Biochemical name of the protein
Tissue or organ expressing the natural allergen
Molecular weight of the mature protein
Posttranslational modifications (i.e., glycosylation)
Recombinant protein expression system, if used
Molecular biology
Nucleotide sequence
Protein sequence
Structure of the protein
Signal sequence; propeptide sequence; mature sequence
Primer sequences if polymerase chain reaction (PCR) strategy was used
Sequence confirmation of protein (i.e., by tandem mass spectrometry [MS/MS])
Allergenicity
Define study population (age, geographical location, etc.)
IgE testing used (i.e., *in vitro* IgE assay; skin test; cellular tests)
If glycosylated, did IgE bind to deglycosylated protein

Note: An allergen must bind IgE from at least five sera from allergic subjects and bind IgE from at least 5% of all tested sera of patients allergic to the allergen source.

Table 17.3 Plant and animal food allergens

Plant food allergens	
Prolamin superfamily	*Examples*
2S albumins	Jug r 1 (walnut); Ara h 2 (peanut)
Nonspecific lipid transfer protein types 1, 2	Ara h 9 (peanut); Sola l 6 (tomato)
Bifunctional α-amylase/protease inhibitors	Sec c 38 (rye)
Cupin superfamily	
Vicilins (also known as 7/8S globulins)	Ara h 1 (peanut); Ses i 3 (sesame)
Legumins (also known as 11S globulins)	Ara h 3 (peanut); Gly m 6 (soybean)
Profilin family	Api g 4 (celery); Pru av 4 (cherry)
Bet v 1 family	Mal d 1 (apple); Ara h 8 (peanut)
Others	Act c 1 (kiwi); Gly m 7 (soybean)
Animal food allergens	
Cow's milk	Bos d 5 (β-lactoglobulin); Bos d 8-12 (caseins)
Egg	Gal d 1 (ovomucoid)
Fish	Gad c 1 (cod parvalbumin)
Shellfish	Pen a 1 (shrimp tropomyosin)
Allergen family chart	
Protein family name	*Number of allergens*
Prolamin superfamily	91
Profilin	53
Tropomyosin	64
EF-hand domain	74
Cupin superfamily	37
Bet v 1–related proteins	29
Lipocalin	25
Expansin, *C*-terminal domain	24
Thaumatin-like proteins	17
α/β Casein	4

and links to the original publications describing and characterizing the allergen. The following information on the various allergens in the eight foods responsible for the majority of allergic reactions, i.e., the "Big 8," was compiled using established literature studies and the http://www.allergen.org database [14]. While these food sources are the most common contributors to allergic reactions in the United States and Europe, differences may exist in other countries depending on the diet of the country, environmental stimuli, and genetic differences among populations.

17.3.1 Cow's milk

A number of milk proteins are allergenic, and patients react to various cow's milk proteins by either skin prick tests or challenge [19]. Caseins (Bos d 8–12) and β-lactoglobulin (Bos d 5) are the major allergens in cow's milk. Casein, a phosphoprotein, is the major protein of bovine milk that exists in equilibrium between soluble and complex colloidal aggregates (micelles). Its heterogeneity consists of α-, β-, and κ-caseins (75%, 22%, and 3%, respectively). The major α- and β-caseins have molecular weights of approximately 23 kDa, and there are several genetic variants of each. β-Lactoglobulin (18 kDa), the most abundant whey protein, also has several genetic variants. α-Lactalbumin (14 kDa) and bovine serum albumin (67 kDa), both whey proteins, are minor cow's milk allergens. The IgE-binding epitopes on the milk caseins, lactalbumin and lactoglobulin, are identified. So too are specific IgE-binding epitopes that may differentiate between patients with persistent and transient cow's milk allergy [20,21].

Confusion can arise in the determination of cow's milk allergy because of the different forms of cow's milk used in challenges, e.g., liquid cow's milk, nonfat dry milk, and infant formula. Similarly, fatal anaphylaxis has resulted from inadvertent or unexpected exposure to different milk proteins in other foods (e.g., casein in sausage). Reliable analytical results for milk allergens (casein, lactalbumin, and lactoglobulin) in nondairy foods are needed for them to be causally associated with milk allergy. Wal's review [19] on the biochemistry and immunochemistry of milk proteins indicates that no single allergen or structure accounts for milk allergenicity or predicts an allergic response. The great variability in the polysensitization and IgE responses to cow's milk and potential immunologic cross-reactions to milk of other species, such as buffalo, goat, sheep, and camel, will vary according to the characteristics of the population studied. Any food that contains native or denatured milk proteins or fragments derived thereof may trigger an allergic reaction.

Approximately 75% of 100 milk allergic subjects tolerated extensively heated or baked milk products in the form of muffins and waffles [22]. These data suggest that there are two distinct phenotypes of milk allergy, one in which subjects tolerant to baked milk have a mild allergy and the second in which subjects intolerant to baked milk have a more severe allergy. Additionally, incorporating these baked forms of milk into the diet appears to accelerate the natural history and allows for earlier tolerance to nonheated milk products [23]. Other treatment strategies that have shown promising improvements in the quality of life in patients with cow's milk allergy include early introduction of cow's milk in infants, oral immunotherapy [24], sublingual immunotherapy (SLIT) [25], and epicutaneous immunotherapy (EPIT) [26].

17.3.2 Eggs

Several studies have identified the major chicken egg allergens [27,28]. Ovomucoid (Gal d 1), a glycoprotein with a molecular weight of 28 kDa and an acidic isoelectric point, is the major egg allergen. In a study of 18 children with egg allergy, ovomucoid was a more potent allergen than purified ovalbumin as determined by skin prick and *in vitro* specific IgE tests [29]. While previous studies indicated that ovalbumin was the major egg allergen, this work demonstrated ovomucoid contamination of the ovalbumin accounted for the discrepancy. Ovalbumin (Gal d 2) is a monomeric phosphoglycoprotein with a molecular weight of 43–45 kDa and an acidic isoelectric point. Purified ovalbumin has three primary variants, A_1, A_2, and A_3. It is difficult to determine the exact role of Gal d 2 because of ovomucoid contamination of ovalbumin [29]. Ovotransferrin (Gal d 3), or conalbumin, has a molecular weight of 78 kDa, an acidic isoelectric point, and antimicrobial activity and iron-binding properties. Lysozyme (Gal d 4) is a lower molecular weight allergen (14.3 kDa) that in some studies appears to be a major allergen but in other studies is a minor allergen. Other minor allergens in eggs include serum albumin (Gal d 5), YGP42 (Gal d 6), myosin light chain 1f (Gal d 7), α-parvalbumin (Gal d 8), β-enolase (Gal d 9), and aldolase (Gal d 10). The carbohydrate portion of the glycoproteins in eggs, particularly in ovomucoid, does not play a primary role in specific IgE binding.

Four sets of distinct egg allergic groups (A, lysozyme and ovalbumin; B, ovomucoid; C, ovomucin; and D, ovotransferrin and the yolk proteins) were demonstrated in 40 subjects based on *in vitro* IgE tests [30]. Both lysozyme and ovomucin bind significant amounts of IgE in the sera of patient groups A and C. Lysozyme-specific IgE was statistically correlated with ovalbumin-specific IgE and was a significant allergen for group A. Other differences in IgE binding were found that may explain why various investigators report different allergens to be important in egg hypersensitivity.

Allen et al. [31] reviewed and identified key points of egg allergy. It primarily affects preschool children. Life-threatening reactions are less common with egg than with peanut or tree nut allergy, and heat and digestion alter the allergenicity of egg proteins. Heating reduces the allergenicity of ovomucoid and ovalbumin but does not affect lysozyme. Ovomucoid allergenicity may also be reduced by gastric pH. It is possible that the age and/or the use of inhibitors of gastric acid secretion in young children promotes egg protein food sensitization. As with baked milk products, baked egg products are tolerated by a majority of egg-allergic patients. Sixty-four of 117 subjects with confirmed egg allergy tolerated baked egg products (muffins or waffles) according to the results of one trial [32]. These clinical findings are consistent with the reduction of egg allergenicity by heating and may reassure select patients of the safety in consuming foods with baked egg.

17.3.3 Peanut

Peanut proteins are customarily classified as albumins (water soluble) and globulins (saline soluble). The albumins include the conglutin family of proteins. The globulin proteins are made up of two major fractions, arachin and conarachin, also known as legumin and vicilin, respectively. Globulin proteins also include the glycinin family of proteins. Arachin in its native state exists as a molecule of at least 600 kDa and readily dissociates into a 340–360 kDa dimer and a monomer of approximately 170–180 kDa. Ultracentrifugation separates conarachin into two fractions, 2S and 8.4S.

Peanut-1 and concanavalin A-reactive glycoprotein were two of the first peanut allergens partially characterized using peanut-specific IgE from allergic subjects. With the advent of more refined methods for allergen purification, allergens were named according to the WHO/IUIS convention. Thus, Ara h 1, a vicilin-type protein (i.e. a conarachin globulin), is a 63.5-kDa glycoprotein identified as the first major peanut allergen using immunoblotting and ELISA [13]. This allergen has an acidic isoelectric point and is relatively resistant to enzymatic degradation. Ara h 1 has at least 23 distinct IgE binding epitopes [33]. In addition to adaptive immune receptor interaction, Ara h 1 has adjuvant activity that promotes Th2-type cellular development [34].

Ara h 2 is a 17-kDa allergen with an acidic isoelectric point that has at least 10 specific-IgE binding epitopes along its amino acid sequence and is a member of the conglutin family (i.e., an albumin) of seed storage proteins [35]. Ara h 6 is a homologue of Ara h 2, and both have a very stable core structure composed primarily of α-helices supported by four disulfide bonds. These 2S albumin allergens are highly resistant to degradation by physiologic enzymes, pepsin and trypsin, which may account for them being highly allergenic [36]. Ara h 2 and 6 are the most potent allergens in functional IgE cross-linking assays using rat basophil cells expressing human IgE receptors primed with human sera from peanut-allergic patients [37]. Ara h 2 and 6 are also critical in anaphylaxis induction in peanut-allergic mice [38].

Ara h 3 is a glycinin seed storage protein (i.e., a globulin) with a molecular weight of 60 kDa and is highly homologous with Ara h 4 (now renamed to Ara h 3.02, an isoallergen of Ara h 3). Approximately 45% of patients with peanut allergy have specific IgE to this allergen [17]. Ara h 9 is a nonspecific lipid transfer protein (LTP) that is 9.8 kDa and is an α-helical folded protein. Ara h 9 is a major allergen in Mediterranean areas [39], whereas its relevance in other populations is likely minor. Ara h 5, a profilin, and Ara h 8 [40], a Bet v 1 homologue, are considered pan-allergens and cross-react with environmental allergens. These proteins can lead to pollen–food allergy syndrome upon ingestion but are easily digested and unlikely to cause systemic allergic symptoms. Altogether, 17 allergens are identified (Ara h 1 to Ara h 17) with Ara h 1, 2, 3, and 6 considered to be the most common allergens in most studies.

17.3.4 Soybean

Globulins are the major proteins of soybean. These globulins can be separated into ultracentrifugation fractions 2S, 7S, 11S, and 15S. Conglutin is a primary protein of the 2S fraction, while β-conglycinin is the primary fraction of the 7S component. The glycinin fraction is the primary component of the 11S ultracentrifugation fraction.

Soybeans, like peanuts, are legumes that contain multiple allergens. When examining specific IgE to ultracentrifugation components, the 2S and 7S fractions contain the primary allergens [41]. Gly m 1 is a 7-kDa allergen that is a component of the 7S fraction. The majority of soybean-allergic patients have soybean-specific IgE to Gly m 1. Gly m 1 has an acidic isoelectric point and sequence homology to a soybean seed 34-kDa oil-body-associated protein, soybean vacuolar protein P34. There are at least 16 distinct soybean-specific IgE binding epitopes along the amino acid sequence of this allergen. The Kunitz soybean trypsin inhibitor is a minor allergen. Gly m 5, β-conglycinin, belongs to the vicilin family of allergens and is thus homologous with peanut Ara h 1. Gly m 6 is a legumin allergen with homology to Ara h 3. Altogether, eight soybean allergens have been identified (Gly m 1 to Gly m 8).

A comprehensive review is available for the identification and characterization of soybean allergens with current techniques to reduce allergenicity, including thermal, enzymatic, chemical, traditional breeding, and genetic modification of the allergens [42].

17.3.5 Tree nuts

Tree nuts cause food-allergic reactions in both children and adults. Just as allergic reactions to fish and peanuts typically persist throughout life, so too can reactions to tree nuts. Hazelnut, walnut, cashew, and almond are the most common tree nuts responsible for allergic reactions with less frequent reactions to pecan, chestnut, Brazil nut, pine nut, macadamia nut, pistachio, and coconut [43]. Clark and Ewan [44] reviewed the development, sensitization, and clinical impact of tree nut allergens, suggesting that multiple nut sensitizations and allergies can take place *in utero* or soon after birth. Findings from the study reveal that a large proportion of children less than 1 year of age were already sensitized (nut specific IgE) to almond, Brazil nut, hazelnut, and walnut. Potential sensitization routes included breast milk, peanut- or soy-containing infant formula, trace contamination of nonformula foods, and use of peanut- or soy-containing eczema creams.

The major tree nut allergens are the seed storage proteins belonging to the 2S albumin, vicilin (i.e., 7S globulin), or legumin (i.e., 11S globulin) families. For example, in English walnuts, the major allergens are a 65-kDa glycoprotein belonging to the vicilin family (Jug r 2), a 2S albumin protein (Jug r 1), and an 11S globulin protein (Jug r 4). The homologous proteins in cashews and almonds are also allergens. Although several different Brazil nut proteins are allergens, the major one, Ber e 1, is a high methionine-containing protein (2S albumin). This 12-kDa protein has two subunits, a 9-kDa and a 3-kDa protein, which have been extensively characterized [45]. Possibly the most interesting finding is that Ber e 1 can skew T-cell responses toward an allergenic phenotype, whereas a homologous 2S albumin from sunflower seeds does not have this property [46]. Additional studies should give insight into what would cause one 2S albumin to be allergenic, while another is not.

17.3.6 Wheat

Wheat and other cereal grains are common food allergens, particularly in children. The proteins of wheat include the water-soluble albumins, the saline-soluble globulins, the aqueous ethanol-soluble prolamines (i.e., gliadins), and the glutelins. Subjects with wheat allergy have specific IgE to wheat fractions of 47 kDa and 20 kDa, proteins not recognized by specific-IgE from subjects with grass allergy [47]. Wheat α-amylase inhibitor (15 kDa) is also a major wheat allergen. This protein does not bind IgE from wheat tolerant control subjects, including those with grass allergy. Battais et al. [48] identified major wheat allergens by IgE-binding studies. IgE from subjects with wheat-dependent exercise-induced anaphylaxis and urticaria react with sequential epitopes (QQX1PX2QQ) in the repetitive domain of gliadins, whereas IgE from atopic dermatitis subjects recognizes conformational epitopes [49].

17.3.7 Fish

The consumption of fish allergens is a common cause of IgE-mediated food reactions. The incidence of fish allergy is much higher in countries where fish consumption is greater. For example, codfish allergy is common in the Scandinavian countries [50]. Red and golden snapper, local species of snapper consumed in Malaysia, commonly cause food allergy in this locale [51].

The canonical fish allergens are the parvalbumins, proteins that control the flow of calcium in and out of cells and are only found in the muscles of amphibians and fish. One of the most comprehensive descriptions of a food allergen is by Apol and Elsayed of codfish allergen, Gad c 1 (originally called Allergen M) [52]. Gad c 1 is a parvalbumin with an acidic isoelectric point and molecular weight of 12 kDa. The tertiary structure of Gad c 1 has three domains. There are at least five IgE-binding sites on the allergen, and the carbohydrate moiety is not likely important in its allergenicity. Gad c 1 is heat stable, as are the major allergens of bhetki and mackerel, whereas other fish allergens are heat labile, such as those from the Indian fish pomfret and hilsa [53], again illustrating that those food allergens can be altered by cooking.

17.3.8 Shellfish

Shrimp is the most studied of the Crustacea allergens, and tropomyosins are the major allergens. Tropomyosin is an actin-binding protein important in regulating muscle contractions. The IgE-binding epitopes of the shrimp allergen Pen a 1, a 36 kDa tropomyosin, are known [54,55]. The deduced amino-acid sequence of 284 amino acids from recombinant allergens and amino acid sequences from allergenic and nonallergenic vertebrate tropomyosins reveal 80%–99% and 51%–58% amino acid sequence homology, respectively. Analysis of the secondary structure of Pen a 1 shows an α-helical conformation that is typical for tropomyosins [56]. Tropomyosin allergens in lobster (Hom a 1) and crab (Cha f 1) have also been identified. Tropomyosin is also a pan-allergen for fish (tilapia, cod, albacore, and swordfish) [57,58] and mollusks (squid [59], oyster [60], and snail [61]). Several other allergens in shrimp and lobster are arginine kinase, myosin light chain 1 and 2, troponin C, and sarcoplasmic calcium-binding protein [14]. Arginine kinase, a major allergen in insect [62] and house dust mite [63] allergy is also a mollusk allergen found in octopus [64], thus causing cross-reactivity [65].

17.4 OTHER FOOD ALLERGENS

Virtually any food can be allergenic and cause symptoms. This section represents a brief review of foods known to cause clinically significant reactions, although at lower frequency than that of the "Big 8" food allergens.

Seeds contain allergenic seed storage proteins similar to peanut and tree nuts. The 2S albumin, vicilin, and legumin proteins in sesame seeds are allergens [66]. Lupin seed, also referred to as lupini bean, is increasingly used as a protein substitute and contains allergens that extensively cross-react with other legume species, particularly peanut proteins [67]. Lentils are another legume associated with allergy. Mustard seeds also have seed storage protein allergens [14]. A seed often used in spicy food, fenugreek, cross-reacts with peanut proteins [68]. Tree nut and sesame seed oil components may also contain major allergens capable of triggering allergic reactions, depending on how the oil is processed [69].

Kiwi allergy is increasing with kiwellin, a cysteine-rich 28-kDa protein, identified as the allergen [70]. Apple peel extract from 10 different apple varieties shows allergenic activity associated with the pollen–food allergy syndrome [71]. An N-linked glycan from oranges has specific IgE binding properties [72]. Celery and peach allergens have also been identified. Food proteins associated with pollen–food allergy syndrome are discussed in a review by Nash and Burks [73].

17.5 α-GAL AS AN ALLERGEN IN RED MEAT

In 2009, delayed anaphylaxis subsequent to ingesting mammalian food products (i.e., beef and pork) was first reported in the United States [74]. Reports from Europe and Australia followed [75]. Symptoms appear to be dose dependent and are not the typical immediate-type reactions induced by classic food allergens (e.g., peanut or egg), instead these symptoms take 3–6 hours to develop. The affected subjects reacted to mammalian meat, but not to fish, chicken, or turkey.

Researchers noticed the similar regional distribution in the southeastern United States of anaphylactic reactions to the monoclonal antibody cetuximab and the delayed anaphylaxis to red meat [75]. Interestingly, the same oligosaccharide, galactose α-1,3-galactose (α-gal), is likely responsible for IgE-mediated reactions both to cetuximab and to mammalian meat [76]. α-Gal is a major blood group substance in nonprimate mammals and is immunogenic in normal individuals as evidenced by the identification of specific-IgG. IgE antibodies specific for α-gal are significantly associated with the syndrome of red meat–induced delayed anaphylaxis.

Several studies report evidence that tick bites may be responsible for the development of α-gal specific IgE. In the United States, the *Amblyomma americanum*, or lone star tick, has been implicated, whereas in France and Australia, the *Ixodes ricinus* and *Ixodes holocyclus*, respectively, are thought to be the culprit species [75]. Case reports of tick bites followed by subsequent reactions to beef, the presence of α-gal IgE, and the regional distribution of the responsible tick has provided convincing, although circumstantial, evidence that tick bites may trigger the production of α-gal IgE, the subsequent red meat allergy syndrome and reactions to cetuximab.

17.6 DIAGNOSIS

Allergic reactions to foods are a common cause of anaphylaxis [77]. Asero et al. [78] in a review of food allergy identified a major problem in the diagnosis of food allergy, i.e., the relatively poor "clinical specificity" of both skin and *in vitro* tests. Another major problem in appropriately diagnosing food allergy is the lack of standardized food allergen extracts. A detailed medical history, physical examination, and appropriate laboratory tests are necessary to diagnose all allergy, including food allergy. Skin prick and *in vitro* specific IgE tests are sensitive indicators of food-specific IgE; however, they are not very predictive of clinical sensitivity. A positive skin test to a food indicates the possibility that the patient has symptomatic reactivity to that specific food, although the positive predictive accuracy is less than 50%. A negative skin test confirms the absence of an IgE-mediated reaction with a negative predictive accuracy of greater than 95%. The definitive diagnosis of food allergy is ultimately based on standardized oral challenges.

Based on previously established 95% predictive decision points for egg, milk, peanut, and fish allergy, greater than 95% of food allergies diagnosed in a prospective study of 100 children were correctly identified by quantifying serum food-specific IgE concentrations using ImmunoCAP methodology [79]. Using allergen-specific IgE values for egg, 6 kUA/L; milk, 32 kUA/L; peanut, 15 kUA/L; and fish, 20 kUA/L as diagnostic decision points, the positive predictive values in this prospective study ranged from 96% to 100%. By using decision points of 100 kUA/L for wheat and 65 kUA/L for soy, the positive predictive values were 100% and 86%, respectively. Using these predictive values, the authors reduced the number of double-blind, placebo-controlled food challenges (DBPCFC) by 40%–50%, since no challenge is administered in those subjects with specific IgE above the diagnostic decision points.

Over 9 years in a tertiary clinic in Australia, large skin prick test wheal (mean size 8–10 mm) in infants and young children was associated with a greater than 95% likelihood of clinical reactivity to cow's milk, egg, and peanut, as confirmed by open food challenges [80]. For each food, a specific size skin wheal diameter predicted a positive reaction: cow's milk, 8 mm; egg, 7 mm; and peanut, 8 mm.

The absence of detectable wheal has a strong negative predictive value but rarely reactions may occur. Therefore, the DBPCFC remains the gold standard to determine food allergy.

Food challenges, when necessary, should be administered with the patient in a fasting state, starting with a challenge dose of the food in question unlikely to provoke symptoms, generally 5 mg of lyophilized food. This dose is then increased every 15–60 minutes, depending on the historical reaction. A similar scheme is followed with the placebo portion of the study. Clinical reactivity can be ruled out when the blinded patient tolerates up to 10 g of lyophilized food in capsules or liquid. If the blinded portion of the challenge is negative, tolerance must be confirmed by an open feeding under observation to rule out rare false-negative challenges.

Novel methods of diagnosis under investigation include epitope microarrays, component-resolved analyses, and basophil degranulation assays (see Table 17.4). Epitope microarrays involve "printing" peptides onto glass slides, such that the entire length of the amino acid sequence of the allergen is printed (i.e., 15 amino acids represent one spot), and assessing which epitopes are recognized by a test subject's IgE [81]. The value of epitope arrays is the ability to evaluate allergen epitope recognition patterns, conformational versus sequential epitopes, number of epitopes recognized, and the intensity of IgE binding to individual epitopes. This information may better predict clinical sensitivity. Component-resolved analyses also hold promise to increase the value of diagnosis based on *in vitro* testing. The idea is to study IgE responses against purified major allergens from foods. This concept is useful in peanut allergy, identifying Ara h 2 as an indicator of severe allergy, whereas other components (e.g., Ara h 8) are associated with sensitization without reactions [40,82].

Basophil activation assays differ from the serologic testing described earlier by using viable basophils to bind IgE molecules from the test subject or basophils from the test subject. This type of assay may be more "functional," but the specific value of cellular assays is not defined. The assay involves using whole blood stimulated with food allergens and assessing CD63 or CD203c on the basophil surface via flow cytometry [83]. Subjects naturally outgrowing milk allergy have decreased basophil reactivity to milk proteins [84]. Another study looked at basophil responses in egg-, milk-, or peanut-allergic patients and determined cut-points for predicting clinical allergy [85].

17.7 THERAPIES

Several groups throughout the United States and Europe are actively conducting clinical trials for food allergies. The most common type of therapy is oral immunotherapy (OIT). OIT involves ingestion of small but increasing amounts of the offending allergen to achieve a state of desensitization. The concept involves initially ingesting doses of allergen below that which would trigger a major allergic reaction, then gradually building up to a maintenance dose in the hundreds of milligrams to gram range. Trials have been conducted for egg [86], milk [87], wheat [88], and peanut allergies [89]. The preliminary success of these trials is demonstrated by the majority of test subjects safely achieving maintenance dosing and tolerance to even larger quantities of the culprit food. However, OIT is limited by allergic side effects and the possibility that the therapy may need to be lifelong, as tolerance induction is not currently understood.

Table 17.5 Novel therapeutic approaches in clinical trials

Oral immunotherapy (OIT)

OIT uses an antigen-specific approach in desensitizing allergic subjects. Trials have targeted egg-, milk-, and peanut-allergic patients. Evidence of clinically important desensitization has been demonstrated in randomized, placebo-controlled trials [86,87,89].

Sublingual immunotherapy (SLIT)

SLIT is an antigen-specific approach to desensitize allergic subjects. Trials with hazelnut, peanut, and cow's milk demonstrate desensitization [91–93].

Epicutaneous immunotherapy (EPIT)

EPIT targets antigen-presenting cells in the superficial layers of the skin. The allergen is delivered via a skin patch. Pilot studies in subjects allergic to cow's milk and peanut showed high safety and tolerability [26,106–108].

Anti-IgE therapy (with or without OIT)

Anti-IgE therapy is an antigen nonspecific approach using the concept that binding circulating IgE will decrease allergic disease. A trial in peanut allergic patients demonstrated efficacy at the highest dose of anti-IgE tested [98]. Anti-IgE therapy may also be used as a pretreatment for OIT to reduce allergic side effects associated with OIT and possibly permit escalation of the antigen dose more quickly [110,111].

Food allergy herbal formula (B-FAHF-2)

B-FAHF-2 is a non-antigen-specific approach to treat food allergies and was originally shown to be effective in peanut allergic mice [109]. Clinical trials are currently underway targeting various food allergies in humans.

Table 17.4 Novel diagnostic approaches used in food allergy research

Component-resolved technology

Based on utilizing purified allergens as opposed to crude extracts of allergenic sources. This approach may be useful in discriminating different phenotypes of peanut allergy (i.e., systemic reactions versus pollen–food allergy syndrome) [82].

Epitope arrays

IgE and IgG binding epitopes can be identified and quantified for allergens with known amino acid sequences. This approach may be useful in determining the severity of reactions for peanut allergy [103], as well as predicting the possibility of outgrowing milk and egg allergies [21,104].

Basophil activation assays

Human basophils in whole blood can be activated *ex vivo* with antigen. Basophil degranulation, as measured by CD63 upregulation, may be useful in determining milk, egg, and peanut allergy [85]; in predicting the development of tolerance to milk allergens [84]; and in measuring desensitization in peanut allergy immunotherapy [105].

Another therapy is sublingual immunotherapy (SLIT), which involves placing small quantities of allergen under the tongue and then swallowing to achieve desensitization. A case report for kiwi allergy demonstrated that SLIT may be applicable to food allergies [90]. A study for hazelnut allergy showed desensitization and some immunologic changes following SLIT [91]. A randomized, placebo-controlled SLIT trial in peanut-allergic subjects in the United States achieved desensitization after 12 months [92]. The advantages of SLIT are the ease of dosing and fewer allergic side effects when compared with OIT. However, SLIT may be less effective in increasing eliciting dose thresholds than OIT, as evidenced by a milk allergy trial comparing SLIT and OIT [93].

Other strategies include intervention prior to the onset of peanut allergy as was studied in the Learning Early about Peanut Allergy (LEAP) trial [94,95]. This approach aimed to exploit oral tolerance induction before peanut allergy developed. The hypothesis that led to the trial is based on the younger age of introduction of peanuts in Israeli versus UK children, and the lower occurrence of peanut allergy in Israel versus the United Kingdom [96]. The LEAP study showed that early introduction of peanut in infants at risk of peanut allergy helped modulate immune responses to peanut and decreased the development of this allergy. Other non-antigen-specific therapies include an herbal formula now in clinical trials in the United States [97] and anti-IgE therapy [98]. Various clinical and preclinical approaches to treat food allergies are summarized in Table 17.5 and reviewed in the literature [99–102].

SALIENT POINTS

- Food allergies affect an estimated 3%–6% of the population in several Westernized societies.
- The major food sources known to cause allergic reactions are cow's milk, eggs, peanuts, soybeans, tree nuts, wheat, fish, and shellfish.
- Food allergens, found in plants and animals, are classified based on their biologic function or protein families.
- Many food allergens occur naturally as dimers or trimers often making their molecular weight 150–200 kDa.
- IgE binding to food allergens occurs at linear, sequential epitopes or at conformational, nonsequential epitopes.
- α-Gal is an allergen in mammalian meats and IgE against α-gal is thought to be induced by tick bites.
- Diagnostics for food allergies may be improved by using purified allergens instead of crude extracts.
- Therapeutic approaches for the treatment of food allergies have shown promise but are not ready for widespread use.

REFERENCES

1. Burks AW. Peanut allergy. *Lancet* 2008; 371(9623): 1538–1546.
2. Fleischer DM, Perry TT, Atkins D et al. Allergic reactions to foods in preschool-aged children in a prospective observational food allergy study. *Pediatrics* 2012; 130(1): e25–e32.
3. King RM, Knibb RC, Hourihane JO. Impact of peanut allergy on quality of life, stress and anxiety in the family. *Allergy* 2009; 64(3): 461–468.
4. Sicherer SH. Epidemiology of food allergy. *J Allergy Clin Immunol* 2011; 127(3): 594–602.
5. Strid J, Hourihane J, Kimber I, Callard R, Strobel S. Epicutaneous exposure to peanut protein prevents oral tolerance and enhances allergic sensitization. *Clin Exp Allergy* 2005; 35(6): 757–766.
6. Berin MC, Sicherer S. Food allergy: Mechanisms and therapeutics. *Curr Opin Immunol* 2011; 23(6): 794–800.
7. Brown SJ, Asai Y, Cordell HJ et al. Loss-of-function variants in the filaggrin gene are a significant risk factor for peanut allergy. *J Allergy Clin Immunol* 2011; 127(3): 661–667.
8. Untersmayr E, Jensen-Jarolim E. The effect of gastric digestion on food allergy. *Curr Opin Allergy Clin Immunol* 2006; 6(3): 214–219.
9. Lemanske RF, Jr., Taylor SL. Standardized extracts, foods. *Clin Rev Allergy* 1987; 5(1): 23–36.
10. Dibbern DA, Jr., Palmer GW, Williams PB, Bock SA, Dreskin SC. RBL cells expressing human FcεRI are a sensitive tool for exploring functional IgE-allergen interactions: Studies with sera from peanut-sensitive patients. *J Immunol Methods* 2003; 274(1–2): 37–45.
11. Untersmayr E, Jensen-Jarolim E. Mechanisms of type I food allergy. *Pharmacol Ther* 2006; 112(3): 787–798.
12. Jenkins JA, Griffiths-Jones S, Shewry PR, Breiteneder H, Mills EN. Structural relatedness of plant food allergens with specific reference to cross-reactive allergens: An *in silico* analysis. *J Allergy Clin Immunol* 2005; 115(1): 163–170.
13. Burks AW, Williams LW, Helm RM, Connaughton C, Cockrell G, O'Brien T. Identification of a major peanut allergen, Ara h I, in patients with atopic dermatitis and positive peanut challenges. *J Allergy Clin Immunol* 1991; 88(2): 172–179.
14. WHO/IUIS official database of named allergens. http://www.allergen.org.
15. Pomés A, Davies JM, Gadermaier G et al. WHO/IUIS allergen nomenclature: Providing a common language. *Mol Immunol* 2018; 100: 3–13.
16. AllFam allergen family chart. http://www.meduniwien.ac.at/allfam/browse.php (accessed Oct 22, 2012).
17. Rabjohn P, Helm EM, Stanley JS et al. Molecular cloning and epitope analysis of the peanut allergen Ara h 3. *J Clin Invest* 1999; 103(4): 535–542.
18. Restani P, Ballabio C, Corsini E et al. Identification of the basic subunit of Ara h 3 as the major allergen in a group of children allergic to peanuts. *Ann Allergy Asthma Immunol* 2005; 94(2): 262–266.
19. Wal JM. Cow's milk proteins/allergens. *Ann Allergy Asthma Immunol* 2002; 89(6 Suppl 1): 3–10.
20. Jarvinen KM, Beyer K, Vila L, Chatchatee P, Busse PJ, Sampson HA. B-cell epitopes as a screening instrument for persistent cow's milk allergy. *J Allergy Clin Immunol* 2002; 110(2): 293–297.
21. Wang J, Lin J, Bardina L et al. Correlation of IgE/IgG4 milk epitopes and affinity of milk-specific IgE antibodies with different phenotypes of clinical milk allergy. *J Allergy Clin Immunol* 2010; 125(3): 695–702, e1–e6.
22. Nowak-Wegrzyn A, Bloom KA, Sicherer SH et al. Tolerance to extensively heated milk in children with cow's milk allergy. *J Allergy Clin Immunol* 2008; 122(2): 342–347, 7.e1–2.
23. Kim JS, Nowak-Wegrzyn A, Sicherer SH, Noone S, Moshier EL, Sampson HA. Dietary baked milk accelerates the resolution of cow's milk allergy in children. *J Allergy Clin Immunol* 2011; 128(1): 125–131.e2.
24. Carraro S, Frigo AC, Perin M et al. Impact and oral immunotherapy on quality of life in children with cow milk allergy: A pilot study 2012; 25(3): 793–798.

25. De Boissieu D, Dupont C. Sublingual immunotherapy for cow's milk protein allergy: A preliminary report. *Allergy* 2006; 61(10): 1238–1239.

26. Dupont C, Kalach N, Soulaines P, Legoue-Morillon S, Piloquet H, Benhamou PH. Cow's milk epicutaneous immunotherapy in children: A pilot trial of safety, acceptability, and impact on allergic reactivity. *J Allergy Clin Immunol* 2010; 125(5): 1165–1167.

27. Anet J, Back JF, Baker RS, Barnett D, Burley RW, Howden ME. Allergens in the white and yolk of hen's egg. A study of IgE binding by egg proteins. *Int Arch Allergy Appl Immunol* 1985; 77(3): 364–371.

28. Hoffman DR. Immunochemical identification of the allergens in egg white. *J Allergy Clin Immunol* 1983; 71(5): 481–486.

29. Bernhisel-Broadbent J, Dintzis HM, Dintzis RZ, Sampson HA. Allergenicity and antigenicity of chicken egg ovomucoid (Gal d III) compared with ovalbumin (Gal d I) in children with egg allergy and in mice. *J Allergy Clin Immunol* 1994; 93(6): 1047–1059.

30. Walsh BJ, Hill DJ, Macoun P, Cairns D, Howden ME. Detection of four distinct groups of hen egg allergens binding IgE in the sera of children with egg allergy. *Allergol Immunopathol* 2005; 33(4): 183–191.

31. Allen CW, Campbell DE, Kemp AS. Egg allergy: Are all childhood food allergies the same? *J Paediatr Child Health* 2007; 43(4): 214–218.

32. Lemon-Mule H, Sampson HA, Sicherer SH, Shreffler WG, Noone S, Nowak-Wegrzyn A. Immunologic changes in children with egg allergy ingesting extensively heated egg. *J Allergy Clin Immunol* 2008; 122(5): 977–983 e1.

33. Shin DS, Compadre CM, Maleki SJ et al. Biochemical and structural analysis of the IgE binding sites on ara h1, an abundant and highly allergenic peanut protein. *J Biol Chem* 1998; 273(22): 13753–13759.

34. Shreffler WG, Castro RR, Kucuk ZY et al. The major glycoprotein allergen from *Arachis hypogaea*, Ara h 1, is a ligand of dendritic cell-specific ICAM-grabbing nonintegrin and acts as a Th2 adjuvant *in vitro*. *J Immunol* 2006; 177(6): 3677–3685.

35. King N, Helm R, Stanley JS et al. Allergenic characteristics of a modified peanut allergen. *Mol Nutr Food Res* 2005; 49(10): 963–971.

36. Koppelman SJ, Hefle SL, Taylor SL, de Jong GA. Digestion of peanut allergens Ara h 1, Ara h 2, Ara h 3, and Ara h 6: A comparative *in vitro* study and partial characterization of digestion-resistant peptides. *Mol Nutr Food Res* 2010; 54(12): 1711–1721.

37. Porterfield HS, Murray KS, Schlichting DG et al. Effector activity of peanut allergens: A critical role for Ara h 2, Ara h 6, and their variants. *Clin Exp Allergy* 2009; 39(7): 1099–1108.

38. Kulis M, Chen X, Lew J et al. The 2S albumin allergens of *Arachis hypogaea*, Ara h 2 and Ara h 6, are the major elicitors of anaphylaxis and can effectively desensitize peanut-allergic mice. *Clin Exp Allergy* 2012; 42(2): 326–336.

39. Krause S, Reese G, Randow S et al. Lipid transfer protein (Ara h 9) as a new peanut allergen relevant for a Mediterranean allergic population. *J Allergy Clin Immunol* 2009; 124(4): 771–778.e5.

40. Asarnoj A, Nilsson C, Lidholm J et al. Peanut component Ara h 8 sensitization and tolerance to peanut. *J Allergy Clin Immunol* 2012; 130(2): 468–472.

41. Ogawa A, Samoto M, Takahashi K. Soybean allergens and hypoallergenic soybean products. *J Nutr Sci Vitaminol (Tokyo)* 2000; 46(6): 271–279.

42. L'Hocine L, Boye JI. Allergenicity of soybean: New developments in identification of allergenic proteins, cross-reactivities and hypoallergenization technologies. *Crit Rev Food Sci Nutr* 2007; 47(2): 127–143.

43. Roux KH, Teuber SS, Sathe SK. Tree nut allergens. *Int Arch Allergy Immunol* 2003; 131(4): 234–244.

44. Clark AT, Ewan PW. The development and progression of allergy to multiple nuts at different ages. *Pediatr Allergy Immunol* 2005; 16(6): 507–511.

45. Moreno FJ, Mellon FA, Wickham MS, Bottrill AR, Mills EN. Stability of the major allergen Brazil nut 2S albumin (Ber e 1) to physiologically relevant *in vitro* gastrointestinal digestion. *FEBS J* 2005; 272(2): 341–352.

46. Kean DE, Goodridge HS, McGuinness S, Harnett MM, Alcocer MJ, Harnett W. Differential polarization of immune responses by plant 2S seed albumins, Ber e 1, and SFA8. *J Immunol* 2006; 177(3): 1561–1566.

47. Jones SM, Magnolfi CF, Cooke SK, Sampson HA. Immunologic cross-reactivity among cereal grains and grasses in children with food hypersensitivity. *J Allergy Clin Immunol* 1995; 96(3): 341–351.

48. Battais F, Pineau F, Popineau Y et al. Food allergy to wheat: Identification of immunogloglin E and immunoglobulin G-binding proteins with sequential extracts and purified proteins from wheat flour. *Clin Exp Allergy* 2003; 33(7): 962–970.

49. Battais F, Mothes T, Moneret-Vautrin DA et al. Identification of IgE-binding epitopes on gliadins for patients with food allergy to wheat. *Allergy* 2005; 60(6): 815–821.

50. Aas K. Studies of hypersensitivity to fish. A clinical study. *Int Arch Allergy Appl Immunol* 1966; 29(4): 346–363.

51. Rosmilah M, Shahnaz M, Masita A, Noormalin A, Jamaludin M. Identification of major allergens of two species of local snappers: *Lutjanus argentimaculatus* (merah/red snapper) and *Lutjanus johnii* (jenahak/golden snapper). *Trop Biomed* 2005; 22(2): 171–177.

52. Elsayed S, Apold J. Immunochemical analysis of cod fish allergen M: Locations of the immunoglobulin binding sites as demonstrated by the native and synthetic peptides. *Allergy* 1983; 38(7): 449–459.

53. Chatterjee U, Mondal G, Chakraborti P, Patra HK, Chatterjee BP. Changes in the allergenicity during different preparations of Pomfret, Hilsa, Bhetki and mackerel fish as illustrated by enzyme-linked immunosorbent assay and immunoblotting. *Int Arch Allergy Immunol* 2006; 141(1): 1–10.

54. Ayuso R, Lehrer SB, Reese G. Identification of continuous, allergenic regions of the major shrimp allergen Pen a 1 (tropomyosin). *Int Arch Allergy Immunol* 2002; 127(1): 27–37.

55. Reese G, Ayuso R, Leong-Kee SM, Plante MJ, Lehrer SB. Characterization and identification of allergen epitopes: Recombinant peptide libraries and synthetic, overlapping peptides. *J Chromatogr B Biomed Sci Appl* 2001; 756(1-2): 157–163.

56. Reese G, Schicktanz S, Lauer I et al. Structural, immunological and functional properties of natural recombinant Pen a 1, the major allergen of brown shrimp, *Penaeus aztecus*. *Clin Exp Allergy* 2006; 36(4): 517–524.

57. Gonzalez-Fernandez J, Alguacil-Guillen M, Cuellar C, Daschner A. Possible allergenic role of tropomyosin in patients with adverse reactions after fish intake. *Immunol Invest* 2018; 47(4): 416–429.

58. Liu R, Holck AL, Yang E, Liu C, Xue W. Tropomyosin from tilapia (*Oreochromis mossambicus*) as an allergen. *Clin Exp Allergy* 2013; 43(3): 365–377.

59. Miyazawa H, Fukamachi H, Inagaki Y et al. Identification of the first major allergen of a squid (*Todarodes pacificus*). *J Allergy Clin Immunol* 1996; 98(5 Pt 1): 948–953.

60. Ishikawa M, Shimakura K, Nagashima Y, Shiomi K. Isolation and properties of allergenic proteins in the oyster. *Crassostrea gigas. Fish Sci* 1997; 63: 610–614.

61. Ishikawa M, Ishida M, Shimakura K, Nagashima Y, Shiomi K. Purification and IgE-binding epitopes of a major allergen in the gastropod *Turbo cornutus. Biosci Biotechnol Biochem* 1998; 62(7): 1337–1343.

62. de Gier S, Verhoeckx K. Insect (food) allergy and allergens. *Mol Immunol* 2018; 100: 82–106.

63. Bi XZ, Chew FT. Molecular, proteomic and immunological characterization of isoforms of arginine kinase, a cross-reactive invertebrate pan-allergen, from the house dust mite, dermatophagoides farinae. *J Allergy Clin Immunol* 2004; 113(2, Suppl): S226.

64. Shen HW, Cao MJ, Cai QF et al. Purification, cloning, and immunological characterization of arginine kinase, a novel allergen of *Octopus fangsiao. J Agric Food Chem* 2012; 60(9): 2190–2199.

65. Ayuso R, Reese G, Leong-Kee S, Plante M, Lehrer SB. Molecular basis of arthropod cross-reactivity: IgE-binding cross-reactive epitopes of shrimp, house dust mite and cockroach tropomyosins. *Int Arch Allergy Immunol* 2002; 129(1): 38–48.

66. Beyer K, Bardina L, Grishina G, Sampson HA. Identification of sesame seed allergens by 2-dimensional proteomics and Edman sequencing: Seed storage proteins as common food allergens. *J Allergy Clin Immunol* 2002; 110(1): 154–159.

67. Magni C, Herndl A, Sironi E et al. One- and two-dimensional electrophoretic identification of IgE-binding polypeptides of *Lupinus albus* and other legume seeds. *J Agric Food Chem* 2005; 53(11): 4567–4571.

68. Vinje NE, Namork E, Lovik M. Cross-allergic reactions to legumes in lupin and fenugreek-sensitized mice. *Scand J Immunol* 2012; 76(4): 387–397.

69. Teuber SS, Brown RL, Haapanen LA. Allergenicity of gourmet nut oils processed by different methods. *J Allergy Clin Immunol* 1997; 99(4): 502–507.

70. Tamburrini M, Cerasuolo I, Carratore V et al. Kiwellin, a novel protein from kiwi fruit. Purification, biochemical characterization and identification as an allergen. *Protein J* 2005; 24(7–8): 423–429.

71. Carnes J, Ferrer A, Fernandez-Caldas E. Allergenicity of 10 different apple varieties. *Ann Allergy Asthma Immunol* 2006; 96(4): 564–570.

72. Ahrazem O, Ibanez MD, Lopez-Torrejon G et al. Orange germin-like glycoprotein Cit s 1: An equivocal allergen. *Int Arch Allergy Immunol* 2006; 139(2): 96–103.

73. Nash S, Burks AW. Oral allergy syndrome. *Curr Allergy Asthma Rep* 2007; 7(1): 1–2.

74. Commins SP, Satinover SM, Hosen J et al. Delayed anaphylaxis, angioedema, or urticaria after consumption of red meat in patients with IgE antibodies specific for galactose-α-1,3-galactose. *J Allergy Clin Immunol* 2009; 123(2): 426–433.

75. Commins SP, Platts-Mills TA. Delayed anaphylaxis to red meat in patients with IgE specific for galactose α-1,3-galactose (α-gal). *Curr Allergy Asthma Rep* 2013 Feb; 13(1): 72–77.

76. Mullins RJ, James H, Platts-Mills TA, Commins S. Relationship between red meat allergy and sensitization to gelatin and galactose-α-1,3-galactose. *J Allergy Clin Immunol* 2012; 129(5): 1334–1342.e1.

77. Bock SA, Munoz-Furlong A, Sampson HA. Fatalities due to anaphylactic reactions to foods. *J Allergy Clin Immunol* 2001; 107(1): 191–193.

78. Asero R, Ballmer-Weber BK, Beyer K et al. IgE-mediated food allergy diagnosis: Current status and new perspectives. *Mol Nutr Food Res* 2007; 51(1): 135–147.

79. Sampson HA. Utility of food-specific IgE concentrations in predicting symptomatic food allergy. *J Allergy Clin Immunol* 2001; 107(5): 891–896.

80. Sporik R, Hill DJ, Hosking CS. Specificity of allergen skin testing in predicting positive open food challenges to milk, egg and peanut in children. *Clin Exp Allergy* 2000; 30(11): 1540–1546.

81. Lin J, Bardina L, Shreffler WG et al. Development of a novel peptide microarray for large-scale epitope mapping of food allergens. *J Allergy Clin Immunol* 2009; 124(2): 315–322, 22.e1–3.

82. Nicolaou N, Poorafshar M, Murray C et al. Allergy or tolerance in children sensitized to peanut: Prevalence and differentiation using component-resolved diagnostics. *J Allergy Clin Immunol* 2010; 125(1): 191–197.e1–13.

83. Shreffler WG. Evaluation of basophil activation in food allergy: Present and future applications. *Curr Opin Allergy Clin Immunol* 2006; 6(3): 226–233.

84. Wanich N, Nowak-Wegrzyn A, Sampson HA, Shreffler WG. Allergen-specific basophil suppression associated with clinical tolerance in patients with milk allergy. *J Allergy Clin Immunol* 2009; 123(4): 789–794.e20.

85. Ocmant A, Mulier S, Hanssens L et al. Basophil activation tests for the diagnosis of food allergy in children. *Clin Exp Allergy* 2009; 39(8): 1234–1245.

86. Burks AW, Jones SM, Wood RA et al. Oral immunotherapy for treatment of egg allergy in children. *N Engl J Med* 2012; 367(3): 233–243.

87. Skripak JM, Nash SD, Rowley H et al. A randomized, double-blind, placebo-controlled study of milk oral immunotherapy for cow's milk allergy. *J Allergy Clin Immunol* 2008; 122(6): 1154–1160.

88. Pacharn P, Vichyanond P. Immunotherapy for IgE-mediated wheat allergy. *Hum Vaccin Immunother* 2017; 13(10): 2462–2466.

89. Varshney P, Jones SM, Scurlock AM et al. A randomized controlled study of peanut oral immunotherapy: Clinical desensitization and modulation of the allergic response. *J Allergy Clin Immunol* 2011; 127(3): 654–660.

90. Kerzl R, Simonowa A, Ring J, Ollert M, Mempel M. Life-threatening anaphylaxis to kiwi fruit: Protective sublingual allergen immunotherapy effect persists even after discontinuation. *J Allergy Clin Immunol* 2007; 119(2): 507–508.

91. Enrique E, Pineda F, Malek T et al. Sublingual immunotherapy for hazelnut food allergy: A randomized, double-blind, placebo-controlled study with a standardized hazelnut extract. *J Allergy Clin Immunol* 2005; 116(5): 1073–1079.

92. Kim EH, Bird JA, Kulis M et al. Sublingual immunotherapy for peanut allergy: Clinical and immunologic evidence of desensitization. *J Allergy Clin Immunol* 2011; 127(3): 640–646.e1.

93. Keet CA, Frischmeyer-Guerrerio PA, Thyagarajan A et al. The safety and efficacy of sublingual and oral immunotherapy for milk allergy. *J Allergy Clin Immunol* 2012; 129(2): 448–455.e5.

94. Du Toit G, Roberts G, Sayre PH et al. Randomized trial of peanut consumption in infants at risk for peanut allergy. *N Engl J Med* 2015; 372(9): 803–813.

95. Du Toit G, Sayre PH, Roberts G et al. Effect of avoidance on peanut allergy after early peanut consumption. *N Engl J Med* 2016; 374(15): 1435–1443.

96. Du Toit G, Katz Y, Sasieni P et al. Early consumption of peanuts in infancy is associated with a low prevalence of peanut allergy. *J Allergy Clin Immunol* 2008; 122(5): 984–991.

97. Wang J, Patil SP, Yang N et al. Safety, tolerability, and immunologic effects of a food allergy herbal formula in food allergic individuals: A randomized, double-blinded, placebo-controlled, dose escalation, phase 1 study. *Ann Allergy Asthma Immunol* 2010; 105(1): 75–84.

98. Leung DY, Sampson HA, Yunginger JW et al. Effect of anti-IgE therapy in patients with peanut allergy. *N Engl J Med* 2003; 348(11): 986–993.

99. Wang J, Sampson HA. Food allergy. *J Clin Invest* 2011; 121(3): 827–835.

100. Pajno GB, Fernandez-Rivas M, Arasi S et al. EAACI guidelines on allergen immunotherapy: IgE-mediated food allergy. *Allergy* 2018; 73(4): 799–815.

101. Dantzer JA, Wood RA. Next-generation approaches for the treatment of food allergy. *Curr Allergy Asthma Rep* 2019; 19(1): 5.

102. Parrish CP, Har D, Andrew Bird J. Current status of potential therapies for IgE-mediated food allergy. *Curr Allergy Asthma Rep* 2018; 18(3): 18.

103. Shreffler WG, Beyer K, Chu TH, Burks AW, Sampson HA. Microarray immunoassay: Association of clinical history, *in vitro* IgE function, and heterogeneity of allergenic peanut epitopes. *J Allergy Clin Immunol* 2004; 113(4): 776–782.

104. Caubet JC, Bencharitiwong R, Moshier E, Godbold JH, Sampson HA, Nowak-Wegrzyn A. Significance of ovomucoid- and ovalbumin-specific IgE/IgG(4) ratios in egg allergy. *J Allergy Clin Immunol* 2012; 129(3): 739–747.

105. Thyagarajan A, Jones SM, Calatroni A et al. Evidence of pathway-specific basophil anergy induced by peanut oral immunotherapy in peanut-allergic children. *Clin Exp Allergy* 2012; 42(8): 1197–1205.

106. Wang J, Sampson HA. Safety and efficacy of epicutaneous immunotherapy for food allergy. *Pediatr Allergy Immunol* 2018; 29(4): 341–349.

107. Sampson HA, Shreffler WG, Yang WH et al. Effect of varying doses of epicutaneous immunotherapy vs placebo on reaction to peanut protein exposure among patients with peanut sensitivity: A randomized clinical trial. *JAMA* 2017; 318(18): 1798–1809.

108. Jones SM, Sicherer SH, Burks AW et al. Epicutaneous immunotherapy for the treatment of peanut allergy in children and young adults. *J Allergy Clin Immunol* 2017; 139(4): 1242–1252.e9.

109. Srivastava KD, Qu C, Zhang T, Goldfarb J, Sampson HA, Li XM. Food allergy herbal formula-2 silences peanut-induced anaphylaxis for a prolonged posttreatment period via IFN-γ-producing CD8+ T cells. *J Allergy Clin Immunol* 2009; 123(2): 443–451.

110. Nadeau KC, Schneider LC, Hoyte L, Borras I, Umetsu DT. Rapid oral desensitization in combination with omalizumab therapy in patients with cow's milk allergy. *J Allergy Clin Immunol* 2011; 127(6): 1622–1624.

111. Lin C, Lee IT, Sampath V et al. Combining anti-IgE with oral immunotherapy. *Pediatr Allergy Immunol* 2017; 28(7): 619–627.

18 Hymenoptera allergens

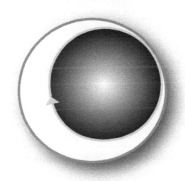

Rafael I. Monsalve
ALK-ABELLO

Te Piao King
Rockefeller University

Miles Guralnick
Independent Scholar (now actively retired)

CONTENTS

18.1 INTRODUCTION

Many insects can cause allergy in man (Table 18.1) [1,2]. People can be exposed to insect body parts or their secretions by inhalation, to their venoms by stinging, and to their salivary gland secretions by biting. Examples of these routes of sensitization are, respectively, allergies to cockroaches of the order Orthoptera; to ants, bees, and vespids of the order Hymenoptera; and to flies and mosquitoes of the order Diptera.

The importance of venoms as the allergen source in Hymenoptera allergy has been known for some time. The majority of known insect venom allergens are proteins of 10–50 kDa containing 100–400 amino acid residues, but there are exceptions. Nearly all these allergens have been sequenced, and their structures are known. Many of them have been expressed in bacteria, insect, or yeast cells.

This chapter reviews the immunochemical properties of some of these known Hymenoptera venom proteins and peptides, and their relevance to our understanding and treatment of insect allergy.

18.2 HYMENOPTERA INSECTS

Essentially all insects responsible for causing insect sting allergic reactions belong to the order Hymenoptera. This is a large and diverse order composed of over 70 families with over 100,000 species. Although many Hymenoptera are capable of stinging, only species from three families sting people with a high degree of frequency. The usual perpetrators are social insects and belong to the Apidae (bees), Formicidae (ants), or Vespidae (wasps). The medically important genera in the United States are outlined in Table 18.2. Four of these insects are shown in Figure 18.1.

Several bee and wasp species listed in Table 18.2 are common in both North America and in Europe. Their closely related species are present in other parts of the world. For example, the vespids of interest in South America include wasps of the genus *Polybia*. The ants of interest in Americas are fire ants, but in Asia they include the Chinese needle ant, *Pachycondyla chinensis*, and the Samsum

Table 18.1 Insects reported to cause allergy in man

Order Coleoptera—beetles
Order Diptera—flies, mosquitoes, gnats, midges
Order Ephemeroptera—mayflies
Order Hemiptera—kissing bugs, bedbugs
Order Hymenoptera—ants, bees, vespids
Order Lepidoptera—moths, caterpillars
Order Orthoptera—cockroaches, grasshoppers
Order Psocoptera—booklice
Order Siphonaptera—fleas
Order Thysanura—firebrats, silverfish
Order Trichoptera—caddisflies

Source: Taken from Golden DB et al. *Ann Allergy Asthma Immunol* 2017; 118(1): 28–54.

ant, *Pachycondyla sennaarensis*; and in Australia they are the jumper ants and the bulldog ants, *Myrmecia* spp. [3]. Nonnative stinging Hymenoptera often become established in new regions as the result of frequent movement of freight from one continent to another. Consequently, fire ants are now established in Asia and Australia, Chinese needle ants are now established in the United States, and the Asian hornet, *Vespa velutina*, is now established in Southern Europe. Another particular case is *Polistes dominula*, which is the predominant *Polistes* species in several European countries [4,5], but that was also introduced in the northeastern part of the United States, and then expanded its distribution to other regions [6–8].

Accurate identification of social stinging Hymenoptera to species level is a difficult task even for most entomologists. Although not definitive, there are several behavioral characteristics that can help provide clues as to a specimen's identity. For example, honeybees have a unique sting anatomy that causes worker bees to leave their sting apparatuses in the victim's skin. Although sting autotomy is almost exclusively attributed to honeybees, other stinging Hymenoptera will occasionally lose their sting. And conversely, honeybees will occasionally sting without autotomizing [9]. Annoying wasps foraging around picnic foods, garbage, or fallen fruit are usually yellow jackets and belong to the genus *Vespula*. Large colonies of wasps living in subterranean nests are also usually of the genus *Vespula* [2], while *Polistes* spp. and *Vespa velutina* usually build hanging nests in trees or buildings. Since there are notable exceptions to these, the only reliable means of obtaining a positive identification is to collect a specimen and have its identity determined by an entomologist with expertise in the social Hymenoptera.

Table 18.2 U.S. geographic distribution and medical importance of some insects of the order Hymenoptera

Family/subfamily	Genus and species	Common name	U.S. geographic distribution	Medical importance
Apidae/Apinae	*Apis mellifera*	Honeybee	Entire United States	Major
	Bombus spp.	Bumblebee	Entire United States	Moderate
Formicidae/ Myrmicinae	*Solenopsis invicta*	Fire ant	Southeast, southwest	Major
	Solenopsis richteri	Fire ant	Mississippi, Alabama	Minor
Vespidae/ Vespinae	*Vespa crabro*	European hornet	Northeast, southeast	Minor
	Dolichovespula maculata	Whitefaced hornet (baldfaced hornet)	Entire United States	Major
	Dolichovespula arenaria	Yellow hornet (aerial yellow jacket)	Northeast, northwest, southwest	Major
	Vespula flavopilosa	Yellow jacket	Northeast, southeast	Major
	Vespula germanica	Yellow jacket	Northeast, northwest	Major
	Vespula maculifrons	Yellow jacket	Northeast	Major
	Vespula pensylvanica	Yellow jacket	Northwest, southwest	Major
	Vespula vulgaris	Yellow jacket	Northeast, northwest, southwest	Major
	Vespula squamosa	Yellow jacket	Northeast, southeast	Major
Vespidae/ Polistinae	*Polistes* spp.	Paper wasp	Entire United States	Major

Note: Only insects with known venom allergens are listed.
Source: Data for geographic distribution and medical importance are taken from Golden DB et al. *Ann Allergy Asthma Immunol* 2017; 118(1): 28–54.

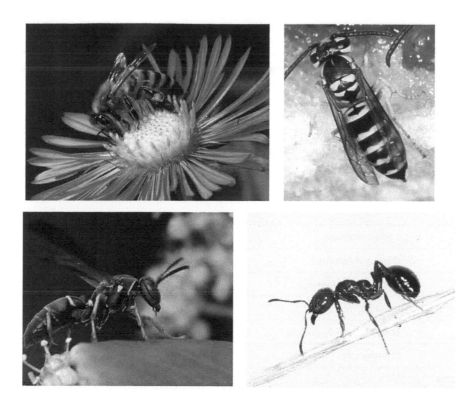

Figure 18.1 Common stinging insects. The photos, starting from top left and going clockwise, show, respectively, honeybee (*Apis mellifera*), yellow jacket (*Vespula maculifrons*), paper wasp (*Polistes fuscatus*), and fire ant (*Solenopsis invicta*). The approximate lengths of these insects in the order given are 16, 10, 19, and 3 mm, respectively. The photos are of different magnifications.

18.3 HYMENOPTERA VENOM ALLERGENS

Table 18.3 lists some of the venom allergens of bees, vespids, and fire ants. A list of known allergens from various sources can be found at the website of the Allergen Nomenclature Sub-Committee of the International Union of Immunological Societies (http://www.allergen.org).

Honeybee venom has 12 known allergens. These allergens differ in their size, biochemical function, and relative abundance. Their size varies from 3 to 200 kDa, and the majority are about 20–40 kDa. As examples, the most abundant ones are Api m 4 (Melittin, a cytolytic peptide) followed by Api m 1 (phospholipase A_2), Api m 2 (hyaluronidase), and Api m 3 (phosphatase); they represent, respectively, about 50%, 12%, 2%, and 1% of venom weight. They also differ in their allergenicity. Nearly all bee-sensitive patients have Api m 1 and 2 specific IgE antibodies, but less than one-third have Api m 4–specific IgE [10]. Homologs of honeybee allergens are present in bumblebees and Asian bees.

Vespid venoms each contain three to six known protein allergens. The most abundant ones are antigen 5, hyaluronidase, and phospholipase A_1. The other three are dipeptidyl peptidase IV [11], protease [12], and vitellogenin [13]. Antigen 5 is of unknown biological function. One antigen 5 homolog from cone snail, *Conus textile*, has protease activity [14], but another from *C. marmoreous* does not [15]. Vespid phospholipase A_1 differs from bee phospholipase A_2 in sequence and enzymatic specificity. Vespid and bee hyaluronidases are homologous with about 55% sequence identity and have identical enzymatic specificity [16]. Homologs of antigen 5, hyaluronidase, and phospholipase A_1 are

found in all vespids studied, for example, the *Vespa* wasps in Asia [17,18] and the *Polybia* wasps from South America [19,20].

Fire ant venom contains four known protein allergens: Sol i 1–4. Sol i 1 is a phospholipase similar to the vespid phospholipase. Sol i 3 is homologous to vespid 5. Sol i 3 and Ves v 5 share a similar structure, but they have limited conservation of surface chemical properties and topology [21]. Studies have been reported with venom allergens of Chinese needle ants [22,23] and jack jumper ants [24]. These ants have components similar to those of fire ant venom together with their own unique components [3].

Several venom allergens have partial sequence identity with other proteins from diverse sources, and this is summarized in Table 18.4. As an example, the sequence identities of three vespid antigen 5s, fire ant antigen 5, human and mouse testis proteins, human glioma protein, and proteins from tomato, nematode, and lizard, in their C-terminal 50-residue region are given in Figure 18.2. These proteins together belong to a protein superfamily known as CAP, the naming due to its main constituents: cysteine-rich secretory proteins, antigen 5, and pathogenesis-related proteins [25].

X-ray crystallography was used to determine the structures of honeybee venom hyaluronidase and phospholipase A_2, and those of antigen 5 and hyaluronidase from yellow jacket, *V. vulgaris*. Also the structure of Sol i 2 has been solved [26]. Vespid phospholipase A_1 has sequence homology with porcine pancreatic lipase. As the structure of porcine lipase is known, the structure of vespid phospholipase can be obtained by modeling. Using the modeling approach, the structures of nearly all the proteins in Table 18.3 can be obtained [27].

Table 18.3 Some known insect venom allergens

Allergen name[a]	Biochemical name	Glycoprotein	Molecular size[b] (kDa)	Structure[c]
Honeybee, *Apis mellifera*				
Api m 1	Phospholipase A_2	Yes	16	Known
Api m 2	Hyaluronidase	Yes	39	Known
Api m 3	Acid phosphatase	Yes	43	Known
Api m 4	Melittin	No	3	Known
Api m 5	Dipeptidyl peptidase IV	Yes	100	
Api m 6	?	No	8	
Api m 7	Serine protease	Yes	39	Modeling
Api m 8	Carboxyl esterase	Yes	70	Modeling
Api m 9	Carboxypeptidase	Yes	60	Modeling
Api m 10	Icarapin	Yes	25	
Api m 11	Major royal jelly protein		50	
Api m 12	Vitellogenin	Yes	200	
Paper wasp, *Polistes annularis*				
Pol a 1	Phospholipase A_1	No	34	Modeling
Pol a 2	Hyaluronidase	Yes	38	Modeling
Pol a 5	Antigen 5	No	23	Modeling
	Protease		28	
Yellow jacket, *Vespula vulgaris*				
Ves v 1	Phospholipase A_1	No	34	Modeling
Ves v 2	Hyaluronidase	Yes	38	Known
Ves v 3	Dipeptidyl peptidase IV	Yes	100	Modeling
Ves v 5	Antigen 5	No	23	Known
Ves v 6	Vitellogenin	Yes	200	
Fire ant, *Solenopsis invicta*				
Sol i 1	Phospholipase A_1	Yes	37	Modeling
Sol i 2			30	Known
Sol i 3	Antigen 5		23	Modeling
Sol i 4			20	

[a] See http://www.allergen.org/.
[b] Several allergens are glycoproteins, and the molecular size given refers to the protein.
[c] Structures were determined directly or by modeling structures of homologous proteins.

18.4 RECOMBINANT HYMENOPTERA VENOM ALLERGENS

Nearly all the allergens in Table 18.3 have been expressed in bacteria, insect, or yeast cells to yield recombinant proteins. The recombinant proteins that are expressed in the cytoplasm of bacteria are usually unfolded as they lack the disulfide bonds of the natural proteins and do not have the native conformation of the natural proteins. The cytoplasm of bacteria is a reducing environment, and any disulfide bonds that do form are reduced through the action of disulfide reducing enzymes. Recombinant proteins from insect or yeast cells have the native conformation of the natural proteins as they are folded during secretion into medium.

Table 18.4 Sequence identity of insect allergens and other proteins

Insect allergens	Other proteins	Residues compared	Percentage (%) identity
Antigen 5 s	Mammalian testis protein	130	35
	Human glioma PR protein	124	23
	Hookworm protein[a]	130	28
	Plant leaf PR protein[b]	130	28
	Mexican lizard toxin	130	28
	Cone snail protease	120	36
	Black fly and midge saliva allergen	170	33
Hyaluronidase	Mammalian sperm protein	331	50
Phosphatase	Mammalian phosphatase	343	16
Phospholipase A$_1$	Mammalian lipases	123	40
Phospholipase A$_2$	Mammalian phospholipases	129	20
Protease	Mammalian acrosin	243	38
	Horseshoe crab enzyme	243	41

[a] Homologous worm proteins are present in other nematodes.
[b] Homologous plant PR proteins are present in tobacco, tomato, barley, and maize.

```
Dol m 5     VGHYTQMVWG KTKEIGCGSI KYIE.DNWYT H....YLVCN YGPGGNDFNQ
Pol a 5     IGHYTQMVWG KTKEIGCGSL KYME.NNMQN H....YLICN YGPAGNYLGQ
Ves v 5     TGHYTQMVWA NTKEVGCGSI KYIQ.EKWHK H....YLVCN YGPSGNFMNE
Sol i 3     VEHYTQIVWA KTSKIGCARI MFKEPDNWTK H....YLVCN YGPAGNVLGA
human tpx   VGHYTQLVWY STYQVGCGIA YCPNQDSLKY .....YYVCQ YCPAGNNMNR
mouse tpx   VGHYTQLVWY SSFKIGCGIA YCPNQDNLKY .....FYVCH YCPMGNNVMK
hum glioma  CGHYTQVVWA DSYKVGCAVQ FCPKVSGFDA LSNGAHFICN YGPGGNYPTW
tomato pr   CGHYTQVVWR NSVRVGCARV QC....NNGG Y....VVSCN YDPPGNYRGE
hookworm    IGHYTQMAWD TTYKLGCAVV FC....NDFT .....FGVCQ YGPGGNYMGH
lizard      IGHYTQVVWY RSYELGCAIA YCPDQPTYKY .....YQVCQ YCPGGNIRSR
```

Figure 18.2 Sequence identity of vespid antigen 5s and other proteins in their C-terminal region. The sequences shown from top to bottom are for antigen 5s from hornet, paper wasp, yellow jacket and fire ant venoms, human and mouse testis specific proteins, human glioma protein, tomato leaf pathogenesis-related protein, hookworm protein, and lizard venom protein, respectively. Bold characters indicate residues identical to those of vespid antigen 5s, and dots indicate blanks added for maximal alignment of sequences. The underlined peptide region was found to contain a dominant T-cell epitope of vespid antigen 5 (see text).

Recombinant allergens have different applications. One obvious application is for use as diagnostic reagents. Several authors have reported the use of venom allergens for improved diagnosis of Hymenoptera hypersensitivity [28–33], and this component-resolved diagnosis (CRD) is certainly of help when determining the correct treatment for patients who cannot always identify the culprit insect. Although purified natural allergens have shown higher sensitivity [32], correctly folded recombinant allergens that are glycoproteins (as shown in Table 18.3) have the advantage in that they can be produced without cross-reacting carbohydrates that can complicate the interpretation of CRD [28]. Venom immunotherapy (VIT) with venom extract is a highly efficacious treatment, mainly due to the advances in the characterization of the venom components as well as the improvements in understanding the mechanism of the treatment [1,30,34,35].

Another application is to prepare allergen hybrids with reduced allergenicity but retain immunogenicity [36,37]. The hybrids contain a small segment of the guest allergen of interest and a large segment of a host protein. The host protein is homologous to the guest allergen, and they are poorly cross-reactive as antigens. The host protein functions as a scaffold to hold the segment of the guest allergen in its native conformation, as homologous proteins of greater than 30% sequence identity can have similar structures. In this way, the hybrids retain the discontinuous epitopes of the guest allergen but at a reduced density.

This approach was demonstrated with hybrids of yellow jacket and wasp antigen 5s [36]. These two antigen 5s have 59% sequence identity, and they are poorly cross-reactive in patients or in animals. Hybrids with one-quarter yellow jacket antigen 5 and three-quarters of wasp antigen 5 showed 10^2- to 10^3-fold reduction in allergenicity when tested by histamine release assay in yellow jacket-sensitive patients. These hybrids retained the immunogenicity of antigen 5 for antibody responses specific for the native protein and for T-cell responses in mice. Therefore, the hybrids might be useful vaccines as they may be used at higher doses than the natural allergen.

18.5 B-CELL EPITOPES OF HYMENOPTERA VENOM ALLERGENS

The entire accessible surface of a protein is believed to represent a continuum of B-cell epitopes [38]. The B-cell epitopes are divided into the continuous and discontinuous types, and their sizes range from 6 to 17 amino acid residues. The continuous type consists of only contiguous amino acid residues in the molecule, while the discontinuous type consists of contiguous as well as noncontiguous residues that are brought together in the folded molecule. The majority of protein-specific antibodies, probably 90% or more, are of the discontinuous type. Studies show that the same B-cell epitopes can induce both IgE and IgG responses.

Data in agreement with this generalization were obtained with vespid allergen-specific mouse antisera, which contain mainly specific IgGs. Vespid allergen-specific mouse antisera bound natural allergens and they bound poorly, if at all, reduced and unfolded allergens that lack the discontinuous epitopes of the folded molecules. This is particularly the case for vespid hyaluronidases and phospholipases [16] and to a lesser extent for vespid antigen 5s [39].

Another general conclusion is that cross-reactivity is readily detectable for homologous venom proteins of greater than 90% sequence identity, and barely detectable for homologous venom proteins of less than 50% sequence identity. Variable extents of cross-reactivity are detectable for homologous proteins with about 50%–90% sequence identity. The variable extents of cross-reactivity of homologous proteins probably reflect the degree and the area of identity on the protein surface.

The continuous B-cell epitopes of a protein can be mapped readily by testing polyclonal antibodies with a series of overlapping peptides of 7–20 residues in length. Multiple epitopes were found for the 204-residue hornet antigen 5, and only one was found for the 26-residue bee venom Melittin [40]. No unusual pattern of amino acid sequence was observed for these B-cell epitopes.

Several insect venom proteins are glycoproteins. Their oligosaccharide side chains have been demonstrated to function as B-cell epitopes for IgE and IgG responses in patients as well as in animals [41]. In contrast to the multitude of amino acid sequences of different insect allergens, the sequence differences in their carbohydrate side chains are limited. The carbohydrate side chain is N-linked to the asparagine residue of the protein by its innermost N-acetylglucosamine residue. The predominant carbohydrate side chain has the sequence of

$$Man\alpha1\rightarrow6(Man\alpha1\rightarrow3)Man\beta1\rightarrow4GlcNАc\beta1\rightarrow4GlcNАc$$

with one or two fucoses (α1,6 and/or α1,3) linked to the innermost N-acetylglucosamine residue. This was shown for bee phospholipase [42] and bee and yellow jacket hyaluronidases [43]. Similar or identical carbohydrate side chains are present in other plant and animal proteins. The glycan in plant proteins contains, in addition to the fucoses, xylose (β1,2) linked to the mannose in the middle position. Tests with patient or animal sera specific for glycans from

different sources suggest that the specificity of the cross-reactive carbohydrate determinant resides mainly in the fucose residues for insect proteins and in the fucose and xylose residues for plant proteins. Indeed, horseradish peroxidase can be used to establish whether patient sera cross-reactive to bees and yellow jackets are due to their cross-reactive carbohydrate determinant [44]. In addition, bromelain and ascorbate oxidase have also been used, in order to avoid false-positive detection in diagnostic methods, as well as their use as cross-reactive carbohydrate determinant (CCD) inhibitors in order to improve interpretation of CRD [28,45].

18.6 T-CELL EPITOPES OF HYMENOPTERA VENOM ALLERGENS

T-cell epitopes are of interest because of the central role of T cells in regulating the antibody class switch event of B cells. They are also of interest as possible reagents for immunotherapy as shown with T-cell peptides of bee venom phospholipase A_2 [46].

T-cell epitopes are peptides of about 15 residues in length formed following intracellular processing of antigens by antigen-presenting cells, and they do not depend on the secondary or tertiary structure of the antigen. This is the case with venom allergens as shown by the identical T-cell stimulating activities of natural or reduced allergens, e.g., vespid antigen 5s, hyaluronidases, and phospholipases A_1 [16].

Bee venom phospholipase A_2 and hornet antigen 5 are found to have multiple T-cell epitopes distributed throughout the entire molecule by tests with a series of overlapping peptides in patients [47,48] or in mice. Because of major histocompatibility complex (MHC) class II restriction, patients of different polymorphic background, or mice of different haplotypes, differ in their pattern of peptide recognition. Nonetheless, both insect allergens were found to have several dominant T-cell epitopes recognized by patients or mice tested.

One of the dominant T-cell epitope peptides of hornet antigen 5 was found to cross-react with paper wasp and yellow jacket antigen 5s as well as with a homologous peptide of a mouse testis protein (Figure 18.2). The cross-reactivity with mouse protein is not reciprocal, as the corresponding peptide from mouse testis protein did not cross-react with hornet antigen 5–specific cells [49].

No unusual features were observed for the dominant T-cell epitope peptides of insect venom allergens. Both normal and atopic people were found to recognize the same T-cell epitope peptides of bee venom phospholipase [48]. Others report similar findings for T-cell epitopes of allergens from grass and tree pollens, cat dander, mites, and ovalbumin [50].

18.7 ANTIGENIC CROSS-REACTIVITY OF HYMENOPTERA VENOMS

Insect-allergic patients often have sensitivity to multiple insects by skin test or radioallergosorbent test with venoms. This multiple sensitivity can be due to exposure to different insects and/or antigenic cross-reactivity of different venoms. This issue of multiple exposure or antigenic cross-reactivity is of importance in the choice of single or multiple venoms for immunotherapy of patients.

Bees, fire ants, and vespids each have unique as well as homologous venom allergens. Two of the known main bee allergens are homologous to vespid allergens—hyaluronidase and protease with about 50% sequence identity. Two of the four fire ant allergens are homologous to vespid allergens, antigen 5, and phospholipase. Fire ant antigen 5 has about 35% sequence identity with vespid antigen 5s. For the vespids, the sequence identity of their homologous antigen 5s, hyaluronidases, and phospholipases range from about 40% to 99% for different species of hornets, yellow jackets, and wasps. Moreover, cross-reactivity of minor components of the venom is also possible, as it has been mentioned for Api m 5 and Ves v 3 (dipeptidyl peptidases IV) [29], or for the Vitellogenis (Api m 12 and Ves v 6) [30]. As noted in Section 16.5, cross-reactivity of B-cell epitopes is readily detectable for homologous venom proteins of greater than 90% sequence identity, and barely detectable for homologous venom proteins of less than 50% sequence identity, and variable extents of cross-reactivity are detectable for homologous proteins with about 50%–90% sequence identity. Attempting to predict cross-reactivity even between distantly related allergenic proteins, the known three-dimensional structure of Api m 2 was successfully used by bioinformatics tools [51]. Recently, knowledge from three-dimensional structures and availability of recombinant proteins has permitted evaluation of cross-reactivity among phospholipases from several Hymenoptera [52].

These considerations would indicate that patients with sensitivity to multiple insects can be due to cross-reactivity of a single allergen, hyaluronidase as in the case for bees and vespids, or of multiple allergens in other cases. For cross-reactivity of fire ants and vespids, or of different vespids, hyaluronidase again has the major role with antigen 5 and phospholipase having secondary roles.

Some insect allergens have common peptide and carbohydrate determinants. However, peptide and carbohydrate determinants differ in their epitope density and in their antibody affinity. For peptide determinants, the entire accessible surface of a protein represents a continuum of epitopes [38]. For carbohydrate determinants, the number of epitopes is restricted to a few potential glycosylation sites, and these sites are not necessarily glycosylated. As an example, yellow jacket hyaluronidase has five potential sites, but only two to three sites are glycosylated [53], being a particular case of a glycoprotein that exhibits high IgE reactivity to CCDs [54].

Mediators are released from IgE-bound mast cells or basophils on allergen challenge. This biological activity requires the allergens to have multiple determinants/epitopes so that they can cross-link the bivalent IgE antibodies. Thus, the low-density carbohydrate determinants are likely to be of less biological importance than are the high-density peptide determinants. Also, the biological activity of allergens to cause mediator release depends on the affinity of allergen-specific IgEs [55]. For these reasons, there is debate as to the importance of glycan-specific IgE in allergic diseases [28,30,54,56,57].

Several authors have reported that a sizable group of normal people who showed no clinical sensitivity to insects tested positive with insect venoms [58]. These false-positive results may possibly represent cross-reactivity of insect venoms with other proteins to which people have been exposed. As noted earlier in Table 18.4, insect allergens have variable extents of sequence identity with proteins from diverse sources.

Investigators have observed that more men than women, in a ratio of about 2 to 1, had insect allergy as judged by their systemic and large local reactions or by their death statistics [59]. It has been assumed that these results were primarily due to greater exposure because of work habits of men and women. Whether or not the partial sequence identity of venom allergens with proteins of male reproductive functions (Table 18.4) plays a role in these observations is not known.

18.8 HYMENOPTERA VENOM PEPTIDES

In addition to proteins, Hymenoptera venoms contain peptides, biogenic amines such as histamine and dopamine, and other low molecular weight components [3,60,61]. The most abundant peptides in bee and vespid venoms are Melittin and mastoparan, respectively, and they have mast cell degranulating activity. Bee venom contains another mast cell degranulating peptide, known as MCD, with a greater mast cell degranulating activity than Melittin.

Melittin and mastoparan are basic peptides with 26 and 14–15 residues, respectively. Both peptides are synthesized in insects as precursor molecules. The precursor is first cleaved by signal peptidase to remove the signal sequence, next cleaved by dipeptidylpeptidase IV to remove the pro sequence to yield the mature peptide [62].

Both peptides are immunogenic in mice for antibody responses [63,64]. Melittin was found to be an allergen but not mastoparan.

Yellow jacket venom was found to be lethal in mice when injected intraperitoneally but not subcutaneously [65]. The toxic action was shown to require the synergistic action of the venom peptide mastoparan and the venom protein phospholipase A_1. This toxin action has also been taken into account in recent studies on the venom components of diverse Hymenoptera [60,66].

18.9 HYMENOPTERA VENOM AS ADJUVANT

Bee and vespid venoms contain hyaluronidase, phospholipase, and proteases as well as bioactive peptides. These biochemicals may function as adjuvant to promote venom allergenicity.

Hyaluronan in skin is a high molecular weight polymer. Normally it does not stimulate inflammatory or immune response because of the presence of specific binding proteins. Bound hyaluronan polymers in skin can be released by venom hyaluronidase. The freed polymers can function as adjuvant to promote IgE and IgG1 response in mice [67]. Bee phospholipase can induce IL-4 release from murine mast cells and induce IgE response in mice [68]. Vespid phospholipase A can induce inflammatory response of murine macrophages with release of prostaglandin E_2 [65]. The biological effect of both bee and wasp phospholipases may enhance hypersensitive reactions [69]. Venom dipeptidyl peptidase IV may also regulate inflammatory and immunological responses. The bioactive peptide Melittin from bee and mastoparan from vespids [70] both can induce release of inflammatory mediators from mast cells and macrophages, and they are reported to have weak adjuvant activity in mice [65].

Venom allergens do not appear to have any special properties to induce IgE and IgG responses in susceptible people. It may be the combined biological properties of these enzymes and bioactive peptides that contribute to the allergenicity of venom.

18.10 STING REACTIONS

There are three types of reactions that individuals may experience from a Hymenoptera sting [1]. The normal response is a *local cutaneous reaction* characterized by redness, swelling, and pain confined to the sting site. This is a toxic response. A *large local reaction* is thought to be IgE mediated and involves an extensive area of warmth, redness, and swelling contiguous with the site of the sting. Large local reactions typically develop in 1–3 days, may involve an entire extremity, and may persist for up to 5 days. An *allergic systemic reaction* usually occurs within half an hour of envenomization and includes symptoms remote from the site of the sting. Systemic allergic reactions may involve the skin, the respiratory system, the vascular system, or any combination thereof.

Minimal treatment is necessary for local cutaneous reactions. The sting site should be kept clean to avoid secondary infections, and ice packs may help to reduce local pain and swelling. Large local reactions may cause considerable discomfort and are frequently treated with analgesics, antihistamines, and glucocorticosteroids. Systemic allergic reactions can be quite serious and occasionally fatal. They can be successfully treated with venom immunotherapy to prevent future reactions (see Chapter 29).

SALIENT POINTS

1. The medically important stinging insects are ants, bees, and vespids (wasps). The vespids include hornets, paper wasps, and yellow jackets.
2. Insect venom allergens are generally proteins of 10–50 kDa. Nearly all known venom allergens have been cloned and expressed as recombinant proteins in different systems. However, some recombinant proteins are not properly folded.
3. Insect venom allergens have different biochemical functions. Their only known common feature is their partial sequence identity with proteins from other sources in the environment.
4. Each of these insect venoms has unique allergen(s) as well as homologous allergen(s) with partial sequence identity.
5. Multiple sensitivity of patients to different insects, or to more closely related vespids can be due to multiple exposures and/or antigenic cross-reactivity of venom allergen(s).
6. Detailed immunochemical knowledge of insect venom allergens is useful for monitoring the quality of insect venoms used for diagnosis and treatment, as well as leading to the development of new immunotherapeutic reagents.

REFERENCES

1. Golden DB, Demain J, Freeman T et al. Stinging insect hypersensitivity: A practice parameter update 2016. *Ann Allergy Asthma Immunol* 2017; 118(1): 28–54.
2. Guralnick M, Benton AW. Entomological aspects of insect sting allergy. In: Levine MI, Lockey RF, editors. *Monograph on Insect Allergy*, 3rd ed. Milwaukee, WI: American Academy of Allergy and Immunology, 1995: 7–20.
3. Hoffman DR. Ant venoms. *Curr Opin Allergy Clin Immunol* 2010; 10(4): 342–346.
4. Fernandez J. Distribution of vespid species in Europe. *Curr Opin Allergy Clin Immunol* 2004; 4(4): 319–324.
5. Severino MG, Campi P, Macchia D et al. European Polistes venom allergy. *Allergy* 2006; 61(7): 860–863.
6. Cervo R, Zacchi F, Turillazzi S. *Polistes dominulus* (Hymenoptera, Vespidae) invading North America: Some hypotheses for its rapid spread. *Insectes Soc* 2000; 47(2): 155–157.
7. Hesler SL. *Polistes dominula* (Christ, 1791) (Hymenoptera: Vespidae: Polistinae) found in South Dakota, U.S.A. *Insecta Mundi* 2010; 145: 1–3.
8. Liebert AE, Gamboa GJ, Stamp NE et al. Genetics, behavior and ecology of a paper wasp invasion: *Polistes dominulus* in North America. *Ann Zool Fennici* 2006; 43: 595–624.
9. Mulfinger L, Yunginger J, Styer W, Guralnick M, Lintner T. Sting morphology and frequency of sting autotomy among medically important vespids (Hymenoptera: Vespidae) and the honey bee (Hymenoptera: Apidae). *J Med Entomol* 1992; 29(2): 325–328.
10. King TP, Sobotka AK, Kochoumian L, Lichtenstein LM. Allergens of honey bee venom. *Arch Biochem Biophys* 1976; 172(2): 661–671.
11. Blank S, Seismann H, Bockisch B et al. Identification, recombinant expression, and characterization of the 100 kDa high molecular weight Hymenoptera venom allergens Api m 5 and Ves v 3. *J Immunol* 2010; 184(9): 5403–5413.
12. Winningham KM, Fitch CD, Schmidt M, Hoffman DR. Hymenoptera venom protease allergens. *J Allergy Clin Immunol* 2004; 114(4): 928–933.
13. Blank S, Seismann H, McIntyre M et al. Vitellogenins are new high molecular weight components and allergens (Api m 12 and Ves v 6) of *Apis mellifera* and *Vespula vulgaris* venom. *PLOS ONE* 2013; 8(4): e62009.
14. Milne TJ, Abbenante G, Tyndall JD, Halliday J, Lewis RJ. Isolation and characterization of a cone snail protease with homology to CRISP proteins of the pathogenesis-related protein superfamily. *J Biol Chem* 2003; 278(33): 31105–31110.
15. Qian J, Guo ZY, Chi CW. Cloning and isolation of a Conus cysteine-rich protein homologous to Tex31 but without proteolytic activity. *Acta Biochim Biophys Sin (Shanghai)* 2008; 40(2): 174–181.
16. King TP, Lu G, González M, Qian NF, Soldatova L. Yellow jacket venom allergens, hyaluronidase and phospholipase: Sequence similarity and antigenic cross-reactivity with their hornet and wasp homologs and possible implications for clinical allergy. *J Allergy Clin Immunol* 1996; 98: 588–600.
17. An S, Chen L, Wei JF et al. Purification and characterization of two new allergens from the venom of Vespa magnifica. *PLOS ONE* 2012; 7(2): e31920.
18. Sukprasert S, Rungsa P, Uawonggul N et al. Purification and structural characterisation of phospholipase A1 (Vespapase, Ves a 1) from Thai banded tiger wasp (*Vespa affinis*) venom. *Toxicon* 2013; 61: 151–164.
19. Pinto JR, Santos LD, Arcuri HA, Dias NB, Palma MS. Proteomic characterization of the hyaluronidase (E.C. 3.2.1.35) from the venom of the social wasp *Polybia paulista*. *Protein Pept Lett* 2012; 19(6): 625–635.
20. Vinzon SE, Marino-Buslje C, Rivera E, Biscoglio de Jimenez BM. A naturally occurring hypoallergenic variant of vespid Antigen 5 from *Polybia scutellaris* venom as a candidate for allergen-specific immunotherapy. *PLOS ONE* 2012; 7(7): e41351.
21. Padavattan S, Schmidt M, Hoffman DR, Markovic-Housley Z. Crystal structure of the major allergen from fire ant venom, Sol i 3. *J Mol Biol* 2008; 383(1): 178–185.
22. Kim SS, Park HS, Kim HY, Lee SK, Nahm DH. Anaphylaxis caused by the new ant, *Pachycondyla chinensis*: Demonstration of specific IgE and IgE-binding components. *J Allergy Clin Immunol* 2001; 107(6): 1095–1099.
23. Lee EK, Jeong KY, Lyu DP et al. Characterization of the major allergens of *Pachycondyla chinensis* in ant sting anaphylaxis patients. *Clin Exp Allergy* 2009; 39(4): 602–607.
24. Street MD, Donovan GR, Baldo BA. Molecular cloning and characterization of the major allergen Myr p II from the venom of the jumper ant *Myrmecia pilosula*: Myr p I and Myr p II share a common protein leader sequence. *Biochim Biophys Acta* 1996; 1305(1-2): 87–97.

25. Gibbs GM, Roelants K, O'Bryan MK. The CAP superfamily: Cysteine-rich secretory proteins, antigen 5, and pathogenesis-related 1 proteins—Roles in reproduction, cancer, and immune defense. *Endocr Rev* 2008; 29(7): 865–897.

26. Borer AS, Wassmann P, Schmidt M et al. Crystal structure of Sol I 2: A major allergen from fire ant venom. *J Mol Biol* 2012; 415(4): 635–648.

27. Hoffman DR. Structural biology of allergens from stinging and biting insects. *Curr Opin Allergy Clin Immunol* 2008; 8(4): 338–342.

28. Altmann F. Coping with cross-reactive carbohydrate determinants in allergy diagnosis. *Allergo J Int* 2016; 25(4): 98–105.

29. Antolin-Amerigo D, Ruiz-Leon B, Boni E et al. Component-resolved diagnosis in hymenoptera allergy. *Allergol Immunopathol* 2017; 46(3): 253–262.

30. Blank S, Bilo MB, Ollert M. Component-resolved diagnostics to direct in venom immunotherapy: Important steps towards precision medicine. *Clin Exp Allergy* 2018; 48(4): 354–364.

31. Mittermann I, Zidarn M, Silar M et al. Recombinant allergen-based IgE testing to distinguish bee and wasp allergy. *J Allergy Clin Immunol* 2010; 125(6): 1300–1307.

32. Monsalve RI, Vega A, Marques L et al. Component-resolved diagnosis of vespid venom-allergic individuals: Phospholipases and antigen 5 s are necessary to identify Vespula or Polistes sensitization. *Allergy* 2012; 67(4): 528–536.

33. Muller U, Schmid-Grendelmeier P, Hausmann O, Helbling A. IgE to recombinant allergens Api m 1, Ves v 1, and Ves v 5 distinguish double sensitization from cross-reaction in venom allergy. *Allergy* 2012; 67(8): 1069–1073.

34. Oppenheimer J, Golden DBK. Hymenoptera venom immunotherapy: Past, present, and future. *Ann Allergy Asthma Immunol* 2018; 121(3): 276–277.

35. Matricardi PM, Kleine-Tebbe J, Hoffmann HJ et al. EAACI molecular allergology user's guide. *Pediatr Allergy Immunol* 2016; 27(Suppl 23): 1–250.

36. King TP, Jim SY, Monsalve RI, Kagey SA, Lichtenstein LM, Spangfort MD. Recombinant allergens with reduced allergenicity but retaining immunogenicity of the natural allergens: Hybrids of yellow jacket and paper wasp venom allergen antigen 5s. *J Immunol* 2001; 166(10): 6057–6065.

37. Tscheppe A, Breiteneder H. Recombinant allergens in structural biology, diagnosis, and immunotherapy. *Int Arch Allergy Immunol* 2017; 172(4): 187–202.

38. Davies DR, Cohen GH. Interactions of protein antigens with antibodies. *Proc Natl Acad Sci USA* 1996; 93(1): 7–12.

39. King TP, Kochoumian L, Lu G. Murine T and B cell responses to natural and recombinant hornet venom allergen, Dol m 5.02 and its recombinant fragments. *J Immunol* 1995; 154: 577–584.

40. King TP, Lu G, Agosto H. Antibody responses to bee melittin (Api m 4) and hornet antigen 5 (Dol m 5) in mice treated with the dominant T-cell epitope peptides. *J Allergy Clin Immunol* 1998; 101(3): 397–403.

41. Altmann F. The role of protein glycosylation in allergy. *Int Arch Allergy Immunol* 2007; 142(2): 99–115.

42. Kubelka V, Altmann F, Staudacher E et al. Primary structures of the *N*-linked carbohydrate chains from honeybee venom phospholipase A2. *Eur J Biochem* 1993; 213(3): 1193–1204.

43. Kolarich D, Leonard R, Hemmer W, Altmann F. The *N*-glycans of yellow jacket venom hyaluronidases and the protein sequence of its major isoform in *Vespula vulgaris*. *Febs J* 2005; 272(20): 5182–5190.

44. Jappe U, Raulf-Heimsoth M, Hoffmann M, Burow G, Hubsch-Muller C, Enk A. *In vitro* hymenoptera venom allergy diagnosis: Improved by screening for cross-reactive carbohydrate determinants and reciprocal inhibition. *Allergy* 2006; 61(10): 1220–1229.

45. Aberer W, Holzweber F, Hemmer W et al. Inhibition of cross-reactive carbohydrate determinants (CCDs) enhances the accuracy of *in vitro* allergy diagnosis. *Allergol Select* 2017; 1(2): 141–149.

46. Muller U, Akdis CA, Fricker M et al. Successful immunotherapy with T-cell epitope peptides of bee venom phospholipase A2 induces specific T-cell anergy in patients allergic to bee venom. *J Allergy Clin Immunol* 1998; 101(6 Pt 1): 747–754.

47. Bohle B, Zwolfer B, Fischer GF et al. Characterization of the human T cell response to antigen 5 from *Vespula vulgaris* (Ves v 5). *Clin Exp Allergy* 2005; 35(3): 367–373.

48. Carballido JM, Carballido-Perrig N, Kagi MK et al. T cell epitope specificity in human allergic and nonallergic subjects to bee venom phospholipase A2. *J Immunol* 1993; 150(8 Pt 1): 3582–3591.

49. King TP, Lu G. Hornet venom allergen antigen 5, Dol m 5: Its T-cell epitopes in mice and its antigenic cross-reactivity with a mammalian testis protein. *J Allergy Clin Immunol* 1997; 99(5): 630–639.

50. van Neerven RJ, Ebner C, Yssel H, Kapsenberg ML, Lamb JR. T-cell responses to allergens: Epitope-specificity and clinical relevance. *Immunol Today* 1996; 17(11): 526–532.

51. Negi SS, Braun W. Cross-react: A new structural bioinformatics method for predicting allergen cross-reactivity. *Bioinformatics* 2017; 33(7): 1014–1020.

52. Perez-Riverol A, Fernandes LGR, Musacchio LA et al. Phospholipase A1-based cross-reactivity among venoms of clinically relevant Hymenoptera from neotropical and temperate regions. *Mol Immunol* 2018; 93: 87–93.

53. Skov LK, Seppala U, Coen JJ et al. Structure of recombinant Ves v 2 at 2.0 Angstrom resolution: Structural analysis of an allergenic hyaluronidase from wasp venom. *Acta Crystallogr D Biol Crystallogr* 2006; 62(Pt 6): 595–604.

54. Jin C, Focke M, Leonard R, Jarisch R, Altmann F, Hemmer W. Reassessing the role of hyaluronidase in yellow jacket venom allergy. *J Allergy Clin Immunol* 2010; 125(1): 184–190.

55. Fromberg J. IgE as a marker in allergy and the role of IgE affinity. *Allergy* 2006; 61(10): 1234.

56. Eberlein B, Krischan L, Darsow U, Ollert M, Ring J. Double positivity to bee and wasp venom: Improved diagnostic procedure by recombinant allergen-based IgE testing and basophil activation test including data about cross-reactive carbohydrate determinants. *J Allergy Clin Immunol* 2012; 130(1): 155–161.

57. van Ree R. Carbohydrate epitopes and their relevance for the diagnosis and treatment of allergic diseases. *Int Arch Allergy Immunol* 2002; 129(3): 189–197.

58. Zora JA, Swanson MC, Yunginger JW. A study of the prevalence and clinical significance of venom-specific IgE. *J Allergy Clin Immunol* 1988; 81(1): 77–82.

59. Settipane GA, Chafee FH, Klein DE, Boyd GK, Sturam JH, Freye HB. Anaphylactic reactions to Hymenoptera stings in asthmatic patients. *Clin Allergy* 1980; 10(6): 659–665.

60. Dos Santos-Pinto JRA, Perez-Riverol A, Lasa AM, Palma MS. Diversity of peptidic and proteinaceous toxins from social Hymenoptera venoms. *Toxicon* 2018; 148: 172–196.

61. Habermann E. Bee and wasp venoms. *Science* 1972; 177(4046): 314–322.

62. Lee VS, Tu WC, Jinn TR, Peng CC, Lin LJ, Tzen JT. Molecular cloning of the precursor polypeptide of mastoparan B and its putative processing enzyme, dipeptidyl peptidase IV, from the black-bellied hornet, *Vespa basalis. Insect Mol Biol* 2007; 16(2): 231–237.

63. Ho CL, Lin YL, Chen WC et al. Immunogenicity of mastoparan B, a cationic tetradecapeptide isolated from the hornet (*Vespa basalis*) venom, and its structural requirements. *Toxicon* 1995; 33(11): 1443–1451.

64. King TP, Kochoumian L, Joslyn A. Melittin-specific monoclonal and polyclonal IgE and IgG1 antibodies from mice. *J Immunol* 1984; 133(5): 2668–2673.

65. King TP, Jim SY, Wittkowski KM. Inflammatory role of two venom components of yellow jackets (*Vespula vulgaris*): A mast cell degranulating peptide mastoparan and phospholipase A1. *Int Arch Allergy Immunol* 2003; 131(1): 25–32.

66. Liu Z, Chen S, Zhou Y et al. Deciphering the venomic transcriptome of killer-wasp *Vespa velutina. Sci Rep* 2015; 5: 9454.

67. King TP, Wittkowski KM. Hyaluronidase and hyaluronan in insect venom allergy. *Int Arch Allergy Immunol* 2011; 156(2): 205–211.

68. Dudler T, Chen WQ, Wang S et al. High-level expression in *Escherichia coli* and rapid purification of enzymatically active honey bee venom phospholipase A2. *Biochim Biophys Acta* 1992; 1165(2): 201–210.

69. Perez-Riverol A, Lasa AM, Dos Santos-Pinto JRA, Palma MS. Insect venom phospholipases A1 and A2: Roles in the envenoming process and allergy. *Insect Biochem Mol Biol* 2019; in press (DOI: 10.1016/j.ibmb.2018.12.011).

70. Wu TM, Chou TC, Ding YA, Li ML. Stimulation of TNF-α, IL-1β and nitrite release from mouse cultured spleen cells and lavaged peritoneal cells by mastoparan M. *Immunol Cell Biol* 1999; 77(6): 476–482.

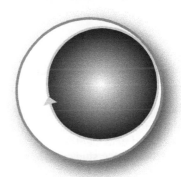

19 Biting insect and tick allergens

Donald R. Hoffman
Brody School of Medicine at East Carolina University

Jennifer E. Fergeson
University of South Florida Morsani College of Medicine

CONTENTS

19.1 INTRODUCTION

Allergic reactions to insect bites are much less common than reactions to insect stings. Several older studies suggest that severe bite reactions occur about 50 times less commonly than severe sting reactions [1]. Many of the clinical aspects of biting insect allergy are thoroughly discussed in a 2003 review [1]. The main focus of this chapter is on which insects are important, the known allergens and salivary components, and the appropriate use of immunotherapy. There are more than 14,000 species from 400 genera of blood-feeding arthropods. The most important hematophagous insects belong to the orders Diptera (flies), Hemiptera (bugs), and Siphonaptera (fleas). Ticks of the order Acarina of the class Arachnida will also be considered, although they are not insects. Some beetles of the order Coleoptera, especially aquatic species, occasionally bite man, but allergic reactions have not been reported. In addition, many insect larval forms may bite, but again allergic reactions to these bites are extremely rare. Rare allergic reactions to bites have been ascribed to bites of spiders and other arachnids, but definitive evidence is lacking of IgE antibodies against spider proteins. Allergic reactions also have been reported from myriapod bites, such as those from centipedes and millipedes, but there are no reported published data identifying the responsible proteins [1–5].

Many of the studies of biting insect allergens predate the era of genomics and proteomics, and many of the allergens have not been completely identified. In this chapter, definitely identified allergens are noted. Many of the specific proteins described are probably allergens.

19.2 TAXONOMY OF BITING INSECTS AND TICKS

19.2.1 Diptera, flies

Many flies are hematophagous. In almost all cases, only the females bite, requiring a blood meal to develop eggs. The more common biting flies are outlined in Table 19.1. A blackfly, deerfly, and horsefly are illustrated in Figures 19.1 through 19.3.

19.2.2 Hemiptera, bugs

There are two important families of biting bugs in North America. The first are variously called kissing bugs, assassin bugs, conenose bugs, vinchucas, or reduviid bugs and are members of the family Reduviidae. There are 39 genera of which the most important in North America are *Triatoma* (Figure 19.4) and *Reduvius*. The genera *Rhodnius* and *Panstrongylus* are important members of this family in South America. The second family of bloodsucking bugs is Cimicidae or bedbugs. There are seven genera, and the species *Cimex lectularius* is the most infamous human bedbug.

19.2.3 Siphonaptera, fleas

The fleas are almost all parasitic insects, with 74% of species associated with rodent hosts and about 6% with avian hosts.

Table 19.1 Biting flies (Diptera)

Common name	Family	Genera
Biting midge	Ceratopogonidae	*Culicoides*, others
Blackfly	Simuliidae	*Simulium, Prosimulium, Cnephia*
Bot and Warble flies	Oestridae	*Dermatobia*, others
Deer fly, Yellow fly	Tabanidae	*Chrysops*
Horse fly	Tabanidae	*Tabanus, Hybomitra*
Mosquito	Culicidae	*Aedes, Culex, Anopheles*, others
Sand fly	Psychodidae (Phlebotominae)	*Lutzomyia, Phlebotomus*
Stable fly	Muscidae	*Stomoxys, Haematobia*
Tsetse fly	Glossinidae (Muscidae)	*Glossina*

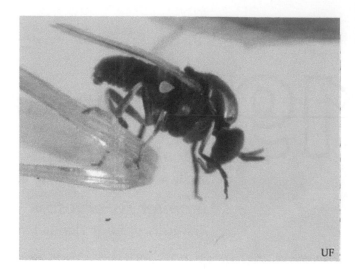

Figure 19.1 A blackfly, *Simulium*; note the humped appearance. (Courtesy of Jerry F. Butler, University of Florida.)

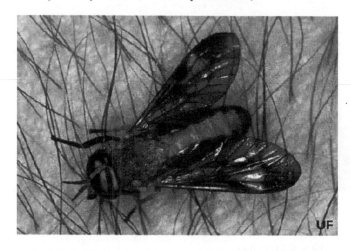

Figure 19.2 A deerfly, *Chrysops*, in biting position. The insect is usually yellow or green, and the bite is painful. (Courtesy of Jerry F. Butler, University of Florida.)

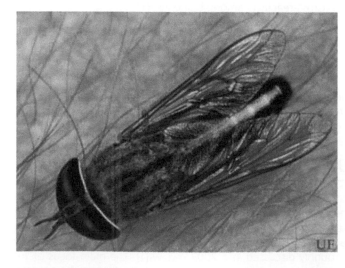

Figure 19.3 A horsefly, *Tabanus*, biting. Horseflies are typically larger than deerflies, have very noisy flight, and the bites are quite painful. (Courtesy of Jerry F. Butler, University of Florida.)

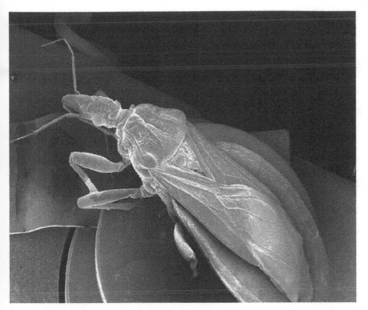

Figure 19.4 Scanning electron micrograph of a kissing bug, *Triatoma protracta*. Bites are painless, typically occurring while sleeping. The insect's definitive host is the wood rat. (Courtesy of C. Demetry and R. Biderman, Worcester Polytechnic Institute.)

The species associated with man are members of the superfamily Pulicoidea, family Pulicidae. The most common are the dog and cat fleas, *Ctenocephalides canis* and *Ctenocephalides felis felis*. *Pulex irritans*, a parasite of carnivores, is sometimes called the human flea. Fleas of the genus *Tunga* are found in Central and South America.

19.2.4 Arachnids

Many species of hard and soft ticks and chiggers bite man. Allergic reactions to these bites are extremely rare, although they are reported [6–9] from many regions.

19.3 IDENTIFYING BITING INSECTS

The identification of a biting insect can be extremely difficult, even with representative specimens. Deerflies, horseflies (see Figure 19.1), and stable flies all cause immediate pain when they bite. Mosquitoes can usually be recognized, but identification of species may require an expert. Identification of flea species is also in the realm of specialists. Kissing bugs typically bite painlessly, most commonly while the victim is sleeping. Useful identification guides with many illustrations are available for hobbyists including Borror and White's *A Field Guide to the Insects*, and the National Audubon Society Field Guides. The much more technical and comprehensive reference *Insects of North America* by Arnett [10] is recommended for those with a serious interest. Keys to various groups are available in the entomology literature and vary widely in quality and usability. Most states employ entomologists, usually within a Department of Agriculture, who can assist with insect identification. There are also entomologists who are willing to assist with insect identification at many land grant universities.

19.4 GEOGRAPHIC DISTRIBUTION OF SOME BITING INSECTS AND TICKS

Mosquitoes are cosmopolitan with species found in almost all land areas of the world. Fleas are found in most areas of the world, except in very dry climates. Blackflies occur in the northern United States and in most of Canada, much of northern and central Europe and Asia; in tropical areas they require the presence of rapidly running water to breed. Horseflies and deerflies are common in most temperate areas of the world. Tsetse flies are only found in tropical Africa and a few laboratories in the United States and Europe. Sand flies and biting midges are also found in many areas, especially around beaches and livestock.

Ticks are found around wooded areas and are commonly carried by dogs, birds, and deer. Various species are distributed in different areas of the world.

Although bugs of the reduviid group are found in many areas, almost all cases of allergic reactions to bites occur in the southwestern United States, Hawaii, Mexico, and Central America. These insects are dependent on the distribution of their hosts, for example, the wood rat in California for *Triatoma protracta*. Other species feed on dogs, cats, mice, opossums, and armadillos.

19.5 SALIVARY COMPONENTS AND ALLERGENS OF BITING INSECTS AND TICKS

The characterization of allergens from saliva of biting insects is very limited; those studies where allergens have been identified typically show that some of the major salivary proteins are allergens. According to Ribeiro, blood feeding evolved independently multiple times among hematophagous arthropods [11]. A variety of anticlotting factors, platelet aggregation antagonists, and vasodilators developed to counter the host's hemostatic and immunomodulatory factors [12]. In addition, arthropod saliva contains digestive enzymes [13] and hyaluronidase. One unsuspected property of some insect saliva is enhancement of infectivity of parasites carried by arthropod vectors [14]. Sand fly saliva decreases the minimum effective dose of *Leishmania major* in mice by several orders of magnitude. In a 2012 review, Mecheri proposed that innate and specific immune responses to *Anopheles* salivary components are important in the pathogenesis of malaria [15]. He provides evidence for the importance of both pro-inflammatory mediators from mast cells and the antigen-specific IgE-mediated response. In 2002 the first complete genome sequence of a biting insect, the malaria mosquito, *Anopheles gambiae*, became available [16]. The set of proteins expressed by the salivary glands has been named the *sialome* by Ribeiro and are mapped for mosquitoes, kissing bugs, and ticks [17–20].

19.5.1 Mosquito

Some of the characterized protein components of mosquito saliva are described in Table 19.2. A number of the proteins appear to be related to either digestive functions, such as maltase, amylase, and esterase, or inhibition of hemostasis, such as tachykinin, factor Xa inhibitor, purine nucleosidase, and apyrase, which is the enzyme

Table 19.2 Selected protein components and known allergens in *Aedes aegypti* mosquito saliva identified by two-dimensional electrophoresis followed by trypsin digestion and mass spectrometry, and also by cDNA expression

Component	GenBank identifier (gi)
Protein D7 (Aed a 2)	159556
Protein D7 (Aed a 3)	2114496
Antigen 5 like protein	18568284
Apyrase (Aed a 1)	556271
Maltase (α-glucosidase) (Aed a 4)	159566
Purine nucleosidase	21654712
Protein disulfide isomerase	94468800
Heat shock protein 70 kDa	94468818
Adenosine triphosphate phosphatase	
Beta unit	94468834
Alpha unit	94468442
Angiopoietin-like protein	1858298
Salivary serpin 1	18568304
Salivary serpin 2	94469320
62 kDa proteins	18568300, 18568302
Amylase	2190949
Adenosine deaminase	18568326
C-type lectins	94468370, 18568318
34 kDa protein 1	94468642
34 kDa protein 2	18568296
Angiopoietin-like protein 2	94468352
30.5 kDa salivary protein	61742033
30 kDa salivary antigen	18568322

Sources: Ribeiro JMC et al. *BMC Genomics* 2007; 8: 6; Peng Z, Simon FER. *Curr Opin Allergy Clin Immunol* 2007; 7: 36–364.

Table 19.3 Molecular weights of IgE-binding components in mosquito extracts from various species

Major allergens[a]				
Aedes aegypti	*Aedes vexans*	*Aedes communis*	*Culex tarsalis*	*Culiseta inornata*
65 kDa	65	36	43	65
48	43	30	17	40
34[b]	38	22	15	34
31				
15				

Note: Allergens have not been purified; data mainly from immunoblot experiments, some, e.g., D7, have been cloned or expressed.
[a] Minor allergens shared by at least three species: 160, 110, 65, 62, 50, 46, 40, 32.5, 24, 17, 15 kDa.
[b] 34 kDa is D7 protein, Aed a 2.

bands are definitively characterized. A 2004 study [22] reported on 14 individuals with acute systemic reactions to mosquito bites; all showed IgE antibodies specific to saliva from at least one of the five species tested.

Cutaneous reactions from mosquito bites may be immediate or delayed, with the former being the most common. Immediate reactions occur within 20–30 minutes following a bite, and delayed reactions occur within 24–36 hours. Lesions typically range between 2 and 10 mm in diameter with surrounding erythema. Some individuals may experience large local reactions characterized by swelling and erythema of about 3 cm or more. This type of reaction is uncommon with one study reporting an incidence of 2.5% [24]. Skeeter syndrome is described as a delayed large local reaction accompanied by fever [25]. Lesions are intensely erythematous, swollen, and painful and may be difficult to differentiate from a bacterial infection of the skin. Anaphylactic reactions from mosquito bites are rare [22]. Some patients with primary or secondary immune deficiencies or hematologic malignancies have severe reactions to insect bites [26].

19.5.2 Blackflies

There are over 18,000 species of *Simulium,* blackflies, identified worldwide. This species is also referred to as the bloodsucking blackfly due to the large amount of bleeding that can occur at the site of the bite. Studies on the saliva of blackflies are limited. Anticoagulation factors against thrombin in blackfly saliva may account for this abnormality in hemostasis [30,31]. Cupp et al. isolated and cloned a major protein of molecular weight 15.35 kDa with strong vasodilator activity manifested by rapid and persistent induction of erythema [31]. The enzyme apyrase is found in blackfly salivary gland secretions. Wirtz demonstrated easily measurable amounts of histamine, putrescine, spermine, *N*-monoacetyl-spermine and spermidine, as well as the presence of proteins with esterase activity in salivary gland secretion [32]. Almost all reactions to blackfly bites are not IgE mediated, and the dermatologic reactions are classified into six forms by Farkas [33]. These include edematous, erythematous-edematous, erysipeloid, inflammatory-indurative, hemorrhagic (plaques, nodules, or vesicles), and allergic.

adenosine triphosphate diphosphohydrolase that inhibits adenosine diphosphate dependent platelet aggregation. Sensory proteins are also important including the protein D7 family, which contains two insect pheromone/odorant binding protein domains and is expressed in a number of different sizes [18,21].

There are numerous published studies of IgE binding components of various mosquito extracts. Some are performed with "saliva," some with salivary gland extract, some with thorax extract, and some with whole-body extract. Numerous species and at least four genera have been investigated. Table 19.3 is a compendium of the major and shared allergens in immunoblot experiments for 5 species and 13 species, respectively [23,27–29]. D7 proteins are important allergens in *Aedes, Culex,* and related mosquitoes, and apyrase is also a significant allergen. None of the other IgE binding

19.5.3 Horseflies and deerflies

Deerfly saliva contains chrysoptin, an inhibitor of ADP-induced platelet aggregation, that interferes with fibrinogen binding to the glycoprotein IIb/IIIa receptor on platelets [34]. The recombinant protein with a molecular mass of 65 kDa, the same as that of the natural protein, is expressed in insect cells. This may be a protein similar to the 69 kDa IgE binding protein found in immunoblots using sera from European patients who experienced anaphylaxis from *Chrysops* bites [35]. In studies of allergic reactions to the Asian horsefly, *Tabanus yao*, three allergens are described, an apyrase, an antigen 5–related protein, and a hyaluronidase [36,37].

19.5.4 Sand flies

Sand fly saliva contains a factor that enhances the infectivity of *Leishmania* by inhibiting the capacity of interferon-γ to activate macrophages. It also reduces nitric oxide production. A delayed-type hypersensitivity reaction to saliva components also may play a role in infectivity and adverse reactions [38,39]. Sand fly saliva contains a potent vasodilator, maxadilan. Other proteins include apyrase, 5′-nucleotidase, and hyaluronidase as well as an anticlotting protein with a carbohydrate-recognition domain and several proteins of unknown function.

19.5.5 Kissing bugs and bedbugs

The major salivary anticoagulant proteins of *Rhodnius prolixus* are called prolixins and consist of four related nitrophorin molecules [40], which are heme proteins that carry nitric oxide. The major component has a molecular weight of 19.69 kDa and inhibits factor VIII–mediated activation of factor X. Two proteins are characterized from the saliva of *Triatoma pallipidipennis,* triabin of 15.62 kDa, an inhibitor of thrombin-based hydrolysis of fibrinogen [41], and pallidipin of 19 kDa, an inhibitor of collagen-induced platelet aggregation [42]. Functional studies of coagulation inhibition suggest that different species of Triatominae have functionally different mechanisms of coagulation inhibition and different sodium dodecyl sulfate polyacrylamide gel electrophoresis (SDS-PAGE) profiles of salivary proteins [43,46]. These proteins, along with proteins having histamine binding, platelet inhibition, anticoagulation, and nitric oxide transport activities, are all members of the lipocalin family [44]. The three-dimensional structures of the nitrophorins NP1, 2, and 4 have been determined by x-ray crystallography. Many important vertebrate-derived allergens are also members of the lipocalin family. An activatable serine protease of 40 kDa named *triapsin*, with an arginine specificity, has been isolated from saliva of *Triatoma infestans* [45].

The major allergenic proteins of *Triatoma protracta* are of 18–20 kDa, and almost all the allergenic activity is found between isoelectric points (pI) 6.7–7.3 and 8.2 [46]. An allergen, a member of the lipocalin family named *procalin*, has been identified, cloned, and expressed in yeast cells [47]. The recombinant procalin reacts in enzyme-linked immunosorbent assay (ELISA) assays with IgE antibodies from allergic patients and cross-reacts with native allergens. Immunohistochemistry with antiserum against procalin localizes procalin to the cytoplasm of cuboidal epithelium and the luminal contents of the salivary glands.

The saliva of the bedbug, *Cimex lectularius*, contains a nitrophorin [48] and is also an inhibitor of the activation of factor X to factor Xa, which does not directly inhibit factor VIII [49]. The apparent molecular weight of this factor is 17 kDa. Bedbug saliva also contains apyrase.

19.5.6 Fleas

Very little work has been done applying contemporary methods to studies of flea saliva. The only characterized proteins in flea saliva are apyrase, which prevents adenosine diphosphate (ADP)–induced platelet aggregation [50], platelet-activating factor acetylhydrolase, and naphthyl esterases.

Diagnostic studies of allergy to flea bites in humans performed by testing with whole-body extracts are complicated by the relatively more common occurrence of inhalant allergy to cat fleas. The major salivary allergen of cat fleas causing allergy in dogs is a protein of 18 kDa and pI 9.3, Cte f 1 [51].

19.5.7 Ticks

There is a great deal of interest in ticks with the recognition of Lyme disease and ehrlichiosis. Allergic reactions to tick bites are usually the result of bites by soft ticks, Ixodiae. Pigeon ticks, *Argas reflexus,* as well as deer ticks and paralysis ticks can cause systemic allergic reactions. Tick salivas contain apyrase and antiplatelet activities [20,52] as well as numerous proteins from 18 to 355 kDa. Several proteins of 15–50 kDa are induced by blood feeding [53].

Five salivary allergens have been isolated from the Australian paralysis tick, *Ixodes holocyclus,* of molecular weights 28, 45, 50, 55, and 355 kDa [54]. The allergens at 28 and 355 kDa react with IgE from most allergic patients, and the protein at 28 kDa (SGA1) is useful for skin prick testing and radioimmunoassay [55].

Soon after cetuximab, a monoclonal antibody, was introduced as an antineoplastic agent, a substantial number of patients experienced anaphylactic reactions on the first administration. The incidence of reactivity was much greater in patients from the southeastern and southcentral United States. Population studies screening for the presence of preformed antibody confirmed the geographical distribution. The specificity of the IgE antibody is against galactose-α-1,3-galactose found in the carbohydrate on the heavy chain of the monoclonal antibody [56]. An IgE antibody of similar specificity occurs in patients who experience anaphylaxis to red meat and gelatin [57,58]. There is significant, although not definitive, evidence that at least some of this presensitization is caused by bites of ticks of the species *Amblyomma americanum* (lone star tick) [59].

19.6 CROSS-REACTIVITY AMONG BITING INSECTS

There are very limited experimental data on IgE cross-reactivity among biting insects. There are some common antigens exhibiting a limited degree of cross-reactivity among mosquito genera and species [23,27,28]. However, typical clinical reactions, including nonallergic responses, are species dependent for most individuals. There may be some cross-reactivity, based on *in vitro* specific IgE testing between horse- and deerflies and sometimes also blackflies [1]. The clinical relevance of this cross-reactivity is unknown. There are antigen-5 related proteins and hyaluronidases in insect saliva [18,37], which could be cross-reactive with vespid venom proteins. There may also be IgE antibodies against fucose-containing cross-reactive carbohydrate determinants (CCD) and galactose-α-1,3-galactose [59].

Allergic reactions to kissing bugs and bedbugs exhibit a strong species dependence, and patients rarely are either skin test positive or *in vitro* specific IgE positive to more than a single species [60].

There are no data on cross-reactivity with fleas in human subjects, but studies with flea-allergic dogs suggest species specificity. Reactions to sand flies, biting midges, ticks, tsetse flies, and other biting arthropods are probably species specific, but experimental data are lacking.

19.7 BITING INSECT CONTROL

The control of biting insects is difficult, as demonstrated by attempts at mosquito vector control in the tropical world. Use of most pesticides, especially large-area spraying, is best left to public health authorities. Spraying of yards usually is not recommended, as this is almost always of limited value and may involve significant risk of pesticide exposure to children and pets.

Control of biting insects in the home should emphasize avoidance. Screens should be used on all doors and windows. Various forms of flypaper traps, with and without attractants, are effective and environmentally friendly. One highly recommended type is clear and is placed on glass doors and windows; another uses 7-W light bulbs. Control of fleas from pets, particularly in warm and humid areas, can be difficult. Veterinarians can recommend several programs, including the use of growth regulators that are fed to dogs and cats to prevent development of adult fleas and substances that are spotted onto the animal and absorbed through the skin or others that are injected. The most effective agent at the present is oral spinosad. The extensive use of conventional antiacetyl cholinesterase pesticides is ineffective and leads to development of resistant fleas. Animals should be regularly washed and carpets and furniture regularly vacuumed to help control fleas.

Bedbug infestations should be eliminated by treatment with appropriate pesticides, preferably by a licensed professional. Reduviid bugs are primarily outdoor insects and are best controlled by eliminating their definitive hosts around houses. *Triatoma protracta* comes from wood rat nests, but other species have varied hosts. Professional assistance is recommended.

Horseflies, deerflies, and blackflies occur primarily around water. They can be extremely difficult to avoid in these areas. The almost ubiquitous mosquito is extremely difficult to avoid. Repellants containing DEET (*N,N'*-diethyl-*m*-toluamide) are the "gold standard" due to broad coverage against various arthropods and duration of efficacy compared to other repellants. Products containing DEET should not be used in infants under 3 months of age due to potential toxicity. Insect repellants containing 10% to 30% DEET are considered safe and effective for infants and older children [62–65]. Covering up as much skin as possible and avoiding outdoor activities at high-risk times, particularly early morning and evening, can help. Avoidance of areas of high mosquito density is recommended. Sources of standing water should be minimized or eliminated. Mosquito netting and the use of citronella candles can also reduce mosquito density. An ultraviolet bug light can also help, particularly

after dark. Both electrocuting and trap models are available. Use of yellow or orange light bulbs outdoors minimizes the attraction of insects to porches and garage. The Centers for Disease Control and Prevention (https:// www.cdc.gov) is an excellent resource for clinicians and patients to refer to for information on protection against mosquitoes, ticks, and other arthropods.

19.8 ALLERGEN IMMUNOTHERAPY

19.8.1 Evidence for efficacy

There is very limited controlled study evidence for the efficacy of allergen immunotherapy in preventing life-threatening systemic allergic reactions to insect bites. There are a significant number of anecdotal reports, most of which describe treatment of variants of large local reactions by subcutaneous immunotherapy. The only challenge-verified trial with an insect salivary-gland derived vaccine was reported in an uncontrolled study with *Triatoma protracta* in 1984 [61]. Subcutaneous immunotherapy provided protection in all five treated patients without significant side effects. Immunologic changes also were observed in parallel with protection as assessed by bite challenge.

A report of treatment with deerfly whole-body vaccine, although not controlled, suggests efficacy for patients with systemic allergic reactions [66]. Subcutaneous immunotherapy with whole-body extracts has been tried in cases of life-threatening allergy to mosquito bites [67]. Results have been mixed with some patients developing the ability to tolerate a larger number of bites and others developing major complications as described later.

It should be noted that in the United States and most other countries, there are no licensed extracts of insect saliva or salivary glands and that most whole-body extracts from biting insects are not approved for use in allergen vaccine therapy. These products should only be used under an investigational new drug (IND) application, as part of a controlled study. One study demonstrated that it is possible to prepare substantially more potent vaccines from biting insects than are available in current commercial products [68]. In some countries, special unlicensed products are prepared for individual patients.

Most cases of severe allergy to mosquito bites are best managed by prophylactic use of the antihistamines. In controlled trials, cetirizine reduced pruritus, significantly decreased large local reactions, and probably reduced the incidence of systemic allergic reactions. Loratadine used prophylactically in children reduced immediate whealing and pruritus from mosquito bites; and it also reduced the size of bite lesions at 24 hours [69–70,72].

19.8.2 Known risks

Rush subcutaneous immunotherapy with mosquito whole-body vaccine has caused local pain, swelling, and redness in a patient who tolerated injections at lower concentrations. Another patient, in the same report, developed arthralgias, fatigue, myalgias, weakness, and swelling of distal extremities, despite treatment with terfenadine, cimetidine, and prednisone during two attempts at rush therapy [67]. Life-threatening anaphylaxis has occurred in studies of experimental vaccines derived from mosquito cell tissue culture [71].

The use of other biting insect vaccines has not been reported to cause unusual reactions, and the experiences reported in the literature correspond to those seen with other allergens routinely used in allergen vaccine therapy.

19.8.3 Potential risks

The existence of species and genus specificity for many biting insect reactions requires the use of more sophisticated diagnostic reagents than are commercially available. There is a risk of using an ineffective preparation and a potential risk of sensitization. Also, many hematophagous insects are vectors for serious diseases (parasitic, viral, rickettsial, and bacterial). Extracts prepared from insect salivary glands must be carefully monitored to be free of infectious agents. The use of biting insect extracts in allergen vaccine therapy is an experimental procedure, and proper safety procedures and regulations are necessary.

SALIENT POINTS

1. There are a large variety of hematophagous insects and arachnids.
2. Many different arthropods can cause bite allergy.
3. Much, if not most, insect bite allergy may be species and/or genus specific.
4. Insect saliva varies widely, but most species contain potent anticoagulants and digestive enzymes.
5. The best diagnostic reagents are insect saliva or salivary gland extract, but none are commercially available or licensed in the United States or in Europe.
6. Subcutaneous immunotherapy is effective to treat systemic allergic reactions to *Triatoma protracta*, deerflies, and mosquitoes in uncontrolled studies.
7. Subcutaneous immunotherapy with mosquito whole-body vaccine is associated with significant side effects.
8. Allergen immunotherapy with biting insect whole-body, salivary gland, and saliva extracts is experimental.
9. Control of many biting insects is difficult, but risk of exposure to bites can be greatly reduced.
10. Reactions to mosquito bites are best managed by prophylaxis with an oral antihistamine.

REFERENCES

1. Hoffman DR. Allergic reactions to biting insects. In: Levine MI, Lockey RF, editors. *Monograph on Insect Allergy*. 4th ed. Milwaukee, WI: American Academy of Allergy, Asthma and Immunology. 2003: 161–173.
2. Singh S, Mann BK. Insect bite reactions. *Indian J Dermatol Venereol Leprol*. 2013; 79: 151–164.
3. Juckett G. Arthropod bites. *Am Fam Physician*. 2013; 88: 841–847.
4. Lee H, Halverson S, Mackey R. Insect allergy. *Prim Care* 2016; 43: 417–431.
5. Golden DB, Demain J, Freeman T et al. Stinging insect hypersensitivity: A practice parameter update 2016. *Ann Allergy Asthma Immunol* 2017; 118: 28–54.
6. Van Nunen SA. Tick-induced allergies: Mammalian meat allergy and tick anaphylaxis. *Med J Aust* 2018; 208: 316–321.
7. Khoury JK, Khoury NC, Schaefer D et al. A tick-acquired red meat allergy. *Am J Emerg Med* 2018; 36: 341.e1–341.e3.
8. Van Wye JE, Hsu Y-P, Lane RS et al. IgE antibodies in tick bite induced anaphylaxis. *J Allergy Clin Immunol* 1991; 88: 968–970.
9. Gauci M, Loh RKS, Stone BF et al. Allergic reactions to the Australian paralysis tick, *Ixodes holocyclus*. Diagnostic evaluation by skin test and radioimmunoassay. *Clin Exp Allergy* 1989; 74: 279–283.
10. Arnett RH. *American Insects*. New York, NY: Van Nostrand Reinhold, 1985.
11. Ribeiro JM. Blood-feeding arthropods: Live syringes or invertebrate pharmacologists? *Infect Agents Dis* 1995; 3: 143–152.
12. Tabachnik WJ. Pharmacological factors in the saliva of blood-feeding insects. *Ann NY Acad Sci* 2000; 916: 444–452.
13. Kerlin RL, Hughes S. Enzymes in saliva from four parasitic arthropods. *Med Vet Entomol* 1992; 6: 121–126.
14. Theodos CM, Ribeiro JM, Titus RG. Analysis of enhancing effect of sand fly saliva on *Leishmania* infection in mice. *Infect Immun* 1991; 59: 1592–1598.
15. Mecheri S. Contribution of allergic inflammatory response to the pathogenesis of malaria disease. *Biochim Biophys Acta* 2012; 1822: 49–56.
16. Holt RA, Subramanian GM, Halpern A et al. The genome sequence of the malaria mosquito *Anopheles gambiae*. *Science* 2002; 298: 129–149.
17. Cantillo JF, Puera L, Puchalska P et al. Allergenome characterization of the mosquito *Aedes aegypti*. *Allergy* 2017; 72: 1499–1509.
18. Ribeiro JMC, Arca B, Lombardo F et al. An annotated catalogue of salivary gland transcripts in the adult female mosquito, *Aedes aegypti*. *BMC Genomics* 2007; 8: 6.
19. Ribeiro JMC, Anderson J, Silva-Neto MAC et al. Exploring the sialome of the blood-sucking bug, *Rhodnius prolixus*. *Insect Biochem Molec Biol* 2004; 34: 61–79.
20. Valenzuela JG, Francischetti IM, Pham VM et al. Exploring the sialome of the tick *Ixodes scapularis*. *J Exp Biol* 2002; 205: 2843–2864.
21. James AA, Blackmer K, Marinotti O et al. Isolation and characterization of the gene expressing the major salivary gland protein of the female mosquito, *Aedes aegypti*. *Mol Biochem Parasitol* 1991; 44: 245–253.
22. Peng Z, Beckett AN, Engler RJ et al. Immune responses to mosquito saliva in 14 individuals with systemic allergic reactions to mosquito bites. *J Allergy Clin Immunol* 2004; 114: 1189–1194.
23. Peng Z, Li HB, Simon FER. Immunoblot analysis of IgE and IgG binding antigens in extracts of mosquitos *Aedes vexans*, *Culex tarsalis* and *Culiseta inornata*. *Int Arch Allergy Immunol* 1996; 110: 46–51.
24. Crisp H, Johnson K. Mosquito allergy. *Ann Allergy Asthma Immunol* 2013; 110: 65–69.
25. Simons FER, Peng Z. Skeeter syndrome. *J Allergy Clin Immunol* 1999; 104: 705–707.
26. Orange J, Song L, Twarog F, Schneider L. A patient with severe black fly (Simullidae) hypersensitivity referred for evaluation of suspect immunodeficiency. *Ann Allergy Asthma Immunol* 2004; 92: 76–80.
27. Li H, Simons FER, Peng Z. Immunoblot analysis of salivary allergens in 10 mosquito species with worldwide distribution and the human IgE responses to these allergens. *J Allergy Clin Immunol* 1998; 101: 498–505.
28. Peng Z, Simons FE. Cross-reactivity of skin and serum specific IgE responses and allergen analysis for three mosquito species with worldwide distribution. *J Allergy Clin Immunol* 1997; 100: 192–198.

29. Brummer-Korvenkonito H, Palusuo T, Francois G et al. Characterization of *Aedes communis, Aedes aegypti* and *Anopheles stephensi* mosquito saliva antigens by immunoblotting. *Int Arch Allergy Immunol* 1997; 112: 169–174.

30. Cupp MS, Ribeiro JM, Cupp EW. Vasodilative activity in black fly salivary glands. *Amer J Trop Med Hyg* 1994; 50: 241–246.

31. Cupp MS, Ribeiro JMC, Champagne DE et al. Analyses of cDNA and recombinant protein for a potent vasoactive protein in saliva of a blood-feeding fly, *Simulium vittatum*. *J Exp Biol* 1998; 201: 1553–1561.

32. Wirtz HP. Bioamines and proteins in the saliva and salivary glands of palaearctic blackflies (Diptera: Simuliidae). *Trop Med Parasitol* 1990; 41: 59–64.

33. Farkas J. Simuliosis. Analysis of dermatological manifestations following blackfly (Simuliidae) bites as observed in the years 1981–1983 in Bratislava (Czechoslovakia). *Derm Beruf Umwelt* 1984; 32: 171–173.

34. Reddy VB, Kounga K, Mariano F et al. Chrysoptin is a potent glycoprotein IIb/IIIa fibrinogen receptor antagonist present in salivary gland extracts of the deerfly. *J Biol Chem* 2000; 275: 15861–15867.

35. Hemmer W, Focke M, Vieluf D et al. Anaphylaxis induced by horsefly bites: Identification of a 69kd IgE-binding salivary gland protein from *Chrysops* spp. (Diptera, Tabanidae) by western blot analysis. *J Allergy Clin Immunol* 1998; 101: 134–136.

36. An S, Ma D, Wei JF et al. A novel allergen Tab y 1 with inhibitory activity of platelet aggregation from salivary glands of horseflies. *Allergy* 2011; 66: 1420–1427.

37. Ma D, Li Y, Dong J et al. Purification and characterization of two new allergens from the salivary glands of the horsefly, *Tabanus yao*. *Allergy* 2011; 66: 101–109.

38. Hall LR, Titus RG. Sand fly vector saliva selectively modulates macrophage functions that inhibit killing of *Leishmania major* and nitric oxide production. *J Immunol* 1995; 155: 3501–3506.

39. Belkaid Y, Valenzuela JG, Kamhawi S et al. Delayed-type hypersensitivity to *Phlebotomus papatasi* sand fly bite: An adaptive response induced by the fly? *Proc Natl Acad Sci USA* 2000; 97: 6704–6709.

40. Champagne DE, Nussenzveig RH, Ribeiro JM. Purification, partial characterization, and cloning of nitric oxide-carrying heme proteins (nitrophorins) from salivary glands of the blood sucking insect *Rhodnius prolixus*. *J Biol Chem* 1995; 270: 8691–8695.

41. Noeske-Jungblut C, Haendler B, Donner P et al. Triabin, a highly potent exosite inhibitor of thrombin. *J Biol Chem* 1995; 270: 28629–28634.

42. Haendler B, Becker A, Noeske-Jungblut C et al. Expression, purification and characterisation of recombinant pallidipin, a novel platelet aggregation inhibitor from the hematophageous triatome bug *Triatoma pallidipennis*. *Blood Coagul Fibrinolysis* 1996; 7: 183–186.

43. Pereira MH, Souza ME, Vargas AP et al. Anticoagulant activity of *Triatoma infestans* and *Panstrongylus megistus* saliva (Hemiptera/Triatominae). *Acta Trop* 1996; 61: 255–261.

44. Montfort WR, Weichsel A, Anderson JF. Nitrophorins and related antihemostatic lipocalins from *Rhodnius prolixus* and other blood-sucking arthropods. *Biochim Biophys Acta* 2000; 1482: 110–118.

45. Amino R, Tanaka AS, Schenkman S. Triapsin an unusual activatable serine protease from the saliva of the hematophagous vector of Chagas' disease *Triatoma infestans* (Hemiptera: Reduviidae). *Insect Biochem Mol Biol* 2001; 31: 465–472.

46. Chapman MD, Marshall NA, Saxon A. Identification and partial purification of species-specific allergens from *Triatoma protracta* (Heteroptera: Reduviidae). *J Allergy Clin Immunol* 1986; 78: 436–442.

47. Paddock CD, McKerrow JH, Hansell E et al. Identification, cloning and recombinant expression of procalin, a major triatomine allergen. *J Immunol* 2001; 167: 2694–2699.

48. Valenzuela JG, Walker FA, Ribeiro JM. A salivary nitrophorin (nitric-oxide-carrying hemoprotein) in the bedbug *Cimex lectularius*. *J Exp Biol* 1995; 198: 1519–1526.

49. Valenzuela JG, Guimaraes JA, Ribeiro JM. A novel inhibitor of factor X activation from the salivary glands of the bed bug *Cimex lectularius*. *Exper Parasit* 1996; 83: 184–190.

50. Ribeiro JM, Vaughn JA, Azad AF. Characterization of the salivary apyrase activity of three rodent flea species. *Comp Biochem Physiol B* 1990; 95: 215–219.

51. McDermott MJ, Weber E, Hunter S et al. Identification, cloning, and characterization of a major cat flea salivary allergen (Cte f 1). *Mol Immunol* 2000; 37: 361–375.

52. Ribeiro JM, Endris TM, Endris R. Saliva of the soft tick, *Ornithodoros moubata*, contains anti-platelet and apyrase activities. *Comp Biochem Physiol A* 1991; 100: 109–112.

53. Sanders ML, Scott AL, Glass GE et al. Salivary gland changes and host antibody responses associated with feeding of male lone star ticks (Acari: Ixodidae). *J Med Entomol* 1996; 33: 628–634.

54. Gauci M, Stone BF, Thong YH. Isolation and immunological characterization of allergens from salivary glands of the Australian paralysis tick *Ixodes holocyclus*. *Int Arch Allergy Appl Immunol* 1988; 87: 208–212.

55. Gauci M, Loh RKS, Stone BF et al. Evaluation of partially purified salivary gland allergens from the Australian paralysis tick, *Ixodes holocyclus* in diagnosis of allergy by RIA and skin prick test. *Ann Allergy* 1990; 64: 297–299.

56. Chung CH, Mirakhur B, Chan E et al. Cetuximab-induced anaphylaxis and IgE specific for galactose-α-1,3-galactose. *N Engl J Med* 2008; 358: 1109–1117.

57. Mullins RJ, James H, Platts-Mills TA et al. Relationship between red meat allergy and sensitization to gelation and galactose-α-1,3-galactose. *J Allerg Clin Immunol* 2012; 129: 1334–1342.

58. Carter MC, Ruiz-Esteves KN, Workman L, Lieberman P et al. Identification of α-gal sensitivity in patients with a diagnosis of idiopathic anaphylaxis. *Allergy* 2018; 73: 1131–1134.

59. Commins SP, James HR, Kelly LA et al. The relevance of tick bites to the production of IgE antibodies to the mammalian oligosaccharide galactose-α-1,3-galactose. *J Allerg Clin Immunol* 2011; 127: 1286–1293.

60. Marshall NA, Chapman MD, Saxon A. Species specific allergens from the salivary glands of Triatominae (Heteroptera: Reduviidae). *J Allergy Clin Immunol* 1986; 78: 430–435.

61. Rohr AS, Marshall NA, Saxon A. Successful immunotherapy for *Triatoma protracta*-induced anaphylaxis. *J Allergy Clin Immunol* 1984; 73: 369–375.

62. Fradin MS, Day JF. Comparative efficacy of insect repellents against mosquito bites. *N Engl J Med* 2002; 347: 13–18.

63. Katz TM, Miller JH, Hebert AA. Insect repellents: Historical perspectives and new developments. *J Am Acad Dermatol* 2008; 58: 865–871.

64. Koren G, Matsui D, Bailey B. DEET-based insect repellents: Safety implications for children and pregnant and lactating women. *CMAJ* 2003; 169: 209–212.

65. Diaz JH. Chemical and plant-based insect repellents: Efficacy, safety, and toxicity. *Wilderness Environ Med* 2016; 27: 153–163.

66. Wilbur RD, Evans R. An immunologic evaluation of deerfly hypersensitivity. *J Allergy Clin Immunol* 1975; 55: 72.

67. McCormack DR, Salata KF, Hershey JN et al. Mosquito bite anaphylaxis: Immunotherapy with whole body extracts. *Ann Allergy Asthma Immunol* 1995; 74: 39–44.

68. Peng ZK, Simon FER. Comparison of proteins, IgE and IgG binding antigens, and skin reactivity in commercial and laboratory-made mosquito extracts. *Ann Allergy Asthma Immunol* 1996; 77: 371–376.

69. Reunala T, Brummer-Korvenkontio H, Karppinen A et al. Treatment of mosquito bites with cetirizine. *Clin Exp Allergy* 1993; 23: 72–75.

70. Karppinen A, Kautianen H, Reunala T et al. Loratadine in the treatment of mosquito-bite-sensitive children. *Allergy* 2000; 55: 668–671.

71. Scott RM, Shelton AL, Eckels KH et al. Human hypersensitivity to a sham vaccine prepared from mosquito cell culture fluids. *J Allergy Clin Immunol* 1984; 74: 808–811.

72. Peng Z, Simons FER. Advances in mosquito allergy. *Curr Opinion Allerg Clin Immunol* 2007; 7: 360–364.

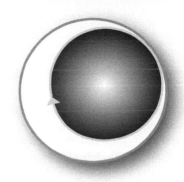

20 Occupational allergens

Loida Viera-Hutchins
Tanner Clinic

Andrew M. Smith
Allergy Associates of Utah

David I. Bernstein
University of Cincinnati College of Medicine

CONTENTS

20.1 INTRODUCTION

Allergen immunotherapy (AIT) is the repeated administration of specific allergens to patients with IgE-mediated diseases, the purpose of which is to provide protection against the allergic symptoms and inflammatory reactions associated with the natural exposure to said allergens [1]. This therapy is efficacious to treat patients with allergic rhinitis due to seasonal pollen allergens [2] (e.g., trees, grasses, and weeds) and for perennial allergic rhinitis induced by house dust mites [3] and cat allergens [4]. Similarly, AIT is effective in treating patients with aeroallergen-induced asthma attributable to sensitization with cat and grass pollens [2,5,6].

AIT is seldom considered in the initial management of workers with occupational rhinitis (OR) or occupational asthma (OA). Environmental control measures to reduce exposures to offending workplace aeroallergens are usually prioritized and emphasized and may account for the lack of published clinical studies about efficacy and safety of AIT in patients with occupational respiratory allergic diseases. However, where appropriate, AIT is considered only in workers in whom specific IgE sensitization to natural protein

allergens is confirmed by skin testing to commercially available extracts or *in vitro* specific IgE tests. Although specific IgE to reactive chemicals known to induce OA is rarely demonstrated, to reactive chemicals known to induce OA [7], AIT with chemical antigens (e.g., hapten-conjugated proteins) cannot be safely recommended or considered due to unknown short-term and long-terms risks of chemical-induced side effects.

The primary treatment of choice for OA or OR remains the elimination or reduction of occupational exposure to causative aeroallergens. Such interventions consist of reassignment to a different low exposure job in the same work facility or job transfer to another workplace where exposure is eliminated or reduced sufficiently to control or prevent work-related allergic respiratory symptoms. Failure to reduce exposure to causative agents in patients with uncontrolled OA can result in disability and even fatal asthma [8,9]. Therefore, pharmacotherapy and AIT should be utilized as ancillary treatments in selected patients but not as substitutes for effective environmental interventions.

There are specific situations in which AIT may be appropriate to treat occupational IgE-mediated respiratory disorders. AIT may be considered in symptomatic workers whose exposure to workplace allergens can be reduced but not entirely eliminated. Workers, recognizing the potential impact of a job change on their income and livelihood, may choose to continue work in a job where there is persistent exposure to an occupational allergen. In these cases, the best possible clinical outcomes may result from a combined approach including institution of personal safety measures (e.g., respirators or masks), pharmacotherapy, and AIT, when appropriate. At the same time, these workers must be medically monitored to assure that persistent exposure does not lead to more severe illnesses or worsening of airway obstruction.

20.2 NATURAL RUBBER LATEX

Natural rubber latex (NRL) is derived from the sap of the rubber tree, *Hevea brasiliensis*, a complex mixture of at least 13 allergenic proteins that bind human IgE antibodies (Hev b allergens) [10]. Hev b 5 and Hev b 6 are the most common allergens identified in the occupational setting, 92% of healthcare workers sensitized to NRL are sensitized to Hev b 5. Hev b 2, 4, 7, and 13 are also considered relevant occupational allergens. Hev b 6, Heb v 6.01, Heb b 6.02, Hev b 6.03, and Hev b 7 have known cross-reactivity with fruits. Hev b 8 (profilin), 11, and 12 (lipid transfer protein) are considered pan-allergens and are usually implicated in latex-fruit syndrome. Hev b 3 is considered the major allergen in individuals with spina bifida who develop latex allergy. Heb v 14 has been identified as a major allergen in the Taiwanese population [11].

NRL gloves are a common source of occupational allergen exposure for healthcare workers and an important cause of allergic occupational disease. An NRL skin test reagent approved by the U.S. Food and Drug Administration (FDA) is not commercially available, although there are FDA-cleared immunoassays to detect NRL-specific IgE in serum [12]. The primary intervention for individuals with established NRL allergy is avoidance of NRL-containing products [13].

The first multicenter, double-blind, placebo-controlled (DBPC) trial with NRL was performed in a French cohort for 1 year in 2000 [14]. Seventeen patients had NRL allergy, defined by a clinical history of rhinitis and conjunctivitis, asthma (9/17), a positive skin prick test with a standardized latex extract (Stallergènes SA, Antony, France), a positive latex conjunctival provocation challenge, and elevated NRL-specific IgE defined as class 2 level or greater (Pharmacia, Uppsala, Sweden).

After 6 months of NRL subcutaneous immunotherapy (SCIT), there were significant improvements in rhinitis symptom scores ($p < .04$) and conjunctivitis symptom scores ($p < .02$) compared with placebo associated with NRL exposure. After 1 year of SCIT, improvement in rhinitis ($p < .05$) and conjunctivitis ($p = .05$) symptoms was maintained with added improvement in cutaneous signs ($p < 0.03$). No effect on work-associated asthma symptoms was demonstrated after 1 year. The mean medication scores with treatment also improved by 79%. Conjunctival challenge with aqueous latex extract was performed pre- and post-SCIT; conjunctival reactivity decreased with active versus placebo treatment ($p < .02$).

Safety was a concern. There was a higher rate of injection-related reactions in the treatment group as compared to placebo, with almost 50% in the treatment group experiencing immediate large local reactions at injection sites. Almost half of actively treated patients (four of nine) had at least one anaphylactic reaction to NRL injections characterized by angioedema, bronchospasm, pharyngeal edema, giant urticaria, or hypotension [14].

Another randomized, DBPC trial of NRL AIT was reported in 2003 [15]. In a 6-month trial with an experimental crude NRL extract, 24 patients were randomized to active NRL SCIT treatment ($n = 16$) or placebo ($n = 8$). This Spanish cohort consisted primarily of healthcare workers with contact urticaria ($n = 24$), rhinitis ($n = 17$), and/or asthma ($n = 15$) related to NRL exposure. Compared to placebo, patients receiving NRL SCIT had a significant decrease in skin prick test (SPT) reactivity to NRL ($p < .01$), decrease in reactions to a latex rubbing test (NRL glove rubbed on wet skin for 30 seconds) ($p = .047$), and in reactions to a glove use test ($p = .046$). However, treatment had no effect on NRL-specific IgE levels, symptoms, or medication scores, methacholine PC20, or the NRL glove exposure time to elicit a 15% decrease in FEV$_1$ by specific inhalation challenge. As in the previous study, a high number of systemic reactions were reported. Of 387 injections, there were 31 mild systemic reactions (8% of doses), with a third of these reactions classified as delayed reactions. These systemic reactions occurred in 11 actively treated patients (68.7%). The authors reported no severe systemic reactions.

Twenty-three patients (6 males and 17 females; mean age: 35 years, range: 24–58 years) with latex hypersensitivity were included in another DBPC study of NRL SCIT [16]. All patients had signs of latex conjunctivitis. Latex allergic rhinitis and cutaneous signs of latex allergy were reported in 22 out of 23. Latex-related asthma (intermittent to chronic moderate) was reported in 20. Treatment comprised a dose progression phase during which latex extract (Stallergènes, Antony, France) was administered in hospital according to a 2-day rush protocol, followed by a 12-month maintenance treatment phase. Change from baseline of rhinitis, conjunctivitis, skin symptoms, asthma symptoms, medication score, and cutaneous reactivity was not significantly different between the two groups. Systemic reactions were much higher in the SCIT than in the placebo group. In the active treatment group, 335 injections were given with 102 systemic reactions (SRs) observed. Nine actively treated patients experienced SRs (81.8% of patients). In the placebo group, 354 injections were given with 9 SRs observed. Two placebo-treated patients experienced SRs (16.7% of patients).

Due to safety concerns with NRL SCIT, sublingual immunotherapy (SLIT) to NRL has been evaluated. Twenty-six patients with symptoms of urticaria, rhinoconjunctivitis, asthma, and/or anaphylaxis associated with NRL exposure were treated with a commercially available sublingual NRL extract (SLIT-LATEX [ALK-Abelló, S.A., Madrid, Spain]) in an open uncontrolled study [17]. After 10 weeks of treatment, 1044 doses were administered. SRs occurred with 38 doses (3.6%) and in 12 patients (46.2%). One patient experienced anaphylaxis. Local oral reactions were reported with 223 doses (21.4%). Compared to baseline, there were decreased symptom scores with the latex glove use test ($p = .0004$) and with the latex glove rubbing test (latex glove rubbed on wet skin for 30 seconds) ($p = .037$).

A nonblinded study evaluated the use of NRL SLIT in 24 patients, including 10 healthcare workers, with symptoms of asthma ($n = 17$), urticaria ($n = 18$), and/or rhinoconjunctivitis ($n = 10$) with NRL exposure [18]. All had a positive SPT to a standardized NRL extract. Twelve underwent a 4-day rush treatment protocol, and 12 others were untreated and served as controls. Two actively treated patients had local reactions in 3 months of treatment with NRL SLIT ($n = 12$). No SRs were reported. Significant improvements in symptom scores with NRL challenge were seen in the treatment group before and after treatment with SLIT. The group treated with SLIT also had significant improvements in symptom scores compared to the untreated control group with sublingual NRL challenge ($p < .001$), with NRL gloved finger in mouth challenge ($p = .0002$), with cutaneous NRL extract challenge ($p < .001$), and with conjunctival NRL challenge ($p < .01$).

Forty patients with latex allergy (11 men and 29 women) aged 18–47 years were enrolled in a DBPC trial of NLR SLIT [19]. At diagnosis, 30 presented with urticaria and 10 with asthma. Treatment consisted of five concentrations of ALK-Abello latex. A 4-day sublingual induction phase was followed by a 12-month maintenance phase (three administrations per week). An improved symptoms score and reduced medication score were seen along with improved bronchial and glove provocation test results (Figures 20.1 and 20.2). Four of 35 patients (11%) (three of 18 in the SLIT group [17%] and one of 17 in the placebo group [6%]) developed adverse reactions during the induction phase. Two patients in the SLIT group reported mouth itching and burning; the third reported an episode of lip swelling.

Twenty-eight adult latex-allergic patients (5 males and 23 females), with a mean age of 39 years (range 24–57) were randomized to receive a NLR SLIT or placebo during one year, followed by another year of open, active therapy [20]. No significant differences in skin prick test, gloves-use score, conjunctival challenge test, total and specific IgE, and adverse reactions were observed between the active and placebo groups at the end of the placebo-controlled phase, and none were observed when each group was compared with their baseline values at the end of the study. During the induction phase, four reactions in the active and five in the placebo group were recorded. During the maintenance phase, two patients dropped out due to pruritus and acute dermatitis.

To overcome safety issues, a final study used a component-resolved approach to treatment, using SLIT with Hev b 6.01, Hev b 2, Hev b 5, Hev b 7, Hev b 2, and hevamine (SLIT-LATEX, ALK-Abelló, SA, Madrid, Spain) [21]. In this prospective, observational, open, case-control study, 18 of 23 children with latex allergy received SLIT. After 12 months of treatment, a cutaneous tolerance index increased by 3.34 times with treatment ($p < .05$), and in-use tests indicated an almost double increased time to elicit pruritus or urticaria with treatment ($p \leq .002$). Conjunctival provocation tests showed an increased response threshold to exposure with treatment ($p = .05$). Compared to previous studies, safety was less of an issue. During initiation, six (33%) developed SRs of oral pruritus (five of six) and atopic dermatitis (one of six). During maintenance, five (28%) developed SRs of oral pruritus.

The aforementioned AIT studies of latex allergy are all considerably underpowered with too few subjects in active treatment and placebo groups to determine clinically meaningful differences in efficacy outcomes. Nevertheless, treatment of NRL allergy with AIT seems to be effective in improving rhinitis symptom scores elicited by NRL exposure. However, proven benefit for asthma or decreased bronchial hyperactivity (specific inhalational challenge) after NRL has not been confirmed. The lack of benefit from AIT may be due to the failure thus far to define optimal latex extract maintenance doses, which is in part due to the unacceptably high risk of SRs. As with clinical trials of grass pollen SLIT, determination of safe and effective treatment doses would first require dose-response studies with well-characterized treatment allergens. Due to reduced rates of SRs, SLIT may be helpful if future evidence from placebo-controlled studies supports its efficacy. Based on the evidence, environmental control of the work environment and avoidance of NRL products remain the primary treatment. Since new cases of NRL allergy are rapidly declining due to widespread introduction of low allergen products used by healthcare professionals, there may be little need to develop AIT products in the future (see Table 20.1).

20.3 WHEAT FLOUR

Bakers and pastry makers exposed to wheat flour, containing high molecular weight protein allergens, often develop occupational rhinitis and bakers' asthma. The prevalence of bakers' asthma is estimated to be 9% among bakery employees, and the incidence of rhinitis ranges from 18% to 29% [22]. The major allergens implicated in bakers' asthma include Tri a 37, Tri a 14 a lipid transfer protein, Tri a Bd36 a peroxidase found in 60% of individuals with bakers asthma, Tri a 25 a thioredoxin, Tri a 39 Serine protease like the inhibitor found in 14%–27% of Spanish patients with baker's asthma, and thaumatin-like proteins that have been found in 30%–45% of Finnish patients with asthma [23].

A case was reported of a 30-year-old baker with asthma symptoms who was found to be sensitized to wheat flour, soybean, rye grain, baker's yeast, and oat grain [24]. Avoidance measures were difficult to implement. Following 12 months of SCIT with the wheat flour extract (Stallergenes SA, Antony, France), asthma symptoms in the workplace significantly decreased to the point where he only rarely required salbutamol for asthma. Follow-up spirometry showed a 30% improvement in FEV_1 compared with baseline spirometry results.

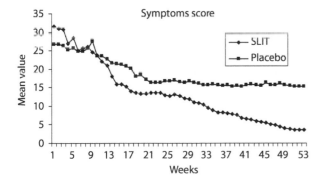

Figure 20.1 Symptoms score in relation to time (53 weeks). (SLIT, sublingual immunotherapy.) (Reprinted from Nettis E et al. *Br J Dermatol* 2007; 156[4]: 674–681.)

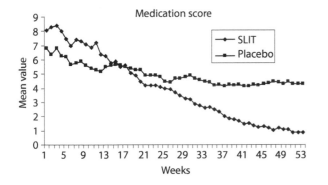

Figure 20.2 Medication score in relation to time (53 weeks). (SLIT, sublingual immunotherapy.) (Reprinted from Nettis E et al. *Br J Dermatol* 2007; 156[4]: 674–681.)

Table 20.1 Natural rubber latex (NRL)

Allergen (route)	Study design	Number studied	Indication	Results	Level of evidence[a]	Reference
NRL (SCIT)	DBPC	17	Rhinitis, asthma, conjunctivitis	• Improvement in rhinitis and conjunctivitis	A	Leynadier et al. [14]
NRL (SCIT)	DBPC	24	Contact urticaria, rhinitis, asthma	• Decrease in SPT reactivity to NRL • Decrease in symptoms with glove use	A	Sastre et al. [15]
NRL (SCIT)	DBPC	23	Urticaria, rhinitis, conjunctivitis, asthma	• No significant change in rhinitis, conjunctivitis, skin, or asthma symptoms	A	Tabar et al. [16]
NRL (SLIT)	Unblinded, no placebo	26	Urticaria, rhinitis, asthma, anaphylaxis	• Improvement of symptom scores with glove use	C	Cisteró Bahima et al. [17]
NRL (SLIT)	Unblinded, placebo controlled	24	Asthma, urticaria, rhinitis, conjunctivitis	• Improvement of symptom scores with NRL challenge	B	Patriarca et al. [18]
NRL (SLIT)	DBPC	40	Asthma, urticaria	• Improvement in symptom score, medication score • Improved bronchial and glove provocation test results	A	Nettis et al. [19]
NRL (SLIT)	Unblinded, placebo controlled	28	Urticaria, conjunctivitis	• No significant change in skin prick test, glove-use score, or conjunctival challenge test	B	Gastaminza et al. [20]
NRL (SLIT)	Unblinded, placebo controlled, observational	23	Urticaria, conjunctivitis	• Improvement in cutaneous tolerance • Decreased conjunctival symptoms on challenge	B	Lasa Luaces et al. [21]

Abbreviations: DBPC, double-blind, placebo-controlled; PEFR, peak expiratory flow rate; SCIT, subcutaneous immunotherapy; SLIT, sublingual immunotherapy; SPT, skin prick test.

[a] Level of evidence: A: Evidence based on randomized controlled trial. B: Evidence based on controlled trial without randomization or other quasi-experimental study design. C: Evidence based on nonexperimental descriptive studies. D: Evidence based on expert opinion.

One DBPC study evaluated 139 patients who worked with wheat flour [22]. Of the 139 subjects, 35 (25%) had a positive SPT with a crude wheat flour extract or elevated *in vitro* specific IgE to wheat flour. Of these, 30 asthmatic patients were selected for the SCIT trial. Eight were treated for 10 months and eight for 20 months with wheat flour extract, and ten received placebo. Four in the active treatment group stopped therapy with resolution of symptoms due to a change of jobs. AIT-treated patients had a significant decrease in wheat flour extract skin prick test sensitivity as determined by the wheal area ($p = .002$) and a significant decrease in bronchial hyperresponsiveness to methacholine ($p < .001$). By 20 months of treatment, there was a significant decrease in wheat flour specific IgE compared to placebo ($p < .005$) and improvement in symptoms associated with exposure to wheat flour compared to placebo ($p < .001$). No severe SRs were reported, although one patient developed transient urticaria after an injection. This study indicates that SCIT with wheat flour extract may be effective in treating bakers' asthma. However, these positive results require confirmation in larger controlled clinical trials (see Table 20.2).

20.4 ANIMAL ALLERGY (MAMMALIAN PROTEINS)

Among animal workers, allergic reactions are an important occupational health problem, with an estimated incidence of 1.32 per 100 person-years and an estimated prevalence of 22% [25]. Of all animal workers, veterinarians are at the greatest risk of developing occupational allergic disorders such as atopic dermatitis, allergic rhinitis, and asthma. In a questionnaire survey of 1416 veterinarians, 38% report rhinitis or conjunctivitis, and 20% report asthma symptoms related to their work environment [25]. Cats are the most commonly reported (58%) animals causing work-related symptoms.

Avoidance of laboratory animals and animal housing facilities is usually recommended in symptomatic workers. However, due to career and job considerations, it is rarely feasible for affected workers to eliminate all exposure to animals. When complete avoidance is not possible, there are reported cases when AIT with laboratory animal allergens has been attempted.

Table 20.2 Wheat flour

Allergen (route)	Study design	Number studied	Indication	Results	Level of evidence[a]	Reference
Wheat flour (SCIT)	Case report	1	Asthma	• Decreased asthma symptoms • Improved FEV1	C	Swaminathan and Heddle [24]
Wheat flour (SCIT)	DBPC	30	Asthma	• Decrease in SPT reactivity to wheat flour • Decrease in bronchial hyperreponsiveness on methacholine challenge • Decrease in wheat flour specific IgE • Improvement of symptoms on exposure	A	Armentia et al. [22]

Abbreviations: DBPC, double-blind, placebo-controlled; PEFR, peak expiratory flow rate; SCIT, subcutaneous immunotherapy; SLIT, sublingual immunotherapy; SPT, skin prick test.

[a] Level of evidence: A: Evidence based on randomized controlled trial. B: Evidence based on controlled trial without randomization or other quasi-experimental study design. C: Evidence based on nonexperimental descriptive studies. D: Evidence based on expert opinion.

SCIT with rodent allergens was utilized in 11 patients with allergic symptoms upon exposure to laboratory animals and compared to a group of matched untreated control patients in an unblinded manner [26]. Laboratory animal allergy was confirmed by intracutaneous skin testing and leukocyte histamine release to animal allergens, such as mouse, rabbit, rat, guinea pig, and hamster. All patients had rhinoconjunctivitis symptoms upon exposure to at least one of these animals, and most had symptoms on exposure to several different species. Nine of 11 patients reported a decrease in symptoms after SCIT. Active treatment was associated with significantly increased titers of blocking antibody determined by serum inhibition of allergen-induced histamine release with relevant laboratory animal allergens in comparison to untreated controls ($p < .0001$). In three of four patients in whom AIT was discontinued, blocking antibodies slowly decreased to pretreatment levels after 16–36 months.

In a second case series, five laboratory animal workers with mouse allergy were evaluated [27]. All workers reported a history of allergic rhinitis. Asthma was reported in two of the five workers. One worker reported anaphylaxis within 10 minutes of a mouse bite at work. Skin prick test to mouse epithelium was positive in four of five workers. Specific IgE to mouse urinary protein was positive in the worker with the negative skin prick test. All of the patients were treated with SCIT with *Mus musculus* allergenic extract from Greer. All patients had a significant improvement in symptoms with immunotherapy. All five patients reported improvement in allergic rhinitis symptoms, assessed by total nasal symptom score. The two patients with asthma reported improvement in asthma symptoms, assessed by the asthma control test. No further bites were reported, so it is unknown if SCIT modified the risk of anaphylaxis.

Both cat-induced allergic rhinitis and asthma have been effectively treated by use of SCIT [28]. In a randomized, DBPC trial, 17 patients with asthma associated with cat exposure were followed [5]. All patients developed cough, wheeze, or shortness of breath with cat exposure and had a positive SPT and bronchial challenge test result to the major cat allergen, Fel d 1. Compared to placebo ($n = 8$), treatment was associated with a significant increase in PD_{20} FEV_1 on bronchial provocation with Fel d 1 ($p < .05$). A higher concentration of allergen was necessary to induce a 3 mm wheal in the treatment versus placebo group on SP titration testing ($p < .01$). The treatment group had increased time to ocular ($p < .05$) and pulmonary ($p < .05$) but not nasal symptoms with cat exposure compared to placebo. Ocular, nasal, and pulmonary symptom scores following

cat exposure ($p \leq .03$) also improved with treatment. Furthermore, active treatment was associated with increased Fel d 1 specific IgG compared to placebo ($p < .001$).

SLIT with cat allergen has also been evaluated. Fifty cat-allergic patients with rhinoconjunctivitis with or without asthma were included in a randomized DBPC trial of cat SLIT over 1 year [29]. Twenty-five patients received active treatment and 25 placebo. Efficacy was assessed by natural exposure challenge to a cat in a cat-room and by skin tests. Thirty-three (66%) out of 50 patients completed the treatment. The cat SLIT group showed a marked reduction (62%) in symptoms during the cat challenge ($p < .001$) with no changes in placebo group. The cat SLIT group also showed a reduced peak expiratory flow (PEF) response to cat exposure ($p < .05$) and a decrease in skin test reactivity to a standardized cat extract ($p < .05$). There were no significant changes in the placebo group. No local or SRs were reported.

One significant barrier to immunotherapy is the prolonged treatment course; therefore, novel approaches are being explored. One approach is to introduce the immunotherapy vaccine through a novel route. Intralymphatic administration was evaluated in one DBPC trial of three injections within 2 months [30]. A novel Fel d 1 fusion protein was used to treat 12 patients. The study included eight control patients. Outcomes were measured within 1 month. Nasal tolerance improved 74-fold with treatment ($p < .001$), and allergen tolerance by SPT improved threefold ($p = .047$). No changes were seen in nasal symptoms. SRs were no higher in the treatment group (five mild, two moderate) as compared to placebo (nine mild, five moderate).

Another approach is to use peptide immunotherapy with synthetic T-cell epitopes derived from major allergens to target induction of T-regulatory cells. A cat-peptide allergen desensitization (Cat-PAD) vaccine was evaluated in a DBPC trial with 202 patients [31]. Patients were treated over 3 months with SCIT and assessed at 12 months. Patients showed a significant improvement in total rhinoconjunctivitis symptom score (-7 for treatment; -3 for placebo; $p = .01$), total nasal symptom score (-3.6 for treatment; -1.6 for placebo; $p = .02$), and total ocular symptom score (-3.4 for treatment; -1.3 for placebo; $p = .01$) with treatment. SRs were similar between the groups: 14 of 66 (21.2%) with treatment including one hypersensitivity reaction and 13 of 69 (18.8%) with placebo. A follow-up study did not show significant long-term benefit for the primary endpoint of mean reduction in total rhinoconjunctivitis symptom score [32].

Table 20.3 Animal allergy (mammalian proteins)

Allergen (route)	Study design	Number studied	Indication	Results	Level of evidence[a]	Reference
Rodent (mouse, rabbit, rat, guinea pig, hamster) (SCIT)	Unblinded, matched-untreated controls	11	Rhinitis, conjunctivitis	• Decrease in symptoms on exposure • Increase in titers of blocking antibodies	B	Wahn and Siraganian [26]
Mouse (SCIT)	Unblinded, no placebo	5	Anaphylaxis, asthma, rhinitis	• Improvement in asthma symptom score • Improvement in allergic rhinitis symptom score	C	Bunyavanich et al. [27]
Fel d1 (SCIT)	DBPC	17	Asthma	• Increase in PD_{20} FEV_1 with bronchial provocation • Decrease in SPT reactivity • Improvement of ocular, nasal, and pulmonary symptom scores	A	Ohman et al. [5]
Fel d1 (SLIT)	DBPC	50	Rhinitis, conjunctivitis, asthma	• Decreased symptoms with cat exposure • Less decrease in peak expiratory flow with cat exposure • Decreased skin test reactivity	A	Alvarez-Cuesta et al. [29]
Fel d 1 fusion (intralymphatic)	DBPC	20	Rhinitis	• Improved nasal tolerance • Decreased skin test reactivity	A	Senti et al. [30]
Fel d 1 peptide (SCIT)	DBPC	200	Rhinitis, conjunctivitis	• Improved total rhinoconjunctivitis, rhinitis, and ocular symptom scores	A	Patel et al. [31]

Abbreviations: DBPC, double-blind, placebo-controlled; PEFR, peak expiratory flow rate; SCIT, subcutaneous immunotherapy; SLIT, sublingual immunotherapy; SPT, skin prick test.

[a] Level of evidence: A: Evidence based on randomized controlled trial. B: Evidence based on controlled trial without randomization or other quasi-experimental study design. C: Evidence based on nonexperimental descriptive studies. D: Evidence based on expert opinion.

Overall, cat immunotherapy is considered safe and effective for the treatment of cat-allergic patients (see Table 20.3).

20.5 SEA SQUIRT

Major allergens from the body fluid of the sea squirt, *Styela plicata*, are the acidic glycoproteins, Gi-rep, Ei-M, and DIIIa. Asthma related to exposure to sea squirt allergens primarily occurs among Japanese oyster-shucking workers. Oyster-shucking workers continuously inhale the sea squirt antigens in the mist of the body fluid of sea squirts. In 1963, the reported prevalence of sea squirt asthma was 36% [33]. With industrial hygiene improvements, the reported prevalence of sea squirt asthma has decreased to 8%, with an incidence of 10.1% [33]. The proportion of serious cases has rapidly decreased as well, from 29.2% of cases in 1963 to 0% after 1984.

A total of 22 females with sea squirt asthma were treated for 2 years with high-concentration purified sea squirt antigen Ei-M [34]. Ages ranged from 22 to 69 years. One patient stopped SCIT, but in the remaining 21 cases, effects were rapidly observed. Treated patients did not develop asthmatic attacks even though they engaged in oyster-shucking work. In addition, serum anti-Ei-M IgG antibody was significantly elevated after the therapy. None of the treated patients developed significant side effects.

In an uncontrolled study, 123 asthmatic patients received SCIT with one of three known major sea squirt allergens, Gi-rep ($n = 47$), Ei-M ($n = 62$), or DIIIa ($n = 14$) [35]. The maximum dose of each AIT injection was 50 µg of antigen. After 1 year of treatment, 72% of those treated with Gi-rep were able to shuck oysters with minimal or no medications. Better results were obtained with Ei-M; 90% of patients reported improved symptoms. DIIIa was the least effective, with only 36% reporting improved symptoms. These results are consistent with a previous study that shows DIIIa is significantly less effective than Gi-rep or Ei-M with AIT [36]. Beneficial effects of AIT were maintained over 5 years of treatment. A significant increase in IgG titer specific for Ei-M occurs within the first year of SCIT and correlates with the therapeutic effect, similar to previous studies [35]. Among Japanese oyster-shucking workers, it has been reported that a significant number are currently treated or have received therapy in the past with SCIT [33]. Between the industrial hygiene improvements and use of SCIT, the Japanese oyster-shucking industry has reduced all cases of occupational asthma reported since 1988 to slight severity (see Table 20.4).

Table 20.4 Sea squirt

Allergen (route)	Study design	Number studied	Indication	Results	Level of evidence[a]	Reference
Gi-rep, Ei-M, DIIIa (SCIT)	Unblinded, no placebo	123	Asthma	• Improvement of asthma symptoms • Decrease in medication use with oyster shucking	C	Jyo et al. [35]
Ei-M (SCIT)	Unblinded, no placebo	22	Asthma	• Improvement of asthma symptoms • Elevated serum anti-Ei-M IgG	C	Jyo et al. [34]

Abbreviations: DBPC, double-blind, placebo-controlled; PEFR, peak expiratory flow rate; SCIT, subcutaneous immunotherapy; SLIT, sublingual immunotherapy; SPT, skin prick test.

[a] Level of evidence: A: Evidence based on randomized controlled trial. B: Evidence based on controlled trial without randomization or other quasi-experimental study design. C: Evidence based on nonexperimental descriptive studies. D: Evidence based on expert opinion.

20.6 HOUSE DUST MITE

House dust mite is the most common indoor allergen [37]. Exposure to house dust mite (DM) allergens occurs in a variety of occupations, including domestic cleaners and janitorial staff personnel. High levels of house dust mite species allergens, *Dermatophagoides pteronyssinus* (Der p1) and *Dermatophagoides farinae* (Der f1), are present in the house dust of rooms with wall-to-wall carpeting.

Several studies evaluated the efficacy of DM AIT, although not specifically in worker cohorts. Twenty-seven patients with a positive skin prick test to Der p1 and/or Der f1 and perennial rhinitis and/or mild asthma received SCIT with aluminum hydroxide adsorbed standardized dust mite extracts (50% Der p1 and 50% Der f1) and were followed yearly for 3 years in a DBPC trial [38]. After 3 years of AIT, there was a significant decrease in medication scores for asthma ($p < .033$) and for rhinitis ($p = .0007$). Subjective symptom scores for asthma were significantly improved after 1 year ($p = .016$) and continued through 3 years of treatment ($p = .0008$). Rhinitis symptom scores were significantly improved at both 2 and 3 years ($p = .0006$). Both skin prick test reactivity and conjunctival reactivity to Der p1 and/or Der f1 significantly decreased over all 3 years ($p < .0001$). Nonspecific bronchial hyperresponsiveness, as measured by methacholine challenge, also improved after 3 years of SCIT as compared to placebo ($p < .0001$). No significant SRs to injections were reported.

In another DPBC study, 29 asthmatic patients with skin prick test positivity to Der p1 were randomized to either SCIT or placebo [39]. After 3 years of SCIT with Der p1 extract, there were no significant differences in the FVC, FEV_1, or FEF25–75. However, there was a significant decrease in the number of annual asthma exacerbations after 1 year of treatment ($p < .01$). Furthermore, there was a significant increase in the number of medication-free days (e.g., bronchodilators or systemic glucocorticoids) between the treatment and placebo groups ($p < .01$). Along with these findings, there was a significant improvement in bronchial hyperresponsiveness to methacholine. As for safety, no major SRs with injections were reported.

A larger randomized, DBPC trial included 95 patients with asthma and percutaneous sensitization to Der p1 and/or Der f1 [40]. SCIT was administered for 3 years using extracts containing Der p1 and/or Der f1 allergens; 72 patients completed the study. There was a significant decrease in percutaneous skin sensitivity to Der p1 and/or Der f1 antigens ($p < .05$) with AIT. Small, but significant improvements were seen in PEF in the AIT group (mean increase of

1.6%–5.5% of predicted from baseline). Asthma symptom scores did not significantly change, but there was an increase in the proportion of patients not requiring use of bronchodilators in the treatment group ($p < .01$). There was no significant change in the FEV_1 or in bronchial hyperresponsiveness to methacholine in the treatment versus the placebo group. Mild bronchospasm after injections was reported on two occasions.

One other study evaluated the effects of rush AIT in 10 Der p1 SPT-positive asthmatic patients to evaluate the underlying immune changes associated with clinical improvement with AIT [41]. While treatment was not blinded, the outcomes were compared 1–2 days prior to the start of rush AIT and 1–2 days after reaching maintenance in a blinded manner. There was a significant decrease in percutaneous reactivity to Der p1 by endpoint skin prick test titration with AIT ($p < .01$). Decreased nasal reactivity to Der p1, symptom scores, and nasal obstruction was found in the AIT-treated versus the placebo group ($p < .01$). A significant increase in anti-Der p1 IgG4 was observed in the AIT-treated group ($p < .01$). There was also a significantly decreased lymphocyte proliferative response to Der p1 after AIT ($p < .05$).

In a randomized DBPC controlled trial, 54 adults with DM-allergic asthma received DM SCIT (Alutard SQ, *Dermatophagoides pteronyssinus*, ALK, Hørsholm, Denmark) or placebo for 3 years [42]. At baseline, and after 1, 2, and 3 years of treatment, the lowest possible inhaled corticosteroid dose required to maintain asthma control was determined, along with determinations of nonspecific and DM-allergen-specific bronchial hyperresponsiveness, immediate and late-phase skin reactions, and immunologic response. DM SCIT provided a statistically significantly higher DM-allergen tolerance ($p < .05$ versus placebo) in terms of a 1.6-fold increase in PD20 (HDM-allergen inhalation challenge) (Figure 20.3), a 60-fold increase in skin test histamine equivalent DM-allergen concentrations, and reduced immediate- and late-phase skin reactions. No life-threatening or other serious adverse events related to treatment were reported.

SLIT with DM has been evaluated in 31 *D. farinae*–sensitive adults with allergic rhinitis with or without mild intermittent asthma [43]. Treatment was with high-dose maintenance ($n = 10$), or low-dose maintenance vaccine ($n = 10$) or placebo ($n = 11$) over 12–18 months. Of the 31 randomized subjects, 4 withdrew because of treatment-ascribed effects: high-dose group, 1 of 10 (gastrointestinal symptoms); low-dose group, 1 of 10 (gastrointestinal symptoms); and placebo group, 2 of 11 (headache and increased nasal symptoms). Eleven of the 21 subjects who completed the study

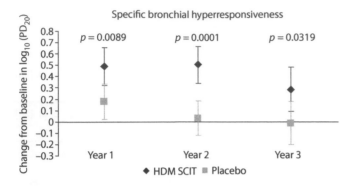

Figure 20.3 The house dust mite (HDM) allergen-specific BHR in terms of change from baseline in log10(PD20); estimate and 95% confidence intervals with p-values for the difference between treatment groups. PD20 is the HDM-allergen dose (SQ-U) causing a 20% decline in FEV_1. Test: ANOVA with change from baseline as response variable, treatment as fixed effect and baseline as covariate. (Reprinted from Blumberga G et al. *Allergy* 2011; 66[2]: 178–185.)

experienced mild to moderate gastrointestinal symptoms, throat irritation, or both (high-dose group, 5/9; low-dose group, 4/7; and placebo group, 2/5). No severe SRs were noted. In the high-dose SLIT group, there was a significant increase in the bronchial threshold to allergen challenge (AgPD20) with *D. farinae*. The AgPD20 value increased from 70 ± 18 cumulative breath units at baseline to 101 ± 13 cumulative breath units ($p = .04$ versus placebo) after treatment (12–18 months). No significant change was found in the placebo or low-dose SLIT groups (see Table 20.5).

A larger study of SLIT with HDM evaluated the efficacy for asthma exacerbations during an inhaled corticosteroid (ICS) reduction period [44]. Treatment was with 12 SQ-HDM ($n = 282$), 6 SQ-HDM ($n = 275$), or placebo ($n = 277$) SLIT tablets. The biological activity of the HDM SLIT tablet is related to the activity of the allergens (*D. farinae* and *D. pteronyssinus*) and is expressed in the unit SQ-HDM. Patients included in the study had HDM allergy-related asthma not well controlled with ICS or combination therapy and with HDM allergy-related rhinitis. Patients were followed for 7–12 months, then ICS reduction was started in October 2012 and

Table 20.5 House dust mite

Allergen (route)	Study design	Number studied	Indication	Results	Level of evidence[a]	Reference
Der p1/Der f1 (SCIT)	DBPC	27	Rhinitis, asthma	• Decrease in medication scores for asthma and rhinitis • Improvement of rhinitis and asthma symptom scores • Decrease in SPT and conjunctival reactivity • Improvement of bronchial hyperresponsiveness by methacholine challenge	A	Pichler et al. [38]
Der p1 (SCIT)	DBPC	29	Asthma	• Decrease in number of annual asthma exacerbations • Increase in medication-free days • Improvement of bronchial hyperresponsiveness by methacholine challenge	A	Pifferi et al. [39]
Der p1/Der f1 (SCIT)	DBPC	95	Asthma	• Decrease in SPT reactivity • Improvement of PEFR • Decrease in use of bronchodilators	A	Maestrelli et al. [40]
Der p1 (Rush SCIT)	Unblinded, no placebo	10	Rhinitis, asthma	• Decrease in SPT reactivity • Decrease in nasal reactivity and obstruction • Decrease in asthma and rhinitis symptom scores	C	Lack et al. [41]
Der p1 (SCIT)	DBPC	54	Asthma	• Improved PD20 on allergen inhalation challenge • Decreased SPT reactivity	A	Blumberga et al. [42]
Der f1 (SLIT)	Unblinded, placebo-controlled	31	Rhinitis, asthma	• Improved PD20 on allergen inhalation challenge	B	Bush et al. [43]
Der p1,2/Der f1,2 (SLIT)	DBPC	834	Asthma	• Decreased moderate or severe asthma exacerbations	A	Virchow et al. [44]

Abbreviations: DBPC, double-blind, placebo-controlled; PEFR, peak expiratory flow rate; SCIT, subcutaneous immunotherapy; SLIT, sublingual immunotherapy; SPT, skin prick test.

[a] Level of evidence: A: Evidence based on randomized controlled trial. B: Evidence based on controlled trial without randomization or other quasi-experimental study design. C: Evidence based on nonexperimental descriptive studies. D: Evidence based on expert opinion.

continued for 6 months. The primary outcome was time to first moderate or severe asthma exacerbation during the ICS reduction period. Among the 693 who completed the study, there were no reports of severe systemic allergic reaction. Both doses of HDM SLIT significantly reduced the risk of a moderate or severe asthma exacerbation compared to placebo (hazard ratio: 0.72 [95% CI, 0.52–0.99] for the 6 SQ-HDM group, $p = .045$, and 0.69 [95% CI, 0.50–0.96] for the 12 SQ-HDM group, $p = .03$).

Based on available data, the 2018 GINA Report includes the recommendation that "For adult patients with allergic rhinitis and sensitized to house dust mite, with exacerbations despite low-high dose ICS, consider adding sublingual allergen immunotherapy (SLIT), provided FEV_1 is >70% predicted" [45].

20.7 HYMENOPTERA VENOM

Stinging insect hypersensitivity is an occupational problem for farm workers, greenhouse workers, forest rangers, biologists, and bee-keepers. Hymenoptera insects in the families Apidae (bees) and Vespidae (wasps) are primarily responsible and include the honey-bee (*Apis melifera*), yellow jacket (*Vespula vulgaris*), wasp (*Polisites annularis*), white-faced hornet *(Dolichovespula maculata)*, and yel-low hornet (*Dolichovespula arenaria*) [46] (see Chapters 18 and 29).

The prevalence of SRs to Hymenoptera stings ranges from 0.8% to 3.3% in the general population [47,48]. Several studies show that the rate of SRs is much higher in beekeepers, between 14% and 35% [49,50]. A prospective evaluation of 35 Greek beekeepers was performed to estimate the incidence of sensitization among previously unsensitized workers [47]. The workers were evaluated by intradermal skin testing every 6 months for the 5 years of the study. During the 5-year period, 10 of 35 beekeepers (28.6%) were sensitized to honeybee venom as compared to 3 of 26 controls (8.3%). While none of the sensitized subjects reported a SR after honeybee stings, 5 of 35 beekeepers (14.3%) experienced large local reactions. Among the beekeepers, the number of stings per year correlated with the probability of sensitization to honeybee venom. In contrast, other studies show that tolerance can be induced by very frequent stings [51,52]. Beekeepers with more than 200 stings per year appear to be protected from systemic sting reactions (no reactions) as compared to beekeepers stung less than 25 times a year (45% with reactions).

SCIT with purified Hymenoptera venoms is the treatment of choice to modify future risk of anaphylactic reactions in workers sensitized to insect venoms. Full protection can be achieved in 83%–95% of patients with a previous history of anaphylactic reactions [50]. Four treatment regimens include conventional (weekly intervals for increasing doses as an outpatient), rush (inpatient induction phase over 4–7 days), ultrarush (reaching maintenance dose in 1–2 days), or cluster (a modified rush approach with a cluster of injections given at the first visit and reaching a maintenance dose within 6 weeks).

Studies demonstrate the efficacy and safety of the rush venom protocols. For example, 97 patients received rush AIT to bee venom, *Vespula* venom, or both [49]. Severe sting-induced allergic reactions were reported in 48 of them. Specific AIT with bee venom alone in 5, *Vespula* venom alone in 73, and with both in 19 was prescribed. The majority of these patients (90) had cutaneous reactions at the injection site. Unusual adverse events included blood pressure elevation in 11 patients, moderate hypotension in 2, and rhinitis in 1. No anaphylaxis was reported, and the protocol was deemed safe by the authors. No evidence of efficacy was presented.

Another study evaluated the safety of rush AIT with Hymenoptera venoms in 101 patients [52]. Bee venom was used in 52 and yellow jacket in 49 patients. Maintenance dose was reached in all but one patient. Bee venom injections induced a higher rate of SR than did yellow jacket. The risk for SRs was 0.79% per injection in the bee venom group as compared to 0.12% with yellow jacket venom. SRs were reported at all stages of the protocol and were generally mild to moderate, with only two severe reactions reported.

The efficacy and safety of the rush protocol also were evaluated prospectively in 18 patients with a history of allergic reactions to Hymenoptera stings [53]. Seven patients were treated with bee venom and seven with yellow jacket venom during a 7-day protocol. After completing 1 year of AIT, there was a significant increase in specific IgG4 levels compared to baseline levels ($p < .05$). There were no changes in specific IgE levels, mean wheal diameter on SPT, or intradermal skin test reactivity after 1 year of AIT. Four SRs were reported for bee venom (1.7%), while none were reported with yellow jacket venom. During the course of AIT, two patients had field sting events, including a beekeeper who was re-stung several times, without consequence.

Another study evaluated 67 patients with confirmed Hymenoptera venom allergy who were treated with an ultrarush protocol [54]. Thirty-four were treated with wasp venom, 20 with honeybee venom, and 13 with both wasp and honeybee venoms. The maintenance dose was reached in 97.5% of the ultrarush courses. Side effects showed no dose dependency and were mainly mild, with 14 (17.5%) patients experiencing allergic reactions. Furthermore, there was no significant difference in the number of SRs in those receiving honeybee (15.2%) versus wasp venom (19.1%).

Venom immunotherapy can be initiated by different schedules. One study compared the safety of two initiation schedules [55]. Patients were randomized to venom immunotherapy initiation by a semirush schedule over 10 visits (9 weeks) or an ultrarush schedule over 3 visits (2 weeks). The primary outcome was the occurrence of one or more objective SRs during venom immunotherapy initiation. Of 213 eligible patients, 93 were randomized to semirush (44 patients) or ultrarush (49 patients) initiation. SRs were more likely during ultrarush initiation (65% versus 29%; $p < .001$) as were severe reactions (12% versus 0%; $p = .029$). Ultrarush initiation appears to increase the risk of SRs.

While bumblebees are generally not very aggressive and allergic reactions are rare, the expanding use of domesticated bumblebees for pollination of crops has resulted in an increased number of reports of occupational allergic reactions [56]. Patients with allergic reactions to bumblebees are treated with honeybee venom because of the high degree of cross-reactivity with this venom. However, case reports indicate that this may not always be effective [57]. Two patients treated with honeybee venom were later stung by a bumblebee at work and developed anaphylactic reactions. Repeat AIT was performed using bumblebee venom. An in-hospital bumblebee sting challenge resulted in a local cutaneous reaction but no SR. Another case series presented seven cases of bumblebee venom allergy among workers on a bumblebee farm, all of whom had anaphylactic reactions to bumblebee stings [58]. They were treated with bumblebee venom specific AIT. During maintenance AIT, at least 36 bumblebee stings were reported, none of which resulted in SRs. Ultrarush AIT with bumblebee venom was evaluated in one case of a biologist with anaphylaxis after bumblebee stings [51]. Two months after reaching maintenance, the patient had another sting at the workplace. Despite the re-sting event, the patient experienced no SR (see Table 20.6).

Table 20.6 Hymenoptera venom

Allergen (route)	Study design	Number studied	Indication	Results	Level of evidence[a]	Reference
Honeybee, *Vespula* sp. (Rush SCIT)	Unblinded, no placebo	97	Anaphylaxis	• Protocol appears safe • No episodes of anaphylaxis	C	Laurent et al. [49]
Honeybee, yellow jacket (Rush SCIT)	Unblinded, no placebo	101	Anaphylaxis	• Higher rate of systemic reactions with honeybee venom versus yellow jacket	C	Sturm et al. [52]
Honeybee, yellow jacket (Rush SCIT)	Unblinded, placebo-controlled	18	Anaphylaxis	• Increase in specific IgG4 • Two field stings without reaction	B	Pasaoglu et al. [53]
Wasp, honeybee (Ultra-rush SCIT)	Unblinded, no placebo	67	Anaphylaxis	• Protocol appears safe • 17.5% with mild allergic reaction during treatment	B	Roll et al. [54]
Myrmecia pilosula (Semirush or ultrarush)	Unblinded, semirush versus ultrarush	93	Anaphylaxis	• Higher rate of systemic reactions with ultrarush initiation	B	Brown et al. [55]
Bumblebee Rush SCIT)	Case reports	2	Anaphylaxis	• In-hospital sting challenge with local reactions only	D	Stern et al. [57]
Bumblebee (Rush SCIT)	Case series	7	Anaphylaxis	• 36 field stings after AIT without systemic reactions	C	Kochuyt et al. [58]
Bumblebee (Ultra-rush SCIT)	Case report	1	Anaphylaxis	• One field sting after AIT without systemic reaction	D	Roll and Schmid-Grendelmeier [51]

Abbreviations: DBPC, double-blind, placebo-controlled; PEFR, peak expiratory flow rate; SCIT, subcutaneous immunotherapy; SLIT, sublingual immunotherapy; SPT, skin prick test.

[a] Level of evidence: A: Evidence based on randomized controlled trial. B: Evidence based on controlled trial without randomization or other quasi-experimental study design. C: Evidence based on nonexperimental descriptive studies. D: Evidence based on expert opinion.

20.8 CONCLUSION

AIT is rarely indicated to treat OR or OA. It should only be considered to modify respiratory allergic symptoms associated with workplace exposure to natural protein allergens; and when commercial extracts are available both to confirm sensitivity by skin test and for treatment. If indicated, AIT should be considered only after all reasonable attempts aimed at cessation or modification of exposure to the offending allergens in the work environment are exhausted. Although there is only modest evidence to support efficacy and safety in worker populations, it appears reasonable to base treatment decisions on data extrapolated from controlled studies of AIT in nonworker populations. SLIT with commercially available treatment allergens may prove to be a potentially safer modality when compared with SCIT in treating appropriately selected workers.

SALIENT POINTS

1. Environmental control measures to reduce workplace exposures constitute the primary intervention in management of occupational asthma (OA) and occupational rhinitis (OR); therefore, allergen immunotherapy (AIT) to offending aeroallergens is seldom initially considered.

2. If appropriate, AIT should be considered in symptomatic workers whose exposure to workplace allergens can be reduced but not eliminated.
3. Although AIT may be considered in workers with sensitization to protein allergens encountered in the workplace, it cannot be safely recommended for chemical sensitizers due to potential toxicity.
4. Although there is sparse evidence proving efficacy and safety in worker populations, rational treatment decisions for individual workers should be based on controlled clinical trials of AIT obtained in nonoccupational study populations.
5. If indicated, AIT should be strongly considered in workers with OA and OR caused by workplace allergens for which commercial and preferably standardized allergens are readily available. Examples include house dust mites in cleaning workers, stinging insect venom in beekeepers, and cat-allergen extracts in veterinary workers.

REFERENCES

1. Joint Task Force on Practice Parameters. Allergen immunotherapy: A practice parameter. American Academy of Allergy, Asthma and Immunology. American College of Allergy, Asthma and Immunology. *Ann Allergy Asthma Immunol Off Publ Am Coll Allergy Asthma Immunol* 2003; 90(1 Suppl 1): 1–40.

2. Calderon MA, Alves B, Jacobson M, Hurwitz B, Sheikh A, Durham S. Allergen injection immunotherapy for seasonal allergic rhinitis. *Cochrane Database Syst Rev* 2007; (1): CD001936.

3. Varney VA, Tabbah K, Mavroleon G, Frew AJ. Usefulness of specific immunotherapy in patients with severe perennial allergic rhinitis induced by house dust mite: A double-blind, randomized, placebo-controlled trial. *Clin Exp Allergy J Br Soc Allergy Clin Immunol* 2003; 33(8): 1076–1082.

4. Varney VA, Edwards J, Tabbah K, Brewster H, Mavroleon G, Frew AJ. Clinical efficacy of specific immunotherapy to cat dander: A double-blind placebo-controlled trial. *Clin Exp Allergy J Br Soc Allergy Clin Immunol* 1997; 27(8): 860–867.

5. Ohman JL, Findlay SR, Leitermann KM. Immunotherapy in cat-induced asthma. Double-blind trial with evaluation of *in vivo* and *in vitro* responses. *J Allergy Clin Immunol* 1984; 74(3 Pt 1): 230–239.

6. Walker SM, Pajno GB, Lima MT, Wilson DR, Durham SR. Grass pollen immunotherapy for seasonal rhinitis and asthma: A randomized, controlled trial. *J Allergy Clin Immunol* 2001; 107(1): 87–93.

7. Bernstein DI, Zeiss CR. Guidelines for preparation and char-acterization of chemical-protein conjugate antigens. Report of the Subcommittee on Preparation and Characterization of Low Molecular Weight Antigens. *J Allergy Clin Immunol* 1989; 84(5 Pt 2): 820–822.

8. Carino M, Aliani M, Licitra C, Sarno N, Ioli F. Death due to asthma at workplace in a diphenylmethane diisocyanate-sensitized subject. *Respir Int Rev Thorac Dis* 1997; 64(1): 111–113.

9. Ehrlich RI. Fatal asthma in a baker: A case report. *Am J Ind Med* 1994; 26(6): 799–802.

10. Sussman GL, Beezhold DH, Kurup VP. Allergens and natural rubber proteins. *J Allergy Clin Immunol* 2002; 110(2 Suppl): S33–S39.

11. Kelly KJ, Sussman G. Latex allergy: Where are we now and how did we get there? *J Allergy Clin Immunol Pr* 2017; (5): 1212–1216.

12. Bernstein DI, Biagini RE, Karnani R et al. *In vivo* sensitization to purified *Hevea brasiliensis* proteins in health care workers sensitized to natural rubber latex. *J Allergy Clin Immunol* 2003; 111(3): 610–616.

13. NIOSH alert: Preventing allergic reactions to natural rubber latex in the workplace. *Hosp Technol Ser* 1997; 16(7): 10–13.

14. Leynadier F, Herman D, Vervloet D, Andre C. Specific immu-notherapy with a standardized latex extract versus placebo in allergic healthcare workers. *J Allergy Clin Immunol* 2000; 106(3): 585–590.

15. Sastre J, Fernández-Nieto M, Rico P et al. Specific immuno-therapy with a standardized latex extract in allergic work-ers: A double-blind, placebo-controlled study. *J Allergy Clin Immunol* 2003; 111(5): 985–994.

16. Tabar AI, Anda M, Bonifazi F et al. Specific immunotherapy with standardized latex extract versus placebo in latex-allergic patients. *Int Arch Allergy Immunol* 2006; 141(4): 369–376.

17. Cisteró Bahima A, Sastre J, Enrique E et al. Tolerance and effects on skin reactivity to latex of sublingual rush immunotherapy with a latex extract. *J Investig Allergol Clin Immunol* 2004; 14(1): 17–25.

18. Patriarca G, Nucera E, Pollastrini E et al. Sublingual desensitization: A new approach to latex allergy problem. *Anesth Analg* 2002; 95(4): 956–960, table of contents.

19. Nettis E, Colanardi MC, Soccio AL et al. Double-blind, placebo-controlled study of sublingual immunotherapy in patients with latex-induced urticaria: A 12-month study. *Br J Dermatol* 2007; 156(4): 674–681.

20. Gastaminza G, Algorta J, Uriel O et al. Randomized, double-blind, placebo-controlled clinical trial of sublingual immunotherapy in natural rubber latex allergic patients. *Trials* 2011; 12: 191.

21. Lasa Luaces EM, Tabar Purroy AI, García Figueroa BE et al. Component-resolved immunologic modifications, efficacy, and tolerance of latex sublingual immunotherapy in children. *Ann Allergy Asthma Immunol Off Publ Am Coll Allergy Asthma Immunol* 2012; 108(5): 367–372.

22. Armentia A, Martin-Santos JM, Quintero A et al. Bakers' asthma: Prevalence and evaluation of immunotherapy with a wheat flour extract. *Ann Allergy* 1990; 65(4): 265–272.

23. Cianferoni A. Wheat allergy: Diagnosis and management. *J Asthma Allergy* 2016; (9): 13–25.

24. Swaminathan S, Heddle RJ. Wheat flour immunotherapy in baker's asthma. *Intern Med J* 2007; 37(9): 663–664.

25. Susitaival P, Kirk JH, Schenker MB. Atopic symptoms among California veterinarians. *Am J Ind Med* 2003; 44(2): 166–171.

26. Wahn U, Siraganian RP. Efficacy and specificity of immunotherapy with laboratory animal allergen extracts. *J Allergy Clin Immunol* 1980; 65(6): 413–421.

27. Bunyavanich S, Donovan MA, Sherry JM, Diamond DV. Immunotherapy for mouse bite anaphylaxis and allergy. *Ann Allergy Asthma Immunol Off Publ Am Coll Allergy Asthma Immunol* 2013; 111(3): 223–224.

28. Kay AB, Larché M. Allergen immunotherapy with cat aller-gen peptides. *Springer Semin Immunopathol* 2004; 25(3–4): 391–399.

29. Alvarez-Cuesta E, Berges-Gimeno P, González-Mancebo E et al. Sublingual immunotherapy with a standardized cat dander extract: Evaluation of efficacy in a double blind placebo controlled study. *Allergy* 2007; 62(7): 810–817.

30. Senti G, Crameri R, Kuster D et al. Intralymphatic immunotherapy for cat allergy induces tolerance after only 3 injections. *J Allergy Clin Immunol* 2012; 129(5): 1290–1296.

31. Patel D, Couroux P, Hickey P et al. Fel d 1–derived peptide antigen desensitization shows a persistent treatment effect 1 year after the start of dosing: A randomized, placebo-controlled study. *J Allergy Clin Immunol* 2013; 131(1): 103–109.e1–7.

32. Couroux P, Patel D, Armstrong K, Larché M, Hafner RP. Fel d 1-derived synthetic peptide immuno-regulatory epitopes show a long-term treatment effect in cat allergic subjects. *Clin Exp Allergy J Br Soc Allergy Clin Immunol* 2015; 45(5): 974–981.

33. Ohtsuka T, Tsuboi S, Katsutani T et al. [Results of 29-year study of hoya (sea-squirt) asthma in Hatsukaichi, Hiroshima prefecture]. *Arerugi [Allergy]* 1993; 42(3 Pt 1): 214–218.

34. Jyo T, Kuwabara M, Kodomari Y et al. [Immunotherapy using high concentration purified antigen showed remarkable effect in all cases]. *Arerugi [Allergy]* 1991; 40(9): 1194–1199.

35. Jyo T, Kodomari Y, Kodomari N et al. Therapeutic effect and titers of the specific IgE and IgG antibodies in patients with sea squirt allergy (hoya asthma) under a long-term hyposensitization with three sea squirt antigens. *J Allergy Clin Immunol* 1989; 83(2 Pt 1): 386–393.

36. Suzuki H, Oka S, Shigeta S, Ono K, Jyo T, Katsutani T. Isolation and characterization of an asthma-inducing sea-squirt antigen. *J Biochem (Tokyo)* 1984; 96(3): 849–857.

37. Platts-Mills TA, Vervloet D, Thomas WR, Aalberse RC, Chapman MD. Indoor allergens and asthma: Report of the Third International Workshop. *J Allergy Clin Immunol* 1997; 100(6 Pt 1): S2–S24.

38. Pichler CE, Helbling A, Pichler WJ. Three years of specific immunotherapy with house-dust-mite extracts in patients with rhinitis and asthma: Significant improvement of allergen-specific parameters and of nonspecific bronchial hyperreactivity. *Allergy* 2001; 56(4): 301–306.

39. Pifferi M, Baldini G, Marrazzini G et al. Benefits of immunotherapy with a standardized Dermatophagoides pteronyssinus extract in asthmatic children: A three-year prospective study. *Allergy* 2002; 57(9): 785–790.

40. Maestrelli P, Zanolla L, Pozzan M, Fabbri LM; Regione Veneto Study Group on the "Effect of immunotherapy in allergic asthma." Effect of specific immunotherapy added to pharmacologic treatment and allergen avoidance in asthmatic patients allergic to house dust mite. *J Allergy Clin Immunol* 2004; 113(4): 643–649.

41. Lack G, Nelson HS, Amran D et al. Rush immunotherapy results in allergen-specific alterations in lymphocyte function and interferon-γ production in CD4+ T cells. *J Allergy Clin Immunol* 1997; 99(4): 530–538.

42. Blumberga G, Groes L, Dahl R. SQ-standardized house dust mite immunotherapy as an immunomodulatory treatment in patients with asthma. *Allergy* 2011; 66(2): 178–185.

43. Bush RK, Swenson C, Fahlberg B et al. House dust mite sublingual immunotherapy: Results of a US trial. *J Allergy Clin Immunol* 2011; 127(4): 974–981.e1–7.

44. Virchow JC, Backer V, Kuna P et al. Efficacy of a house dust mite sublingual allergen immunotherapy tablet in adults with allergic asthma: A randomized clinical trial. *JAMA* 2016; 315(16): 1715–1725.

45. 2018 GINA Report: Global Strategy for Asthma Management and Prevention [Internet]. Global Initiative for Asthma—GINA. https://ginasthma.org/2018-gina-report-global-strategy-for-asthma-management-and-prevention/

46. Moffitt JE, Golden DBK, Reisman RE et al. Stinging insect hypersensitivity: A practice parameter update. *J Allergy Clin Immunol* 2004; 114(4): 869–886.

47. Kalogeromitros D, Makris M, Gregoriou S, Papaioannou D, Katoulis A, Stavrianeas NG. Pattern of sensitization to honeybee venom in beekeepers: A 5-year prospective study. *Allergy Asthma Proc* 2006; 27(5): 383–387.

48. King TP, Spangfort MD. Structure and biology of stinging insect venom allergens. *Int Arch Allergy Immunol* 2000; 123(2): 99–106.

49. Laurent J, Smiejan JM, Bloch-Morot E, Herman D. Safety of Hymenoptera venom rush immunotherapy. *Allergy* 1997; 52(1): 94–96.

50. Lerch E, Müller UR. Long-term protection after stopping venom immunotherapy: Results of re-stings in 200 patients. *J Allergy Clin Immunol* 1998; 101(5): 606–612.

51. Roll A, Schmid-Grendelmeier P. Ultrarush immunotherapy in a patient with occupational allergy to bumblebee venom (*Bombus terrestris*). *J Investig Allergol Clin Immunol* 2005; 15(4): 305–307.

52. Sturm G, Kränke B, Rudolph C, Aberer W. Rush Hymenoptera venom immunotherapy: A safe and practical protocol for high-risk patients. *J Allergy Clin Immunol* 2002; 110(6): 928–933.

53. Pasaoglu G, Sin BA, Misirligil Z. Rush hymenoptera venom immunotherapy is efficacious and safe. *J Investig Allergol Clin Immunol* 2006; 16(4): 232–238.

54. Roll A, Hofbauer G, Ballmer-Weber BK, Schmid-Grendelmeier P. Safety of specific immunotherapy using a four-hour ultra-rush induction scheme in bee and wasp allergy. *J Investig Allergol Clin Immunol* 2006; 16(2): 79–85.

55. Brown SGA, Wiese MD, van Eeden P et al. Ultrarush versus semirush initiation of insect venom immunotherapy: A randomized controlled trial. *J Allergy Clin Immunol* 2012; 130(1): 162–168.

56. de Groot H, de Graaf-in 't Veld C, van Wijk RG. Allergy to bumblebee venom. I. Occupational anaphylaxis to bumblebee venom: Diagnosis and treatment. *Allergy* 1995; 50(7): 581–584.

57. Stern A, Wüthrich B, Müllner G. Successful treatment of occupational allergy to bumblebee venom after failure with honeybee venom extract. *Allergy* 2000; 55(1): 88–91.

58. Kochuyt AM, Van Hoeyveld E, Stevens EA. Occupational allergy to bumble bee venom. *Clin Exp Allergy J Br Soc Allergy Clin Immunol* 1993; 23(3): 190–195.

Section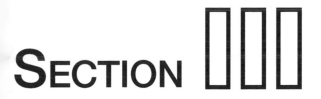

Immunotherapy techniques: Production, preparation and administration of allergen immunotherapy

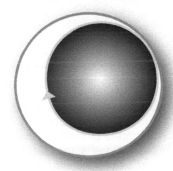

21 Manufacturing pollen and fungal extracts

Robert E. Esch
Lenoir-Rhyne University

Rosa Codina
Allergen Sciences & Consulting
University of South Florida Morsani College of Medicine

Fernando Pineda and Ricardo Palacios
Diater, S.A.

CONTENTS

21.1 INTRODUCTION

Many types of natural allergen extracts are available on the market to diagnose and treat allergic diseases. The commercially available, nonstandardized allergen extracts that have been used for years may not have been subjected to rigorous studies supporting their efficacy. Therefore, it is often difficult for the clinician to select the most appropriate extracts to use in daily practice. A critical element to make such decisions is to know how allergen extracts are manufactured. Available scientific information regarding the topic is

scarce and almost limited to a series of articles prepared as a part of a task force to inform the clinician about the subject [1–9].

Because pollen and fungal raw materials are utilized to manufacture medicinal products for animal use, they are considered active pharmaceutical ingredients (APIs). APIs that are produced by chemical synthesis, extraction or recovery from natural products, cell culture or fermentation, recombinant DNA technology, or any combination of these processes are regulated by the U.S. Food and Drug Administration (FDA) and the Center for Biologics Evaluations and Research (CBER) in the United States [10]. The main regulatory agencies in Europe include the European Medicines Agency (EMA) in compliance with the European Pharmacopoeia (EP) [11,12], although other entities operate in particular countries.

Among the factors responsible for the composition and quality of allergen extracts, the raw materials used to make them and their processing play an important role in assuring that the final products are safe and efficacious as well as that the lot-to-lot consistency is maximized to the best possible extent [13,14]. The use of natural products poses various challenges to allergen manufacturing companies and regulatory entities. For example, phylogenetically and nonphylogenetically related pollen and fungal taxa often cross-react, and this phenomenon should receive appropriate attention to assure that the materials contain clinically relevant, nonredundant allergens, and that they are obtained from the appropriate genera and/or species.

Other selective challenges associated with the procurement of natural allergenic raw materials exist. For example, pollen is exposed to the outdoor environment, and thus natural and man-made contaminants might impact the product [1,2]. Fungi are organisms that mutate, potentially changing their allergenic characteristics; they can produce mycotoxins and other metabolites that must be removed during processing. Therefore, the careful selection of fungal strains as well as the validation of cultivation, harvesting, and processing steps are critical parameters to obtain appropriate fungal raw materials [3].

The objective of this chapter is to describe how pollen and fungal allergen extracts are manufactured, from the procurement of appropriate allergenic raw materials until the derived extracts are vialed and made available to the clinician. Practical recommendations and future directions to improve the quality and consistency of pollen and fungal extracts are also discussed. This chapter does not reiterate information associated with the topic, presented in detail in other sections of this book. It is beyond the scope of this chapter to describe how purified or recombinant allergens are obtained and converted into vaccines. It is expected that the information presented will assist the clinician in selecting appropriate pollen and fungal extracts for use in daily practice.

The published literature regarding portions of the topics presented in this chapter is scarce. Therefore, we have utilized personal experience and expertise in making it as informative and useful as possible.

21.2 POLLEN AND FUNGAL RAW MATERIALS USED TO PREPARE ALLERGEN EXTRACTS

As discussed in other chapters of this book (see Chapters 10, 11, 12, and 13), exposure to pollen and fungal allergens can cause hypersensitivity diseases, including allergic rhinoconjunctivitis and asthma, in genetically predisposed individuals. Many plant taxonomic groups produce allergenic pollen (see Chapters 10, 11, and 12 of this book). In addition, fungi are recognized etiologic agents of other hypersensitivity illnesses, such as hypersensitivity pneumonitis (extrinsic allergic alveolitis), fungal allergic sinusitis, bronchopulmonary mycoses, and atopic dermatitis [3]. The fungi associated with hypersensitivity reactions belong to different taxonomic groups, including Ascomycetes, Basidiomycetes, and Zygomycetes. Among them, the asexual or mitotic forms of Ascomycetes, known as mitosporic fungi, comprise most of the culprit genera (see Chapter 13).

While exposure to pollen allergens occurs mainly outdoors, people can be exposed to fungal allergens and antigens both outdoors and indoors [15–18]. The environmental parameters responsible for fungal growth include moisture, a source of nutrients, oxygen, and particular temperature and light conditions. However, because fungi have evolved to colonize different habitats, the combination of the conditions for fungi to grow can fluctuate within ample ranges. Fungi are cosmopolitans and are present everywhere on Earth, except in areas with permanent ice covers.

The pollen and fungal raw materials used to produce allergen extracts are obtained from different sources, have selective characteristics, and pose diverse challenges during their procurement and processing. The most distinctive feature between pollen and fungal raw materials is their respective origins. While pollen is obtained from nature, fungal materials are derived from laboratory cultures [3], except for spores from Basidiomycetes and Ascomycetes, which are very difficult to harvest in sufficient quantities to prepare allergen extracts. This is the reason why allergen extracts derived from these fungal groups are not commercially available.

21.2.1 Pollen raw materials

Plant biodiversity is responsible for the pollen genera and species present in particular locations, which are collected for the production of allergen extracts. The factors responsible for plant and pollen biodiversity can be classified as natural or associated with human activities. Both factors interact and should be considered to properly evaluate the clinical relevance of different pollen genera/species and obtain the appropriate products to produce clinically relevant allergen extracts.

Plants selectively colonize particular ecological niches based on their genetic makeup. For example, 10 major floristic zones have been described in the United States, and many of the pollen genera/species in these zones are allergenic [19]. The United States is a large nation, with the approximate size of all combined European countries. Therefore, climatic gradients exist among different geographic areas, including subtropical, polar, temperate, and desert environments. These gradients result in a larger botanical biodiversity compared to that existing in each European country. This fact is partially responsible for the manufacture of many pollen allergen extracts derived from local species in the United States to satisfy the needs of local allergists, who have traditionally preferred these extracts rather than those derived from cross-reactive species or even families. This perception contributes to the fact that an excessive number of pollen extracts are available on the U.S. market.

Climate gradients analogous to those existing in the United States also exist in Europe, where different floristic zones have been described. They include Boreal, Alpine, Atlantic, Continental, Mediterranean, and Subtropical [19–21].

Geographic location, local weather, and soil composition are responsible for plant growth and nutrition, which affect the qualitative and quantitative allergenic composition of pollen. For example, a study that investigated the Amb a 1 content of short ragweed (*Ambrosia artemisiifolia*) pollen collected from the same location over a 30-year time span indicates that the concentration of this allergen can vary by 10-fold, as assessed by quantitative immunochemical tests [13] (Figure 21.1). Pollen collection and storage also can affect the allergenic composition of pollen [22]. While it is possible to address and monitor some of these variables,

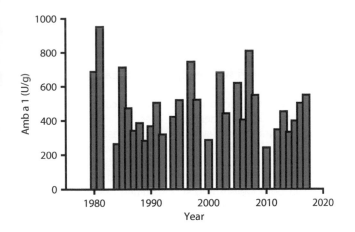

Figure 21.1 Amb a 1 content detected in *Ambrosia artemisiifolia* pollen collected from the same location over 30 years.

it is not possible to control all of them, in particular, the weather and soil composition where individual plants grow and where the pollen is collected from.

Many genetic varieties of botanical species exist due to agricultural practices and natural hybridization. Different plant varieties of the same species often produce pollen with distinctive allergenic characteristics. For example, a study that investigated the allergenicity of pollen derived from six different varieties of olive trees (*Olea europaea*) identified large differences in allergenicity, as determined by various chemical and immunochemical tests [23]. This phenomenon implies that an extensive level of control should be ideally implemented at the manufacturing level to assure the consistency of the final extracts to the best possible extent.

The pollen derived from many plant families, genera, and species often contain cross-reacting allergens belonging to conserved allergen families, e.g., pathogenesis-related proteins and profilins, which are also present in fruits and vegetables [24–26]. This explains why some subjects who are allergic to particular pollen species also experience allergic symptoms following ingestion of particular fruits and vegetables. For example, subjects allergic to short ragweed (*Ambrosia artemisiifolia*) pollen often react to bananas and melons. Similarly, subjects with clinical sensitivity to birch (*Betula* spp.) pollen might also experience symptoms following the ingestion of apples and peaches.

The cross-reactivity phenomenon described is relevant to prepare allergen extracts for diagnosis and allergen immuno-therapy (AIT). While cross-reactive allergen extracts can be used for diagnostic purposes, the sensitizing extracts are the election of choice for AIT.

Another consideration is the fact that because pollen is exposed to the outdoor environment, naturally occurring biological contaminants can impact pollen. For example, fungal spores and associated structures, bacteria, pollen grains derived from other species, plant debris, algae, and insect debris can potentially contaminate pollen.

The application of molecular engineering techniques since 1996 has steadily increased to obtain crops with certain desirable characteristics [27,28]. Today, more than 50% of crops in the United States are transgenic [29]. In some cases, allergen extracts are prepared from pollen derived from transgenic plants due to the difficulty of obtaining sufficient quantities of pollen derived from wild-type plants. These plants include many grasses and some tree species, for example, corn (*Zea mays*) and olive tree (*Olea europaea*), respectively.

Both the U.S. Environmental Protection Agency (EPA) and the U.S. FDA generally share responsibilities of regulating the safety of foods for the consumer, including those obtained from genetically modified crops [30]. However, a clear opinion regarding the safety of products derived from transgenic plants for pharmaceutical applications has not been disclosed. In Europe, European regulatory agencies approve the use of pollen derived from transgenic plants if its use is appropriately justified [11]. Scientific evidence, obtained from risk-analysis evaluations, is lacking to preclude the use of such pollen for pharmaceutical applications due to potential health concerns [31–34].

Another aspect regarding the impact of human activities on pollen is associated with environmental contamination. The use of fossil fuels, fertilizers, and pesticides causes the release of chemical products into the environment. The potential effects of these components on pollen are largely unknown. However, there is ample evidence that increasing levels of carbon dioxide in the atmosphere could augment the allergenicity of short ragweed and other pollen species [35,36]. In addition, several observations suggest that pollen collected from areas with high levels of air pollution have greater pro-inflammatory properties than pollen obtained from nonpolluted locations [21,35,36]. This effect on the pollen collected for manufacturing purposes should be investigated.

Human activities also affect plant distribution, pollination seasons, and the allergenic relevance of different pollen species For example, urbanization alters the distribution of native plants by reducing the sizes and locations of their ecological habitats. On the contrary, plants that produce highly allergenic pollen are often introduced into urban areas because of man-made changes to the landscape [37]. Short ragweed (*Ambrosia artemisiifolia*), a weed native to the United States, was introduced into Europe years ago and now is becoming a relevant source of seasonal allergies in many European countries [36,39]. A gradual increase in the global ambient temperature or global warming, and associated changes in rainfall is another phenomenon resulting from a long-term impact of human activities on the planet, reportedly to affect plant distribution, pollen allergenicity, and pollination patterns [34–41].

21.2.2 Pollen collection and cleaning practices

Pollen collection is tedious and requires a high level of specialization. The pollination seasons associated with botanical species typically vary depending on climate and geographic location. In addition, many pollen species often need to be collected over short time intervals and at specific times of the day due to rapid fluctuations of particular environmental parameters, e.g., ambient humidity, which affects pollen release.

A few large pollen collection producers utilize their own land to cultivate the desired plants for pollen collection, under conditions that minimize exposure to man-made pollutants. However, this is an emerging strategy and often does not result in sufficient quantities of pollen necessary for manufacturers who produce pollen extracts. Therefore, pollen also is collected from naturally growing plants that are not planted for the specific purpose of pollen collection.

Many small family-owned pollen collection entities also obtain pollen for pharmaceutical use. A close collaboration between pollen collection entities and allergen manufacturing companies is essential to maximize the efficacy of the collection activities and assure that sufficient quantities of the necessary pollen genera or species are obtained.

Three general main methods used to collect pollen from wind-pollinated plants are used; first, the water-set; second, the vacuum; and third, the cut/dry/sieve. While many pollen species can be collected using any of these three methods, the decision as to which collection practice is utilized depends on the expertise of particular collectors and the resources they have available. Each of the three collection methods has advantages and disadvantages.

The water-set method consists of placing plant parts containing mature anthers on trays of water. As the anthers open, pollen falls onto a clean surface from which it is collected (Figure 21.2). The main advantage of this method is that it results in very clean pollen. On the contrary, it is very labor intensive, requires large facilities, and the resulting pollen can be affected by moisture and subsequent microbial growth.

The vacuum method is recommended for collecting pollen from plants that grow in pure strands, such as most grasses and some weeds. As soon as the plants begin to bloom, the pollen is collected. Before beginning this process, the field is carefully inspected to remove any infected or different plants that bloom simultaneously. The main advantage of this method is that it is relatively simple to perform. The main problem is that the resulting pollen often contains high levels of biological contaminants, which can be difficult to remove.

The cut/dry/sieve method is extensively used to collect pollen from plants that produce male catkins such as oak (*Quercus* spp.) and birch (*Betula* spp.). The advantage of this method is that it allows for the collection of large quantities of pollen. The catkins are removed from the trees as they begin to open and are placed on clean surfaces in a heated room (Figure 21.3). However, the resulting pollen needs extensive cleaning, comparable to pollen obtained by vacuuming.

Regardless of the collection method, the pollen is then dried to reduce moisture content and prevent microbial growth and potential allergen biodeterioration. This activity is usually performed in moisture-controlled environments.

When the pollen is sufficiently dry, plant parts, fungal spores, insect fragments, and foreign pollen grains are removed. The two primary methods to clean pollen are mechanical gradation sieving and air classification, both described later.

Mechanical gradation sieving is the simplest and most widely used method to clean pollen because sieving with various micron-sized meshes can remove biologic contaminants that differ in size (Figure 21.4). The air classification method can separate particles that differ in both weight and size, resulting in very clean pollen. However, air classification equipment is costly, and the cleaning process often disrupts pollen, making its allergenic quality difficult to assess. Some cytoplasmic material containing allergens can be lost during this cleaning process. Another strategy to clean pollen is the use of organic solvents, although this procedure alone might not be efficient to obtain pollen with the purity required for further manufacturing, and it is typically performed later after pollen has been cleaned using other methods.

The procedures utilized to clean pollen depend on the resources available at pollen collection sites. The utilization of particular collection and cleaning methods is not associated with one particular pollen species versus another or with standardized or nonstandardized allergen extracts [1,14,42]. The final goal is to obtain large quantities of pure pollen regardless of their final applications. Allergen manufacturing companies use the pollen available at a given time regardless of the methods used to collect and purify it.

Established programs to qualify pollen collection entities and/or individual collectors are lacking in both the United States and Europe. Therefore, allergen manufacturing companies usually propose the criteria for approval of pollen collection entities and individual collectors.

21.2.3 Pollen identification and evaluation of biological contaminants

The identity of the pollen species collected to manufacture allergen extracts must be verified. Pollen collectors are requested to provide portions of the plants to verify plant identity from which pollen is obtained. Allergen manufacturing companies ideally should employ expert botanists to perform this task.

Pollen microscopic analysis is performed to further verify pollen identity and assess its purity (Figure 21.5). Pollen purity assessments include counting and identifying biological components contaminating the pollen. However, this method of evaluating pollen purity may not permit assessment of the potential clinical relevance or amounts of specific contaminants compared to the pollen in the final sample. While the potential relevance of many pollen contaminants is unknown, volumetric counting instead of particle counting could provide a better estimation of the amount of foreign biological materials contained in the collected pollen. However, standardized and approved methods to perform this evaluation are lacking.

For the purpose of microscopic pollen identity and purity evaluations, samples are stained and examined under various magnifications, even though the staining cannot selectively differentiate viable from nonviable pollen grains. The detection of nonviable pollen grains could indicate that the pollen has

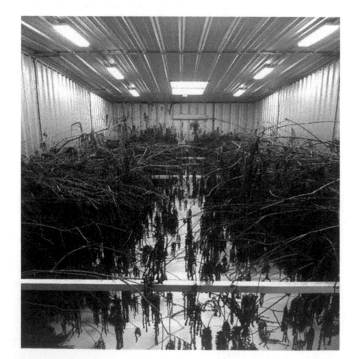

Figure 21.2 Pollen being collected using the water-set method. (Photo courtesy of copyright owner, Stallergenes Greer.)

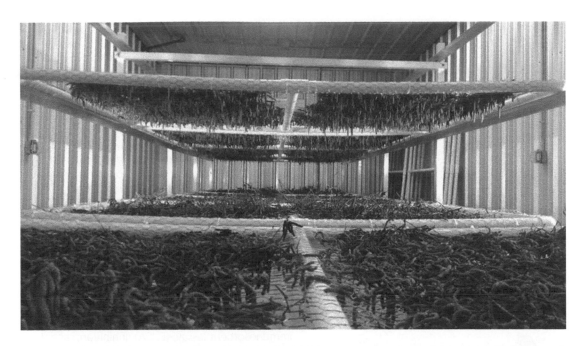

Figure 21.3 Pollen being collected using the cut, dry, and sieve method. (Photo courtesy of copyright owner, Stallergenes Greer.)

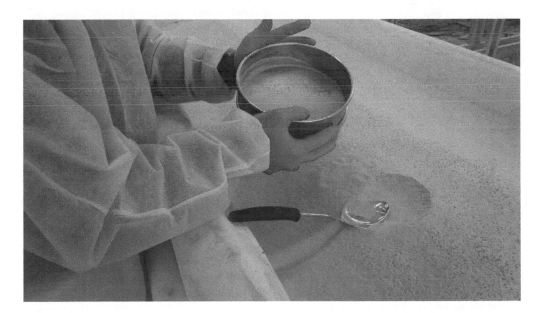

Figure 21.4 Pollen being cleaned by mechanical gradation sieving. (Photo courtesy of copyright owner, Stallergenes Greer.)

been impacted by air pollution, and that therefore its use for the production of allergen extracts should be reconsidered.

Staining solutions able to differentiate viable from nonviable pollen are available, mainly for agricultural purposes [43,44]. Currently, these solutions are not used to evaluate the quality of the pollen collected for pharmaceutical applications because it is assumed that both viable and nonviable pollen are equally allergenic. Nevertheless, this assumption may not be true because pollen allergenicity may be compromised under conditions that render pollen nonviable, for example, exposure to high temperatures during transportation and processing.

Microscopic pollen analysis also can provide valuable information regarding pollen quality. For example, the presence of many plant parts and a variety of miscellaneous fungal spores generally indicates that the pollen is not sufficiently clean and that additional activities to remove biological contaminants are necessary. On the contrary, the presence of large amounts of one single spore type, hyphae, or sporulating structure indicates that fungi have infested the pollen for a period, most likely because of excessive moisture.

21.2.4 Fungal raw materials

The role of fungi in allergic diseases is established [3,14,42], but major clinical problems still exist in defining to what extent an allergic patient's symptoms can be attributed to specific fungal species.

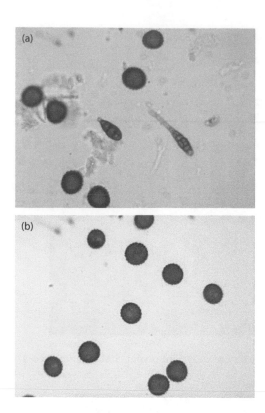

Figure 21.5 Microphotograph of *Ambrossia artemisiifolia* pollen before (a) and after (b) cleaning.

As compared to pollen exposure, typically seasonal, patients may be exposed to outdoor fungal spores and other fungal products throughout the year. Indoor fungal products may also be present throughout the year. The types and levels of these components to which people are exposed through different routes on any given day depends on their home or work environment as well as their daily activities.

Over decades, several attempts were made among allergists to build lists of allergenic fungi for use in diagnosis and treatment. The first of such attempts in the United States was made by the Association of Allergists for Mycological Investigations in the 1960s. The "MMP Molds" named for three of its members, Morrow, Meyer, and Prince, served as the framework on which the practicing allergist could add or delete, depending on location or clinical judgement [45–47]. For example, the 10 most common allergenic fungal genera, based on prevalence and on skin sensitization among allergic subjects in the southeastern United States are *Alternaria*, *Helminthosporium*, *Cladosporium*, *Aspergillus*, *Penicillium*, *Epicoccum*, *Fusarium*, *Stemphylium*, *Botrytis*, and *Curvularia* [48]. A thorough clinical history with indoor environmental assessments may be sometimes useful in clinical diagnoses, but additional obstacles still exist [49]. Fungi adapt by modifying their metabolism to changing environments and can mutate at a high rate. Thus, natural variants of a single species are innumerable, and the differences between these variants range from indistinguishable to great. It is worth noting that investigators studying fungal allergens have reported greater differences among strains of the same species than among genera [50–52]. IgE cross-reactivity among different related fungal taxa is common (see Chapter 13). For example, *Alternaria* spp., *Stemphylium* spp., and *Ulocladium* spp. produce allergens homologous to Alt a 1, the major allergen from *Alternaria alternata* [53]. In some cases, it has been observed that extracts

derived from *Stemphylium* spp. or *Ulocladium* spp. contain greater concentrations of Alt a 1 than *A. alternata* extracts.

Fungi obtained from well-characterized pure seed cultures are grown under defined laboratory conditions to control the quality of the source materials used to produce allergen extracts [3,14,42]. More than 200 different fungal allergen extracts are produced and marketed by U.S.-licensed manufacturers. The strains used for this purpose are selected and maintained under particular conditions that minimize the occurrence of the spontaneous genetic mutations that could potentially alter the identity and/or quality of the raw material. For example, fungal source materials used to produce allergen extracts should ideally yield particular amounts and types of clinically relevant allergens and contain limited quantities of nonallergenic products and/or secondary metabolites. The culture medium should be devoid of potentially allergenic substances if not removed during processing. The relative importance of spores, mycelial fractions, and filtrates of fungal cultures have been evaluated for some fungi [52,54–56]. Bisht et al. [52] compared culture filtrate (CF) to mycelium (M)-spore(S) extracts prepared from *Epicoccum nigrum* cultures using sodium dodecyl sulfate polyacrylamide gel electrophoresis (SDS-PAGE) and immunoblotting, enzyme-linked immunosorbent assay (ELISA) inhibition, and by skin testing in patients sensitized to this fungus. Although the CF and M-S extracts showed comparable skin reactivity in sensitized patients, there were qualitative and quantitative differences between the two extracts, suggesting the need to combine CF and M-S antigens to produce a complete and more representative *E. nigrum* allergen product. Similar results were obtained when evaluating *Fusarium solani* CF, M, and S extracts. Verma and Gangal [54] showed increased overall potency in *F. solani* CF extracts and major allergen content by immunoblot and ELISA-inhibition testing. Most of the IgE-binding components detected in M and S extracts were also detected in the CF extract. However, due to the presence of unique IgE-binding components in the M and S extracts, the authors recommended combining the three fractions. Martinez et al. [57,58] identified a difference between the concentration of Alt a 1 in a CF extract, compared to M and S extracts, particularly when *Alternaria* spp. was grown in protein-rich media. Similarly, Arruda et al. [55] compared Asp f I levels in *A. fumigatus* S, M, and CF fractions to determine the kinetics of allergen production. The ratio of Asp f 1:protein was found to be 100-fold lower in M than in CF, suggesting the need to include CF fractions in *A. fumigatus* allergen extracts to supply a product with a suitable Asp f 1 content. Nissen et al. [56] evaluated cellular and CF extracts from *Candida albicans*, *Fusarium moniliforme*, *Penicillium notatum*, *Malassezia furfur* (*Pityrosporum ovale*), and *Trichophyton rubrum* cultures by IgE-immunoblotting using sera from atopic dermatitis patients, histamine release, and skin testing. Patients produced IgE antibodies recognizing allergens present in both CF and cellular fractions from multiple fungal sources. Overall, IgE binding was more frequent and pronounced toward CF preparations, but differences were not significant when considering their relative reactivities in histamine release and skin testing. These experiments suggest that excluding culture filtrate, mycelia, or spores as source materials for the production of fungal extracts could reduce their suitability for use in some patients. Since different patients respond to selective arrays of allergens in any given extract, the goal should be to produce extracts with a complete repertoire of allergens consistently, not to maximize the concentration of a few major ones. Thus, an optimal composition of the fungal raw materials used to manufacture allergen extracts may depend on multiple factors including the characteristics of

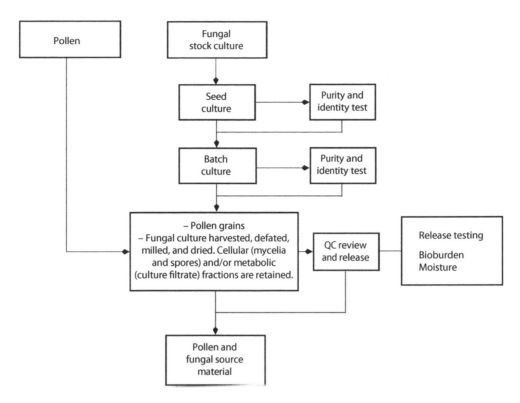

Figure 21.6 Flowchart outlining the general steps involved in the production of allergen extracts. (Adapted from Hauck PR, Williamson S. *Clin Rev Allergy Immunol* 2001; 21: 93–110.)

particular fungi, as well as the specific patients' sensitization profiles and types of immune responses, which are unique for each patient.

Each manufacturer utilizes different strains as well as different techniques and equipment for their cultivation, harvesting, and processing. Some manufacturers may use particular culture conditions to maximize sporulation, while others may optimize those that promote the production of both mycelia and spores. For these reasons, variability exists among manufacturers' products that may be labeled with the same fungal genera and species [59–61].

Licensed manufacturers must have a separate facility dedicated for culturing and processing fungi [42]. While the specific methods used to produce fungal source materials may vary among manufacturers, the general process is analogous in concept (Figure 21.6).

The seed cultures are inspected regularly for identity and purity by morphologic tests, then used to inoculate batch cultures. These cultures are grown until they are ready for harvesting and further processing.

The growth conditions, including grow medium, temperature, humidity, pH, cultivation time, photoperiod, and aeration are controlled to maximize the product quality and yield. The culture is rendered nonviable, usually by the addition of phenol prior to harvesting. This is required for the safety of manufacturing personnel and to prevent contamination of the manufacturing environment with viable spores and other fungal products. The fungal cells, mycelia, and spores are harvested, generally by separating the pellicle from the culture followed by homogenization, acetone treatment, drying, and milling. The spent medium, which contains secreted allergens, may also be harvested and processed to remove low molecular weight substances including media components. There has been no systematic clinical study evaluating compositional differences or their

impact on diagnostic or therapeutic efficacy [62]. With the exception of a few allergenic fungal species, specific fungal allergens have not been identified and characterized (see Chapter 13). Thus, to date, no fungal allergen products have been standardized in the United States or Europe. Each manufacturing company performs internal standardization by establishing manufacturing and quality controls to ensure lot-to-lot consistency and reproducibility of its allergenic extracts to the best possible extent. Some fungal standardization approaches have been suggested in the past, including pooling selected relevant strains to ensure an adequate composition of the derived raw materials [63,64].

21.3 HOW POLLEN AND FUNGAL EXTRACTS ARE MADE

21.3.1 General measures to assure quality of pollen and fungal raw materials from procurement to extraction

As previously discussed in this chapter, natural allergenic raw materials, particularly pollen and fungi, are complex because several genetic and environmental factors account for a large lot-to-lot qualitative and quantitative variation of their composition. This is responsible for the fact that in the United States, allergenic raw materials are not required to meet particular specifications because it is difficult, if not impossible, to control them. It is assumed that the manufacturing process will assure that the final extracts are appropriate for human use. Therefore, stability studies to justify assigned expiration and retest dates are primarily conducted on the final extracts and intermediate products and not on the raw materials [65–67]. In the United States, nonstandardized extracts and extract mixtures lacking standards of potency are exempt from this requirement [68,69]. For extracts formulated in at least 50% glycerin and stored at 2°C–8°C, the expiratory dating is a maximum of 6 years—no more than 3 years in manufacturer's storage, and no more than 3 years after the product is distributed by the manufacturer. For extracts formulated in less than 50% glycerin, and for alum-precipitated extracts, the dating is a maximum of 3 years—no more than 18 months in manufacturer's storage and no more than 18 months after distribution by the manufacturer. In Europe, it is mandatory to control the quality of both the raw materials and the derived extracts [11,12].

While it is not possible to control all the genetic and environmental factors that affect allergenic raw materials, it is critical to store them properly after they are obtained to assure that their allergenic activity is not compromised before extraction. While the FDA has not proposed expiration dates for raw materials, European regulatory agencies indicate that stability must be adequately justified with the corresponding stability programs. However, these programs have not been established.

A pilot study that investigated the stability of two grass pollen and one fungal species (*Phleum pratense, Cynodon dactylon,* and *Alternaria alternata*, respectively) stored under different temperature and moisture conditions over a 10-year period, indicates that no obvious allergen degradation occurred, as determined by the parameters tested, if the products were properly dried and stored

under particular temperatures [22]. Table 21.1 summarizes the results of this study.

Real-time stability studies are necessary to perform, generally following proposed guidelines. The information derived from the completion of these studies would likely identify selective expiration dates for different pollen and fungal raw materials, as expected, due to their diverse nature. However, such guidelines for allergenic raw materials have not been proposed in the United States or in Europe.

Quality guidelines for herbal drugs and foods are used to propose limits for potential contaminants in pollen and fungal raw materials, particularly in the European Union [11,12] where it is an ongoing requirement to test pollen for the presence of various heavy metals, residuals solvents, and many pesticides even though many of them are no longer in use.

In the United States, the use of products for pest control (including herbicides, insecticides, and fungicides) is regulated by the EPA, according to the directions of the Federal Insecticide, Fungicide, and Rodenticide Act (FIFRA) to reinforce regulations regarding pesticide use in this country. In Europe, analogous regulations are managed by the European Commission, European Food Safety Authority (EFSA), European Chemical Agency (ECHA) in cooperation with the European Union Member States. In addition, the European Pharmacopoeia establishes the limits of pesticides for pharmaceutical products according to general and individual monographs [70–72].

Analogously, fungal raw materials must be tested for the potential presence of various mycotoxins, derived from various fungi. The threshold limits for the detected concentrations of

Table 21.1 Stability results of two pollen (*Phleum pratense* and *Cynodon dactylon*) and one fungal (*Alternaria alternata*) species stored under various temperatures and moisture conditions for a maximum of 10 or 8 years

| Raw material | Assay | Years stable under each storage condition | | | | | |
| | | <0°C | | | 20°C–25°C | | |
		<5% RH	7%–8% RH	>10% RH	<5%RH	7%–8% RH	>10% RH
Phleum pratense (timothy grass)	Total protein content	>10	>10	6 to <10	6 to 10	NT	NT
	Relative potency	>10	>10	6 to <10	6 to 10	NT	NT
	SDS-PAGE	>10	>10	6 to <10	6 to 10	NT	NT
	SDS-PAGE/Western blot	>10	>10	6 to <10	6 to 10	NT	NT
Cynodon dactylon (Bermuda grass)	Total protein content	>8	>8	3 to 8	3 to 8	NT	NT
	Relative potency	>8	>8	3 to 8	3 to 8	NT	NT
	SDS-PAGE	>8	>8	>8	38	NT	NT
	SDS-PAGE/Western blot	>8	>8	>8	3 to 8	NT	NT
Alternaria alternata	Total protein content	>10	>10	>10	>10	>10	>10
	Relative potency	>10	>10	>10	>10	>10	>10
	SDS-PAGE	>10	>10	>10	>10	>10	>10
	SDS-PAGE/Western blot	>10	>10	>10	>10	>10	>10
	Major allergen (Alt a1)	>10	>10	>10	>10	6 to 10	6 to 10

Abbreviations: NT, not tested due to loss of stability detected at the previous testing interval; RH, relative humidity; SDS-PAGE, sodium dodecyl sulfate polyacrylamide gel electrophoresis.

those components must be less than proposed levels in foods or herbal drugs, according to toxicologic assays on animal models (LD_{50} results may be misleading due to the physiologic differences between mice, rats, and humans) after gastrointestinal exposure and these laid on general and individual monographs. [72]

The need for testing allergenic raw materials in the European Community has expanded because of the demands of regulatory entities, and a number of laboratories specialized in such testing have emerged in Europe but not in other areas of the world.

Another essential measure to assure the quality of allergenic raw materials is to properly train and qualify the personnel involved in performing different tasks associated with the process. Currently, this training is internally provided at allergen manufacturing companies because accredited programs in that regard are lacking.

It is important to perform all activities associated with each type of raw material, including pollen and fungi, in dedicated areas of allergen manufacturing companies where other types of materials are not present. Maximizing proper ventilation, maximizing cleanliness, and avoiding passive transport of allergens are necessary to prevent potential cross-contamination among different products. The specific measures to avoid potential passive cross-contamination generally vary among allergen manufacturing companies. However, universal guidelines mandate that the personnel involved in the processing of allergenic raw materials and manufacture of allergen extracts use personal protective equipment, not only to protect themselves from exposure to allergens but also to minimize potential cross-contamination among different products, including those transported by humans into a building. Toward these ends, manufacturers conduct cleaning and process validation studies to assure that their source materials maintain their identity, purity, and potency throughout the manufacturing process [73,74]. Furthermore, pollen and fungal source materials have unique attributes as source materials, and validation studies are designed to address these issues [75].

21.3.2 General manufacturing overview

Several steps are involved in the processing of raw materials to convert them into allergen extracts (Figure 21.7). Some of the steps apply to any type of raw material, others are selective, and a few are exclusive depending on the specific material that needs to be extracted.

It is routine to defat allergenic source materials using diethyl ether or acetone to remove lipids and to facilitate the extraction of proteins. The amount of lipids in pollen and fungal source materials varies widely depending on species and growth conditions. The selection and use of optimal extraction procedures are based on variables of temperature, time, extraction fluid, and ratio [42]. The final form of the extract, whether aqueous, glycerinated, lyophilized, or alum-precipitated, will also be a factor. Large-scale extractions performed by commercial manufacturers can impose limitations on process variables. For example, short extraction times are difficult to replicate due to the length of time necessary to mix large quantities of source materials with extraction fluid and to complete solid/liquid separation by filtration or centrifugation. Regardless of the extraction parameters selected, they must be based on internal validation work conducted by each manufacturer.

After the extract is separated from the pellet, some products may undergo additional processing, e.g., dialysis, concentration, addition of preservatives, and alum precipitation, prior to final

aseptic filtration to render the product sterile. Critical process parameters for each step must be studied as part of the process validation. For example, the microbial bioburden prior to aseptic filtration must be studied to validate that the filtering process is suitable under the "worst-case" conditions. The sterile bulk product is tested and released for commercial distribution as a "stock concentrate" or compounded with other bulk products to produce "stock mixtures." These stock concentrates and mixtures are used to prepare individual prescriptions by compounding pharmacies or practicing allergists. The policies and regulations pertaining to the mixing, diluting, and repackaging of licensed allergenic products for individual prescriptions are addressed in an FDA guidance [76] and in the U.S. Pharmacopeia General Chapter <797> [77].

Most allergen extracts in the United States, including those derived from pollen and fungi, are available in both aqueous and glycerinated forms. Extracts used for diagnostic prick testing are exclusively used in glycerinated form, while both aqueous and glycerinated extracts are used to compound immunotherapy formulations. In Europe, most aeroallergen extracts for subcutaneous immunotherapy (SCIT) are adsorbed to depot materials (aluminum hydroxide) to facilitate their slow release. Allergoids are allergen extracts that have been chemically modified to reduce their allergenicity while preserving the antigenicity. They have reduced IgE binding capacity and are also used for SCIT purposes in Europe [78].

Perhaps the most distinct feature between the types of allergen extracts available in the United States and Europe is associated with the regulatory guidelines in place in each area of the world. For example, in Europe, the EMA regulations are based on the concept of "homologous groups," which permits the extrapolation of quality data internally obtained by each manufacturing company among products classified in the same group [79]. On the contrary, in the United States, quality data are obtained with references manufactured and supplied by the FDA. In addition, the EMA includes guidelines for allergenic substances that are not licensed in the United States, such as recombinant allergens, synthetic peptides, and allergoids.

21.4 NUMBER OF POLLEN AND FUNGAL ALLERGEN EXTRACTS AVAILABLE ON THE MARKET: HOW MANY ARE NECESSARY TO DIAGNOSE AND TREAT THE ALLERGIC PATIENT?

A consideration regarding the large number of pollen and fungal extracts available on the U.S. market is associated with biogeography and the perspectives that allergists have had for years regarding allergen extracts, based on particular preferences. However, because it is clear that a high level of allergenic cross-reactivity among closely related and distant phylogenetic groups exists, perspectives are evolving to reflect a better scientific understanding with practical applications in the allergy practice.

Years ago, CBER created a committee to review scientific data about the safety and efficacy of nonstandardized allergen extracts. Such extracts were classified into various categories according to the level of scientific information available and safety considerations to justify their use [80]. CBER proposed to remove all products with

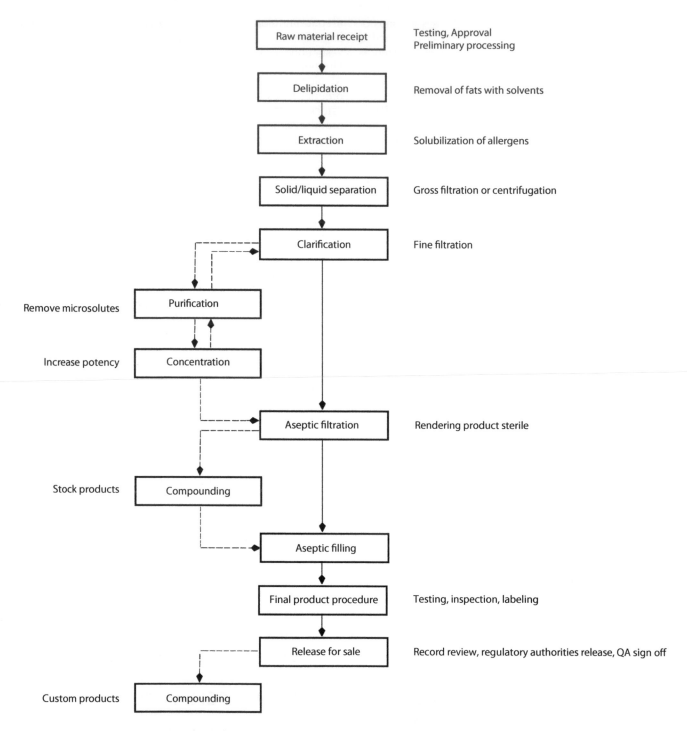

Figure 21.7 Flowchart outlining the general steps to convert pollen and fungal raw materials into allergen extracts.

potential safety concerns or lack of therapeutic value (Docket #FDA-2011-N-599). While this activity is taking place slowly, the number of pollen and fungal extracts currently available on the market likely will be reduced considerably. This should be the first step to select additional allergen extracts for standardization, although the high level of effort and cost requires a thorough evaluation of the potential benefits of this process.

The current perspective in the European Community is different because of the increasing regulatory requirements regarding allergenic raw materials and extracts. The concept of

"homologous groups" is based on similar biochemical composition and homology/cross-reactivity of allergens or allergen sources. European regulatory agencies adopted this concept and require that allergen manufacturing companies obtain quality data for representative allergen sources classified in each homologous group, seven of which represent pollen species [81]. In addition, the European Directive 2001/83 incorporates the concept of industrial allergens and seeks to regularize their commercialization, based on quality, safety, and efficacy, both in fixed formulations and in named-patient products. No homologous group has been formed for fungi, so a justification would be required according similar stability if it was necessary.

European regulatory agencies also have proposed norms to reduce the number of allergenic preparations available on the market. These approximations are analogous in concept to that proposed by CBER in the United States, but are generally more rigorous, and the number of allergen extracts permitted are fewer than those currently available in the United States.

21.5 REGULATORY ASPECTS

Allergen manufacturing companies in the United States must comply with CBER regulations for pollen allergen extracts, particularly with mandated limits for relative potency or major allergen concentrations of standardized pollen allergen extracts [80]. However, regulations or guidelines for nonstandardized extracts are lacking. In addition, the organization has not proposed regulations for pollen raw materials because it is assumed that the manufacturing process will assure that the final extracts are appropriate for human use.

In Europe, regulatory agencies control the quality of both the raw materials and the finished products. Therefore, European allergen manufacturing companies must comply with general regulatory guidelines for pollen and fungal raw materials [11,12]. These regulations sometimes are specific to each country [82].

All guidance documents are subjected to interpretations that can differ among allergen manufacturing companies. Companies are responsible for justifying internal interpretations and documenting compliance. As expected, these guidance documents are continually being revised.

In summary, there are some differences between regulatory agencies. In Europe, allergen manufacturing companies use internal reference standards. In the United States, standardized allergen extracts have a reference to maintain a constant potency among U.S. manufacturers. The FDA allows the use of properly calibrated in-house reference preparations (IHRPs) according to the U.S. reference standards for this purpose (Table 21.2).

Table 21.2 General comparison of the regulatory focus between the United States and Europe

Concept	United States	Europe
Regulatory focus	Final allergen extracts	Both raw materials and allergen extracts
Number of pollen species available on the market	Extensive	Limited
Limits for biological contaminants	Internally proposed by companies	Proposed by regulatory agencies
Limits for man-made contaminants	Not proposed	Testing required
Recommendations to avoid man-made contaminants	Avoid exposure	Avoid exposure and perform testing

SALIENT POINTS

1. Proper understanding of the processes associated with the collection and processing of pollen and fungal raw materials and the regulations in place in different areas of the world are essential to improve the quality of the finished products.
2. The number of pollen and fungal allergen extracts commercially available, particularly in the United States, should be reduced. This action would allow for the selection of fungal allergen extracts as candidates for standardization.
3. Programs and guidelines to train pollen collectors and the personnel involved in processing allergenic raw materials are necessary. These programs and guidelines should be harmonized for worldwide use and developed by manufacturers in collaboration with regulatory entities.
4. The strict European regulations regarding the quality of allergenic raw materials, including those derived from pollen and fungi, are generally based on the "worst-case scenario" and not on appropriate scientific principles. This practice could limit the availability of clinically relevant allergens in the future.
5. The selection of appropriate allergen extracts for diagnosis and treatment should be based on various considerations, among which general understanding of cross-reactivity principles deserves particular attention.

REFERENCES

1. Codina R, Crenshaw RC, Lockey RF. Considerations about pollen used for the production of allergen extracts. *J Allergy Clin Immunol Pract* 2015; 3: 676–682.
2. Codina R, Lockey RF. Pollen used to produce allergen extracts. *Ann Allergy Asthma Immunol* 2017; 118: 148–153.
3. Esch RE, Codina R. Fungal raw materials used to produce allergen extracts. *Ann Allergy Asthma Immunol* 2017; 118: 399–405.
4. Carnes J, Iraola V, Cho S, Esch RE. Mite allergen extracts and clinical practice. *Ann Allergy Asthma Immunol* 2017; 118: 249–256.
5. Fernández-Caldas E, Cases B, El-Qutob D, Cantillo JF. Mammalian raw materials used to produce allergen extracts. *Ann Allergy Asthma Immunol* 2017; 119: 1–8.
6. Plunkett G, Jacobson RS, Golden DBK. Hymenoptera venoms used to produce allergen extracts. *Ann Allergy Asthma Immunol* 2017; 118: 649–654.
7. Khurana T, Bridgewater JL, Rabin JL. Allergenic extracts to diagnose and treat sensitivity to insect venoms. *Ann Allergy Asthma Immunol* 2017; 118(5): 531–536.
8. David NA, Penumarti A, Burks AW, Slater JE. Food allergen extracts to diagnose food-induced diseases. How they are made. *Ann Allergy Asthma Immunol* 2017; 119: 101–107.
9. Curin M, Garib V, Valenta R. Single recombinant and purified major allergens and peptides. How they are made and how they change allergy diagnosis and treatment. *Ann Allergy Asthma Immunol* 2017; 119: 201–209.
10. Manual of Compliance Policy Guides, 2018. https://www. fda. gov/ICECI/ComplianceManuals/CompliancePolicyGuidance Manual/ucm200364.htm. Accessed on May 30, 2018.
11. European Medicines Agency (EMA), Committee for Medical Products for Human Use and Biologics Working Party. Draft guideline on allergen products: Production and quality issues, 2008; EMEA/CHMP/BWP/304831/2007.

12. Allergen Products. EP1063, 01/2010:1063.
13. Esch RE. Allergen source materials and quality control of allergenic extracts. *Meth Enzymol* 13: 2–13.
14. Slater JE, Esch RE. Preparation and standardization of allergen extracts. In: Adkinson NF, Bochner BS, Burks W, Busse WW, Holgate ST, Lemanske Jr RF, O'Hehir R, editors. *Allergy: Principles and Practice*, 8th ed. Philadelphia, PA: Mosby, 2014: 470–481.
15. Codina R, Fox RW, Lockey RF, DeMarco P, Bagg A. Typical levels of airborne fungal spores in houses without obvious moisture problems during a rainy season in Florida, USA. *J Investig Allergol Clin Immunol* 2008; 18: 156–162.
16. Horner WE, Worthan AG, Morey PR. Air- and dust-borne mycoflora in houses free of water damage and fungal growth. *Appl Environ Microbiol* 2004; 70: 6394–6400.
17. Nielsen KF, Thrane U. *Mould Growth on Building Materials: Secondary Metabolites, Mycotoxins, and Biomarkers*. Lyngby: Biocentrum-DTU, Technical University of Denmark, 2002.
18. Flannigan B, Miller JD. Microbial growth in indoor environments. In: Flannigan B, Samson RA, Miller JD, editors. *Microorganisms in Home and Indoor Work Environments: Diversity, Health Impacts, Investigation and Control*. London: Taylor & Francis Group, CRC Press, 2011.
19. Weber RW. Floristic zones and aeroallergen diversity. *Immunol Allergy Clin N Am* 2003; 23: 357–369.
20. Bohn U, Zazanashvili N, Nakhutsrishvili G. The map of the natural vegetation of Europe and its application in the Caucasus Ecoregion. *Bull Georg Natl Acad Sci* 2007; 175.
21. D'Amato G, Cecchi L, Bonini S, Nunes C, Annesi-Maesano I, Behrendt H, Liccardi G, Popov T, van Cauwenberge P. Allergenic pollen and pollen allergy in Europe. *Allergy* 2007; 62(9): 976–990.
22. Codina R, LeFevre DM, Duncan EA et al. Stability of allergen source materials stored under various temperature and moisture conditions over several years. *28th Annual Meeting of the European Academy of Allergology and Clinical Immunology*. Warsaw, Poland, June 2009.
23. Fernandez-Caldas E, Carnes J, Iraola V, Casanovas M. Comparison of the allergenicity and Ole e 1 content of 6 varieties of *Olea europaea* pollen collected during 5 consecutive years. *Ann Allergy Asthma Immunol* 2007; 98; 464–470.
24. Migueres M, Davila I, Frati F et al. Types of sensitization to aeroallergens: Definitions, prevalences and impact on the diagnosis and treatment of allergic respiratory diseases. *Clin Transl Allergy* 2014; 1: 4–16.
25. Weber RW. Cross-reactivity of pollen allergens: Impact on allergen immunotherapy. *Curr Allergy Asthma Rep* 2008; 8: 413–417.
26. Hoffmann A, Burks AW. Pollen food syndrome: Update on allergens. *Curr Allergy Asthma Rep* 2008; 8: 413–417.
27. Tandang-Silvas MR, Tecson-Mendoza EM, Mikami B et al. Molecular design of seed storage proteins for enhanced food physicochemical properties. *Annu Rev Food Sci Technology* 2011; 2: 59–73.
28. Cominelli E and Tonelli C. Transgenic crops coping with water scarcity. *J Biotechnol* 2010; 27: 473–477.
29. Schlundt J. Food Safety Department, World Health Organization (WHO). Pan American Health Organization and World Health Organization. *14th inter-American meeting, at the ministerial level, on health and agriculture*.
30. U.S. regulation of Genetically Modified Crops. https://fas.org/biosecurity/education/dualuse-agriculture/2.-agricultural-biotechnology/us-regulation-of-genetically-engineered-crops.html. Accessed in June 7, 2018.
31. Fresco LO. The GMO stalemate in Europe. *Science* 2013; 339: 883.
32. *Fourth Assessment Report of the Intergovernmental Panel on Climate Change (IPCC), Climate Change 2007: Synthesis Report*. Cambridge, UK: Cambridge University Press, 2007.
33. *Safety aspects of genetically modified foods of plant origin. Food and Agriculture Organization of the United Nations*. Geneva, Switzerland: World Health Organization, May–June 2000.
34. *Modern Food Biotechnology, Human Health and Development: An Evidence-Based Study. Food Safety Department*. Geneva, Switzerland: World Health Organization, 2005.
35. Alfaya T, Feo Brito F, García Rodríguez C, Pineda F, Lucas JA, Gutiérrez Mañero FJ, Guerra F. *Lolium perenne* pollen from a polluted city shows high allergenic potency and increased associated Enterobacteriaceae counts. *J Investig Allergol Clin Immunol* 2014; 24(2): 132–134.
36. Buters J, Alberternst B, Nawrath S, Wimmer M, Traidl-Hoffmann C, Starfinger U, Behrendt H, Schmidt-Weber C, Bergmann KC. *Ambrosia artemisiifolia* (ragweed) in Germany—Current presence, allergological relevance and containment procedures. *Allergo J Int* 2015; 24: 108–120.
37. Barnes CS, Alexis NE, Bernstein JA et al. Climate change and outdoor environment: The effect on respiratory and allergic disease. *J Allergy Clin Immunol Pract* 2013; 1: 137–141.
38. Thompson JL, Thompson JE. The urban jungle and allergies. *Immunol Allergy Clin N Am* 2003; 23: 371–387.
39. Smith M, Cecci L, Skjoth CA et al. Common ragweed a threat to environmental health in Europe. *Environ Int* 2013; 61: 115–126.
40. Kelly FJ, Fussell JC. Air pollution and airway disease. *Clin Exp Allergy* 2011; 41: 1057–1071.
41. Convention on Biological Diversity. Metalink: P4.ENV.CBD. GMO. http://www.fao.org. Accessed on August 31, 2018.
42. Hauck PR, Williamson S. The manufacture of allergenic extracts in North America. *Clin Rev Allergy Immunol* 2001; 21: 93–110.
43. Alexander MP. Differential staining of aborted and non-aborted pollen. *Biotech Histochemistry* 1969; 44: 117–122.
44. Peterson R, Slovin JP, Chen C. A simplified method for differential staining of aborted and non-aborted pollen grains. *Int J Plant Biol* 2010; 1: e13.
45. Prince HE, Morrow MB. Mold fungi in the etiology of respiratory allergic diseases. XV. Selection of molds for therapy. *Ann Allergy* 1954; 12: 253–260.
46. Morrow MB, Meyer GH, Prince HE. A summary of air-borne mold surveys. *Ann Allergy* 1964; 22: 575–587.
47. Prince HE, Morrow MB. A logical approach to mold allergy. *Ann Allergy* 1969; 27: 79–86.
48. Esch RE. Selection of allergen products for skin testing. *Immunol Allergy Clinics North Amer* 2001; 21: 251–261.
49. Aukrust L. Selections of source materials for reference preparations of molds. *Arb Paul Ehrlich Insitut* 1985; 80: 7–13.
50. Steringer I, Aukrust L, Einarsson R. Variability of antigenicity/allergenicity in different strains of *Alternaria alternata*. *In Arch Allergy Appl Immunol* 1987; 84: 190–197.
51. Wallenbeck I, Aukrust L, Einarsson R. Antigenic variability of different strains of *Aspergillus fumigatus*. *Int Arch Allergy Appl Immunol* 1984; 73: 166–172.

52. Bisht V, Singh BP, Kumar R et al. Culture filtrate antigens and allergens of *Epicoccum nigrum* cultivated in modified semi-synthetic medium. *Med Microbiol Immunol* 2002; 191: 11–15.

53. Moreno A, Pineda F, Alcover J, Rodríguez D, Palacios R, Martínez-Naves E. Orthologous allergens and diagnostic utility of major allergen Alt a 1. *Allergy Asthma Immunol Res* 2016; 8(5): 428–437.

54. Verma J, Gangal SV. *Fusarium solani*: Immunochemical characterization of allergens. *Int Arch Allergy Immunol* 1994; 104: 175–183.

55. Arruda LK, Mann BJ, Chapman MD. Selective expression of a major allergen and cytotoxin, Asp f I, in *Aspergillus fumigatus*. Implications for the immunopathogenesis of *Aspergillus*-related diseases. *J Immunol* 1992; 149: 3354–3359.

56. Nissen D, Petersen LJ, Esch R et al. IgE-sensitization to cellular and culture filtrates of fungal extracts in patients with atopic dermatitis. *Ann Allergy Asthma Immunol* 1998; 81: 247–255.

57. Martínez J, Gutiérrez A, Postigo I, Cardona G, Guisantes J. Variability of Alt a 1 expression by different strains of *Alternaria alternata*. *Allergy Asthma Immunol Res* 2015; 7(3): 205–220.

58. Martínez J, Martínez A, Gutiérrez G, Llamazares A, Palacios R, Sáenz de Santamaría M. Influencia del proceso de obtención en la actividad alergénica y rendimiento de extractos de *Alternaria alternata*. *Revista Iberoamericana de Micología* 1994; 11: 10–13.

59. Agarwal MK, Jones RT, Yunginger JW. Immunochemical and physiochemical characterization of commercial *Alternaria* extracts: A model for standardization of mold allergen extracts. *J Allergy Clin Immunol* 1882; 70: 432–436.

60. Kespohl S, Maryska S, Zahradnik E et al. Biochemical and immunological analysis of mould skin prick test solution: Current status of standardization. *Clin Exp Allergy* 2013; 43: 1286–1296.

61. Vailes L, Sridhara S, Cromwell O et al. Quantitation of the major fungal allergens, Alt a 1 and Asp f 1, in commercial allergenic products. *J Allergy Clin Immunol* 2001; 107: 641–646.

62. Twaroch TE, Curin M, Valenta R, Swoboda I. Mold allergens in respiratory allergy: From structure to therapy. *Allergy Asthma Immunol Res* 2015; 7(3): 205–220.

63. Portnoy J, Pacecho F, Barnes C, Upadrastita B, Crenshaw R, Esch R. Selection of representative *Alternaria* strain groups on the basis of morphology, enzyme profile, and allergen content. *J Allergy Clin Immunol* 1993; 91: 773–782.

64. Steringer I, Aukrust L, Einarsson R. Variability of antigenicity and allergenicity in different strains of *Alternaria alternata*. *Int Arch Allergy Appl Immunol* 1987; 84: 190–197.

65. Esch RE, Grier TG. Allergen compatibilities in extract mixtures. *Immunol Allergy Clinics North Amer* 2011; 31: 227–239.

66. Plunkett G. Stability of allergen extracts used in skin testing and immunotherapy. *Curr Opin Otolaryngol Head Neck Surg* 2008; 16: 285–291.

67. U.S. Department of Health and Human Services, FDA, CBER. Guidance for Industry: Testing Limits in Stability Protocols for Standardized Grass Pollen Extracts. September 2000.

68. Code of Federal Regulations (CFR) Title 21 Part 680.3 Additional standards for miscellaneous products: Tests.

69. Code of Federal Regulations (CFR) Title 21 Part 610.53 Dating periods for licensed biological products.

70. European Pharmacopoeia 9.5. Pesticides residues, 2.8.13.

71. Commission Regulation (EC) 396/2005.

72. European Pharmacopoeia 9.5. Heavy metals in herbal drugs and herbal drug preparations, 2.4.27.

73. U.S. Department of Health and Human Services, FDA, CBER. Draft Guidance for Industry: On the content and format of chemistry, manufacturing and controls information and establishment description for an allergenic extract or allergen patch test. April 1999.

74. European Medicines Agency (EMEA), Committee for Medicinal Products for Human Use (CHMP), and Biologics Working Party (BWP). Draft Guideline on allergen products: Production and quality issues. 2007; EMEA/CHMP/BWP/304831/2007.

75. Esch RE. Allergen source materials: State of the art. *Arb Paul Ehrlich Institut* 2009; 96: 5–11.

76. U.S. Department of Health and Human Services, FDA, CDER/CBER. Mixing, Diluting, or Repackaging Biological Products Outside the Scope of an Approved Biologics License Application: Guidance for Industry. January 2018.

77. U.S. Pharmacopeia. General Chapter <797> Pharmaceutical compounding—Sterile preparations. June 1, 2008.

78. Cox L, Jacobsen L. Comparison of allergen immunotherapy practice patterns in the United States and Europe. *Ann Allergy Asthma Immunol* 2009; 103: 451–460.

79. Lorenz AR, Luttkopf D, May D et al. The principle of homologous groups in regulatory products—A proposal. *Int Arch Allergy Immunol* 2009; 148: 1–17.

80. Slater JE, Menzies SL, Bridgewater J et al. The U.S. Food and Drug Administration review of the safety and effectiveness on non-standardized allergen extracts. *J Allergy Clin Immunol* 2012; 129: 1014–1019.

81. Lorenz AR, Lüttkopf D, Seitz R, Vieths S. The regulatory system in Europe with special emphasis on allergen products. *Int Arch Allergy Immunol* 2008; 147: 263–275.

82. De Blair F, Doyen V, Bloch-Morot E et al. French application of the European guidelines for regulation of allergenic extracts. *J Allergy Clin Immunol* 2013; 131: 1435–1437.

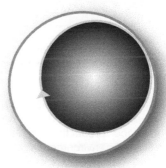

22 Manufacturing arthropod and mammalian allergen extracts

Enrique Fernández-Caldas
Inmunotek S.L.
University of South Florida Morsani College of Medicine

Eva Abel Fernández and Jonathan Kilimajer
Inmunotek S.L.

Seong H. Cho
University of South Florida Morsani College of Medicine

CONTENTS

22.1 INTRODUCTION

In the eighteenth century, Carolus Linnaeus developed a system for classifying living organisms into specialized subdivision groups depending on their specific characteristics. Currently there are five kingdoms into which all living organisms are divided: Monera Kingdom, Protist Kingdom, Fungi Kingdom, Plant Kingdom, and Animal Kingdom. The Animal Kingdom is, in turn, subdivided in three phyla that include three groups: Chordata (vertebrates such as mammals, birds, amphibians, and reptiles), Arthropods, and Annelids. The most extended group, including more than 85% of all known animal species, is the phylum Arthropods, along with a great diversity of animals with hard exoskeletons and jointed appendages such as Insects, Arachnids (spiders, mites, and scorpions), Myriapods (centipedes and millipedes), and Crustaceans (salters, prawn, crabs) [1]. The organisms in this phylum make up more than 75% of all the life on Earth. This phylum includes insects like butterflies and beetles, crustaceans like crabs and lobsters, and chelicerates like spiders and scorpions. Arthropods are found in all parts of the world in a wide variety of environments. Over 800,000 species have been identified. The word *arthropod* is a combination of two Greek words: *arthro* meaning "jointed" and *pod* meaning "foot" [2].

The presence of arthropod pests in the urban environment results in a variety of medical problems. These organisms may also be vectors of bacterial, prion [3], and viral infections [4]. Exposure to arthropod allergens is more extensive in the domestic as compared to the occupational environment. The main reasons may be that humidity is generally higher in the domestic environment due to a higher water vapor production and that the exposure period is longer in the domestic environment as compared to the occupational domain. Furthermore, indoor exposure to arthropod allergens has increased in the last 20 years due to energy-saving campaigns, leading to less ventilation and resulting in improved conditions for arthropods [5]. A recent study surveyed the complete arthropod fauna of the indoor biome in 50 houses in North Carolina. We discovered high diversity, with a conservative estimate range of 32–211 species, and 24–128 arthropod families per house. The majority (73%) consisted of true flies (Diptera), spiders (Araneae), beetles (Coleoptera), cockroaches, wasps, and ants [6].

Allergy to arthropods is a major social, economic, and medical concern. Arthropods are sources of potent allergens that sensitize and induce IgE-mediated allergic reactions in humans. Important allergen sources from arthropods include Hymenoptera venoms, edible crustaceans and body secretions, saliva, excreta, exoskeletons, and disintegrating bodies and body parts, of nonparasitic insects and mites. They contain immunogenic, immune-modulating, and other pharmacologically active molecules [7]. Sensitization to arthropod allergen sources such as cockroaches, ticks, storage mites, spiders, mosquitos, red chironomid larvae, silverfish, and ladybugs, as well as a variety of storage pests [8] has been described. Table 22.1 contains a list of the main species of Arthropods to which allergic sensitization has been shown. A novel IgE antibody response to a mammalian oligosaccharide epitope, galactosealpha-1,3-galactose (α-gal) has been described. IgE to α-gal has been associated with a delayed onset anaphylaxis 3–6 hours after ingestion of mammalian food products, such as beef and pork. Several studies have shown that tick bites are the main cause of IgE antibody responses to α-gal in the United States, Europe, Australia, and parts of Asia [9,10].

Approximately 5450 species of mammals have been described. They are characterized by the presence of mammary glands and a neocortex. They represent an important source of allergens and are considered an important risk factor for the development of allergy [11]. Mammalian allergens belong to a few protein families, and lipocalins represent the largest group. An important number of them are classified as major allergens. These proteins are odorant and pheromone-binding proteins that carry small hydrophobic molecules in their internal binding pocket and are present in urine, saliva, and animal dander. Serum albumins are the second most frequent allergen present as a major component in animal and human plasma. They are also present in animal dander and fluid such as urine, saliva, and milk [12].

The inhalation of skin-derived mammalian allergens is a common cause of allergic sensitization and allergic respiratory symptoms worldwide [13]. Their sensitization may occur at home by allergens derived from cats, dogs, horses, cows, and rodents present in up to 35% of European and 60% of U.S. households. In Sweden, in an unselected population including more than 4000 children, a significant increase in the rate of sensitization to cat, dog, and horse has been reported [14]. Mammalian allergens also play an important role in occupational settings, where veterinarians and laboratory animal workers, among others, may be exposed to large and small mammals and rodents, such as guinea pigs, rabbits, mice, and rats. In these settings, sensitization to rodents may affect between 11% and 44% of the exposed personnel. Sensitivity to mouse dander and urine is also common in inner-city children with asthma in the United States. It has been reported that mouse allergens are detectable in dust and bedrooms of an important population of atopic children. By contrast, several studies have indicated

that early pet keeping could protect the infant from later allergy development. In a cross-sectional cohort in Sweden, allergy decreased from 49% in those with no pets, to 0% in those with five or more pets [15]. Sensitization to animals, as well as pollens, also decreased with an increasing number of animals in the household.

The introduction of exotic pets has also increased the number of mammalian species to which allergic sensitization may occur, such as new furry pets including prairie dogs, chinchillas, guinea pigs, gerbils, hamsters, ferret, hedgehogs, rabbits, hares, and monkeys; sensitization to sheep and goats and cross-reactivity among different ungulate species (deer, cow, horse, goat, and roe deer) have also been described and could be attributable to the presence of lipocalins. It is important to note that mammalian allergens can be present in the meat, milk, and milk derivatives.

In this chapter, various methods of manufacturing arthropod and mammalian allergen extracts for respiratory and food allergy are discussed. Their clinical implications are also addressed.

22.2 MANUFACTURING OF ALLERGEN EXTRACTS

Allergen extracts are complex mixtures of allergenic and nonallergenic substances, including proteins, glycoproteins, polysaccharides, lipids, nucleic acids, low molecular weight metabolites, salts, and pigments. Most allergens are proteins or glycoproteins with a molecular weight between 5 and 100 kDa. In theory, all foreign proteins, or chemicals, are potential allergens, although only certain proteins are confirmed to be allergenic in humans. So far, no structural properties have been identified that distinguish allergenic from nonallergenic proteins, although there is evidence that certain protein structures are more allergenic than others [15]. Current evidence suggests that allergen extracts contain cross-reactive and species-specific allergens in arthropods, as well as in mammalian extracts.

Allergen products are pharmaceutical preparations derived from extracts of naturally occurring source materials containing allergens, which are substances that cause or provoke allergic (hypersensitivity) disease. The manufacturing process development of allergen extract is based on the manufacturing experience in allergen products by different industrial and research settings.

Allergen source materials are obtained from controlled and audited suppliers with a certificate of analysis confirming collection methods and sources. An expiration date should be assigned to the source materials based on stability studies and a code should be received to enable testing and tracking according to Good Manufacturing Practice (GMP) requirements. Pollen source materials are collected by specialized companies and are subjected to strong quality regulations and processes, and they include purity, foreign contaminations, and stability data [16]. Raw materials from mites are grown in specialized facilities and are also subject to regulatory controls [17,18]. Animal dander is collected from housed animals and is accompanied with a certificate from a veterinary doctor stating that the animals are healthy and free of infectious and contagious agents [19]. In most European countries, allergen production is regulated mainly by the Guideline on Allergen Products: Production and Quality Issues [20] and the Monograph on Allergen Extracts of the European Pharmacopoeia [21].

The first step in the preparation of allergen extract is the careful selection of the raw source materials. The quality of allergen products is a key issue for both diagnosis and therapy, and the standardization of allergen extracts is thus of primary importance. Effective diagnosis, using skin test reagents, requires the optimal

Table 22.1 Species of insects identified as allergenic sources

Cat fleas			*Ctenocephalides felis*
Mosquitoes			*Aedes* sp. (*A. aegypti, A. communis, A. vexans, A. albopictus, A. togoi, A. triseratus*)
			Anopheles sp. (*A. sinensis, A. gambiae*)
			Calliphora sp. (*C. stygia, C. augar*)
			Culex sp. (*C. pipiens, C. quinquifasciatus, C. tarsalis*)
			Forcipomyia taiwana
			Glossina morsitans (Savannah Tsetse fly)
House flies			*Chrysomya bezziana*
			Cochliomyia hominivorax (=*americana*) (Coquerel)
			Culiseta inornata
			Lucilia cuprina
			Musca domestica
			Parasarcophaga sp.
Nonbiting midges			*Chironomus* sp. (*C. thummi thummi, C. annularius, C. tentans, C. tepperi, C. lewisi, C. plumosus, C. salinaris, C. calipterus, C. yoshimatsui, C. kiiensis*)
			Cladotanytarus lewisi
			Cricotopus sylvestris
			Polypedilum kyotoense
			Tokunagayusurica akamusi
Confused flour beetles			*Tribolium confusum*
Rice weevils			*Sitophilus granarius*
Stinging insects	Apids		*Apis* sp. (*A. mellifera* (honeybee), *A. cerana* (Asiatic honeybee), *A. dorsata* (giant honeybee)
			Bombus pennsylvanicus (bumblebee), *Bombus terrestris*
	Vespids	Hornets	*Dolichovespula* sp. (*D. maculata* [white-faced hornet], *D. arenaria* [yellow hornet])
			Vespa crabro (European hornet), *V. magnifica* (hornet), *Vespa mandarinia* (giant Asian hornet)
		Wasps	*Polistes* sp. (*P. annularis* [paper wasp], *P. dominulus, P. exclamans, P. fuscatus, P. gallicus, P. metricus*)
			Polybia paulista, Polybia scutellaris
		Yellow jackets	*Vespula* sp. (*V. vulgaris, V. flavopilosa, V. germanica, V. maculifrons, V. pensylvanica, V. squamosa, V. vidua*)
	Fire ants	Fire ants	*Solenopsis* sp. (*S. invicta, S. richteri, S. geminata, S. saevissima*)
		Harvester ants	*Euprenolepis procera*
Silkworms			*Bombyx mori* (silk moth)
Cockroaches			*Blattella* sp. (*B. asahinai* [Asian cockroach], *B. germanica* [German cockroach])
			Blatta orientalis (Oriental cockroach)
			Periplaneta americana (American cockroach)
			Supella longipalpis (brown-banded cockroach)

(Continued)

Table 22.1 (*Continued*) Species of insects identified as allergenic sources

Miscellaneous insects	Ants	*Myrmecia pilosula* (Australia jumper ant)
		Pachycondyla chinensis (Asian needle ant)
	Beetles	*Callosobruchus maculatus* Fabricius (Bruchid beetle)
		Tenebrio molitor Linnaeus (common meal beetle)
		Trogoderma angustum Solier (Berlin carpet beetle)
	Asian ladybeetle	*Harmonia axyridis*
	Kissing bugs	*Triatoma* sp. (*T. protracta, T. rubra*)
	Silverfish	*Lepisma saccharina*
		Cyenolepism longicaudata
	Caddisflies	*Macronema radiatum*
	Locusts	*Locusta migratoria* Linnaeus (migratory locust)
		Schistocerca gregaria Forskal (desert locust)
	Moths	*Ephestia* sp. (*E. cautella* [warehouse moth], *E. kuehniella* [Mediterranean flour moth])
		Galleria mellonella (Linnaeus) (large bee moth)
		Plodia interpunctella (Indianmeal moth)
		Tineola bisselliella (clothes moth)
	Bedbugs, deerflies, and other flies	*Cimex* sp. (bedbugs)
		Ephemera danica Muller (mayfly)
		Psychoda alternata Latreille (sewer fly)
		Tabanus yao (horsefly)
	Caterpillars	*Thaumetopoea pityocampa* (Pine processionary)
	House cricket	*Acheta domesticus* (Linnaeus)
	Lesser mealworm	*Alphitobius diaperinus* (Panzer)
	Water flea	*Daphnia pulex* (De Geer)
	Dust (book) louse	*Liposcelis bostrichophil* (Booklouse)
	Mexican bean weevil	*Zabrotes subfasciatus* (Boheman)
	Pigeon tick	*Argas reflexus*
	Formosan subterranean termite	*Coptotermes formosanus*

concentration of allergens and an adequate composition including the most relevant allergens.

Allergen extracts are usually prepared by aqueous extraction of allergenic source materials obtained from natural sources. Recombinant allergens are not contemplated in the current regulations and require a different type of registration in Europe and in the United States. The composition and biological properties of the allergen extracts may be influenced by the quality and purity of the source material, as well as their processing, extraction, and storage conditions. A general scheme of the preparation of allergen extracts is shown in Figure 22.1.

22.3 PREPARATION OF ARTHROPOD EXTRACTS

22.3.1 Special considerations for mites

The allergenicity of house dust has been known for many years. However, it was not until the mid-1960s that it became clear that house dust mites were the main source of house dust mite allergens [22]. *Dermatophagoides pteronyssinus* and *D. farinae* are considered the most important house dust mite species and

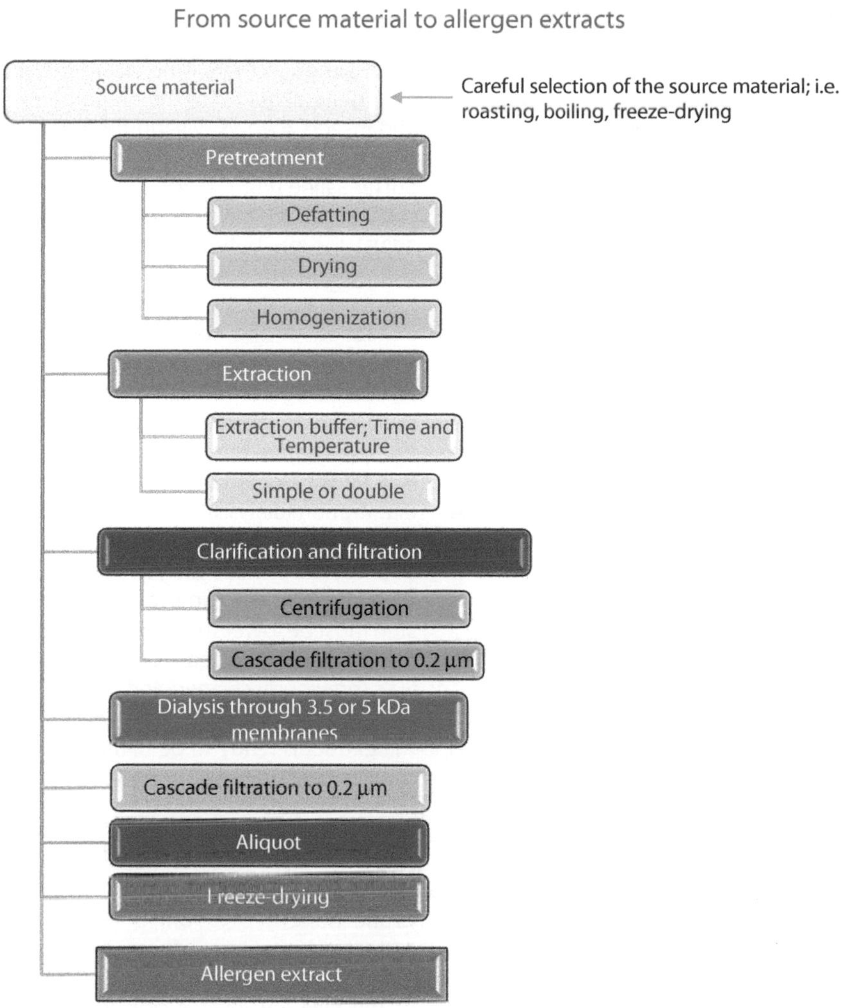

From source material to allergen extracts

Figure 22.1 General scheme of the preparation of allergen extracts.

have a global distribution. The allergenicity of other species, such as *Blomia tropicalis*, *Lepidoglyphus destructor*, and *Tyrophagus putrescentiae*, has also been demonstrated. Extracts of these species are also commercially available in many countries. It is now firmly established that *D. pteronyssinus* and *D. farinae* are some of the most important sources of clinically relevant allergens worldwide. The material harvested from large-scale cultures is used to prepare mite extracts for diagnosis and immunotherapy of mite-allergic individuals. Kilogram quantities of mite cultures are harvested yearly, and millions of individuals are diagnosed with allergen extracts and treated with mite vaccines worldwide.

Although there are some general recommendations on the subject, mite cultures may be used as whole cultures, thus containing more fecal material, or sieved, containing more purified mites. Both raw materials are used. Currently, there is a clear trend toward using more purified cultures to avoid the presence of food medium [23]. Mites were first grown on human skin scales collected from barber shops, and on yeast [24]; other food media used included fish food flakes, dried Daphnia, dog food, rodent chow, several cereal preparations, and even mold cultures [25]. Due to their position in the trophic chain, mites mainly feed on proteins found in house and mattress dust. A supplement of yeast is also important to complement the intake of micronutrients. The ingestion of a high-protein diet is a common determinant and is needed for their proliferation. Several food media are currently being used to grow mites. There are general recommendations to avoid the use of human- and other animal-derived proteins. Food media currently used in Europe and the United States include autoclaved pork liver powder and yeast, brine shrimp eggs and yeast, and wheat germ. Other companies produce mites grown on wheat germ, supplemented with amino acids (resembling the composition of human *stratum corneum*) and baker's yeast [27,28]. The use of a well-defined nonallergic medium is warranted.

In general, the diet influences allergen composition and growth rate of the mite cultures, and this fact may be of significant importance in the preparation of allergen extracts [26]. A study by Avula-Poola et al. demonstrated that *D. farinae* and *D. pteronyssinus* grow at different rates and that the rates of accumulation and of group 1 and group 2 allergen production and the levels of endotoxin in mite cultures are influenced by the foods on which the mites are grown. Ecological and laboratory studies have shown that the two species behave differently in the environment. Similar results have also been observed in longitudinal studies [27]. Thus, diet should be an important consideration when culturing mites and comparing allergen data of mite extracts from different sources and in standardizing and characterizing mite extracts [28,29]. Population and age of the cultures also seem to influence the microbiome profiles of house dust mites [30].

For the preparation of mite allergen extracts, the U.S. Food and Drug Administration (FDA) only allows mite cultures containing more than or at least 99% pure mites. In Europe, there are also recommendations by the European Medicines Agency [31] stating: "The cultivation method and the composition of the cultivation medium as well as the media components should be described. Details on the composition of the cultivation medium and the media components should be submitted. Synthetic and consequently free of animal-derived material and allergen-free media should be preferably used. The conditions of culture and the time of harvest should be described, and the corresponding crucial parameters defined. It should be indicated which part of the culture is used for further processing, e.g. mites, mite feces only or the whole mite culture or mixes thereof." Therefore, consecutive batches of the mite source materials should be similar in composition to assure the consistency and allergen composition of the produced vaccines. A recent review on mite allergen extracts describes the different steps involved in the preparation of mite source materials [32].

22.3.2 Special considerations for whole-body insects

The optimal source for insect allergens depends on the natural route of exposure, i.e., inhalation or injection (bite/sting). If whole insects or insect debris is inhaled, the whole insect body is selected as the allergen source. For biting or stinging insects, saliva or venom should be selected as the allergen source. Live insects are stored in deep freezers, lyophilized, and crushed to be further used for antigen preparation [33,34]. The preparation of insect body allergens follows a similar scheme as for mite allergen extracts, i.e., an aqueous extraction of water-soluble proteins. Cockroaches are grown in a closed, moist container. The whole bodies, along with their secretions and excretions, are collected and killed by freezing. The killed frozen insect bodies are the source material for allergen extraction. After thawing, the bodies are milled to a fine powder [35]. As in the case for mites, raw materials to be extracted should be defatted before the extraction process in acetone or anhydrous ether, and extracted as suggested before.

Insects commonly used for skin testing, such as the cockroach species, *Blatella germanica*, *Periplaneta americana*, and *Blatta orientalis*, are grown in specialized laboratories on defined diets. Wild cockroaches cannot be used for commercial extraction purposes due to a potential colonization by pathogenic agents. Several suppliers of allergen source material produce cockroaches, and other insects, such as mosquitoes, for the preparation of allergen extracts.

Allergy to species of the mosquito genera *Aedes*, *Culex*, and *Anopheles* has been reported worldwide [36]. It is now well established that mosquitoes may sensitize individuals through inhalation and/or bites. Generally, mosquito extracts are made of whole bodies that contain salivary and nonsalivary proteins. Living mosquitoes are captured to obtain fresh saliva, and their proboscises are inserted into collection tubes. Salivation is stimulated by applying malathion to thoraces. The saliva is collected, pooled, and lyophilized [36]. In recent years, several somatic and salivary mosquito allergens have been described [37], and cross-reactivity between mosquitoes and other arthropods has also been demonstrated [38]. Furthermore, it has been shown that mosquito and mite tropomyosin cross-react at the cellular and humoral levels

[39]. This may suggest that individuals who are allergic to dust mites may have a higher risk to develop allergic reaction to mosquito bites, although there is no clear clinical evidence yet.

A general guide for the preparation of allergen extracts of mites and insects follows: Weigh the desired amount of source material in a 1:20 weight/volume ratio of a specific buffer, i.e., phosphate buffer saline (PBS), at 4°C for 4–8 hours under continuous stirring conditions. Other weight/volume ratios can also be used. Afterward, adjust the pH between 7.5 and 8.5 by the addition of NaOH or HCl. The careful selection of the extraction buffer is a key issue, as has been previously demonstrated [40]. In some cases, a double extraction of the source material can be performed. Once the extraction is completed, centrifuge the recovered extract volume in a centrifuge at 10,000 rpm for 30 minutes at 4°C (the centrifuge must be cooled down in advance). Afterward, carefully separate the supernatant and discard the pellet. Filtrate the obtained extract in a filter cascade until going through a 0.2 μm pore size filter. A diafiltration (dialysis) step is now performed in a Pellicon tangential flow filtration system (Pellicon, Merck Millipore), using a cassette of 5 kDa cutoff. The dialysis process should be performed with five times the same volume of ultrapure. The conductivity in the last step must be lower than 500 ppm (approximately 800 μS/cm). Once the extract is dialyzed, aliquot the extract in 50 mL freeze-drying vials (previously cleaned and labeled) and freeze-dry it according to the program selected. After the freeze-drying cycle is completed, the extract is ready to be diluted to the desired concentration, and after several manufacturing steps, it is ready to be used.

22.3.3 Special considerations for venoms

Crude honeybee venom is used in the manufacture of allergen extracts. Honeybee venom is usually collected by applying an electric shock through a grid that is placed adjacent to the entrance of the hive and over a collection apparatus (a polyethylene sheet stretched over a glass plate). The honeybees then sting the grid and eject venom into the collecting apparatus. After 15–20 minutes, the venom is collected from the glass plate and polyethylene sheet. After ultrafiltration, the honeybee venom is freeze-dried [36,41].

The allergen manufacturing process of yellow jacket (*Vespula* spp.) and paper wasp (*Polistes* spp.) starts with the collection of live insects from their nests. After collection, the insects are frozen. Once frozen, they are thawed for the removal of the venom sac. The collected venom sacs are crushed and filtered to purify the venom and then are freeze-dried and stored in a freezer.

22.3.4 Special considerations for seafood extracts

Humans have eaten seafood since prehistoric times. Crustaceans such as crab, lobster, and shrimp may induce sensitization and clinical symptoms upon ingestion, or inhalation, in sensitized individuals. Workers involved in manual or automated processing of crabs, prawns, and fishmeal are exposed to various seafood aerosols during the cooking, or general processing. Aerosolization of seafood and cooking fluid are potential occupational situations that could result in sensitization through inhalation [42,43]. Several allergens have been described, which include heat-labile as well as heat-sensitive molecules [44,45]. Seafood extracts can be made of boiled or raw source materials. Generally, extracts should be made with source materials that resemble the way in which they are eaten, i.e., raw or cooked. They are commonly prepared by homogenizing in a blender peeled, raw, or boiled crustaceans (prawns, scampi, shrimps, crabs, lobster, etc.). The extraction process is performed in PBS or similar buffer and follows the main scheme described earlier. After a clarification (centrifugation step) and filtration, extracts are filtered and dialyzed in dialysis membranes with a nominal cutoff pore size of 3–5 kDa. Afterward, the extract is sterile filtered and freeze-dried.

22.4 PREPARATION OF MAMMALIAN EXTRACTS

22.4.1 Special considerations for inhalant allergens

Special precautions should be considered for the preparation of mammalian extracts. In recent years, there has been concern about the spread of bovine spongiform encephalopathy (BSE) across Europe and the United States and the potential contamination of skin-derived allergen extracts. Precautions must be taken to avoid the presence of infectious agents in these extracts. The European Pharmacopoeia, 5th edition, volume 1, contains a section (Section 5.2.8) entitled: "Minimising the risk of transmitting animal spongiform encephalopathy agents via human and veterinary medicinal products." In this section, it is clearly stated that "derivatives of wool and hair of ruminants, such as lanolin, and wool alcohols derived from hair shall be considered in compliance with this chapter, provided the wool and hair are sourced from live animals" [46]. The hair samples should be shipped to the laboratory together with a certificate of analysis in which a doctor in veterinary medicine states that the hair was collected from healthy animals free of infectious diseases and infectious agents. When the hair is collected from cows, sheep, goats, or other ungulates, it should be done from herds in which no BSE had been declared previously.

Hair should be collected from live animals using an electric razor. The collected hair is stored in sealed plastic bags until further analysis. Afterward, the hair is defatted with acetone (1:40 wt/vol) for 16 hours and the dander separated after sequential sieving, using vacuum, through a stainless steel, 1 mm mesh size sieve and a Whatman number 1 filter. This procedure is repeated several times. The dander collected on the filters is air dried.

22.4.2 Special considerations for food allergens

Mammalian-derived food allergens are mainly derived from the meat and milk of mammalians. Foods are normally processed raw or boiled. The extraction process of the meat is the same as outlined previously. Basically, meats are processed in a blender at the desired speed and in contact with the extraction buffer (i.e., PBS or another buffer). After approximately 5 minutes, the extract is removed from the blender and placed in a cool chamber at 4°C for the desired length of time. Afterward, the extracts are centrifuged and filtered through a 0.2 μm filter. A dialysis step is conducted to remove salts, and afterward, the extract is freeze-dried.

Cow's milk contains approximately 30–35 g of proteins per liter and includes more than 25 different proteins. However, only a few are known to be allergenic. Raw skim milk is acidified to pH 4.6 at 20°C,

and two fractions are obtained: the coagulum containing the casein proteins which account for 80% and the lactoserum (whey proteins) representing 20% of the total milk proteins [47]. These two fractions are further processed, extracted, sterile filtered, and freeze-dried.

SALIENT POINTS

1. Allergy to arthropods is a major social, economic, and medical concern.
2. Arthropods are sources of potent allergens that sensitize and induce IgE-mediated allergic reactions in humans.
3. Important allergen sources from arthropods include Hymenoptera venoms, edible crustaceans and body secretions, and disintegrating bodies and body parts of nonparasitic insects and mites.
4. Allergen extracts are complex mixtures of allergenic and nonallergenic substances, including proteins, glycoproteins, polysaccharides, lipids, nucleic acids, low molecular weight metabolites, salts, and pigments.
5. Most allergens are proteins or glycoproteins with a molecular weight between 5 and 100 kDa.
6. Allergen products are pharmaceutical preparations derived from extracts of naturally occurring source materials containing allergens, which are substances that cause or provoke allergic (hypersensitivity) disease.
7. Special precautions should be considered for the preparation of mammalian extracts.
8. Precautions must be taken to avoid the presence of infectious agents in these extracts.
9. Mammalian-derived food allergens are mainly derived from the meat and milk of mammalians.
10. Mammalian derived food extracts are normally processed raw or boiled.

REFERENCES

1. Thorp H, Rogers J, Christopher D. Introduction to the phylum arthropoda. In: Thorp JH, Christopher Rogers D (eds.). *Thorp and Covich's Freshwater Invertebrates: Ecology and General Biology*, 4th ed, 2015: 591–597.
2. Arthropoda—Crustaceans, Insects. https://nhpbs.org/wild/arthropoda.asp
3. Lupi O. Could ectoparasites act as vectors for prion diseases? *Int J Dermatol* 2003; 42(6): 425–429.
4. Van Lynden-Van Nes AMT, Koren LGH, Snijders MCL, Van Bronswijk JEMH. In: Wildey KB, (ed.). *Proceedings of the Second International Conference on Urban Pests*. 1996.
5. Wickman M, Nordvall S, Pershagen G, Korsgaard J, Johansen N. Sensitization to domestic mites in a cold temperate region. *Am Rev Respir Dis* 1993; 148: 58–62.
6. Bertone MA, Leong M, Bayless KM, Malow TLF, Dunn RR, Trautwein MD. Arthropods of the great indoors: Characterizing diversity inside urban and suburban homes. *PeerJ* 2016; 4: e1582.
7. Arlian L. Arthropod allergens and human health. *Annu Rev Entomol* 2002; 47: 395–433.
8. Hilger C, Kuehn A, Raulf M, Jakob T. Cockroach, tick, storage mite and other arthropod allergies: Where do we stand with molecular allergy diagnostics? Part 15 of the Series Molecular Allergology. *Allergo J Int* 2014; 23: 172–178.

9. Commins SP, Platts-Mills TA. Tick bites and red meat allergy. *Curr Opin Allergy Clin Immunol* 2013; 13(4): 354–359.

10. Steinke JW, Platts-Mills TA, Commins SP. The α-gal story: Lessons learned from connecting the dots. *J Allergy Clin Immunol* 2015; 135(3): 589–596.

11. Vaughan TA, Ryan JM, Czaplewski NJ. "*Classification of Mammals*". *Mammalogy*, 6th ed. Burlington, MA: Jones and Bartlett Learning, 2013.

12. Zahradnik E, Raulf M. Animal allergens and their presence in the environment. *Front Immunol* 2014; 5: 76.

13. Fernández-Caldas E, Cases B, El-Qutob D, Cantillo JF. Mammalian raw materials used to produce allergen extracts. *Ann Allergy Asthma Immunol* 2017; 119(1): 1–8.

14. Hilger C, Van Hage M, Kuehn A. Diagnosis of allergy to mammals and fish: Cross-reactive vs. specific markers. *Curr Allergy Asthma Rep* 2017; 17(9): 64.

15. Jenkins JA, Breiteneder H, Clare Mills EN. Evolutionary distance from human homologs reflects allergenicity of animal food proteins. *J Allergy Clin Immunol* 2007; 120: 1399–1405.

16. Pollens for allergen products. European Pharmacopoeia 9.0; 01/2017:2627; 3362-3363.

17. Mites for allergen products. Acari ad producta allergenica. European Pharmacopoeia 9.0; 01/2017:2625; 3077-3078.

18. Fernández-Caldas E. Towards a more complete standardization of mite allergen extracts. *Int Arch Allergy Immunol* 2013; 160(1): 1–3.

19. Animal epithelia and outgrowths for allergen products. European Pharmacopoeia 9.0; 01/2017:2621; 1736-1737.

20. Guideline for Allergen Products: Production and Quality Issues (EMEA/CHMP/BWP/304831/2007).

21. European Directorate for the Quality of Medicines (EDQM). *Monograph: Allergen Products—Producta Allergenica* 01/2010:1063. In: Council of Europe editor. 6th ed. Strasbourg: European Pharmacopoeia, 2010, supplement 6, pp. 679–680, as implemented of 01. 01. 2010.

22. Voorhorst R, Spieksma-Boezeman MI, Spieksma FT. Is a mite (Dermatophagoides SP.) the producer of the house-dust allergen? *Allerg Asthma (Leipz)* 1964; 10: 329–334.

23. Henmar H, Frisenette SM, Grosch K et al. Fractionation of source materials leads to a high reproducibility of the SQ house dust mite SLIT-tablets. *Int Arch Allergy Immunol* 2016; 169(1): 23–32.

24. Spieksma FHM, Spieksma-Boezeman MIM. The mite fauna of house dust with particular reference to the house-dust mite *D. pteronyssinus* (Trt.) (Psoroptidae:Sarcoptiformes). *Acarologia* 1967; 9: 226–241.

25. Colloff MJ. *Dust Mites*. Collingwood, Australia: CSIRO Publishing; Dordrecht: Springer, 2009: 268–271.

26. Avula-Poola S, Morgan MS, Arlian LG. Diet influences growth rates and allergen and endotoxin contents of cultured *Dermatophagoides farinae* and *Dermatophagoides pteronyssinus* house dust mites. *Int Arch Allergy Immunol* 2012; 159(3): 226–234.

27. Fernández-Caldas E, Andrade J, Trudeau WL, Souza Lima E, Souza Lima I, Lockey RF. Serial determinations of Der p 1 and Der f 1 show predominance of one *Dermatophagoides* species. *J Investigational Allergol Clin Immunol* 1998; 8(1): 27–29.

28. Casset A, Mari A, Purohit A et al. Varying allergen composition and content affects the *in vivo* allergenic activity of commercial *Dermatophagoides pteronyssinus* extracts. *Int Arch Allergy Immunol* 2012; 159(3): 253–262.

29. Vidal-Quist JC, Ortego F, Rombauts S, Castañera P, Hernández-Crespo P. Dietary shifts have consequences for the repertoire of allergens produced by the European house dust mite. *Med Vet Entomol*. 2017;31(3):272–280.

30. Hubert J, Nesvorna M, Kopecky J, Erban T, Klimov P. Population and culture age influence the microbiome profiles of house dust mites. *Microb Ecol* 2019; 77(4): 1048–1066.

31. Guideline on Allergen Products: Production and Quality Issues. *Committee for Medicinal Products for Human Use (CHMP)*. London: European Medicines Agency Evaluation of Medicines for Human Use, 20 November 2008, EMEA/CHMP/BWP/304831/2007.

32. Carnés J, Iraola V, Cho SH, Esch RE. Mite allergen extracts and clinical practice. *Ann Allergy Asthma Immunol* 2017; 118(3): 249–256.

33. Singh AB. Allergen Preparation and Standardization: An Update. https://juniperpublishers.com/gjo/pdf/GJO.MS.ID.555968.pdf

34. Larsen JN, Dreborg S. Standardization of allergen extracts. *Methods Mol Med* 2008; 138: 133–145.

35. Khurana T, Bridgewater JL, Rabin RL. Allergenic extracts to diagnose and treat sensitivity to insect venoms and inhaled allergens. *Ann Allergy Asthma Immunol* 2017; 118(5): 531–536.

36. Cantillo JF, Fernández-Caldas E, Puerta L. Immunological aspects of the immune response induced by mosquito allergens. *Int Arch Allergy Immunol* 2014; 165(4): 271–282.

37. Cantillo JF, Puerta L, Puchalska P, Lafosse-Marin S, Subiza JL, Fernández-Caldas E. Allergenome characterization of the mosquito *Aedes aegypti*. *Allergy* 2017; 72(10): 1499–1509.

38. Cantillo JF, Puerta L, Lafosse-Marin S, Subiza JL, Caraballo L, Fernandez-Caldas E. Allergens involved in the cross-reactivity of *Aedes aegypti* with other arthropods. *Ann Allergy Asthma Immunol* 2017; 118(6): 710–718.

39. Cantillo JF, Puerta L, Fernandez-Caldas E et al. Tropomyosins in mosquito and house dust mite cross-react at the humoral and cellular level. *Clin Exp Allergy* 2018; 48(10): 1354–1363.

40. Jeong KY, Choi SY, Lee JH et al. Standardization of house dust mite extracts in Korea. *Allergy Asthma Immunol Res* 2012; 4(6): 346–350.

41. Eskridge EM, Elliott WB, Elliott AH et al. Adaptation of the electrical stimulation procedure for the collection of vespid venoms. *Toxicon* 1981; 19: 893–897.

42. Weytjens K, Cartier A, Malo JL et al. Aerosolized snow-crab allergens in a processing facility. *Allergy* 1999; 54(8): 892–893.

43. Jeebhay MF, Robins TG, Lehrer SB, Lopata AL. Occupational seafood allergy: A review. *Occup Environ Med* 2001; 58(9): 553–562.

44. Carnés J, Ferrer A, Huertas AJ, Andreu C, Larramendi CH, Fernández-Caldas E. The use of raw or boiled crustacean extracts for the diagnosis of seafood allergic individuals. *Ann Allergy Asthma Immunol* 2007; 98(4): 349–354.

45. Liu GM, Cheng H, Nesbit JB, Su WJ, Cao MJ, Maleki SJ. Effects of boiling on the IgE-binding properties of tropomyosin of shrimp (*Litopenaeus vannamei*). *J Food Sci* 2010; 75(1): T1–T5.

46. Council of Europe, European Pharmacopoeia Commission Staff. 5.2. General texts on vaccines: 5.2.8. Minimising the risk of transmitting animal spongiform encephalopathy agents via human and veterinary medicinal products. In *European Pharmacopoeia*. Vol 1. 5th ed. Strasbourg, France: Council of Europe, 2005: 463–471.

47. Hochwallner H, Schulmeister U, Swoboda I, Spitzauer S, Valenta R. Cow's milk allergy: From allergens to new forms of diagnosis, therapy and prevention. *Methods* 2014; 66(1): 22–33.

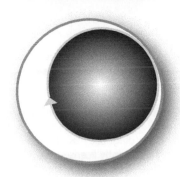

23 Manufacturing food extracts

Natalie A. David
U.S. Food and Drug Administration

Anusha Penumarti
University of North Carolina

Jay E. Slater
U.S. Food and Drug Administration

CONTENTS

23.1 INTRODUCTION

Humans consume a wide variety of foods in their daily diet, and virtually any of these foods can induce an allergic reaction. Food allergy is a nonprotective immune response induced by exposure to certain foods or food additives [1]. In the United States, the most common allergenic foods are milk, eggs, fish, crustacean shellfish, tree nuts, peanuts, wheat, and soybeans [2–6]. Worldwide, differences in food allergies exist based on factors including, but not limited to, geographic location, age, genetic variation, and dietary habits. For example, sesame is a common food and food allergy in Israel, while buckwheat and the edible nest of swiftlets, called "bird's nest," are common food allergens in Japan and Singapore, respectively [7–9]. In addition, some studies have shown that the incidence of food allergy is higher in infants and toddlers when compared to adults and adolescents, indicating that the prevalence of food allergy slightly decreases with age [2,10]. Despite this overall trend, allergies to certain foods, fish and shellfish in particular, become more common during adolescence and adulthood [11].

Age may also predict the allergen(s) to which an individual might become sensitized. For example, although allergies to cow's milk, egg, soy, and wheat are more prevalent in infants and children, peanut, tree nut, fish, and shellfish allergies typically persist in adolescents and adults [2,12,13].

Although treatments are available for food-induced allergic reactions, the only way to prevent adverse reactions is to avoid the problematic food. The offending food can be identified using skin prick testing (SPT) with allergen extracts, SPT using fresh foods ("prick-and-prick" method), specific IgE testing, or double-blind, placebo-controlled food challenges (DBPCFCs). SPTs with commercially available food allergen extracts are reliable for foods with stable proteins. Allergens in many fruits and vegetables are more labile, and prepared extracts may give more false-negative SPT results. In these cases, the prick-and-prick method or SPT with a slurry of food and sterile saline may be more informative [14].

Allergen extracts have been used since the early twentieth century for the diagnosis and treatment of allergic diseases. Historically, extracts were prepared by individual allergists in their practices, but production soon transitioned to commercial allergen extract manufacturers. Unlike most allergen extracts, which are approved for both diagnostic use and for use in subcutaneous immunotherapy (SCIT), currently licensed food allergen extracts are not approved for the treatment of food allergy [2,15]. Here we describe the selection of source materials, manufacturing procedures, relevant regulations, and standardization efforts for food allergen extracts as well as challenges associated with developing allergen extracts for particular foods.

23.2 MANUFACTURING FOOD EXTRACTS

23.2.1 Methods of collecting, identifying, and processing food source materials

The appropriate selection of the starting source material and all subsequent manufacturing steps contribute to the final quality of an allergen extract. Once the optimal conditions are established, deviations in any of these procedures may result in increased heterogeneity of allergen extracts between manufacturers or even between production lots of a single manufacturer.

Some allergen extract manufacturers purchase source materials from source material suppliers who have already processed foods from vendors into a form ready to use in manufacturing, while others maintain divisions dedicated to acquiring source materials directly from food vendors and processing the materials themselves [16–18]. Food source material may be obtained in powdered, liquid, or freeze-dried forms, but processing should be minimal. Ideally, food sources should be fresh or frozen and should be of a quality suitable for human consumption [19,20]. Careful consideration of the origin of source materials may be important to preserve lot-to-lot consistency of the final product [21]. Controlled collection, storage, and processing of the raw materials also enhances consistency [22]. Storage temperature and controlled atmosphere conditions are known to affect allergen levels in fruits [23]. Overall apple allergenicity is reduced with cold storage at 3°C under controlled atmospheric conditions [24]. The apple allergen Mal d 3 is reduced with cold storage conditions, particularly when stored under controlled atmosphere conditions [25]. Another apple allergen, Mal d 1, increases with both cold storage and modified atmosphere packaging [26,27].

Changes in cultivars, climate, timing of source material collection, geography, or environmental conditions may produce inconsistent levels of specific allergens in source materials [18,28]. Timing of source material collection determines the harvest maturity of the collected food. For citrus, allergen expression generally decreases as the fruits progress from underripe to overripe [29]. However, these results are not generalizable across all citrus allergens and cultivars. Harvest maturity is also an important factor in the allergenicity of apples. Mal d 1 increases with increasing ripeness [30]. Manufacturers may align their production schedules with the harvest season of a particular food or may freeze or freeze-dry it for storage upon receipt of the fresh food [31].

Special attention should also be paid to identification and purity of source materials to minimize heterogeneity [21]. For food allergies, misidentification of source material may result in the production of an improperly labeled allergen extract and incorrect diagnoses for patients. Inaccurate diagnosis of food allergy, based on skin testing alone, may cause patients to avoid foods they are able to tolerate, while causing them to inadvertently fail in avoiding truly problematic foods. Surveys show that certain foods, particularly fish, may be

mislabeled by U.S. wholesalers, restaurants, and grocery stores; a 2016 review of studies published since 2014 revealed a normalized average rate of seafood fraud of 28% in the United States [32]. In a 2014 study conducted by the U.S. Food and Drug Administration's (FDA) Center for Food Safety and Applied Nutrition (CFSAN), 15% of tested fish samples ($n = 174$) across 14 states were not labeled in accordance with the FDA Seafood List [33].

Considering these findings, it is important that source materials be properly identified. Although definitive chemical or biochemical identification procedures are not used at this time in the United States [18,34], most foods can be identified definitively by gross appearance. In particular, fish and other seafood may be identified with reasonable certainty by visual appearance alone if the whole organism is purchased rather than fillets or fragments. When whole organisms are unavailable, manufacturers can consult the FDA's Regulatory Fish Encyclopedia (RFE), which includes high-resolution photographs of fish fillets, as well as isoelectric focusing (IEF) and electrophoresis tissue protein patterns and mitochondrial DNA sequencing information. By sequencing a 600 base-pair segment of the highly polymorphic mitochondrial gene cytochrome oxidase I (COI), an organism can be taxonomically identified. This approach is called DNA barcoding [35]. In addition, databases such as the Fish Barcode of Life (FISH-BOL) initiative, Catalog of Fishes, and FishBase may assist in seafood identification.

23.2.2 Regulatory considerations for source materials (see also Chapters 25 and 26)

Regulation of source materials is the responsibility of the FDA and the European Medicines Agency (EMA) and European Pharmacopoeia (EP) in Europe. Requirements for source materials used in the production of allergen extracts licensed in the United States are specifically addressed in 21 C.F.R. §680. The FDA requires that licensed extract manufacturers provide a listing of the manufacturer's source material suppliers [36]. Manufacturers are responsible for ensuring that suppliers of source materials are qualified and that procedures for collection and identification of source materials are appropriate. In addition, animals used as food source materials must have been in good health [37], and source materials must be used fresh or appropriately stored [38].

The 1999 FDA guidance document for allergenic product manufacturers provides additional information recommended for products licensed in the United States [19]. Manufacturers should identify source materials by genus, species, common name, and microscopic and macroscopic characteristics [19,39]. For foods, the guidance specifies that canned and processed foods are not to be used as source materials. Additionally, the batch production record includes the packaging label from the store where the food is purchased. If no packaging label is available, the location and identity of the supplying store are identified.

Regulation of source materials in Europe is similar: control methods, acceptance criteria for identity and purity, and controlled storage conditions are particularly important. In addition, information detailing source material suppliers, specifications, quality control methods, storage conditions, and identification are provided. The origin of food source materials is maintained constant to provide uniformity of the licensed product [39]. The procedure for any source materials that have been pretreated (e.g., flour, spices) is described. For meat, fish, and seafood, any veterinary and microbiological controls to which the animal or source material was subjected are indicated. If certain part(s) of the animal are used, the procedure for its isolation and treatment is included [40].

23.2.3 Manufacturing allergen extracts

Although the scale and available technologies for extract preparation have changed dramatically since the process was first described, many of the manufacturing steps remain unchanged [41,42]. In general, the following procedures apply to the preparation of food

Table 23.1 Manufacturing workflow for food allergen extracts

Selection of source materials

Foods for use as source materials should be fresh or frozen. Consideration of cultivar, climate, geography, and environmental conditions may be made.

Collection of source materials

Controlled collection conditions, including timing, may increase consistency of the final product.

Identification of source materials

Foods are usually definitively identified by gross appearance alone. Biochemical methods may be used to complement this approach.

Storage

Foods are stored under controlled conditions. Harvested food source materials are frozen or freeze-dried if not immediately proceeding to extraction.

Grinding

Grinding increases surface area of the source material prior to extraction.

Defatting

Defatting source materials with organic solvents removes fats, oils, and/or waxes and improves extraction efficiency.

Extraction

Extraction solubilizes the allergens from the source material in a buffered aqueous solution.

Clarification

Clarification removes solid source materials through a series of filtration steps.

Sterilization

Allergen extracts are sterilized using a 0.2 μm filter.

Product evaluation

Manufacturers test the final allergen extract for sterility, general safety, pH, and preservative content.

Source: Adapted from David NA et al. *Ann Allergy Asthma Immunol* 2017; 119: 101–107, with permission from Elsevier.

extracts: grinding, defatting, extraction, clarification, sterilization, and product testing (Table 23.1) [31,41]. Following careful selection and preservation of the allergen source material, foods may undergo preliminary processing such as grinding or blending, which increases the surface area of the material prior to extraction. Defatting, the removal of fats, oils, and/or waxes using solvents, may be performed. Manufacturers remove these substances to improve exposure of allergenic proteins and extraction efficiency and to remove components insoluble in water [31]. Foods with high water content (such as fruits and vegetables) are usually not defatted; meats, fish, and nuts are often defatted [42].

Grinding and defatting are followed by extraction, which solubilizes the allergens in the source material into an extracting fluid. Extraction procedures can vary considerably: the extraction ratio (weight of raw material to volume of extracting fluid), extraction time, extraction temperature, and composition of the extraction solution all determine the yield of the allergen in solution. Extraction generally takes place in a buffered, slightly alkaline solution [31]; optimal allergen extraction is buffer dependent, and extraction buffers should ideally be individually optimized for each allergenic food [43]. The solution used for extraction is determined by the desired final product formulation. For aqueous extracts, a buffered saline solution with preservatives such as phenol or glycerin is used for extraction [31,44]; in some protocols, glycerin is added after extraction. Allergen extracts may also be distributed as lyophilized products. However, no lyophilized food allergen extracts are licensed for distribution in the United States.

After extraction, the solid source materials are removed through the process of clarification. The extract is clarified using a succession of increasingly fine filters [31]. The selected filters must be compatible with the extract, not leach chemicals into the product, and not adsorb the extracted allergens [31]. Some manufacturers may use additional steps such as dialysis or ultrafiltration to further clarify the extract or remove low molecular weight compounds. The final manufacturing steps for allergen extracts are sterilization and product testing. Allergen extracts are thermolabile and must be sterilized using aseptic filtration, using a 0.2 μm pore sterilizing filter [31,41]. Final product evaluation by manufacturers includes testing for sterility (for both anaerobic and aerobic microorganisms), general safety, pH, and preservative content [31].

Because no food allergen extracts have been standardized, manufacturers label the final product with either protein nitrogen units (PNUs), a measure of total protein content, or extraction ratio (w/v) to reflect how the product is manufactured. In Europe, qualitative profiling for allergen content may be performed using electrophoretic methods [44]. In addition, consistency and composition of manufactured food allergen extracts may be assessed through the use of in-house references.

23.2.4 Regulatory considerations for manufacturing procedures (see also Chapters 25 and 26)

In the United States, manufacturing requirements for allergen extracts are described in 21 C.F.R. §600, 610, and 680. A specific emphasis is placed on manufacturing procedures for product consistency, particularly because no potency or composition standards exist for food allergen extracts. Manufacturers provide written standard operating procedures in their biologic product license file. These procedures include information regarding extraction solutions and their components; complete details of the production; all quality control tests and release limits; procedures for packaging and labeling; storage temperatures and systems for controlling them; expiration dating information; product release procedures; shipping procedures; and records preparation, verification, and retention. Manufacturers also test products for identity, potency, and sterility [45]. Product labeling is consistent with FDA regulations to ensure that the labeling contains the essential scientific information for the safe and effective use of the product [46]. Correct and consistent nomenclature must be used for licensed allergen extracts [47].

EMA and EP maintain similar standards for allergen extract manufacturers [39,48]. EP requires manufacturers to report the extraction ratio, use manufacturing conditions designed to minimize enzymatic degradation, design purification procedures to remove irritants and nonallergenic components, and justify the addition of any antimicrobial preservatives. It also requires that extract identity be confirmed using an in-house reference preparation. The finished product is tested for water content (lyophilized products), sterility, microbial contamination, protein content, and protein profile. Some additional tests may be applied, including aluminum and calcium content, allergen profile, total allergenic activity, and individual allergen content.

EMA Directive 81/852/EEC, amended by Directive 92/18/EEC, applies to allergen extracts. EMA also provides additional guidance information for manufacturers submitting marketing authorization applications for these products. Like the FDA, EMA states that manufacturers should describe the production process, step by step, using a diagram. Each manufacturing step should be clearly explained and the point at which aseptic precautions are introduced should be identified. In-process controls, purification methods, and fractionation methods should also be reported. Production, characterization, and use of an in-house reference preparation should be described. Appropriate use of an in-house reference is essential for batch-to-batch consistency. In these applications, manufacturers include safety, efficacy, and stability data as well. Total allergenic activity of the finished allergen extract is measured and reported. Sterility testing is performed in accordance with EP. In addition, EMA's Committee for Medicinal Products for Human Use (CHMP) has issued a document for allergen products which provides further elaboration on this guidance [40].

23.2.5 Food processing and allergenicity

In the United States, all food allergen extracts are manufactured from raw food source materials, based on the frequent observation that thermal and nonthermal processing reduce the allergenicity of foods and thus result in a less potent extract. The nonthermal process of peeling fruits, for example, reduces the allergenicity of *Rosaceae* family members [49]. The peels of peach and apple, which are typically consumed, are enriched in certain allergens compared to the pulps of these fruits [50,51]. For some non-*Rosaceae* family members, like citrus, only the pulp of the fruit is edible. Transcriptional data show that citrus allergens Cit s 1.01 and Cit s 3.01 are more highly expressed in the peel than in the pulp [29]. A peeled orange allergen extract would be more representative of the portion of the fruit typically consumed, the pulp, though potentially less allergenic for diagnostic use.

There is evidence that, for some foods, certain thermal processes may enhance allergenicity (Table 23.2) [52]. This is an important consideration given that many foods for which extracts are

Table 23.2 Effects of heating on the allergenicity of certain foods

Food	Thermostable allergens	Thermolabile allergens	Tolerance to ingestion of heated food
Milk	Caseins	Whey proteins (α-lactalbumin, β-lactogloblin)	Some patients can tolerate baked milk.
Egg		OVM, OVT, OVA, α-levitin	Some patients can tolerate baked or heated egg.
Peanut	All		Roasting peanuts increases allergenicity, but boiling or frying reduces allergenicity.
Tree nuts	Almond (amandin), walnut, hazelnut, Brazil nut, pecan, pistachio (dry roasted)	Almond (lower MW allergens), cashew, pistachio (steam roasted), cashew, pistachio (boiled)	No
Wheat	Most		No
Soybean	Gly m 7	Gly m Bd 30K	Boiling decreases the allergenicity of soybeans.
Shellfish	Tropomyosin		Boiling generally increases the allergenicity of shrimp but is highly species specific.
Fish	Parvalbumins		Canned fish demonstrates reduced allergenicity.

Source: Adapted from David NA et al. *Ann Allergy Asthma Immunol* 2017; 119: 101–107, with permission from Elsevier.
Abbreviations: MW, molecular weight; OVA, ovalbumin; OVM, ovomucoid; OVT, ovotransferrin.

available are commonly consumed following thermal processing. The same food may also not be subject to a uniform type of thermal processing globally: peanuts are commonly roasted or fried in the United States and Europe, whereas they are more commonly boiled in China. To the degree that processing might enhance allergenicity of a food, processing of the food source material prior to extraction could be expected to increase the likelihood of IgE reactivity with the allergen extract. It is challenging to generalize the results of published studies regarding the effects of thermal processing on allergenicity because of the varying cooking methods employed as well as the different time-temperature combinations used. Thermal processing may involve any combination of baking, roasting, frying, boiling, pressure cooking, and microwave heating. The IgE-binding capacity of an allergen may be unchanged following heating, particularly for linear epitopes. In contrast, heating may bring about substantial changes in allergenicity by altering the protein and/or glycoprotein structure of relevant epitopes, thereby modulating the IgE-binding capacity [11,53]. Existing IgE-reactive epitopes may be destroyed, or neoallergen epitopes may be revealed through heating [54]. In addition to the more predictable changes in protein structure following heating, proteins in processed food may also interact with other components such as other proteins, fats, and sugars, resulting in a matrix effect. The resulting matrix effect reduces the ability of allergenic proteins to interact with the immune system and results in a decrease in allergenicity. For example, heating of the milk allergen β-lactoglobulin decreases its allergenicity due to the formation of intermolecular disulfide bonds and its complex formation with other food proteins [55]. Following is a brief overview on the effects of common food processing on the allergenic nature of the most common food allergens.

23.2.5.1 MILK

Milk allergy is one of the most common food allergies in infants but is usually outgrown by adulthood [2]. The known allergens of cow milk are caseins and globular whey proteins (α-lactalbumin and β-lactoglobulin) [56]. Caseins lack a three-dimensional structure, instead forming micelles in solution, and are heat stable. IgE from milk-allergic patients demonstrates preferential binding to the linear epitopes of caseins, thus providing further evidence that IgE binding to caseins is not sensitive to denaturation [57]. In fact, pasteurized and homogenized milk, which is readily commercially available and commonly consumed, is more allergenic than raw milk in allergic individuals [58].

In contrast, the binding of human IgE to α-lactalbumin and β-lactoglobulin is reduced when milk is heated to higher temperatures, above 90°C, than those used for pasteurization [59,60]. Protein denaturation and aggregation with other milk components are both hypothesized to contribute to the decreased allergenicity of milk heated to these temperatures [61]. In clinical studies, baked milk products containing wheat are shown to be tolerated by 75% of children with milk allergy [62]. Furthermore, the introduction of baked milk in the diet of children allergic to milk appears to accelerate the development of tolerance to raw milk when compared to strict avoidance [63]. The IgE-binding capacity and stability of milk proteins are largely dependent on temperature and duration of thermal processing, pH, and food matrix effect and can also be greatly variable among patients.

23.2.5.2 EGG

The primary chicken egg allergens, ovomucoid (OVM or Gal d 1), ovalbumin (OVA or Gal d 2), ovotransferrin (OVT or Gal d 3), and lysozyme (LYS or Gal d 4), are present in egg white [64]. Egg yolk contains the allergen α-levitin (Gal d 5), also known as chicken serum albumin, and displays low levels of allergenicity [64,65]. In vitro studies show that heating egg decreases the IgE-binding capacity of OVM, OVT, and OVA, thus reducing its allergenicity [66]. The allergenicity of α-levitin was reported to be significantly decreased but not completely eliminated by heating [67]. In some

cases of egg allergy, children tolerate baked or heated forms of egg better than its raw form [68]. Furthermore, introduction of baked egg in the diet of allergic children may accelerate the development of tolerance to regular egg, compared to strict avoidance [69].

23.2.5.3 PEANUTS

The major allergens in peanut are vicilin seed storage protein (Ara h 1) and conglutin (Ara h 2). The minor peanut allergens include glycinin (Ara h 3, previously Ara h 4), profilin (Ara h 5), other conglutin family members (Ara h 6, 7), and peanut agglutinin (Ara h agglutinin). Changes in peanut allergenicity with thermal processing can be divided into two categories: dry heating (roasting) and wet heating (boiling and frying). Temperatures achieved using roasting can be higher than in frying or boiling [70]. Roasting peanuts decreases the solubility of the major peanut allergens, while IgE-binding remains unchanged [71] or increases [72]. Maleki et al. show that roasted peanuts have increased allergenicity, approximately 90-fold higher than raw peanuts, and that the protein modifications caused by the Maillard reaction contribute to this effect [72]. The Maillard reaction is a form of nonenzymatic browning in which amino acids react with reducing sugars. In addition, boiling or frying peanuts significantly decreases the IgE-binding of Ara h 1, Ara h 2, and Ara h 3 when compared to raw or roasted peanuts [73]. This finding is recapitulated in a mouse model of allergy using Ara h 2 purified from heat-treated peanuts [74]. Finally, a study of peanut-allergic patients shows that the SPT wheal sizes and IgE-binding properties of peanut protein extracts are significantly lower when extracts were made from boiled compared to raw peanuts and when extracts from raw, fried, and roasted peanuts are subjected to specific conditions of heat and pressure compared to their untreated forms [75].

23.2.5.4 TREE NUTS

Tree nuts include almond, cashew, walnut, hazelnut, Brazil nut, pecan, and pistachio. Allergens in most tree nuts, including almond (amandin, Pru du 6) [76], walnut [77], hazelnut [78], Brazil nut [79], pecan [80], and pistachio (dry roasted) [81] nuts demonstrate antigenic stability following heating in in vitro studies, but binding to human IgE is reduced following heating for almond (lower molecular weight allergens) [76], cashew [82], and pistachio (steam roasted) [81] nuts. Boiled cashews and boiled pistachios have decreased basophil degranulation in vitro as well [83]. In a DBPCFC study, the allergenicity of roasted hazelnut is considerably reduced compared to raw hazelnut, but clinical symptoms are not reduced in all patients. Thus, roasted hazelnut cannot be reliably consumed by hazelnut-allergic patients [84]. In order to further evaluate the effects of heating on the allergenicity of other tree nuts, future studies using DBPCFCs are warranted.

23.2.5.5 WHEAT

While some allergenic wheat proteins are destroyed by baking, others remain stable. In addition, some proteins become more resistant to digestion with pepsin following heat treatment [85]. This decreased protein digestibility is the result of protein modifications that involve not only protein breakdown, but also aggregation, cross-linking, and Maillard-type reactions. Since the crust is subjected to higher temperatures than the crumb during baking, protein aggregation is also greater in the crust, and the solubility and allergenicity of these protein aggregates are different from those found in the crumb [85].

23.2.5.6 SOYBEANS

Soybean allergens include prolamin, cupin, profilin, and oleosin superfamily members [86]. These allergens do not respond uniformly to heating. The soybean allergen Gly m Bd 30K (protein P34) has decreased IgE reactivity with boiling [87], whereas the same treatment does not reduce the IgE reactivity of Gly m 7 [88]. As with Gly m Bd 30K, overall IgE reactivity to soybean is reduced with increasing boiling times. Boiled soybean extracts also demonstrate reduced allergenicity through reduced wheal size on SPT [89]. Processing of soybeans into soy sauce through the fermentation attenuates but does not completely eliminate their allergenicity as measured by radioallergosorbent test (RAST) inhibition [90].

23.2.5.7 FISH AND SHELLFISH

The allergens in fish are the calcium-binding parvalbumins (e.g., Gal c 1). The allergenicity of fish proteins is not affected by heat treatment such as boiling or frying [91]. However, the IgE-binding activity is significantly reduced in canned fish due to the extreme temperature and pressure used during canning [92]. Tropomyosin, the major allergen present in shellfish, is thermostable [93], although cooked extracts demonstrate significantly higher IgE reactivity than raw extracts [94]. Boiling extracts increases the allergenicity of prawn (*Penaeus* spp.) as assessed using wheal size on SPT [95]. Results from a more recent study from Thailand using different varieties of shrimp have shown conflicting results. Raw *Penaeus monodon* (black tiger prawn) extracts induce larger wheal sizes than boiled extracts, but there is no difference between boiled and raw *Macrobrachium rosenbergii* (freshwater prawn) extracts [96]. PBMCs isolated from crustacean-allergic individuals do not show significant differences in proliferation or cytokine production when stimulated with cooked extracts compared to raw extracts [94]. These studies suggest that allergen thermostability data may be highly species-specific for crustaceans.

23.2.6 Relevance of pan-allergens and cross-reactivity considerations

Each food contains several glycoproteins that are potential allergens. These glycoproteins have specific physicochemical properties and are broadly divided into two classes: class 1 and class 2 allergens [97]. Class 1 (complete) food allergens range from 10 to 70 kDa in size, are water-soluble, resistant to heat and gastric digestion, and are not affected by food processing or preparation. They are capable of inducing IgE sensitization following absorption through the gastrointestinal mucosa [97] and are typically responsible for systemic allergic reactions [98,99]. In contrast, class 2 (incomplete) food allergens (also known as cross-reacting allergens) are sensitive to heat and gastric digestion and do not cause gastrointestinal sensitization, but they are capable of producing allergic reactions in patients already sensitized through the respiratory route to cross-reactive aeroallergens [99,100]. Cross-reactive ubiquitous allergens belonging to widely different protein families, well preserved throughout various species and able to trigger IgE antibody binding, are known as pan-allergens [101]. Because of protein homologies, cross-reactivity among the different tree nuts and between tree nuts and pollens is common. For example, the birch pollen allergen Bet v 1, a PR-10 family member, is cross-reactive with the hazelnut allergen Cor a 1 [102]. A 2009 study in mice showed a high level of cross-reactivity between cashew and walnut but a weaker cross-reactivity between cashew and peanut [103]. Although such cross-reactivity may be demonstrated *in vitro* or with SPT, it may not always be evident clinically [104]. Other reports on tree nut cross-reactivity indicate that patients allergic to one nut should avoid all nuts as they are likely to react to others [105]. Finally, consistent clinical reports of cosensitization to latex, banana, avocado, chestnut, and kiwi appear to be due to cross-reactivity of specific latex and fruit allergens, a so-called latex-fruit allergy syndrome; primary sensitization is usually to the latex protein [106].

23.2.7 Fruit and vegetable allergy associated with pollenosis

Allergies to uncooked fruits and vegetables usually arise from prior sensitization to pollen aeroallergens through respiratory exposure. This phenomenon is known as oral allergy syndrome (OAS) or pollen-associated food allergy syndrome (PFAS) [100]. The high degree of structural similarity of allergenic molecules derived from closely related or functionally similar molecules within the same protein family may lead to IgE cross-reactivity [107]. For example, patients allergic to the birch pollen allergen Bet v 1 may develop allergies to fruits in the *Rosaceae* family (e.g., apple, strawberry, peach, plum, pear) and vegetables in the *Apiaceae* family (e.g., carrot, celery) [14]. Other examples of PFAS include sensitization to profilins, associated with grass pollens, leading to reactions to tomato and peach [108] as well as sensitization to cross-reacting carbohydrate determinants (CCD), leading to reactions to vegetables in the *Cucurbitaceae* family (e.g., pumpkin, melon, squash, cucumber) [109]. Other instances of cross-reactivity between aeroallergens and fruit and vegetable allergens are documented [100]. This knowledge is of great clinical importance in order to individualize treatment and instruct patients to avoid foods that have potentially cross-reactive proteins.

23.2.8 Standardization considerations (see also Chapters 25 and 26)

The inherent variability of complicated biologic products such as allergen extracts presents a considerable challenge for standardization efforts. Variations in source material selection and extraction procedure, among other variables, contribute to the potential for substantial heterogeneity among products from different manufacturers and even between production lots of a single manufacturer. In most cases, the identity of the active ingredients is uncertain. This presents a particular problem to regulatory agencies tasked with the responsibility of ensuring the efficacy, safety, and consistency of these products. Historically, a number of approaches have been used to address such concerns; an international scientific consensus has not been achieved.

In the United States, nonstandardized allergen extracts, including all food extracts, are labeled with either the extraction ratio or with protein nitrogen units ([PNU]/mL) using the Kjeldahl method [22]. Neither designation is particularly informative nor strongly correlates with the overall biological potency of allergen products. The Center for Biologics Evaluation and Research (CBER) at the FDA maintains a reference standard for 19 standardized allergen extracts and designates procedures to compare a manufactured product to the reference. The reference extract is assigned a particular unitage, and the manufactured extract is therefore assigned a relative potency in relation to the standard. Bioequivalent allergen units (BAUs) are assigned based on a quantitative intradermal skin test titration in highly allergic subjects; other standardized units include allergen-specific unitage (Amb a 1 or Fel d 1 units), AU/mL, and mass units, as appropriate [22,110]. Release limits are set such that the manufactured extract must be statistically equivalent to the reference extract at a specified confidence level [22]. Proteomic profile comparison of the manufactured extract to the reference standard may also be part of the assessment of standardized extracts.

The approach to standardization is considerably different outside of the United States. Rather than complying with a single reference standard, the European method is based on comparing manufactured products to in-house reference preparations, which are unique to each manufacturer. Another challenge is that Europe lacks a common label for allergenicity. Most manufacturers follow one skin test–based protocol (the Nordic system) for biological standardization, but other manufacturers apply the FDA's $ID_{50}EAL$ protocol [110,111]. Applying these two approaches can lead to very different results.

There are several novel approaches on the horizon for standardization of allergen extracts. The European Union CREATE project worked to develop certified recombinant reference materials and validated monoclonal antibody–based immunoassays for measurement of specific allergens [111]. Other researchers have developed additional assays for quantification of major allergens; examples include assays for Ara h 1 and Ara h 2 [112]. Another potential method for standardization would utilize tandem mass spectrometry (MS/MS). MS/MS-based approaches have the advantage of simultaneous detection of many allergens and their unique isoforms [28]. The multiplex allergen extract potency assay has only been applied to aeroallergens so far but may be applied to complex food allergens as well [113].

Ultimately, regulatory authorities must balance two competing priorities. They must consider the need for increased regulatory requirements for product safety and efficacy and public health. However, they must not make regulatory demands so arduous to manufacturers that these companies become limited in their ability to offer a wide range of food allergen extracts [114]. Maintaining a diverse portfolio of these products is important for accurate diagnosis of food allergy in clinical practice.

23.3 CONCLUSION

Allergen extracts are used for the diagnosis and sometimes the treatment of allergic diseases. For food allergies, allergen extracts are used for testing to identify the offending foods. As there is no cure for food allergy, strict avoidance of allergenic foods is employed to prevent food allergy–induced adverse reactions. Unlike some allergies, SCIT using allergen extracts is not licensed for the treatment of food allergy, though other routes of immunotherapy administration (e.g., oral/sublingual and epicutaneous) are under investigation. In addition, experienced practitioners and investigators have long been aware of the limitations in using food allergen extracts, all of which are nonstandardized, for accurate diagnosis and management. Variability among manufacturers, and between lots of a given manufacturer, raise the possibility that specific allergens within a food allergen extract will be underrepresented or missing in the extract used for testing, rendering the test results

unreliable [115]. In the case of fruit and vegetable allergy diagnosis, commercially prepared extracts may lack specificity and sensitivity in SPT [116]. Direct use of the unprocessed foods ("prick-and-prick" method) has been proposed as an alternative to the use of licensed extracts in the diagnosis of fruit and vegetable allergy [117]. Investigational attempts at molecular-based diagnostics combined with recombinant allergens or hypoallergens represent efforts to confront these issues [118,119].

SALIENT POINTS

1. Food allergen extracts are only approved for diagnostic use, not therapeutic use, in the United States.
2. Currently (2019), there are no standardized food allergen extracts approved in the United States.
3. Quality of source materials determines the quality of the allergen extract.
4. Thermal processing can change the allergenicity of some common food allergens, but only unprocessed foods are used in the manufacture of food allergen extracts in the United States.
5. Pan-allergens may result in cross-reactivity in skin testing, which may or may not correlate with clinical cross-reactivity.
6. Cross-reactivity between pollen allergens and food allergens may lead to oral reactivity to uncooked fruits and vegetables in individuals sensitized to pollen.

REFERENCES

1. Burks W, Ballmer-Weber BK. Food allergy. *Mol Nutr Food Res* 2006; 50(7): 595–603.
2. Sicherer SH, Sampson HA. Food allergy. *J Allergy Clin Immunol* 2010; 125(Suppl 2): S116–S125.
3. Rona RJ, Keil T, Summers C et al. The prevalence of food allergy: A meta-analysis. *J Allergy Clin Immunol* 2007; 120(3): 638–646.
4. Sicherer SH, Muñoz-Furlong A, Sampson HA. Prevalence of seafood allergy in the United States determined by a random telephone survey. *J Allergy Clin Immunol* 2004; 114(1): 159–165.
5. Sicherer SH, Muñoz-Furlong A, Godbold JH, Sampson HA. US prevalence of self-reported peanut, tree nut, and sesame allergy: 11-year follow-up. *J Allergy Clin Immunol* 2010; 125(6): 1322–1326.
6. Zuidmeer L, Goldhahn K, Rona RJ et al. The prevalence of plant food allergies: A systematic review. *J Allergy Clin Immunol* 2008; 121(5): 1210–1218.e1214.
7. Akiyama H, Imai T, Ebisawa M. Japan food allergen labeling regulation—History and evaluation. *Adv Food Nutr Res.* 2011; 62: 139–171.
8. Dalal I, Binson I, Reifen R et al. Food allergy is a matter of geography after all: Sesame as a major cause of severe IgE-mediated food allergic reactions among infants and young children in Israel. *Allergy* 2002; 57(4): 362–365.
9. Goh DL, Lau YN, Chew FT, Shek LP, Lee BW. Pattern of food-induced anaphylaxis in children of an Asian community. *Allergy* 1999; 54(1): 84–86.
10. Sicherer SH, Sampson HA. Food allergy: Recent advances in pathophysiology and treatment. *Annu Rev Med* 2009; 60: 261–277.

11. Kosti RI, Triga M, Tsabouri S, Priftis KN. Food allergen selective thermal processing regimens may change oral tolerance in infancy. *Allergol Immunopathol (Madr)* 2013; 41(6): 407–417.

12. Lee LA, Burks AW. Food allergies: Prevalence, molecular characterization, and treatment/prevention strategies. *Annu Rev Nutr* 2006; 26: 539–565.

13. Savage JH, Kaeding AJ, Matsui EC, Wood RA. The natural history of soy allergy. *J Allergy Clin Immunol* 2010; 125(3): 683–686.

14. Sampson HA, Aceves S, Bock SA et al. Food allergy: A practice parameter update-2014. *J Allergy Clin Immunol* 2014; 134(5): 1016–1025.e1043.

15. Lemanske RF, Jr., Taylor SL. Standardized extracts, foods. *Clin Rev Allergy* 1987; 5(1): 23–36.

16. Allergon. Food Allergens. http://www.allergon.com/products/food/. Published 2019. Accessed 11 December 2019.

17. Stallergenes-Greer. Source Materials- What We Offer. https://www.stagrsourcematerials.com/what-we-offer/. Accessed 11 December 2019.

18. Grier T. Allergenic source materials—Considerations and challenges for biopharmaceutical product or assay development. *Pharm Process* 2007: 18–20.

19. CBER F. "Guidance for Industry: On the Content and Format of Chemistry, Manufacturing and Controls Information and Establishment Description Information for an Allergenic Extract or Allergen Patch Test"; Availability. Food and Drug Administration, HHS. Notice. *Fed Regist* 1999; 64(78): 20006–20007.

20. Biological Products; Allergenic Extracts; Implementation of Efficacy Review; Proposed Rule.21 *Federal Register* 600, 610, and 680, 23 January 1985: 3082–3288.

21. Esch RE. Allergen source materials and quality control of allergenic extracts. *Methods* 1997; 13(1): 2–13.

22. Morrow KS, Slater JE. Regulatory aspects of allergen vaccines in the US. *Clin Rev Allergy Immunol* 2001; 21(2-3): 141–152.

23. Wang J, Vanga SK, Raghavan V. Effect of pre-harvest and post-harvest conditions on the fruit allergenicity: A review. *Crit Rev Food Sci Nutr* 2019; 59(7): 1027–1043.

24. Bolhaar ST, van de Weg WE, van Ree R et al. *In vivo* assessment with prick-to-prick testing and double-blind, placebo-controlled food challenge of allergenicity of apple cultivars. *J Allergy Clin Immunol* 2005; 116(5): 1080–1086.

25. Sancho AI, Foxall R, Rigby NM et al. Maturity and storage influence on the apple (*Malus domestica*) allergen Mal d 3, a nonspecific lipid transfer protein. *J Agric Food Chem* 2006; 54(14): 5098–5104.

26. Hsieh LS, Moos M, Jr., Lin Y. Characterization of apple 18 and 31 kd allergens by microsequencing and evaluation of their content during storage and ripening. *J Allergy Clin Immunol* 1995; 96(6 Pt 1): 960–970.

27. Sancho AI, Foxall R, Browne T et al. Effect of postharvest storage on the expression of the apple allergen Mal d 1. *J Agric Food Chem* 2006; 54(16): 5917–5923.

28. Burastero S. *Allergen Extract Analysis and Quality Control.* InTech, 2011, Quality Control of Herbal Medicines and Related Areas.

29. Wu J, Chen L, Lin D, Ma Z, Deng X. Development and application of a multiplex real-time PCR assay as an indicator of potential allergenicity in citrus fruits. *J Agric Food Chem* 2016; 64(47): 9089–9098.

30. Schmitz-Eiberger M, Matthes A. Effect of harvest maturity, duration of storage and shelf life of apples on the allergen Mal d 1, polyphenoloxidase activity and polyphenol content. *Food Chem* 2011; 127(4): 1459–1464.

31. Hauck PR, Williamson S. The manufacture of allergenic extracts in North America. *Clin Rev Allergy Immunol* 2001; 21: 93–110.

32. Warner K, Mustain P, Lowell B, Geren S, Talmage S. *Deceptive Dishes: Seafood Swaps Found Worldwide.* Washington, DC: Oceana, 2016.

33. U.S. Food and Drug Administration. FY12-FY13 CFSAN Sampling for Seafood Species Labeling in Wholesale and Imported Seafood. 2014.

34. 21 C.F.R. §610.14.

35. Hebert PD, Cywinska A, Ball SL, deWaard JR. Biological identifications through DNA barcodes. *Proc Biol Sci* 2003; 270(1512): 313–321.

36. 21 C.F.R. §680.1(c).

37. 21 C.F.R. §680.1(b)(3)(i)-(iv), (vi).

38. 21 C.F.R. §680.1 (b)(3)(v),(vi).

39. *Specific Requirements for the Production and Control of Allergen Products.* European Medicines Agency, 1994.

40. *Guideline on Allergen Products: Production and Quality Issues.* European Medicines Agency CHMP, 2008.

41. Sheldon JM, Lovell RG, Mathews KP. *A Manual of Clinical Allergy.* Philadelphia, PA: W.B. Saunders Company, 1953.

42. Strauss MB, Siegel BB, Blumstein GI. Allergenic food extracts. I. Methods of preparation. *J Allergy* 1958; 29(2): 173–180.

43. Westphal CD, Pereira MR, Raybourne RB, Williams KM. Evaluation of extraction buffers using the current approach of detecting multiple allergenic and nonallergenic proteins in food. *J AOAC Int* 2004; 87(6): 1458–1465.

44. Grier TJ. Laboratory methods for allergen extract analysis and quality control. *Clin Rev Allergy Immunol* 2001; 21(2-3): 111–140.

45. 21 C.F.R. §680.3.

46. 21 C.F.R. §610.60-68.

47. 21 C.F.R. §610.60.

48. Allergen Products (producta allergenica). *European Pharmacopoeia* 2014; 8(2): 3945–3947.

49. Fernandez-Rivas M, Cuevas M. Peels of Rosaceae fruits have a higher allergenicity than pulps. *Clin Exp Allergy* 1999; 29(9): 1239–1247.

50. Ahrazem O, Jimeno L, Lopez-Torrejon G et al. Assessing allergen levels in peach and nectarine cultivars. *Ann Allergy Asthma Immunol* 2007; 99(1): 42–47.

51. Marzban G, Puehringer H, Dey R et al. Localisation and distribution of the major allergens in apple fruits. *Plant Sci* 2005; 169(2): 387–394.

52. Besler M, Steinhart H, Paschke A. Stability of food allergens and allergenicity of processed foods. *J Chromatogr B Biomed Sci Appl* 2001; 756(1–2): 207–228.

53. Sathe SK, Teuber SS, Roux KH. Effects of food processing on the stability of food allergens. *Biotechnol Adv* 2005; 23(6): 423–429.

54. Leduc V, Moneret-Vautrin D-A, Guerin L, Morisset M, Kanny G. Anaphylaxis to wheat isolates: Immunochemical study of a case proved by means of double-blind, placebo-controlled food challenge. *J Allergy Clin Immunol* 2003; 111(4): 897–899.

55. Thomas K, Herouet-Guicheney C, Ladics G et al. Evaluating the effect of food processing on the potential human allergenicity of novel proteins: International workshop report. *Food Chem Toxicol* 2007; 45(7): 1116–1122.

56. Wal JM. Bovine milk allergenicity. *Ann Allergy Asthma Immunol* 2004; 93(5 Suppl 3):S2–11.

57. Kohno Y, Honma K, Saito K et al. Preferential recognition of primary protein structures of α-casein by IgG and IgE antibodies of patients with milk allergy. *Ann Allergy* 1994; 73(5): 419–422.

58. Host A, Samuelsson EG. Allergic reactions to raw, pasteurized, and homogenized/pasteurized cow milk: A comparison. A double-blind placebo-controlled study in milk allergic children. *Allergy* 1988; 43(2): 113–118.

59. Bloom KA, Huang FR, Bencharitiwong R et al. Effect of heat treatment on milk and egg proteins allergenicity. *Pediatric Allergy Immunol* 2014; 25(8): 740–746.

60. Ehn BM, Ekstrand B, Bengtsson U, Ahlstedt S. Modification of IgE binding during heat processing of the cow's milk allergen β-lactoglobulin. *J Agric Food Chem* 2004; 52(5): 1398–1403.

61. Golkar A, Milani JM, Vasiljevic T. Altering allergenicity of cow's milk by food processing for applications in infant formula. *Crit Rev Food Sci Nutr* 2019; 59(1): 159–172.

62. Nowak-Wegrzyn A, Bloom KA, Sicherer SH et al. Tolerance to extensively heated milk in children with cow's milk allergy. *J Allergy Clin Immunol* 2008; 122(2): 342–347, 347.e341–342.

63. Kim JS, Nowak-Wegrzyn A, Sicherer SH, Noone S, Moshier EL, Sampson HA. Dietary baked milk accelerates the resolution of cow's milk allergy in children. *J Allergy Clin Immunol* 2011; 128(1): 125–131.e122.

64. Mine Y, Yang M. Recent advances in the understanding of egg allergens: Basic, industrial, and clinical perspectives. *J Agric Food Chem* 2008; 56(13): 4874–4900.

65. Anet J, Back JF, Baker RS, Barnett D, Burley RW, Howden ME. Allergens in the white and yolk of hen's egg. A study of IgE binding by egg proteins. *Int Arch Allergy Appl Immunol* 1985; 77(3): 364–371.

66. Mine Y, Zhang JW. Comparative studies on antigenicity and allergenicity of native and denatured egg white proteins. *J Agric Food Chem* 2002; 50(9): 2679–2683.

67. Quirce S, Maranon F, Umpierrez A, de las Heras M, Fernandez-Caldas E, Sastre J. Chicken serum albumin (Gal d 5ᵂ) is a partially heat-labile inhalant and food allergen implicated in the bird-egg syndrome. *Allergy* 2001; 56(8): 754–762.

68. Leonard SA, Nowak-Wegrzyn AH. Baked milk and egg diets for milk and egg allergy management. *Immunol Allergy Clin North Am* 2016; 36(1): 147–159.

69. Leonard SA, Sampson HA, Sicherer SH et al. Dietary baked egg accelerates resolution of egg allergy in children. *J Allergy Clin Immunol* 2012; 130(2): 473–480.e471.

70. Cabanillas B, Jappe U, Novak N. Allergy to peanut, soybean, and other legumes: Recent advances in allergen characterization, stability to processing and IgE cross-reactivity. *Mol Nutr Food Res* 2018; 62(1).

71. Koppelman SJ, Bruijnzeel-Koomen CA, Hessing M, de Jongh HH. Heat-induced conformational changes of Ara h 1, a major peanut allergen, do not affect its allergenic properties. *J Biol Chem* 1999; 274(8): 4770–4777.

72. Maleki SJ, Chung SY, Champagne ET, Raufman JP. The effects of roasting on the allergenic properties of peanut proteins. *J Allergy Clin Immunol* 2000; 106(4): 763–768.

73. Beyer K, Morrow E, Li XM et al. Effects of cooking methods on peanut allergenicity. *J Allergy Clin Immunol* 2001; 107(6): 1077–1081.

74. Zhang W, Zhu Q, Zhang T, Cai Q, Chen Q. Thermal processing effects on peanut allergen Ara h 2 allergenicity in mice and its antigenic epitope structure. *Food Chem* 2016; 212: 657–662.

75. Cabanillas B, Cuadrado C, Rodriguez J et al. Potential changes in the allergenicity of three forms of peanut after thermal processing. *Food Chem* 2015; 183: 18–25.

76. Venkatachalam M, Teuber SS, Roux KH, Sathe SK. Effects of roasting, blanching, autoclaving, and microwave heating on antigenicity of almond (*Prunus dulcis* L.) proteins. *J Agric Food Chem* 2002; 50(12): 3544–3548.

77. Su M, Venkatachalam M, Teuber SS, Roux KH, Sathe SK. Impact of γ-irradiation and thermal processing on the antigenicity of almond, cashew nut and walnut proteins. *J Sci Food Agric* 2004; 84(10): 1119–1125.

78. Müller U, Lüttkopf D, Hoffmann A et al. Allergens in raw and roasted hazelnuts (*Corylus avellana*) and their cross-reactivity to pollen. *Eur Food Res Technol* 2000; 212(1): 2–12.

79. Koppelman SJ, Nieuwenhuizen WF, Gaspari M et al. Reversible denaturation of Brazil nut 2S albumin (Ber e1) and implication of structural destabilization on digestion by pepsin. *J Agric Food Chem* 2005; 53(1): 123–131.

80. Venkatachalam M, Teuber SS, Peterson WR, Roux KH, Sathe SK. Antigenic stability of pecan [*Carya illinoinensis* (Wangenh.) K. Koch] proteins: Effects of thermal treatments and *in vitro* digestion. *J Agric Food Chem* 2006; 54(4): 1449–1458.

81. Noorbakhsh R, Mortazavi SA, Sankian M et al. Influence of processing on the allergenic properties of pistachio nut assessed *in vitro*. *J Agric Food Chem* 2010; 58(18): 10231–10235.

82. Mattison CP, Bren-Mattison Y, Vant-Hull B, Vargas AM, Wasserman RL, Grimm CC. Heat-induced alterations in cashew allergen solubility and IgE binding. *Toxicol Rep* 2016; 3: 244–251.

83. Sanchiz A, Cuadrado C, Dieguez MC et al. Thermal processing effects on the IgE-reactivity of cashew and pistachio. *Food Chem* 2018; 245: 595–602.

84. Hansen KS, Ballmer-Weber BK, Luttkopf D et al. Roasted hazelnuts—Allergenic activity evaluated by double-blind, placebo-controlled food challenge. *Allergy* 2003; 58(2): 132–138.

85. Simonato B, Pasini G, Giannattasio M, Peruffo AD, De Lazzari F, Curioni A. Food allergy to wheat products: The effect of bread baking and *in vitro* digestion on wheat allergenic proteins. A study with bread dough, crumb, and crust. *J Agric Food Chem* 2001; 49(11): 5668–5673.

86. Cabanillas B, Jappe U, Novak N. Allergy to peanut, soybean, and other legumes: Recent advances in allergen characterization, stability to processing and IgE cross-reactivity. *Mol Nutr Food Res* 2017; 62(1): 1700446.

87. Wilson S, Martinez-Villaluenga C, De Mejia EG. Purification, thermal stability, and antigenicity of the immunodominant soybean allergen P34 in soy cultivars, ingredients, and products. *J Food Sci* 2008; 73(6):T106–T114.

88. Riascos JJ, Weissinger SM, Weissinger AK, Kulis M, Burks AW, Pons L. The seed biotinylated protein of soybean (*Glycine max*): A boiling-resistant new allergen (Gly m 7) with the capacity to induce IgE-mediated allergic responses. *J Agric Food Chem* 2016; 64(19): 3890–3900.

89. Cabanillas B, Cuadrado C, Rodriguez J, Dieguez MC, Crespo JF, Novak N. Boiling and pressure cooking impact on IgE reactivity of soybean allergens. *Int Arch Allergy Immunol* 2018; 175(1–2): 36–43.

90. Hefle SL, Lambrecht DM, Nordlee JA. Soy sauce retains allergenicity through the fermentation/production process. *J Allergy Clin Immunol* 2005; 115(2):S32.

91. Mondal G, Chatterjee U, Samanta S, Chatterjee BP. Role of pepsin in modifying the allergenicity of bhetki (*Lates calcarifer*) and mackerel (*Rastrelliger kanagurta*) fish. *Indian J Biochem Biophys* 2007; 44(2): 94–100.

92. Bernhisel-Broadbent J, Strause D, Sampson HA. Fish hypersensitivity. II: Clinical relevance of altered fish allergenicity caused by various preparation methods. *J Allergy Clin Immunol* 1992; 90(4 Pt 1): 622–629.

93. Leung PS, Chu KH, Chow WK et al. Cloning, expression, and primary structure of *Metapenaeus ensis* tropomyosin, the major heat-stable shrimp allergen. *J Allergy Clin Immunol* 1994; 94(5): 882–890.

94. Abramovitch JB, Lopata AL, O'Hehir RE, Rolland JM. Effect of thermal processing on T cell reactivity of shellfish allergens—Discordance with IgE reactivity. *PLOS ONE* 2017; 12(3): e0173549.

95. Carnes J, Ferrer A, Huertas AJ, Andreu C, Larramendi CH, Fernandez-Caldas E. The use of raw or boiled crustacean extracts for the diagnosis of seafood allergic individuals. *Ann Allergy Asthma Immunol* 2007; 98(4): 349–354.

96. Pariyaprasert W, Piboonpocanun S, Jirapongsananuruk O, Visitsunthorn N. Stability and potency of raw and boiled shrimp extracts for skin prick test. *Asian Pac J Allergy Immunol* 2015; 33(2): 136–142.

97. Sampson HA. Update on food allergy. *J Allergy Clin Immunol* 2004; 113(5): 805–819; quiz 820.

98. Breiteneder H, Ebner C. Molecular and biochemical classification of plant-derived food allergens. *J Allergy Clin Immunol* 2000; 106(1 Pt 1): 27–36.

99. Han Y, Kim J, Ahn K. Food allergy. *Korean J Pediatr* 2012; 55(5): 153–158.

100. Popescu FD. Cross-reactivity between aeroallergens and food allergens. *World J Methodol* 2015; 5(2): 31–50.

101. Hauser M, Roulias A, Ferreira F, Egger M. Panallergens and their impact on the allergic patient. *Allergy Asthma Clin Immunol* 2010; 6(1): 1–1.

102. Hofmann C, Scheurer S, Rost K et al. Cor a 1-reactive T cells and IgE are predominantly cross-reactive to Bet v 1 in patients with birch pollen-associated food allergy to hazelnut. *J Allergy Clin Immunol* 2013; 131(5): 1384–1392.e1386.

103. Kulis M, Pons L, Burks AW. *In vivo* and T cell cross-reactivity between walnut, cashew and peanut. *Int Arch Allergy Immunol* 2009; 148(2): 109–117.

104. Liu M, Burks AW, Green TD. Tree nut allergy: Risk factors for development, mitigation of reaction risk and current efforts in desensitization. *Expert Rev Clin Immunol* 2015; 11(5): 673–679.

105. Clark AT, Ewan PW. The development and progression of allergy to multiple nuts at different ages. *Pediatr Allergy Immunol* 2005; 16(6): 507–511.

106. Pollart SM, Warniment C, Mori T. Latex allergy. *Am Fam Physician* 2009; 80(12): 1413–1418.

107. Canonica GW, Ansotegui IJ, Pawankar R et al. A WAO-ARIA-GA(2)LEN consensus document on molecular-based allergy diagnostics. *World Allergy Organ J* 2013; 6(1): 1–17.

108. Sankian M, Varasteh A, Pazouki N, Mahmoudi M. Sequence homology: A poor predictive value for profilins cross-reactivity. *Clin Mol Allergy* 2005; 3: 13.

109. Reindl J, Anliker MD, Karamloo F, Vieths S, Wuthrich B. Allergy caused by ingestion of zucchini (*Cucurbita pepo*): Characterization of allergens and cross-reactivity to pollen and other foods. *J Allergy Clin Immunol* 2000; 106(2): 379–385.

110. Turkeltaub PC. Use of skin testing for evaluation of potency, composition, and stability of allergenic products. *Arb Paul Ehrlich Inst Bundesamt Sera Impfstoffe Frankf A M.* 1994; 87: 79–117.

111. Becker W-M, Vogel L, Vieths S. Standardization of allergen extracts for immunotherapy: Where do we stand? *Curr Opin Allergy Clin Immunol* 2006; 6(6): 470–475.

112. Schmitt DA, Cheng H, Maleki SJ, Burks AW. Competitive inhibition ELISA for quantification of Ara h 1 and Ara h 2, the major allergens of peanuts. *J AOAC Int* 2004; 87(6): 1492–1497.

113. Khurana T, Dobrovolskaia E, Shartouny JR, Slater JE. Multiplex assay for protein profiling and potency measurement of German cockroach allergen extracts. *PLOS ONE* 2015; 10(10):e0140225.

114. Klimek L, Hoffmann HJ, Renz H et al. Diagnostic test allergens used for *in vivo* diagnosis of allergic diseases are at risk: A European Perspective. *Allergy* 2015; 70(10): 1329–1331.

115. Vieths S, Hoffmann A, Holzhauser T, Muller U, Reindl J, Haustein D. Factors influencing the quality of food extracts for *in vitro* and *in vivo* diagnosis. *Allergy* 1998; 53(46 Suppl): 65–71.

116. Ortolani C, Ispano M, Pastorello EA, Ansaloni R, Magri GC. Comparison of results of skin prick tests (with fresh foods and commercial food extracts) and RAST in 100 patients with oral allergy syndrome. *J Allergy Clin Immunol* 1989; 83(3): 683–690.

117. Dreborg S, Foucard T. Allergy to apple, carrot and potato in children with birch pollen allergy. *Allergy* 1983; 38(3): 167–172.

118. Kazemi-Shirazi L, Niederberger V, Linhart B, Lidholm J, Kraft D, Valenta R. Recombinant marker allergens: Diagnostic gatekeepers for the treatment of allergy. *Int Arch Allergy Immunol* 2002; 127(4): 259–268.

119. Valenta R, Lidholm J, Niederberger V, Hayek B, Kraft D, Gronlund H. The recombinant allergen-based concept of component-resolved diagnostics and immunotherapy (CRD and CRIT). *Clin Exp Allergy* 1999; 29(7): 896–904.

120. David NA, Penumarti A, Burks AW, Slater JE. Food allergen extracts to diagnose food-induced allergic diseases: How they are made. *Ann Allergy Asthma Immunol* 2017; 119(2): 101–107.

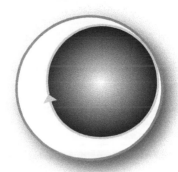

24 Regulation of allergen extracts in the United States*

Jennifer L. Bridgewater, Jay E. Slater, and Ronald L. Rabin
U.S. Food and Drug Administration

CONTENTS

24.1 INTRODUCTION

Allergen extracts and other biologics were first regulated by the Hygienic Laboratory of the Public Health and Marine Hospital Service. In 1930, the Hygienic Laboratory was renamed the National Institute (singular) of Health (NIH). The NIH continued to regulate biologics (beginning in 1955, through its Division of Biologics Standards) for over 40 years. In 1972, regulatory authority over biologics was transferred to the Bureau of Biologics at the U.S. Food and Drug Administration (FDA). In 1982, the FDA merged the Bureau of Biologics and the Bureau of Drugs into a single National Center for Drugs and Biologics; 5 years later, the entities that regulated drugs and biologics were once again separated, and the Center for Biologics Evaluation and Research (CBER) assumed responsibility for regulation of allergenic extracts [1,2].

CBER's authority to regulate allergen extracts is derived from two federal laws, the Food, Drug, and Cosmetic Act of 1938 and the Public Health Service Act of 1944, as amended. The specific regulations that govern CBER's regulation of allergens appear in part 680 of Title 21 of the Code of Federal Regulations (21 CFR 680), although other parts of 21 CFR also apply to allergen regulation. Over the past several decades, two features of CBER's regulatory program have had a significant impact on allergen manufacturers and enhanced the safety of allergen extracts marketed to the American public. The first is the enforcement in the 1960s of current Good Manufacturing Practice (cGMP) standards (21 CFR 210, 211, and 600–680) on the manufacture of allergen products. cGMPs include requirements regarding organization and personnel, buildings and facilities, equipment, control of components and drug product containers and closures, production and process controls, holding and distribution, quality control, laboratory controls, and records and reports.

The second feature of significant impact is allergen standardization. 21 CFR 680.3(e) specifies that when a potency test exists for a specific allergenic product, and when CBER has notified manufacturers that the test exists, manufacturers will be required to determine the potency of each lot of the product prior to release. Since the 1980s, 19 allergen extracts have been standardized (see Table 24.1). What follows is a discussion of the regulation of allergen extracts in the United States, with a special focus on standardized products and the tests that are used to ascertain extract potency.

---

* This chapter is an informal communication and represents the best judgment of the authors. These comments do not bind or obligate the U.S Food and Drug Administration.

Table 24.1 Standardized allergen extracts currently licensed in the United States

Allergen extract	Current lot release tests	Labeled unitage
Dust mite (*Dermatophagoides farinae*)	Competition ELISA	AU/mL (equivalent to BAU/mL)
Dust mite (*Dermatophagoides pteronyssinus*)	Protein[a]	
Cat pelt (*Felis domesticus*)	Fel d 1 (RID)	BAU/mL
Cat hair (*Felis domesticus*)	IEF	
	Protein	5–9.9 Fel d 1 U/mL = 5000 BAU/mL
		10–19.9 Fel d 1 U/mL = 10,000 BAU/mL
Bermuda grass (*Cynodon dactylon*)	Competition ELISA	BAU/mL
Red top grass (*Agrostis alba*)	IEF	
June (Kentucky blue) grass (*Poa pratensis*)	Protein[a]	
Perennial ryegrass (*Lolium perenne*)		
Orchard grass (*Dactylis glomerata*)		
Timothy grass (*Phleum pratense*)		
Meadow fescue grass (*Festuca elatior*)		
Sweet vernal grass (*Anthoxanthum odoratum*)		
Short ragweed (*Ambrosia artemisiifolia*)	Amb a 1 (RID)	Amb a 1 units
Yellow hornet (*Vespa* spp)	Hyaluronidase and phospholipase activity	μg protein
Wasp (*Polistes* spp)		
Honeybee (*Apis mellifera*)		
White-faced hornet (*Vespa* spp)		
Yellow jacket (*Vespula* spp.)		
Mixed vespid (*Vespa* + *Vespula* spp)		

Abbreviations: IEF, isoelectric focusing; RID, radial immunodiffusion.
[a] Test for informational purposes only.

24.2 ALLERGEN EXTRACTS CURRENTLY ON THE MARKET (STANDARDIZED AND NONSTANDARDIZED)

Allergen extracts are manufactured and sold worldwide for the diagnosis and treatment of IgE-mediated allergic disease. These extracts are complex mixtures of natural biomaterials. Each extract contains proteins, carbohydrates, enzymes, and pigments of which the allergens—presumably the active ingredients—may constitute only a small proportion [3]. Traditionally, allergen extracts have been labeled either with a designation of extraction ratio (weight to volume, or w/v) or with a protein unit designation that is determined using the Kjeldahl method (protein nitrogen units/mL) [4]. However, there is little correlation between these two designations and biological measures of allergen potency.

The extraction processes employed for nonstandardized and standardized extracts are essentially identical. The primary difference at the extraction stage is the approach to formulation. Nonstandardized extracts are formulated based on w/v or protein content, while standardized extracts are formulated based on potency test results from the source material or small-scale extractions. Optimal conditions for extraction must be considered, especially when the allergens are heat-labile or protease-sensitive. Therefore, extractions may be performed either at reduced temperatures or in the presence of additives that suppress microbial growth (e.g., 0.4% phenol, 50% glycerin). Slightly alkaline buffers such as bicarbonate buffer (pH 8) are usually preferred for increasing protein and allergen yields. Prolonged processing times may increase total protein recovery from source materials but may denature the allergens, which can diminish allergenic potency. *In-process testing* for specific allergen content or marker proteins can be used to monitor processing steps and ensure a reproducible and high-quality product. The bulk intermediate may be adjusted based on results of in-process chemistry or potency tests. Dialysis or ultrafiltration may also be used to remove low molecular weight (<5 kD) nonantigenic substances. After sterile filtration, quality control testing is performed to insure the quality, safety, and sterility of the bulk. Since standardized allergen extracts have unitage based on biological potency, quality control testing includes assessment of potency either in-process or at the sterile bulk release stage. Sterile bulk extracts may be stored at 2°C–8°C, freeze-dried, or used directly to fill final containers.

All allergen extracts for injection must be sterile. Sterilization is accomplished by filtration through a sterilizing filter with a nominal

0.2 μm pore size. Requirements for sterility testing are specified in U.S. regulations (21 CFR 610.12). Sterility testing may be performed in accordance with the *U.S. Pharmacopeia* General Chapter <71> or an alternate validated method. Allergen extracts in multiple-dose vials must contain a preservative unless the extract contains 50% or more v/v glycerin (21 CFR 610.15). Most manufacturers use phenol at a concentration of 0.4% as a preservative either with or without 50% glycerin. Allergen extracts for sublingual tablets are not required to be sterile but are required to meet limits for total organisms and specified microorganisms (USP <61> and <62>).

Quality control tests vary by manufacturer, product characteristics, and regulatory requirements. Measurements of total protein content, specific allergen content, protein and allergen profile, and allergenic activity all contribute to the quality control process. Since standardized allergen extracts have unitage based on biological potency, quality control tests include assessments for potency during and after manufacture. All quality control assays must be demonstrated as suitable for their intended use. In the United States, lot release testing for standardized extracts is performed using a single national potency standard or reference preparation. In contrast, lot release testing in the European countries employs the manufacturer's in-house reference preparation derived from a production run according to the validated and licensed manufacturing process.

In the absence of a concerted effort to maintain product consistency, lot-to-lot variations in allergen content may be considerable. Differences in consistency among allergenic extracts may reflect the inherent nature of the raw materials. For example, pollen and pure mite extracts [5] generally have greater lot-to-lot consistency than mold, house dust, and insect extracts [6]. Manufacturers can increase the consistency of their products by controlled collection, storage, and processing of the raw materials; by reproducible and optimized extraction and manufacturing techniques; and by applying expiration dates that are based on real-time stability data. However, consistency can only be assured by measuring the potency of each lot of extracts, and by marketing only those lots whose potency falls within an acceptable range.

The purpose of allergen standardization is to characterize the potency of allergen extracts and minimize the variation between lots of allergen extracts, even among different manufacturers. Once standardized, patients and their physicians can switch from one manufacturer's product to another with minimized risk of causing an adverse reaction. To that end, 21 CFR 680.3 establishes a U.S. standard of potency for each standardized product and mandates that once an appropriate potency test exists, manufacturers must test each lot of an allergen extract for potency and state the potency on the label of each vial sold.

For each of the 19 standardized allergen extracts available from U.S. manufacturers, there is a U.S. standard of potency to which each lot of the extract is compared prior to release for sale to the public. The potency measurements and the assays used to determine these values are specified in the approved product license applications of each manufacturer for each product. Manufacturers may measure potency of extracts using the methods described used by CBER's Laboratory of Immunobiochemistry (see later in this chapter), or may seek approval to use alternative test methods that provide equally reliable measures of product potency and meet regulatory requirements.

The level of quality control for the 19 standardized allergen extracts is the exception rather than the rule. *In vitro* potency tests that correlate with *in vivo* clinical responses have not been developed for the hundreds of nonstandardized extracts available in the United States. Therefore, consistency cannot be ensured by potency testing for most allergen extracts.

24.2.1 Alternate formulations

In the United States, the primary marketed formulations of currently licensed allergen extracts are sterile extracts for subcutaneous or intradermal injection. These extracts include aqueous and glycerinated standardized and nonstandardized extracts, and a small number of acetone precipitated or alum adsorbed nonstandardized allergen extracts. More recently, the FDA has approved license applications for new allergen extracts in sublingual tablet formulations [7–10]. The potencies of these products were established by each manufacturer during clinical studies performed in support of their license application. Therefore, these products are not classified as standardized or nonstandardized. Formulations under investigation that are combination products, such as transdermal epicutaneous systems or prefilled syringes, are also subject to certain regulatory requirements for devices.

24.3 BASIS OF ALLERGEN STANDARDIZATION IN THE UNITED STATES

In the United States, allergen standardization comprises two important components: the selection of a reference preparation of allergenic extract and the selection of the procedures to compare manufactured products to the reference extract [11–13]. The use of a biological model of allergen standardization has permitted the assignment of bioequivalent allergen units for most standardized allergens [12]. Once a specific unitage is assigned to a reference, then all allergen extracts from the same source can be assigned units based on the relative potency (RP) with respect to the reference using the established quantitative in vitro potency method [14].

In contrast to the United States, commercial allergens in the European Union are labeled in disparate manufacturer-specific units, and products are standardized using manufacturers' in-house references [15]. While earlier European efforts to establish biological standards were similar to those in the United States, the Europeans now focus on the validation of major allergens to facilitate studies that will establish whether the amounts of these molecules can be used as the sole potency label [16,17].

In theory, standardizing an allergen extract requires purifying each allergen in the extract and precisely establishing the importance of each of these allergens. However, most allergen extracts are complex mixtures of several relevant allergens for which immunodominance is uncertain. In addition, an individual allergen may be less "allergenic" (in other words, may have lost affinity for IgE) in an individual manufactured lot due to instability or denaturation.

The choice of the best potency test depends on the allergen extract to be standardized. For two allergen extracts (short ragweed pollen and cat hair), data support using measurements of a single immunodominant allergen (Amb a 1 and Fel d 1, respectively). For cat pelt and Hymenoptera venoms, the presence of two allergens (Fel d 1 and albumin for cat pelt; hyaluronidase and phospholipase A2 for Hymenoptera venoms) is verified for each lot. In the absence of data supporting the potency designations based on single allergen content, a measure of "overall allergenicity" may be a better predictor of safe and effective dosing. This is the case for dust mites and grass pollen extracts.

For initial assessment of overall allergenicity, CBER developed a method of serial intradermal testing of highly allergic individuals that uses the size of erythema in response to intradermal injection. Intradermal injection was chosen over prick/puncture testing to achieve greater dosing accuracy; erythema size was chosen over wheal size to achieve greater accuracy in reaction measurements [18]. This method is called "IntraDermal dilution for 50 mm sum of Erythema determines the bioequivalent ALlergy units" ($ID_{50}EAL$), and it can be used to compare the allergenicity of extracts regardless of source. Subsequent comparisons of extracts from the same source material are made by a variant analysis called the parallel line bioassay. Both of these methods are discussed briefly later.

In the $ID_{50}EAL$ method, allergenic extracts are evaluated in subjects maximally reactive to the respective reference concentrates. Each subject is tested with serial threefold dilutions of the reference extract. After 15 minutes, the sum of the longest and midpoint orthogonal diameters of erythema (ΣE) is determined at each dilution, and the log dose producing a 50 mm ΣE response (D_{50}) is calculated [14]. Extracts that produce similar D_{50} responses are considered bioequivalent and are assigned similar units, the bioequivalent allergy unit (BAU). Because the modal D_{50} of a series of extracts was 14 (a 3^{-14} or 1:4.8 million dilution), extracts with a mean D_{50} of 14 were arbitrarily assigned the value of 100,000 BAU/mL [11]. Thus, the following is the formula for the determination of potency from the D_{50} [19,20]:

$$\text{Potency} = 3^{-(14 - \text{mean D50})} * 100,000 \text{ BAU/mL}$$

By a similar technique and analysis, bioequivalent doses of test extracts from the same source as the reference extract can be determined by the parallel-line bioassay [21]. The inverse ratio of the doses of test extract required to produce identical D_{50} responses to a reference extract is the relative potency (RP) of that extract. This analysis requires that the log dose-response curves of the test extract and the reference extract are parallel. If the two dose-response lines are not parallel, then the ratio of skin test doses for identical responses—and the RP—will vary with the dose because the distance between the two lines is different at each dose and a meaningful RP cannot be determined [11,21] (Figure 24.1). This situation strongly suggests that there are compositional differences between the two extracts.

In the original protocol, the D_{50} for the extract was determined by the mean D_{50} from 15 highly allergic individuals. To test the arbitrary choice of a sample size of 15, Rabin et al. [22] applied the following formula for the number of study subjects, n, that would be required:

$$n = 2\left(\frac{\sigma}{\delta}\right)^2 (z_{1-\alpha} + z_{1-\beta/2})^2$$

where σ is the standard deviation of the measurement, δ is the acceptable difference in D_{50}s of two equivalent products, and the z values are the critical values from the cumulative normal distribution table for a significance level α and a power of $1 - \beta$ [23]. From this formula, n is a function of the *squares* of σ and δ. The value of n depends on the particular allergen to be tested but, as may be seen in sample calculations represented in Table 24.2, n, the sample size

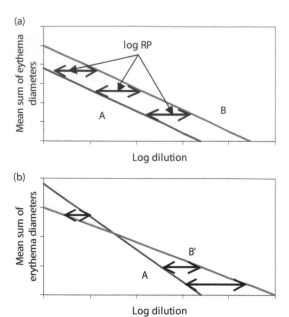

Figure 24.1 Hypothetical parallel line bioassay curves. (a) The bioassay curves are parallel, and the difference of log dilutions resulting in the same diameters is constant at all diameters. The log relative potency (log RP) of test sample B compared to reference A is represented by the difference. (b) The curves are not parallel, and the differences vary with the strength of the reaction. Thus, the log RP of B' compared to A cannot be calculated.

to determine the D_{50} of an allergenic product, usually must be larger than 15 subjects.

Although skin testing is an essential component of the allergen standardization program, it is not intended for routine use in the testing of manufactured lots of extracts prior to release. For that purpose, surrogate *in vitro* potency assays that accurately predict the *in vivo* activity of extracts have been developed [21]. Surrogate

Table 24.2 Estimates of sample size n from the formula $n = 2\left(\dfrac{\sigma}{\delta}\right)^2 (z_{1-\alpha} + z_{1-\beta/2})^2$ to demonstrate equivalence at the $\alpha = 0.05$ level by the two one-sided test formalism for a variety of β, tolerance intervals δ, and standard deviations σ ($z_{0.975} = 1.96$; $z_{0.95} = 1.645$; $z_{0.90} = 1.282$)

σ/δ	β	n
1.0	0.05	26
	0.10	22
	0.20	18
1.5	0.05	59
	0.10	49
	0.20	39
2.0	0.05	104
	0.10	87
	0.20	69

methods can be based on quantitation of the total protein content (Hymenoptera venoms), the specific allergen content within the allergen extracts (short ragweed pollen and cat), or the inhibition of the binding of IgE from pooled allergic sera to reference allergen (grasses, mites) [24]. In addition to total protein, the potency of Hymenoptera venom allergen extracts is also based on the content of the known principal allergens within the extract, hyaluronidase and phospholipase, both of which are determined by enzyme activity (see Table 24.1).

The potency units for short ragweed pollen extracts were originally assigned based on their Amb a 1 content. Subsequent data suggest that 1 unit of Amb a 1 is equivalent to 1 μg of Amb a 1, and while 350 Amb a 1 units/mL is equivalent to 100,000 BAU/mL, the original unitage of Amb a 1 units has been retained. Grass pollen extracts are labeled in BAU/mL, based on $ID_{50}EAL$ testing.

In some cases, the assignment of potency units to standardized allergenic extracts in the United States has changed as bioequivalence data have become available [14]. Cat extracts were originally standardized based on their Fel d 1 content, with arbitrary unitage (called "allergy units," or AU/mL) tied to the Fel d 1 determinations. Subsequent $ID_{50}EAL$ testing resulted in the assignment of 10,000 BAU/mL unitage to cat extracts, which contained 10–19.9 Fel d 1 U/mL [25]. In addition, 20% of individuals allergic to cat were found to have antibody to non-Fel d 1 proteins [26]. Consequently, the presence of a band on isoelectric focusing (IEF) showing that the extract contains albumin (Fel d 2), which was added as a requirement for cat pelt extracts. Dust mite extracts were originally standardized (in AU/mL) based on radioallergosorbent test (RAST) inhibition assays. Since subsequent $ID_{50}EAL$ testing indicated that the arbitrary unitage was statistically bioequivalent to BAU/mL [27], the original unitage of AU/mL was retained [28].

In addition to these quantitative measurements of potency, the identity of an allergen extract may be verified by visualizing the separated allergen proteins based on their size and isoelectric points [3]. IEF is an important safety test in the lot release of grass pollen and cat extracts. The patterns produced by the crude allergen mixtures are reproducible enough to consistently indicate the presence of known allergens, to identify possible contaminants present in the extracts, and to check lot-to-lot variation in the extracts [29,30]. IEF is also used to verify the presence of Fel d 2 (albumin) in cat pelt extracts.

24.4 POTENCY TESTS CURRENTLY APPLIED TO STANDARDIZED ALLERGENS

Several *in vitro* tests have been established for testing the potency and identity of standardized allergens (Table 24.1). Tests for potency include assays for the specific allergen content, for the RP, and for the enzyme activity of allergenic extracts. (The full protocols for these assays may be obtained by emailing the authors.)

24.4.1 Radial immunodiffusion assay

This assay is used to determine the potencies of short ragweed pollen and cat allergenic extracts, products in which the immunodominant allergens (Amb a 1 and Fel d 1, respectively) have been identified and defined. In this assay, antiserum specific for the dominant allergen is added to an agar solution, which then solidifies. Wells are then punched into the agar, and test allergen is placed in the wells. As the specific allergen diffuses out of the wells and into the agar, a precipitin ring forms that delineates the equivalence zone for antigen-antibody binding. Since the antiserum concentration in the agar is constant, the allergen concentration decreases with increasing size of the precipitin ring. The diameter of the precipitin ring is proportional to the log of the concentration of the allergen, which is determined by placing the value of the ring diameter on a standard curve derived from measurement of multiple concentrations of a reference extract. CBER's Laboratory of Immunobiochemistry is working on an improved approach, using simpler technology and more durable critical reagents, to measure these allergens [31].

24.4.2 Enzymatic assays

The allergen content of Hymenoptera venoms is based on the two most important glycoprotein enzymes, hyaluronidase and phospholipase A2. These venom allergen extracts are standardized using enzymatic assays that estimate hyaluronidase and phospholipase content based on their enzymatic activity. In these assays, an agar solution is prepared with the appropriate enzymatic substrate, and test samples are then added to wells in the agar. As the enzyme present in the sample diffuses into the agar, it digests the substrate, forming clearing zones around the wells. The radius of the clear zones is then measured and calculated as the log of the concentration of the enzyme present in the sample.

24.4.3 Competition enzyme-linked immunosorbent assay

This assay is used for standardized allergen extracts (grass pollens, dust mites) for which there is no consensus regarding the immunodominant components. Potency is determined by comparing the overall binding to human IgE in pooled sera from highly allergic subjects and comparing to a reference extract. After coating the wells of the polystyrene microtiter plate with the reference allergen extract, a mixture of the allergen extract that is being tested and the pooled sera is added to the wells. The test extract in solution competes for the IgE in the pooled sera with the bound reference allergen such that the more immunoreactive allergen in the mix, the less IgE antibody from the sera will bind to the immobilized allergen on the plate. Once again, the concentration of the allergens in the allergen extract is determined by comparison to the reference allergen extract. However, since this assay does not explicitly measure a specific allergen, the allergen concentration is expressed as relative potency (RP), with the reference extract assigned an arbitrary RP of 1.0. RP assigned by titration skin testing correlates well with RP determined by both RAST inhibition (used initially by CBER) [12] and competition ELISA [29].

24.5 HOW SHOULD RELEASE LIMITS BE CHOSEN?

Fundamental to the standardization process is establishing an acceptable range of comparability or equivalence. Limits that are too broad lead to unacceptable risk to patients (anaphylaxis when the physician changes from one bottle to another, or changes to a different manufacturer), while limits that are too narrow lead to unacceptable risk for manufacturers (the rejection of a large percentage of safe and effective lots of product). In the competition ELISA, potency limits have been set according to the precision of the test; the candidate extracts are expected to be *statistically equivalent to the reference extract*, at a specified level of confidence with a specified test. Mite and grass pollen extracts are currently expected to be equivalent to the reference at the 98% confidence level, using three replicates of a validated competition ELISA; the standard deviation σ in $\log_{10}$ RP for a single replicate is 0.1375 [30]. The 98% confidence interval is given by $10^{\pm 2.326\sigma/\sqrt{3}}$, such that when the RP of a lot falls in the range 0.654–1.530, it is within the 98% confidence interval and is approved for release. This criterion also implies that an average of 2% of lots that have a potency equivalent to the reference extract will fall outside of the release limits, and that although lots that are not identical to the reference will fail at predictably higher rates, a small fraction of those will pass release testing as well.

An alternative approach would be to base the potency limits on acceptable ranges established in clinical studies. Three criteria would appear to be important. The first, *therapeutic equivalence,* addresses the efficacy of allergen extracts for immunotherapy. Thus, an RP range will have the property of therapeutic equivalence if, for the allergen extract in question, lots with RPs anywhere in that range have an equal likelihood of effecting clinical improvement in an immunotherapy trial. Likewise, *diagnostic equivalence* addresses the efficacy of allergen extracts for *in vivo* diagnostics. Finally, *safety equivalence* reflects the likelihood of the safe administration of the extract for either diagnostic or therapeutic indications. The acceptable limits should fall within the narrowest of the equivalence ranges established by these criteria.

The aggregate consistency of manufactured lots might also be considered when developing testing methods and limits. For example, if typical lot-to-lot consistency is very high and well within clinical limits, then testing protocols could be adjusted to eliminate outliers while rarely failing lots whose RP is close to 1. On the other extreme, if the distribution of lots is broad, equivalence to the reference would be imposed. This would narrow the distribution, but at a cost: at 95% equivalence, 5% of lots whose RP = 1 would fail release.

In an analysis of studies using ragweed and dust mite allergens [5], the range of therapeutic equivalence was at least 10-fold, and the ranges of diagnostic equivalence and safety equivalence were approximately fourfold. In the same study, the lot-to-lot consistency of 412 lots of grass pollen extracts and 91 lots of dust mite extracts were analyzed. The variability of the samples was comparable to the assay variability. Furthermore, the mean ratio (in RP) of two randomly selected lots of allergen would be 1.12 (for mites) and 1.18 (for grass pollen). The calculated 95th percentile ratios were 1.48 and 1.8, respectively. Thus, the equivalence ranges appear to be considerably broader than the current lot release limits (twofold) and the expected variations in product potency using current manufacturing and quality control practices. Based on these estimates, CBER broadened the internal release limits for standardized dust mite and grass pollen allergen extracts to 0.5–2.0 [32].

24.6 FUTURE DIRECTIONS

The effort to standardize allergens in the United States has resulted in the development of a core group of highly used allergen extracts that are better characterized and more consistent than their nonstandardized predecessors. Most allergens marketed in the United States, however, remain unstandardized. Ideally, all allergen extracts will be subject to potency testing and compared to a reference extract, whether manufacturer specific, industry-wide, national, or international. To date, we are far from reaching that goal.

The current approach toward allergen standardization in the United States is binomial: either according to an immunodominant allergen, or to overall potency that is established with the $ID_{50}EAL$ method. Standardizing to an immunodominant allergen is restricted by the limited number of allergens for which there is uniform consensus of an immunodominant allergen. But overall potency fails to account for the explosive body of literature in which many allergenic proteins have been defined and categorized.

In consideration of these limitations, CBER researchers have been developing novel approaches to allergen extract potency determinations to assess the overall potency of complex allergen mixtures as the integral of multiple discrete allergen assays [33–36]. These approaches remain investigational.

SALIENT POINTS

1. Allergen standardization in the United States is currently based on skin test responses in highly allergic individuals.
2. Most allergen extracts in the United States are not standardized.
3. Nonstandardized allergens are labeled in units (PNU/mL or w/v) that may be unrelated to potency.
4. All U.S. allergen extracts, whether standardized or nonstandardized, must be manufactured in accordance with current Good Manufacturing Practices (cGMPs).
5. The number of individuals needed to establish the potency of a product by skin testing is related to the *square of the ratio* of the standard deviation (σ) of the skin test results and the acceptable difference (δ) in potency between two identically labeled products.
6. The unitage adopted for standardized allergens in the United States is based on the best available scientific understanding of the specificity of responses in allergic individuals.
7. The potencies of individual lots of standardized allergen extracts are determined by specific surrogate *in vitro* tests that have been determined to correlate with the skin test results. In some cases, the potencies are based on specific allergen determinations.
8. Release limits for lots of standardized allergens are established based on manufacturing capabilities, potency assay performance, and clinical data.

REFERENCES

1. Harden VA. A short history of the National Institutes of Health. http://history.nih.gov/exhibits/history/ Accessed July 19, 2018.
2. History of FDA's Centers and Offices. https://www.fda.gov/AboutFDA/History/FOrgsHistory/HistoryofFDAsCentersand-Offices/default.htm. Accessed July 19, 2018.
3. Yuninger JW. Allergenic extracts: Characterization, standardization and prospects for the future. *Pediatr Clin North Am* 1983; 30: 795–805.
4. Bonertz A, Roberts G, Slater JE et al. Allergen manufacturing and quality aspects for allergen immunotherapy in Europe and the United States: An analysis from the EAACI AIT Guidelines Project. *Allergy* 2018; 73(4): 816–826.

5. Slater JE, Pastor RW. The determination of equivalent doses of standardized allergen vaccines. *J Allergy Clin Immunol* 2000; 105(3): 468–474.

6. Patterson ML, Slater JE. Characterization and comparison of commercially available German and American cockroach allergen extracts. *Clin Exp Allergy* 2002; 32: 721–727.

7. Prescribing information, GRASTEK, https://www.fda.gov/downloads/BiologicsBloodVaccines/Allergenics/UCM393184.pdf. Accessed July 19, 2018.

8. Prescribing information, ORALAIR, https://www.fda.gov/downloads/BiologicsBloodVaccines/Allergenics/UCM391580.pdf. Accessed July 19, 2018.

9. Prescribing information, ODACTRA, https://www.fda.gov/downloads/BiologicsBloodVaccines/Allergenics/UCM544382.pdf. Accessed July 19, 2018.

10. Prescribing information, RAGWITEK, https://www.fda.gov/downloads/BiologicsBloodVaccines/Allergenics/UCM393600.pdf. Accessed July 19, 2018.

11. Turkeltaub PC. In-vivo standardization. In: Middleton EJ, Reed CE, Ellis EF, editors. *Allergy, Principles and Practice*. St. Louis, MO: C.V. Mosby Co., 1988, pp. 388–401.

12. Turkeltaub PC. Biological standardization of allergenic extracts. *Allergol Immunopathol (Madr)* 1989; 17(2): 53–65.

13. Turkeltaub PC. Biological standardization. *Arb Paul Ehrlich Inst Bundesamt Sera Impfstoffe Frankf A M* 1997; 91: 145–156.

14. Turkeltaub PC. Allergen vaccine unitage based on biological standardization. Clinical significance. In: Lockey R, Bukantz SC, editors. *Allergens and Allergen Immunotherapy*. New York, NY: Marcel Dekker, 1999: 321–340.

15. Bonertz A, Roberts GC, Hoefnagel M et al. Challenges in the implementation of EAACI guidelines on allergen immunotherapy: A global perspective on the regulation of allergen products. *Allergy* 2018; 73(1): 64–76.

16. van Ree R, Chapman MD, Ferreira F et al. The CREATE project: Development of certified reference materials for allergenic products and validation of methods for their quantification. *Allergy* 2008; 63: 310–326.

17. Committee for Medicinal Products for Human Use. *Guideline on Allergen Products: Production and Quality Issues*. London: European Medicines Agency, November 2008. http://www.emea.europa.eu/docs/en_GB/document_library/Scientific_guideline/2009/09/WC500003333.pdf. Accessed July 19, 2018.

18. Turkeltaub PC, Rastogi SC, Baer H et al. A standardized quantitative skin-test assay of allergen potency and stability: Studies on the allergen dose-response curve and effect of wheal, erythema, and patient selection on assay results. *J Allergy Clin Immunol* 1982; 70(5): 343–352.

19. James R, Mitchell H, Gergen PJ et al. Statistical analysis of ID50EAL data. *Arb.Paul Ehrlich Inst.Bundesamt Sera Impfstoffe Frankf.A.M* 2006; 95: 117–127.

20. Slater JE, James R, Pongracic JA et al. Biological potency of German cockroach allergen extracts determined in an inner city population. *Clin Exp Allergy* 2007; 37(7): 1033–1039.

21. Turkeltaub PC. *In vivo* methods of standardization. *Clin Rev Allergy* 1986; 4: 371–387.

22. Rabin RL, Slater JE, Lachenbruch P et al. Sample size considerations for establishing clinical bioequivalence of allergen formulations. *Arb Paul Ehrlich Inst Bundesamt Sera Impfstoffe Frankf A M* 2003; 94: 24–33.

23. Schuirmann DJ. A comparison of the two one-sided tests procedure and the power approach for assessing the equivalence of average bioavailability. *J Pharmacokinet Biopharm* 1987; 15(6): 657–680.

24. Platts-Mills TAE, Rawle F, Chapman MD. Problems in allergen standardization. *Clin Rev Allergy* 1985; 3: 271–290.

25. Matthews J, Turkeltaub PC. The assignment of biological allergy units (AU) to standardized cat extracts. *J Allergy Clin Immunol* 1992; 89: 151.

26. Turkeltaub PC, Matthews J. Determination of compositional differences (CD) among standardized cat extracts by *in vivo* methods. *J Allergy Clin Immunol* 1992; 89: 151.

27. Turkeltaub PC, Anderson MC, Baer H. Relative potency (RP), compositional differences (CD), and assignment of allergy units (AU) to mite extracts (Dp and Df) assayed by parallel line skin test (PLST). *J Allergy Clin Immunol* 1987; 79: 235.

28. Turkeltaub PC. Use of skin testing for evaluation of potency, composition, and stability of allergenic products. *Arb Paul Ehrlich Institut* 1994; 87: 79–87.

29. Yuninger JW, Adolphson CR. Standardization of allergens. In: Rose NR, de Macario EC, Fahey JL, Friedman H, Penn GM, editors. *Manual of clinical laboratory immunology*. Washington, DC: American Society for Microbiology, 1992: 678–684.

30. Lin Y, Miller CA. Standardization of allergenic extracts: An update on CBER's standardization program *Arb Paul Ehrlich Inst Bundesamt Sera Impfstoffe Frankf A M* 1997; 91: 127–130.

31. Rabin RL. Proposed Change of Potency Assay to be used by CBER for Standardized Short Ragweed Pollen and Cat Allergen Extracts. Presented at Allergenic Products Advisory Committee. March 18, 2009. https://wayback.archive-it.org/7993/20170111224206/http://www.fda.gov/AdvisoryCommittees/CommitteesMeetingMaterials/BloodVaccinesandOtherBiologics/AllergenicProductsAdvisoryCommittee/ucm129361.htm. Accessed January 4, 2018.

32. Guidance for Reviewers: Potency Limits for Standardized Dust Mite and Grass Allergen Vaccines: A Revised Protocol. November 2000. https://www.fda.gov/downloads/BiologicsBloodVaccines/GuidanceComplianceRegulatoryInformation/Guidances/Allergenics/UCM078624.pdf. Accessed July 19, 2018.

33. deVore NC, Huynh S, Dobrovolskaia EN et al. Multiplex microbead measurements for the characterization of cat and ragweed allergen extracts. *Ann Asthma All Immunol* 2010; 105: 351–358.

34. Khurana T, Dobrovolskaia E, Shartouny JR, Slater JE. Multiplex assay for protein profiling and potency measurement of German cockroach allergen extracts. *PLOS ONE* 2015; 10(10): e0140225.

35. Mindaye ST, Spiric J, David NA, Rabin RL, Slater JE. Accurate quantification of five German cockroach (GCr) allergens in complex extracts using multiple reaction monitoring mass spectrometry (MRM MS). *Clin Exp Allergy* 2017; 47(12): 1661–1670.

36. Slater JE. A global view of allergenic product potency. *Arb Paul Ehrlich Inst Bundesamt Sera Impfstoffe Frankf AM* 2009; 96: 178–185.

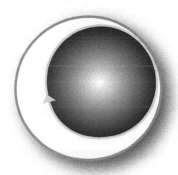

25 Manufacturing and standardizing allergen extracts in Europe

Jørgen Nedergaard Larsen, Christian Gauguin Houghton, Manuel Lombardero Vega, and Hendrik Nolte
ALK A/S

Henning Løwenstein
Henning Løwenstein APS

CONTENTS

25.1 INTRODUCTION

25.1.1 History of standardization in Europe

Specific allergy treatment, i.e., specific immunotherapy or specific allergy vaccination, has been performed for more than a century, since it was first described by Noon in 1911 [1]. The discovery in 1966 of the IgE molecule [2], and the central role of IgE in allergy, has facilitated a better understanding of the immunologic mechanisms of allergic disease and has led to improvement of diagnostic tools and consolidation of the concept of specific allergy diagnosis and treatment. Scientific methods were introduced to standardize allergen extracts in the 1970s and 1980s [3] and, in combination with gradual improvement of the clinical procedures, established specific allergy treatment as a scientifically based, reproducible, and safe treatment for allergic diseases.

The first international initiative on allergen standardization was based on the Danish Allergen Standardization 1976 program [4], which was published as part of the Nordic Guideline in 1989 [5]. The Nordic Guideline established the first regulatory requirements for allergen extracts. The guideline introduced the biological unit (BU), based on skin testing, for potency measures. Each manufacturer was instructed to produce an in-house reference preparation (IHRP), adjust the potency in BU, and use the IHRP for batch-to-batch control using scientifically based laboratory testing. The significance of using the major allergen content for the biological activity was recognized in the early 1990s and was established in the World Health Organization (WHO) Guideline [6]. Current regulation and requirements for authorization are described in the European Pharmacopoeia, Monograph on Allergen Products [7], and in the European Medicines Agency's Guideline on Allergen Products [8]; an overview can be found in Zimmer et al. [9]. This chapter describes important issues in the control of source materials and in the preparation of extracts as part of the standardization process the way it is performed in Europe. Procedures differ from those used in the United States, as does the selection of extracts for vaccination in common allergy practice (see Chapter 24).

25.1.2 Standardization of allergen extracts

Allergen extracts/vaccines are used for specific diagnoses and treatments of allergic diseases and indirectly for the detection of environmental allergens. Allergen extracts are aqueous solutions of allergenic source materials, such as pollen, animal hair and dander, dust mite bodies or cultures, insect venoms, or mold mycelia and spore particles. Since no structural feature defining an allergen has hitherto been described, the definition of an allergen is based on the functional criterion of being able to elicit an IgE response in susceptible individuals. All allergens are proteins, and they are readily soluble in water. Airborne allergens are carried by particles in the micrometer (μm) range, a characteristic that is compatible with the concept that the particle carrying the allergen is inhaled and the allergen is deposited on the mucosal surface of the airways, thereby stimulating the immune system. The allergen is thus defined by the immune system of the individual patient.

By this definition, any immunogenic protein (antigen) has allergenic potential, even though most allergic patients have IgE specific for a relatively limited number of "major" allergens. Analysis of a larger number of patients leads to the identification of still more IgE binding proteins (Figure 25.1). Thus, the number of allergens in a given source material converge toward the total number of antigens, and any antigen has the potential to elicit an IgE response.

The antigen composition of the allergenic source materials must be reflected in the allergen extract, and moreover, need the composition to be consistent across batches. Therefore, all aspects of the manufacturing procedures from selection, collection, and purification of allergenic source materials to extraction, purification, and stabilization impact the quality of the extract. Combined with adequate quality control of the allergen extract itself, i.e., verification of the protein and allergen composition and quantification of the total and major allergen activity potency, it makes up the backbone in standardization of allergen extracts. The standardization procedure has distinct importance for the quality of allergen extracts/vaccines in diagnosis as well as treatment.

25.2 PREPARATION OF ALLERGEN EXTRACTS

25.2.1 Source materials

Inhalant allergens are present in airborne particles derived from natural allergen sources. The particles are inhaled and constitute the material to which humans are exposed. The most important allergen sources are found among the particles most frequently inhaled. Table 25.1 lists the most important allergen extracts in Europe and the United States.

The aim of selecting source materials for allergen extract production is to gather materials containing all relevant active allergens in a manageable form. In most cases, the optimal source material is rather obvious, but in some cases, the allergen source is still debated, i.e., cat saliva/pelt/hair and dander or mouse urine/hair and dander. The source materials should be selected with attention to the need for specificity and for inclusion of all relevant allergens in sufficient amounts [10].

Since January 2017, production of the most important source materials for allergen extracts have been regulated by specific monographs in the European Pharmacopoeia, including pollens [11], mites [12], animal epithelia [13], Hymenoptera venoms [14], and molds [15]. The general aspects of the production of source materials described in the five monographs are identical, and they are described here, whereas specific aspects of source material production are mentioned later.

25.2.1.1 GENERAL ASPECTS OF SOURCE MATERIAL PRODUCTION

25.2.1.1.1 Production process

The collection of the source materials should be performed by qualified personnel, and reasonable measures must be employed by the producer of allergen extracts to assure that collector qualifications and collection procedures are appropriate to verify the identity and quality of the source materials. This means that only specifically identified allergenic source materials that do not contain avoidable foreign substances should be used in the manufacture of allergen extracts. Means of identification and contents of foreign materials and other types of impurities should meet established acceptance criteria for each source material, ensuring consistency from qualitative and quantitative points of view. Where identity and purity cannot be determined by direct examination of the source materials, other appropriate methods should be applied to trace the materials from their origin. This includes complete identity labeling and certification from competent collectors. Major changes to the production process must be qualified.

The processing and storage of source materials should be performed in a way to ensure that no unintended substances are introduced into the materials, and such that consistent quality is ensured from batch to batch. Allergenic source materials are stored under controlled conditions justified by stability data. Records should describe source materials in as much detail as possible, including the particulars of collection, purification, pretreatment, and storage.

Microbial contamination may be unavoidable and should be monitored on a representative number of batches according to a justified sampling plan, and repeated each time a new supplier and/or a new process for production is introduced. Microbial contamination values and potential increases during storage are monitored in the context of stability studies.

25.2.1.1.2 Reference standard

An appropriate reference batch is established for each species. The nature of the reference depends on the testing performed to verify batch-to-batch consistency and establish acceptable quality. Characterization of the reference must be described, depending on the knowledge of allergenic components and availability of suitable reagents. The reference batch is stored under controlled conditions ensuring its stability.

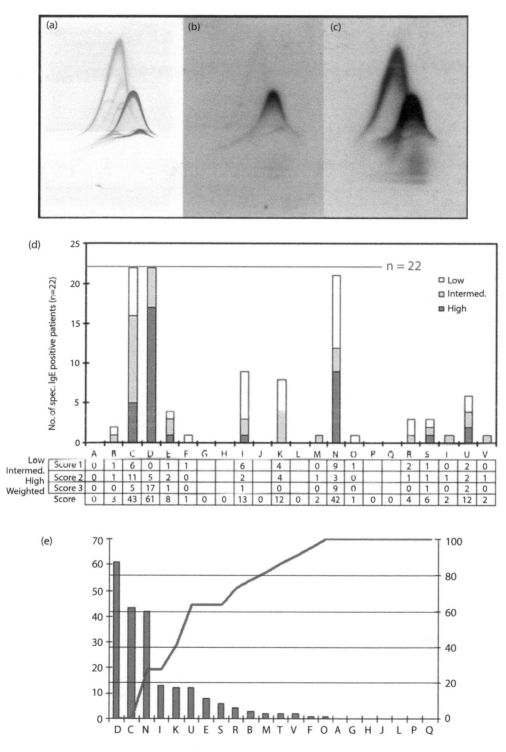

The table in panel (d):

		A	B	C	D	E	F	G	H	I	J	K	L	M	N	O	P	Q	R	S	T	U	V
Low	Score 1	0	1	6	0	1	1			6		4		0	9	1			2	1	0	2	0
Intermed.	Score 2	0	1	11	5	2	0			2		4		1	3	0			1	1	1	2	1
High	Score 3	0	0	5	17	1	0			1		0		0	9	0			0	1	0	2	0
Weighted	Score	0	3	43	61	8	1	0	0	13	0	12	0	2	42	1	0	0	4	6	2	12	2

Figure 25.1 Complexity of patients' responses to allergen extracts. (a) Crossed immunoelectrophoresis (CIE) with blue-stained bell-shaped antigen-antibody precipitates. Each precipitate represents one antigen. (b and c) Crossed radioimmunoelectrophoresis (CRIE) with x-ray chromatograms of radio-staining of IgE from individual patients. Each stained precipitate represent reactivity with an allergen that can be identified by comparison with (a). (d) An allergogram illustrating the number of patients with IgE reactivity toward each of the precipitates identified in (a). Precipitates are arbitrarily labeled in alphabetical order from left to right. The total number of patients in the analysis is $n = 22$. The IgE binding score for each allergen is calculated as the sum of the weighted scores for each patient. Arbitrary weights are assigned as follows: 1 = low IgE binding, 2 = intermediate IgE binding, and 3 = high IgE binding. (e) Accumulated reactivity to common allergens. On the basis of the allergogram in (d), the precipitates are ordered according to their relative importance in terms of IgE binding score. The blue bars represent the sum of a graduated score of the IgE binding of each of the 22 patients. The red line represents the percentage of patients having all their IgE reactivities covered by the allergens to the left of the point. NOTE: (1) None of the patients have all their IgE reactivity covered by the two most important allergens. (2) In order to cover all IgE reactivity in half of the patients, six allergens are needed.

Table 25.1 Most important allergen extracts

Europe		North America	
Temperate grasses	*Lolium perenne*	House dust mites	*Dermatophagoides pteronyssinus*
	Phleum pratense		*Dermatophagoides farinae*
	Poa pratensis		
	Festuca pratensis		
	Dactylis glomerata		
	Secale sereale		
House dust mites	*Dermatophagoides pteronyssinus*	Temperate and subtropical grasses	*Lolium perenne*
	Dermatophagoides farinae		*Phleum pratense*
			Poa pratensis
			Festuca pratensis
			Dactylis glomerata
			Cynodon dactylon
Trees	*Alnus glutinosa*	Ragweed	*Ambrosia* spp.
	Betula verrucosa		
	Corylus avellana		
Parietaria	*Parietaria* spp.	Cat	*Felis domesticus*
Olive	*Olea europea*	Dog	*Canis familiaris*
Yellow jacket	*Vespula* spp.	Lambs quarter	*Chenopodium* spp.
Mugwort	*Artemisia vulgaris*	Mugwort	*Artemisia* spp.
Molds	*Alternaria* spp.	Pigweed	*Amranthus* spp.
	Cladosporium spp.		
	Aspergillus spp.		
	Penicillium spp.		
Cat	*Felis domesticus*	Plantain	*Plantago* spp.
Honeybee	*Apis mellifera*	Molds	*Alternaria* spp.
			Cladosporium spp.
			Aspergillus spp.
			Penicillium spp.
Dog	*Canis familiaris*	Hymenoptera venoms	*Apis mellifera*
			Vespula spp.

Note: The two most important allergen sources in the world are the house dust mites and the grass pollens. Patients often cross-react between the two important mite species, i.e., *D. pteronyssinus* and *D. farinae*, and between several species of the grasses. Commercial extracts are often based on mixtures of species within these groups. Important worldwide are also the indoor allergens from cat, dog, and molds, as well as the extracts derived from Hymenoptera venoms. In local regions, other species may dominate. Examples are ragweed in large parts of the United States, birch in Northern Europe, and *Parietaria* and olive in Southern Europe.

25.2.1.1.3 Batch-to-batch consistency

To establish batch-to-batch consistency, one or more of the following tests are performed on each batch. The choice of test(s) must be justified.

- Total protein
- Protein profile by suitable electrophoresis methods
- Allergen profile based on identification of relevant allergenic components by allergen-specific antibody reagents
- Major allergen content by suitable immunochemical method, such as enzyme-linked immunosorbent assay (ELISA) [16]
- Total allergenic activity by IgE inhibition or suitable equivalent *in vitro* method
- Possible specific test for the source material in question mentioned in the monograph

25.2.1.2 SPECIFIC ASPECTS OF SOURCE MATERIAL PRODUCTION

25.2.1.2.1 Pollens

The natural source of inhalant allergens from plants is pollen. Pollens for allergen products are defined by their species and geographic location, which must be documented for each batch. Species identification is performed in the original plant from which the pollen is collected. The identity of the pollen is confirmed by macroscopic and microscopic inspection in comparison with an IHRP. Protein analysis may supplement tests for identity. Pollen may be obtained by collection either in nature or from cultivated fields or greenhouses. Where pollens are collected from wild species, the nature of the collection area is specified. The methods of collection are described and must ensure the origin, quality, consistency, and traceability of the pollen.

The collection may be performed by several methods, such as vacuuming or drying flower heads followed by grinding. Where applicable, reference is made to good agricultural and collection practice (GACP). Pollens are typically cleaned using various separation techniques, e.g., by sieving and/or by means of fluid bed separation. For some pollen, a waxy layer covering the exterior surface of the pollen grain is removed by extraction in organic solvent. Finally, pollen are dried under controlled conditions and stored in sealed containers at temperatures below 5°C. The content of pesticides, heavy metals, microbial contamination, and residual solvent is monitored and determined on a number of batches according to a justified sampling plan. The maximum level of accepted contamination with pollen from other species is 1%, and 0.5% of any individual pollen as determined by microscopic examination. It should also be devoid of flower and plant debris, with a limit of 10% by weight. Pollen may show some variation in relative composition depending on cultivar, season, and location of growth. Established criteria for collection and production as well as handling must be qualified in order to achieve a consistent composition from batch to batch.

Regulatory requirements for the use of pollen in allergen product manufacturing are listed in the European Pharmacopoeia [11].

25.2.1.2.2 Mites

House dust mites for the production of allergen extracts are cultivated under controlled temperature and humidity conditions in pure cultures. Critical cultivation parameters, e.g., temperature and humidity, are monitored and controlled. Constituents of the culture medium should be devoid of contaminating substances from other allergen sources, and control methods and acceptance criteria relating to identity and purity of the mites must be established. Recently, genetic identification of mite species has been described, allowing identification of the mite species from mite fragments and even fecal particles [17]. Appropriate measures should be taken to avoid contamination with other mites, and mite cultures should be free of visible traces of molds.

Source materials from mites are either whole mite cultures (WMCs) or purified mite fractions, e.g., mite bodies and fecal particles, which can be prepared prior to the manufacture of the active substance. As bodies are rich in group 2 major allergen, and fecal particles are rich in group 1 allergen, quantitative assessment of major allergens in each fraction and subsequent mixing of the fractions can yield a product with constant ratio between the major allergens, and a very consistent composition with respect to all allergens [18]. The purification process should be qualified, and the purity of the fractions should meet predefined specifications. Regulatory requirements for the use of mites in allergen product manufacturing are listed in the European Pharmacopoeia [12].

25.2.1.2.3 Animal epithelia

Allergens of animal origin may emanate from various sources, i.e., hair, dander, fragments of epithelia, feathers, serum, saliva, or urine. The allergens to which humans are exposed depend on the normal behavior of the animal. Therefore, the optimal source of allergens cannot be generalized, but most allergens are present in the epidermis of the animal. Source materials should be collected only from animals that are declared overtly healthy by a veterinarian or other qualified person at the time of collection. Foreign matter,

defined as vermin (e.g., mites and fleas), dirt, and foreign animal epithelia and outgrowths, has to be determined by suitable assays (microscopy, ELISA, etc.) and meet predefined acceptance criteria. Established procedures should minimize the risk of inclusion of zoonoses, i.e., diseases that can be transmitted from animals to humans. Animal epithelia and outgrowths may be processed (e.g., cut or washed) using qualified methods.

Regulatory requirements for the use of animal epithelia and outgrowths in allergen product manufacturing are listed in the European Pharmacopoeia [13].

25.2.1.2.4 Insects

The optimal source for insect allergens is dependent on the natural route of exposure, i.e., inhalation, bite, or sting. Where whole insects or insect debris are inhaled, the whole insect body is selected as allergen source. In the case of stinging insects, venom is the ideal allergen source. With biting insects, saliva would be ideal since it contains the relevant allergens.

The collection of source material for Hymenoptera venom allergen product manufacturing is quite different for bees and wasps. Bees are kept in hives, and they can be electrostimulated to deliver venom when entering the hive. Wasps and yellow jackets, on the contrary, need to be dissected manually after freezing in dry ice to yield a few microliters of venom per insect. Wasps and yellow jackets are typically caught by using vacuum devices where they appear from their natural habitats in cracks in masonry, nests, or holes in the ground.

The species is specified by morphologic features, and the method of collection and venom extraction is described and must ensure that the venom is of appropriate quality. Control methods and acceptance criteria relating to identity and purity of the Hymenoptera venom source material are established. The identity of the Hymenoptera venom source material is confirmed by protein analysis and enzyme activity assays, e.g., hyaluronidase and phospholipase activity, in comparison with an IHRP. Crude Hymenoptera venoms can be further processed (dissolution, filtration, drying, etc.) using validated methods.

Regulatory requirements for the use of Hymenoptera venoms in allergen product manufacturing are listed in the European Pharmacopoeia [14].

25.2.1.2.5 Molds

Source materials for manufacturing of mold or yeast allergen products are obtained by growing the mold under controlled conditions in pure culture. The identity of the mold source material must be confirmed by macroscopic and microscopic inspection and protein analysis in comparison with an IHRP. The harvested source materials consist of mycelia and spores as well as constituents released into the culture medium. Due to difficulties in maintaining a constant composition of mold cultures, an extract should be derived from at least five independent cultures of the same species. Production of the source material should be conducted under aseptic conditions to reduce the risk of contamination by microorganisms or other fungi. The inoculum should be obtained from established fungal culture banks, i.e., American Type Culture Collection (ATCC) available through LCG Standards' offices in Europe (http://www.lgcstandards-atcc.org/) or Centraalbureau voor Schimmelcultures (CBS), Utrecht, The Netherlands (http://www.cbs.knaw.nl/). The cultivation medium should be synthetic or at least devoid of antigenic constituents, i.e., proteins. The method of cultivation, inactivation, harvesting, and postharvesting must be described and must ensure the quality, homogeneity, and traceability of the mold. Critical cultivation parameters such as temperature and humidity are controlled and monitored. Appropriate measures must be taken to avoid contamination by foreign species, and controls must document the absence of suspected toxins. Regulatory requirements for the use of molds in allergen product manufacturing are listed in the European Pharmacopoeia [15].

25.2.1.2.6 Foods

Foods constitute a diversified area, and the market for standardized allergen extracts is scarce. Foods are often derived from various cultivars and subspecies grown under a broad variety of conditions reflecting geographic regions worldwide. In addition, foods are often cooked prior to ingestion, and cooking unpredictably affects the allergenicity of the foods. Consequently, the source of allergen exposure, qualitative as well as quantitative, is highly variable [19].

Ideally, source materials for food allergen extracts should reflect local subspecies, conditions, and habits for the cultivation, harvesting, storing, and cooking of the foods. However, ingested foods are increasingly derived from distant parts of the world. The best solution to these problems may be to combine materials from as many sources as possible to reflect variation in as many parameters as possible. The quality of the source material should be suitable for human consumption, and the origin and identity of the raw material should be documented.

For some plant foods, differences in tissue distribution and solubility properties of individual allergens may prevent optimal yields in a single extraction procedure [20]. In such cases, an optimal extract may be derived only by combining extracts produced using different buffers and different parts of the plant, i.e., peel and pulp for fruits, as raw material.

A further challenge in food allergen extract production is the presence in many foods of natural or microbial toxins, pesticides, antibiotics, preservatives, and other additives that may be concentrated in the allergen extract manufacturing process. In general, the use of organic source material should be preferred.

Source materials for the manufacture of food-derived allergen products are not regulated by a specific monograph in the European Pharmacopoeia.

25.2.2 Aqueous allergen extracts

25.2.2.1 PREPARATION OF AQUEOUS ALLERGEN EXTRACTS

The production process of allergen extracts imposes a number of constraints on both selection of source materials and the physicochemical conditions used during the extraction procedure. The process must be gentle and neither denature the proteins/allergens nor significantly alter the composition, including the quantitative ratio between soluble components. The extraction should be performed under conditions resembling the physiologic conditions in the human airways, i.e., pH and ionic strength, and suppressing possible proteolytic degradation and microbial growth [21]. The optimal extraction time is always a compromise between yield and degradation/denaturation of the specific allergens.

Low molecular weight materials (below 5000 Da) often include irritants, such as histamine, and should be removed from the final extract. This can be accomplished by dialysis, ultrafiltration, or size

exclusion chromatography. Any substance excluded from the final extract should be verified nonallergenic. The production procedure should include assessment of known toxins, viral particles, microorganisms, and free histamine, and where relevant, verifying their concentration below defined thresholds.

The final extract should be stored under conditions that impede deterioration of the allergenic activity either by lyophilizing or by storing it at low temperatures (−20°C to −80°C), possibly in the presence of stabilizing agents such as 50% glycerol or a nonallergenic protein, such as certified human serum albumin.

The most widely used extraction media are aqueous buffer systems of pH 6–9 and ionic strength 0.05–0.2. In general, nonaqueous solvents should be avoided due to the risk of protein denaturation.

Critical steps of the manufacturing process are validated, and acceptable process variation limits are established to secure a robust manufacturing process.

25.2.3 Modified allergen extracts/vaccines

25.2.3.1 INTRODUCTION

The efficacy of allergen-specific immunotherapy, i.e., specific allergen vaccination, is related to the dose of vaccine administered, but the inherent allergenic properties of the vaccine imply a limitation due to the risk of inducing anaphylaxis. The risk of allergic side effects is minimized by administering repeated injections of increasing dose over time. Physical or chemical modification of the extract can further reduce this risk. Physical modification involves adsorption of the allergens to inorganic gels, such as aluminum hydroxide or alum, for the purpose of attaining a depot effect characterized by a slow release of the allergens. Chemical modification includes cross-linking of the allergens by treatment with aldehydes, such as formaldehyde or glutaraldehyde, for the purpose of reducing allergenic reactivity. Modified allergen vaccines are used for allergy vaccination but are not used for diagnosis since they were intentionally modified to reduce interaction with IgE.

25.2.3.2 PHYSICAL MODIFICATION OF ALLERGENS

Physical modification of allergens involves adsorption of the allergen extract with insoluble complexes of inorganic salts, such as aluminum hydroxide or calcium phosphate. Aluminum hydroxide, $Al(OH)_3$, is especially useful for vaccination purposes and is used in both human and veterinary medicine [22]. Its advantages are based on two characteristics of the complexes, the depot effect and the adjuvant effect. The allergens bind firmly to the inorganic complexes, giving rise to slow release of the proteins, thereby lowering the concentration of allergen in the tissue and reducing the risk of systemic side effects. Furthermore, the depot effect reduces the number of injections needed in the course of specific allergy vaccination. Although the significance of the adjuvant effect is unclear, higher levels of IgG antibodies are observed when alum-adsorbed vaccines are used in specific allergy vaccination, as compared to aqueous vaccine [23]. Compared to aqueous vaccines, patients receiving depot preparations seem to experience fewer systemic side effects [24], particularly severe early reactions. The frequency of late reactions, which seem to be milder and can be managed by the patient at home, are reduced to a lesser extent, especially in asthmatic patients [25].

25.2.3.2.1 Preparation of aluminum hydroxide-adsorbed extract

Aluminum hydroxide is available as a stable viscous homogeneous gel with a high capacity for noncovalent coupling of proteins. The adsorption is performed simply by mixing the aqueous extract and the gel. After a few minutes at room temperature, the adsorption is complete. Buffer conditions need to be controlled, as the binding capacity varies with buffer composition, ionic strength, pH, and additives [26].

Standardization of the allergen extract must be completed prior to adsorption, as the insoluble complex is difficult to analyze. Therefore, it is difficult to verify the amount of protein adsorbed. Manufacturers must specify criteria to withdraw batches above certain thresholds, as different allergens are bound to the complex with different efficiency. Thus, if a large fraction of the allergen extract is unbound, the relative composition of the vaccine may not reflect the composition of the standardized extract. In each case, the binding capacity has to be empirically determined [27]. The EMA Guideline requires unbound protein to be documented at release and at the end of the shelf-life period [8].

25.2.3.3 CHEMICALLY MODIFIED ALLERGENS

The theory behind chemical modification of allergen extracts is based on the observation that successful allergy vaccination is accompanied by an increase in allergen-specific IgG. Thus, if the allergen could be modified in such a way as to reduce allergenic reactivity, i.e., IgE binding, while preserving immunogenicity, higher doses could be administered without the risk of systemic reactions, leading to higher levels of allergen specific IgG and improved outcome of specific allergy vaccination [28].

Formaldehyde had been used for extract development in detoxification of bacterial toxins, when Marsh and coworkers in 1970 applied formaldehyde treatment of allergens for allergy vaccination [28]. The allergens are incubated with formaldehyde yielding "allergoids," high molecular weight covalently coupled allergen complexes. Compounds with similar immunological properties can be produced using glutaraldehyde instead of formaldehyde. The rationale behind the reduced allergenicity of allergoids is threefold: (1) the large polymeric structures would contain concealed antigenic determinants (epitopes) unable to react with IgE; (2) polymeric antigens would have a lower "epitope concentration" and thus reduced ability to cross-link IgE on mast cells; and (3) high molecular weight polymers would diffuse more slowly through tissue.

25.2.3.3.1 Preparation of chemically modified allergens

Several allergens are heat labile and thus not readily applicable to the standard procedure of incubation with formaldehyde at elevated temperatures. Instead, a two-step procedure has been applied [29]: The first step is incubation with 2 M formaldehyde at 10°C in aqueous buffer at pH = 7.5 yielding a stabilized intermediate. After 16 days, the reaction is diluted fourfold and incubated another 16 days at 32°C. The first step at low temperature results in limited inter- and intramolecular cross-linking, thus stabilizing the allergen complex. The intermediate can be cross-linked further at elevated temperature. Residual formaldehyde is removed by dialysis, and the allergoid is distributed stabilized by addition of 50% glycerol, lyophilized, or coupled to aluminum hydroxide.

25.2.3.4 OTHER MODIFICATIONS

Approaches have been taken to reduce the allergenicity of allergen extracts by disruption of the tertiary structure of allergen molecules using denatured or degraded antigens or peptides, however, with reduced efficacy in allergy vaccination as compared to native allergens. Such molecules do have reduced IgE binding activity but also substantially reduced immunizing capacity leading to insufficient stimulation of a protective immune response.

The employment of structural and molecular biology has revealed molecular details to the atomic level of several important major allergens. Biotechnology and epitope engineering may facilitate the development of safer allergen molecules in the form of mutated recombinant allergens [30], which can be standardized as chemical entities, obviating the problems of current allergen standardization [31].

25.2.3.5 STANDARDIZATION OF MODIFIED ALLERGEN EXTRACTS

Most of the techniques used to characterize and standardize aqueous allergen extracts are not applicable to modified ones. It is therefore recommended that standardization be completed using the intermediate allergen preparation (IMP) prior to modification, and the reproducibility of the modification process be documented by methods specific to the procedure in question. Standardization of aqueous allergen extracts is discussed elsewhere in this chapter. A brief discussion of the methods suitable for the documentation of the modification processes in aluminum hydroxide-adsorbed and aldehyde-treated allergen extracts follows.

Protein content is used to document the dose strength of the aluminum hydroxide-adsorbed product, and it can be a useful measure in terms of normalization of other activities; for example, radioallergosorbent test (RAST) inhibition capacity per Lowry unit of protein. Determination of the reduction in primary amino groups is a good indication of the degree of modification in aldehyde-treated allergen extracts, since aldehydes react preferentially with primary amino groups. This measure can also be used for stability monitoring of the allergoid, as a reversal of the coupling will lead to an increase in the number of primary amino groups.

It is essential to verify that all protein is bound for adsorbed allergen vaccines. The acceptable level of allergen in the supernatant following centrifugation should be considerably below the initial dose used in the updosing schedule of allergy vaccination. Protein content in the supernatant is also used to monitor stability of the adsorbed complex.

Electrophoretic techniques, such as acrylamide gel electrophoresis [32] and isoelectric focusing [33] possibly combined with immunoblotting [34], are widely used for allergen characterization. For analysis of allergens liberated from adsorbed complexes, acrylamide gel electrophoresis is preferred. However, for "allergoids," acrylamide gel electrophoresis is not useful because of the high molecular weight. As formaldehyde preferentially reacts with primary amino groups, the pI of the allergoid is more acidic relative to the allergens. The shift in pI can be monitored by isoelectric focusing. Size exclusion chromatography, preferably conducted by high-performance liquid chromatography (HPLC), is suited to control for the increase in molecular weight of allergoids relative to the allergens.

Crossed (radio-) immunoelectrophoresis [35] cannot be used to analyze modified allergen extracts. RAST inhibition [36] or related techniques, however, are readily applicable to both alum-adsorbed allergen extracts and allergoids for the purpose of assessing the reduction in allergenicity. These methods are also suited for stability studies.

In vivo testing in patients to standardize modified allergen vaccines is theoretically attractive; however, it is not practical. First, it would not be ethically acceptable to base production of all batches of extracts on routine *in vivo* assays. There are also large differences in the immune responses of individual patients necessitating large patient panels for such assays. Second, *in vivo* tests are expensive in terms of labor, time, and money.

25.2.3.6 COMPARISON OF MODIFIED EXTRACTS

Allergen extracts contain a variety of enzymatic activities, including proteolytic activities, resulting in reduced stability of aqueous extracts if stored in solution. Both chemical and physical modification enhances the stability of allergoid preparations; however, the chemical modification process is slow and may permit proteolytic breakdown before completion. In addition, both physical (aluminum hydroxide) and chemical (formaldehyde or glutaraldehyde) modification result in reduced allergenicity.

Acquired immune responses are driven by contact with epitopes, which are structural elements of the allergens (antigens). T-cell epitopes are linear fragments of its polypeptide chain, whereas B-cell epitopes (antibody binding epitopes) are sections of the surface structure present only in the native conformation of the allergen (Figures 25.2 and 25.3). Both T- and B-cell epitopes are essential for effective initiation and stimulation of immune responses; however, the repertoire of epitopes functional in any individual is highly heterogeneous [37,38].

Whereas the modification introduced by aluminum hydroxide adsorption is biologically reversible, the chemical modification of individual amino acids will irreversibly inactivate B-cell (mainly) and T-cell epitopes. This chemical effect decreases immunogenicity explaining why higher doses of allergoid are needed to achieve clinical efficacy as compared to native allergen extract. The chemical modifications are not randomly distributed, as ε-amino groups on lysine residues are preferentially modified. Some epitopes are consequently more sensitive to modification than others, which may enhance the patient-to-patient variation when allergoids are used for allergy vaccination.

Contrary to expectation, however, allergoids are not safer in practical allergy vaccination compared to native allergens. This

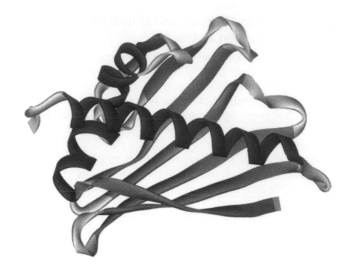

Figure 25.2 Molecular structure of the major allergen from Birch, Bet v 1. The main feature of the structure is a 25 amino acid long α-helix surrounded by a seven stranded antiparallel β-sheets. A most unusual feature of the structure is a large internal cavity with three openings to the surface. This is the first experimentally determined structure of a clinically important inhalant major allergen [68].

was documented in a report from the German Federal Agency for Sera and Vaccines which analyzed all reported adverse reactions to allergen vaccines over a 10-year period, 1991 to 2000, including 555 life-threatening, nonfatal events [39].

Commercial allergoid products are difficult to compare by laboratory methods as concentrations differ widely between manufacturers, but studies comparing IgE binding in recommended maintenance doses of commercial products show that allergoid based on formaldehyde modification did not show reduced IgE binding compared to intact allergen as did allergoids based on glutaraldehyde modification [40]. Results vary widely between allergoids, and it may not be meaningful to speak about allergoids as a homologous group. All investigated allergoids did show reduced capacity to induce an immune response as compared to intact allergens [40]. Other studies have excluded differences based on the composition of the allergen extract, as the same extract was compared with or without chemical modification [41]. One study compared the same extract modified with formaldehyde and glutaraldehyde, respectively, to confirm that glutaraldehyde is superior to formaldehyde in reducing IgE binding [42].

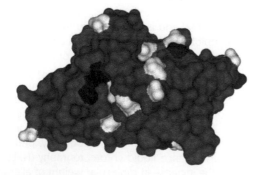
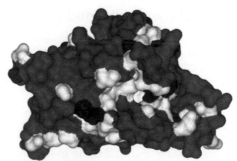

Figure 25.3 The molecular basis of cross-reactivity. Front and back views of the molecular structure of Bet v 1. Gray patches represent areas on the surface completely conserved among the homologous major allergens of alder, birch, and hazel. Conservative substitutions occur in dark gray areas. The conserved areas represent potential highly cross-reactive IgE epitopes on the protein surface.

In conclusion, allergoid products currently available on the market in Europe do not fulfill the allergoid concept as originally formulated by Marsh [28], as not all allergoids show reduced IgE binding, and none of the allergoids show enhanced immunogenicity compared to intact allergen extracts.

25.3 STANDARDIZATION OF ALLERGEN EXTRACTS

Allergen extracts are complex mixtures of antigenic components. They are produced by extraction of naturally occurring source materials known to vary considerably in composition depending on time and place. Without intervention, this variation would be reflected in the final products.

The purpose of standardization is to minimize the variation in composition, qualitative as well as quantitative, of the final products for the purpose of obtaining a higher level of safety, efficacy, accuracy, and simplicity for allergy diagnosis and allergen vaccination. Standardization of allergen extracts can never be absolute; standardization should be progressively improved as new methodologies and technologies are developed and the understanding of the properties of the allergens and of the immune responses of allergic patients increases. The benefits for the clinician from improved standardization of allergen vaccines include easier differentiation between allergic and nonallergic subjects, a more precise definition of the specificity and degree of allergy, and a more reliable and reproducible outcome of specific allergy vaccination.

Standardization of allergen extracts is complicated due to their complexity, the allergen molecules, and their epitopes. Allergens are complex mixtures of isoallergens and variants, differing in amino acid sequence (Figure 25.4). Some allergens are composed of two or more subunits, the association and dissociation of which will affect IgE binding. In addition, partial denaturation or degradation, which may be imposed by physical or chemical conditions in the production process, is difficult to assess and has a significant effect on the IgE binding activities of the allergens. The B-cell epitopes that bind to IgE are largely conformational by disposition, meaning that they will be missing from the extract if the allergens are irreversibly denatured.

Another complicating aspect is the complexity of the immune responses of individual patients. Patients respond individually to allergen sources with respect to both specificity and potency. Allergens are proteins, and all proteins are potential allergens. A major allergen is defined as an allergen that is frequently recognized by patients' serum IgE when a large panel of patient sera is analyzed. A minor allergen binds IgE less frequently (below 50%) [43]. Furthermore, patients respond individually to B- and T-cell epitopes and hence to isoallergens and variants.

A major objective of allergen extract standardization is to ensure an adequate complexity in their composition. Knowledge of all essential allergens is a precondition for the safety of ensuring their presence in the final products (Figure 25.5).

The other important aspect of standardization is the control of the total allergenic potency. The total IgE binding activity is intimately related to the content of major allergen [44], and for an optimal standardization procedure, control of the content of major allergen is essential.

A variety of techniques are available to assess allergen extract complexity and potency. Most techniques use antibodies as reagents, adding another level of complexity to the standardization procedure. Both human IgE and antibodies raised by immunization

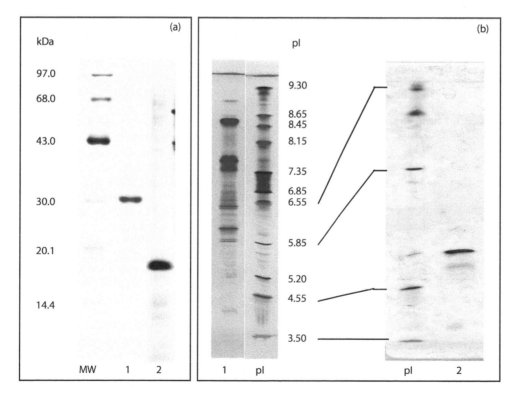

Figure 25.4 Isoallergenic variation. Allergens are mixtures of isoallergenic variants differing in amino acid sequence, whereas recombinant allergens are homogenous. (a) A silver-stained SDS gel, lane MW: molecular weight markers, lane 1: purified natural Phl p 1, lane 2: purified recombinant Bet v 1. (b) Silver-stained isoelectric focusing gels of pI markers, and the same preparations of purified allergens (lanes 1 and 2).

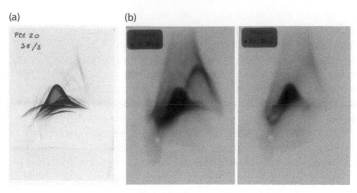

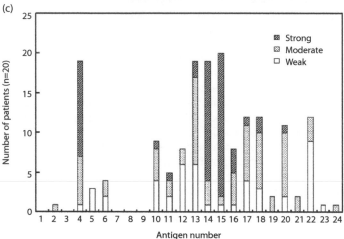

Figure 25.5 Complexity of allergen extracts. Crossed (radio)-immunoelectrophoresis used for the determination of important allergens. (a) A crossed immunoelectrophoresis plate of a *Dermatophagoides pteronyssinus* allergen extract. Each bell-shaped precipitate represents the reaction of an antigen in the extract with the corresponding antibody present in a rabbit antiserum, raised by repeated immunization with the extract. (b) An autoradiogram of similar plates after incubation with patient's serum and a radiolabeled anti-IgE antibody. Stained precipitates represent allergens. Precipitates from (a) are arbitrarily numbered, and the number of sera in a patient panel showing IgE reactivity with each precipitate is recorded and displayed in an allergogram (c). Der p 1 corresponds to antigen number 15, Der p 2 to antigen 14.

of animals are subject to natural variation and, in addition, may change over time.

These problems are handled by the establishment of reference and control extracts. International collaboration is necessary to ensure that manufacturers, government authorities, clinicians, and research laboratories worldwide can refer to the same preparations when comparing the results of quality control studies and potency estimates for different allergen extracts. Ideally, standards for reagents should also be established to promote and assist international collaboration.

25.3.1 Standards, references, and controls

25.3.1.1 ESTABLISHMENT AND USE OF INTERNATIONAL STANDARDS

Guidelines for the establishment of international standards (IS) were formulated by a subcommittee under the International Union of Immunological Societies (IUIS) in 1980–1981. It was assumed that the collaboration and joint authority of the WHO would be essential for international acceptance. In the following years, the subcommittee selected, characterized, and produced international standards in the form of allergen extracts from several allergenic sources. These included *Ambrosia artemisiifolia* (short ragweed) [45], *Phleum pratense* (timothy grass) [46], *Dermatophagoides pteronyssinus* (house dust mite) [47], *Betula verrucosa* (birch) [48], and *Canis familiaris* (dog) [49]. Additional standards were planned for the *Alternaria alternata* (a mold) [50], *Cynodon dactylon* (Bermuda grass) [51] and *Lolium perenne* (ryegrass) [52], *Felis domesticus* (cat), and *Dermatophagoides farinae* (house dust mite). This initiative failed because of a lack of consensus and acceptance, primarily due to the differences in practical standardization between Europe and the United States (see Section 25.3.7). Although not supported by regulatory authorities, the standards can still be useful in practical allergen standardization.

International standards can be obtained from the National Institute of Biological Science and Control (NIBSC), Herts, United Kingdom.

25.3.1.2 PURIFIED ALLERGENS AS INTERNATIONAL STANDARDS

From November 2001 to April 2005, the European Commission funded an allergen standardization project entitled "Development of Certified Reference Materials for Allergenic Products and Validation of Methods for their Quantification" or in short, the CREATE project [53]. The two major objectives of the project were evaluation of the potential use of purified recombinant allergens as certified reference materials (CRMs) and evaluation of available ELISA assays for measurement of major allergens using the candidate CRM as a standard [53]. The allergens included were major inhalant allergens in Europe, i.e., Bet v 1 from birch pollen, Phl p 1 and Phl p 5 from grass pollen, Ole e 1 from olive pollen, and Der p 1, Der p 2, Der f 1, and Der f 2 from house dust mites. The result of the CREATE project was the establishment of the basis for the first two recombinant allergens as CRMs: rBet v 1 and rPhl p 5.01 (also called Phl p 5a). Both rBet v 1 and rPhl p 5.01 were found to be correctly folded molecules, and they fulfilled the necessary stability requirements and were similar to their natural counterparts with respect to immunologic characteristics [54]. For each CRM, two ELISA assays were identified with potential for future use as reference methods. A follow-up study of CREATE, BSP090, was approved in 2005 under the auspices of the European Directorate of the Quality of Medicines (EDQM, http:// www.edqm.eu). The goals of this project were the establishment of rBet v1 and rPhl p 5.01 as European Pharmacopoeia reference standards and validation of the candidate ELISAs for the measurement of the two allergens in a true ring trial. The two standards were adopted in October 2012 by the European Pharmacopoeia Commission as Recombinant Major Allergen rBet v 1 Chemical Reference Substance (CRS) and Recombinant Major Allergen rPhl p 5a CRS, respectively [55]. They are intended for use as reference preparations for determination of the Bet v 1 and Phl p 5.01 content, respectively, in allergen extracts and recombinant Bet v 1 and Phl p 5.01 preparations by ELISA. The standards are available from the EDQM under catalog number Y0001565 for rBet v 1 CRS and Y0001566 for rPhl p 5a CRS. Regarding the ELISA methods, one candidate assay was selected and proposed as the future European Pharmacopoeia standard method for Bet v 1 quantification [56]. The assay for Phl p 5 quantification is still under validation.

The existence and availability of purified allergen references will enable the assignment of a major allergen content in mass units to the internal reference preparations (see the next section), which are in use in different laboratories of manufacturers, allergen research groups, or control authorities. Furthermore, the references can be used for standardizing major allergen content in batch-to-batch standardization.

25.3.1.3 ESTABLISHMENT AND USE OF IN-HOUSE REFERENCE PREPARATIONS

Having established a production process including control of raw materials, batch-to-batch standardization is performed relative to an IHRP. The IHRP must be thoroughly characterized by *in vitro* laboratory methods to demonstrate an adequate complexity as well as an appropriate content of relevant major allergen(s). The potency of the IHRP must be determined by *in vivo* methods, such as skin testing, and ideally the content of major allergen(s) should be determined in absolute amounts. Furthermore, the IHRP should prove efficacious in clinical trials of specific allergy vaccination.

The IHRP serves as a blueprint of the allergy extract to be matched in all aspects by every following batch. The IHRP can be renewed by selecting a new batch as IHRP, and in this situation, *in vitro* methods may substitute for *in vivo* methods for the determination of the relative potency between the two; however, special care needs to be exerted to ensure that the new IHRP matches the old IHRP in all possible aspects.

25.3.2 Strategy for standardization

It is impossible to assess the clinical efficacy of every batch in the production of routine batches of allergen extracts. In practice, the batches are compared to the IHRP using a combination of different *in vitro* techniques to achieve a uniform composition, content of major allergen, and potency of extracts. The batch-to-batch standardization can be performed using the following three-step procedure:

1. Determination of allergen composition to ensure that all important allergens are present
2. Quantification of specific allergens to ensure that essential allergens are present in constant ratios
3. Quantification of the total allergenic activity to ensure that the overall potency of the extract is constant (*in vivo* and/or *in vitro*)

25.3.3 Methods for assessment of allergen extract quality

The quality of an allergen extract is a measure of the complexity of the composition, including the concentration of each constituent. Having established careful control of raw materials and a robust production process, a relatively constant ratio between individual components can be achieved independently by quantifying only one or two components, i.e., the major allergens.

The complexity of the composition of allergen extracts can be assessed by several techniques. These techniques are standard biochemical and immunochemical separation techniques. Polyacrylamide gel electrophoresis with sodium dodecyl sulfate (SDS-PAGE) [32] is a widely used high-resolution technique available in rapid and partly automated systems. The proteins are separated, but only after denaturation, according to size. Densitometric scanning has been reported, but this technique is not quantitative due to differences in staining intensities. It should only be used for a qualitative assessment of the allergen extract. In combination with electroblotting [57], the proteins can be immobilized on protein-binding membranes, such as nitrocellulose, and stained using a variety of dyes or labeled antibodies (immunoblotting), thereby considerably increasing the sensitivity. Some allergens, however, are irreversibly denatured by SDS treatment and may escape detection by IgE immunoblotting [34].

Isoelectric focusing (IEF) [33] is a qualitative electrophoretic technique that separates proteins according to charge (isoelectric points [pI]). Individual allergens are difficult to identify as many proteins form several bands due to charge differences between isoallergens and variants (Figure 25.4).

Crossed immunoelectrophoresis (CIE) [58] is a technique by which individual antigens are distinguished in agarose gels in the form of bell-shaped antigen-antibody precipitates. The technique is dependent on the availability of broadly reactive polyspecific rabbit antibodies, but the method yields information on the relative concentrations of several important antigens in a single experiment. In crossed radioimmunoelectrophoresis (CRIE) [35], the plates are incubated with patient serum for the identification of allergens.

Methods based on HPLC [59] (Figure 25.6) and mass spectrometry (MS) [60] (Figure 25.7) are being evaluated for use in allergen standardization. Both methods have the potential of generating both qualitative and quantitative information on individual components in a complex mixture.

25.3.4 Quantification of specific allergens

Having determined an adequate complexity in composition, an allergen extract may still theoretically be deficient in the content of major allergen (Figure 25.8). It is important to independently assess the content of major allergen(s), especially for allergen vaccines used for allergy vaccination, as the maintenance dose in effective allergy vaccination contains a defined amount of major allergen. The optimal dose may differ between sublingual and subcutaneous immunotherapy, but the major allergen content is still a usable measure relating vaccine potency and therapeutic effect. Table 25.2 lists major allergen content for optimal subcutaneous immunotherapy.

The significance of controlling individual allergens in extracts is gaining more importance among government regulators and clinicians. Allergen extract manufacturers today have access to the published purification procedures of most major allergens. The purified major allergens can be used to produce antibodies for independent quantification, even in complex mixtures, such as allergen extracts. Polyspecific or monospecific polyclonal rabbit antibodies or murine monoclonal antibodies are most often used for this purpose.

Several immunoelectrophoretic techniques might be applied for the quantitative determination of individual allergens. These techniques are referred to as quantitative immunoelectrophoresis (QIE) [58], and they are convenient and reliable techniques to measure allergen concentrations relative to an in-house standard.

The area of a diffusion ring formed by the precipitated antigen in the monospecific antibody-containing gel can be correlated to the amount of antigen applied in single radial immunodiffusion (SRID),

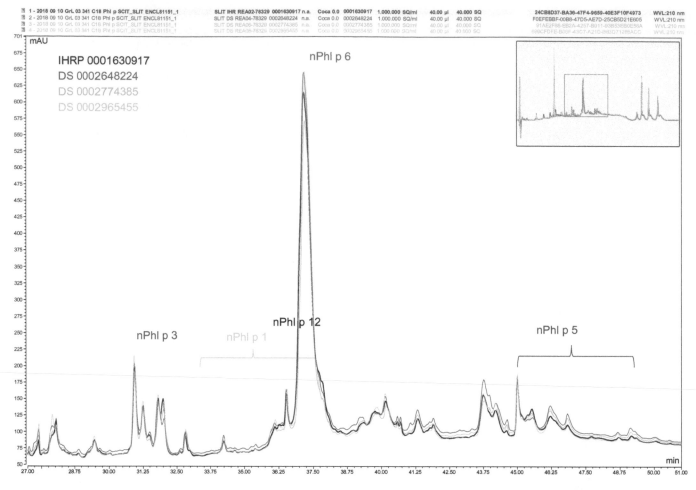

Figure 25.6 High-performance liquid chromatography (HPLC). Experimental characterization of a timothy grass (*Phleum pratense*) in-house reference preparation (IHRP) in black, and three different batches of drug substance (DS) in color illustrating the potential for using HPLC in allergen standardization. Peaks in the chromatogram representing identified major allergens are labeled.

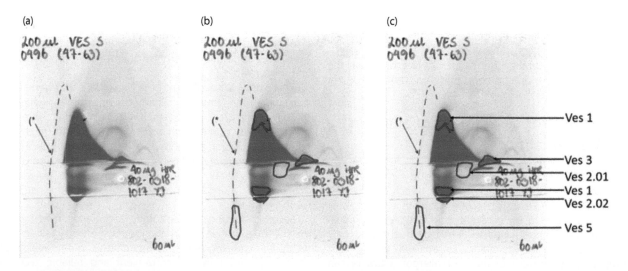

Figure 25.7 Identification of allergens by mass spectrometry. Mass spectrometry used for identification of wasp species' (mix of five *Vespula* species) wasp venom major allergens represented by precipitation arcs in crossed immunoelectrophoresis (CIE). (a) CIE pattern of wasp species' allergen extract; (b) fragments of gel excised (red silhouette) for identification; (c) CIE pattern labeled with identified allergen designations.

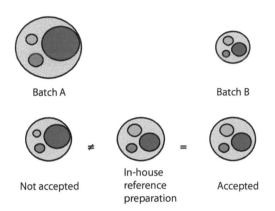

Batch A   Batch B

Not accepted ≠ In-house reference preparation = Accepted

Figure 25.8 Standardization of allergen extracts. Complexity of allergen extracts represented by a model with three major allergens. The area of shaded circles represents the relative potency of individual components. The area of outer circles represents the total allergenic potency of the extracts. The total allergenic potency of batches A and B may be adjusted by dilution or concentration, but the composition of the extracts still may vary, accentuating the significance of the measurement of individual components.

also known as the Mancini technique. The area of the precipitate, alternatively, the height of the precipitate, formed by electrophoresis of the antigen into the agarose gel containing the monospecific antibody, is proportional to the antigen concentration in rocket immunoelectrophoresis (RIE) or quantitative CIE. Both SRID and RIE are dependent on monospecific antibodies, whereas CIE is dependent on polyspecific antibodies.

The ELISA technique [16], in which the allergen is directly bound to a microtiter plate or captured using a monoclonal or polyclonal, monospecific antiserum coated to the plate, and subsequently detected using monoclonal or polyclonal, monospecific antiserum, is a technique offering the possibility of multisample testing and partial automation. When optimized properly, the technique is very accurate. Monoclonal antibody-based ELISA is the most widely used technique for allergen measurement in mass units [61], and a number of validated ELISA assays for major allergens from the main allergenic sources are available. One ELISA method for determination of the major birch pollen allergen, Bet v 1, is now approved by the European Pharmacopoeia Commission as a reference method.

The standard ELISA format is a two-site sandwich assay. An allergen-specific mAb is coated to the microtiter plate and, upon incubating the allergen vaccine, the allergen molecules are captured and subsequently detected using a second mAb or a polyclonal antiserum. An in-house reference, calibrated against a purified allergen preparation or CRS if available, is used as standard. The advantages of mAb based ELISA assays are their suitability for automation, well-defined specificity and an inexhaustible reagent supply, precise quantification in mass units of allergen, detection limits in the range of 0.1–5 ng/mL, and good reproducibility (intra-assay coefficient of variation in the 10%–15% range).

A potential problem of mAb-based ELISA assays is the specificity of the mAb(s) used. Allergens are heterogeneous mixtures of isoallergens and variants, and in some cases, it has been shown that specific mAb reacts to individual subsets of isoallergens [62], introducing a bias in the allergen measurement. A solution to this problem is to use a cocktail of mAbs on the solid phase of the ELISA and a polyclonal antibody as the second reagent.

In the future, absolute quantification of allergens without the use of antibody reagents may become available by mass spectrometry (Figure 25.9).

Table 25.2 Maintenance doses in effective specific allergy vaccination

Allergen source	Major allergen	Major allergen in maintenance dose	Approximate equivalent U.S. Food and Drug Administration potency	Reference
Cat				[69–72]
Felis domesticus	Fel d 1	14.6 µg	2,500 BAU	
House dust mite				[73,74]
Dermatophagoides pteronyssinus	Der p 1	9.8 µg	740 AU	
Dermatophagoides farinae	Der f 1	13.8 µg	2,628 AU	
Ragweed				[75]
Ambrosia artemisiifolia	Amb a 1	10.0 µg	3,000 AU	
Grasses				[76–79]
Lolium perenne	Lol p 5	12.5 µg	3,948 BAU	
Phleum pratense	Phl p 5	20.2 µg	5,220 BAU	
Dactylis glomerata	Dac g 5	12.0 µg	2,956 BAU	
Festuca pratense	Fes p 5	18.6 µg	12,568 BAU	

Note: Discrepancy between diagnostic and therapeutic potency illustrated by the recommended maintenance doses of various clinical studies. For the average patient, the recommended maintenance dose contains 5–20 µg of major allergen.

Absolute allergen quantification using mass spectrometry

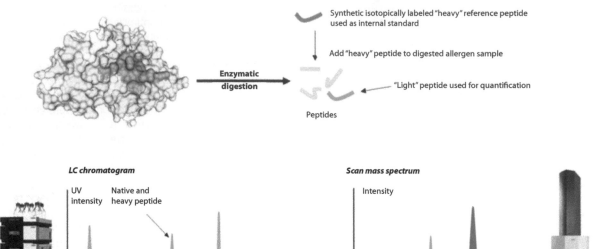

Figure 25.9 Quantification of individual allergens by mass spectrometry. Example illustrating the use of mass spectrometry for absolute quantification of individual allergen molecules in a complex mixture [60].

25.3.5 Allergen extract potency

The potency of an allergen extract is the total allergen activity, i.e., the sum of the contribution to allergenic activity from any individual IgE molecule specific for any epitope on any molecule in the allergen extract. It follows that potency measures will always depend on the serum pool or patient panel selected as well as the methodology used. The potency of an allergen extract may be expressed mathematically as shown in Equation 25.1:

$$a = \sum_{i=1}^{n} f_i c_i \qquad (25.1)$$

Allergen extract potency is the sum of the activities of all individual allergens, where a is the total allergen activity, and c_i and f_i are the concentration and activity coefficients, respectively, of molecule number i.

Methods used for the assessment of allergen extract potency may be divided in two: *in vitro* or *in vivo* techniques. The classic *in vitro* technique for the estimation of relative allergenic potency is RAST inhibition [36] or related solid-phase immunoassays. A standardized reference extract is coupled to a solid phase, paper discs, sepharose gels, or magnetic particles. A serum pool is added, and bound IgE is detected using labeled anti-IgE. In RAST inhibition, the binding of IgE to the solid phase is inhibited by the simultaneous addition of a dilution series of the allergen extract subject to testing. The activity is determined relative to the reference extract itself; parallel inhibition curves indicate similar composition, whereas nonparallel curves indicate that the extracts differ both qualitatively and quantitatively. Techniques based on ELISA [16] using the extract coated onto the microtiter plastic well as a solid phase may be applied using the same principles.

The serum pool is a critical reagent and should be established for batch-to-batch control and for the qualification of individual IHRP. The EMA guideline on allergen products [8] lists specific regulation on the preparation of the pool. The pool should contain sera from 10 to 15 individuals with clinical history of allergy to the allergen substance in question and with no previous vaccination with the corresponding or cross-reactive allergen vaccine. In addition, the patients should come from different areas to minimize the problem of different sensitization patterns depending on the geographical area. Sera containing IgE directed against carbohydrate epitopes (CCD) should not be used to prepare the pool. In addition, sera with IgE to the blocking protein used in the immunoassay (bovine serum albumin, milk proteins, or gelatin) could cause nonspecific binding and should be avoided. Specifications should be set for the reactivity profile of the serum pool. Thus, the frequency of IgE recognition of different allergens and the level of IgE should be considered when preparing the pool. Tests of histamine release from washed human leukocytes utilize the quantification of histamine liberated from allergic patients' leukocytes upon stimulation with allergen [63]. The tests are dependent on freshly drawn blood samples from a panel of allergic individuals, thus limiting the practical applicability in routine allergen extract potency determination.

Direct skin testing of human allergic subjects is the main *in vivo* method to assess allergen extract potency [64]. It is impractical to use *in vivo* testing as a routine assay for production batch release; however, production batches can be compared by suitable *in vitro* methods to internal reference extracts, the *in vivo* activity of which has been already established. Patient selection criteria for *in vivo* assays are important since all *in vivo* methods will ultimately depend on the selected patient panel.

Skin testing in humans is the principle underlying the establishment of biological units of allergen extract potency. Several units are used. In Europe, the potency unit is based on the dose of allergen that results in a wheal comparable in size to the wheal produced by a given concentration of histamine. This unit was originally called histamine equivalent prick (HEP). The Nordic Guidelines introduced the biological unit (BU) [5]. One thousand BU is the equivalent of 1 HEP.

25.3.6 Determination of clinical efficacy

The potency of allergen extracts used for specific allergy vaccination should ideally be expressed in units describing clinical efficacy, since there is no relationship between therapeutic dose and skin-test potency. Approaches to relate extract potency and clinical efficacy have been performed in the United States and Europe and commented on by the WHO. For several standardized vaccines, various trials have established an optimal maintenance dose when used for subcutaneous treatment. This dose corresponds to 5–20 μg of major allergen (Table 25.2), which is different for other administration routes, such as sublingual treatment.

However, determinations of clinical efficacy are extremely laborious. They can only be performed by using highly standardized vaccines, which have been described in detail with respect to composition and *in vitro* and *in vivo* potency.

More recent developments of tablets for sublingual allergy vaccination have been conducted in large, properly designed development programs comprising phase I tolerability trials, phase II dose-response studies, and large, double-blinded and placebo-controlled phase III confirmatory trials with several hundreds of patients in each randomized trial. For some of these sublingual immunotherapy (SLIT) tablets, an optimal maintenance dose, which is product specific, has been established in large, randomized dose-response studies [65].

25.3.7 Standardization and allergy vaccination in Europe and in the United States

Standardization of allergy extracts in Europe is regulated by the European Pharmacopoeia and the EMA guideline on Allergen Products [66]. This regulation is different from that in the United States, where regulation is enforced by the Food and Drug Administration (FDA). Whereas allergen extract consistency in Europe is maintained primarily through the use of in-house standards and international references, this goal is achieved by the FDA by mandating detailed standardization procedures and reagents for use by all manufacturers. An advantage of the European system is that it provides options for the doctor to choose from different products and for manufacturers to continuously improve quality and incorporate new methodology in analysis and control of the extracts. However, allergen medicinal products in the European Union are regulated differently across the different Member States, and different standards do exist [67]. The advantage of the American system is that it results in a higher degree of consistency of extracts among manufacturers. Another difference between Europe and the United States is in the formulation of the extracts used for allergy vaccination. Physicians in the United States primarily use aqueous vaccines, whereas in Europe, alum-adsorbed vaccines, either chemically modified or native, are most often used (Table 25.3).

Table 25.3 Major differences between the United States and Europe in allergen vaccine standardization and performing of specific allergy vaccinations

United States	Europe
Standardization of allergen vaccines	
U.S. Food and Drug Administration (FDA) selects representative extract as FDA reference (FDAR)	Manufacturer selects representative extract as in-house reference preparation (IHRP) according to the European Pharmacopoeia
Biological activity (*in vivo* and *in vitro* potency/total allergen activity) relative to FDAR	Biological activity (*in vivo* and *in vitro* potency/total allergen activity) relative to IHPR
Concentration of major allergen molecules (FDA optional) relative to FDA major allergen reference	Concentration of major allergen molecules (cf. World Health Organization recommendations) relative to IHPR
Methods and reagents selected and distributed by the FDA	Methods and reagents selected and developed by manufacturer
Performing specific allergy vaccination	
Predominantly aqueous vaccines	Predominantly aluminum hydroxide adsorbed vaccines
Nonmodified vaccine	Nonmodified or chemically modified vaccines
Vaccines are mixed for multiallergic patients	Vaccines are predominantly used separately

Source: See Bonertz A et al. *Allergy* 2018; 73(4): 816–826 for a complete comparison.

25.4 CONCLUSION

In Europe, each manufacturer uses individual biological units for the measure of allergen extract potency. This may cause confusion but is enforced by differences in allergen extract composition hampering direct comparison. Furthermore, biological units in current use are based primarily on skin reactivity measurements, which may not be relevant for therapeutic efficacy. Since there is a remarkable coherence between the content of major allergen in the optimal maintenance dose comparing various allergen sources, the content of major allergen for many allergen extracts could be used as a marker relating vaccine potency to therapeutic efficacy. The provision of certified standards and assays for convenient major allergen determination facilitates comparison of the major allergen content of different extracts. However, major allergen content alone does not completely determine potency of current allergen vaccines, since other allergens, which may vary between extracts, also contribute to their biological potency. It is therefore necessary to assess biological potency to avoid the misunderstanding that extracts/vaccines having equal major allergen content are interchangeable.

SALIENT POINTS

1. All allergens are proteins, and all water-soluble proteins are potential allergens.
2. Allergen extracts are complex, biological mixtures, and standardization is essential to ensure safety and efficacy of diagnosis and treatment.
3. The process of extraction is highly dependent on physicochemical conditions. Extreme conditions are likely to destroy allergen epitopes and affect activity.
4. Statistically, patients' IgE binds to some antigens more frequently than to others, thereby defining major allergens.
5. The effective maintenance dose in specific allergy vaccination for the average patient is proportional to the content of major allergen in an allergen vaccine, but different for different administration routes.
6. Major allergen content alone is not a sufficient measure of extract potency.
7. Chemically modified allergen extracts are deficient in specific epitopes.
8. The existence and use of internal as well as external standards are essential for standardization and control of allergen extracts.
9. The quality of an allergen extract is dependent on the qualitative as well as quantitative composition.
10. The potency of an allergen extract is determined by the combination of the concentration of one or more major allergens and the composition, qualitative as well as quantitative, of the allergen extract.

REFERENCES

1. Noon L. Prophylactic inoculation against hay fever. *Lancet* 1911; 177(4580): 1572–1573.
2. Ishizaka K, Ishizaka T, Hornbrook MM. Physico-chemical properties of human reaginic antibody. IV. Presence of a unique immunoglobulin as a carrier of reaginic activity. *J Immunol* 1966; 97(1): 75–85.
3. Løwenstein H. Characterization and standardization of allergen extracts. In: Bergmann K-C, Ring J, editors. *History of Allergy*. Volume 100. Basel: Karger, 2014: 323–332.
4. Løwenstein H. Physico-chemical and immunochemical methods for the control of potency and quality of allergenic extracts. *Arb Paul Ehrlich Inst* 1980; 75: 122–132.
5. Nordic Council on Medicines. *Registration of Allergen Preparations: Nordic Guidelines*. NLN Publication 1989; No 23: 1–34.
6. Bousquet J, Lockey RF, Malling HJ. (eds.) *WHO Position Paper—Allergen Immunotherapy: Therapeutic Vaccines for Allergic Diseases*. Geneva, Switzerland: January 27–29, 1997. Allergy 1998; 53(Suppl. 44): 1–42.
7. Monograph on Allergen Products, European Pharmacopoeia 01/2019:1063.
8. European Medicines Agency. *Committee for Medicinal Products for Human Use (CHMP) and Biologics Working Party (BWP): Guideline on Allergen Products: Production and Quality Issues (EMEA/CHMP/BWP/304831/2007)*. London, 2008.
9. Zimmer J, Vieths S, Kaul S. Standardization and regulation of allergen products in the European Union. *Curr Allergy Asthma Rep* 2016; 16(21): 1–11.
10. Løwenstein H. Selection of reference preparation. IUIS reference preparation criteria. *Arb Paul Ehrlich Inst* 1987; 80:75–78.
11. Monograph on Pollens for Allergen Products. European Pharmacopoeia 01/2017:2627.
12. Monograph on Mites for Allergen Products. European Pharmacopoeia 01/2017:2625.
13. Monograph on Animal Epithelia and Outgrowths for Allergen Products. European Pharmacopoeia 01/2017:2621.
14. Monograph on Hymenoptera Venoms for Allergen Products. European Pharmacopoeia 01/2017:2623.
15. Monograph on Moulds for Allergen Products. European Pharmacopoeia 01/2017:2626.
16. Aydin S. A short history, principles, and types of ELISA, and our laboratory experience with peptide/protein analysis using ELISA. *Peptides* 2015; 72: 4–15.
17. Beroiz B, Couso-Ferrer F, Ortego F et al. Mite species identification in the production of allergenic extracts for clinical use and in environmental samples by ribosomal DNA amplification. *Med Vet Entomol* 2014; 28(3): 287–296.
18. Henmar H, Frisenette SM, Grosch K et al. Fractionation of source materials leads to a high reproducibility of the SQ house dust mite SLIT-tablets. *Int Arch Allergy Immunol* 2016; 169(1): 23–32.
19. Lemanske RF, Taylor SL. Standardized extracts, foods. *Clin Rev Allergy* 1987; 5(1): 23–36.
20. Ahrazem O, Jimeno L, López-Torrejón G et al. Assessing allergen levels in peach and nectarine cultivars. *Ann Allergy Asthma Immunol* 2007; 99(1): 42–47.
21. Løwenstein H, Marsh DG. Antigens of *Ambrosia elatior* (short ragweed) pollen. I. Crossed immunoelectrophoretic analyses. *J Immunol* 1981; 126(3): 943–948.
22. Butler NR, Voyce MA, Burland WL, Hilton ML. Advantages of aluminium hydroxide adsorbed combined diphtheria, tetanus and pertussis vaccines for the immunization of infants. *Br Med J* 1969; 1(5645): 663–666.
23. Norman PS, Lichtenstein LM. Comparisons of alum-precipitated and unprecipitated aqueous ragweed pollen extracts in the treatment of hay fever. *J Allergy Clin Immunol* 1978; 61(6): 384–389.
24. Mellerup MT, Hahn GW, Poulsen LK, Malling H. Safety of allergen-specific immunotherapy. Relation between dosage regimen, allergen extract, disease and systemic side-effects during induction treatment. *Clin Exp Allergy* 2000; 30(10): 1423–1429.

25. Tabar AI, Garcia BE, Rodriguez A, Olaguibel JM, Muro MD, Quirce S. A prospective safety-monitoring study of immunotherapy with biologically standardized extracts. *Allergy* 1993; 48(6): 450–453.

26. al-Shakhshir RH, Regnier FE, White JL, Hem SL. Contribution of electrostatic and hydrophobic interactions to the adsorption of proteins by aluminium-containing adjuvants. *Vaccine* 1995; 13(1): 41–44.

27. Weeke B, Weeke E, Løwenstein H. The adsorption of serum proteins to aluminium hydroxide gel examined by means of quantitative immunoelectrophoresis. In: Axelsen NH, editor. *Quantitative Immunoelectrophoresis, New Developments and Applications. Scand J Immunol* 1975; (Suppl 2): 149–154.

28. Marsh DG, Lichtenstein LM, Campbell DH. Studies on "allergoids" prepared from naturally occurring allergens. I. Assay of allergenicity and antigenicity of formalinized rye group I component. *Immunol* 1970; 18(5): 705–722.

29. Marsh DG, Norman PS, Roebber M, Lichtenstein LM. Studies on allergoids from naturally occurring allergens. III. Preparation of ragweed pollen allergoids by aldehyde modification in two steps. *J Allergy Clin Immunol* 1981; 68(6): 449–459.

30. Akdis CA, Blaser K. Regulation of specific immune responses by chemical and structural modifications of allergens. *Int Arch Allergy Immunol* 2000; 121(4): 261–269.

31. Løwenstein H, Larsen JN. Recombinant allergens/allergen standardization. *Curr Allergy Asthma Rep* 2001; 1(5): 474–479.

32. Laemmli UK. Cleavage of structural proteins during the assembly of the head of bacteriophage T4. *Nature* 1970; 227 (5259): 680–685.

33. Brighton WD. Profiles of allergen extract components by isoelectric focussing and radioimmunoassay. *Dev Biol Stand* 1975; 29: 362–369.

34. Ipsen H, Larsen JN. Detection of antigen-specific IgE antibodies in sera from allergic patients by SDS-PAGE immunoblotting and crossed radioimmunoelectrophoresis. In: Bjerrum O, Heegaard NHH, editors. *Handbook of Immunoblotting of Proteins*, Volume II. Boca Raton, FL: Chemical Rubber Company, 1988: 159–166.

35. Weeke B, Søndergaard I, Lind P, Aukrust L, Løwenstein H. Crossed radio-immunoelectrophoresis (CRIE) for the identification of allergens and determination of the antigenic specificities of patients' IgE. In: Axelsen NH, editor. *Handbook of Immunoprecipitation-in-Gel Techniques, Scand J Immunol* 1983; 17(Suppl. 10): 265–272.

36. Ceska M, Eriksson R, Varga JM. Radioimmunosorbent assay of allergens. *J Allergy Clin Immunol* 1972; 49(1): 1–9.

37. Larsen JN. Isoallergens—Significance in allergen exposure and response. *ACI News* 1995; 7:141–146.

38. van Neerven RJJ, Ebner C, Yssel H, Kapsenberg ML, Lamb JR. T-cell responses to allergens: Epitope-specificity and clinical relevance. *Immunol Today* 1996; 17(11): 526–532.

39. Lüderitz-Püchel U, Keller-Stanislawski B, Haustein D. Neubewertung des Risikos von Test- und Therapieallergenen. *Bundesgesundheitsbl-Gesundheitsforsch-Gesundheitsschutz* 2001; 44: 709–718.

40. Lund L, Henmar H, Würtzen PA, Lund G, Hjortskov N, Larsen JN. Comparison of allergenicity and immunogenicity of an intact allergen vaccine and commercially available allergoid products for birch pollen immunotherapy. *Clin Exp Allergy* 2007; 37(4): 564–571.

41. Würtzen PA, Lund L, Lund G, Holm J, Millner A, Henmar H. Chemical modification of birch allergen e11xtract leads to a reduction in allergenicity as well as immunogenicity. *Int Arch Allergy Immunol* 2007; 144: 287–295.

42. Heydenreich B, Bellinghausen I, Lorenz S et al. Reduced *in vitro* T-cell responses induced by glutaraldehyde-modified allergen extracts are caused mainly by retarded internalization of dendritic cells. *Immunology* 2012; 136(2): 208–217.

43. King TP, Hoffman D, Løwenstein H, Marsh DG, Platts-Mills TAE, Thomas W. Allergen nomenclature. *J Allergy Clin Immunol* 1995; 96(1): 5–14.

44. Dreborg S, Einarsson R. The major allergen content of allergenic preparations reflects their biological activity. *Allergy* 1992; 47(4 Pt 2): 418–423.

45. Helm RM, Gauerke MB, Baer H et al. Production and testing of an international reference standard of short ragweed pollen extract. *J Allergy Clin Immunol* 1984; 73(6): 790–800.

46. Gjesing B, Jäger L, Marsh DG, Løwenstein H. The international collaborative study establishing the first international standard for timothy (*Phleum pratense*) grass pollen allergenic extract. *J Allergy Clin Immunol* 1985; 75(2): 258–267.

47. Ford A, Seagroatt V, Platts-Mills TAE, Løwenstein H. A collaborative study on the first international standard of *Dermatophagoides pteronyssinus* (house dust mite) extract. *J Allergy Clin Immunol* 1985; 75(6): 676–686.

48. Arntzen FC, Wilhelmsen TW, Løwenstein H et al. The international collaborative study on the first international standard of birch (*Betula verrucosa*) pollen extract. *J Allergy Clin Immunol* 1989; 83(1): 66–82.

49. Larsen JN, Ford A, Gjesing B et al. The collaborative study of the international standard of dog, *Canis domesticus*, hair/dander extract. *J Allergy Clin Immunol* 1988; 82(3 Pt 1): 318–330.

50. Helm RM, Squillace DL, Yunginger JW. Members of the international collaborative trial. Production of a proposed international reference standard *Alternaria* extract II. Results of a collaborative trial. *J Allergy Clin Immunol* 1988; 81(4): 651–663.

51. Baer H, Anderson MC, Helm RM et al. The preparation and testing of the proposed international reference (IRP) Bermuda grass (*Cynodon dactylon*)-pollen extract. *J Allergy Clin Immunol* 1986; 78(4 Pt 1): 624–631.

52. Stewart GA, Turner KJ, Baldo BA et al. Standardization of ryegrass pollen (*Lolium perenne*) extract. An immunochemical and physicochemical assessment of six candidate international reference preparations. *Int Arch Allergy Appl Immunol* 1988; 86(1): 9–18.

53. van Ree R, CREATE Partnership. The CREATE project: EU support for the improvement of allergen standardization in Europe. *Allergy* 2004; 59(6): 571–574.

54. Fernandez-Rivas M, Aalbers M, Fötisch K et al. Immune reactivity of candidate reference materials. *Arb Paul Ehrlich Inst* 2006; 95: 84–88.

55. Vieths S, Barber D, Chapman M et al. Establishment of recombinant major allergens Bet v 1 and Phl p 5a as Ph.Eur. reference standards and validation of ELISA methods for their measurement. *Pharmeuropa Bio&SN* 2012; 8: 118–134.

56. Kaul S, Zimmer J, Dehus O et al. Standardization of allergen products: 3. Validation of candidate European Pharmacopoeia standard methods for quantification of major birch allergen Bet v 1. *Allergy* 2016; 71(10): 1414–1424.

57. Kyhse-Andersen J. Electroblotting of multiple gels: A simple apparatus without buffer tank for rapid transfer of proteins from polyacrylamide to nitrocellulose. *J Biochem Biophys Methods* 1984; 10(3–4): 203–209.

58. Løwenstein H. Quantitative immunoelectrophoretic methods as a tool for the analysis and isolation of allergens. *Prog Allergy* 1978; 25: 1–62.

59. Corran PH. Reversed-phase chromatography of proteins. In: Oliver RWA, editor. *HPLC of Macromolecules, a Practical Approach.* Oxford: IRL Press, 1989: 127–156.

60. Seppälä U, Dauly C, Robinson S, Hornshaw M, Larsen JN, Ipsen H. Absolute quantification of allergens from complex mixtures: A new sensitive tool for standardization of allergen extracts for specific immunotherapy. *J Proteome Res* 2011; 10(4): 2113–2122.

61. Carreira J, Lombardero M, Ventas P. New developments in *in vitro* methods. Quantification of clinically relevant allergens in mass units. *Seventh International Paul-Ehrlich-Seminar,* Langen, Germany, September 9–11, 1993.

62. Park JW, Kim KS, Jin HS et al. Der p 2 isoallergens have different allergenicity, and quantification with 2-site ELISA using monoclonal antibodies is influenced by the isoallergens. *Clin Exp Allergy* 2002; 32(7): 1042–1047.

63. Siraganian RP. Automated histamine analysis for *in vitro* allergy testing. II. Correlation of skin test results with *in vitro* whole blood histamine release in 82 patients. *J Allergy Clin Immunol* 1977; 59(3): 214–222.

64. Platts-Mills TAE, Chapman MD. Allergen standardization. *J Allergy Clin Immunol* 1991; 87(3): 621–625.

65. Larsen JN, Broge L, Jacobi H. Allergy immunotherapy: The future of allergy treatment. *Drug Discov Today* 2016; 21(1): 26–37.

66. Zimmer J, Bonertz A, Vieths S. Quality requirements for allergen extracts and allergoids for allergen immunotherapy. *Allergol Immunopathol* 2017; 45(S1): 4–11.

67. Timón M. Proposals for harmonization of allergens regulation in the European Union. *Allergol Immunopathol* 2017; 45(S1): 1–3.

68. Gajhede M, Osmark P, Poulsen FM et al. X-ray and NMR structure of Bet v 1, the origin of birch pollen allergy. *Nat Struct Biol* 1996; 3(12): 1040–1045.

69. Sundin B, Lilja G, Graff-Lonnevig V et al. Immunotherapy with partially purified and standardized animal dander extracts. I. Clinical results from a double-blind study on patients with animal dander asthma. *J Allergy Clin Immunol* 1986; 77(3): 478–487.

70. van Metre TE, Marsh DG, Adkinson NF et al. Immunotherapy for cat asthma. *J Allergy Clin Immunol* 1988; 82(6): 1055–1068.

71. Hedlin G, Graff-Lonnevig V, Heilborn H et al. Immunotherapy with cat- and dog-dander extracts V. Effects of 3 years of treatment. *J Allergy Clin Immunol* 1991; 87(5): 955–964.

72. Hedlin G, Heilborn H, Lilja G et al. Long-term follow-up of patients treated with a three-year course of cat or dog immunotherapy. *J Allergy Clin Immunol* 1995; 96(6 Pt 1): 879–885.

73. Wahn U, Schweter C, Lind P, Løwenstein H. Prospective study on immunologic changes induced by two different *Dermatophagoides pteronyssinus* extracts prepared from whole mite culture and mite bodies. *J Allergy Clin Immunol* 1988; 82(3 Pt 1): 360–370.

74. Haugaard L, Dahl R, Jacobsen L. A controlled dose-response study of immunotherapy with standardized, partially purified extract of house dust mite: Clinical efficacy and side effects. *J Allergy Clin Immunol* 1993; 91(3): 709–722.

75. Creticos PS, Reed CE, Norman PS et al. Ragweed immunotherapy in adult asthma. *N Engl J Med* 1996; 334(8): 501–506.

76. Østerballe O. Immunotherapy in hay fever with two major allergens 19, 25 and partially purified extract of timothy grass pollen. *Allergy* 1980; 35(6): 473–489.

77. Varney VA, Gaga M, Frew AJ, Aber VR, Kay AB, Durham SR. Usefulness of immunotherapy in patients with severe summer hay fever uncontrolled by antiallergic drugs. *Br Med J* 1991; 302(6771): 265–269.

78. Durham SR, Walker SM, Varga EM et al. Long-term clinical efficacy of grass-pollen immunotherapy. *N Engl J Med* 1999; 341(7): 468–475.

79. Frew AJ, Powell RJ, Corrigan CJ, Durham SR; UK Immunotherapy Study Group. Efficacy and safety of specific immunotherapy with SQ allergen extract in treatment-resistant seasonal allergic rhinoconjunctivitis. *J Allergy Clin Immunol* 2006; 117(2): 319–325.

80. Bonertz A, Roberts G, Slater JE et al. Allergen manufacturing and quality aspects for allergen immunotherapy in Europe and United States: An analysis from the EAACI AIT guidelines project. *Allergy* 2018; 73(4): 816–826.

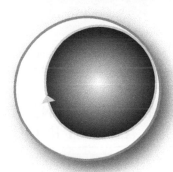

26 Indications for and preparing and administering subcutaneous allergen vaccines

Harold S. Nelson

National Jewish Health
University of Colorado Denver School of Medicine

CONTENTS

26.1 INDICATIONS FOR SUBCUTANEOUS ALLERGY IMMUNOTHERAPY

Subcutaneous immunotherapy (SCIT) may be considered for patients with allergic rhinitis (AR) and/or asthma who demonstrate specific IgE sensitization by *in vivo* or *in vitro* testing to allergens to which they are significantly exposed and whose pattern of occurrence corresponds to that of the patient's symptoms. The allergic respiratory disease should be of sufficient severity and duration to warrant the inconvenience and expense of SCIT. It is particularly indicated in patients whose symptoms do not respond sufficiently to or who do not tolerate pharmacotherapy. However, subjects controlled on pharmacotherapy may choose to receive SCIT for its disease-modifying effect in preventing progression to asthma and in providing persisting relief after discontinuation. There are also studies that suggest SCIT may be of benefit in selected patients with atopic dermatitis, although this remains controversial [1,2].

The other approaches to treatment of allergic respiratory disease are allergen avoidance and pharmacotherapy. Avoidance is of limited usefulness for seasonal exposures, but pet, rodent, and cockroach elimination are effective, and the results with house dust mite control measures are favorable in patients with house dust mite sensitization and exposure [3]. The usual first approach to treating allergic respiratory disease is pharmacotherapy. Whether or not it is fully effective, if it is elected to treat the patient with SCIT, pharmacotherapy should be continued until no longer needed to control symptoms.

26.1.1 Subcutaneous or sublingual allergy immunotherapy?

An alternative treatment to SCIT in these patients is sublingual immunotherapy (SLIT). The choice will usually be made by discussion between the physician and the patient. An important consideration is the greater safety of SLIT, allowing home administration. In favor of SCIT, however, is the lack of defined doses of liquid extracts for SLIT [4], the lack of studies supporting the use of multiple allergen mixes by SLIT [5], and the apparent greater efficacy, at least in the first year, with SCIT compared to SLIT [6,7].

26.1.2 Contraindications for SCIT

European Academy of Allergy and Clinical Immunology (EAACI) guidelines list as absolute contraindications for SCIT uncontrolled or severe asthma, active systemic autoimmune disorders, active malignant neoplasms and pregnancy, and conditions where benefits must outweigh potential risk, such as partially controlled asthma, β-blocker therapy, severe cardiovascular disease, systemic autoimmune disorders in remission, severe psychiatric disorders, poor adherence, primary and secondary immunodeficiencies, and a history of serious systemic reaction to AIT [8]. The U.S. Practice Parameters generally concur, although autoimmune conditions are only a relative contraindication, and they state that AIT should be initiated only if the patient's asthma is stable with pharmacotherapy [9].

26.2 EVIDENCE OF EFFICACY OF SCIT

26.2.1 Allergic rhinitis

Two U.S. healthcare agencies commissioned systematic reviews of the medical literature on the use of AIT in AR [10,11]. The first found highly significant differences in favor of SCIT over placebo for improvement of symptoms and medication use and improved rhinitis quality of life [10]. The second found high-quality evidence for SCIT, compared to placebo, for improving rhinitis and rhinoconjunctivitis symptoms and quality of life and moderate quality of evidence for reduction in medication used for treating AR [11].

26.2.2 Allergic asthma

The 2010 Cochrane systematic review of randomized, placebo-controlled studies of SCIT for allergic asthma included 88 clinical trials, 42 with house dust mite extracts, 27 with pollen extracts, 10 with animal dander extracts, but only 2 with fungal extracts and none with cockroach extracts [12]. Overall SCIT significantly reduced asthma symptoms and medication scores, as well as both specific and nonspecific bronchial hyperresponsiveness [12].

26.2.3 Atopic dermatitis

A systematic review of six randomized controlled trials of SCIT concluded that it had a significant positive effect in selected patients with atopic dermatitis [1]. However, a Cochrane systematic review of 12 randomized controlled trials of which 6 were with SCIT concluded that the results provided little support for the use of AIT to treat atopic dermatitis [2].

26.2.4 A note of caution

The studies reviewed in the previous section employed, almost without exception, single allergen extracts. Although the meta-analyses indicate that SCIT is effective, this conclusion should be limited to the products actually tested in the clinical trials. This caution applies to those modified extracts that were not studied, to most fungal extracts, and to cockroach extracts.

26.3 MANAGEMENT OF POLYALLERGIC PATIENTS

Most patients with allergic respiratory disease are sensitized to multiple allergens (polysensitized). When polysensitization is accompanied by symptoms to multiple allergens, patients are termed *polyallergic*. The management of polyallergic patients differs between U.S and European allergists. SCIT, with mixtures of unrelated allergen extracts, is the rule in the United States [13], although the U.S. Practice Parameters caution that patients should be treated only with relevant allergens [9]. European guidelines, however, do not recommend the use of mixtures [8,14,15]. They recommend that only the most clinically important allergen extract be administered or, if two extracts containing unrelated allergens are of equal importance, that they be given on alternative days or during the same visit in the left and right arms with at least a 30-minute interval between injections [8,14,15]. They consider the requirement for more than two extracts to be exceptional [15].

26.4 DISEASE MODIFICATION BY SCIT

SCIT tends to reverse the T-helper-2 (TH_2) bias underlying the allergic response (see Chapter 5). This results in improvement in the allergic disease under treatment that persists after SCIT is discontinued, but also, in patients with only AR, reduces the likelihood of the patient developing asthma. The persisting improvement after 3 years of SCIT has been demonstrated in several studies [16–18]. However, when patients with grass pollen–induced AR received 2 years of treatment with either conventional doses of timothy SCIT or placebo, symptomatic improvement in the SCIT group that was present at the end of the 2 years of treatment was lost at the end of 1-year follow-up [6].

Reduction in the risk of patients with only rhinitis developing asthma was demonstrated in children with AR due to grass, birch, or both who received 3 years of SCIT with one or both allergen extracts and were followed a total of 10 years [19]. The odds ratio for not developing asthma in the treated group, compared to the control group, was approximately 2.5 throughout the follow-up period. Data from the German National Health Insurance were used to follow patients with AR for 6 years who had been started on AIT (84% SCVIT) in 2006 [20]. After adjusting for markers of AR severity, the risk of incident asthma was significantly lower in patients receiving SCIT (relative risk 0.57) despite the fact that more than half continued on SCIT for less than 3 years.

26.5 PREPARATION OF ALLERGEN VACCINES

26.5.1 Commercially available allergy extracts

Allergen immunotherapy is appropriately performed with vaccines of inhalant allergens and the venom or in some cases the whole-body extract from stinging insects. The term *vaccine* is used to designate the solution administered to the patient. The materials used to prepare the vaccine are referred to as extracts. In the United States, allergen extracts are either standardized or nonstandardized and are available in a variety of formulations: lyophilized, adsorbed to aluminum, or as aqueous or 50% glycerin solutions. Potency is expressed as allergen units (AUs), bioequivalent allergen units (BAUs), content of the major allergen, weight by volume (w/v), or protein nitrogen units (PNUs).

26.5.1.1 STANDARDIZED EXTRACTS

The manufacturing and sale of allergen extracts in the United States are regulated by the Center for Biologics Evaluation and Research (CBER) of the Food and Drug Administration (FDA) [21]. CBER has established reference extracts and reference serum pools to be used by extract manufacturers to standardize certain allergen extracts. The potency of some of the CBER standard extracts was established by titrated intradermal skin testing. For these extracts, allergen extract companies compare their extract to the CBER reference using enzyme-linked immunosorbent assay (ELISA) inhibition, and a potency is assigned. In contrast, the extracts of cat and short ragweed are standardized by their content of the major allergen, expressed in FDA units, rather than quantitative skin testing [21].

The inhalant allergen extracts that are currently standardized are house dust mites (*Dermatophagoides pteronyssinus* and *Dermatophagoides farinae*), cat hair (which is low in cat serum albumin) and cat pelt (which contains substantial amounts of cat albumin), short ragweed (*Ambrosia elatior*), and eight grasses (Bermuda, June, meadow fescue, orchard, red top, rye, sweet vernal, and timothy). For further details see Chapter 24.

A second group of standardized extracts are the venoms of the stinging Hymenoptera. These are standardized on the basis of a venom protein content of 100 mcg/mL for all the individual species, or 300 mcg/mL for the mixed vespids. For further details see Chapter 29.

26.5.1.2 PHYSICAL FORM AND DILUENT OF AVAILABLE ALLERGEN EXTRACTS

Standardized extracts are available in a lyophilized state (Hymenoptera venoms), in 50% glycerin-saline (grasses, short ragweed, cat, house dust mites) and in aqueous solution or glycerin-saline (short ragweed). Nonstandardized extracts are available in either a 50% glycerin or an aqueous solution. The 50% glycerin contains equal parts of glycerin and normal saline. The aqueous extract consists of normal saline and 0.4% phenol. Glycerin at 50% concentration inhibits microbial growth and maintains the potency of allergenic extracts. Phenol, which is added to aqueous extracts to inhibit bacterial and fungal growth, has an adverse effect on the potency of stored extracts. The choice between the two extracting and diluting fluids would favor glycerin were it not for the discomfort associated with injection of 50% glycerin [22].

A limited number of pollen extracts are available adsorbed to aluminum to delay their absorption from the injection site. When the initial extraction is performed with aqueous extracting fluids and the aluminum is subsequently added, the resulting vaccine is equally efficacious compared to aqueous vaccines [23] but is associated with a decreased incidence of systemic allergic reactions (SARs) [24].

26.5.1.3 EXPRESSED EXTRACT POTENCY

The traditional expressions of extract potency are weight by volume (w/v) and PNUs. Neither provides precise information regarding the allergenic potency of the extract. However, it is likely that within broad limits many extracts obtained from the same commercial supplier have reasonable reproducible batch-to-batch potency [25]. Thus, it is possible, as a general practice, to refill allergy treatment vaccines with new lots of the same stated potency from the same manufacturer without untoward reactions by reducing the first injection from the new vial by approximately one-third to one-half of the previous dose.

Weight by volume (w/v) is the simplest way to express the potency of allergen extracts. It is only necessary to weigh the material to be extracted and measure the volume of extracting fluid. Thus, 10 g of pollen extracted in 100 mL of extracting solution yields a final concentration of 1:10 w/v. One advantage of this method of expressing potency is that the extract need not be further diluted to achieve the desired level of potency.

PNUs were introduced in an attempt to more accurately express the allergen content of extracts [26]. First, the protein nitrogen content is determined, and then the content is converted to units (one unit equal to 0.00001 mg of protein nitrogen). The major allergens usually represent only a few percent of the total protein content of allergen extracts. Therefore, PNU offers little advantage as an expression of allergenic potency over w/v. The distinct disadvantage of PNU is that extracts are commercially available in specific concentrations (e.g., 20,000–40,000 PNU/mL). This requires that the extract be diluted from the strength obtained during the extraction process; therefore, the most potent PNU extract available will be weaker than the most concentrated weight/volume for any given allergen.

The CBER BAU is used to express the potency of the eight standardized grasses, cat hair, and cat pelt. An equivalent AU is used to designate the potency of the house dust mites *Dermatophagoides pteronyssinus* and *Dermatophagoides farinae*. The potency of the grasses and house dusts mites is based on quantitative intradermal skin testing.

The CBER standardization method for cat hair and cat pelt is the content of Fel d 1 expressed in FDA units (each unit equals 2–4 µg of Fel d 1). Short ragweed is available with a w/v designation of potency but with the content of Amb a 1 expressed as FDA units listed on the label. An FDA unit of Amb a 1 is roughly equivalent to 1 µg. An extract with 350 FDA units of Amb a 1/mL is considered to be equivalent to 100,000 BAU/mL [9]. The CBER standardization method is more reproducible when content of major allergen is used as a basis.

26.6 ADEQUATE DOSING FOR DEMONSTRATED EFFICACY

26.6.1 Studies with vaccines prepared from standardized extracts

One of the major advantages of using standardized vaccines is that effective treatment regimens from placebo-controlled studies can be more accurately applied by physicians to their clinical practices. There are a number of randomized, double-blind studies in which the effective dose is expressed in terms of the major allergen administered at maintenance (Table 26.1). In some instances, only one concentration was employed, but the clinical benefit was demonstrable within a few months to a year and was clinically relevant. In other studies, more than one dose was employed so, for those vaccines, both an effective and a suboptimal dose have been defined (Table 26.1). It is apparent that the dose response to SCIT is steep, and a dose one-tenth to one-twentieth of the effective dose produces suboptimal results. To allow application of this information to extracts available in the United States, values for the major allergen content of standardized and some nonstandardized extracts from one manufacturer are given in Table 26.2. Standardized extracts labeled with the same BAU/AU potency may contain different amounts of the major allergens whether produced by the same or different extract manufacturers.

26.6.1.1 HOUSE DUST MITES

The study by Ewan [27] demonstrated that a maintenance dose containing 11.9 µg Der p I reduced symptoms and objective responses significantly after only 3 months, but with a high incidence of SARs (approximately 15% of injections). The dose-response study by Haugaard [28] demonstrated that there was marginal reduction in bronchial reactivity to mite allergen after 2 years of treatment with a maximum dose containing 0.7 µg Der p I, but the reduction with a dose containing 7 µg was significantly greater. A higher dose (21 µg) did not result in any additional benefit

but caused more than twice as many SARs per injection as the 7 µg dose (7.1% versus 3.3%). Therefore, the investigators conclude that a maintenance dose containing 7 µg Der p I/injection appears to be optimal based on benefit/risk considerations. Olsen treated 23 adult subjects with asthma for 1 year with a maintenance dose of 7.0 µg Der p I or 10.0 µg Der f I [29]. Compared to subjects who received placebo, those treated with mite vaccines had significantly decreased symptoms of asthma and required less β-adrenergic agonists and inhaled corticosteroids.

26.6.1.2 CAT DANDER

Four studies demonstrate significant improvement employing a narrow range of doses. Van Metre's [30] treatment with a maintenance dose containing 13.8 µg of Fel d I reduced both bronchial and skin reactions to cat dander extract. Alvarez-Cuesta [31], treating with a maximum dose containing 11.3 µg/injection Fel d 1 for 1 year, also noted decreased skin, conjunctival, and bronchial sensitivity, as well as a 90% reduction in symptom medication scores. Hedlin [32], treating with a maximum dose containing 17.3 µg/injection Fel d 1 for 3 years, observed not only a reduced bronchial sensitivity to cat dander, but also a significantly reduced response to bronchial challenge with histamine. Varney's subjects, treated to a maintenance dose containing 15 µg/injection Fel d I for only 3 months, had significantly reduced symptoms on exposure in a house contaminated with cat dander [33].

Ewbank [34] compared the clinical response shortly after achieving maintenance doses, by a cluster buildup, of vaccines containing 0.6 µg Feld 1, 3.0 µg Fel d 1, or 15 µg Fel d 1. Both higher doses of vaccine produced significant decreases in prick skin test sensitivity and increases in cat-specific IgG_4, but only the vaccine containing a dose of 15 µg/injection Fel d 1 produced a significant reduction in the percent of $CD4^+/IL4^+$ peripheral blood mononuclear cells. This study was duplicated in 28 additional cat-allergic subjects, and outcomes were assessed both after reaching maintenance and again after 1 year of maintenance injections [35]. Again there was a dose-related suppression of prick skin tests. Cat-specific IgG_4 was significantly increased with the two higher doses, but only the dose containing 15 µg/injection of Fel d 1 produced sustained reduction in symptoms on nasal challenge. The conclusion of these two studies is that a maintenance dose of cat vaccine containing 15 µg of Fel d 1 is superior to one containing 3 µg of Fel d 1, while the results with a maintenance dose containing only 0.6 µg/injection is similar to placebo.

26.6.1.3 DOG DANDER

Although dog dander extracts are not standardized in the United States, the major allergen of dog, Can f 1, can be measured in dog allergen extracts. Most of the commercial dog dander extracts contain very low levels of Can f 1; however, the acetone precipitated (A-P) dog 1:100 w/v manufactured by Hollister-Stier contains an average of 140 µg/mL Can f 1. A study, similar in design to those conducted with cat extract by Ewbank and Nanda, compared the response to Hollister-Stier A-P dog vaccine containing 0.6 µg/injection, 3.0 µg/injection, or 15 µg/injection of Can f 1 to placebo [36]. There was a dose-related rise in dog-specific IgG_4, suppression of the titrated prick skin test, and reduction of in vitro secretion of TNF-α from allergen-stimulated lymphocytes. The conclusion was that the greatest and most consistent response was seen with a dose of dog extract containing 15 µg of Can f 1.

Table 26.1 Effective maintenance subcutaneous immunotherapy doses expressed as major allergen content

Allergen	Author	Effective dose	Suboptimal dose
Dermatophagoides	Ewan [27]	11.9 µg *Der p I*	
	Haugaard [28]	7.0 µg *Der p I*	0.7 µg *Der p 1*
	Olsen [29]	7.0 µg *Der p I*, 10.0 µg *Der f I*	
Cat dander	Van Metre [30]	13.8 µg *Fel d*	
	Alvarez-Cuesta [31]	11.3 µg *Fel d I*	
	Hedlin [32]	17.3 µg *Fel d 1*	
	Varney [33]	15 µg *Fel d I*	
	Ewbank [34]	15 µg *Fel d 1*	3 µg *Fel d 1*
	Nanda [35]	15 µg *Fel d 1*	3 µg *Fel d 1*
Dog dander	Lent [36]	15 µg *Can f 1*	3 µg *can f 1*
Grass	Varney [37]	18.6 µg *Phl p*	
	Dolz [38]	15 µg *Dac g 5 +* *Lol p 5 + Phl p 5*	
	Walker [39]	20 µg *Phl p 5*	
	Frew [40]	20 µg *Phl p 5*	2 µg *Phl p 5*
	Möller [41]	20 µg *Phl p 5*	
Short ragweed	Van Metre [42]	11. µg *Amb a I*	
	Creticos [43]	12.4 µg *Amb a I*	0.6 µg *Amb a 1*
	Creticos [44]	6 µg *Amb a I*	
	Furin [45]	24 µg *Amb a 1*	2 µg *Amb a 1*
Parietaria	Polosa [46]	4.8 µg *Par j 1*	
Birch	Möller [41]	12 µg *Bet v 1*	
	Kinchi [47]	3.3 µg *Bet v 1*	
	Bodtiger [48]	12 µg *Bet v 1*	
Alternaria	Horst [49]	1.6 µg *Alt a 1*	
	Kuna [50]	8.0 µg *Alt a 1*	

26.6.1.4 GRASS POLLEN

Varney conducted a preseasonal, double-blind trial of AIT with timothy pollen vaccine in subjects with seasonal, grass-pollen AR [37]. A maintenance dose containing 18.6 µg/injection *Phl p 5* reduced symptoms and medication use each by more than 50% compared to placebo. This treatment also reduced conjunctival sensitivity and the late skin test response to timothy grass extract. Dolz treated allergic subjects for 3 years with a vaccine containing 15 µg/injection of the major allergens of a grass mixture [38]. There was a progressive decrease in ocular, nasal, and pulmonary symptoms over the 3 years of the study. Walker treated subjects with both seasonal AR and asthma with a timothy vaccine containing, at maintenance, 20 µg of *Phl p 5* [39]. AIT not only diminished symptoms of rhinitis but also markedly reduced chest symptoms and blocked the seasonal increase in methacholine sensitivity. Frew conducted a trial of a single year of treatment with either placebo or timothy grass vaccine containing a maintenance dose of either 20 or 2 µg of *Phl p 5* in 347 subjects with AR [40]. Compared to placebo, symptom and medication scores during the peak pollen season were reduced 32% and 41% in the high-dose cohort versus 19% and 14% in those on the low dose. Möller treated children with grass and/or birch AR for 3 years, with the dose of timothy at 20 µg Phl p 5. SCIT reduced rhinitis symptoms and also decreased the risk of developing asthma for up to 10 years [41].

Table 26.2 Representative values for major allergen content of U.S. standardized allergen extracts

Allergen extract	Expressed potency	Major allergen	Mean content major allergen	Minimum content major allergen U.S. extracts	Maximum content major allergen U.S. extracts
Timothy	100,000 BAU/mL	*Phl p 5*	620 µg/mL[a]	354 µg/mL[b]	1336 µg/mL[b]
Kentucky Bluegrass	100,000 BAU/mL	*Poa p 5*	270 µg/mL[c]	190 µg/mL[b]	330 µg/mL[b]
Bermuda	10,000 BAU/mL	*Cyn d 1*	200 µg/mL[a]	125 µg/mL[b]	449 µg/mL[b]
Short Ragweed	1:10 w/v	*Amb a 1*	500 µg/mL[a]		
D. pteronyssinus	10,000 AU/mL	*Der p 1*	62 µg/mL[c]	38 µg/mL[b]	98 µg/mL[b]
		Der p 2	63 µg/mL[c]	28 µg/mL[b]	104 µg/mL[b]
D. farinae	10,000 AU/mL	*Der f 1*	73 µg/mL[c]	21 µg/mL[b]	140 µg/mL[b]
		Der f 2	85 µg/mL[c]	51 µg/mL[b]	140 µg/mL[b]
Cat hair	10,000 BAU/mL	*Fel d 1*	40 µg/mL[a]	26 µg/mL[b]	44 µg/mL[b]

[a] Plunket G. Major allergens and allergenic extracts. ALK Technical Memo June 2013.
[b] Based on multiple allergen extracts from multiple companies manufactured in the United States provided in footnotes a and c.
[c] Based on multiple lots of extracts manufactured by a single manufacturer between 2001 and 2011. (Data provided by G Plunket. PhD, ALK-Abello' Inc. Round Rock, TX.)

In summary, grass pollen vaccines containing 15–20 µg of major grass allergen are effective, but there was only marginal improvement compared to placebo when the maintenance dose contained only 2 µg of major allergen.

26.6.1.5 RAGWEED POLLEN

The most extensive experience with vaccines containing known amounts of the major allergens is with ragweed. Studies at Johns Hopkins have included both single and multiple maintenance doses. However, the dose studies have involved either progressively increasing doses in the same individuals or administering different doses for a different number of years. There have been no studies in which groups of subjects receive different maximum doses for the same duration of treatment. Nevertheless, the data show that clinical and objective benefits occur within months and are maintained with maximum maintenance doses containing 11 µg [42] to 24.8 µg [43] of the major ragweed allergen, *Amb a* I. Similar benefits were observed in a group that received a maintenance dose of 6 µg *Amb a* I for 3–5 years [44]. However, the response to doses containing 0.6 µg [43] or to 2 µg [45] was inconsistent and less than the response to higher doses.

26.6.1.6 *PARIETARIA* POLLEN

Treatment for 3 years with a *Parietaria* pollen vaccine with a maintenance dose containing 4.8 µg of *Par j 1* reduced symptom and medication scores in subjects with AR [46].

26.6.1.7 BIRCH POLLEN

In two 1-year studies of SCIT with birch pollen vaccine, a maintenance dose containing 3.3 µg of *Bet v 1* reduced AR symptoms to one-third those with placebo [47], while treatment with a maintenance dose of 12 µg of *Bet v 1* significantly reduced rhinitis and asthma symptoms, reduced medication score, and increased the general well-being of the treated subjects [48]. Möller treated children with grass and/or birch AR for 3 years; the dose of birch pollen vaccine was 12 µg *Bet v 1* [41]. SCIT significantly reduced rhinitis symptoms and also decreased the risk of developing asthma for up to 10 years.

26.6.1.8 *ALTERNARIA*

Two studies assessed the response to SCIT with a standardized *Alternaria alternata* vaccine [49,50]. After 1 year of SCIT with a maintenance dose containing 1.6 µg *Alt a 1*, global symptom/medication scores were significantly reduced, and there was a significant increase in the mean provocative dose on nasal allergen challenge [49]. In a 3-year study of SCIT in children with asthma and/or rhinitis by Kuna, there was a progressive decrease in combined symptom/medication scores, with reduction, compared to placebo of 38.7% in the second and 63.5% in the third year [50].

26.6.1.9 HYMENOPTERA VENOM VACCINES

Immunotherapy in insect-sensitive patients with Hymenoptera venom is effective in reducing reactions to intentional sting challenge [51] (see Chapter 29).

26.7 CONSIDERATIONS IN FORMULATING AN ALLERGEN VACCINE FOR TREATMENT

The first consideration in formulating an allergen vaccine for immunotherapy is inclusion of an adequate dose of each extract in a vaccine to achieve an optimal response. If, as is most often true in the United States, the patient is to receive a mixture of unrelated extracts, then (1) utilization of allergenic relationships and cross-allergenicity to achieve similar effective doses for non-cross-reacting and cross-reacting allergens; (2) avoidance of a combination of extracts that will degrade other components; and (3) selection of the type of diluent become important considerations.

26.7.1 Adequate doses of each allergen

The maintenance doses expressed as major allergen content effective in placebo-controlled studies are listed in Table 26.1, and the approximate content of these major allergens in the U.S. standardized extracts are provided in Table 26.2. It is possible to estimate the amount of each extract that should be added to the maintenance vial in order to deliver an effective dose from this information (Table 26.3). The major allergen content of U.S. standardized extracts varies substantially, even in cat and short ragweed, which are standardized based on major allergen content. It is best to use the mean value in the absence of specific information on the major allergen content of a specific vial (Table 26.2). The amount of major allergen will differ not only with different sources of the same extract but also between different allergens, as is suggested by different maximum BAU/mL and AU/mL values (e.g., grasses 100,000 BAU/mL, house dust mites 10,000 AU/mL).

To formulate a 10 mL maintenance vaccine, the effective dose expressed as its major allergen content is multiplied by 20. This amount is then divided by the major allergen content per milliliter in the concentrated extract to give the amount of the concentrated extract to be added to the maintenance vial. Representative amounts of the standardized extracts to be added to a 10 mL maintenance vial are provided in Table 26.3.

What of the majority of allergens for which there is no information about optimal doses and no standardized extracts? Here it is necessary to work with the best clinical information available. Limited data on major allergen content of nonstandardized pollen extracts suggests a range of major allergen content similar to that of standardized pollens (Table 26.4). The Immunotherapy Practice Parameters (IPP), third update, recommend for nonstandardized

pollen extracts that at a maintenance dose of 0.5 mL, the vaccine should contain a 1:10 dilution of the maximum concentration commercially available (see Table 26.5) [9]. Extracts that are less potent cannot be diluted to the same degree. In the case of the very

Table 26.3 Representative amounts to add to prepare an effective maintenance-dose vaccine using U.S. standardized extracts

Extract	Concentration	Effective dose expressed as major allergen content	Amount to be added to a 10 mL vial with maintenance dose 0.5 mL
Timothy	100,000 BAU/mL	18.6 cg Phl p 5	0.6 mL
Short ragweed	1:10 w/v	12 mcg Amb a 1	0.5 mL
D. pteronyssinus	10,000 AU/mL	3.5 mcg Der p 1	1.75 mL
D. farinae	10,000 AU/mL	5 mcg Der f 1	1.4 mL
Cat dander	10,000 BAU/mL	15 mcg Fel d 1	7.5 mL

Note: These recommendations are based on the mean documented effective doses (Table 26.1) and the mean content of major allergens contained in U.S. standardized extracts (Table 26.2). The amount for the two house dust mite extracts is reduced to one-half to allow for significant cross-allergenicity; if only one is used, the amount should be doubled. Major allergen content will vary from lot to lot from the same manufacturer and among different manufacturers for extracts of the same labeled potency.

Table 26.4 Representative values for major allergen content of nonstandardized U.S. extracts

Allergen	Expressed concentration	Major allergen	Major allergen concentration	Range
Black birch	1:10 w/v	Bet v 1	415 µ/mL[a]	234–688 µ/mL[b]
Olive	1:10 w/v	Ole e 1	>350 µ/mL[c]	
Sage/mugwort	1:10 w/v	Art v 1	3000 µ/mL[c]	
Brome grass	1:10 w/v	Group 5	135 µ/mL[c]	
Dog	1:10 w/v	Can f 1	5.4 µ/mL[a]	0.5 to 7.2 µ/mL[b]
AP Dog	1:100 w/v	Can f 1	140 µg/mL[d]	90–225 µg/mL[d]
Alternaria alternata	1:10 and 1:20 w/v, 50% glycerin	Alt a 1	1.4 µ/mL [52]	<0.01–6.1 µ/mL [52]
Alternaria alternata	1:5–1:20 w/v	Alt a 1	0.98 (0.04–2.75) µ/mL [53]	0.04–2.75 µ/mL [53]
Aspergillus fumigatus	1:10 and 1:20 w/v, 50% glycerin	Asp f 1	16.3 (4–64.0) µ/mL [52]	4–64.0 µ/mL [52]
German cockroach	1:10–1:20 w/v 50% glycerin (?)	Bla g 1	44 µ/mL [54]	

[a] Based on multiple lots of extracts manufactured by a single manufacturer between 2001 and 2011. (Data provided by G Plunket. PhD, ALK-Abello' Inc. Round Rock, TX.)
[b] AP, acetone precipitated. (Assays performed by Hollister-Stier Laboratories, Spokane, WA.)
[c] Plunket G. Major allergens and allergenic extracts. ALK Technical Memo, June 2013.
[d] Based on multiple allergen extracts manufactured by multiple companies in the United States as cited in footnotes a and c.

Table 26.5 Representative amounts to add to prepare an effective maintenance vaccine using nonstandardized extracts

Extract	Concentration	Amount to be added to a 10 mL vial with maintenance dose 0.5 mL
Birch, Olive, Oak	1:10 w/v	1 mL
Sage	1:10 w/v	1 mL
Kochia*	1:10 w/v	0.5 mL
Russian thistle*	1:10 w/v	0.5 mL
Giant ragweed	1:10 w/v	1.0 mL

Note: The final concentration for each nonstandardized allergen group is approximately 1:100 w/v. Those extracts marked with an (*) are included in reduced amounts to compensate for significant cross-allergenicity [31]. The rationale for a target of 1:100 w/v or a 10-fold dilution from the strongest available stock extract is by analogy with clinical studies on standardized ragweed [7].

weak, nonstandardized extracts, such as dog dander (other than A-P dog) and various fungi and cockroach (Table 26.4), it would be very difficult to deliver a major allergen dose in the range shown to be clinically effective for other allergen extracts (Table 26.1). The IPP suggest, for fungal and cockroach vaccines, that only glycerinated extracts be employed and to consider administering the maximum tolerated dose [9]. Representative amounts of some nonstandardized extracts to be added to a 10 mL maintenance vial are given in Table 26.5.

26.7.2 Botanical relationships and cross-allergenicity

In the example of representative dosing for a maintenance vaccine (Table 26.3), the recommended amount of each dust mite is reduced by half. This reflects the high degree of cross-allergenicity between these two species of *Dermatophagoides*. Cross-allergenicity among closely related plant pollen is also the rule (see Table 26.6). If these relationships are not recognized, an allergen vaccine may contain excessive amounts of some groups of allergens. This is most likely to occur with the grasses, since most of the prevalent species in the United States fall into two non-cross-reacting botanical subfamilies [55]: northern pasture grasses typified by timothy and Bermuda and related grasses. Other important cross-reacting groups are the individual members of the *Ambrosia* subtribe; the *Artemisia* genus; the Chenopod-Amaranth families of weeds; and members of certain tree groups, such as the genus *Populus* containing aspen, poplar, and cottonwood species, and the junipers and cedars of the family *Cupressaceae* [55].

Table 26.6 Patterns of botanical cross-allergenicity [55]

There is rarely significant cross-allergenicity between families.
There is generally a degree of cross-allergenicity between tribes or genera of a family, but this is variable.
There is generally a high degree of cross-allergenicity between species of the same genus.

26.7.2.1 PATTERNS OF CROSS-ALLERGENICITY

26.7.2.1.1 Trees

Among the trees, there are a few cases of cross-allergenicity sufficiently strong to restrict inclusion to only one representative in an allergen vaccine mix. These are listed in Table 26.7.

26.7.2.1.2 Grasses

Two non-cross-reacting subfamilies of grasses are recognized. They are represented by the northern pasture grasses and Bermuda. Each should be treated as a separate allergen group, using either timothy or a mixture for the northern pasture grasses for one and Bermuda for the other. If more than one member of each of these subfamilies of grasses is to be included in a vaccine, the amount of each grass should be reduced to compensate for the marked cross-allergenicity.

There are also some regional grasses such as Bahia and Johnson that are in distinct subfamilies (Table 26.8). Although they share some allergenicity with the northern pasture grasses, if locally important, they should be added as an additional component of the vaccine.

Table 26.7 Patterns of significant cross-allergenicity among the tree pollen [55]

Birch Family [56]:
  Birch
  Alder
  Hazelnut
  Hornbeam

Olive Family [57]:
  European olive
  Ash
  Privet
  Russian olive (unrelated)

Cupressaceae (cypress) Family [55]:
  Cedar
  Cypress
  Juniper
  Arbor vitae

Fagaceae Family [55]
  Beech-oak

Genus Carya [55]
  Pecan-hickory

Genus Populus [55]
  Poplar-aspen-cottonwood

Table 26.8 Botanical and allergenic relationships among the grasses [55]

Festucoideae: Northern pasture grasses: orchard, timothy, June, red top, etc.

Eragrostoideae: Bermuda grass, grama, several western prairie grasses

Pancoideae: Bahia, Johnson

26.7.2.1.3 Weeds

There are three major groups of weeds (Table 26.9). Two are in the Composite family, the *Ambrosia,* which includes the ragweeds and related species, and the *Artemisia,* which includes the sages, wormwoods, and mugworts. The Chenopod-Amaranth families include many of the prominent weeds of the Western United States. The major ragweeds (short, giant, and western) are strongly cross-reactive, and an experimental *Amb a 1* extract inhibited the binding of serum sIgE to the three major and seven minor ragweed species by 98%–100% suggesting strong cross-reactivity [58]. The locally most important of the three major ragweeds or a mixture should be used for treatment. There is no clinically important cross-allergenicity of the ragweeds with other members of the *Ambrosia* tribe, such as cocklebur and burweed, nor is there significant cross-reactivity between ragweeds and the other clinically significant group in the Composite family, the *Artemisia* [59]. Within the *Artemisia,* however, there is strong cross-reactivity, and one representative species should suffice for treatment [59]. The Chenopod-Amaranth families, which share some allergenicity, are best viewed as three groups: the *Atriplex* and the Amaranths, both of which are strongly cross-reactive, and the Chenopods, which share some allergens. If several species

Table 26.9 Botanical and allergenic relationships among the weeds [55]

Ambrosia
Ragweeds
Cocklebur
Burweed
Artemisia
Sages
Wormwood
Mugworts
Chenopods
Russian thistle
Kochia (burning bush)
Lambs quarters
Atriplex
Amaranths
Pigweed
Palmer's amaranth
Western water hemp

of Chenopods are locally important (e.g., Russian thistle and *Kochia*), it is better to include them as a mix rather than use one representative species to cover the whole family. Locally important weeds such as sorrel, dock, and plantain should be treated as distinct allergens [55].

House dust mites. The house dust mites, *Dermatophagoides pteronyssinus* and *Dermatophagoides farinae,* are strongly cross-reactive [60]. A mix of both major species is probably best employed if both are locally important.

26.7.3 Components of allergen vaccines that may have a deleterious effect on other extracts with which they are mixed in a vaccine

Some extracts of pollen [61,62] contain enzymes that may cause autodigestion and contribute to loss of potency. Extracts of a number of fungi (molds) and insects contain proteases that are capable of degrading allergenic proteins in other extracts with which they may be mixed in a vaccine [63–66] (Table 26.10). Major allergens in American cockroach and house dust mites are gut derived and very likely are digestive enzymes [63,67]. However,

Table 26.10 Protease content of allergen extracts

Extract	Protease content[a]	Potency of ryegrass extract mixed with extract
Pollen		
Sagebrush	<1	1.18
Ragweed	<1	0.70
Oak	<1	0.89
Epithelia		
Cat epithelia	<1	0.95
Dog epithelia	<1	0.90
Insects/mites		
D. pteronyssinus	<5[b]	
D. farinae	<5[b]	
P. americana	168	0.17
Fungi		
Alternaria alternata	29	0.22
Penicillium notatum	242	0.19

Source: Adapted from Esch RE. *Role of Proteases on the Stability of Allergenic Extracts.* Arbeiten aus dem Paul-Ehrlich-Institut. Stuttgart: Gustav Fischer Verlag, 1991: 171–179.

Note: The extract listed in the first column was mixed with perennial ryegrass extract and stored at 4°C for 1 month. Potency of the ryegrass extract was compared to a reference preparation of 1. Potency of ryegrass was determined by IgE ELISA inhibition.

[a] mcg trypsin equivalent units/mL.

[b] U.S. house dust mite extracts are derived from washed mite bodies without spent culture medium and contain less protease activity than is typical for European extracts. (Personal communication Robert Esch, Greer Laboratories.)

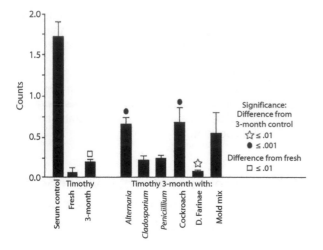

Figure 26.1 Stability of timothy grass alone and in mixtures. The potency of a 10-fold dilution of timothy grass stored under differing conditions was compared by enzyme-linked immunosorbent assay inhibition to that of a freshly diluted aliquot. After 3 months, the diluted timothy extract had a significant decrease in potency compared to the fresh. In addition, those aliquots of timothy stored in combination with *Alternaria*, cockroach, and the mixture of *Alternaria*, *Cladosporium*, *Penicillium*, and cockroach all showed significantly greater loss of potency than the timothy extract stored alone.

protease activity is lower in American house dust mite extracts than in European, since only mite bodies are extracted and not spent culture medium containing fecal particles (Personal communication,

Robert Esch, Greer laboratories). Detectable trypsin-like proteolytic activity is absent from extracts derived from animal dander and pollen [63] (Table 26.10).

Grass pollen extracts are uniquely susceptible to these proteolytic enzymes (Figure 26.1) [63,65,66,68]. In a systematic assessment (Table 26.11), there were a number of pollen and animal dander extracts that lost potency when mixed with one or more protease-containing extracts, while others are quite resistant (Figure 26.2) [68]. *Alternaria* significantly reduced the potency of five of eight extracts, cockroach reduced the potency of three of eight, and *Cladosporium* reduced the potency of only one extract. *Cladosporium* and cockroach reduced the potency of some extracts that were not affected by *Alternaria*. Furthermore, the effect of *Alternaria* extracts was inconsistent from lot to lot, suggesting varying quantities of protease activity were present in different lots of *Alternaria* extract [68].

The extracts that have been shown to have deleterious effects on the potency of other extracts include *Alternaria* [68,69], *Cladosporium* [68,69], cockroach [65,68,69], *Helminthosporium* [65], *Penicillium* [63,69], *Aspergillus* [63,69], *Fusarium* [66], *Bipolaris* [69], and *Epicoccum* [69]. House dust mite extracts have had no effect on other extracts [68,69]. This possibly results from their having low protease activity and having been tested in a diluent containing glycerin [68,69]. While no single inhibitor will protect against all proteases [64], glycerin has been shown to have protective effects against some [63,69].

The degree of loss of potency due to mixing extracts in a vaccine may be marked. Allergenic activity of perennial ryegrass was reduced to 4% by mixing with *Helminthosporium* and to 11%

Table 26.11 Effects of mixing extracts on allergen vaccines

Extract		Alt	Clad	PCN	CR	Mix	Mite	Overall *p*
Timothy		+	−	−	+	+	−	<0.0001
Bermuda		+	−	−	−	−	−	<0.0001
Short ragweed		−	−	−	−	−	−	0.64
Rus thistle	1st	−	−	−	+	+	−	<0.0001
	2nd	−	−	−	−	+	−	<0.01
White oak	1st	+	−	−	−	−	−	<0.01
	2nd	−	−	−	−	+	−	<0.02
Box elder	1st	+	−	−	+	+	−	<0.0001
	2nd	−	−	−	−	−	−	0.02
D. farinae	1st	−	−	−	−	−	−	<0.01
	2nd	−	ND	−	ND	ND	ND	0.49
Cat	1st	−	+	−	−	−	−	<0.002
	2nd	+	−	ND	ND	ND	ND	<0.001

Source: Adapted from Nelson HS et al. *J Allergy Clin Immunol* 1996; 98: 382–388.

Note: The reference extracts listed on the ordinate were stored at a 10-fold dilution of the most concentrated available for 3 months either diluted in HSA-saline or combined with the extracts listed across the top of the table. After 3 months, the residual allergenic activity of the reference allergen extract in the mixes was compared to that of the same extract stored alone. The *p* value is the overall difference among the seven conditions of storage (alone and six different combinations with other allergenic extracts). A (+) indicates significant degradation of the reference allergen extract due to mixing.

Abbreviations: Alt, *Alternaria*; Clad, *Cladosporium*; CR, cockroach; Mix, mixture of Alt, Clad, PCN, and CR; Mite, house dust mite; PCN, *Penicillium*; 1st, first of two studies with the same combinations; 2nd, second study; +, *P* < .05; −, *P* > .05; ND, not done.

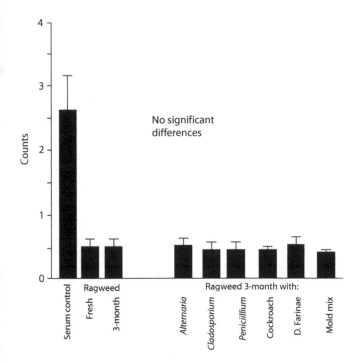

Figure 26.2 Stability of short ragweed alone and in mixtures. The potency of a 10-fold dilution of short ragweed stored under differing conditions was compared by enzyme-linked immunosorbent assay inhibition to that of a freshly diluted aliquot. After 3 months, the diluted short ragweed extract and those aliquots of ragweed stored in combination with *Alternaria*, *Penicillium*, *Cladosporium*, and cockroach alone and in combination were all equal in potency to the freshly diluted aliquot of short ragweed.

by mixing with cockroach [65]. Over 50% of timothy grass extract potency was lost within 3 days of being mixed with *Fusarium* [66]. Birch pollen lost 70% of its allergenic potency over a period of 60 days when mixed with *Fusarium* [66]. Some allergenic activity always remains, suggesting that not all allergens in these extracts are susceptible to proteolytic digestion. On mixing with *Fusarium*, *Bet v* 6 and *Phl p* 5 were almost entirely degraded, while *Bet v* 1 and *Phl p* 1 remained relatively stable [66]. However, even though there may be a significant amount of overall allergenic activity remaining, the selective reduction in certain allergens will make the vaccine less suitable for treatment and may place the patient at risk when being treated with a freshly prepared vaccine that contains allergens no longer present in the mix that they had been receiving for immunotherapy. The results of testing of the effects of mixing extracts is not always consistent. Thus, ragweed is reported to be resistant [66] and susceptible [69] and cat dander susceptible [68] and resistant [69] when mixed with *Fusarium*. These differing results may reflect the marked variability in the composition of fungal and cockroach extracts and differing methods of assessing loss of potency.

In summary, many pollen and animal dander extracts are susceptible to accelerated loss of potency when mixed in a vaccine with protease containing extracts. Despite the variable reports, the safest practice is to not include pollen and dander extracts in a vaccine with cockroach or fungal extracts. House dust mite extracts in 10% glycerin appear to be neither susceptible to exogenous proteases nor to cause loss of potency due to their protease content [68,69]. Degradation of *Alternaria alternata* and

German cockroach allergens by mixture with other fungal and insect extracts was examined [70]. Mixing *Alternaria* extract with several other fungal extracts did not cause loss of potency, and mixing cockroach and imported fire ant extracts did not cause loss of potency. However, mixing *Alternaria* extract with insect extracts or German cockroach extract with fungal extracts, even in 10%–25% glycerin, led to marked loss of some allergens in both extracts [70]. Similar results are reported with mixing *Aspergillus* and other fungal extracts with American cockroach [71].

26.7.4 Diluents employed in mixing allergen vaccines

Because allergen extracts tend to lose potency with time, an effect that is enhanced by storing at higher temperatures and greater dilutions, a number of substances have been added to extracts both to preserve potency and prevent growth of microorganisms. The most effective preservation of extract integrity and potency is not by adding a preservative but by lyophilization [72,73]. This is not routinely employed because the lyophilization process adds to the cost of the extracts.

26.7.4.1 GLYCERIN

Glycerin is the most effective preservative for allergen extracts [74]. It is very effective at a 50% concentration. At this concentration, it inhibits some but not all proteolytic enzymes [63,66,73]. This may contribute to but does not completely explain its effectiveness as a preservative. Decreasing effectiveness of glycerin as a preservative occurs with 25% and 10% concentrations of glycerin [69,74,75]. However, even 10% glycerin is as effective as 0.03% human serum albumin (HSA) in preserving extract potency. It is possible that the presence of glycerin accounts for the lack of proteolytic degradation of pollen extracts by the house dust mite extracts in several mixing studies [65,68,69].

26.7.4.2 HUMAN SERUM ALBUMIN

The preservative effect of HSA is largely due to reduction of adsorption of allergenic proteins to the vial surface [76] and protection of allergenic proteins from phenol denaturation [77]. Human serum albumin does not have protective effects against proteolytic enzymes [63]. Similar degrees of preservative effect were found with concentrations of 0.03%, 0.1%, and 1.0% HSA [74].

Concern has been expressed that patients may become sensitized by repeated injections of HSA; however, no sensitization to HSA in allergen vaccines has been reported, and one study that looked for evidence of positive skin tests or IgG antibodies directed toward human serum albumin was negative [78].

26.7.4.3 PHENOL

Phenol is added to multidose vials of allergen extracts to prevent growth of microorganisms. Phenol denatures proteins, including those in allergen extracts [72], and the deleterious effect of phenol increases with greater allergen dilutions [74]. Phenol degrades allergens in vaccines that are in 50% glycerin solutions [77,79]. HSA is relatively more protective than glycerin against the effect of phenol on extract potency [77,79].

26.7.4.4 OTHERS

A number of other approaches to preserve extract potency have been suggested but have not found wide acceptance. Siliconization of vials has been suggested to decrease adsorption of proteins to their surface. Testing this method revealed it to be without effect [74]. Polysorbate 80 in concentrations of 0.002%–0.2% had a slight effect in preserving potency, but it was less effective than human serum albumin [74].

Epsilon-aminocaproic acid (EACA) has been suggested as a preservative [80], since pollens are known to contain enzymatic activity that may contribute to their loss of potency, and EACA is a potent enzyme inhibitor. However, EACA was found to be ineffective against a variety of fungal proteases [63]. EACA was found to be less effective than glycerin or human serum albumin in preserving extract potency [80]. This observation may be due to human serum albumin reducing adsorption of allergenic proteins to the walls of the vial, whereas EACA provides protection from prolonged thermal denaturation [80].

In the absence of preservatives, extracts stored in saline buffered with bicarbonate lost potency to a greater extent than those stored in phosphate-buffered saline or normal saline [73,75].

26.7.4.5 MIXING EXTRACTS TO CONSTITUTE A VACCINE

Extracts that are stored combined with several other extracts retain their potency to a greater extent than the same extract, at the same dilution, stored alone [75]. This preservative effect is probably related to total protein content. In this instance, the proteins in the other extracts are functioning in a manner analogous to HSA in decreasing adsorption to the surface of the vial.

26.7.5 Special considerations in preparation of an allergen vaccine

26.7.5.1 QUALIFICATION OF VACCINE PREPARATION PERSONNEL

The Immunotherapy Practice Parameters state that a physician with training and expertise in allergen immunotherapy should be responsible for ensuring that the compounding personnel are instructed and trained in preparation of immunotherapy vaccine using aseptic technique and that they meet the requirements of the guidelines [9]. The qualifications of the vaccine preparation personnel include the following: (1) be trained in preparation of allergenic products; (2) pass a written test on aseptic technique and extract preparation; (3) be able to correctly identify, measure, and mix ingredients; (4) be able to demonstrate understanding of antiseptic hand cleaning and disinfection of mixing surfaces; and (5) annually pass a media-fill test [9]. The American College of Allergy Asthma and Immunology provides much of the training and materials needed to meet these requirements, including a Physician Instruction Guide, an Allergen Extract Mixing Quiz, and sources for the Media-fill test (https://education.acaai.org) and (https://education.acaai.org/allergenextractquiz). The American Academy of Allergy Asthma and Immunology provides similar information in the form of an Allergen Immunotherapy Extract Preparation Manual at (https://www.aaaai.org/PM%20Resource%20Guide/Ch-9-allergen-immunotherapy).

26.8 CONDITIONS OF STORAGE

Maintenance of potency of a therapeutic allergen vaccine is a function of the dilution, the diluent, the effectiveness of preservatives, the temperature of storage, and the presence of proteolytic enzymes. The processes that lead to loss of vaccine potency and the measures that can be used to reduce the effect are listed in Table 26.12.

26.8.1 Temperature

Allergen extracts and vaccines are susceptible to loss of potency if maintained at room rather than refrigerator temperature [75,79]. Loss of activity with storage at room temperatures is likely caused by the proteases [72], while loss of potency with brief exposure to higher temperatures is probably related to heat lability of some of the allergenic proteins [81]. Some extracts, such as cat [79], are relatively resistant to this thermal lability effect. Other extracts, including white ash, elm, orchard grass, Bermuda grass [82], ragweed [81], and house dust mites [79] lose potency at high temperature (25°C–100°C). Since the loss of potency is a result of either protease-susceptible or heat-labile proteins, the stored extract will have an altered pattern of specificity due to the preferential persistence of the resistant proteins, resulting in an altered pattern of skin test reactivity and potential therapeutic efficacy [81].

Less extreme temperature exposure of allergen extracts and vaccines, such as exposure to room temperature for 13 hours per week, resulted in significant loss of potency [75]. However, summer mailing, between Texas and Arizona, taking 12 days, did not result in significant loss of potency of a 100,000 BAU/mL timothy extract, although there was a 25% decline in potency of a 10,000 BAU/mL extract [83]. The effect on allergen potency of repeated freezing and thawing has not been extensively studied, but the reduction in the potency of ragweed [61] and dilute *Lolium perenne* [80] extracts has been reported.

26.8.2 Dilution

Extracts and vaccines are more susceptible to loss of potency when stored diluted rather than concentrated [68,74] The increased susceptibility of diluted extract is likely the result of lesser protein content and, hence, relatively greater adsorption of allergens to the container wall [72,75,76]. However, the addition of human serum

Table 26.12 Mechanisms of loss of potency of allergenic extracts

Mechanism	Favored by	Avoidance by
Adsorption	High dilution; high surface-to-volume ratio	Human serum albumin or glycerin
Thermal denaturation	High temperature	Storage at 4°C–8°C
Enzymatic autodigestion	Enzymes in extract	Glycerin and/or storage at 4°C–8°C

Table 26.13 Stability of major allergens in dilute solutions (% of original potency) [84]

Extract	Diluent	1:125 v/v			1:625 v/v		
		3 months	6 months	12 months	3 months	6 months	12 months
Grass	HAS	60	76	51	79	74	54
	NSP	54	60	16	29	24	6
Bermuda	HAS	73	67	43	68	51	34
	NSP	62	53	9	26	16	0
Birch	HAS	93	79	75	76	63	49
	NSP	82	41	34	41	21	13

Abbreviations: HAS, human albumen saline; NSP, normal saline with phenol.

albumen does not completely prevent this loss, and all allergen extracts are not equally susceptible to this effect [68], suggesting that other factors may be involved. One study compared the retained potency of two dilutions of grass, Bermuda, and birch extracts in normal saline with phenol or normal saline with 0.03% HSA for periods up to 12 months (Table 26.13) [84]. The superiority of HSA was evident, but there was loss of potency over time with both extracts.

Loss of potency is related to the total protein content of the extract or vaccine. Not entirely filling a vial with extract enhances loss of potency due to the greater surface area relative to the volume of solution from which protein is available for adsorption. This effect is diminished by including other extracts in a vaccine, thus increasing the total protein content [75]. The same protective effect can be achieved by added extraneous protein, such as HSA [75,76].

26.9 PATTERNS OF LOSS OF POTENCY

26.9.1 Assessment

A variety of methods are employed to assess the residual potency of allergenic extracts [74]. The two approaches most commonly employed, the ELISA inhibition [75] and skin testing [85], yield similar results. In occasional studies, residual activity is greater by skin testing than by RAST inhibition [72,73]. However, a careful comparison of titrated intradermal skin testing and ELISA inhibition yields similar results with multiple allergen extracts [65], suggesting that, properly done, the results with the two methods are comparable.

26.9.2 Individual allergens

The stability of allergen extracts and vaccines to degradation can vary due to differing heat susceptibility of their components, different total protein content affecting the percent adsorbed to the container wall, and the content of proteolytic enzymes which may cause autodigestion (Figures 26.3 and 26.4). Stability varies with the addition of phenol as well as the presence of proteases in extracts used for the vaccine. As expected, studies show

differing loss of potency for different extracts stored under similar conditions. Therefore, it is best to follow general principles that protect the potency of the most susceptible extracts. These include the following: (1) avoiding mixing fungal and insect extracts with pollen, house dust mite, and dander extracts or with each other in formulating a vaccine; (2) keeping the total protein content high by using concentrated extracts and adding human serum albumin to dilutions; and (3) keeping the extracts and vaccines at refrigerator temperatures except when actually being used (for dilute vaccines left at room temperature consider using a refrigerated tray when exposed to room temperatures).

With attention to these details, some diluted vaccines will still lose potency even after 3 months at concentrations used for maintenance immunotherapy (Figures 26.1 and 26.3), whereas others will not lose any potency at the same dilution over a year (Figures 26.2 and 26.4). Full-strength extracts and vaccines are probably stable at refrigerator temperatures for their stated shelf-life. Full-strength extracts in 50% glycerin, as used for prick skin testing, are consistently stable until their expiration date [74]. Diluted

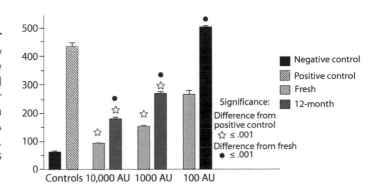

Figure 26.3 The potencies of Bermuda grass extract stored at 4°C in concentrations of 100 AU/mL, 1000 AU/mL, and 10,000 AU/mL were compared after 12 months by enzyme-linked immunosorbent assay inhibition to freshly diluted aliquots of the same Bermuda extract. There was, as indicated, significant loss of potency after 12 months in all dilutions. Negative control contained the Bermuda disc but no serum. Positive control contained Bermuda disc and mixed grass-allergic patients' serum, but no Bermuda extract, while the tested aliquot contained Bermuda disc, Bermuda-allergic serum, and dilutions of Bermuda extract.

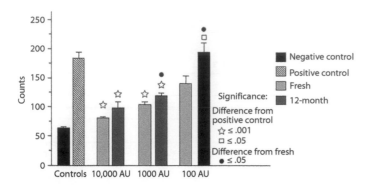

Figure 26.4 The potencies of short ragweed extract stored at 4°C in concentrations of 100 AU/mL, 1000 AU/mL, and 10,000 AU/mL were compared after 12 months by enzyme-linked immunosorbent assay inhibition to freshly diluted aliquots of the same short ragweed extract. There was no loss of potency after 12 months in the 10,000 AU/mL aliquot, but there was a significant loss of potency in the other two dilutions. Negative control contained the short ragweed disc but no serum. Positive control contained short ragweed disc and mixed ragweed-allergic patients' serum, but no short ragweed extract, while the tested aliquots contained short ragweed disc, ragweed-allergic serum, and dilutions of short ragweed extract.

extracts, used for intradermal skin testing, are stable for prolonged periods by some investigators [79] but not by others (Table 26.13) [74]. Some allergen extracts are susceptible to rapid loss of potency at high temperatures (25°C–100°C) [79,80,81], but the loss with exposure to room temperature is not rapid [75].

26.10 ADMINISTRATION OF ALLERGEN VACCINES BY SCIT

Because of the risk of SARs, SCIT should be administered only in a medical facility where prompt recognition and treatment of anaphylaxis are assured, and the patient should remain under observation for 30 minutes after receiving the injection [9]. (See Chapter 34 for further discussion on the safety of SCIT.)

Injections should be given subcutaneously in the lateral or posterior medial portion of the arm using a calibrated small volume syringe with a 26–27 gauge, 3/8 to 1/2 inch safety-engineered sharp injury protection needle [9]. Injections should be administered under the direct supervision of an appropriately trained physician or qualified physician extender [9].

26.10.1 Dosing schedules

SCIT is customarily initiated at a 1000- or 10,000-fold dilution of the maintenance concentration [9]. Conventionally, doses are increased with weekly (occasionally more often) injections over a period of months to a maintenance dose that is administered at 2- to 4-week (usually 4-week) intervals for 3–5 years. The buildup may be conservative [9] (30 injections, Table 26.14) in patients at increased risk, e.g., patients with multiple large skin test reactions, persistent asthma, or a history of SARs to previous immunotherapy, or it may be more rapid (18 injections, Table 26.15) in patients without these risk factors [34–36].

Table 26.14 Subcutaneous immunotherapy injection schedule for patients at increased risk of a systemic allergic reaction [9]

Concentration: 1:1000 dilution of maintenance vial
Dose
0.05 mL
0.10 mL
0.20 mL
0.40 mL

Concentration: 1:100 dilution of maintenance vial
Dose
0.05 mL
0.10 mL
0.20 mL
0.30 mL
0.40 mL
0.50 mL

Concentration 1:10 dilution of maintenance vial
Dose
0.05 mL
0.07 mL
0.10 mL
0.15 mL
0.25 mL
0.35 mL
0.40 mL
0.45 mL
0.50 mL

Maintenance concentration
Dose
0.05 mL
0.07 mL
0.10 mL
0.15 mL
0.20 mL
0.25 mL
0.3 mL
0.35 mL
0.40 mL
0.45 mL
0.50 mL

Note: A 30-injection subcutaneous immunotherapy (SCIT) schedule recommended for patients at increased risk for systemic allergic reaction (SAR), e.g., patients with multiple large skin test reactions, persistent asthma, or a history of SARs to previous immunotherapy.

Table 26.15 Subcutaneous immunotherapy injection buildup for patients not at increased risk for systemic allergic reaction and for cluster buildup [34–36]

Visit and dose	Concentration (dilution of maintenance)
Visit 1	
0.10 mL	1:1000 (Vial 4)
0.40 mL	1:1000 (Vial 4)
0.10 mL	1:100 (Vial 3)
Visit 2	
0.20 mL	1:100 (Vial 3)
0.40 mL	1:100 (Vial 3)
0.07 mL	1:10 (Vial 2)
Visit 3	
0.10 mL	1:10 (Vial 2)
0.15 mL	1:10 (Vial 2)
0.25 mL	1:10 (Vial 2)
Visit 4	
0.35 mL	1:10 (Vial 2)
0.50 mL	1:10 (Vial 2)
Visit 5	
0.07 mL	1:1 (Vial 1)
0.10 mL	1:1 (Vial 1)
Visit 6	
0.15 mL	1:1 (Vial 1)
0.20 mL	1:1 (Vial 1)
Visit 7	
0.30 mL	1:1 (Vial 1)
0.40 mL	1:1 (Vial 1)
Visit 8	
0.50 mL	1:1 (Vial 1)

Note: An 18-injection cluster subcutaneous immunotherapy schedule that allows achievement of maintenance dosing in 4 weeks if visits are twice-weekly. These same incremental doses may be given once-weekly in patients without increased risk for systemic allergic reaction.

Alternatives to conventional dosing are cluster and rush immunotherapy schedules. Cluster treatment involves two or more injections per visit, but visits less often than daily. Several studies suggest that SARs are not more frequent with cluster than with conventional dosing [86,87]. An example of a cluster schedule is in Table 26.15. Rush SCIT, which involves multiple injections per day on consecutive days, is regularly associated with an increased incidence of SARs, even with extensive premedication [88,89].

Table 26.16 Adjustments in subcutaneous immunotherapy dosing for gaps in treatment [9]

Buildup phase	
Up to 7 days late	Continue buildup as scheduled
8 to 13 days late	Repeat previous dose
14–21 days late	Reduce dose 25%
21 to 287 days late	Reduce dose 50%
Maintenance phase	
2 to 4 weeks late	Reduce dose 75%
>4 weeks late	Reduce by one or more dilutions depending on length of time and patient sensitivity

26.10.2 Dosing adjustments

It may be necessary to make adjustments in the dosing schedule because of missed doses, large local or SARs to an injection, or replacement with a new vial of vaccine. There are no studies to provide guidance for dose adjustments when patients have unscheduled gaps in immunotherapy. A suggested schedule of adjustments was provided in the Practice Parameters, third update (Table 26.16) [9]. In patients who had received 3–4 years of grass pollen SCIT with good response but subsequently relapsed, immunotherapy was safely reinstituted with a buildup of 11 weekly injections [17]. New vials of allergen vaccine will generally be more potent than the one being replaced due to gradual loss of potency that occurs in vaccines over time. With a new vial employing the same extracts from the same physician, it is customary to reduce the dose by one-third to one-half and build back up to maintenance. If it is necessary to change the supplier of the extracts, it is recommended that the dose of vaccines containing standardized extracts should be reduced to 1/5, those containing nonstandardized pollen to 1/10, and those containing cockroach or fungi to 1/100th of the previous dose.

26.11 DURATION OF SCIT

Several studies show persisting improvement of symptoms of rhinitis and asthma following 3 years of SCIT [15–17]. The response to 3 or 5 years of SCIT with house dust mite extract was compared [90]. After 3 years, rhinitis, asthma, and rhinitis and asthma quality of life scores were all significantly improved [90]. Two further years of SCIT produced a further reduction in rhinitis scores; however, the authors conclude that 3 years of treatment may be sufficient [90]. However, when a 2-year course of timothy SCIT was compared to placebo, there was significant improvement in symptoms on nasal challenge and during the grass pollen season, but there was no significant persistence of improvement 1 year after stopping SCIT [6]. These results support the general recommendation that SCIT be continued for a total of 3–5 years. During the period of treatment, it is recommended that the patients be seen every 6–12 months to review progress in buildup, adherence, clinical response, adjustments in dosing or allergen content, and safety measures [9].

SALIENT POINTS

1. AIT is an effective treatment for allergic rhinitis (AR) and allergic asthma and should be considered in patients with those conditions who are sensitized to and exposed to an aeroallergen whose pattern of occurrence corresponds to that of the patient's symptoms.

2. Although sublingual immunotherapy (SLIT) is safer than subcutaneous immunotherapy (SCIT), several other factors favor SCIT, such as lack of defined liquid SLIT doses, lack of studies supporting use of multiple allergen mixes by SLIT, and apparent greater efficacy, at least in the first year, with SCIT.

3. Practices diverge between U.S. and European allergists/immunologists in their approach to the polyallergic patient. U.S. allergists commonly treat with multiallergen SCIT vaccines, while European allergists/immunologists predominantly treat with one, or at the most two different allergen vaccines, each containing a single allergen extract.

4. An attractive feature of SCIT is modification of the underlying disease when adequate dosing and duration are applied. This reduces the risk of patients with AR developing asthma and provides persisting benefit after completion of treatment.

5. Standardized extracts of cat pelt and hair, house dust mites, short ragweed, eight grasses, and the venoms of four Hymenoptera are commercially available in the United States.

6. Neither of the two expressions for potency used for nonstandardized extracts, weight by volume (w/v) or protein nitrogen units (PNUs), adequately reflects allergenic potency of a vaccine.

7. Placebo-controlled studies that demonstrated clinical effectiveness have been performed for the allergens that are standardized in the United States (house dust mites, cat dander, grass, and ragweed) and for birch, *Parietaria*, dog dander, and *Alternaria*. In each instance, the effective dose of major allergen is in the range of 7–20 mcg (Table 26.1).

8. Examples of representative values for the major allergen content of U.S. standardized vaccines are listed in Table 26.4. However, the major allergen contents in Table 26.4 are only representative, and the values may vary significantly from lot to lot and from one manufacturer to another.

9. The information in Tables 26.1 and 26.2 allows formulation of an allergen vaccine mixture containing concentrations of the major allergens that approximate those proven to be clinically effective (Table 26.3).

10. Vaccines should contain effective quantities of each aeroallergen. If two or more components of the allergen mixture cross-react, the amount of each should be decreased so that the sum of the cross-reacting aeroallergens is equal to the optimal effective dose for a single allergen of the mixture.

11. Most fungal and cockroach extracts contain proteases capable of degrading allergenic proteins contained in other extracts when combined in a vaccine. Therefore, mixing fungal and cockroach extracts with pollen or dander extracts or mixing fungal with cockroach or fire ant extracts in a vaccine is to be avoided.

12. Vaccines containing multiple component extracts are the rule in the United States. Their use is supported by four randomized controlled studies demonstrating efficacy in both AR and allergic asthma.

13. It is the physician's responsibility to ensure that personnel preparing vaccines are adequately trained. Qualifications for vaccine preparation personnel include a written test on aseptic technique and vaccine preparation and an annual test of their ability to make sterile dilutions, the media-fill test.

14. Degradation of allergen extracts and vaccines is increased by dilution and by the time they are maintained at room temperature.

15. Glycerin is the most effective preservative but is poorly tolerated by injection at 50% solution. Ten percent and 20% glycerin solutions cause some brief discomfort but are usually tolerated. Human serum albumin is less effective than 50% glycerin but is well tolerated. Glycerin or human serum albumin should be included in all dilute vaccines.

16. SCIT should be administered only in a medical facility where prompt recognition and treatment of anaphylaxis are assured, and the patient should remain under observation for 30 minutes following the injection.

17. For patients at increased risk of a SAR, a 30-incrementally increasing dosing schedule may be used to reach the maintenance dose. In other patients, an 18-incrementally increasing schedule may be safe and provides more rapid attainment of maintenance dosing. The same 18-injection schedule can be given twice weekly in a cluster regimen and maintenance reached in 4 weeks.

18. Rush SCIT can achieve maintenance dosing within a few days but is associated with an increased incidence of SARs even with premedication.

19. SCIT at adequate doses for 3 years produces persisting benefit. There is some further improvement if treatment is continued for 5 years. However, 2 years of SCIT proved inadequate for even 1 year of persisting benefit.

REFERENCES

1. Bae JM, Choi YY, Park CO, Chung KY, Lee KH. Efficacy of allergen-specific immunotherapy for atopic dermatitis: A systematic review and meta-analysis of randomized controlled trials. *J Allergy Clin Immunol* 2013; 132: 110–117.

2. Tam HH, Calderon MA, Manikam L et al. Specific allergen immunotherapy for the treatment of atopic eczema: A Cochrane systematic review. *Allergy* 2016; 71: 1345–1356.

3. Matsui EC, Abramson SL, Sandel MT. Indoor environmental control practices and asthma management. *Pediatrics* 2016; 138: e20162589.

4. Larenas-Linnemann D, Mösges R. Dosing of European sublingual immunotherapy maintenance solutions relative to monthly recommended dosing of subcutaneous immunotherapy. *Allergy Asthma Proc* 2016; 37: 50–56.

5. Amar SM, Harbeck RJ, Sills M, Silveira LJ, O'Brien H, Nelson HS. Response to sublingual immunotherapy with grass pollen extract monotherapy versus combination in a multiallergen extract. *J Allergy Clin Immunol* 2009; 124: 150–156.

6. Scadding GW, Calderon MA, Shamji MH et al. Effect of 2 years of treatment with sublingual grass pollen immunotherapy on nasal response to allergen challenge at 3 years among patients with moderate to severe seasonal allergic rhinitis: The GRASS randomized clinical trial. *JAMA* 2017; 317: 615–625.

7. Aasbjerg K, Backer V, Lund G et al. Immunological comparison of allergen immunotherapy tablet treatment and subcutaneous immunotherapy against grass allergy. *Clin Exp Allergy* 2014; 44: 417–428.

8. Roberts G, Pfaar O, Akdis CA et al. EAACI guideline on allergen immunotherapy: Allergic rhinoconjunctivitis. *Allergy* 2018; 73(4): 765–798.

9. Cox L, Nelson H, Lockey R. Allergen immunotherapy: A practice parameter third update. *J Allergy Clin Immunol* 2011; 127(1, Suppl): S1–S55.

10. Meadows A, Kaambwa B, Novielli N et al. A systematic review and economic evaluation of subcutaneous and sublingual allergen immunotherapy in adults and children with seasonal allergic rhinitis. *Health Technol Assess* 2013; 17: 1–322.

11. Lin SY, Erekosima N, Sarez-Cuervo C et al. *Allergen-Specific Immunotherapy for the Treatment of Allergic Rhinoconjunctivitis and/or Asthma: Comparative Effectiveness Review [Internet].* Rockville, MD: Agency for Healthcare Research and Quality, March 2013.

12. Abramson MJ, Puy RM, Winer JM. Injection allergen immunotherapy for asthma. *Cochrane Database Syst. Rev.* 2010; (8): CD001186.

13. Esch RE. Specific immunotherapy in the U.S.A.: General concept and recent initiatives. *Arb Paul Ehrlich Inst Bundesamt Sera Impfstoffe Frankf AM.* 2003; 94: 17–22.

14. Zuberbier T, Bachert C, Bousquet PJ et al. GA²LEN/EAACI pocket guide for allergen-specific immunotherapy for allergic rhinitis and asthma. *Allergy* 2010; 65: 1525–1530.

15. Demoly P, Passalacqua G, Pfaar O, Sastre J, Wahn U. Management of the polyallergic patients with allergy immunotherapy: A practice-based approach. *Allergy Asthma Clin Immunol* 2016; 12(2). doi: 10.1186/s13223-015-0109-6.

16. Des Roches A, Paradis L, Knani J et al. Immunotherapy with a standardized *Dermatophagoides pteronyssinus* extract: V. Duration of the efficacy of immunotherapy after its cessation. *Allergy* 1996; 51: 430–433.

17. Durham S, Walker SM, Varga EM et al. Long-term clinical efficacy of grass-pollen immunotherapy. *N Engl J Med* 1999; 3341: 468–475.

18. Ebner C, Kraft D, Ebner H. Booster immunotherapy (BIT). *Allergy* 1994; 49: 38–42.

19. Jacobsen L, Niggemann B, Dreborg S et al. Specific immunotherapy has long-term preventive effect on seasonal and perennial asthma: 10-years follow-up on the PAT study. *Allergy* 2007; 62: 943–948.

20. Schmitt J, Schwarz K, Stadler E, Wüstenberg EG. Allergy immunotherapy for allergic rhinitis effectively prevents asthma: Results from a large retrospective cohort study. *J Allergy Clin Immunol* 2015; 136: 1511–1516.

21. Cox L, Jacobsen L. Comparison of allergy immunotherapy practice patterns in the United States and Europe. *Ann Allergy Asthma Immunol* 2009; 103: 451–460.

22. Van Metre TE JR, Rosenberg GL, Vaswani SK, Ziegler SR, Adkinson NF Jr. Pain and dermal reaction caused by injected glycerin in immunotherapy solutions. *J Allergy Clin Immunol* 1996; 97: 1033–1039.

23. Norman PS, Winkenwerder WL, Lichtenstein LM. Trials of alum-precipitated pollen extracts in the treatment of hay fever. *J Allergy Clin Immunol* 1972; 50: 31–44.

24. Nelson HS. Long-term immunotherapy with aqueous and aluminum-precipitated grass extracts. *Ann Allergy* 1980; 45: 333–337.

25. Sherman WB. *Hypersensitivity: Mechanisms and Management.* Philadelphia, PA: WB Saunders, 1968. Table 38-1 page 422.

26. Stull A, Cooke RA, Tennant J. The allergic content of pollen extracts: Its determination and its deterioration. *J Allergy* 1933; 4: 455–467.

27. Ewan, PW, Alexander MM, Snape C, Ind PW, Agrell B, Dreborg S. Effective hyposensitization in allergic rhinitis using a potent partially purified extract of house dust mite. *Clin Allergy* 1988; 18: 501–508.

28. Haugaard L, Dahl R, Jacobsen L. A controlled dose-response study of immunotherapy with standardized, partially purified extract of house dust mite: Clinical efficacy and side effects. *J Allergy Clin Immunol* 1993; 91: 709–722.

29. Olsen OT, Larsen KR, Jacobsen L, Svendsen UG. A 1-year, placebo-controlled double-blind house dust mite immunotherapy study in asthmatic adults. *Allergy* 1997; 52: 853–859.

30. Van Metre TE Jr, Marsh DG, Adkinson NF Jr et al. Immunotherapy for cat asthma. *J Allergy Clin Immunol* 1988; 82: 1055–1068.

31. Alvarez-Cuesta E, Cuesta-Herranz J, Puyana-Ruiz J, Cuesta-Herranz C, Blanco-Quiros A. Monoclonal antibody-standardized cat extract immunotherapy: Risk benefit effects from a double-blind placebo study. *J Allergy Clin Immunol.* 1994; 93: 556–566.

32. Hedlin G, Graff-Lonnevig V, Heilbron H et al. Immunotherapy with cat- and dog-dander extracts. V. Effects of 3 years of treatment. *J Allergy Clin Immunol* 1991; 87: 955–964.

33. Varney VA, Edward J, Tabbah K et al. Clinical efficacy of specific immunotherapy to cat dander, a double-blind, placebo-controlled trial. *Clin Exp Allergy* 1997; 27: 860–867.

34. Ewbank PA, Murray J, Sanders K, Curran-Everett D, Dreskin S, Nelson HS. A double-blind, placebo-controlled immunotherapy dose-response study with standardized cat extract. *J Allergy Clin Immunol* 2003; 111: 155–161.

35. Nanda A, O'Connor M, Anand M et al. Does dependence and time course of the immunologic response to administration of standardized cat allergen extract. *J Allergy Clin Immunol* 2004; 14: 1339–1344.

36. Lent AM, Harbeck R, Strand M et al. Immunologic response to administration of standardized dog allergen extract at differing doses. *J Allergy Clin Immunol* 2006; 118: 1249–1256.

37. Varney VA, Gaga M, Frew AJ, Aber VR, Kay AB, Durham SR. Usefulness of immunotherapy in patients with severe summer hay fever uncontrolled by antiallergic drugs. *Br Med J* 1991; 302: 530–531.

38. Dolz I, Martinez-Cocera C, Barlolome JM, Cimarra M. A double-blind, placebo-controlled study of immunotherapy with grass pollen extract Alutard SQ during a three-year period with initial rush immunotherapy. *Allergy* 1996; 51: 489–500.

39. Walker SM, Pajno GB, Torres Lima M, Wilson DR, Durham SR. Grass pollen immunotherapy for seasonal rhinitis and asthma: A randomized, controlled trial. *J Allergy Clin Immunol* 2001; 107: 87–93.

40. Frew AJ, Powell RJ, Corrigan CJ, Durham SR. Efficacy and safety of specific immunotherapy with SQ allergen extract in treatment-resistant seasonal allergic rhinoconjunctivitis. *J Allergy Clin Immunol* 2006; 117: 319–325.

41. Möller C, Dreborg S, Ferdousi HA et al. Pollen immunotherapy reduces the development of asthma in children with seasonal rhinoconjunctivitis (the PAT-study). *J Allergy Clin Immunol* 2002; 109: 251–256.

42. Van Metre TE Jr, Adkinson NF, Amodio FJ et al. A comparative study of the effectiveness of the Rinkel method and the current standard method of immunotherapy for ragweed pollen hay fever. *J Allergy Clin Immunol* 1979; 66: 500–513.

43. Creticos PS, Marsh DG, Proud D et al. Responses to ragweed-pollen nasal challenge before and after immunotherapy. *J Allergy Clin Immunol* 1989; 84: 197–205.

44. Creticos PS, Adkinson NF Jr, Kagey-Sobotka A et al. Nasal challenge with ragweed pollen in hay fever patients: Effect of immunotherapy. *J Clin Invest* 1985; 76: 2247–2253.

45. Furin MJ, Norman PS, Creticos PS et al. Immunotherapy decreases antigen-induced eosinophil cell migration into the nasal cavity. *J Allergy Clin Immunol* 1991; 88: 27–32.

46. Polosa R, Li Gotti F, Mangano G et al. Effect of immunotherapy on asthma progression, BHR and sputum eosinophils in allergic rhinitis. *Allergy* 2004; 59: 1224–1228.

47. Khinchi MS, Poulsen LK, Carat F, André, Hansen AB, Malling HJ. Clinical efficacy of sublingual and subcutaneous birch pollen allergen-specific immunotherapy: A randomized, placebo-controlled, double-blind, double-dummy study. *Allergy* 2004; 59: 45–53.

48. Bodtger U, Poulsen LK, Jacobi HH, Malling HJ. The safety and efficacy of subcutaneous birch pollen immunotherapy—A one-year, randomized, double-blind, placebo-controlled study. *Allergy* 2002; 57: 297–303.

49. Horst M, Hejjaoui A, Horst V, Michel FB, Bousquet J. Double-blind, placebo-controlled rush immunotherapy with a standardized *Alternaria* extract. *J Allergy Clin Immunol* 1990; 85: 460–472.

50. Kuna P, Kaczmarek J, Kupczyk M. Efficacy and safety of immunotherapy for allergies to *Alternaria alternata* in children. *J Allergy Clin Immunol* 2011; 127: 502–508.

51. Hunt KJ, Valentine MD, Sobotka AK, Benton AW, Amodio FJ, Lichtenstein LM. A controlled trial of immunotherapy in insect hypersensitivity. *N Engl J Med* 1978; 299: 157–161.

52. Vailes L, Sridhara S, Cromwell O, Weber B, Breitenbach M, Chapman M. Quantitation of the major fungal allergens, Alt a 1 and Asp f1, in commercial allergenic products. *J Allergy Clin Immunol* 2001; 107: 641–646.

53. Esch RE. Manufacturing and standardizing fungal allergen products. *J Allergy Clin Immunol* 2004; 113: 210–215.

54. Patterson ML, Slater JE. Characterization and comparison of commercially available German and American cockroach allergen extracts. *Clin Exp Allergy* 2002; 32: 721–738.

55. Weber RW. Patterns of pollen cross-allergenicity. *J Allergy Clin Immunol* 2003; 112: 229–239.

56. Valenta R, Breiteneder H, Pettenburger K et al. Homology of the major birch-pollen allergen, Bet v I with the major pollen allergens of alder, hazel, and hornbeam at the nucleic acid level as determined by cross-hybridization. *J Allergy Clin Immonol* 1991; 87: 677–682.

57. Kernerman SM, McCullough J, Green J, Ownby DR. Evidence of cross-reactivity between olive, ash, privet and Russian olive tree pollen allergens. *Ann Allergy* 1992; 69: 493–496.

58. Christensen LH, Ipsen H, Nolte H et al. Short ragweeds is highly cross-reactive with other ragweeds. *Ann Allergy Asthma Immunol* 2015; 115: 490–495.

59. Weber R. Cross-reactivity of pollen allergens: Recommendations for immunotherapy vaccines. *Cur Opin Allergy Clin Immunol* 2005; 5: 563–569.

60. Heymann PW, Chapman MD, Aalberse RC, Fox JW, Platts-Mills TAE. Antigenic and structural analysis of group II allergens (Der f II and Der p II) from house dust mites (*Dermatophagoides* spp). *J Allergy Clin Immunol* 1989; 83: 1055–1067.

61. Center JG, Shuller N, Zeleznick LD. Stability of antigen E in commercially prepared ragweed pollen extracts. *J Allergy Clin Immunol* 1974; 54: 305–310.

62. Bousquet J, Marty JP, Coulomb Y, Robinet-Levy M, Cour P, Michael FB. Enzyme determination and RAST inhibition assays for orchard grass (*Dactylis glomerata*): A comparison of commercial pollen extracts. *Ann Allergy* 1978; 41: 164–169.

63. Esch RE. *Role of Proteases on the Stability of Allergenic Extracts.* Arbeiten aus dem Paul-Ehrlich-Institut. Stuttgart: Gustav Fischer Verlag, 1991: 171–179.

64. Wongtim S, Lehrer SB, Salvaggio JE, Horner WE. Protease activity in cockroach and basidiomycete allergen extracts. *Allergy Proc* 1993; 14: 263–268.

65. Kordash TR, Amend MJ, Williamson SL, Jones JK, Plunkett GA. Effect of mixing allergenic extracts containing *Helminthosporium*, *D. farinae*, and cockroach with perennial ryegrass. *Ann Allergy* 1993; 71: 240–246.

66. Haff M, Krail M, Kastner M, Haustein D, Vieths S. *Fusarium culmorum* causes strong degradation of pollen allergens in extract mixtures. *J Allergy Clin Immunol* 2002; 109: 96–101.

67. Stewart GA, Ward LD, Simpson RJ, Thompson PJ. The group III allergen from the house dust mite *Dermatophagoides pteronyssinus* is a trypsin-like enzyme. *Immunol* 1992; 75: 29–35.

68. Nelson HS, Ikle D, Buchmeier A. Studies of allergen extract stability: The effects of dilution and mixing. *J Allergy Clin Immunol* 1996; 98: 382–388.

69. Grier TJ, LeFevre DM, Duncan EA, Esch RE. Stability of standardized grass, dust mite, cat and short ragweed allergens after mixing with mold or cockroach extracts. *Ann Allergy Asthma Immunol* 2007; 99: 151–160.

70. Grier TJ, LeFevre DM, Duncan EA, Esch RE, Coyne TC. Allergen stabilities and compatibilities in mixtures of high-protease fungal and insect extracts. *Ann Allergy Asthma Immunol* 2012; 108: 439–447.

71. Grier TJ, Hal DM, Duncan EA, Coyne TC. Mixing compatibilities of Aspergillus and American cockroach allergens with other high-protease fungal and insect extracts. *Ann Allergy Asthma Immunol* 2015; 114: 233–239.

72. Ayuso R, Rubio M, Herrera T, Gurbindo C, Carreira J. Stability of *Lolium perenne* extract. *Ann Allergy* 1984; 53: 426–431.

73. Anderson MC, Baer H. Antigenic and allergenic changes during storage of a pollen extract. *J Allergy Clin Immunol* 1982; 69: 3–10.

74. Nelson HS. The effect of preservatives and dilution on the deterioration of Russian thistle (*Salsola pestifer*), a pollen extract. *J Allergy Clin Immunol* 1979; 63: 417–425.

75. Nelson HS. Effect of preservatives and conditions of storage on the potency of allergy extracts. *J Allergy Clin Immunol* 1981; 67: 64–69.

76. Norman PS, Marsh DG. Human serum albumin and Tween 80 as stabilizers of allergen solutions. *J Allergy Clin Immunol* 1978; 62: 314–319.

77. Naerdal A, Vilsvik JS. Stabilization of a diluted aqueous mite allergen preparation by addition of human serum albumin. An intracutaneous test study. *Clin Allergy* 1983; 13: 149–153.

78. Brown JS, Ledoux R, Nelson HS. An investigation of possible immunologic reactions to human serum albumin used as a stabilizer in allergy extracts. *J Allergy Clin Immunol* 1985; 76: 808–812.

79. Niemeijer NR, Kauffman HF, van Hove W, Dubois AEJ, de Moncy GR. Effect of dilution, temperature, and preservatives on the long-term stability of standardized inhalant allergen extracts. *Ann Allergy, Asthma, Immunol* 1996; 76: 535–540.

80. Van Hoeyveld EM, Stevens EAM. Stabilizing effect of ε-aminocaproic acid on allergenic extracts. *J Allergy Clin Immunol* 1985; 76: 543–550.

81. Baer H, Anderson MC, Hale R, Gleich GJ. The heat stability of short ragweed pollen extract and the importance of individual allergens in skin reactivity. *J Allergy Clin Immunol* 1980; 66: 281–285.

82. Hale R, Grater WC, Haykik IB, McConnell LH, Santilli J Jr, Scherr MS, Zitt MJ. Report of the Committee on Standardization of Allergenic Extracts: A study of the heat stability of white oak, elm, orchard grass, and Bermuda grass. *Ann Allergy* 1985; 55: 86–87.

83. Moore M, Tucker M, Grier T, Quinn J. Effects of summer mailing on *in vivo* and *in vitro* relative potencies of standardized timothy grass extract. *Ann Allergy Asthma Immunol* 2010; 104: 147–151.

84. Plunkett G. Stability of allergen extracts used in skin testing and immunotherapy. *Curr Opin Otolaryngol Head Neck Surg* 2008; 16: 285–291.

85. Bousquet J, Djoukadar F, Hewitt B, Guerin B, Michel F-B. Comparison of the stability of a mite and a pollen extract stored in normal conditions of use. *Clin Allergy* 1985; 15: 29–35.

86. Tabar A, Echechipía S, García, Olaguibel JM et al. Double-blind comparative study of cluster and conventional immunotherapy schedules with *Dermatophagoides pteronyssinus*. *J Allergy Clin Immunol* 2005; 116: 109–118.

87. Winslow AW, Turbyville JC, Sublett JW, Sublett JL, Pollard SJ. Comparison of systemic reactions in rush, cluster, and standard-build aeroallergen immunotherapy. *Ann Allergy Asthma Immunol* 2016; 117: 542–545.

88. Hejjaoui A, Dhivert H, Michel FB, Bousquet J. Immunotherapy with a standardized *Dermatophagoides pteronyssinus* extract. IV. Systemic reactions according to the immunotherapy schedule. *J Allergy Clin Immunol* 1990; 85: 473–479.

89. Portnoy J, Bagstad K, Kanarek H, Pacheco F, Hall B, Barnes C. Premedication reduces the incidence of systemic reactions during inhalant rush immunotherapy with mixtures of allergenic extracts. *Ann Allergy*. 1994; 73(5): 409–418.

90. Tabar A, Arroabarren E, Echechipía S, Garcia BE, Martin S, Alvarez-Puebla MJ. Three years of specific immunotherapy may be sufficient in house dust mite respiratory allergy. *J Allergy Clin Immunol* 2011; 127: 57–63.

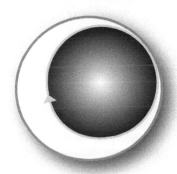

27 Preparing and administering sublingual allergen vaccines

Miguel Casanovas and *Jonathan Kilimajer*
Inmunotek S.L.

Enrique Fernández-Caldas
University of South Florida, Morsani College of Medicine

CONTENTS

27.1 INTRODUCTION

The oral route for allergen immunotherapy (AIT) was suggested in 1900 [1]. Clinical attempts to determine the best dose and route for AIT increased dramatically in the 1920s and 1930s [2]. Clinical use of sublingual immunotherapy (SLIT), as currently practiced, was published for food in 1969 by David Morris [3] and for inhalant allergens in 1970 [4]. In the 1980s, SLIT was proposed as an alternative to the traditional subcutaneous route of administration to provide a more convenient (suitable for home treatment) and safer therapeutic intervention [5]. In 1998 and 2009, the World Health Organization (WHO) recognized the efficacy and safety of SLIT, concluding that SLIT was an acceptable method of AIT administration. In addition, in 2018, the European Academy of Allergy and Clinical Immunology (EAACI) published guidelines on

AIT (SCIT and SLIT) in order to inform and facilitate high-quality clinical practice for both types of treatment [6]. Furthermore, in recent years, several studies have been conducted showing more information on mechanisms of action and short- and long-term effects. The results of preventive intervention studies provide evidence on the effective role of AIT in changing the natural history of allergic respiratory diseases, although it is not clear how long this benefit is maintained. Evidence is also available in favor of a reduced risk for developing new sensitizations in patients who are already sensitized to one allergen [7].

Mucosal immunization, especially through the oral/sublingual mucosa, has attracted much interest for the following reasons: as a means for eliciting protective immunity for infection and as a possible approach for immunologic treatment of various diseases caused by an aberrant immune response associated with tissue-damaging inflammation (e.g., allergy, rheumatoid arthritis, inflammatory bowel diseases, Bechet's disease, and systemic lupus erythematosus) [8].

Most exogenous agents that contact and/or enter into the body, including particulate and soluble antigens and microbes, interact with mucosal membranes rather than just the skin. The epithelial lining of mucous membranes covers an area of several hundred square meters in an adult and is approximately 200 times larger than the skin [9]. These mucosal membranes are endowed with effective mechanical and chemical cleansing mechanisms. In addition, a large and highly specialized innate and adaptive mucosal immune system protects these surfaces. In a healthy human adult, this local immune system contributes almost 80% of all immunocytes [10]. These cells are in transit between, or accumulate in, various mucosa-associated lymphoid tissues (MALTs), which together form the largest mammalian lymphoid organ system [11].

The sublingual route has been used for many years to deliver low molecular weight drugs into the bloodstream [12,13]. Small immunogenic peptides administered through this route induce systemic immune responses [14]. Furthermore, the delivery of antigens using this route is thought to be effective for suppressing systemic antibody responses, including IgE responses, and is being exploited for the treatment of IgE-dependent allergy [15].

Immune tolerance predominates in the oral/sublingual mucosa, and the antigen-presenting cells, such as dendritic cells and various T-cell subtypes, serve as key players in oral mucosal tolerance induction [16]. In mice, immunohistologic analyses of the sublingual mucosa show that there is a dense network of dendritic-like (DC) cells, located both in lamina propria and in the epithelial compartment. These DCs share phenotypical characteristics with epidermal Langerhans cells and appear mainly composed of transitional DCs [17]. In humans, Allam et al. [18] showed that mucosal regions, such as the vestibule of the mouth, or cheek mucosa (vestibulum or bucca), have a high density of oral Langerhans cells and high FcεRI expression on these cells. These findings suggest these sites could be an appropriate application site, with potent allergen uptake, for SLIT.

27.2 REGULATORY REQUISITES FOR SUBLINGUAL IMMUNOTHERAPY

Mucosal vaccines have advantages from production and regulatory perspectives when compared with injected vaccines [19,20]. Preparations intended for oral/sublingual administration do not require extensive purification from bacterial by-products, as the oral mucosa is already populated by bacteria, whereas the same preparation intended for parenteral injection would be unacceptable. Preparations produced for SLIT only require the bioburden test. Bioburden is normally defined as the number of bacteria living on a surface that has not been sterilized. Bioburden testing, also known as microbial limit test, is performed on pharmaceutical and medical products for quality control. Bioburden of raw materials and finished pharmaceutical products helps to determine whether the product complies with the requirements of the European Union (EU) or the U.S. Pharmacopeia.

In terms of vaccination, mucosal vaccines are practical due to the ease of administration and the possibility that they can be delivered by personnel without medical training, or even by the patient. This is viewed as a benefit of mucosal vaccine strategies [21,22]. However, in accordance with the current regulations [23], the presence of certain microorganisms in nonsterile preparations may have the potential to reduce, or even inactivate, the therapeutic activity of the product and may have the potential to adversely affect the health of the patient. Manufacturers therefore must ensure a low bioburden of finished dosage forms by implementing current guidelines on Good Manufacturing Practice (GMP) during the manufacturing process, storage, and distribution of pharmaceutical preparations [24]. That means that these preparations must be handled by qualified personnel in adequate facilities.

27.3 SUBLINGUAL IMMUNOTHERAPY IN EUROPE AND THE UNITED STATES

SLIT was successfully introduced in Europe in the 1990s [25]. Its rapid success was mainly due to safety concerns associated with subcutaneous immunotherapy (SCIT).

SLIT use has attracted increasing interest in the United States. Physicians may use the allergen extract sublingually rather than subcutaneously, the formula of which is called off-label use. Off-label use means that the medication is being used in a manner not specified in the U.S. Food and Drug Administration's (FDA)-approved packaging label or insert [26,27]. Every prescription drug marketed in the United States carries an individual, FDA-approved label. This label is a written report that provides detailed instructions regarding the approved uses and doses, which are based on the results of clinical studies that the drug maker submitted to the FDA. However, most physicians are uncomfortable prescribing and compounding SLIT for their patients until the FDA approves the products. The main hurdles are related to the establishment of the optimal dose, the safety of a treatment administered at home, compliance issues, medical legal risk, and lack of billing codes. This subject has been recently reviewed [28].

SLIT constitutes the preferred route of administration of AIT for respiratory allergies in some European countries, including France and Italy, and SLIT is now approved for treatment in the United States [5], where there are two forms of SLIT utilized, i.e., tablets and use of "off-label" aqueous solution (which involves the use of allergens approved for SCIT in an off-label form of administration, as there are no aqueous products specifically approved by the FDA for sublingual use in the United States) [29]. Because of this lack of approval from the FDA, insurance plans often do not reimburse for SLIT in the United States. Important differences exist between the EU and the United States regarding SLIT. These differences include allergen extract regulation, standardization, formulation, types of allergen extracts, routes of administration, approval status, and reimbursement. Currently, most SLIT used in the United States is formulated in the offices of allergists. In April 2014, the FDA approved the first sublingual allergen tablet, GRASTEK (Merck Sharp & Dohme Corp), for the treatment of respiratory allergies. Subsequently, they approved ORALAIR (Stallergènes S.A.), ODACTRA (Merck Sharp & Dohme Corp.), and RAGWITEK (Merck Sharp & Dohme Corp.).

In Europe, SLIT is formulated by extract manufacturers, and some preparations were licensed as drugs in September 2009 [5]. SLIT represents a significant percentage of SIT treatment in Europe; however, a relatively small percentage of U.S. allergists prescribe it [30]. Nevertheless, the number of prescribers appears to have doubled in a 4-year period, from 5.9% in 2007 to 11.4% in 2011 [31]. In a survey published in 2014 among U.S. allergists, it was stated that, if approved, 80% would consider using it for allergic rhinitis, 56.3% for mild asthmatics, 37.1% for moderate to severe asthmatics, and 20.2% for food allergy [31].

In Europe, the product is prescribed by the physician, prepared in a GMP licensed pharmaceutical laboratory, and delivered to a pharmacy, to be acquired by the patient, as with other pharmaceuticals. These vaccines are supplied in one vial, containing a standard, single maintenance concentration, or several vials of increasing concentrations. The biological potency of these extracts is expressed in different units, and in some cases, major allergen content is also provided [32]. Other formulations of allergens, besides the conventional aqueous, glycerinated liquid extracts are produced as SLIT tablets (also approved in the United States) [7]. SLIT is administered by the patient at home, although the first dose can be given in a clinic under a physician's supervision. Due to the nature of this treatment, which requires daily or alternative day use, application is usually done at home.

A special consideration when prescribing SLIT is adherence, a common problem, in general, for prolonged medical treatment. Insufficient duration of AIT prevents the occurrence of the immunologic changes that produce clinical efficacy [33]. Analysis of the rate of spontaneous discontinuation in SLIT treatments of two large manufacturers in Italy, over a 3-year period, demonstrated a decrease from 100% to 43.7% in the first year, to 27.7% in the second year, and to 13.2% in the third year [34].

27.4 PREPARING, MIXING, AND LABELING SUBLINGUAL IMMUNOTHERAPY IN THE UNITED STATES

Allergen products are pharmaceutical preparations derived from extracts of naturally occurring source materials containing allergens, which are substances that cause or provoke allergic (hypersensitivity) disease. Allergen source materials are obtained from controlled, audited suppliers and are obtained with a certificate of analysis confirming collection methods and source. Pollens from trees, weeds, and grasses are collected under controlled conditions by certified suppliers; quality and purity must be documented. Source materials should be assigned an expiration date based on stability studies and receive a code to enable testing and tracking according to GMP requirements. Pollen source materials are collected by specialized companies and are subjected to strong quality regulations and processes, and include purity, foreign contaminations, and stability data [35]. Raw materials from mites and molds are grown in specialized facilities and also are subject to regulatory controls [36–38]. Animal dander is collected from housed animals and is accompanied with a certificate from a veterinary doctor stating that the animals are healthy and free of infectious and contagious agents [39]. In most European countries, national regulations allow marketing of allergen products as "Named Patient Preparations" (NPPs), although in the last few years, registration procedures have begun. NPPs are industrially prepared allergen vaccines following the prescription issued by an allergy specialist. They are regulated mainly by the Guideline on Allergen Products: Production and Quality Issues [40] and the Monograph on Allergen Extracts of the European Pharmacopoeia [41]. European

manufacturers of allergen extracts develop their own methods and in-house reference preparations for standardization. In the United States, the FDA Center for Biologics Evaluation and Research (CBER) reference preparations, standardized by approved methods, are used. Consistent SLIT preparations rely on the availability of standardized products formulated at an optimum concentration and manufactured following validated processes.

If physicians in the United States do not use the currently approved SLIT tablets, they may prepare the vaccines for the patients and adjust the doses as needed [42]. In this case, the main requisites for the preparation of allergen vaccines in clinical practice are the qualifications, knowledge, and experience of the clinician; the quality of the allergen extracts; the compatibility of allergen extracts in a mixture; an allergen immunotherapy prescription containing the percentages of each allergen extract; and efficient labeling.

When SLIT vaccines are utilized, the allergist is responsible for establishing the optimal dose, based on the medical literature and clinical experience. The personnel involved in these preparations should pass a written test on aseptic techniques and extract preparation and be trained in the preparation of allergenic products. Furthermore, they must annually pass a media-fill test for subcutaneous vaccine preparation (may be necessary for sublingual vaccines), demonstrate understanding of antiseptic hand cleaning and disinfection of mixing surfaces, and be able to identify, measure, and mix allergenic extracts.

Ideally, a specific site should be chosen for mixing vaccines where personnel traffic is restricted. The preparation area must be sanitized with 70% isopropanol or equivalent. The personnel should thoroughly wash hands to wrists with detergent or soap. The necks of the ampules and stoppers of vials to be punctured must be sanitized before use, as is done for the subcutaneous preparations. The use of a laminar flow hood is not mandatory but is a consideration.

Allergen immunotherapy prescriptions must specify the precise content of an individual treatment set. Each prescription should contain two patient identifiers (e.g., name and date of birth), name of the preparer, date of preparation, concentration and volume of each allergen extract, type and volume of diluents, and expiration date. The source or manufacturer of the allergen extract should also be mentioned. A consistent uniform labeling system should be used for AIT treatment vials.

Allergenic extracts available for the preparation of sublingual vaccine administration may be aqueous, glycerinated, or lyophilized. Allergen extracts that have been used for SLIT include pollens, mites, epithelia, and molds. Allergen extract dilutions should be in a bacteriostatic solution. The choice of diluents is also important, since diluents are solutions used to keep the allergens stable and preserved. The diluents most commonly used are saline, human serum albumin, and/or glycerin with phosphate-buffered saline.

A sublingual mixing protocol should be established, and an allergen extract mixing location selected prior to formulating SLIT vaccines. A supervising physician ideally should be present in the same building or immediately accessible. An aseptic work environment must be maintained. Vial labels should be prepared in accordance with prescription and verified for accuracy. Treatment set vials should be labeled according to the previously mentioned protocols.

The preparation of new stock vials should be done as follows: Use new empty sterile vials and label according to the requisites;

use the stock extracts stored in the refrigerator, and note expiration dates of stock allergen extracts. Use a new syringe for each stock allergen extract to avoid cross-contamination and to maintain aseptic conditions. Afterward, aspirate the correct amount of each antigen and diluents according to the prescription and inject into the labeled treatment vial. Conduct a final quality assurance check after mixing is completed.

Several points are critical and should always be kept in mind. Contamination is prevented by use of aseptic techniques and adequate training. Accurate labels are critical to prevent errors. Quality assurance checks should be made throughout the mixing and dilution process. The expiration dates on all products should also be routinely checked.

If SLIT is prescribed off-label, patients should be specifically informed during the risk/benefit discussion. Informed consent is needed. Physicians who prescribe SLIT, regardless of whether it is FDA approved or off-label, also need to provide their patients with specific instructions regarding the management of adverse reactions, unplanned interruptions in treatment, and situations during which they should withhold SLIT [43].

27.5 PROTECTIVE AGENTS IN SUBLINGUAL VACCINES

Allergen extracts used for SLIT originate from different allergen sources. Besides microbial contamination and long-term stability, other issues such as degradation and loss of biological potency should be minimized.

27.5.1 Glycerol

Published reports describe the antimicrobial and antiviral effects of glycerol [44,45], which are dependent on concentration and temperature [46]. The capacity of glycerol, and other polyhydric alcohols, to confer stability on complex biological materials is recognized [47]. Glycerol is widely used as a preservative in allergen extracts due to proven inhibition of proteolytic activity [48] and of protein aggregation [49]. Glycerin is a neutral, sweet-tasting, colorless, thick liquid that freezes to a gummy paste and has a high boiling point (290°C or 554°F). Glycerin readily dissolves in water or alcohol. Other important properties of glycerin are its hygroscopicity (the power to absorb and retain moisture and act as a humectant) and its viscosity, which provide a means of prolonging the contact of antigens with surfaces [50]. Fifty percent glycerol in normal saline or phosphate-buffered saline is usually used as the diluent in the preparation of allergen vaccines.

27.5.2 Phenol

This compound is often used in allergenic preparations for preventing the growth of microorganisms in multidose vials, although it may have some deleterious effects on allergen extracts [27]. When used in preparations intended for sublingual administration, phenol has an unpleasant "metallic" taste. However, since glycerol has antimicrobial and antiviral effects [23–25], and the life cycle of a vial intended for sublingual administration is short (1–2 months), the use of phenol can be omitted.

Table 27.1 Different constituents of sublingual vaccines of various companies

Company	Diluent	Phenol	Flavoring agent	Buildup	Delivered as
A	PBS	No	No	Yes	Drops
B	PBS	No	Yes	Yes	Drops
C	Saline	Yes	No	No	Pump
D	Saline	Yes	No	Yes	Spray
E	PBS	No	Yes	No	Drops
F	Saline	No	Yes	No	Spray
G	PBS	Yes	No	No	Drops
H	Saline	No	No	Si	Drops

27.5.3 Flavors

Some companies provide SLIT with different flavors, including strawberry and pineapple (Table 27.1). These flavors are accepted by the pharmaceutical and food industries and do not interact with the active ingredients (allergens) in the extracts. A common source is International Flavors and Fragrances [51].

27.6 DEVICES

Several types of devices are used to deliver the allergen extract onto the mucosal surface of the sublingual region or to other oral mucosal regions that have a high density of antigen-presenting cells [10]. The most widely used devices administer drops of the allergen vaccines (see Figure 27.1). One of these is the vial and the drop dispenser used for skin-prick tests. Other devices are vials with a pump that dispense drops or a spray or disposable single-dose preparations. Usually the dose administered by a drop dispenser is approximately 40–50 μL/drop. The administration of drops allows deposition of the extract in a selected region (e.g., sublingual, vestibular). It requires the active cooperation of the patient to maintain the liquid for a period of time (1–2 minutes) and to dispense the correct number of drops in order to deliver an appropriate, consistent volume of vaccine.

Other devices are the "spray." Usually the volume administered per spray is approximately 100 μL. The advantage of these devices is that the extract may be applied to a large surface of the sublingual, vestibular, or buccal mucosa, allowing a greater surface area to contact between the vaccine and the mucosa.

27.7 DIFFERENT PRESENTATIONS OF SUBLINGUAL IMMUNOTHERAPY

Table 27.1 shows the main characteristics of the most commonly used sublingual preparations in Europe [52]. Preparations containing 50% glycerol are stable in cool conditions (41° ± 37.4°F, or 5° ± 3°C) for an extended time period. Furthermore, these preparations are also stable at 77°F or 25°C for 2–3 months.

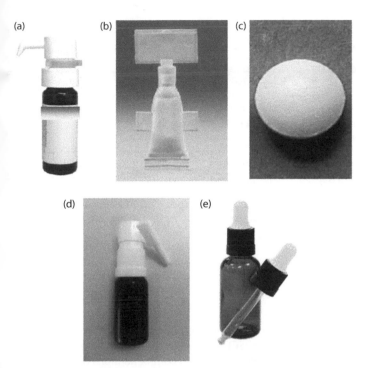

Figure 27.1 Several delivery systems commonly used for sublingual immunotherapy. (a) Automated dropper bottle. (b) Individual dose. (c) Allergen tablet. (d) Spray bottle. (e) Dropper bottle.

27.7.1 Tablets

Tablets are an alternative to sublingual sprays and drops. They are distributed and prescribed as a final registered product, approved in Europe and the United States. Two companies are manufacturing these tablets, i.e., ALK/Merck and Stallergènes. The main excipients in these preparations are mannitol, microcrystalline cellulose, croscarmellose sodium, silica colloidal anhydrous, magnesium stearate, and lactose monohydrate. Other tablets contain gelatin (fish source) and sodium hydroxide.

In the United States, four tablet formulations of SLIT are available for clinical use: dust mite, ragweed, timothy grass, and grass mix [29]. Birch and cedar SLIT tablets are in phase III studies. Due to the expense of developing and obtaining registration for these products, it will be difficult to produce SLIT tablets for most of the allergens treated with AIT in the United States [54]. In general, safety and efficacy results are similar to those obtained in multiple European studies with tablets [31].

27.8 DOSES AND SCHEMES

The maximum monthly dose and efficacy studies of maintenance SLIT vaccines range from 2 to 375 times the usual SCIT monthly dose [55–57]. This dose variability is one of the major questions not totally resolved about SLIT. One drop of SLIT contains approximately 50 microliters (μL) of the allergen vaccine, and since the treatment is usually administered daily, the usual SLIT dose is 1/10 to 10 times the monthly SCIT dose. SLIT buildup can be given in the clinical practice utilizing the 1:10 dilution of stock allergen extracts commonly used for SCIT. A 1:10 to a 1:100 dilution of the maintenance dose of SCIT may be used with the following dosing scheme: day 1: one drop;

day 2: two drops; day 3: three drops; day 4: four drops; and day 5: five drops. Once this maximum dose is achieved without adverse reactions, this can be maintained for a period (1–4 weeks) before switching to the next concentration or the maintenance vaccine. An example of a maintenance dust mite vaccine would be a 1:5 dilution of 10,000 AUs/mL to a final concentration of 2000 AUs/mL. The maintenance dosing would be given as one or two drops daily (50–100 AU) or at 2-day intervals. The duration of the treatment is for approximately 3–5 years or longer. An example of a dosing scheme is provided in Table 27.2 and is based on different commercial companies in Europe.

Another approach is to initiate treatment with a maintenance vial and accept that the local and gastrointestinal side effects will be greater. There is no consensus on the need of a buildup versus starting with maintenance. Thus, there is variability in the approach, with some clinicians starting at a dose that does not result in an intradermal or epicutaneous positive skin test response and increase to maintenance, whereas others start with a dilution of 1:5–1:100 of the intended maintenance concentration. There is no general recommendation to vary the dose based on the patient's weight.

The effective dose regimes for SLIT tablets, such as the five-grass product, is available in two strengths (100 and 300 IR). The dose is increased during the first 3 days ("updosing"); on day 1, a 100-IR tablet; on day 2, two 100-IR tablets; and on day 3 and after, the 300-IR tablet. For the ragweed and timothy grass products, a single-dose tablet is administered daily over the prescribed time period, without updosing. Treatment with the ragweed and timothy products is initiated at least 12 weeks before the expected onset of the season and continued throughout the season. The treatment with the five-grass product is initiated 16 weeks before the expected onset of the season and continued throughout the season, i.e., a "pre-coseasonal" regimen. The time suggested for this treatment is for 3 consecutive years. The published optimal maintenance doses of major allergens based on dose-ranging studies vary from 15 μg of Phl 5/day (timothy grass tablet) to 25 μg/mL group 5/day for the five-grass mix tablets. The ragweed tablet contains 12 μg of Amb a 1/day, and the major mite allergen content for one of the tablets is 28 μg of Der p 1 and 120 μg of Der f 1 (500 IR). Other doses are expressed in arbitrary units (6 SQ-HDM) [58].

27.9 STORAGE

SLIT vials should be stored in a refrigerator at 5°C–6°C. and kept safe from access by children. Sublingual preparations containing glycerol may be stable for several months at room temperature; nevertheless, refrigeration is recommended. For SLIT tablets, no refrigeration is needed.

27.10 SAFETY

One of the advantages of SLIT over SCIT is greater safety [59]. Fatal reactions to SLIT have not been reported to date, although cases of anaphylaxis have occurred. Mild side effects, such as an itchy mouth, occur in the majority of treated people, and moderate side effects occur once in approximately every 12,000 doses. These moderate side effects include lip, mouth, and tongue irritation; eye itching, redness, and swelling; nausea, vomiting, abdominal cramping, and diarrhea; sneezing, nasal itching, and congestion;

Table 27.2 Possible administration schemes of sublingual immunotherapy

Vial number (letter)	Dilution	Number of drops	Dose per drop	Total dose per day
A (1) Maintenance	1:5 of 10,000 AU (2 000 AU/mL)	Maintenance: 1, or 2 drops daily	100 AU per drop (50 µL)	100–200 AU daily
B (2)	1:5 of 2000 (400 AU/mL)	1 drop the first day, increasing to up to 5 drops per day in 5 days. Then switch to vial A (1)	20 AU per drop (50 µL)	20, 40, 60, 80, *100 AU (5th day)*
C (3)	1:5 of 400 AU/mL (80 AU/mL)	1 drop the first day, increasing to up to 5 drops per day in 5 days. Then switch to vial B (2)	4 AU per drop (50 µL)	4, 8, 12, 16, *20 AU (5th day)*
D (4) Initiation	1:5 of 80 AU/mL (16 AU/mL)	1 drop the first day, increasing to up to 5 drops per day in 5 days. Then switch to vial C (3)	0.8 AU per drop (50 µL)	0.8, 1.6, 3.2, *4 AU (5th day)*

Note: This scheme should be adapted for each patient and does not represent a universal dosing scheme. Discontinue treatment if severe local or generalized adverse reactions occur.

asthma symptoms; generalized urticaria; and angioedema. A review of adverse effects of SLIT revealed that in approximately 1,181,000 doses given to 4378 patients, there were no fatalities or events described as anaphylaxis, although there were 14 probable, serious adverse events (7 were asthma reactions) [46]. Oral-mucosal reactions, considered a SLIT local reaction, were relatively common, affecting up to 75% of patients and occurring most frequently in the buildup phase. The severity of these tends to be mild. In the studies that specified the type of reaction, 169 of 314,959 (0.056% of doses administered) were classified as serious reactions. There were 244 moderately severe adverse events requiring dose adjustment or causing withdrawal from the study in 2939 patients treated for 4586 treatment years with 810,693 doses of SLIT (50 studies) [46]. Most of these reactions were gastrointestinal symptoms, rhinoconjunctivitis, urticaria, or some combination of these. Subsequently, there have been several reports of SLIT-associated anaphylaxis using different allergen extracts with different indications [59–62]. Likewise, SLIT tablets administered with the appropriate scheme and formulation have been shown to be safe in adult and pediatrics populations in a large number of randomized, double-blind, placebo-controlled trials [53].

27.11 CONCLUSION

Sublingual immunotherapy has been used for more than 100 years. There is increased interest in SLIT due to its growing use in Europe and other parts of the world, including the United States. The main constraints for its widespread use remain dose adjustments, safety issues and definition of the optimal dose, and treating multisensitized subjects with SLIT versus SCIT. Important differences exist between Europe and the United States. These include allergen extract regulation, standardization, formulation, types of allergen extracts, routes of administration, and reimbursement.

Physicians preparing SLIT are responsible for establishing the optimal dose for standardized and nonstandardized allergen extracts, based on the medical literature and clinical experience. The personnel involved in these preparations should pass a written test on aseptic techniques and extract preparation and be trained

in the preparation of allergenic products. Overall, the safety record of SLIT is better than SCIT. However, SLIT is not free of risk, and patients should closely follow the recommendations of the allergist when using this treatment at home.

SALIENT POINTS

1. Studies demonstrate the efficacy of sublingual immunotherapy (SLIT) in the treatment of allergic rhinitis and asthma.
2. Mucosal allergic vaccines have advantages from production and regulatory perspectives when compared with injected vaccines.
3. Allergenic extracts available for the preparation of sublingual vaccine administration may be aqueous, glycerinated, or lyophilized. Allergen extracts that have been used for SLIT include pollens, mites, epithelia, and molds. Allergen extract dilutions should be in a bacteriostatic solution. The choice of diluents is also important, since diluents are solutions used to keep the allergens stable and preserved. The diluents most commonly used are saline, human serum albumin, and/or glycerin with phosphate-buffered saline.
4. Several types of devices are used to deliver the allergenic extract sublingually.
5. Several allergen tablets are now available in the U.S. and European markets. They offer advantages of simplicity, consistent dose delivery, and possibly enhanced efficacy.
6. Physicians who prescribe SLIT, regardless of whether it is FDA approved or off-label, need to provide their patients with specific instructions regarding the management of adverse reactions, unplanned interruptions in treatment, and situations during which they should withhold SLIT.
7. Adherence to the SLIT treatment is poor.

This sublingual immunotherapy scheme is based on a compilation from different companies. Treatment is started with vial D (4) (0.8 AU/drop). Dose should be adjusted individually. The table only provides a general dilution scheme. Stop if local or generalized adverse reactions occur. The authors are not responsible for any adverse reaction.

REFERENCES

1. Curtis HH. The immunizing cure of hayfever. *Med News (NY)* 1900; 77: 16–18.

2. Black JH. The oral administration of pollen. *J Lab Clin Med* 1927; 12: 1156.

3. Morris D. Use of sublingual antigen in diagnosis and treatment of food allergy. *Ann Allergy* 1969; 27(6): 289–294.

4. Morris D. Treatment of respiratory disease with ultra-small doses of antigens. *Ann Allergy* 1970; 28(10): 494–500.

5. Arasi S, Passalacqua G , Caminiti L, Crisafulli G, Fiamingo C, Battista Pajno G. Efficacy and safety of sublingual immunotherapy in children. *Exp Rev Clin Immunol* 2015; 12(1): 49–56.

6. Muraro A, Roberts G, Halken S et al. EAACI Guidelines on allergen immunotherapy: Executive statement. *Allergy*. Recent guidelines informing and facilitating high quality clinical practice for AIT. 2018; 73(4). https://doi.org/10.1111/all.13420

7. Porcaro F, Corsello G, Battista Pajno G. SLIT's prevention of the allergic march. *Curr Allergy Asthma Rep* 2018; 18(5): 31.

8. Holmgren J, Czerkinsky C, Eriksson K, Mharandi A. Mucosal immunisation and adjuvants: A brief overview of recent advances and challenges. *Vaccine* 2003; 21: S89–S95.

9. Brandtzaeg P. Mucosal immunity: Induction, dissemination, and effector functions. *Scand J Immunol* 2009; 70(6): 505–515.

10. McKenzie BS, Brady JL, Lew AM. Mucosal immunity: Overcoming the barrier for induction of proximal responses. *Immunol Res* 2004; 30(1): 35–71.

11. Holmgren J, Czerkinsky C. Mucosal immunity and vaccines. *Nature Med* 2005; 11(Suppl 4): S45–S53.

12. American Academy of Pediatrics. Committee on Drugs. Alternative routes of drug administration—Advantages and disadvantages (subject review). *Pediatrics* 1997; 100(1): 143–152.

13. Zhang H, Zhang J, Streisand JB. Oral mucosal drug delivery: Clinical pharmacokinetics and therapeutic applications. *Clin Pharmacokinet* 2002; 41(9): 661–680.

14. BenMohamed L, Belkaid Y, Loing E, Brahimi K, Gras-Masse H, Druilhe P. Systemic immune responses induced by mucosal administration of lipopeptides without adjuvant. *Euro J Immunol* 2002; 32(8): 2274–2281.

15. Passalacqua G, Canonica GW. Sublingual immunotherapy: Update 2006. *Curr Opin Allergy Clin Immunol* 2006; 6(6): 449–454.

16. Novak N, Haberstok J, Bieber T, Allam JP. The immune privilege of the oral mucosa. *Trends Mol Med* 2008; 14(5): 191–198.

17. Çuburu N, Kweon M-N, Song J-H et al. Sublingual immunization induces broad-based systemic and mucosal immune responses in mice. *Vaccine* 2007; 25(51): 8598–8610.

18. Allam JP, Stojanovski G, Friedrichs N et al. Distribution of Langerhans cells and mast cells within the human oral mucosa: New application sites of allergens in sublingual immunotherapy? *Allergy* 2008; 63(6): 720–727.

19. Levine MM. Immunogenicity and efficacy of oral vaccines in developing countries: Lessons from a live cholera vaccine. *BMC Biol* 2010; 8: 129.

20. Walker RI. Considerations for development of whole cell bacterial vaccines to prevent diarrheal diseases in children in developing countries. *Vaccine* 2005; 23(26): 3369–3385.

21. Levine MM, Dougan G. Optimism over vaccines administered via mucosal surfaces. *Lancet* 1998; 351(9113): 1375–1376.

22. Yuki Y, Kiyono H. Mucosal vaccines: Novel advances in technology and delivery. *Exp Rev Vaccin* 2009; 8(8): 1083–1097.

23. USP 30-NF25 (1111). Microbiological examination of nonsterile products: Acceptance criteria for pharmaceutical preparations and substances for pharmaceutical use.

24. ISPE. Good Manufacturing Practice (GMP) resources. https://ispe.org/initiatives/regulatory-resources/gmp

25. Incorvaia C, Di Rienzo A, Celani C, Makrì E, Frati F. Treating allergic rhinitis by sublingual immunotherapy: A review. *Ann Ist Super Sanita* 2012; 48(2): 172–176.

26. Stafford RS Regulating off-label drug use—Rethinking the role of the FDA. *N Engl J Med* 2008; 358(14): 1427–1429.

27. Stafford RS. Off-label use of drugs and medical devices: A review of policy implications. *Clin Pharmacol Ther* 2012; 91(5): 920–925.

28. Pitsios C, Dietis N. Ways to increase adherence to allergen immunotherapy. *Curr Med Res Opin* 2019; 35(6): 1027–1031.

29. Lin SY, Azar A, Suarez-Cuervo C et al. Role of sublingual immunotherapy in the treatment of asthma: An updated systematic review. *Int Forum Allergy Rhinol* 2018; 8; 982–992.

30. Cox L, Jacobsen L. Comparison of allergen immunotherapy practice patterns in the United States and Europe. *Ann Allergy Asthma Immunol* 2009; 103(6): 451–459; quiz 459-61.

31. Cox L. Sublingual immunotherapy for aeroallergens: Status in the United States. *Allergy Asthma Proc* 2014; 35(1): 34–42.

32. Larenas-Linnemann D, Esch R, Plunkett G et al. Maintenance dosing for sublingual immunotherapy by prominent European allergen manufacturers expressed in bioequivalent allergy units. *Ann Allergy Asthma Immunol* 2011; 107(5): 448–458.

33. Incorvaia C, Mauro M, Leo G, Ridolo E. Adherence to sublingual immunotherapy. *Curr Allergy Asthma Rep* 2016; 16: 12.

34. Manzotti G, Riario-Sforza GG, Dimatteo M et al. Comparing the compliance to a short schedule of subcutaneous immunotherapy and to sublingual immunotherapy during three years of treatment. *Eur Ann Allergy Clin Immunol* 2016; 48(6): 224–227.

35. Pollens for allergen products. European Pharmacopoeia 9.0; 01/2017; 2627: 3362–3363.

36. Mites for allergen products. Acari ad producta allergenica. European Pharmacopoeia 9.0; 01/2017; 2625: 3077–3078.

37. Fernández-Caldas E. Towards a more complete standardization of mite allergen extracts. *Int Arch Allergy Immunol* 2013; 160(1): 1–3.

38. Moulds for allergen products. European Pharmacopoeia 9.0; 01/2017: 2626; 3094–3095.

39. Animal epithelia and outgrowths for allergen products. European Pharmacopoeia 9.0; 01/2017: 2621; 1736–1737.

40. Guideline for Allergen Products: Production and Quality Issues (EMEA/CHMP/BWP/304831/2007).

41. European Directorate for the Quality of Medicines (EDQM). Monograph: Allergen products. In: Council of Europe editor. *Producta Allergenica 01/2010:1063*. 6th ed. Strasbourg: European Pharmacopoeia, 2010, supplement 6: pp. 679–680, as implemented of 01. 01. 2010.

42. Sanchez JG, Garcia Ibanez R. Efficacy of sublingual immunotherapy in a typical American practice. *J Allergy Clin Immunol* 2012; 129(2): AB192.

43. Cox L, Compalati E, Canonica W. Will sublingual immunotherapy become an approved treatment method in the United States? *Curr Allergy Asthma Rep* 2011; 11(1): 4–6.

44. Saegeman VS, Ectors NL, Lismont D, Verduyckt B, Verhaegen J. Short- and long-term bacterial inhibiting effect of high concentrations of glycerol used in the preservation of skin allografts. *Burns* 2008; 34(2): 205–211.

45. van Baare J, Buitenwerf J, Hoekstra MJ, du Pont JS. Virucidal effect of glycerol as used in donor skin preservation. *Burns* 1994; 20(Suppl 1): S77–S80.

46. Marshall L, Ghosh MM, Boyce SG, MacNeil S, Freedlander E, Kudesia G. Effect of glycerol on intracellular virus survival: Implications for the clinical use of glycerol-preserved cadaver skin. *Burns* 1995; 21(5): 356–361.

47. Bradbury SL, Jakoby WB. Glycerol as an enzyme-stabilizing agent: Effects on aldehyde dehydrogenase. *Proc Natl Acad Sci USA* 1972; 69(9): 2373–2376.

48. Nelson H. Preparing and Mixing Allergen Vaccines. In: Lockey RF, Bukantz, SC, editor. *Allergens and Allergen Immunotherapy*. 2nd ed. New York, NY: Marcel Decker, 1999: 401–422.

49. Vagenende V, Yap MG, Trout BL. Mechanisms of protein stabilization and prevention of protein aggregation by glycerol. *Biochemistry* 2009; 48(46): 11084–11096.

50. Pennington AK, Ratcliffe JH, Wilson CG, Hardy JG. The influence of solution viscosity on nasal spray deposition and clearance. *Int J Pharm* 1988; 43: 221–224.

51. IFF. http://www.iff.com/

52. Immunotherapy Committee of the Spanish Society of Allergy and Clinical Immunology. 2013. https://www.vacunasalergia.es/vademecum.php.

53. Poddighe D, Licari A, Caimmi S, Marseglia GL. Sublingual immunotherapy for pediatric allergic rhinitis: The clinical evidence. *World J Clin Pediatr* 2016 8; 5(1): 47–56.

54. Nelson HS. Current and future challenges of subcutaneous and sublingual allergy immunotherapy for allergists in the United States. *Ann Allergy Asthma Immunol* 2018; 121(3): 278–280.

55. Lin SY, Erekosima N, Kim JM et al. Sublingual immunotherapy for the treatment of allergic rhinoconjunctivitis and asthma: A systematic review. *JAMA* 2013; 309(12): 1278–1288.

56. Canonica GW, Passalacqua G. Noninjection routes for immunotherapy. *J Allergy Clin Immunol* 2003; 111: 437–449.

57. Bousquet J, Van Cauwenberge P, Khaltaev N. Allergic rhinitis and its impact on asthma. *J Allergy Clin Immunol* 2001; 108: S147–S334.

58. Li JT, Bernstein D, Calderon MA et al. Sublingual grass and ragweed immunotherapy: Clinical considerations-a PRACTALL consensus report. *J Allergy Clin Immunol* 2016; 137(2): 369–376.

59. Dunsky EH, Goldstein MF, Dvorin DJ, Belecanech GA. Anaphylaxis to sublingual immunotherapy. *Allergy* 2006; 61: 1235.

60. Eifan AO, Keles S, Bahceciler NN, Barlan IB. Anaphylaxis to multiple pollen allergen sublingual immunotherapy. *Allergy* 2007; 62: 567–568.

61. Antico A, Pagani M, Crema A. Anaphylaxis by latex sublingual immunotherapy. *Allergy* 2006; 61: 1236–1237.

62. Blazowski L. Anaphylactic shock because of sublingual immunotherapy overdose during third year of maintenance dose. *Allergy* 2008; 63: 374.

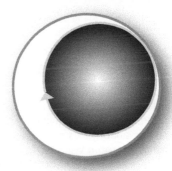

28 Sublingual and oral food immunotherapy: Indications, preparation, and administration

Whitney Block, Sayantani B. Sindher, Vanitha Sampath, and Kari C. Nadeau
Stanford University

CONTENTS

28.1 INTRODUCTION

28.1.1 Food allergy

The prevalence of allergies, including food allergies, has continued to increase rapidly over the past decades, and food allergy is an increasingly significant health burden. Food allergies are now estimated to affect 6%–13% of the global population, depending on methodology of identification, sex, age, population studied, allergen, and geography [1–9]. Approximately 40% of children with food allergies are allergic to more than one allergen [10]. Additionally, comorbid atopic diseases, such as atopic dermatitis, allergic rhinoconjunctivitis, and allergic asthma, are common in those with food allergy [11]. Food allergy prevalence can be attributed to both genetic and environmental factors. The current hypotheses are that in those genetically predisposed to allergy, lifestyle and environmental factors, such as increased hygiene, use of antibiotics, and exposure to environmental pollutants, mediate food allergy [12]. The diagnosis of food allergy leads to a decreased quality of life by imposing dietary restrictions, increasing anxiety, and limiting social activities [13]. In severe cases, it can result in systemic anaphylaxis and, rarely, even death. The number of U.S. emergency room visits for food-induced anaphylaxis has increased to approximately 200,000/year and continues to rise, posing a significant burden to our healthcare system [14,15].

Currently, no drugs have been approved by the U.S. Food and Drug Administration (FDA) for the treatment of food allergy. The current standard of care remains avoidance of allergenic foods and management of acute allergic reactions with antihistamines and epinephrine auto-injectors [16]. With food allergies, even with increased vigilance, accidental exposures are common [17]. The increased prevalence of food allergies has spurred research in the area leading to considerable insight into the basic mechanisms of food allergy and tolerance. Allergen immunotherapy (AIT) for food allergy has been studied for a number of years, and many AIT clinical trials are in advanced phase 3 studies. Additionally, in recent years, biologics for food allergy are also in development. Most biologics are in preclinical development, although a few such as dupilumab (Dupixent; Sanofi and Regeneron Pharmaceuticals) and etokinab (AnaptysBio), which block key cytokines involved in food allergy, are now in phase 2 clinical trials for food allergy. This chapter focuses on AIT for food allergy, specifically oral immunotherapy (OIT) and sublingual immunotherapy (SLIT), which are the most commonly studied.

28.1.2 Basic mechanisms of food allergy, tolerance, and desensitization with allergen immunotherapy

Tolerance to innocuous foods is an active process, and food allergy is due to dysfunction of tolerogenic pathways. Disruption of the epithelium in response to inflammation or injury at barrier surfaces, such as the skin, gastrointestinal tract, or the respiratory tract [18,19], is a first step in the predisposition toward allergic sensitization. Disrupted epithelial cells produce pro-inflammatory cytokines, such as interleukin (IL)-25, IL-33, and TSLP [20]. These epithelial cytokines (alarmins) mediate T-cell activation and skew naïve T cells toward a Th2-type profile with subsequent release of pro-inflammatory type 2 cytokines, such as IL-4, IL-5, IL-9, and IL-13. Together, these type 2 cytokines lead to IgE class switching by B cells and IgE binding to FcεRI receptors on mast cells or basophils. These cells with IgE bound FcεRI receptors are primed and sensitized to the allergen. On subsequent encounters with allergen, the FcεRI-bound IgE antibodies cross-link and mediate degranulation and release of allergic mediators such as histamine, leukotrienes, and prostaglandins into the surrounding tissue, resulting in allergic reactions, characterized by eosinophil infiltration, mucous production, dilation of blood vessels, and smooth muscle contraction.

T cells play a central and pivotal path in food allergy. In natural tolerance and desensitization with immunotherapy, naïve T cells skew toward T-regulatory and Th1 subtypes rather than a Th2 subtype as seen with allergy. Overall, natural tolerance or desensitization with immunotherapy is due to one or more of the following mechanisms: suppression of T_H2 cells, decreased production of IgE by B cells, increased IgA and IgG_4 production by B cells, induction of IL-10, and suppression of basophil, eosinophil, and mast cell activation [21]. A major clinical difference between naturally acquired clinical unresponsiveness to allergens and that brought about by

immunotherapy is durability. While natural tolerance is a permanent state, current data indicate that in the majority of patients, clinical unresponsiveness achieved after successful immunotherapy is a temporary state. Patients often became resensitized on discontinuation of regular consumption of the food allergen. This temporary clinically unresponsive state, which requires continued ingestion of food allergen to maintain unresponsiveness, is termed *desensitization* and differs from the permanent unresponsive state of *tolerance* as seen in healthy nonallergic individuals [22]. With immunotherapy, the exact mechanism of desensitization is not known but is likely due to deviation of Th2-type responses to a Th1-type response (immune deviation), induction of Treg cells (immune regulation), deletion of Th2 cells (apoptosis), or anergy of Th2 cells (unresponsiveness to antigen) (Figure 28.1) [21]. Key research questions that are now the focus of AIT research are the maintenance food dose required after successful desensitization to maintain desensitization and whether alterations in allergen dose, type, duration, and method of administration can increase durability of desensitization toward a permanent state of tolerance or sustained unresponsiveness. Biomarkers for determining prognosis and progression of AIT are also areas of active research.

28.2 ALLERGEN IMMUNOTHERAPY FOR FOOD ALLERGY

28.2.1 Indications for food AIT

OIT and SLIT are the most common forms of AIT. Although there have been only a few studies using epicutaneous immunotherapy, recent studies indicate that this mode of therapy may also be safe and efficacious. Initial clinical trials of subcutaneous immunotherapy for food allergies indicated that it was efficacious, but it was largely abandoned due to serious safety concerns [23]. Here, we limit our discussion to OIT and SLIT, as these are the best-studied AIT treatments for food allergy.

Food allergy diagnosis is complex, and there is no single universal method that meets the criteria of safety, sensitivity, and specificity to diagnose a food allergy. A diagnosis of food allergy often requires consideration of patient clinical history, measurement of specific IgE, elimination diets, and food challenges. Both skin prick wheal size and serum IgE levels assist in the diagnosis of allergy, but they have high sensitivities and low specificities and are associated with a high number of false positives [16,24,25]. At the current time, the double-blind, placebo-controlled food challenge (DBPCFC) remains the gold standard for diagnosing an IgE-mediated food allergy; however, it is resource consuming and carries with it the risk of severe reaction during challenge [24].

AIT procedures have varied in dose, duration of therapy, route of administration, and adjunctive therapy, if any. The goal of immunotherapy also varies in different protocols. The goal of some protocols is to increase the threshold dose of allergen that can be safely consumed before the onset of an allergic reaction so as to prevent problems following accidental consumption. Other protocols aim to further increase the threshold dose of the food allergen, but these increases are still less than that consumed in normal diets. There is still considerable debate whether benefits of therapeutic intervention with OIT or SLIT outweigh the burden of avoidance of allergen. Currently, benefits should be weighed

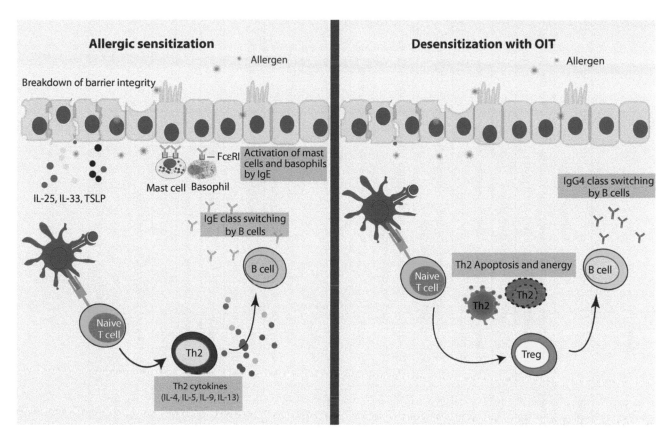

Figure 28.1 Mechanisms underlying allergic sensitization and desensitization with immunotherapy. (OIT, oral immunotherapy; Th2, type 2 T-helper cells; Treg, T-regulatory cells; TSLP, thymic stromal lymphopoietin.)

against risks on a case-by-case basis [26]. Limitations of therapy are the risk of adverse reaction during therapy, impermanence of desensitization, and lengthy treatment period.

Due to safety considerations, diagnosis of food allergy and initiation of OIT and SLIT should be conducted in an allergist's office or clinic with trained staff who can recognize and quickly treat symptoms of allergic reactions.

28.3 ORAL IMMUNOTHERAPY FOR FOOD ALLERGY

Food allergen–specific immunotherapy has been investigated for over 100 years, with the first successful report of OIT performed in a child with egg-induced anaphylaxis published in 1908 [27]. OIT clinical trials primarily have been for peanut, egg, milk, and multiple, coincident food allergies (Table 28.1). Some OIT clinical trials are now in phase 2 or 3 [28]. OIT is mostly conducted in research centers; however, as OIT uses common food items as therapy, which do not require FDA approval, private and academic practices also offer OIT for food allergies. Treatments among centers, however, vary widely, as there is no single, standardized protocol. As mentioned earlier, limitations of therapy are the risk of adverse reaction during therapy, impermanence of desensitization, and lengthy treatment period. Risks of reactions during treatment are being addressed by the use of adjuvants before and during therapy. As biomarkers to assess tolerance are unavailable and long-term

data are limited, durability of desensitization is generally assessed as *sustained unresponsiveness* (SU), which is defined as unresponsiveness to the allergen after a predetermined period of allergen discontinuation following successful OIT for a period of time (generally a few weeks). Further, preliminary data suggest that longer periods of treatment with OIT may increase durability of SU.

28.3.1 Preparing foods for OIT

As opposed to subcutaneous or SLIT immunotherapy for inhalant allergy, which typically uses aqueous, bulk medical extracts for therapy, most clinicians currently offering OIT in their practice use commercially available food flours or powders. There is currently no FDA-approved drug for therapeutic use. There is debate about whether the food flours or powders used for OIT should be considered food or drug. Currently, the FDA approves drugs, devices, electronic products, cosmetics, veterinary products, and tobacco products [29]. Food products sold in the United States are held to strict FDA regulations but are not granted official FDA approval. Food flours and powders are highly variable with regard to protein content and type, containing both allergenic (associated with varying severity) and nonallergenic proteins. When using commercially available food flours, patients are instructed not to bake the food to limit the risk of altering the allergenic protein content. Egg and milk proteins in particular are heat-labile proteins that denature when baked. At the current time, with the exception of AR101, food allergens tested in clinical trials use commercially available food flours or powders. AR101

Table 28.1 Examples of oral immunotherapy clinical trials

Allergen	Study (year)	Adjuvant therapy	N	Participant age (years)	Maintenance dose	Primary outcome
Egg	Pérez-Rangel et al. [75]	None	33	6–16	2808 mg every other day	A 5-day rush oral immunotherapy followed by every other day dosing for 5 months desensitized 94% to 2808 mg
Egg	Akashi et al. [76]	None	36	3–15	4 g	57% passed 4 g OFC after 6 months
Egg	Jones et al. [36]	None	55	5–18	2 g	50% achieved sustained unresponsiveness by year 4 (4–6 week discontinuation)
Egg	Escudero et al. [77]	None	61	5–17	2808 mg every other day	37% achieved sustained unresponsiveness after 3 months on therapy followed by 1 month avoidance
Egg	Caminiti et al. [78]	None	31	4–11	4 g	31% achieved sustained unresponsiveness after 10 months on therapy followed by 3-month avoidance
Egg	Burks et al. [35]	None	40	5–11	1.6 g	75% passed 10 g OFC; 28% SU (6- to 8-week discontinuation)
Egg	Vickery et al. [79]	None	8	3–13	0.3–3.6 g	75% passed OFC 1 month after stopping OIT
Egg	Buchanan et al. [80]	None	7	1–16	0.3 g	57% passed 8 g OFC
Microwave-heated milk	Takahashi et al. [81]	Omalizumab	16	6–14	200 mL	100% achieved desensitization to 200 mL fresh cow's milk after 24 weeks of OIT (8 weeks after discontinuing omalizumab)
Milk	Wood et al. [82]	Omalizumab	57	7–32	3.8 g	48.1% achieved sustained unresponsiveness after discontinuing the maintenance dose for 4 months
Milk	Keet et al. [61]	None	20	6–17	1–2 g	70% desensitized to 8 g OFC, SU in 40% after 6 weeks
Milk	Martorell et al. [39]	None	30	2–3	200 mL	90% showing complete desensitization
Milk	Nadeau et al. [83]	Omalizumab	11	7–17	2 g	90% reached the maximum daily dose of 2000 mg milk
Milk	Pajno et al. [84]	None	15	4–10	200 mL	67% tolerant to 200 mL of cow's milk
Multiple	Andorf et al. [48]	Omalizumab	48	4–15	2 g per allergen	83% passed OFC to 2 g for two or more of their offending foods at week 36 (20 weeks after discontinuing omalizumab)

(Continued)

Table 28.1 (*Continued*) Examples of oral immunotherapy clinical trials

Allergen	Study (year)	Adjuvant therapy	N	Participant age (years)	Maintenance dose	Primary outcome
Multiple	Begin et al. [85]	Omalizumab	25	4+	4 g per allergen	401 reactions/7530 home doses (5.3%); median of 3.2 reactions per 100 doses; 94% of reactions were mild; one severe reaction occurred
Multiple and peanut	Begin et al. [86]	None	15, peanut; 25, multiple	4+	4 g	Rates of reaction per dose did not differ significantly between single or multiple allergen therapy
Peanut: AR101	Bird et al. [87]	None	55	4–26	300 mg	62% AR101 participants tolerated ≥443 mg at the exit DBPCFC by 20–36 weeks
Peanut: in capsule	Fauquert et al. [88]	None	30	12–18	400 mg	81% of participants achieved desensitization to 400 mg of peanut protein
Peanut	Blumchen et al. [89]	None	62	3–17	250 mg	74.2% children tolerated at least 300 mg peanut protein at final OFC after 16 of OIT
Peanut	MacGinnitie et al. [90]	Omalizumab	37	7–25	4 g	79% tolerated 2 g 6 weeks after stopping omalizumab
Peanut	Tang et al. [51]	Probiotics	62	1–10	2 g	82.1% achieved sustained unresponsiveness 2–5 weeks after stopping maintenance dosing
Peanut	Anagnostou et al. [91]	None	39	7–16	800 mg	62% tolerated 1400 mg challenge
Peanut	Narisety et al. [92]	None	16	7–13	2 g	OIT greater than SLIT in OFC threshold, low rate of SU
Peanut	Vickery et al. [37]	None	24	1–16	4 g	50% SU to 5000 mg OFC after 4-week avoidance
Peanut	Schneider et al. [66]	Omalizumab	13	7–25	4 g	100% reached the 500 mg peanut flour dose on the first day (cumulative dose, 992 mg) with minimal or no symptoms

Abbreviations: DBPCFC, double-blind, placebo-controlled food challenge; OFC, oral food challenge; OIT, oral immunotherapy; SLIT, sublingual immunotherapy; SU, sustained unresponsiveness.

is a drug developed by Aimmune Therapeutics (Brisbane, California) to address variability of allergenic proteins in foods. AR101 is a highly characterized, pharmaceutical-grade, peanut OIT formulation that is designed to provide consistent dosing of peanut allergens. It is standardized to Ara h1, h2, and h6, the three major allergenic proteins in peanuts. Results of a phase 3 trial of AR101 in peanut-allergic children and adolescents found that patients could ingest higher doses of peanut protein without dose-limiting symptoms [28].

28.3.2 Administering OIT

OIT is generally conducted for one allergen, but OIT to multiple allergens simultaneously is also an option. OIT typically consists of three to four phases (Figure 28.2) [30]. The first phase is the *screening phase* during which the patient is evaluated by a medical professional to determine which food(s) should be included in therapy and ensure key eligibility criteria are met. The next phase is the *buildup phase* that can last as little as 8 weeks but may extend to years depending on number of allergens, allergen type, and use, if any, of adjuvants. The third phase, typically the last phase, is the *maintenance phase*. This is the phase in which the allergen dose is not increased but rather is maintained at a constant amount. At the end of a specified maintenance phase (weeks to years), a food challenge is conducted to assess desensitization. Some trials add a fourth phase called the *tolerance phase*, to determine SU [31]. Current OIT research is focused on understanding rates of SU, and the molecular mechanisms that mediate desensitization and potentially a more permanent state of tolerance.

28.3.2.1 SCREENING

The screening phase typically includes collecting medical history, including food allergen reaction history and other aeroallergen history, spirometry testing to ensure asthma is controlled (if

applicable), a physical examination, and a review of key inclusion and exclusion criteria (Box 28.1). Before initiation of treatment, there should be a discussion on risks of adverse reactions and a consent form signed, documenting understanding of the risks and benefits of treatment. Sometimes the screening phase will require skin prick testing, blood specific-IgE levels, and/or oral food challenges (OFCs) to prove a certain food should or should not be included in OIT. To participate in OIT, a patient must be compliant with the dosing regimen, willing to use reaction medications appropriately, and have an IgE-mediated allergy to the foods that are to be included in therapy. Food allergies are commonly associated with other allergic disorders. There appears to be a natural progression of these diseases, with eczema generally occurring first, followed by food allergies, asthma, and hay fever. The natural progression of these atopic diseases is termed the "Allergic or Atopic March" [32]. All other allergic disorders should be well controlled prior to starting OIT and should be managed optimally throughout OIT.

28.3.2.2 BUILDUP PHASE

The buildup phase of OIT starts with the initial dose escalation day (IDED) (Figure 28.3). A patient should be in good health; free from illness, asthma, and eczema flares; and should have eaten a meal prior to dosing. In our experience, we find that a high-carbohydrate diet before dosing is preferable. On this day, the allergenic food(s) is (are) typically administered by mixing a small amount of food flour or powder into a vehicle of the patient's choosing (applesauce, pudding, etc.), with dosing approximately every 30 minutes followed by at least 2 hours of observation. OIT dosing starts at about 1 mg protein and gradually builds up to about 6 mg protein during IDED. The decision to stop dose escalation and the amount of protein to be consumed for the first home dose is based on the type and severity of the initial allergic reaction (Box 28.2). If there are no symptoms with IDED, the first home dose will be the highest dose ingested that day. Some clinicians may choose to have their patients

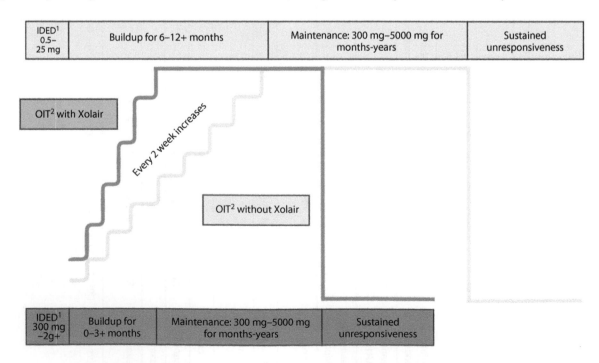

Figure 28.2 Oral immunotherapy phases with and without adjuvant omalizumab. (1, Initial dose escalation day. 2, Oral immunotherapy.)

Box 28.1 Key inclusion and exclusion criteria for oral immunotherapy

Inclusion criteria

- IgE-mediated food allergy as determined by either recent history, positive results on oral food challenge (OFC), skin prick tests (SPTs), or specific IgE (sIgE).
- Willingness to adhere to protocol.

Exclusion criteria

- Unwilling to carry and use (if necessary) epinephrine auto-injector
- Unwilling to comply with home dosing instructions and home dosing requirements
- Pregnant or planning to get pregnant during buildup oral immunotherapy (OIT)
- History consistent with poorly controlled persistent asthma
- Patients with unstable angina, significant arrhythmia, uncontrolled hypertension, chronic sinusitis, or other chronic or immunologic diseases that, in the judgment of the clinician, might interfere with the evaluation or administration of OIT or pose additional risk to the patient (e.g., gastrointestinal or gastroesophageal disease, chronic infections, scleroderma, hepatic and gallbladder disease, chronic nonallergic pulmonary disease)
- Patient taking certain medications, such as angiotensin-converting enzyme (ACE) inhibitors and β-blockers
- Patients with a diagnosis of symptomatic eosinophilic esophagitis, eosinophilic colitis, or eosinophilic gastritis

return to the clinic the next day for their first dose after IDED prior to starting home dosing without medical supervision. For mild symptoms, the action should be to continue IDED in 30–60 minutes depending on the clinician's discretion. For moderate symptoms, the action should be to discontinue IDED and administer rescue medications. If symptoms resolve quickly, the first home dose may be the current dose or a one-step reduction at the discretion of the clinician. For severe symptoms, the action should be to discontinue IDED and administer rescue medications. The first home dose may be a one- or two-step reduction at the discretion of the clinician.

After IDED, the patient is sent home with the highest tolerated dose achieved at the IDED along with home dosing instructions

(Box 28.2) and advised to return in approximately 2 weeks for a dose escalation (DE). Pre-dosing about 30–60 minutes with an appropriate dose of cetirizine (or equivalent) and/or famotidine (or equivalent) prior to home OIT dosing is discussed with the patient. Pre-dosing, along with following all the home dosing instructions, may minimize allergic discomfort during OIT (especially oral pruritus and/or mild abdominal pain). At each DE appointment, the previous 2 weeks of home dosing are discussed and the patient is assessed for reactions, symptoms, and concerns with the OIT dosing; a physical examination is performed to ensure the patient is in good health and

Box 28.2 Example home-dosing instructions for oral immunotherapy (OIT)

- Be awake and monitored for about 1 hour after each dose.
- Try to make sure dosage is taken around the same time every day.
- Never take two doses in one day; each dose should be at least 12 hours apart.
- Take the dose with a meal or snack preferably containing carbohydrates (rice, pasta, bread, cereal, oatmeal).
- Mix the dosage with an appropriate vehicle (applesauce, yogurt, juice, chocolate pudding).
- Do not do any significant exercise for 2 hours after the dose and 1 hour prior to the dose.
- Avoid hot baths or showers or heat for 2 hours after the dose.

DO NOT MISS ANY DOSES, BUT IF YOU DO:

- *IF YOU MISS 1–2 days*: Take the next dose at your next normal dosage time. There should be at least 12 hours between doses.
- *IF YOU MISS 3 days or more*: Contact your OIT provider as soon as you can to schedule a visit to the office. Do NOT take the dose at home as you may have a severe allergic reaction since desensitization may have been lost.
- *When you travel by plane*: Skip your dose on days with plane travel. Never take your dose within 2 hours of going up in the air.

WHAT TO DO IF YOU ARE ILL:

- *If you have a fever (≥100°F)*: DO NOT take your dose. Contact your primary care physician if your fever lasts more than 3 days for advice and possible evaluation.
- *If you have cold symptoms (but no fever)*: Decrease the dose by one-half until symptoms have resolved and do the following:
  - If you took the half-dose for 1–2 days, then you may go back up to the full dose on day 3 on your own at home.
  - If you took the half-dose for 3 or more days, notify your OIT provider for further instructions.
  - If you have gastrointestinal symptoms (vomiting/diarrhea) related to an illness: Do NOT take the dose. If the symptoms have resolved and you have missed 1–2 days, then resume the full dose at your normally scheduled time. If you have missed 3 days, then call your OIT provider right away as you will need to return to the office to receive the next dose.

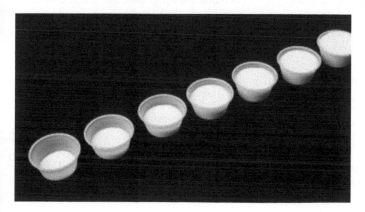

Figure 28.3 An example of updosing with liquid milk during oral immunotherapy.

- If you have asthma symptoms:
  - Less than 2 hours after taking the dose, give epinephrine immediately, call 911/go to emergency room, and then call OIT clinic.
  - NOT within 2 hours after taking the dose, then use two puffs albuterol and follow your asthma action plan. You may continue the normal dosage as long as your symptoms have resolved. *If you have a cold that is triggering asthma, also follow the instructions for cold symptoms noted previously.
- Always follow your food allergy action plan. Administer epinephrine right away if indicated and then call 911. Do NOT wait to call your OIT provider before giving epinephrine.

all other allergic disorders are in control. Then, the next dose in the schedule is given followed by 1–2 hours of observation to ensure the dose is tolerated. If the patient has symptoms during the observation period, the dose may need to be adjusted back to the previous dose or a multiple dose step reduction to ensure safety when dosing at home. For mild symptoms, the action should be to send home with the escalated dose for 2 weeks (with or without instructions to administer an antihistamine prior to the dose) or send home with the prior (nonescalated) dose at the discretion of the clinician. For moderate symptoms, the action should be to send home with old (nonescalated) dose or a one-step reduction at the discretion of the

clinician. For severe symptoms, the action should be to send home with one- or two-step reduction at the discretion of the clinician (Table 28.2).

DE appointments are repeated approximately every 2 weeks until the maintenance dose is achieved. For single-food OIT, the dose escalation phase lasts approximately 6–8 months, but with multiple foods and/or with high maintenance doses, the phase may last 1 year or more. Withdrawal rates generally vary between 10% and 20%, but rates as high as 36% have been reported [30]. The most common reasons for withdrawal are adverse events (especially gastrointestinal), noncompliance, and/or patient preference.

28.3.2.3 MAINTENANCE PHASE

Maintenance doses of up to 300 mg to 5 g of protein per allergen are used in OIT trials [33]. It was hypothesized that high maintenance doses might enable patients to eat a full serving or more of their allergens, have a greater impact on the immune system, and provide greater safety from accidental exposures. It soon became clear that many patients, even after desensitization to the food, did not like the taste of their allergens. For many, the primary goal of therapy was absence of an allergic reaction on accidental consumption and higher quality of life, rather than eating full servings of their allergens. Research has shown that a lower maintenance dose (i.e., 300 mg protein) allows many patients to pass challenges to higher amounts of their allergenic foods (i.e., 2 g–5 g protein) without continuing the higher dose of maintenance OIT. Additionally, one study found that there were no differences in T-cell or basophil

Table 28.2 Symptom severity and appropriate dosing actions

Symptoms	First home dose determination after IDED	Dose determination after in-clinic dosing escalation visit
No symptoms	Highest dose tolerated during IDED	New escalated dose
For *mild symptoms*, defined as: • Skin—limited or localized hives, swelling or redness, skin flushing or pruritus • Respiratory — rhinorrhea or sneezing, nasal congestion, occasional cough, throat discomfort • GI — mild abdominal	For mild symptoms, the action should be to continue IDED in 30–60 minutes depending on the clinician's discretion.	For mild symptoms, the action should be to send home with escalated dose for 2 weeks (with or without instructions to administer an antihistamine prior to the dose) or send home with old (nonescalated) dose at the discretion of the clinician.
For *moderate symptoms*, defined as: • Skin—systemic hives or swelling • Respiratory—throat tightness without hoarseness, persistent cough • GI—persistent moderate abdominal pain/cramping/nausea, vomiting	For moderate symptoms, the action should be to discontinue IDED and administer rescue medications. If symptoms resolve quickly, the first home dose may be the current dose or a one-step reduction at the discretion of the clinician.	For moderate symptoms, the action should be to send home with old (nonescalated) dose or a one-step reduction at the discretion of the clinician.
For *severe symptoms*, defined as: • Respiratory—laryngeal edema, throat tightness with hoarseness, wheezing with or without dyspnea • GI—significant severe abdominal pain/cramping/repetitive vomiting • Neurologic—change in mental status • Circulatory—hypotension	For severe symptoms, the action should be to discontinue IDED and administer rescue medications. The first home dose may be a one- or two-step reduction at the discretion of the clinician.	For severe symptoms, the action should be to send home with one-step reduction or two-step reduction at the discretion of the clinician.

responses between patients on low-dose or high-dose maintenance OIT [34]. The maintenance phases during clinical trials vary widely (weeks to years). However, data indicate that continued indefinite ingestion of allergen as a maintenance dose may be necessary for the majority of patients to maintain desensitization. More research is underway to determine the minimal maintenance dose needed to remain desensitized to various amounts of allergenic food or whether alterations in OIT protocols can increase durability of desensitization.

28.3.2.4 TOLERANCE PHASE

After reaching a maintenance dose, some studies have explored SU which involves discontinuing the patient's maintenance dose for a predetermined period of time and then performing food challenges to determine if the allergy has resolved or is persistent. Although SU has been achieved for some, rates in trials vary from 28% to 78% of subjects passing an OFC after avoiding their maintenance dose for 2–4 weeks [35–38]. More research is underway to determine which patients are most likely to benefit and how SU can be achieved.

28.3.3 Safety of OIT dosing

OIT dosing is generally well tolerated but does come with a risk of side effects ranging from mild allergic reactions to severe anaphylaxis, as well as the risk of eosinophilic esophagitis (EoE). The most commonly observed symptoms with OIT are mild to moderate, typically involving oropharyngeal pruritus or transient abdominal pain that is either self-limited or easily treated with antihistamines. Moderate and severe reactions do occur. In one study of milk OIT, 47% of participants had moderate reactions over the course of treatment [39]. Many patients may benefit from pretreatment with H_1 antagonists, H_2 antagonists, or both, although research publications on this are limited. Although severe reactions most often occur during the buildup phases, they can occur during the maintenance phase as well. Often, but not always, a severe reaction is associated with cofactors such as infection, exercise, menstruation, or alcohol consumption. Exercise and alcohol consumption should be minimized or avoided for several hours following home dosing.

Another major concern is the presence of EoE in some subjects undergoing OIT [40]. Clinical symptoms may include reflux-like symptoms, abdominal pain, vomiting that is refractory to reflux treatment, dysphagia, or food impaction in conjunction with histologic evidence of dense eosinophilic infiltration of the mucosa (greater than 15 eosinophils per high-power field [eos/hpf]) [41]. A meta-analysis [42] and a review [43] estimate the incidence of EoE during OIT varies from 2.7% to 5.3%, respectively. Some authorities suggest that subjects with OIT-induced EoE may have preexisting, subclinical disease [44]. This is supported by estimates that EoE prevalence in patients with food allergy is 125 times more common than in the general population [45].

28.3.4 Adjuvant therapy with OIT

Omalizumab (Xolair; Genentech, South San Francisco, California), a monoclonal humanized anti-IgE antibody, has been utilized in food OIT with the rationale that blocking food-specific IgE antibodies might facilitate reduction in food allergy OIT symptoms. Omalizumab is thought to form immune complexes with circulating free IgE, preventing IgE from interacting with high-affinity IgE receptors, which are expressed on dendritic cells, mast cells, and basophils. Omalizumab also results in downregulation of the same high-affinity receptors. This action may suppress cellular response by inhibiting antigen presentation by these cells, allowing for more rapid OIT [46,47]. A double-blind, placebo-controlled trial comparing multiple allergen OIT with omalizumab, found that 83% of the omalizumab-treated patients versus 33% of the placebo-treated arm passed a DBPCFC to 2 g protein for two or more of their offending foods [48]. In August 2018, the FDA granted Genentech breakthrough therapy designation to expedite the development and review for omalizumab for food allergies.

Toll-like receptor ligands and bacterial adjuvants have been hypothesized to complement OIT treatment. Furthermore, gut microbiota may aid in polarization of T cells. In a mouse model, administration of a *Lactobacillus* spp. was associated with generation of $CD4^+CD8\alpha\alpha^+$ T-cell receptor $\alpha\beta$ T cells (also termed double-positive intraepithelial lymphocytes), resulting in regulatory and tolerogenic properties to the culprit food [49,50]. A double-blind, placebo-controlled, randomized controlled trial (DBPCRCT) of the probiotic *Lactobacillus rhamnosus* plus peanut protein OIT (PPOIT) versus placebo (maltodextrin, brown food coloring, and peanut essence) implemented a buildup dosing protocol every 2 weeks over 8–12 months followed by a 2 g peanut protein maintenance dose for 10 months (total 18–22 months of OIT), followed by an oral peanut DBPCFC to a cumulative 4000 mg peanut protein to assess peanut desensitization. Subjects who passed the OFC subsequently underwent a second DBPCFC 2 weeks or more after completing study treatment, while on a peanut elimination diet. Eighty-two percent (82%) of the PPOIT cohort versus 3.6% of the placebo group passed the OFC suggesting that the PPOIT group had achieved SU. However, a major weakness of the study was the lack of a probiotic alone control group; therefore, the individual contributions of the probiotic and of the OIT (or the combination) cannot be assessed [51].

Dupilumab (Dupixent, Sanofi, Regeneron) is a recombinant human IgG4 antibody that blocks IL-4 and IL-13 receptors [52]. IL-4 stimulates IgE production from B cells. Expression of IL-13 correlates with disease severity and asthma and atopic dermatitis flares. Dupilumab is FDA approved for the treatment of atopic dermatitis and asthma. Clinical trials of dupilumab as adjuvant therapy with OIT for food allergies are currently being investigated in clinical trials [53].

28.3.5 OIT flour and powder types and storage

Commercially available food flours and powders sold in the United States must be manufactured and labeled according to FDA standards. Studies show that 69%–83% of cow's milk allergic children can tolerate baked cow's milk, and 63%–83% of egg-allergic children can tolerate baked egg [54]. Since egg and milk proteins are heat labile, meaning the protein denatures when heated, OIT for milk and egg is typically done with powders in the unbaked/heated form. Most other food flours and powders are not heat labile and should be stored as stated in the product label recommendation. Once a maintenance dose is achieved (and sometimes sooner), a patient may switch from the food flour or powder to the protein equivalent of the whole food (i.e., peanut flour to a whole peanut). For standardization purposes, most OIT research trials use food flours or powders throughout the trial.

28.4 SUBLINGUAL IMMUNOTHERAPY FOR FOOD ALLERGY

SLIT was first used in 1990 in patients with allergic rhinitis secondary to grass or dust mite [55]. In this form of food immunotherapy, the extract of food protein is delivered sublingually, held for 2 minutes, and then swallowed. The efficacy of SLIT is limited by the volume of liquid that can be held sublingually and low concentration of available extracts [56]. The lower dosing associated with SLIT improves its safety profile [57]. Local dendritic cells (predominantly Langerhans cells) take up antigen and migrate to local lymph nodes, where they present antigen to naïve T cells and mediate the formation of T-regulatory cells [58,59]. SLIT differs from OIT in that the dendritic cells encounter intact food protein, rather than digested proteins.

28.4.1 Preparing SLIT

Typical doses for SLIT are much lower than in OIT, starting in microgram (of protein) and increasing to milligram doses at maintenance. Most clinicians currently offering SLIT use medically available aqueous food extracts and dilute them as needed. In a 2006 study, cow's milk SLIT was administered by having the patients place milk in their mouth for 2 minutes (0.1 mL for the first 2 weeks, increasing by 0.1 mL every 15 days until 1 mL/day) [60]. Current studies generally use commercially available extracts. Keet et al. used commercial glycerinated cow's milk extract in prefilled vials that dispensed a set amount of liquid per squirt [61]. Studies by Kim et al. [62] and by Burks et al. [63] used commercially available aqueous peanut extracts (in 50% glycerin) made from the edible portions of whole, nonroasted peanut using 0.5% sodium chloride and 0.54% sodium bicarbonate (pH 6.8–8.4). Placebo extracts were prepared from a glycerinated saline solution plus phenol with caramel coloring. The standard concentration (1:20 wt/vol) was 3300 μg/mL, and dilutions were shipped in prepacked vials with 50 or 140 μL actuators. Commercialized peach extracts enriched in Pru p 3 were used in a clinical trial of SLIT for peach allergy [64]. Sanofi is in the process of developing a drug to be used for peanut SLIT, which is currently used in research trials (Clinicaltrials.gov; NCT03463135).

28.4.2 Administering SLIT

Clinical trials on SLIT for food allergy are limited and include hazelnut [65], cow's milk [60,61], peach [64], peanut [62,63,67], and kiwi [68]. Similar to OIT, SLIT is administered in the same phases: screening, buildup, maintenance, and tolerance. The screening phase is similar to OIT with the primary purpose of determining which food(s) will be included in therapy and assessing key inclusion and exclusion criteria that are practically the same as for OIT. It is unclear whether SLIT food allergens can be mixed (i.e., multiple allergens at once), as some studies suggest a saturation effect on the local immune environment under the tongue with mixing sublingual allergens in aeroallergen SLIT [69].

The buildup phase for SLIT starts with an IDED with gradually increasing doses (Table 28.3) given every 30 minutes followed by 2 hours of observation. The patient is then sent home with home dosing instructions (Box 28.3) and instructed to return approximately every 2 weeks for DE appointments until a

Table 28.3 Example of sublingual immunotherapy (SLIT) dosing steps without adjuvant therapy

Microgram (mcg) protein	SLIT phase
10	
20	
40	Initial dose escalation
80	day (IDED)
160	
320	
1280	Buildup
2560	
5120	Maintenance

maintenance dose is achieved. Maintenance dosing is variable and ranges from 1.3 to 7 mg. Due to fewer studies being conducted on SLIT, data on withdrawal rates are sparse. One trial reported greater than 50% withdrawal rate due to dosing symptoms, noncompliance, and patients feeling that the daily dosing was too difficult to maintain [63].

Because the maintenance dose is significantly lower than OIT, it is difficult to determine the clinical significance of SLIT once maintenance is achieved. To determine effectiveness, many trials have done food challenges at some point during the maintenance phase. Results show that allergen SLIT is more effective than placebo. Peanut SLIT studies show that after maintaining for approximately 1 year, patients pass food challenges with up to 496–1710 mg peanut protein without reaction [70].

Box 28.3 Example home-dosing instructions for sublingual immunotherapy (SLIT)

Try to make sure dosage is taken around the same time every day.

Never take two doses in one day; each dose should be at least 12 hours apart.

Withhold the dose in the following circumstances:

- In the presence of oropharyngeal infection
- In the case of major dental surgery
- Acute gastroenteritis
- Exacerbation of the asthma
- Peak expiratory flow rate (PEFR) less than 80% of personal best value
- Simultaneous administration of viral vaccines

Do not miss any doses, but

- IF YOU MISS 1–6 days, then take the next dose at your next normal dosage time. There should be at least 12 hours between doses.
- IF YOU MISS 7 days or more, contact your allergist as soon as you can to schedule a visit to the office. Do NOT take the dose at home as you may have a severe allergic reaction since desensitization may have been lost.

28.4.3 Safety of SLIT

SLIT likely has a better safety profile than OIT [61,71]. Side effects tend to be localized to the mouth, and systemic reactions and anaphylaxis are rare [61,63,65,67,72]. SLIT likely also has a lower risk for EoE. Keet et al. compared OIT and SLIT for cow's milk allergy and found that the overall reaction rate was similar (23 versus 29%, respectively); however, the reactions during OIT were more likely to be systemic [61]. EoE has not been observed with food allergen SLIT but has been reported in aeroallergen SLIT [73].

28.4.4 Adjuvant therapy with SLIT

Sanofi has an ongoing study to assess peanut extract SLIT adjuvanted with glucopyranosyl lipid A (GLA) in peanut-allergic adolescents and adults. GLA is a potent toll-like receptor-4 (TLR4) ligand that induces Th1-promoting cytokines, thereby enhancing the antigen-specific immune responses compared to immunization with antigen alone.

In vitro studies show that GLA also induces the tolerogenic and antiproliferative cytokine IL-10 in peripheral blood mononuclear cells from peanut allergic patients, thereby suppressing allergic T-effector cells (Clinicaltrials.gov; NCT03463135).

28.4.5 Storing SLIT

SLIT extracts are typically stored in the refrigerator. It should always be stored and handled according to manufacturer labels. SLIT extracts should never be baked or mixed with another vehicle.

28.5 CROSS-REACTIVITY OF ALLERGENS

There are well-known cross-reactive patterns among tree nuts, such as between cashew and pistachio or pecan and walnut [74]. OIT with one food in the pair, in conjunction with omalizumab, was associated with passing an OFC with the counterpart tree nut allergen after 36 weeks of treatment. All subjects treated with walnut who passed walnut OFC, also passed an OFC with pecan. Eighty-three percent of patients treated with cashew and who passed a cashew challenge also passed a pistachio OFC [48].

28.6 CONCLUSION

OIT clinical trials for food allergy demonstrate efficacy; but the lengthy treatment period, frequent in-clinic visits, high rates of resensitization after a period of allergen discontinuation, and risk of allergic reaction during active treatment and on maintenance dosing are concerns. Adjuvants such as omalizumab and probiotics with OIT show promise in mitigating some of these concerns, but further studies are needed. The use of adjuvant omalizumab with OIT has enabled treatment of patients with multiple food allergies with multiple allergens simultaneously. Although there are a relatively fewer number of SLIT clinical trials for food allergy, studies show that food SLIT is safe and efficacious. As the allergen dose in SLIT is log-fold lower than in OIT and is associated with fewer systemic reactions, it may be useful as initial treatment in highly

sensitive individuals before OIT. Further investigation is needed to define optimal protocols for both OIT and SLIT, and the potential for combining the two treatment methods remains to be explored. More DBPCRT, head-to-head clinical trials are necessary for a direct comparison. More data are needed for the long-term outcome as well, since very little is known about the effects of brief lapses in exposures, even after many years of therapy.

SALIENT POINTS

1. There are currently no FDA-approved drugs for treatment of food allergy.
2. The current standard of care remains avoidance of allergenic foods and management of acute allergic reactions with antihistamines and epinephrine auto-injectors.
3. Oral immunotherapy (OIT) and sublingual immunotherapy (SLIT) are the most common forms of allergen immunotherapy (AIT). Clinical trials of OIT and SLIT show safety and efficacy for the treatment of food allergy.
4. Limitations of therapy are the risk of adverse reaction during therapy, impermanence of desensitization, and lengthy treatment period.
5. OIT and SLIT typically consist of three phases (screening, buildup, and maintenance). Some studies include a fourth phase (tolerance phase) to determine sustained unresponsiveness.
6. To address some of the limitations of OIT, adjuvants such as omalizumab and probiotics have been used along with OIT.
7. SLIT has a better safety profile than OIT as it is associated with fewer systemic reactions but is less efficacious. SLIT may be useful as initial treatment in highly sensitive individuals before OIT.

REFERENCES

1. Jackson KD, Howie LD, Akinbami LJ. Trends in allergic conditions among children: United States, 1997–2011. *NCHS Data Brief* 2013; 121: 1–8.
2. Nwaru BI, Hickstein L, Panesar SS, Roberts G, Muraro A, Sheikh A. Prevalence of common food allergies in Europe: A systematic review and meta-analysis. *Allergy* 2014; 69: 992–1007.
3. Osborne NJ, Koplin JJ, Martin PE et al. Prevalence of challenge-proven IgE-mediated food allergy using population-based sampling and predetermined challenge criteria in infants. *J Allergy Clin Immunol* 2011; 127: 668–676.
4. Rinaldi M, Harnack L, Oberg C, Schreiner P, St Sauver J, Travis LL. Peanut allergy diagnoses among children residing in Olmsted County, Minnesota. *J Allergy Clin Immunol* 2012; 130: 945–950.
5. Sicherer SH, Munoz-Furlong A, Godbold JH, Sampson HA. US prevalence of self-reported peanut, tree nut, and sesame allergy: 11-year follow-up. *J Allergy Clin Immunol* 2010; 125: 1322–1326.
6. Soller L, Ben-Shoshan M, Harrington DW et al. Overall prevalence of self-reported food allergy in Canada. *J Allergy Clin Immunol* 2012; 130: 986–988.
7. Gupta RS. Estimates of the distribution, determinants, and severity of food allergies among US adults. *JAMA Netw Open* 2019; 2(1): e185630.
8. Tang ML, Mullins RJ. Food allergy: Is prevalence increasing? *Intern Med J* 2017; 47: 256–261.
9. Kattan J. The prevalence and natural history of food allergy. *Curr Allergy Asthma Rep* 2016; 16: 47.

10. Gupta RS, Warren CM, Smith BM et al. The public health impact of parent-reported childhood food allergies in the United States. *Pediatrics* 2018; 142(6). pii: e20181235.

11. Hill DA, Grundmeier RW, Ram G, Spergel JM. The epidemiologic characteristics of healthcare provider-diagnosed eczema, asthma, allergic rhinitis, and food allergy in children: A retrospective cohort study. *BMC Pediatr* 2016; 16: 133.

12. Sicherer SH, Sampson HA. Food allergy: Epidemiology, pathogenesis, diagnosis, and treatment. *J Allergy Clin Immunol* 2014; 133: 291–307.

13. Sicherer SH, Noone SA, Munoz-Furlong A. The impact of childhood food allergy on quality of life. *Ann Allergy Asthma Immunol* 2001; 87: 461–464.

14. Clark S, Espinola J, Rudders SA, Banerji A, Camargo CA, Jr. Frequency of US emergency department visits for food-related acute allergic reactions. *J Allergy Clin Immunol* 2011; 127: 682–683.

15. Dyer AA, Lau CH, Smith TL, Smith BM, Gupta RS. Pediatric emergency department visits and hospitalizations due to food-induced anaphylaxis in Illinois. *Ann Allergy Asthma Immunol* 2015; 115: 56–62.

16. Boyce JA, Assa'ad A, Burks AW et al. Guidelines for the diagnosis and management of food allergy in the United States: Report of the NIAID-sponsored expert panel. *J Allergy Clin Immunol* 2010; 126: S1–S58.

17. Vander Leek TK, Liu AH, Stefanski K, Blacker B, Bock SA. The natural history of peanut allergy in young children and its association with serum peanut-specific IgE. *J Pediatr* 2000; 137: 749–755.

18. Chinthrajah RS, Hernandez JD, Boyd SD, Galli SJ, Nadeau KC. Molecular and cellular mechanisms of food allergy and food tolerance. *J Allergy Clin Immunol* 2016; 137: 984–997.

19. Berin MC. Pathogenesis of IgE-mediated food allergy. *Clin Exp Allergy* 2015; 45: 1483–1496.

20. Lozano-Ojalvo D, Berin C, Tordesillas L. Immune basis of allergic reactions to food. *J Investig Allergol Clin Immunol* 2019; 29(1): 1–14.

21. Yu W, Freeland DMH, Nadeau KC. Food allergy: Immune mechanisms, diagnosis and immunotherapy. *Nat Rev Immunol* 2016; 16: 751–765.

22. Sampath V, Tupa D, Graham MT, Chatila TA, Spergel JM, Nadeau KC. Deciphering the black box of food allergy mechanisms. *Ann Allergy Asthma Immunol* 2017; 118: 21–27.

23. Nelson HS, Lahr J, Rule R, Bock A, Leung D. Treatment of anaphylactic sensitivity to peanuts by immunotherapy with injections of aqueous peanut extract. *J Allergy Clin Immunol* 1997; 99: 744–751.

24. Gomes-Belo J, Hannachi F, Swan K, Santos AF. Advances in food allergy diagnosis. *Curr Pediatr Rev* 2018; 14: 139–149.

25. Sicherer SH, Sampson HA. Food allergy: A review and update on epidemiology, pathogenesis, diagnosis, prevention, and management. *J Allergy Clin Immunol* 2018; 141: 41–58.

26. Bird JA. Food oral immunotherapy is superior to food avoidance. *Ann Allergy Asthma Immunol* 2019; 122(6): 566–568.

27. Schofield A. A case of egg poisoning. *The Lancet* 1908; 171.

28. Palisade Group of Clinical Investigators, Vickery BP, Vereda A et al. AR101 Oral immunotherapy for peanut allergy. *N Engl J Med* 2018; 379: 1991–2001.

29. What does FDA regulate? 2018. https://www.fda.gov/aboutfda/transparency/basics/ucm194879.htm

30. Wood RA. Oral immunotherapy for food allergy. *J Investig Allergol Clin Immunol* 2017; 27: 151–159.

31. Freeland DMH, Manohar M, Andorf S, Hobson BD, Zhang W, Nadeau KC. Oral immunotherapy for food allergy. *Semin Immunol* 2017; 30: 36–44.

32. Hill DA, Spergel JM. The atopic march: Critical evidence and clinical relevance. *Ann Allergy Asthma Immunol* 2018; 120: 131–137.

33. Bluemchen K, Eiwegger T. Oral peanut immunotherapy—How much is too much? How much is enough? *Allergy* 2019; 74(2): 220–222.

34. Kulis M, Yue X, Guo R et al. High- and low-dose oral immunotherapy similarly suppress pro-allergic cytokines and basophil activation in young children. *Clin Exp Allergy* 2019; 49(2): 180–189.

35. Burks AW, Jones SM, Wood RA et al. Oral immunotherapy for treatment of egg allergy in children. *N Engl J Med* 2012; 367: 233–243.

36. Jones SM, Burks AW, Keet C et al. Long-term treatment with egg oral immunotherapy enhances sustained unresponsiveness that persists after cessation of therapy. *J Allergy Clin Immunol* 2016; 137: 1117–1127.e10.

37. Vickery BP, Scurlock AM, Kulis M et al. Sustained unresponsiveness to peanut in subjects who have completed peanut oral immunotherapy. *J Allergy Clin Immunol* 2014; 133: 468–475.e6.

38. Syed A, Garcia MA, Lyu SC et al. Peanut oral immunotherapy results in increased antigen-induced regulatory T-cell function and hypomethylation of forkhead box protein 3 (FOXP3). *J Allergy Clin Immunol* 2014; 133: 500–510.

39. Martorell A, De la Hoz B, Ibanez MD et al. Oral desensitization as a useful treatment in 2-year-old children with cow's milk allergy. *Clin Exp Allergy* 2011; 41: 1297–1304.

40. Burk CM, Dellon ES, Steele PH et al. Eosinophilic esophagitis during peanut oral immunotherapy with omalizumab. *J Allergy Clin Immunol Pract* 2017; 5: 498–501.

41. Atkins D, Kramer R, Capocelli K, Lovell M, Furuta GT. Eosinophilic esophagitis: The newest esophageal inflammatory disease. *Nat Rev Gastroenterol Hepatol* 2009; 6: 267–278.

42. Lucendo AJ, Arias A, Tenias JM. Relation between eosinophilic esophagitis and oral immunotherapy for food allergy: A systematic review with meta-analysis. *Ann Allergy Asthma Immunol* 2014; 113: 624–629.

43. Petroni D, Spergel JM. Eosinophilic esophagitis and symptoms possibly related to eosinophilic esophagitis in oral immunotherapy. *Ann Allergy Asthma Immunol* 2018; 120: 237–240.e4.

44. Wright BL, Fernandez-Becker NQ, Kambham N et al. Baseline gastrointestinal eosinophilia is common in oral immunotherapy subjects with IgE-mediated peanut allergy. *Front Immunol* 2018; 9: 2624.

45. Hill DA, Dudley JW, Spergel JM. The prevalence of eosinophilic esophagitis in pediatric patients with IgE-mediated food allergy. *J Allergy Clin Immunol Pract* 2017; 5: 369–375.

46. Labrosse R, Graham F, Des Roches A, Begin P. The use of omalizumab in food oral immunotherapy. *Arch Immunol Ther Exp (Warsz)* 2017; 65: 189–199.

47. Lieberman JA, Chehade M. Use of omalizumab in the treatment of food allergy and anaphylaxis. *Curr Allergy Asthma Rep* 2013; 13: 78–84.

48. Andorf S, Purington N, Block WM et al. Anti-IgE treatment with oral immunotherapy in multifood allergic participants: A double-blind, randomised, controlled trial. *Lancet Gastroenterol Hepatol* 2018; 3: 85–94.

49. Cervantes-Barragan L, Chai JN, Tianero MD et al. *Lactobacillus reuteri* induces gut intraepithelial CD4+CD8αα+ T cells. *Science* 2017; 357: 806–810.

50. Sujino T, London M, Hoytema van Konijnenburg DP et al. Tissue adaptation of regulatory and intraepithelial CD4+ T cells controls gut inflammation. *Science* 2016; 352: 1581–1586.

51. Tang ML, Ponsonby AL, Orsini F et al. Administration of a probiotic with peanut oral immunotherapy: A randomized trial. *J Allergy Clin Immunol* 2015; 135: 737–744.e8.

52. Chang HY, Nadeau KC. IL-4Rα inhibitor for atopic disease. *Cell* 2017; 170: 222.

53. Sastre J, Davila I. Dupilumab: A new paradigm for the treatment of allergic diseases. *J Investig Allergol Clin Immunol* 2018; 28: 139–150.

54. Leonard SA. Debates in allergy medicine: Baked milk and egg ingestion accelerates resolution of milk and egg allergy. *World Allergy Organ J* 2016; 9: 1.

55. Tari MG, Mancino M, Monti G. Efficacy of sublingual immunotherapy in patients with rhinitis and asthma due to house dust mite. A double-blind study. *Allergol Immunopathol (Madr)* 1990; 18: 277–284.

56. Gernez Y, Nowak-Wegrzyn A. Immunotherapy for food allergy: Are we there yet? *J Allergy Clin Immunol Pract* 2017; 5: 250–272.

57. Sindher S, Fleischer DM, Spergel JM. Advances in the treatment of food allergy: Sublingual and epicutaneous immunotherapy. *Immunol Allergy Clin North Am* 2016; 36: 39–54.

58. Feuille E, Nowak-Wegrzyn A. Allergen-specific immunotherapies for food allergy. *Allergy Asthma Immunol Res* 2018; 10: 189–206.

59. Akdis CA, Barlan IB, Bahceciler N, Akdis M. Immunological mechanisms of sublingual immunotherapy. *Allergy* 2006; 61(Suppl 81): 11–14.

60. De Boissieu D, Dupont C. Sublingual immunotherapy for cow's milk protein allergy: A preliminary report. *Allergy* 2006; 61: 1238–1239.

61. Keet CA, Frischmeyer-Guerrerio PA, Thyagarajan A et al. The safety and efficacy of sublingual and oral immunotherapy for milk allergy. *J Allergy Clin Immunol* 2012; 129: 448–455, 55.e1–5.

62. Kim EH, Bird JA, Kulis M et al. Sublingual immunotherapy for peanut allergy: Clinical and immunologic evidence of desensitization. *J Allergy Clin Immunol* 2011; 127: 640–646.e1.

63. Burks AW, Wood RA, Jones SM et al. Sublingual immunotherapy for peanut allergy: Long-term follow-up of a randomized multicenter trial. *J Allergy Clin Immunol* 2015; 135: 1240–1248.e1–3.

64. Gomez F, Bogas G, Gonzalez M et al. The clinical and immunological effects of Pru p 3 sublingual immunotherapy on peach and peanut allergy in patients with systemic reactions. *Clin Exp Allergy* 2017; 47: 339–350.

65. Enrique E, Pineda F, Malek T et al. Sublingual immunotherapy for hazelnut food allergy: A randomized, double-blind, placebo-controlled study with a standardized hazelnut extract. *J Allergy Clin Immunol* 2005; 116: 1073–1079.

66. Schneider LC, Rachid R, LeBovidge J, Blood E, Mittal M, Umetsu DT. A pilot study of omalizumab to facilitate rapid oral desensitization in high-risk peanut-allergic patients. *J Allergy Clin Immunol* 2013; 132: 1368–1374.

67. Fleischer DM, Burks AW, Vickery BP et al. Sublingual immunotherapy for peanut allergy: A randomized, double-blind, placebo-controlled multicenter trial. *J Allergy Clin Immunol* 2013; 131: 119–127.e1–7.

68. Mempel M, Rakoski J, Ring J, Ollert M. Severe anaphylaxis to kiwi fruit: Immunologic changes related to successful sublingual allergen immunotherapy. *J Allergy Clin Immunol* 2003; 111: 1406–1409.

69. Lawrence MG, Steinke JW, Borish L. Basic science for the clinician: Mechanisms of sublingual and subcutaneous immunotherapy. *Ann Allergy Asthma Immunol* 2016; 117: 138–142.

70. Wood RA. Food allergen immunotherapy: Current status and prospects for the future. *J Allergy Clin Immunol* 2016; 137: 973–982.

71. Le UH, Burks AW. Oral and sublingual immunotherapy for food allergy. *World Allergy Organ J* 2014; 7: 35.

72. Fernandez-Rivas M, Garrido Fernandez S, Nadal JA et al. Randomized double-blind, placebo-controlled trial of sublingual immunotherapy with a Pru p 3 quantified peach extract. *Allergy* 2009; 64: 876–883.

73. Miehlke S, Alpan O, Schroder S, Straumann A. Induction of eosinophilic esophagitis by sublingual pollen immunotherapy. *Case Rep Gastroenterol* 2013; 7: 363–368.

74. Smeekens JM, Bagley K, Kulis M. Tree nut allergies: Allergen homology, cross-reactivity, and implications for therapy. *Clin Exp Allergy* 2018; 48: 762–772.

75. Perez-Rangel I, Rodriguez Del Rio P, Escudero C, Sanchez-Garcia S, Sanchez-Hernandez JJ, Ibanez MD. Efficacy and safety of high-dose rush oral immunotherapy in persistent egg allergic children: A randomized clinical trial. *Ann Allergy Asthma Immunol* 2017; 118: 356–364.e3.

76. Akashi M, Yasudo H, Narita M et al. Randomized controlled trial of oral immunotherapy for egg allergy in Japanese patients. *Pediatr Int* 2017; 59: 534–539.

77. Escudero C, Rodriguez Del Rio P, Sanchez-Garcia S et al. Early sustained unresponsiveness after short-course egg oral immunotherapy: A randomized controlled study in egg-allergic children. *Clin Exp Allergy* 2015; 45: 1833–1843.

78. Caminiti L, Pajno GB, Crisafulli G et al. Oral immunotherapy for egg allergy: A double-blind placebo-controlled study, with post-desensitization follow-up. *J Allergy Clin Immunol Pract* 2015; 3: 532–539.

79. Vickery BP, Pons L, Kulis M, Steele P, Jones SM, Burks AW. Individualized IgE-based dosing of egg oral immunotherapy and the development of tolerance. *Ann Allergy Asthma Immunol* 2010; 105: 444–450.

80. Buchanan AD, Green TD, Jones SM et al. Egg oral immunotherapy in nonanaphylactic children with egg allergy. *J Allergy Clin Immunol* 2007; 119: 199–205.

81. Takahashi M, Soejima K, Taniuchi S et al. Oral immunotherapy combined with omalizumab for high-risk cow's milk allergy: A randomized controlled trial. *Sci Rep* 2017; 7: 17453.

82. Wood RA, Kim JS, Lindblad R et al. A randomized, double-blind, placebo-controlled study of omalizumab combined with oral immunotherapy for the treatment of cow's milk allergy. *J Allergy Clin Immunol* 2016; 137: 1103–1110.e11.

83. Nadeau KC, Schneider LC, Hoyte L, Borras I, Umetsu DT. Rapid oral desensitization in combination with omalizumab therapy in patients with cow's milk allergy. *J Allergy Clin Immunol* 2011; 127: 1622–1624.

84. Pajno GB, Caminiti L, Ruggeri P et al. Oral immunotherapy for cow's milk allergy with a weekly up-dosing regimen: A randomized single-blind controlled study. *Ann Allergy Asthma Immunol* 2010; 105: 376–381.

85. Begin P, Dominguez T, Wilson SP et al. Phase 1 results of safety and tolerability in a rush oral immunotherapy protocol to multiple foods using Omalizumab. *Allergy Asthma Clin Immunol* 2014; 10: 7.

86. Begin P, Winterroth LC, Dominguez T et al. Safety and feasibility of oral immunotherapy to multiple allergens for food allergy. *Allergy Asthma Clin Immunol* 2014; 10: 1.

87. Bird JA, Spergel JM, Jones SM et al. Efficacy and safety of AR101 in oral immunotherapy for peanut allergy: Results of ARC001, a randomized, double-blind, placebo-controlled phase 2 clinical trial. *J Allergy Clin Immunol Pract* 2018; 6: 476–485.e3.

88. Fauquert JL, Michaud E, Pereira B et al. PITA Group Peanut Gastro-Intestinal Delivery Oral Immunotherapy in Adolescents: Results of the build-up phase of a randomized, double-blind, placebo-controlled trial (PITA study). *Clin Exp Allergy* 2018; 48: 862–874.

89. Blumchen K, Trendelenburg V, Ahrens F et al. Efficacy, safety, and quality of life in a multicenter, randomized, placebo-controlled trial of low-dose peanut oral immunotherapy in children with peanut allergy. *J Allergy Clin Immunol Pract* 2019; 7(2): 479–491.

90. MacGinnitie AJ, Rachid R, Gragg H et al. Omalizumab facilitates rapid oral desensitization for peanut allergy. *J Allergy Clin Immunol* 2016; 139: 873–881.e8.

91. Anagnostou K, Islam S, King Y et al. Assessing the efficacy of oral immunotherapy for the desensitisation of peanut allergy in children (STOP II): A phase 2 randomised controlled trial. *Lancet* 2014; 383: 1297–1304.

92. Narisety SD, Frischmeyer-Guerrerio PA, Keet CA et al. A randomized, double-blind, placebo-controlled pilot study of sublingual versus oral immunotherapy for the treatment of peanut allergy. *J Allergy Clin Immunol* 2015; 135: 1275–1282.e1–6.

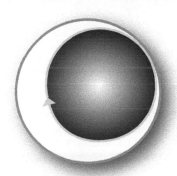

29 Indications for and preparing and administering Hymenoptera vaccines

David B.K. Golden
Johns Hopkins University

Farnaz Tabatabaian
University of South Florida Morsani College of Medicine

Ulrich Müller-Gierok (Retired)

Richard F. Lockey
University of South Florida Morsani College of Medicine

CONTENTS

29.1 INTRODUCTION

Insect stings, especially by Hymenoptera of the families *Apidae* (the honeybee and the bumblebee), *Vespidae* (wasps, yellow jackets, and hornets) with the species *Vespula, Dolichovespula, Vespa,* and *Polistes*), and in some regions also *Formicidae/Myrmicidae* (the ants), are one of the major causes of severe, generalized, IgE-mediated hypersensitivity reactions, which may be fatal. According to the registered data of the Swiss Statistical Department, 148 individuals died from Hymenoptera stings in Switzerland between 1962 and 2010, an average of 2.9 per year. Extrapolation of the Swiss data (population 7.8 million) to the European Union (population about 500 million), these data indicate about 200 yearly fatalities from Hymenoptera stings in the European Union. Government statistics

423

in the United States show at least 40 deaths each year from insect stings, although it is likely that many others are not reported.

The first attempts at immunotherapy for subjects allergic to Hymenoptera stings were made at the end of the 1920s. Insect venom or venom sac vaccines were used at first, but the high frequency of side effects with these vaccines, and the report of the successful treatment of a beekeeper with whole-body extract (WBE) of bees, led to the worldwide use of WBE. The results of immunotherapy with these preparations were favorable in uncontrolled studies [1,2]. It was only in the late 1960s and 1970s of the last century that venoms were shown to be superior to whole-body extracts for diagnosis, and controlled studies documented the superiority of venoms over whole-body vaccines for immunotherapy for individuals allergic to Hymenoptera venom [3,4]. Venoms obtained by electrostimulation or by venom sac extraction were commercially introduced in 1979 and are now used worldwide successfully for immunotherapy of subjects allergic to stings by *Apidae* and *Vespidae*. Venom preparations are as yet not commercially available for ants (*Formicidae, Myrmicidae*). Various aspects of immunotherapy for Hymenoptera sting hypersensitivity are reviewed in the following sections. The last section considers new approaches to venom immunotherapy. Details of the taxonomy of stinging Hymenoptera and their venom allergens are outlined in Chapter 18.

29.2 INDICATIONS

29.2.1 History

The indications for venom immunotherapy (VIT) include two factors: a history of systemic allergic reaction (SAR) to a sting and positive diagnostic tests [5,6]. The history is especially important because diagnostic tests with venoms are positive in 10%–20% of asymptomatic individuals. There is an absolute need to correlate the history with the test results [7–9].

SAR to stings consist of any one or more of the signs and symptoms of anaphylaxis or may be limited to cutaneous manifestations; such cutaneous systemic reactions (cSR) are more common in children (60%) than in adults (15%) [10]. Respiratory or cardiovascular symptoms are present in up to 85% of adults, although individual symptoms are present in only a portion of those (e.g., hypotension/dizziness in 30%–40%, throat/respiratory in 40%–50%). By contrast, hypotension/dizziness is present in only 10% of children, but throat/respiratory symptoms are present in 40%. It is sometimes difficult to be certain whether symptoms are truly consistent with a SAR because they may result from anxiety, pain, or toxic effects of stings, especially when several stings occur at the same time. It is most helpful when objective signs of a SAR (or anaphylaxis) are noted, e.g., generalized urticaria, angioedema, documented hypotension, wheezing, reduced air flow, or oxygen desaturation. The severity of a SAR is one of the most important factors determining the need for VIT, the duration of treatment, and the risk of adverse reactions to injections [11]. Although identification of the stinging insect by subjects and physicians is unreliable, the identity of the culprit insect is important because honeybee venom allergy is associated with greater risks and less reliable treatment efficacy [12]. In the absence of a history of a sting-induced SAR, sensitization by an asymptomatic sting is reported to be associated with a 5%–17% chance of a SAR to a future sting but is not considered an indication for VIT, especially since

asymptomatic sensitivity is transient in many cases [8,9]. For this reason, venom allergy testing and treatment are not recommended when requested by some individuals without history of SAR, out of fear alone, e.g., because a family member has had a very severe or even fatal reaction to a sting.

Contraindications for VIT are the same as for inhalant allergen immunotherapy but are relative in nature because of the lifesaving potential of therapy. The relative contraindications include severe immunodeficiency, autoimmune and neoplastic diseases, and chronic infections. Elderly individuals with cardiovascular disease are at increased risk to develop severe or even fatal sting reactions. Treatment with β-blockers may increase the severity of a SAR when patients are re-stung. Many patients, by necessity, are on a β-blocker and VIT is often indicated in these subjects [13]. Although one large study found that angiotensin-converting enzyme (ACE) inhibitor therapy is associated with an increased risk of severe anaphylaxis [14], another study found no such correlation [15].

VIT should not be started during pregnancy unless under extenuating circumstances, such as a beekeeper or a beekeeper's spouse, but continuation of maintenance VIT during pregnancy is thought to be safe [16]. Sting reactions such as Henoch-Schöenlein syndrome, vasculitis, acute disseminated encephalomyelitis, or interstitial nephritis are not IgE mediated and should not be treated by VIT, while subjects who developed a cerebrovascular accident or a myocardial infarction during anaphylaxis and have positive tests should not be excluded from such therapy [17,18].

29.2.2 Diagnostic testing: Skin tests and *in vitro* serum IgE

The decision to begin venom immunotherapy requires confirmation of allergic sensitivity to venom allergens by positive venom skin tests or detection of venom-specific IgE antibodies in the serum (Table 29.1).

The standard skin test utilizes the intradermal test technique with commercially available Hymenoptera venom preparations. For Hymenoptera venom testing, prick tests at 0.1–100 μg/mL may

Table 29.1 Clinical recommendations based on history of sting reactions and results of venom skin or serum IgE test

Reaction to previous sting	Skin or serum test	Risk of systemic reaction	Clinical advice
No reaction	Positive	5%–15% (<3% anaphylaxis)	Avoidance
Large local	Positive	5%–10% (<3% anaphylaxis)	Avoidance
Cutaneous only	Positive	10%–15% (<3% anaphylaxis)	Avoidance
Anaphylaxis (respiratory, cardiovascular)	Positive	40%–75%[a]	Venom immunotherapy
	Negative	2%–5%	Repeat skin or serum IgE test

[a] According to controlled studies.

be used initially for subjects with a history of a severe SAR [5,19]. Aqueous venom preparations are used for intradermal tests, usually beginning with concentrations of 0.001–0.01 µg/mL and increasing, as necessary, to 1.0 µg/mL to find the minimum concentration causing a positive reaction. When desired, intradermal skin tests can be safely performed using only the 1.0 mcg/mL concentration (without prior testing at lower concentrations) [20,21]. Honeybee venom is somewhat more irritating and can induce weak positive reactions in nonallergic individuals. Yellow jacket (*Vespula*) venom may cause false-positive reactions at the 10 µg/mL concentration in up to 10% of nonallergic subjects.

Most subjects with a convincing history of insect allergy have positive venom tests, but some are skin-test negative (Table 29.2). Negative skin tests can be due to loss of sensitivity and can also occur in up to 50% during the refractory period of 4–6 weeks following a sting reaction. They may also result from the use of concomitant antihistamines and certain neuroleptic and antidepressant medications. When there is a history of a severe SAR (anaphylaxis) and venom skin tests are negative, *in vitro* tests for venom-specific IgE antibodies should be obtained, and the patient should continue avoidance precautions. In many cases like this, the *in vitro* test may be positive. Some cases of apparent sting-induced SARs are thought to be non-IgE mediated, which would account for the negative *in vivo* and *in vitro* test results. Mast cell disorders should be suspected in such cases.

The detection *in vitro* of allergen-specific IgE antibodies is useful. A high level of venom-specific IgE is usually diagnostic but must be correlated with the history. A low level of venom-IgE is more difficult to interpret. Even a very low level of venom-IgE can be associated with near-fatal anaphylaxis. The venom skin test and *in vitro* test results may not correlate as the *in vitro* test results are negative in approximately 15% of skin-test positive subjects [22–25]. Therefore, skin tests are preferred clinically for their greater sensitivity. The converse is also true: approximately 5%–10% of skin-test negative subjects have a positive *in vitro* test. Therefore, European allergists/immunologists recommend skin testing and estimation of venom-specific IgE in all individuals with a history of a SAR. If both tests are negative in the presence of a strong history, cellular tests like CAST (cellular antigen stimulation test) or BAT (basophil activation test), although more expensive, may be useful [26,27]. A positive result with these tests may also point to a non-IgE-mediated mast cell activation mechanism. Neither the degree of skin-test sensitivity nor the titer of specific IgE correlate reliably with the severity of the SAR. Subjects who have had only large local reactions may have very high levels of sensitivity of both skin and *in vitro* tests but are a very low risk for a SAR, whereas some subjects who have had an abrupt and near-fatal anaphylactic reaction have only weak skin-test or serologic positivity. In fact, almost 25% of subjects presenting for evaluation of a SAR to stings are skin-test

Table 29.2 Diagnosis of insect allergy in subjects with a positive history of systemic reaction

Skin-test positive	68%
Skin-test negative/serum IgE positive	14%
Skin-test negative/serum IgE negative	18%
Sting challenge negative	17%
Sting challenge positive	1%

positive only at the 1.0 µg/mL concentration, demonstrating the importance of testing with the full diagnostic range of venoms. Again, these points emphasize the importance of the history in making the correct diagnosis, assessing prognosis, and instituting appropriate treatment.

Another diagnostic option is a supervised live sting challenge. The history and test results help identify subjects at high risk, but even subjects with previous severe SARs only have a 50%–75% chance of reacting to a future sting. The sting challenge helps select subjects who will most likely have another SAR to a field sting [28]. However, even a negative sting challenge does not rule out future reactions, because 20% of subjects who did not react to one challenge react to a repeat challenge sting [29]. Others consider the diagnostic sting challenge to be unnecessary and even unethical and recommend it only as a test to evaluate the efficacy of VIT [30].

Some subjects with positive venom skin tests have a low risk of a SAR, including those with no history of allergic sting reaction (asymptomatic sensitization), with large local reactions, and who had a cSR. Subsequent stings usually cause no SAR or a reaction that tends to be equal to, or less severe than the previous reactions. In both children and adults with a cSR, less than 3% had a more severe reaction to subsequent stings [28,31,32]. In a 15- to 20-year follow-up study of field stings in children, 87% of those with a history of cSR who were stung had no SAR, 7% had another mild cSR, and 6% a moderate SAR. None had a more severe SAR (anaphylaxis) [31]. The authors pointed out several significant types of selection bias in their survey and estimated that the true risk of anaphylaxis is less than 3% in children with a cSR. The two prospective studies of sting challenge in adults that included subjects with cSR showed a similarly low risk of anaphylaxis. Therefore, VIT is generally not recommended for subjects with cSR. However, it may be considered for highly exposed individuals or those with a severely impaired quality of life that does not always improve with a prescription for an epinephrine auto-injector and an admonition to carry it with them [33].

Individuals who have positive venom skin tests but have never developed a SAR from a sting have a relatively low risk of a SAR to a future sting [8,9]. Most subjects with large local reactions have positive venom skin tests. Children and adults with a large local but no SAR have a 4%–10% chance of a subsequent SAR, but less than half are severe [34]. Therapy is not usually recommended for subjects with a history of a large local reaction, but such therapy may be helpful in heavily exposed individuals such as farmers, gardeners, or beekeepers and their families. There is evidence from a controlled study that VIT effectively reduces the size and duration of large local reactions [35].

Subjects with systemic mastocytosis are at even higher risk to develop a severe SAR (anaphylaxis) [36–38]. Several studies indicate that reactions with hypotension are associated with an elevated baseline serum tryptase (>11.4 ng/mL) in up to 25% of such patients, perhaps as a result of the increased risk for life-threatening sting reactions that is associated with an increased number of mast cells [39–41]. Therefore, a routine baseline serum tryptase test is recommended for all subjects with a SAR. With an elevated baseline serum tryptase, especially above 20 ng/mL, the patient should be evaluated for systemic mastocytosis. Patients with known mastocytosis should be tested for venom allergy, and when positive, should be treated with VIT, even if they have no history of a sting-induced SAR [38]. Patients with elevated baseline serum tryptase but no symptoms or diagnosis of mastocytosis have not been fully characterized but are considered to have abnormally high risk similar to those with mastocytosis. Mastocytosis cannot be excluded without bone marrow biopsy as it is often asymptomatic in these patients.

29.2.3 Selection of venoms

The selection of venom vaccines for immunotherapy is dependent on the venom skin-test reaction and presence of serum-specific IgE antibodies. North American allergists/immunologists recommend that all venoms resulting in positive tests be included for VIT because preventing future sting reactions is not possible without specific therapy. Some investigators recommend treatment only with the venom of the suspected insect culprit [42]. When vespids are involved, the most common practice is to treat with *Vespula* venom alone or, in North America, with the mixed vespid venom preparation. It contains equal parts of yellow jacket (*Vespula* spp.), yellow hornet (*Dolichovespula arenaria*) and white-faced hornet (*Dolichovespula maculata*). The *Dolichovespula* venoms are not available in Europe. Although *Dolichovespula* are by no means rare, they are responsible for only a small percentage of vespid stings. These insects do not forage on human food and, therefore, almost exclusively sting in the proximity of their nests. The same is true for the European hornet, *Vespa crabro*. Moreover, European *Dolichovespula*, in contrast to American *D. maculata*, only can be distinguished from *Vespula* by those trained to do so. Finally, *in vitro* studies demonstrate ample cross-reactivity among venoms of *Vespula*, *Dolichovespula*, and *Vespa*. Therefore, vespid-allergic European patients are treated with *Vespula* venom alone, effective in more than 95% of subjects.

The skin test is also positive to wasp (*Polistes*) venoms in at least 50% of vespid-allergic subjects. When positive, it is usually included in therapy as a separate injection, at least in areas where *Polistes* is prevalent, such as in the U.S. Gulf states and the European Mediterranean countries. Therapy with *Vespula* or mixed vespid venoms protects against *Polistes* stings, but this only occurs in subjects whose *Polistes*-specific IgE antibodies completely cross-react with *Vespula* venom as assessed by the degree of radioallergosorbent test (RAST) inhibition [43].

Dual positivity of diagnostic tests with *Vespula* and honeybee venom is commonly observed in areas where bee stings are as frequent as vespid stings. The history sometimes helps to identify the culprit insect, since vespid stings are less frequent in spring and most species do not, in contrast to the honeybee, leave the stinger in the skin. However, in the United States, *V. maculifrons* is one of the most common causes of severe sting reactions and is known to leave the stinger in 30%–50% of cases [44]. The limited cross-reactivity based on peptide analysis between protein allergens of *Vespula* and honeybee venoms is largely confined to hyaluronidase and dipeptidyl-peptidase. Double positivity is often due to cross-reactive carbohydrate determinants (CCDs), which are present not only in insect venoms but also in various plants and pollens and are probably of no clinical relevance [45]. When tests are positive with the two venoms, both should be included for VIT, unless complete cross-reactivity can be demonstrated by serum IgE measurement with whole venoms and CCDs. Component-resolved diagnosis (CRD) utilizes recombinant species-specific allergens without CCDs. CRD with Api m 1 for bee venom and Ves v 5 for *Vespula* venom is helpful to distinguish cross-reactivity versus true double sensitization [46–48]. The accuracy of CRD to identify cross-reactivity distinct from dual sensitization is limited but can be improved by adding

additional relevant recombinant species-specific allergens like Ves v 1 and Api m 10 [49,50]. There is not yet a similar option to distinguish true dual sensitization to yellow jacket and Polistes wasp from cross-reactivity. However, a RAST inhibition test can be helpful for this purpose [43]. This test can be ordered from the DACI Reference Laboratory (Robert Hamilton, PhD, Director).

29.3 EFFICACY, SAFETY, AND MONITORING OF VENOM IMMUNOTHERAPY

The recommended maintenance dose is 100 μg of venom, both in children and adults. This dose originally was believed to be equivalent to two stings. This is true for honeybee stings but may be closer to 10 *Vespula* stings. Doses lower than 100 μg are not reliably effective in adults [51]. Immunotherapy with honeybee venom gives full protection in 80%–85% of cases, whereas immunotherapy with *Vespula* venom is 95%–98% effective [12]. When treatment with 100 μg is not effective, subjects may be given a higher dose such as 200 μg [52]. Studies also suggest that 50 mcg may be an effective maintenance dose in children [53,54].

Venom immunotherapy is safe. SARs were expected to be more frequent or severe when VIT was first introduced; however, that has not been confirmed by decades of experience. The incidence of adverse reactions to venom is similar to that reported for inhalant allergen immunotherapy [55]. For unexplained reasons, SARs are considerably more frequent with honeybee venom [12]. Systemic symptoms occur in 5%–15% of subjects on vespid venoms and 20%–40% on honeybee venom, most often during the first weeks of treatment, regardless of the immunotherapy protocol used. Most reactions are mild. In the unusual case of recurrent venom-induced SARs, therapy may be streamlined using the most appropriate single venom given in divided doses, 30 minutes apart (cluster immunotherapy). Rush VIT, using a 2- to 3-day regimen, is effective in subjects with recurrent SARs to VIT, and in the few who continue to have reactions, omalizumab treatment is effective in facilitating maintenance treatment [56,57]. Premedication with antihistamines reduces systemic side effects and may even improve efficacy [58]. Premedication with montelukast may also reduce large local reactions to VIT [59]. SAR side effects occur more frequently in subjects with an elevated baseline serum tryptase and systemic mastocytosis [60]. Large local reactions, which may be larger (>10 cm) than are generally accepted as a side effect from inhalant allergen immunotherapy, occur in up to 50% of subjects, especially during updosing (20–50 μg range). Large local reactions, however, are not predictive of a SAR to subsequent injections and should not prevent achieving the maintenance target dose of VIT.

Annual visits with the allergist/immunologist are indicated to review the treatment plan and assure that there are no new medications that would possibly augment a SAR and to review outcomes of therapy. There is no need for annual skin or blood tests, although repeat skin tests every few years to identify subjects with negative tests is recommended. If all evidence of venom-specific IgE disappears, it may be possible to stop VIT. The venom-specific IgE levels and skin-test sensitivity usually increase during the first months of therapy, return to baseline after 12 months, and then steadily decline during VIT maintenance. This decline continues even after a sting or after therapy is discontinued (Figure 29.1) [61]. Less than 20% of VIT patients become skin-test negative after

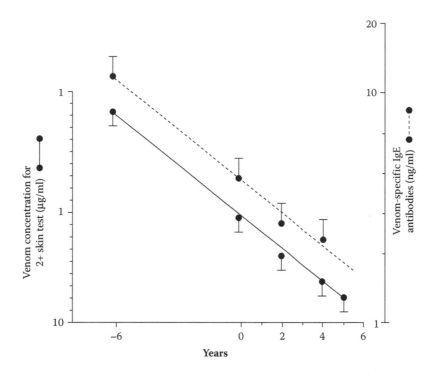

Figure 29.1 Mean venom skin test sensitivity (concentration in µg/mL for 2 or more reactions) and venom-specific IgE antibody level (in ng/mL) shown before venom immunotherapy (time, −6 years), after a mean of 6 years of treatment (time 0), and 2, 4, and 5 years after stopping therapy. (From Golden DBK et al. Discontinuing venom immunotherapy: Outcome after five years. *J Allergy Clin Immunol* 1996; 97: 579; with permission.)

5 years; however, 50%–60% become negative after 7–10 years [62]. Specific IgE may persist at very low levels even when venom skin tests become negative [63].

Venom-specific IgG antibodies, especially IgG4, are high in beekeepers, and passive immunotherapy with beekeeper γ-globulin protects bee venom-specific individuals against sting-induced SARs [64]. Assays for venom-specific IgG correlate with clinical protection but cannot accurately predict the outcome of stings in every individual. The test may be used to confirm protective levels after initiating VIT and subsequently to verify that the venom-IgG level remains adequate when the patient is treated at longer maintenance intervals. In one study, the IgG level of greater than 3 µg/mL was considered protective during the first 4 years of maintenance therapy, but protection became independent of the IgG after 4 years of treatment, presumably because of other protective mechanisms that come into play [65]. Venom immunotherapy is associated with profound changes in T-cell reactivity to venom stimulation in venom-allergic subjects, with a shift from a TH2 to a TH1 or TH0 pattern and induction of IL-10 producing T-regulatory cells [66].

29.4 IMMUNOTHERAPY PROTOCOLS

The starting dose of VIT is between 0.001 and 1.0 µg, injected subcutaneously. The recommended maintenance dose is 100 µg of venom protein, corresponding to two bee stings and 5–10 *Vespula* stings [5,6,67]. Higher maintenance doses (200 µg or more) are recommended for beekeepers [68], who may be stung by several insects at the same time, as well as in treatment failures [52]. The success rate increases with these higher maintenance doses.

A number of protocols are utilized for the buildup phase, some of which are summarized in Table 29.3 (conventional,

cluster, rush, or ultrarush protocols) [69–72]. However, there is no consistent definition of these regimens among the published studies. The consensus is that the 100 mcg maintenance dose is achieved in a period of months with the conventional, weeks for the modified-rush or cluster, days for rush, and hours with the ultrarush regimens. Many allergists/immunologists in Europe use aluminum hydroxide adsorbed venom for conventional protocols, while others use aqueous preparations for the buildup with accelerated protocols and then change to aluminum hydroxide adsorbed venoms, which have a comparable efficacy to aqueous venoms but are somewhat safer for maintenance VIT [73]. Only aqueous preparations are available in the United States. Rush and ultrarush protocols result in more rapid protection and therefore are recommended in highly exposed at-risk individuals, especially during the height of the Hymenoptera season. Moreover, the number of visits during the buildup phase is greatly reduced, which is a significant advantage in locales where extended travel is needed to access specialized medical care. However, the side effects are higher with the most rapid buildup protocols, especially in individuals allergic to bee venom [12], and with high cumulative daily dose protocols [69]. Ultrarush regimens carry more risk of a SAR, but 3-day vespid regimens appear to be as safe as a 9-week regimen [70]. The interval between injections is extended to 4 weeks in the first year and to 6–8 weeks during the second year of immunotherapy, if VIT is tolerated. A longer interval is not recommended for subjects allergic to honeybee venom since beekeepers with less than 10 stings a year develop a SAR most frequently [68]. With *Vespula* VIT, the maintenance interval may be increased to 12 weeks after 4 years of treatment. The buildup phase of VIT should usually be performed by a specialist; however, injections can be continued by general physicians once the maintenance is tolerated and achieved.

Table 29.3 Treatment protocols for venom immunotherapy

Protocol					Dose in µg venom	
Day	Hour	Ultrarush	Rush	Cluster	Conventional	Al-hydroxide adsorbed
1	0	0.1	0.01	0.001	0.01	0.02
	0.5	1	0.1	0.01	0.1	
	1	10	1	0.1		
	1.5	20				
	2.5	30	2			
	3.5	40				
2	0		4			
	1		8			
	2		10			
	3		20			
3	0		40			
	1		60			
	2		80			
4	0		100			
8	0		100	1	1	0.04
	1			5	2	
	2			10		
15	0	50	100	20	4	0.08
	1	50		30	8	
22	0	100		50	10	0.2
	1			50	20	
29			100	100	40	0.4
36				100	60	0.8
43		100	100		80	2
50					100	4
57					100	6
64				100		8
71		100	100		100	10
78						20
85					100	40
92				100		60
99		100	100			80
106					100	100

Note: Further injections of the maintenance dose of 100 mg every 4 weeks during the first year, every 6 weeks during further years of venom allergen-specific immunotherapy.

29.5 DURATION OF VENOM IMMUNOTHERAPY

When VIT was introduced in 1979, the recommendation was to continue treatment for life, or at least until both skin- and venom-specific IgE tests become negative. However, even after prolonged VIT, only a small proportion of subjects develop negative tests, and VIT compliance often decreases [61,74].

A number of studies address the protection rate after stopping VIT. In one study, the reaction to a sting challenge (CH) 1–3 years after discontinuation resulted in continued protection in 83%–100% of subjects. Results are somewhat more favorable in individuals allergic to *Vespula* versus bee venom and in children versus adults (Table 29.4) [75].

Long-term protection for up to 13 years after discontinuing VIT (Table 29.5) is analyzed in five studies [61–63,76,77]. Reisman observed relapses following a field sting for up to more than 5 years after discontinuing VIT in 10 of 113 (9%) mostly *Vespula* venom–allergic subjects [77]. Golden followed 74 predominantly *Vespula* venom–allergic subjects for 5 years after stopping VIT of at least 5 years duration with a sting challenge every year (29 subjects), every second year (25 subjects), or only after 2 years (20 subjects) [61]. Seven (9.5%) developed at least one generalized mild SAR. The same group (51) observed a SAR to a field sting in 5 of 26 (19%) subjects who were stung (out of 125 total) when followed up to 7 years after VIT, and some of these reactions were severe [62]. Lerch reported on 358 subjects up to 7 years after stopping successful VIT [76]. Two-hundred were reexposed by either a field sting or a challenge, and 25 (12.5%) developed a SAR. Fourteen developed a cSR, while 8 had respiratory symptoms, and 3 had cardiovascular symptoms; SARs occurred only after the second sting after stopping VIT in 8 of the 11 subjects with respiratory or cardiovascular symptoms. These three studies found relapses to be somewhat more frequent than earlier, shorter, follow-up studies. Still, the great majority, 80% or more, remain protected when restung up to 13 years after VIT is discontinued. Of note is that the chance of a reaction to each sting is unpredictable and can occur with one sting and not another. Patients who have several stings during the 5–10 years after stopping treatment have more chances that one of those stings will cause a

Table 29.4 Prospective studies with sting provocation test after stopping venom immunotherapy of short duration (1–3 years)

Author	Number of patients	Insect	Sting challenge (CH) After years	Number with SAR (%)
Urbanek (60)	29	Honey bee	1	1 (3)
(mostly children)	14		2	2 (14)
Golden (61)	29	m *Vespula*	1	0
Müller (62)	86	Honeybee	1	15 (17)
Haugaard (63)	25	*Vespula*	2	0
Keating (64)	51	m *Vespula*	1	2 (4)
Van Halteren (65)	75	*Vespula*	1–3	6 (8)

Abbreviations: CH, sting challenge; m *Vespula*, mostly *Vespula*; SAR, systemic allergic reaction.

Table 29.5 Long-term protection after discontinuation of venom immunotherapy

Author	Patients	Insect	Observation Years after stop	Reexposure	SAR (%)
Reisman (66)	113	mV	1–5 or more	FS	10 (9)
Golden (50)	74	mV	1–5	CH	7 (9.5)
Golden (51)	26	mV	3–7	FS	5 (19)
Golden (52)		mV	3–13	FS	
Lerch (67)	120	B	3–7	FS/CH	19 (15.8)
	80	V	3–7	FS/CH	6 (7.5)

Abbreviations: B, honeybee; CH, sting challenge; FS, field sting; mV, mostly *Vespula*; SAR, systemic allergic reaction; V, *Vespula*.

SAR. For this reason, the cumulative relapse rate (SAR after stopping VIT) was more than 17% [63].

A number of risk factors for a Hymenoptera sting induced SAR recurrence following discontinuation of VIT include the following:

Age: Children generally have a more favorable prognosis than adults, both without VIT and after discontinuing VIT [10]. Urbanek [75] saw relapses in only 3% of children allergic to bee venom (BV), whereas Müller [78] observed 17% in 86 mostly adult subjects after BV-immunotherapy. Lerch recorded 8.3% relapses in 24 children as compared to 13.1% in 176 adults who were reexposed up to 7 years after stopping VIT [76]. Golden reported sustained unresponsiveness in 83% of adults and 95% of children [10,63].

Insect: Analysis of the results presented in Table 29.5 as well as the recurrence rates after VIT reported by Lerch of 7.5% for *Vespula* venom and 15.8% for bee venom–treated subjects indicate a higher risk of relapse in subjects allergic to bee versus *Vespula* venom [76]. The reason for this difference is not clear [12,30].

Severity of pretreatment reaction: Relapses were observed in 5 (4.1%) of 123 with mild but 38 (14.5%) of 263 with severe pretreatment SAR ($X^2 = 9.128$, $p < .01$) in four prospective studies involving 386 subjects [76,77,79,80]. In addition, there is also a higher risk that a recurring reaction after stopping VIT in these subjects will be more severe than in those with milder pretreatment reactions.

Safety and efficacy of VIT: Subjects who develop SARs to VIT injections have a relapse risk of 38%, whereas those who do not have a relapse risk of 7% [81]. Similarly, incomplete protection with a re-sting during VIT is associated with an increased risk of relapse [61].

Duration of VIT: The risk of a relapse seems to be reduced with more prolonged VIT. Only 4.8% of 82 subjects with a VIT duration of 50 months or more, as opposed to 17.8% of 118 with a VIT duration of 33–49 months, developed SARs when re-stung after discontinuation ($X^2 = 7.382$; $p < .01$) [76]. VIT for 5 years gave greater suppression of venom-IgE and lower relapse rate than 3 years [80].

Elevated basal serum tryptase, mastocytosis: Insect venom allergy in patients with urticaria pigmentosa and systemic mastocytosis is most often associated with a severe SAR or anaphylaxis [38,39,82]. Two female patients with urticaria pigmentosa and *Vespula* venom sensitivity died from a re-sting 1.3 and 9 years after stopping venom immunotherapy [83]. One additional fatal sting reaction occurred in a patient with systemic mastocytosis. This patient was successfully treated with VIT for 4 years for severe anaphylaxis following bee stings but died 15 years later when he was stung by a yellow jacket [84]. Up to one-quarter of subjects with anaphylaxis following Hymenoptera stings have an elevated baseline serum tryptase level [39,40]. Patients with mastocytosis and/or elevated baseline serum tryptase are at increased risk to develop severe or even fatal sting reactions. VIT in such patients should be continued for life [5,38,39].

Repeated reexposure after stopping VIT: About half of the relapses occur after the first, the other half with subsequent re-stings [63,76]. The risk of a SAR increases significantly with repeated re-stings. Golden et al., also described an increased frequency of SARs 4 years versus the first 1–2 years after stopping VIT [61]. This was also the case in subjects who developed SARs after VIT for 7–13 years [63]. This occurred despite no reaction to a previous sting during the first few years after discontinuing VIT. This gives additional credence to the concept that a sting challenge is not recommended after stopping VIT.

High sensitivity according to diagnostic testing: There may be an association of re-sting reactions with a persistent high degree of sensitivity using intradermal skin testing [63]. Others are unable to confirm this observation indicating that specific serum IgE and IgG-antibodies, per se, do not predict the re-sting risk following discontinuation of VIT [76]. Diagnostic tests currently utilized are of limited value to predict long-term protection following VIT

Most patients with Hymenoptera venom sensitivity remain protected following discontinuation of VIT for at least 3–5 years. An even longer treatment program should be considered in the high-risk situations as discussed earlier. About one-third of patients on VIT have one of the high-risk factors discussed, and collectively they have about 45% frequency of relapse after stopping VIT. About two-thirds of patients on VIT have none of these high-risk factors and have less than 3% chance of anaphylaxis to a sting after stopping VIT. Because of the small but relevant risk of re-sting reactions, the relative cost and benefit of epinephrine for self-administration should be considered for subjects stopping VIT.

29.6 ANT HYPERSENSITIVITY

29.6.1 Classification

Ants are among the most biodiverse organisms worldwide with approximately 26,854 species, 489 genera, and 21 subfamilies described to date (https://antweb.org). The majority of ants are rarely aggressive. Fire ants, common in various parts of the world, are aggressive and bite their victims, including humans. They are included in the order Hymenoptera, family Formicidae, and a variety of different subfamilies, the primary ones of which are *Pachycondyla*, *Myrmecia*, *Solenopsis*, and *Pogonomyrmex* [85,86]. Human reactions to these ants, as to other Hymenoptera insects, can be self-limited local reactions to life-threatening SARs and anaphylaxis. Grades 1, 2, and 3 are SARs; grades 4 and 5 are anaphylaxis [5,87]. The majority of adverse reactions in the United States and other parts of the world, such as some parts of South America, are due to two members of the Myrmicinae subfamily, genus *Solenopsis* (*S.*) (Figure 29.2). The first, *Solenoposis richteri*, is native to the Mato Grosso of South America and was introduced into the United States

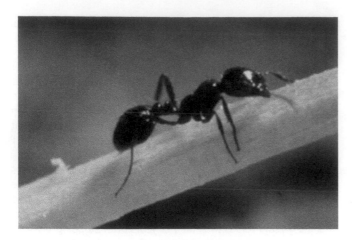

Figure 29.2 Imported fire ant (*Solenopsis invicta*).

in 1918 in Mobile, Alabama. The second, *Solenopsis invicta,* which is also native to the Mato Grosso, was introduced in the 1930s. It is the dominant species of IFA found in the United States and throughout the world [5,85]. These ants build nests that vary in size, sometimes 0.3–0.6 meters in diameter and up to 15–30 centimeters high, depending on the type of soil in which they live. When their nest are

disturbed, they aggressively and repeatedly sting by first biting the skin and then rotating in a circular fashion, leaving a telltale pustule which develops over 24–48 hours [5,89]. The U.S. Department of Agriculture (USDA) estimates that the IFA currently infest more than 367 million acres in states that occupy the southeast, south central, and southwest part of the United States (Alabama, Arkansas, California, Florida, Georgia, Louisiana, Mississippi, New Mexico, North Carolina, Oklahoma, South Carolina, Tennessee, Texas, and Virginia) (Figure 29.3). They also have been found in Puerto Rico and other parts of the world, e.g., Australia [90].

Other ants can also sting and cause local reactions or SARs in humans.

Harvester ants in the genus *Pogonomyrmex* live in the arid grasslands and deserts of the western United States. The red harvester ant, *Pogonomyrmex barbatus*, is found in various other parts of the United States, predominately east of the Mississippi River. While these ants are not aggressive, the sting is painful and associated with local reactions as well as SARs [91]. Two deaths allegedly from harvester ants and stings were reported in Oklahoma [92] and four severe systemic allergic reactions in Arizona [93]. Another ant, the Chinese needle ant, *Pachycondyla chinensis*, is found in the southeastern parts of the United States and causes SARs [90,94]. SARs also have been reported in 2.1% of *P. chinensis* sting victims living in South Korea [94].

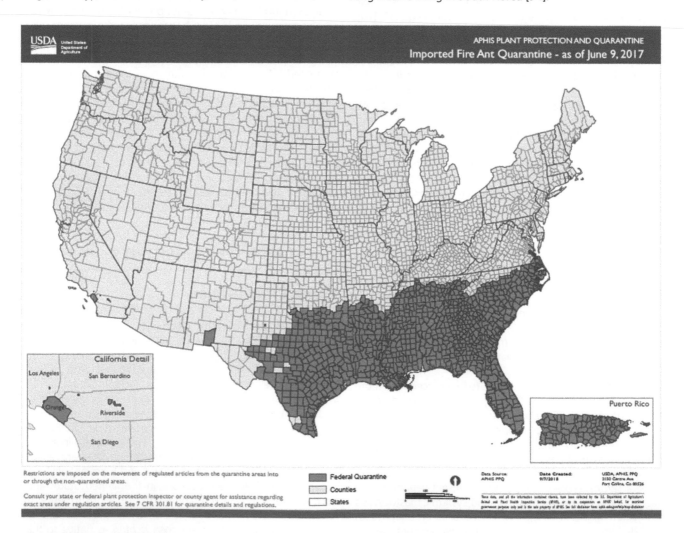

Figure 29.3 Distribution of imported fire ants in the United States.

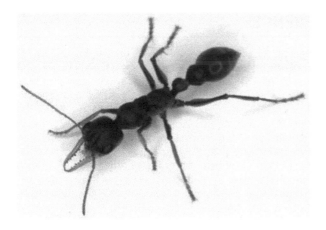

Figure 29.4 Jack jumper ant (*Myrmecia pilosula*).

Other species of stinging ants can cause SARs in other parts of the world. The greenhead ant, *Rhytidoponera metallica*, causes SARs in various regions of Australia. However, the jack jumper (*Myrmecia pilosula*) and bulldog ants (*Myrmecia gulosa*), genus *Myrmecia*, are a more common etiology for such reactions in this country (Figure 29.4) [91]. Ant stings were the most common cause of a SAR (30%), exceeding cases attributed to other Hymenoptera, antibiotics, or foods in an Australian emergency room [95]. The jack jumper ant (Figure 29.4) is reported to be responsible for two-thirds of all SARs treated in some parts of Australia [95].

Another ant, *Pachycondyla sennaarensis*, subfamily Ponerinae, referred to as the Samsum ant, causes SARs in the Middle East [97]. In Qatar, 23.5% of all-cause "anaphylaxis" cases in emergency departments were attributed to bites by this ant. A number of other species of ants from this subfamily, including *Odontomachus bauri*, *Hypoponera punctissima*, and *Dinoponera gigantea*, are also known to bite humans and cause allergic reactions [92]. Several species of ants from the subfamily Pseudomyrmicinae, including *Pseudomyrmex ejectus*, cause SARs. Details of the taxonomy of stinging ants and their worldwide significance in Hymenoptera venom allergy are outlined earlier in this chapter.

29.6.2 Clinical presentation of reactions

IFAs in the United States could build over 500 mounds per acre with multiple queens in each colony. However, since South American predators for IFAs have been introduced into the United States, the proliferation of these ants has been severely limited. Because of these natural predators, such colonies are no longer common. However, IFA colonies are found both in cities, i.e., lawns, playgrounds, under pavements, next to buildings, and in the country. Disturbing the colony results in activation of the worker ants that sting the cause for the disturbance. The IFA attaches to the skin by means of a powerful mandible and stings, releasing venom that produces a characteristic "fire-like" pain. If not removed, the IFA will continue to rotate in a pivotal fashion, repeatedly injecting small amounts of venom. An initial local reaction begins as a 25–50 mm erythematous flare. This is followed a few minutes later by a larger wheal, and within the next 24 hours, an umbilicated pustule forms which usually remains for 3–10 days, later rupturing and leaving a residual macule, nodule, or scar. Immediate sting effects are caused by toxic alkaloids present in more than 95% of ant venom. The allergic reaction is due to venom proteins that make up about 5% of the aqueous venom solution [96,98].

Stings of the IFA commonly produce large local reactions that are similar to those induced by stings of flying Hymenoptera. Following an initial wheal-and-flare, a large local reaction may develop several hours later. This includes erythema and edema that extend more than 10 cm from the initial sting site. This reaction is thought to occur in up to 17%–50% of IFA stings lasting 24–72 hours [99]. A pustule associated with the wheal-and-flare reaction is a diagnostic finding.

Symptoms of a SAR include generalized erythema, urticaria and pruritus, angioedema, nausea, vomiting, diarrhea, laryngeal edema, asthma, as well as shock. The IFA sting–induced SARs are thought to occur in up to 1% of IFA stings [100]. A survey of 29,300 physicians in 1989 reported a total of 32 deaths thought to be secondary to anaphylaxis induced by ant stings [101]. Although the species of ant was not identified in most cases, *Solenopsis* and *Pogonomyrmex* species were implicated in these deaths. Postmortem case reports of deaths following IFA stings describe findings of acute pulmonary changes and cerebral vascular congestion compatible with shock due to anaphylaxis. Neurologic sequelae due to the IFA are rare but include mononeuropathy and focal motor and grand mal epileptic seizures [102].

29.6.3 Allergens of the imported fire ant

The venom of the IFA is unique when compared to other Hymenoptera. The venom of the IFA, unlike other Hymenoptera venoms, has a low protein content in the aqueous fraction, less than 0.1%, with a prominence of toxic alkaloids. The aqueous component contains the allergenic proteins. Alkaloids comprise 95% and the aqueous 5% of the venom. The alkaloids are responsible for the hemolytic, bactericidal, and cytotoxic properties that result in formation of a sterile pustule. This alkaloid portion, however, is nonallergenic [100,103]. The venom of the harvester ant, *Pogonomyrmex*, more closely resembles that of the flying Hymenoptera and consists of 73% protein. *Solenopsis* and *Pogonomyrmex* proteins do not cross-react [100]. IFA WBE, unlike the WBE of other members of Hymenoptera, contains the clinically important allergens responsible for hypersensitivity [85]. Both IFA WBE and venom produce positive skin tests in sensitized individuals. Skin testing with IFA venom is more sensitive and specific than IFA WBE. The venom is also thought to be 10 times more potent and better tolerated for skin testing and RAST testing with IFA venom more sensitive than WBE. IFA venom, however, is not commercially produced, leaving IFA WBE as the only available option for testing and immunotherapy. Similarly, WBE and not venoms are available for *Pogonomyrmex* species [5,85].

29.6.4 Diagnosis

There is a high rate of false-positive results when skin testing is performed on subjects in endemic regions. Therefore, only subjects who have experienced a SAR following an ant sting should undergo skin testing with IFA WBE. Skin testing should be done at least 30 days after the SAR. A prick-puncture test with IFA WBE is performed first, and if negative, followed by serial intradermal testing beginning with a 1:1,000,000 weight/volume (w/v) dilution. A great majority of subjects who are sensitive react before reaching a 1:500 w/v dilution [5]. Complimentary diagnostic testing via *in vitro* tests (or Immunocap blood test) for IFA IgE should be obtained in subjects with a positive history of SAR following an ant sting who had a negative skin test.

29.6.5 Allergen immunotherapy

As with other Hymenoptera (honeybee, wasp, hornet, and yellow jacket), children or adults who have only had a cutaneous systemic reaction (cSR) are not usually candidates for AIT [5]. However, some physicians place patients with such reactions on AIT because there are no data to indicate that children and adults who have only had a cSR to an IFA bite will not have a more serious SAR with subsequent stings.

IFA AIT is begun with 0.05 mL of the highest dilution of WBE that produces a positive skin test (usually 1:10,000 or 1:100,000 w/v). The dose is increased with each injection, either weekly or twice weekly during a buildup. Once a maximum tolerated dose or 0.5 mL of a 1:100 w/v is achieved, the interval between injections is extended to every 4–6 weeks [5].

A 2-day rush protocol for IFA AIT has been studied in a small population of subjects and shown to be safe and efficacious [5,95]. Of 58 subjects, only 3 (5.2%) experienced a mild SAR during the 2-day rush protocol, a final dose of 0.3 mL of 1:100 w/v. When 56 subjects (total of 112 stings) had sting challenges on day 22, all (98.2%) tolerated the sting except one. He complained of light-headedness, which resolved without intervention. Prophylactic pretreatment with H1 and H2 antihistamines and glucocorticosteroids did not reduce the SAR rate associated with rush immunotherapy [95].

IFA AIT can be discontinued when the individual becomes negative on repeat skin testing. Otherwise, the decision to discontinue such therapy after 5 years is determined by the physician in consultation with the patient, since no data exist when IFA AIT can be discontinued when skin tests remain positive.

Only WBEs are used for AIT. However, a double-blind placebo-controlled crossover study on venom AIT in subjects allergic to the jack jumper ant, *Myrmecia pilosula*, was reported from Tasmania, Australia [95]. Of 29 subjects on placebo, 21 (72%) developed a cSR skin reaction, while only one of the 35 (3%) on ant venom developed a mild urticarial reaction when purposely stung. When the placebo group switched to venom AIT, all 26 subjects, except one, tolerated a sting challenge. Ant venom AIT to the jack jumper ant, *Myrmecia pilosula*, could offer some benefit to prevent life-threatening sting anaphylaxis in southeastern Australia. Such impressive evidence of the efficacy of venom AIT to the jack jumper ant, *Myrmecia pilosula*, supports more research investment in this area [88]. Currently, ant venom products are not commercially available for AIT.

SALIENT POINTS

1. Venom allergen immunotherapy (AIT) is highly effective for Hymenoptera venom allergy.
2. Indication for venom AIT is based on a history of systemic allergic reactions (SARs) to Hymenoptera stings and positive diagnostic tests.
3. Rush and ultrarush protocols for AIT provide more rapid protection than conventional protocols but may be associated with more side effects.
4. Most subjects remain protected for many years after stopping venom immunotherapy (VIT) of 3–5 years' duration.
5. AIT with whole-body vaccines of the fire ant (*Solenopsis invicta*) and probably other ants appears to be effective, in contrast to other Hymenoptera, where only venoms induce protection.

REFERENCES

1. Benson R, Semenov H. Allergy in its relation to bee sting. *J Allergy Clin Immunol* 1930; 1: 105–111.
2. Insect Allergy Committee, American Academy of Allergy. Insect sting allergy, cooperative study. *JAMA* 1965; 193: 115–120.
3. Hunt KJ, Valentine MD, Sobotka AK, Benton AW, Amodio FJ, Lichtenstein LM. A controlled trial of immunotherapy in insect hypersensitivity. *N Engl J Med* 1978; 299: 157–161.
4. Muller U, Thurnheer U, Patrizzi R, Spiess J, Hoigne R. Immunotherapy in bee sting hypersensitivity: Bee venom versus whole-body extract. *Allergy* 1979; 34: 369–378.
5. Golden DB, Demain J, Freeman T et al. Stinging insect hypersensitivity: A practice parameter update 2016. *Ann Allergy Asthma Immunol* 2017; 118(1): 28–54.
6. Sturm GJ, Varga EM, Roberts G et al. EAACI guidelines on allergen immmunotherapy: Hymenoptera venom allergy. *Allergy* 2018; 73: 744–764.
7. Bilo MB, Bonifazi F. The natural history and epidemiology of insect venom allergy: Clinical implications. *Clin Exp Allergy* 2009; 39: 1467–1476.
8. Golden DBK, Marsh DG, Freidhoff LR et al. Natural history of Hymenoptera venom sensitivity in adults. *J Allergy Clin Immunol* 1997; 100: 760–766.
9. Sturm GJ, Kranzelbinder B, Schuster C et al. Sensitization to Hymenoptera venoms is common, but systemic sting reactions are rare. *J Allergy Clin Immunol* 2014; 133: 1635–1643.
10. Golden DBK, Kagey-Sobotka A, Norman PS, Hamilton RG, Lichtenstein LM. Outcomes of allergy to insect stings in children with and without venom immunotherapy. *N Engl J Med* 2004; 351: 668–674.
11. Reisman RE. Natural history of insect sting allergy: Relationship of severity of symptoms of initial sting anaphylaxis to re-sting reactions. *J Allergy Clin Immunol* 1992; 90: 335–339.
12. Muller U, Helbling A, Berchtold E. Immunotherapy with honeybee venom and yellow jacket venom is different regarding efficacy and safety. *J Allergy Clin Immunol* 1992; 89: 529–535.
13. Muller U, Haeberli G. Use of β-blockers during immunotherapy for Hymenoptera venom allergy. *J Allergy Clin Immunol* 2005; 115: 606–610.
14. Rueff F, Przybilla B, Bilo MB et al. Predictors of severe systemic anaphylactic reactions in patients with Hymenoptera venom allergy: Importance of baseline serum tryptase—A study of the EAACI Interest Group on Insect Venom Hypersensitivity. *J Allergy Clin Immunol* 2009; 124: 1047–1054.
15. Stoevesandt J, Hain J, Kerstan A, Trautmann A. Over- and underestimated parameters in severe Hymenoptera venom-induced anaphylaxis: Cardiovascular medication and absence of urticaria/angioedema. *J Allergy Clin Immunol* 2012; 130: 698–704.
16. Schwartz HJ, Golden DBK, Lockey RF. Venom immunotherapy in the Hymenoptera-allergic pregnant patient. *J Allergy Clin Immunol* 1990; 85: 709–712.
17. Muller UR. Cardiovascular disease and anaphylaxis. *Curr Opin Allergy Clin Immunol* 2007; 7: 337–341.
18. Reisman RE. Unusual reactions to insect stings. *Curr Opin Allergy Clin Immunol* 2005; 5: 355–358.
19. Bilo BM, Rueff F, Mosbech H, Bonifazi F, Oude-Elberink JNG, EAACI. Diagnosis of Hymenoptera venom allergy. *Allergy* 2005; 60: 1339–1349.

20. Quirt JA, Wen X, Kim J, Herrero AJ, Kim HL. Venom allergy testing: Is a graded approach necessary? *Ann Allergy Asthma Immunol* 2016; 116: 49–51.

21. Strohmeier B, Aberer W, Bokanovic D, Komericki P, Sturm GJ. Simultaneous intradermal testing with Hymenoptera venoms is safe and more efficient than sequential testing. *Allergy* 2013; 68: 542–544.

22. Day J, Buckeridge D, Welsh A. Risk assessment in determining systemic reactivity to honeybee stings in sting-threatened individuals. *J Allergy Clin Immunol* 1994; 93: 691–705.

23. Golden DBK, Kagey-Sobotka A, Hamilton RG, Norman PS, Lichtenstein LM. Insect allergy with negative venom skin tests. *J Allergy Clin Immunol* 2001; 107: 897–901.

24. Hunt KJ, Valentine MD, Sobotka AK, Lichtenstein LM. Diagnosis of allergy to stinging insects by skin testing with Hymenoptera venoms. *Ann Intern Med* 1976; 85: 56–59.

25. Schwartz HJ, Lockey RF, Sheffer AL, Parrino J, Busse WW, Yuninger JW. A multicenter study on skin test reactivity of human volunteers to venom as compared with whole body Hymenoptera antigens. *J Allergy Clin Immunol* 1981; 67: 81–85.

26. Hamilton RG. Clinical laboratory assessment of immediate-type hypersensitivity. *J Allergy Clin Immunol* 2010; 125: S284–S296.

27. MacGlashan DWJ. Basophil activation testing. *J Allergy Clin Immunol* 2013; 132: 777–787.

28. vanderLinden PG, Hack CE, Struyvenberg A, vanderZwan JK. Insect-sting challenge in 324 subjects with a previous anaphylactic reaction: Current criteria for insect-venom hypersensitivity do not predict the occurrence and the severity of anaphylaxis. *J Allergy Clin Immunol* 1994; 94: 151–159.

29. Franken HH, Dubois AEJ, Minkema HJ, van der Heide S, deMonchy JGR. Lack of reproducibility of a single negative sting challenge response in the assessment of anaphylactic risk in patients with suspected yellow jacket hypersensitivity. *J Allergy Clin Immunol* 1994; 93: 431–436.

30. Rueff F, Przybilla B, Muller U, Mosbech H. The sting challenge test in Hymenoptera venom allergy. *Allergy* 1996; 51: 216–225.

31. Golden DBK, Breisch NL, Hamilton RG et al. Clinical and entomological factors influence the outcome of sting challenge studies. *J Allergy Clin Immunol* 2006; 117: 670–675.

32. Valentine MD, Schuberth KC, Kagey-Sobotka A et al. The value of immunotherapy with venom in children with allergy to insect stings. *N Engl J Med* 1990; 323: 1601–1603.

33. Oude-Elberink JNG, van der Heide S, Guyatt GH, Dubois AEJ. Immunotherapy improves health-related quality of life in adult patients with dermal reactions following yellow jacket stings. *Clin Exp Allergy* 2009; 39: 883–889.

34. Graft DF, Schuberth KC, Kagey-Sobotka A et al. The development of negative skin tests in children treated with venom immunotherapy. *J Allergy Clin Immunol* 1984; 73: 61–68.

35. Golden DBK, Kelly D, Hamilton RG, Craig TJ. Venom immunotherapy reduces large local reactions to insect stings. *J Allergy Clin Immunol* 2009; 123: 1371–1375.

36. Muller UR. Elevated baseline serum tryptase, mastocytosis and anaphylaxis. *Clin Exp Allergy* 2009; 39: 620–622.

37. Niedoszytko M, Bonadonna P, Oude-Elberink JNG, Golden DBK. Epidemiology, diagnosis, and treatment of Hymenoptera venom allergy in mastocytosis patients. *Immunol Allergy Clin North Am* 2014; 34: 365–381.

38. Vos BJPR, Anrooij BV, Doormaal JJV, Dubois AEJ, Oude-Elberink JNG. Fatal anaphylaxis to yellow jacket stings in mastocytosis: Options for identification and treatment of at risk patients. *J Allergy Clin Immunol Pract* 2017; 5: 1264–1271.

39. Bonadonna P, Perbellini O, Passalacqua G et al. Clonal mast cell disorders in patients with systemic reactions to Hymenoptera stings and increased serum tryptase levels. *J Allergy Clin Immunol* 2009; 123: 680–686.

40. Haeberli G, Bronnimann M, Hunziker T, Muller U. Elevated basal serum tryptase and hymenoptera venom allergy: Relation to severity of sting reactions and to safety and efficacy of venom immunotherapy. *Clin Exp Allergy* 2003; 33: 1216–1220.

41. Ludolph-Hauser D, Rueff F, Fries C et al. Constitutively raised serum concentration of mast cell tryptase and severe anaphylactic reactions to Hymenoptera stings. *Lancet* 2001; 357: 361.

42. Reisman RE. Venom hypersensitivity. *J Allergy Clin Immunol* 1994; 94: 651–658.

43. Hamilton RH, Wisenauer JA, Golden DBK, Valentine MD, Jr NFA. Selection of Hymenoptera venoms for immunotherapy based on patients' IgE antibody cross-reactivity. *J Allergy Clin Immunol* 1993; 92: 651–659.

44. Greene A, Breisch NL, Golden DB, Kelly D, Douglass LW. Sting embedment and avulsion in yellowjackets (Hymenoptera:Vespidae): A functional equivalent to autotomy. *American Entomologist* 2012; 58: 50–57.

45. Hemmer W, Frocke M, Kolarich K et al. Antibody binding to venom carbohydrates is a frequent cause for double positivity to honeybee and yellow jacket venom in patients with stinging insect allergy. *J Allergy Clin Immunol* 2001; 108: 1045–1052.

46. Eberlein B, Krischan L, Darsow U, Ollert M. Double positivity to bee and wasp venom: Improved diagnostic procedure by recombinant allergen-based IgE testing and basophil activation test including data about cross-reactive carbohydrate determinants. *J Allergy Clin Immunol* 2012; 130: 155–161.

47. Muller UR, Johansen N, Petersen AB, Fromberg-Nielsen J, Haeberli G. Hymenoptera venom allergy: Analysis of double positivity to honey bee and Vespula venom by estimation of IgE antibodies to species-specific major allergens Api m1 and Ves v5. *Allergy* 2009; 64: 543–548.

48. Sturm GJ, Hemmer W, Hawranek T et al. Detection of IgE to recombinant Api m 1 and rVes v 5 is valuable but not sufficient to distinguish bee from wasp venom allergy. *J Allergy Clin Immunol* 2011; 128: 247–248.

49. Blank S, Seismann H, Michel Y et al. Api m 10, a genuine A. mellifera venom allergen, is clinically relevant but underrepresented in therapeutic extracts. *Allergy* 2011; 66: 1322–1329.

50. Muller UR, Schmid-Grendelmeier P, Hausmann O, Helbling A. IgE to recombinant allergens Api m 1, Ves v 1, and Ves v 5 distinguish double sensitization from cross-reaction in venom allergy. *Allergy* 2012; 67: 1069–1073.

51. Golden DBK, Kagey-Sobotka A, Valentine MD, Lichtenstein LM. Dose dependence of Hymenoptera venom immunotherapy. *J Allergy Clin Immunol* 1981; 67: 370–374.

52. Rueff F, Wenderoth A, Przybilla B. Patients still reacting to a sting challenge while receiving conventional Hymenoptera venom immunotherapy are protected by increased venom doses. *J Allergy Clin Immunol* 2001; 108: 1027–1032.

53. Houliston L, Nolan R, Noble V et al. Honeybee venom immunotherapy in children using a 50-mcg maintenance dose. *J Allergy Clin Immunol* 2011; 127: 98–99.

54. Konstantinou GN, Manoussakis E, Douladiris N et al. A 5-year venom immunotherapy protocol with 50 mcg maintenance dose: Safety and efficacy in school children. *Pediatr Allergy Immunol* 2011; 22: 393–397.

55. Lockey RF, Turkeltaub PC, Olive ES, Hubbard JM, Baird-Warren IA, Bukantz SC. The Hymenoptera venom study III: Safety of venom immunotherapy. *J Allergy Clin Immunol* 1990; 86: 775–780.

56. Galera C, Soohun N, Zankar N, Caimmi S, Gallen C, Demoly P. Severe anaphylaxis to bee venom immunotherapy: Efficacy of pretreatment with omalizumab. *J Investig Allergol Clin Immunol* 2009; 19: 225–229.

57. Goldberg A, Confino-Cohen R. Rush venom immunotherapy in patients experiencing recurrent systemic reactions to conventional venom immunotherapy. *Ann Allergy* 2003; 91: 405–410.

58. Muller UR, Jutel M, Reimers A et al. Clinical and immunologic effects of H1 antihistamine preventive medication during honeybee venom immunotherapy. *J Allergy Clin Immunol* 2008; 122: 1001–1007.

59. Wohrl S, Gamper S, Hemmer W, Heinze G, Stingl G, Kinaciyan T. Premedication with montelukast reduces large local reactions of allergen immunotherapy. *Int Arch Allergy Immunol* 2007; 144: 137–142.

60. Rueff F, Przybilla B, Bilo MB et al. Predictors of side effects during the buildup phase of venom immunotherapy for Hymenoptera venom allergy: The importance of baseline serum tryptase. *J Allergy Clin Immunol* 2010; 126: 105–111.

61. Golden DBK, Kwiterovich KA, Kagey-Sobotka A, Valentine MD, Lichtenstein LM. Discontinuing venom immunotherapy: Outcome after five years. *J Allergy Clin Immunol* 1996; 97: 579–587.

62. Golden DBK, Kwiterovich KA, Addison BA, Kagey-Sobotka A, Lichtenstein LM. Discontinuing venom immunotherapy: Extended observations. *J Allergy Clin Immunol* 1998; 101: 298–305.

63. Golden DBK, Kagey-Sobotka A, Lichtenstein LM. Survey of patients after discontinuing venom immunotherapy. *J Allergy Clin Immunol* 2000; 105: 385–390.

64. Muller UR, Morris T, Bischof M, Friedli H, Skarvil F. Combined active and passive immunotherapy in honeybee-sting allergy. *J Allergy Clin Immunol* 1986; 78: 115–122.

65. Golden DBK, Lawrence ID, Kagey-Sobotka A, Valentine MD, Lichtenstein LM. Clinical correlation of the venom-specific IgG antibody level during maintenance venom immunotherapy. *J Allergy Clin Immunol* 1992; 90: 386–393.

66. Jutel M, Akdis CA. Immunological mechanisms of allergen-specific immunotherapy. *Allergy* 2011; 66: 725–732.

67. Hoffman DR, Jacobson RS. Allergens in Hymenoptera venom. XII. How much protein is in a sting? *Ann Allergy* 1984; 52: 276–278.

68. Muller U. Bee venom allergy in beekeepers and their families. *Curr Opin Allergy Clin Immunol* 2005; 5: 343–347.

69. Birnbaum J, Charpin D, Vervloet D. Rapid Hymenoptera venom immunotherapy: Comparative safety of three protocols. *Clin Exp Allergy* 1993; 23: 226–230.

70. Brown SG, Wiese MD, vanEeden P et al. Ultrarush versus semirush initiation of insect venom immunotherapy: A randomized controlled trial. *J Allergy Clin Immunol* 2012; 130: 162–168.

71. Confino-Cohen R, Rosman Y, Goldberg A. Rush venom immunotherapy in children. *J Allergy Clin Immunol Pract* 2017; 5: 799–803.

72. Golden DBK. Rush venom immunotherapy: Ready for prime time? *J Allergy Clin Immunol Prac* 2017; 5: 804–805.

73. Rueff F, Wolf H, Schnitker J, Ring J, Przybilla B. Specific immunotherapy with honey bee venom: A comparative study using aqueous and aluminum hydroxide adsorbed preparations. *Allergy* 2004; 59: 589–595.

74. Muller UR, Ring J. When can immunotherapy for insect allergy be stopped? *J Allergy Clin Immunol Pract* 2015; 3: 324–328.

75. Urbanek R, Forster J, Kuhn W. Discontinuation of bee venom immunotherapy in children and adolescents. *J Pediatr* 1985; 107: 367–371.

76. Lerch E, Muller U. Long-term protection after stopping venom immunotherapy. *J Allergy Clin Immunol* 1998; 101: 606–612.

77. Reisman RE. Duration of venom immunotherapy: Relationship to the severity of symptoms of initial insect sting anaphylaxis. *J Allergy Clin Immunol* 1993; 92: 831–836.

78. Muller U, Berchtold E, Helbling A. Honeybee venom allergy: Results of a sting challenge 1 year after stopping venom immunotherapy in 86 patients. *J Allergy Clin Immunol* 1991; 87: 702–709.

79. Golden DBK, Johnson K, Addison BI, Valentine MD, Kagey-Sobotka A, Lichtenstein LM. Clinical and immunologic observations in patients who stop venom immunotherapy. *J Allergy Clin Immunol* 1986; 77: 435–442.

80. Keating MU, Kagey-Sobotka A, Hamilton RG, Yunginger JW. Clinical and immunologic follow-up of patients who stop venom immunotherapy. *J Allergy Clin Immunol* 1991; 88: 339–348.

81. Golden DBK, Addison BI, Gadde J, Kagey-Sobotka A, Valentine MD, Lichtenstein LM. Prospective observations on patients who discontinue venom immunotherapy. *J Allergy Clin Immunol* 1989; 84: 162–167.

82. Fricker M, Helbling L, Schwartz L, Muller U. Hymenoptera sting anaphylaxis and urticaria pigmentosa: Clinical findings and results of venom immunotherapy in ten patients. *J Allergy Clin Immunol* 1997; 100: 11–15.

83. Oude-Elberink J, deMonchy J, Kors J, vanDoormaal J, Dubois A. Fatal anaphylaxis after a yellow jacket sting despite venom immunotherapy in two patients with mastocytosis. *J Allergy Clin Immunol* 1997; 99: 153–154.

84. Reimers A, Muller U. Fatal outcome of a Vespula sting in a patient with mastocytosis after specific immunotherapy with honey bee venom. *J WAO Org* 2005; 17: 69–70.

85. Hoffman DR. Ant venoms. *Curr Opin Allergy Clin Immunol* 2010; 10(4): 342–346.

86. Kim SS, Park HS, Kim HY, Lee SK, Nahm DH. Anaphylaxis caused by the new ant, *Pachycondyla chinensis*: Demonstration of specific IgE and IgE-binding components. *J Allergy Clin Immunol* 2001; 107(6): 1095–1099.

87. Cox LS, Sanchez-Borges M, Lockey RF. World allergy organization systemic allergic reaction grading system: Is a modification needed? *J Allergy Clin Immunol Pract* 2017; 5(1): 58–62.e5.

88. Wanandy T, Wilson R, Gell D et al. Towards complete identification of allergens in Jack Jumper (*Myrmecia pilosula*) ant venom and their clinical relevance: An immunoproteomic approach. *Clin Exp Allergy* 2018; 48(9): 1222–1234.

89. Steigelman DA, Freeman TM. Imported fire ant allergy: Case presentation and review of incidence, prevalence, diagnosis, and current treatment. *Ann Allergy Asthma Immunol* 2013; 111(4): 242–245.

90. Available at https://www.aphis.usda.gov. Accessed April 4, 2019.

91. Schmidt JO. Clinical consequences of toxic envenomations by Hymenoptera. *Toxicon* 2018; 150: 96–104.

92. Klotz JH, deShazo RD, Pinnas JL et al. Adverse reactions to ants other than imported fire ants. *Ann Allergy Asthma Immunol* 2005; 95(5): 418–425.

93. Weber RW. Allergen of the month-harvester ant. *Ann Allergy Asthma Immunol* 2013; 111(3): A19.

94. Nelder MP, Paysen ES, Zungoli PA, Benson EP. Emergence of the introduced ant *Pachycondyla chinensis* (Formicidae: Ponerinae) as a public health threat in the southeastern United States. *J Med Entomol* 2006; 43(5): 1094–1098.

95. Brown SG, van Eeden P, Wiese MD et al. Causes of ant sting anaphylaxis in Australia: The Australian Ant Venom Allergy Study. *Med J Aust* 2011; 195(2): 69–73.

96. Tankersley MS. The stinging impact of the imported fire ant. *Curr Opin Allergy Clin Immunol* 2008; 8(4): 354–359.

97. Dib G, Guerin B, Banks WA, Leynadier F. Systemic reactions to the Samsum ant: An IgE-mediated hypersensitivity. *J Allergy Clin Immunol* 1995; 96(4): 465–472.

98. Zamith-Miranda D, Fox EGP, Monteiro AP et al. The allergic response mediated by fire ant venom proteins. *Sci Rep* 2018; 8(1): 14427.

99. Stafford CT. Hypersensitivity to fire ant venom. *Ann Allergy Asthma Immunol* 1996; 77(2): 87–95; quiz 6–9.

100. deShazo RD, Butcher BT, Banks WA. Reactions to the stings of the imported fire ant. *N Engl J Med* 1990; 323(7): 462–466.

101. Rhoades RB, Stafford CT, James FK, Jr. Survey of fatal anaphylactic reactions to imported fire ant stings. Report of the Fire Ant Subcommittee of the American Academy of Allergy and Immunology. *J Allergy Clin Immunol* 1989; 84(2): 159–162.

102. Candiotti KA, Lamas AM. Adverse neurologic reactions to the sting of the imported fire ant. *Int Arch Allergy Immunol* 1993; 102(4): 417–420.

103. Touchard A, Aili SR, Fox EG et al. The biochemical toxin arsenal from ant venoms. *Toxins* 2016; 8(1).

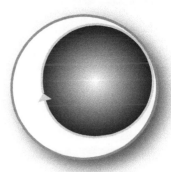

30 Recombinant and modified vaccines and adjuvants used for allergen immunotherapy

Jeffrey Stokes
Washington University School of Medicine

Thomas B. Casale
University of South Florida Morsani School of Medicine

CONTENTS

30.1 INTRODUCTION

Novel agents are being developed to treat allergic diseases based on expanding knowledge of innate and adaptive responses of the immune system on a molecular level. Allergen immunotherapy (AIT) is the only form of immunomodulation shown to induce immune tolerance for allergic diseases that persists after its discontinuation. There is also the potential benefit to prevent new sensitization to additional aeroallergens and to prevent asthma in high-risk children. Despite the benefits of AIT, improvement is not universal, and there is the risk of severe adverse reactions. Immunomodulators and novel forms of immunotherapy, which may be safer and more effective, are being developed to hopefully improve immunogenicity without increasing allergenicity. Novel forms of AIT seek to lessen the TH2 responses to allergens by altering the allergen vaccine or changing the mode by which the allergen vaccine is delivered. Other approaches include the use of adjuvants or vaccines that are nonallergen specific, such as toll-like receptor ligands (Figure 30.1 and Table 30.1).

30.2 RECOMBINANT VACCINES

Recombinant allergens are molecules with biological, immunologic, and molecular qualities that are well characterized [1]. They can be produced as either recombinant wild-type allergens, where the molecules mimic exactly the properties of natural allergen, or as modified variants with the desired properties to increase immunogenicity and/or decrease

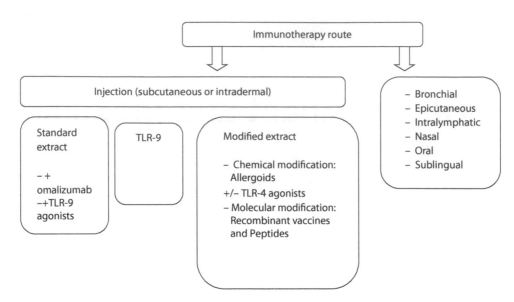

Figure 30.1 Potential immunotherapy approaches in development. (Modified from Casale TB, Stokes JR. Future forms of immunotherapy. *J Allergy Clin Immunol.* 2011; 127: 8–15.)

Table 30.1 Current and future forms of immunotherapy for allergic diseases

Treatment	Allergens	Diseases
SCIT	Pollen, mold, dust mite, animals, venom	Allergic rhinitis, asthma, Hymenoptera allergy
SLIT	Pollen, mold, dust mite, animals, venom	Allergic rhinitis, asthma, Hymenoptera allergy
Oral immunotherapy	Food	Food allergy
Wild-type recombinant vaccines	Grass, tree, cat	Allergic rhinitis
Hypoallergenic recombinant vaccines	Tree, grass, dust mite, venom	Allergic rhinitis, Hymenoptera allergy
Immunostimulatory DNA sequences (CpG)	Ragweed	Allergic rhinitis, asthma
CpG 1 and VLP	Dust mite, pollen	Allergic rhinitis, asthma
Allergoid modification	Grass, tree, dust mite	Allergic rhinitis, asthma
Allergoid 1 and TLR-4 agonist	Grass, tree, ragweed	Allergic rhinitis
Peptide	Animals, venom, grass, dust mite, weed	Allergic rhinitis, Hymenoptera allergy
Addition of omalizumab	Ragweed, birch, cat, dog, dust mite	Allergic rhinitis, asthma

Source: Modified from Casale TB, Stokes JR. Future forms of immunotherapy. *J Allergy Clin Immunol.* 2011; 127: 8–15.

allergenicity. They can also be produced as hybrid molecules resembling epitopes of multiple allergens including the relevant epitopes of complex allergens [2]. Recombinant allergens can obviate the potential problems of allergen extract contamination and inconsistency, for they contain specific molecules free of undesired components. Additionally, they have the potential to be tailor-made based on an individual's sensitization profile [3].

30.2.1 Genetically modified recombinant vaccines

Genetically modified recombinant vaccines are engineered to exhibit reduced allergenic activity. Bet v 1 is the major birch pollen allergen, and a hypoallergenic derivative of this allergen has been

manufactured and studied. In one of the initial clinical trials, a randomized, double-blind, placebo-controlled study, 124 birch-allergic patients received one preseasonal course of a mixture of two recombinant Bet v 1 fragments (rBet v 1) or a recombinant trimer of Bet v 1 adsorbed to aluminum hydroxide [4]. Preclinical testing previously had shown that rBet v 1 fragments and rBet v 1 trimer reduced allergenic activity 100-fold compared to Bet v 1 [3]. The hypoallergenic nature of the derivatives resulted in high dose tolerance with most patients reaching cumulative doses of greater than 150 µg of active treatment within an 8- to 16-week treatment duration.

In a clinical trial, patients received only one preseasonal treatment course but developed robust IgG1, IgG2, and IgG4 antibody responses against natural Bet v 1, Bet v 1–related allergens, allergens from alder (Aln g1) and hazel (Cor a 1), and cross-reactive food allergens, such as apple, carrot, and celery. One treatment course was enough to suppress the seasonal pollen exposure-induced increase in allergen-specific IgE in both active treatment groups versus the placebo group. Patients treated with the trimer showed a decrease in Bet v 1–specific TH2 responses, thought to be secondary to the high-treatment Bet v 1 trimer dose, and a greater allergen-specific TH1 response than that produced by the recombinant wild-type allergen [5,6].

Bet v 1 fragments or Bet v 1 trimers are less allergenic compared to wild-type recombinant birch pollen extracts when comparing skin test results in birch-allergic patients. In a small group of patients with birch allergy who were treated with Bet v 1 fragments and Bet v 1 trimers, nasal secretion of Bet v 1 IgG4 increased, while nasal provocation responses decreased to birch pollen [7].

In a small study performed in oral allergy patients treated with rBet v 1 fragments and rBet v 1 trimers, improvements in oral allergy syndrome symptoms were noted in 7 of 25 patients in the treatment group compared to only one patient in the placebo group. A year after treatment, rBet v 1 therapy decreased the seasonal rise in antigen-specific IgE levels [8].

Recombinant allergens developed to date include dust mite, cat, timothy grass, ragweed, and birch. Specific immunotherapy with recombinant allergens appears to be safe and effective.

30.2.2 Recombinant wild-type vaccines

Recombinant wild-type vaccines are formulated based on recombinant allergens that are equivalent to the natural allergens in molecular, immunologic, and biological characteristics. A combination of five different recombinant allergens of timothy grass (Ph1 p 1, Ph 1 p2, Ph1 p5a, Ph1 p 5b, and Ph1 p6) adsorbed onto aluminum hydroxide was administered to 62 patients with grass pollen allergic rhinitis in a randomized, double-blind, placebo-controlled trial. Patients received subcutaneous injections over an 18-month period. There was a 36% decrease in both medication use and symptoms during the grass season in the treated versus the placebo groups. Additionally, there was improvement in quality-of-life scores in the initial pollen season in patients receiving active treatment with significant improvements in several additional domains noted in the second pollen season. An increase in grass-specific IgG1 levels and a 4000-fold increase in IgG4 levels were found in the active treatment group. Systemic reactions including generalized urticaria, asthma exacerbation, and rhinoconjunctivitis were noted in 1% of the active treatment group [9].

In a multicenter, randomized, double-blind, placebo-controlled trial, wild-type recombinant birch pollen allergen vaccine, Bet v 1a, Bet v 1, and standard birch pollen extract were compared to placebo [10]. Over 2 years, 134 patients with birch allergy were treated with subcutaneous injections. All three treatment groups showed equivalent improvements in symptoms, medication use, and decreased skin test reactivity in both the initial and second pollen seasons compared with the placebo group. There was a greater rise in Bet v 1–specific IgG levels and a statistically significant greater level of reduction in skin-test reactivity in the recombinant allergen treatment group compared to either the standard or purified-extract treated groups.

In another multicenter, randomized, double-blind, placebo-controlled trial, 124 birch-allergic patients were treated with a trimer of rBet v 1a (three copies of the same gene sequence), Bet v 1 fragments (two recombinant peptides), or placebo for 4–5 months

prior to the birch season. Patients with active treatments had 100-fold increases in their IgG1 and IgG4 to Bet v 1 compared to placebo. Despite this, no significant improvement was noted in combined symptom-medication scores, skin-test reactivity, or nasal challenge [11].

Recombinant major cat dander allergen Fel d 1 was fused to a translocation sequence (TAT) and to part of the human invariant chain, generating a modular antigen transporter (MAT) vaccine (MAT–Fel d 1). In this first-in-human clinical study, intralymphatic immunotherapy (ILIT) with MAT–Fel d 1 was safe and induced allergen tolerance after three injections [12]. It elicited no adverse events. Three placebo injections given within 2 months increased nasal tolerance less than threefold, whereas three intralymphatic injections with MAT– Fel d 1 increased nasal tolerance 74-fold. ILIT with MAT–Fel d 1 stimulated regulatory T-cell responses and increased cat dander–specific IgG4 levels by almost sixfold; this change positively correlated with IL-10 production [12].

30.3 TOLL-LIKE RECEPTOR AGONISTS

Toll-like receptors (TLRs) are intracellular or cell surface receptors that recognize molecular patterns of pathogens such as in bacteria, viruses, and certain fungi. When agonists bind to TLRs on antigen-presenting cells, such as macrophages and dendritic cells, they initiate both innate and adaptive immune responses and induce both TH1 and regulatory T-cell responses [13]. Theoretically, TLR agonists can shift the cytokine balance from TH2 to TH1, thus improving allergic diseases. Eleven TLRs occur in humans and agonists for four (TLR-1, TLR-4, TLR-8, and TLR 9) have been studied in humans to treat allergic diseases.

30.3.1 TLR-9 agonists

TLR-9 recognizes unmethylated CpG DNA exposed in bacteria engulfed by endosomes after proteolytic degradation or produced *de novo* with the intracellular persistence of these pathogens. CpGs, which are often found in bacterial DNA, are commonly suppressed by methylation in eukaryotic DNA. The highest concentrations of TLR-9 are expressed in plasmacytoid dendritic cells (pDCs) and B cells. When TLR-9 is activated, pDCs release interferon α (IFN-α), which results in the subsequent activation of monocytes, natural killer T cells, and neutrophils. B cells stimulated via TLR-9 produce interleukin-6 (IL-6) and interleukin-10 (IL-10), thus inducing the differentiation of B cells into plasma cells with IgG isotype switching and production of antibodies. TLR agonists act via these mechanisms to activate both the innate and adaptive immune systems.

The three known classes of immunostimulatory CpG oligodeoxynucleotides (ISS-ODNs) are labeled A, B, and C. They differ in motif, length, and the immune responses they elicit. A and B classes have been studied as adjuvants in AIT, and B and C classes have been studied for treatment of malignancies and prevention of infectious diseases.

When the ISS is covalently bonded to an allergen, such as ragweed antigen Amb a 1, it modifies the antibody response to the allergen by reducing allergenicity and increasing immunogenicity [14]. *In vitro* studies with CpG ISSs Amb a1 reversed the ragweed-induced TH2 profile with decreased IL-5 secretion and increased IFN-γ production from peripheral blood mononuclear cells (PBMCs) [15]. A subsequent *in vivo* study showed that TH2 responses (induced by ragweed) were shifted toward TH1 with an increase in

IFN-γ [16]. TOLAMBA (Dynavax Technologies, Berkeley, California) is an example of a class B ISS-ODN covalently linked to Amb a 1. Six weekly subcutaneous escalating doses of TOLAMBA or placebo were administered in a phase 2 clinical trial conducted in 25 ragweed-sensitive adult subjects with allergic rhinitis. The group that received TOLAMBA versus placebo reported statistically significant improvement in quality-of-life scores and reduced rhinitis symptoms. Amb a 1–specific IgE antibody levels were suppressed for both seasons, while a transient rise in Amb a 1–specific IgG level was noted only during the first ragweed season [17]. A prior clinical study conducted in ragweed-sensitive patients who received six escalating doses of TOLAMBA or placebo before the ragweed season showed that only treated patients had markedly reduced increases in eosinophil and IL-4 mRNA positive cell numbers and increased number of IFN-γ mRNA positive cells compared at 4 and 5 months posttreatment. Symptom improvement was noted during the second but not during the initial ragweed season [18].

The development of TOLAMBA was discontinued after a large multicenter trial failed to demonstrate a difference in total nasal symptom scores in the active versus the placebo treated subjects, most likely because the symptom scores were too low in both the treatment and placebo groups to detect a treatment benefit. However, the study showed that patients from areas with high ragweed counts, such as the U.S. Midwest, experienced a reduction in the total nasal symptom scores compared to placebo [19].

Treatment with an inhaled form of ISS-1018 in atopic asthmatic patients showed significant increases in both IFN-γ and IFN-γ-inducing genes but did not modify early phase or late-phase asthmatic responses to allergen challenge [20]. There was also a nonsignificant reduction in sputum eosinophils and TH2-related gene expression.

Another therapeutic option with A-type ISS-ODNs involves packaging them in virus-like particles (VLPs), thus protecting them against proteases and endonucleases, reducing adverse reactions, and improving uptake by antigen-presenting cells. ODN phosphodiester backbones make them labile until stabilized by association to virus-like particles such as bacteriophage Qβ protein (Qb).

A phase I/IIa study of A-type ISS-ODN contained in the VLP, Qb 10, mixed with house dust mite (HDM) extract injected subcutaneously over a 10-week period in 20 patients with perennial HDM allergic rhinitis reduced skin-test reactivity to HDM [21]. The effect lasted for up to 38 weeks after treatment was discontinued. There was a median individual rise in conjunctival allergen provocation dose of 100-fold or greater after treatment. After the 10-week treatment period, patients were nearly symptom free, and a clinical benefit was noted up to 38 weeks posttreatment.

A subsequent phase II trial, which was randomized, double-blind, and placebo-controlled, was conducted in patients with mild to moderate perennial allergic rhinoconjunctivitis. Patients were treated weekly for a period of 6 weeks with CYT003-QbG10 alone (Cytos Biotechnology, Zurich, Switzerland) or placebo. There was improvement in both total rhinoconjunctivitis and asthma symptoms in the treatment group. Median allergen tolerance on nasal allergen provocation was enhanced 100-fold. In another phase 2 trial of 63 subjects with persistent allergic asthma treated with inhaled corticosteroids (ICS), subjects received either seven subcutaneous injections of CYT003-QbG10 or placebo and were followed for 12 weeks. All were stabilized on an ICS (beclomethasone); 4 weeks later, the dose of ICS was decreased by 50% and reduced to zero in the subsequent 4 weeks, as tolerated [22]. During weeks 6–12, the treatment group reported significantly improved symptom and medication scores compared to placebo. At the 12-week mark, the treatment group had significantly better forced expiratory volume in 1 second (FEV$_1$) values compared to placebo. The average ACQ score was significantly improved in patients treated with QbG10 versus placebo from week 4 until week 12 and remained below 0.75 (improved) during all but 1 week, despite ICS reduction at week 4 and ICS withdrawal at week 8.

CYT003-QbG10 was injected weekly over 6 weeks in a double-blind, placebo-controlled, randomized phase II b trial with 299 subjects with HDM allergy. Two different doses were compared against placebo, and the higher-dose treatment group reported improved rhinoconjunctivitis symptoms, reduced medication use, and better quality-of-life scores [23]. There also was a 10-fold increase in allergen tolerance in the higher-dose group versus the placebo group in the conjunctival provocation test. These data point to a non-allergen-specific TLR-9 treatment causing an allergen-specific therapeutic benefit.

A subsequent double-blind phase 2b study assessed the efficacy and safety of CYT003 in subjects with persistent, moderate-to-severe allergic asthma not sufficiently controlled on standard inhaled glucocorticosteroid therapy with or without long-acting β-agonists (LABAs) [24]. Toll-like receptor-9 stimulation with CYT003 showed no additional benefit in subjects with uncontrolled or partially controlled moderate-to-severe allergic asthma receiving standard inhaled glucocorticosteroid therapy with or without LABAs. Further development of this approach has been discontinued.

30.3.2 TLR-4 agonists

TLR-4 is expressed on immune cell surfaces. Endotoxins, such as lipopolysaccharides (LPSs) found on gram-negative bacteria, are TLR-4 receptor agonists [25]. TLR-4 when combined with the adaptor molecule CD 14 can bind LPS and lead to a proinflammatory TH1 response.

Pollinex Quattro (Allergy Therapeutics, West Sussex, United Kingdom) is a modified pollen extract, available as grass, tree, *Parietaria*, or ragweed. It is chemically modified by glutaraldehyde and adsorbed onto L-tyrosine in combination with the TLR-4 agonist monophosphoryl lipid A (MPL), which is derived from an active component of LPS of *Salmonella minnesota* R595 [26]. Trials of Pollinex Quattro in both pediatric and adult patients with allergic rhinitis, allergic conjunctivitis, and allergic asthma to various trees (e.g., birch), grass, and ragweed have been conducted. It has been used as preseasonal short-course immunotherapy administered as four subcutaneous injections over a period of at least 3–4 weeks annually in Europe and Canada and decreases skin prick test reactivity and seasonal rises in allergen-induced IgE levels [27]. In 141 subjects with grass pollen allergic rhinitis, nasal, ocular, and combined symptom/medication scores were reduced with four injections prior to the grass season [28]. In a survey conducted in over 3000 patients who received a total of 21,428 Pollinex Quattro injections over 3 years, 93% reported improvement in allergic rhinitis symptoms, while 75% reported a reduction in medication use. Local reactions were noted after 6.3% of injections, while systemic reactions, usually rhinitis symptoms, occurred in 0.5%. There were no reports of anaphylaxis or other serious reactions [29]. Similarly, 400 pediatric patients reported a response as good or very good in 94% with rescue medication use decreasing from 83% to 24% after the initial treatment course, with a further decrease to 13% after a second treatment course.

A prospective study was conducted in patients with seasonal grass pollen allergic rhinitis where Pollinex Quattro-Grass was administered for two seasons. Grass-specific total IgG and IgG4 levels increased minimally during the initial season but increased significantly after the second season. There was also an increase in FoxP3 + regulatory T cells, suggesting that at least two seasonal immunotherapy courses would be required to achieve tolerance [30].

A nonrandomized, prospective, cross-sectional case-control study of 68 subjects with allergic rhinitis to grass pollen, compared outcomes in patients treated with Pollinex-Quattro-Grass (four injections prior to grass season for 3 years), after cessation of treatment 3–6 years later, and an untreated control group. Allergen immunotherapy with Pollinex-Quattro significantly reduced nasal and ocular symptoms when compared with controls without AIT. Despite the clinical improvement, T-regulatory cells and TH1/TH2 cytokine patterns did not differ among the three patient groups [31]. No significant differences in symptom improvement were noted between the AIT group immediately following immunotherapy and the group off immunotherapy for 3–6 years.

A recent phase IIb study evaluated 228 patients treated with four weekly injections of a L-tyrosine absorbed ragweed extract combined with MPL or placebo. An environmental exposure chamber was used to demonstrate decreased total nasal and nonnasal symptom scores [32].

CRX-675 is an aqueous formulation of MPL lipid A, aTLR-4 agonist that induces a TH1 response. A single-center, randomized, double-blind, placebo-controlled trial was conducted in subjects with ragweed allergic rhinitis who received differing doses of 2, 20, 100, and 200 μg of intranasal CRX-675 24 hours before an intranasal allergen challenge. There was no clear trend in the ability of CRX-675 to reduce allergen challenge responses; however, nasal symptom scores were improved in the 100 μg group only [33].

A controlled field study conducted in 29 patients with seasonal *Parietaria* allergies who underwent MPL-adjuvanted subcutaneous immunotherapy showed improvement in asthma and rhinoconjunctivitis symptoms after 3 years of immunotherapy that persisted for 5 years following discontinuation. However, there was no improvement in pulmonary function measurements [34].

Trials for both grass and ragweed Pollinex-Quattro were positive in the United States, but studies were suspended due to a report of transverse myelitis in one patient. It was subsequently determined that the transverse myelitis likely was unrelated to the immunotherapy.

A study assessed the effects of MPL on safety/tolerability and clinical and immunologic efficacy when combined with grass pollen sublingual immunotherapy (SLIT) in subjects with seasonal allergic rhinitis. Eighty grass pollen–sensitive subjects were randomized into four groups of 20 subjects to receive daily treatment for 8 weeks in this double-blind, placebo-controlled, phase I/IIa study. Sixteen subjects per group received SLIT, and four received placebo. The formulation given to each group varied with respect to grass pollen extract and MPL content. There were no differences in adverse effects between the treatment groups. Patients in the two groups given SLIT containing the highest amounts of monophosphoryl lipid A had the highest proportion of negative nasal challenge tests after 10 weeks of treatment (47% and 44%, versus 20% with placebo). These subjects also showed earlier and greater increases in specific IgG and smaller increases in IgE levels than those receiving other formulations [35].

Overall, these data suggest that TLR agonists in combination with allergen-specific immunotherapy might represent a viable approach to treatment with allergic respiratory diseases.

30.4 ALLERGOIDS

Allergoids are allergens modified with glutaraldehyde or formaldehyde. This chemical process causes irreversible molecular polymerizations of the proteins at the primary amino groups in the amino-terminus or at the amino acid lysine. Allergoids have reduced IgE reactivity and allergenic activity while preserving T-cell epitopes [36,37]. Thus, allergoids might allow faster and higher updosing with preserved or even improved immunogenicity because of formation of higher molecular weight complexes after modification [37].

Allergovit (Allergopharma KG, Reinbek, Germany) is a compound composed of six grass pollen allergens adsorbed onto aluminum hydroxide. In a double-blind, placebo-controlled study of allergic rhinoconjunctivitis subjects conducted over 2 years, Allergovit reduced both symptom and medication scores while increasing grass-specific IgG1 and IgG4 levels [38]. Allergen tolerance was increased as determined by conjunctival provocation testing. There were additional improvements in quality-of-life and medication and symptom scores after the third year of treatment [39]. One year of Allergovit treatment of children decreased in seasonal grass-specific IgE levels, reduced the production of IL-4 and decreased skin test and nasal reactivity.

Depogoid (LetiPharma GmbH, Witten, Germany) is a tree pollen allergoid. Depogoid treatment improved rhinoconjunctivitis and medication scores compared with placebo with a 64% response to therapy [40]. Studies in asthmatic children with allergoid SCIT showed improved peak flows in the morning and reduction in inhaled corticosteroid dose compared with placebo [41].

Pollinex Quattro is another unique allergoid manufactured with the addition of the TLR-4 agonist MPL and was discussed earlier.

There is concern that the reduced allergenicity of allergoids compared to standard extracts may be associated with reduced immunogenicity. However, this form of immunotherapy remains an appealing alternative to traditional SCIT [37]. The U.S. Food and Drug Administration had theoretical concerns that the glutaraldehyde and formaldehyde treatment could increase risk of malignancy in treated subjects. This concern has limited the development of allergoids in the United States but has not been an impediment in Europe.

30.5 PEPTIDES

Peptide fragments made of corresponding T-cell epitopes of specific allergens have decreased ability to cross-link allergen-specific IgE on mast cells by virtue of their small size [42]. Initial studies of Fel d 1 peptide therapy were performed using two peptides that were 27 amino acids long (Allervax Cat; Circassia, Oxford, United Kingdom). Subcutaneous injections of three differing doses of peptides were given weekly for a period of 4 weeks in 95 subjects with cat allergy [43]. After cat room exposure, only high-dose therapy was effective in reducing nasal and respiratory symptoms. Immediate hypersensitivity reactions occurred one or more hours after the initial high-dose injections in 16 of 24 subjects. Additionally, in the active treatment group, subjects experienced more frequent pruritus, allergic rhinitis, and asthma symptoms a few hours after administration. In patients treated with either the medium- or high-dose Allervax Cat injections, methacholine challenge responses improved. IL-4 was the only cytokine found to decline, and this change was noted only in the high-dose treatment group. In subsequent studies, decreases in IL-4 or other cytokines have not been reliably found.

A large, randomized, double-blind, placebo-controlled study of Allervax Cat therapy was performed in 133 cat-allergic patients who had previously undergone unsuccessful cat immunotherapy. Allervax Cat therapy was given twice a week for 2 weeks and repeated 4 months later for a total of eight treatments. Subjects in the active treatment group experienced improvement in tolerance of cat exposure. However, only patients who received high-dose peptide injections showed a significant improvement in FEV_1 after 3 weeks of therapy. Adverse reactions were noted in all groups but were more frequent in the Allervax Cat treatment group, with three subjects in that group requiring epinephrine [44].

Studies have been performed using smaller Fel d 1 peptides (approximately 16–17 amino acids in length) and a larger number of peptides (12 compared to 2 peptides) administered intradermally. It was postulated that larger peptides were more likely to cross-link IgE and cause immediate allergic reactions. However, late responses were still noted with the smaller peptides. Late asthmatic reactions were noted in 9 of 40 subjects in cat-allergic subjects treated with peptide therapy even though no visible early or late cutaneous responses were detected. Postulates to explain this phenomenon include initiation of a T-cell-dependent late asthmatic reaction without prior induction of an early IgE or mast cell–dependent response [45]. The 12 peptide vaccine of Fel d 1 is known as Cat-PAD (also known as ToleroMune Cat [Circassia Limited, Oxford, UK]). In the dose ranging phase IIa clinical trial, the single administration was well tolerated with the most effective dose being 3 nmol [46]. In a randomized, double-blind, placebo-controlled, parallel group study, cat-allergic adults were exposed to cat allergen in an environmental exposure chamber (EEC) before and after treatment with two regimens of Cat-PAD (either eight doses of 3 nmol or four doses of 6 nmol) given intradermally over a 3-month period. The administration of four doses of a 6 nmol preparation 4 weeks apart led to a persistent improvement in rhinoconjunctivitis symptoms lasting at least 1 year after the start of treatment [47]. In the follow-up study, 51 of the 86 subjects who completed the 1-year follow-up were evaluated with EEC cat exposure 2 years after initial therapy. Subjects treated with 6 nmol of Cat-PAD continued to demonstrate a decrease in rhinoconjunctivitis symptoms after initial therapy [48].

In a phase III study of Cat-PAD versus placebo, both active treatment regimens and placebo greatly and equally reduced subjects' combined allergy symptom and rescue medication use scores from baseline. As a result of the very marked placebo effect, the treatment did not meet the study's primary endpoint. The treatment was well tolerated with a highly favorable safety profile [49]. The results from a phase IIb trial for HDM allergy immunotherapy using a similar approach also failed. Although the treatment greatly reduced allergy symptoms in the patients, so did the placebo [50]. Subsequent development of peptide immunotherapy by Circassia has ceased.

Patients with bee venom allergy have been treated with peptides derived from major allergens Api m 1 and phospholipase A_2 (PLA_2) with promising results. In a small study, three out of five patients who received a mixture of 3 PLA_2 peptides were completely protected after bee sting challenge, while the other two patients experienced only mild systemic allergic reactions [51]. There were marked rises in serum levels of allergen-specific IgG4 and IgE after sting challenge, while the ratio of PLA_2-specific IgE to IgG4 was reduced. Sixteen subjects underwent peptide rush immunotherapy in another study where three larger peptides were used to represent the entire Api m 1 antigen. Except for injection site erythema, which occurred more than 2 hours after administration in two subjects, bee venom peptide immunotherapy was well tolerated. Additionally, the peptide therapy increased IL-10 and IFN-γ secretion and allergen-specific IgG4 levels from stimulated T cells [52]. Studies utilizing the binding affinity of PLA_2 peptides for commonly expressed HLA-DRB1 molecules on antigen-presenting cells show that in those peptide-treated subjects, late-phase IL-13 and IFN-γ production decreases while IL-10 production increases in PLA_2-stimulated PBMCs compared to placebo. A reduction in late-phase cutaneous reactions and transient rises in bee venom IgG4 levels were also noted with peptide treatment [53].

Vaccines composed of nonallergenic peptides with lengths ranging from 20 to 35 amino acids derived from conformational IgE epitopes have been chemically coupled to carrier proteins. The aim is to direct blocking IgG antibodies at sequences within conformational IgE epitopes to induce immunologic tolerance and reduce allergenicity. A vaccine consisting of hepatitis B–derived PreS domain as the carrier protein fused to two nonallergenic Fel d 1–derived peptides has been developed. The recombinant fusion proteins did not show associated IgE activity and exhibited a 1000-fold reduction in allergenic activity in basophil activation tests. Immunization of mice and rabbits subcutaneously with the fusion proteins induced Fel d 1– specific IgG antibodies that inhibited binding of human IgE to the allergen [54]. These results show promise as a safe vaccine for cat allergy. Current studies are ongoing looking at peptide immunotherapy for dust mite and tree pollen [55].

30.6 ADDITION OF OMALIZUMAB TO IMMUNOTHERAPY

Another approach has been to add omalizumab to immunotherapy. Pretreatment with omalizumab prior to SCIT improves its safety and tolerability during buildup, ability to reach maintenance, and overall effectiveness [56,57]. Omalizumab's added effects have been noted in patients with allergic rhinitis, asthma, Hymenoptera allergy, and food allergy.

30.7 OTHER MODES OF DELIVERY OF IMMUNOTHERAPY

Other modes of delivery have been investigated and include oral, nasal, bronchial, epicutaneous, intraepithelial, and as previously mentioned, intralymphatic. Intranasal and intrabronchial immunotherapy are not currently used because of local symptoms associated with administration. Sublingual and oral immunotherapy are commonly used in Europe, and there are four products approved for use in the United States (see Chapters 27 and 28).

30.8 CONCLUSION

AIT has been in use for over 100 years. In the first 75 years of its existence, there was not much change in how it was delivered. However, in the last two decades, there has been a renaissance in efforts to improve the safety and efficacy of AIT including alternative approaches to traditional SCIT. Multiple approaches to increase regulatory T-cell and TH1 cytokine levels while reducing TH2 cytokine production are at the forefront of these efforts. The addition of omalizumab appears to improve the safety and efficacy of SCIT and OIT. The use of TLR agonists either alone or with allergens appears to skew the immune response away from a TH2 response, but this approach has had variable results. The modification of allergens chemically or molecularly might make a more focused immunogenic and less allergenic vaccine. Although the studies so far have not shown universal efficacy or safety, as more is discovered about the pathogenesis of allergic diseases and the immunologic changes induced by standard immunotherapy, better ways to modify allergic diseases using novel immunotherapy approaches likely will be found.

SALIENT POINTS

1. Recombinant allergens are specific molecules with unique biological, immunologic, and molecular qualities. They can be produced as either recombinant wild-type allergens, where the molecules mimic exactly the properties of natural allergen, or modified variants with the desired properties to increase immunogenicity and/or decrease allergenic activity.
2. Recombinant allergens can obviate the potential problems of allergen extract contamination and inconsistency.
3. Recombinant allergens developed to date include dust mite, cat, timothy grass, ragweed, and birch. Specific immunotherapy, with recombinant allergens, appears to be safe and effective.
4. Toll-like receptor (TLR) agonists can shift the cytokine balance from TH2 to TH1, thus improving allergic diseases. Eleven TLRs have been identified in humans, and agonists for TLR-1, TLR-4, TLR-8, and TLR-9 have been studied to treat allergic diseases.
5. Pollinex Quattro is a pollen extract available as grass, tree, *Parietaria*, or ragweed. It is chemically modified by glutaraldehyde and adsorbed onto L-tyrosine in combination with the TLR-4 agonist monophosphoryl lipid A.
6. Allergoids are allergens modified with glutaraldehyde or formaldehyde, which irreversibly polymerizes the proteins. Allergoids have reduced IgE reactivity and allergenic activity while preserving T-cell epitopes.
7. Allergoids might allow faster and higher updosing with preserved or even improved immunogenicity because of formation of higher molecular weight complexes after modification. Examples of allergoids are Allegovit (six grass pollen allergens adsorbed onto aluminum hydroxide), Depogoid, and Pollinex Quattro.
8. Peptide fragments made of corresponding T-cell epitopes of specific allergens have decreased ability to cross-link allergen-specific IgE on mast cells by virtue of their small size but theoretically retain immunogenicity.
9. Recombinant peptides of 13–17 amino acids in length for cat, ragweed, HDM, and grass have been investigated in clinical trials. The lack of B-cell epitopes in these peptides avoids cross-linking of mast cells, thereby eradicating the necessity for dose escalation.

REFERENCES

1. Larche M, Akdis CA, Valenta R. Immunological mechanisms of allergen-specific immunotherapy. *Nat Rev Immunol* 2006; 6: 761–771.
2. Valenta R, Ferreira F, Focke-Tejkl M et al. From allergen genes to allergy vaccines. *Annu Rev Immunol* 2010; 28: 211–241.
3. Valenta R, Niederberger V. Recombinant allergens for immunotherapy. *J Allergy Clin Immunol* 2007; 119: 826–830.
4. Niederberger V, Horak F, Vrtala S et al. Vaccination with genetically engineered allergens prevents progression of allergic disease. *Proc Natl Acad Sci USA* 2004; 101(Suppl 2): 14677–14682.
5. Pauli G, Purohit A, Oster JP et al. Comparison of genetically engineered hypoallergenic rBet v 1 derivatives with rBet v 1 wild-type by skin prick and intradermal testing: Results obtained in a French population. *Clin Exp Allergy* 2000; 30: 1076–1084.
6. Gafvelin G, Thunberg S, Kronqvist M et al. Cytokine and antibody responses in birch-pollen-allergic patients treated with genetically modified derivatives of the major birch pollen allergen Bet v 1. *Int Arch Allergy Immunol* 2005; 138: 59–66.
7. Reisinger J, Horak F, Pauli G et al. Allergen-specific nasal IgG antibodies induced by vaccination with genetically modified allergens are associated with reduced nasal allergen sensitivity. *J Allergy Clin Immunol* 2005; 116: 347–354.
8. Niederberger V, Reisinger J, Valent P et al. Vaccination with genetically modified birch pollen allergens: Immune and clinical effects on oral allergy syndrome. *J Allergy Clin Immunol* 2007; 119(4): 1013–1016.
9. Jutel M, Jaeger L, Suck R, Meyer H, Fiebig H, Cromwell O. Allergen-specific immunotherapy with recombinant grass pollen allergens. *J Allergy Clin Immunol* 2005; 116: 608–613.
10. Pauli G, Larsen TH, Rak S et al. Efficacy of recombinant birch pollen vaccine for the treatment of birch-allergic rhinoconjunctivitis. *J Allergy Clin Immunol* 2008; 122: 951–960.
11. Purohit A, Niederberger V, Kronqvist M et al. Clinical effects of immunotherapy with genetically modified recombinant birch pollen Bet v 1 derivatives. *Clin Exp Allergy* 2008; 38: 1514–1525.
12. Senti G, Crameri R, Kuster D et al. Intralymphatic immunotherapy for cat allergy induces tolerance after only 3 injections. *J Allergy Clin Immunol* 2012; 129: 1290–1296.
13. Racila DM, Kline JN. Perspectives in asthma: Molecular use of microbial products in asthma prevention and treatment. *J Allergy Clin Immunol* 2005; 116: 1202–1205.
14. Higgins D, Rodriguez R, Milley R et al. Modulation of immunogenicity and allergenicity by controlling the number of immunostimulatory oligonucleotides linked to Amb a 1. *J Allergy Clin Immunol* 2006; 118: 504–510.
15. Marshall JD, Abtahi S, Eiden JJ et al. Immunostimulatory sequence DNA linked to the Amb a 1 allergen promotes T(H)1 cytokine expression while downregulating T(H)2 cytokine expression in PBMCs from human patients with ragweed allergy. *J Allergy Clin Immunol* 2001; 108: 191–197.
16. Simons FE, Shikishima Y, Van Nest G, Eiden JJ, HayGlass KT. Selective immune redirection in humans with ragweed allergy by injecting Amb a 1 linked to immunostimulatory DNA. *J Allergy Clin Immunol* 2004; 113: 1144–1151.
17. Creticos PS, Schroeder JT, Hamilton RG et al. Immunotherapy with a ragweed–toll-like receptor 9 agonist vaccine for allergic rhinitis. *N Engl J Med* 2006; 355: 1445–1455.
18. Tulic MK, Fiset PO, Christodoulopoulos P et al. Amb a 1-immunostimulatory oligodeoxynucleotide conjugate immunotherapy decreases the nasal inflammatory response. *J Allergy Clin Immunol* 2004; 113: 235–241.
19. Casale TB, Stokes JR. Future forms of immunotherapy. *J Allergy Clin Immunol* 2011; 127: 8–15; quiz 6–7.

20. Gauvreau GM, Hessel EM, Boulet LP, Coffman RL, O'Byrne PM. Immunostimulatory sequences regulate interferon-inducible genes but not allergic airway responses. *Am J Respir Crit Care Med* 2006; 174: 15–20.

21. Senti G, Johansen P, Haug S et al. Use of A-type CpG oligodeoxynucleotides as an adjuvant in allergen-specific immunotherapy in humans: A phase I/IIa clinical trial. *Clin Exp Allergy* 2009; 39: 562–570.

22. Beeh KM, Kanniess F, Wagner F et al. The novel TLR-9 agonist QbG10 shows clinical efficacy in persistent allergic asthma. *J Allergy Clin Immunol* 2013; 131: 866–874.

23. Klimek L, Willers J, Hammann-Haenni A et al. Assessment of clinical efficacy of CYT003-QbG10 in patients with allergic rhinoconjunctivitis: A phase IIb study. *Clin Exp Allergy* 2011; 41: 1305–1312.

24. Casale TB, Cole J, Beck E et al. CYT003, a TLR9 agonist, in persistent allergic asthma—A randomized placebo-controlled phase 2b study. *Allergy* 2015; 70: 1160–1168.

25. Tulic MK, Fiset PO, Manoukian JJ et al. Role of toll-like receptor 4 in protection by bacterial lipopolysaccharide in the nasal mucosa of atopic children but not adults. *Lancet* 2004; 363: 1689–1697.

26. Gawchik SM, Saccar CL. Pollinex Quattro Tree: Allergy vaccine. *Expert Opin Biol Ther* 2009; 9: 377–382.

27. McCormack PL, Wagstaff AJ. Ultra-short-course seasonal allergy vaccine (Pollinex Quattro). *Drugs* 2006; 66: 931–938.

28. Drachenberg KJ, Wheeler AW, Stuebner P, Horak F. A well-tolerated grass pollen-specific allergy vaccine containing a novel adjuvant, monophosphoryl lipid A, reduces allergic symptoms after only four preseasonal injections. *Allergy* 2001; 56: 498–505.

29. Zielen S, Metz D, Sommer E, Scherf HP. Short-term immunotherapy with allergoids and the adjuvant monophosphoryl lipid A. Results from a 3-year post-marketing surveillance study. *Allergologie* 2007; 30: S1–S8.

30. Rosewich M, Schulze J, Eickmeier O et al. Tolerance induction after specific immunotherapy with pollen allergoids adjuvanted by monophosphoryl lipid A in children. *Clin Exp Immunol* 2010; 160: 403–410.

31. Zielen S, Gabrielpillai J, Herrmann E, Schulze J, Schubert R, Rosewich M. Long-term effect of monophosphoryl lipid A adjuvanted specific immunotherapy in patients with grass pollen allergy. *Immunotherapy* 2018; 10: 529–536.

32. Patel P, Holdich T, Fischer von Weikersthal-Drachenberg KJ, Huber B. Efficacy of a short course of specific immunotherapy in patients with allergic rhinoconjunctivitis to ragweed pollen. *J Allergy Clin Immunol* 2014; 133: 121–129.e2.

33. Casale TB, Kessler J, Romero FA. Safety of the intranasal toll-like receptor 4 agonist CRX-675 in allergic rhinitis. *Ann Allergy Asthma Immunol* 2006; 97: 454–456.

34. Musarra A, Bignardi D, Troise C, Passalacqua G. Long-lasting effect of a monophosphoryl lipid-adjuvanted immunotherapy to *Parietaria*. A controlled field study. *Eur Ann Allergy Clin Immunol* 2010; 42: 115–119.

35. Pfaar O, Barth C, Jaschke C, Hörmann K, Klimek L. Sublingual allergen-specific immunotherapy adjuvanted with monophosphoryl lipid A: A phase I/IIa study. *Int Arch Allergy Immunol* 2011; 154: 336–344.

36. Marsh DG, Lichtenstein LM, Campbell DH. Studies on "allergoids" prepared from naturally occurring allergens. I. Assay of allergenicity and antigenicity of formalinized rye group I component. *Immunology* 1970; 18: 705–722.

37. Henmar H, Lund G, Lund L, Petersen A, Wurtzen PA. Allergenicity, immunogenicity and dose-relationship of three intact allergen vaccines and four allergoid vaccines for subcutaneous grass pollen immunotherapy. *Clin Exp Immunol* 2008; 153: 316–323.

38. Corrigan CJ, Kettner J, Doemer C, Cromwell O, Narkus A. Efficacy and safety of preseasonal-specific immunotherapy with an aluminium-adsorbed six-grass pollen allergoid. *Allergy* 2005; 60: 801–807.

39. Williams A, Henzgen M, Rajakulasingam K. Additional benefit of a third year of specific grass pollen allergoid immunotherapy in patients with seasonal allergic rhinitis. *Eur Ann Allergy Clin Immunol* 2007; 39: 123–126.

40. Pfaar O, Robinson DS, Sager A, Emuzyte R. Immunotherapy with depigmented-polymerized mixed tree pollen extract: A clinical trial and responder analysis. *Allergy* 2010; 65: 1614–1621.

41. Zielen S, Kardos P, Madonini E. Steroid-sparing effects with allergen-specific immunotherapy in children with asthma: A randomized controlled trial. *J Allergy Clin Immunol* 2010; 126: 942–949.

42. Larche M. Update on the current status of peptide immunotherapy. *J Allergy Clin Immunol* 2007; 119: 906–909.

43. Norman PS, Ohman JL, Jr., Long AA et al. Treatment of cat allergy with T-cell reactive peptides. *Am J Respir Crit Care Med* 1996; 154: 1623–1628.

44. Maguire P, Nicodemus C, Robinson D, Aaronson D, Umetsu DT. The safety and efficacy of ALLERVAX CAT in cat allergic patients. *Clin Immunol* 1999; 93: 222–231.

45. Haselden BM, Larche M, Meng Q, et al. Late asthmatic reactions provoked by intradermal injection of T-cell peptide epitopes are not associated with bronchial mucosal infiltration of eosinophils or T(H)2-type cells or with elevated concentrations of histamine or eicosanoids in bronchoalveolar fluid. *J Allergy Clin Immunol* 2001; 108: 394–401.

46. Worm M, Lee HH, Kleine-Tebbe J et al. Development and preliminary clinical evaluation of a peptide immunotherapy vaccine for cat allergy. *J Allergy Clin Immunol* 2011; 127: 89–97, e1–14.

47. Patel D, Couroux P, Hickey P et al. Fel d 1–derived peptide antigen desensitization shows a persistent treatment effect 1 year after the start of dosing: A randomized, placebo-controlled study. *J Allergy Clin Immunol* 2013; 131: 103–109.e7.

48. Couroux P, Patel D, Armstrong K, Larché M, Hafner RP. Fel d 1-derived synthetic peptide immuno-regulatory epitopes show a long-term treatment effect in cat allergic subjects. *Clin Exp Allergy* 2015; 45: 974–981.

49. Circassia. Circassia announces top-line results from cat allergy phase III study. June 20, 2016. https://www.circassia.com/wp/wp-content/uploads/2016/06/CIR-PR-17_CATALYST-results-final.pdf. Accessed December 21, 2018.

50. Circassia. Circassia announces top-line results from house dust mite allergy field study. April 18, 2017. https://www.circassia.com/wp/wp-content/uploads/2017/04/CIR-PR-20_HDM-SPIRE-results.pdf. Accessed December 21, 2018.

51. Muller U, Akdis CA, Fricker M et al. Successful immunotherapy with T-cell epitope peptides of bee venom phospholipase A2 induces specific T-cell anergy in patients allergic to bee venom. *J Allergy Clin Immunol* 1998; 101: 747–754.

52. Fellrath JM, Kettner A, Dufour N et al. Allergen-specific T-cell tolerance induction with allergen-derived long synthetic peptides: Results of a phase I trial. *J Allergy Clin Immunol* 2003; 111: 854–861.

53. Tarzi M, Klunker S, Texier C et al. Induction of interleukin-10 and suppressor of cytokine signalling-3 gene expression following peptide immunotherapy. *Clin Exp Allergy* 2006; 36: 465–474.

54. Niespodziana K, Focke-Tejkl M, Linhart B et al. A hypoallergenic cat vaccine based on Fel d 1-derived peptides fused to hepatitis B PreS. *J Allergy Clin Immunol* 2011; 127: 1562–1570.e6.

55. David C, Selene B, Lucia C, Blanca C. New treatments for allergy: Advances in peptide immunotherapy. *Curr Med Chem* 2018; 25: 2215–2232.

56. Casale TB, Busse WW, Kline JN et al. Omalizumab pretreatment decreases acute reactions after rush immunotherapy for ragweed-induced seasonal allergic rhinitis. *J Allergy Clin Immunol* 2006; 117: 134–140.

57. Massanari M, Nelson H, Casale T et al. Effect of pretreatment with omalizumab on the tolerability of specific immunotherapy in allergic asthma. *J Allergy Clin Immunol* 2010; 125: 383–389.

SECTION IV

Clinical application of allergen immunotherapy and biological therapy for allergic diseases

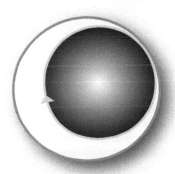

31 Adherence and cost-effectiveness of subcutaneous immunotherapy and sublingual immunotherapy

Dana V. Wallace
Nova Southeastern University College of Allopathic Medicine

John Oppenheimer
UMDNJ-Rutgers

CONTENTS

31.1 INTRODUCTION

Allergen immunotherapy (AIT), used for the treatment of allergic rhinitis (AR), allergic conjunctivitis, asthma, stinging insect hypersensitivity, and atopic dermatitis for over 100 years, has been slow to gain universal acceptance. With the publication in 1998 of the "WHO Position Paper, Allergen Immunotherapy," which summarized the scientific evidence for the efficacy and long-term benefit of this therapy, it has become a more accepted and respected modality

of treatment [1]. AIT is recommended for patients with moderate to severe AR who remain symptomatic despite maximum, feasible allergen avoidance and pharmacotherapy, who experience adverse effects from pharmacotherapy, or who choose to avoid long-term pharmacotherapy [2,3]. Subcutaneous immunotherapy (SCIT) and sublingual immunotherapy (SLIT) reduce symptoms of AR, decrease medication use, and may prevent the development of asthma and new allergen sensitizations [2,4–7]. Furthermore, it is recognized that AIT is the only treatment modality capable of bringing about

449

immunologic changes that can modify the underlying allergic disease. Following an adequate course of treatment, with 3 years usually considered the minimum, AIT has the potential to alter the natural history of disease with significant AR symptom reduction for several years following discontinuation of AIT and to prevent the development of asthma for up to 2 years post-AIT [8]. However, only a small proportion of appropriately selected candidates for AIT elect to initiate treatment. Of those who start AIT, a high percentage are nonadherent to the recommended treatment schedule, often discontinuing therapy before completion of the recommended 3–5 years required to achieve sustained clinical benefit [9–11]. In this chapter, we explore adherence both in terms of inconsistency with the administration of the allergy injections for SCIT or the sublingual tablets for SLIT, as well as nonpersistence, the premature discontinuation of AIT. While efficacy studies rely on rigorous controlled trials delivered in a standardized, uniform fashion to a narrowly defined, homogeneous population, effectiveness trials examine whether an intervention provides more harm than good, examining a heterogeneous population in which the intervention is delivered under real-world conditions [12]. "Effectiveness" in AIT incorporates the concept of being "worth the cost" to the patient, to third-party providers, and to policy makers. With the inherent cost of AIT, both the patient and third-party payors need assurance that AIT is efficacious in the short term, has long-term benefit, and is cost-effective. The limited data available on AIT cost-effectiveness are also reviewed.

31.2 DEFINITION AND PREVALENCE OF NONADHERENCE

Adherence and compliance are often used interchangeably; however, compliance is following or yielding to the proposed treatment plan that has been prescribed by the physician. Adherence differs from compliance, as adherence requires the patient's agreement to the recommendation; patients should be active, informed participants in the medical decision under consideration, e.g., to start AIT [13]. The World Health Organization (WHO) defines adherence as "the extent to which a person's behavior—taking medication (including AIT), following a diet, and or executing lifestyle changes—corresponds with the agreed recommendations of a provider" [14]. When the physician and patient have participated in shared decision-making, there is better patient engagement, the building of a stronger physician-patient trust, and usually, better disease outcome [15]. While the perception is that shared decision-making alone improves adherence, it is only one component of a complex intervention strategy that involves many additional elements, e.g., incorporating structured disease state and disease management education, often using a variety of patient decision aids; teaching self-management skills; and using frequent and consistent reminder systems [16]. The WHO has reported that only about 50% of patients with chronic illnesses take their medication as prescribed, even for diseases such as cardiovascular disease and diabetes mellitus, where the mortality rate is nearly double for nonadherent subjects [14,17]. For children with asthma and adults with chronic obstructive pulmonary disease, long-term, full adherence to prescribed medications does not exceed 25% [18,19]. Unfortunately, for most chronic diseases, even when specific interventions improve short- to medium-term adherence, this may not be enough. Adherence alone is often not enough to change disease outcome as other factors, e.g., lifestyle

choices, disease progression, and comorbidities have not changed. Therefore, patients and third-party payors are reluctant to allocate the time and financial resources required to improve adherence [16]. When looking broadly at the components of and obstacles to medication adherence, patients' perceptions, beliefs, and attitudes toward taking their medication often have more impact on their actions than age, cost, inconvenience, or adverse effects [20].

31.3 ECONOMIC IMPACT OF MEDICATION NONADHERENCE

The economic impact of medication nonadherence is documented. Estimates are that the U.S. annual cost due to medication nonadherence ranges from $100 to $290 billion [21]. In a systematic review of 79 individual studies, the annual cost of "all causes" nonadherence ranged from $5,271 to $52,341 per person [22]. Unfortunately, the current research assessing the economic impact of medication nonadherence has failed to impact healthcare policy, largely due to the varying quality of the research and to the use of nonstandardized methods of measuring adherence [22]. Nonadherence is often treated as a disease, perhaps explaining the fact that policy makers in the United States disallow increased premiums to be charged by third-party payors, including employers, for nonadherence [23].

31.4 ALLERGEN IMMUNOTHERAPY ADHERENCE: PERSISTENCE AND CONSISTENCY

What constitutes adherence or nonadherence has not been uniformly or operationally defined for most medical treatments, and certainly not for AIT, be it in research or in "real life." Nonadherence could be failing to keep the prescribed schedule of AIT treatments, e.g., daily administration of tablets for SLIT or obtaining weekly to monthly allergy injections for SCIT. Nonadherence could also refer to stopping AIT short of some defined period of time, usually the 3-year minimum discussed earlier. And unfortunately, nonadherence is often defined differently for SCIT than for SLIT. SCIT nonadherence is usually reported as attrition rates, e.g., the absence of a SCIT allergy injection for 3–6 months within 2 years of starting AIT [24,25]. However, SLIT nonadherence, similar to the criteria used for oral medication nonadherence, is often based on failure to take at least 80% of the recommended dosages of tablets or liquid. To arrive at a fair comparison of nonadherence for SCIT versus SCIT, one needs to evaluate these two modalities of AIT in terms of both attrition (discontinuation) of AIT, and the number of doses taken/received within a specific period of time [26]. However, some published articles that discuss the number of doses taken define this in terms of "compliance," while in other literature the number of doses taken is often referred to as "adherence." To avoid confusion of these closely related terms, for this review, "adherence" will incorporate both "persistence" and "consistency" of AIT. "Persistence" will refer to the degree to which the patient adheres to a 3-year minimum course of AIT, with "nonpersistence" also referred to as "discontinuation." "Consistency" will refer to the degree to which all scheduled SCIT injections or SLIT tablets or liquids are actually taken.

31.5 LITERATURE REVIEW OF PERSISTENCE OF AIT

The most relevant studies to determine adherence to AIT in clinical practice are derived from real-life studies and not controlled studies, e.g., randomized double-blind, placebo-controlled (DBPC) trials that require careful screening of participants, have clinical research personnel to assist physicians and patients, often incentivize patients, mandate closer patient follow-up, and routinely use standardized instruments to measure results. Therefore, achieving a nonadherence rate of 14%, as was reported in a SLIT meta-analysis of well-conducted research studies [27], is likely to be unachievable in clinical practice. For this review, all studies selected are considered "real life," followed patients long enough for them to have completed 3 years of therapy, and provided enough treatment and outcome data for meaningful comparison with other studies. Therefore, a set of inclusion and exclusion criteria as outlined in the footnotes to Table 31.1 were used for article selection.

The most meaningful studies are those that compare SCIT and SLIT head-to-head in the same study. While ideal inclusion and exclusion criteria were set *a priori*, some had to be loosely followed due to the incompleteness of the data reported, e.g., many studies failed to indicate the reason(s) that AIT was initiated and failed to provide the reason(s) for discontinuation of AIT. Nine studies, comparing persistence of SCIT to that of SLIT for a minimum of 3 years, published in 2001–2018, fulfilled, for the most part, the inclusion/exclusion criteria [26,28–35]. In these nine studies, 105,292 patients were included (SCIT: 96,297; SCIT: 8913; lymph node injection therapy [LNIT]: 82). For SCIT, the nonpersistence rate varied from 11% to 95% and for SLIT from 22% to 97%. Not factoring in study size, the mean nonpersistence rate was 54% for SCIT and 58% for SLIT. Three studies, published in 1999–2008 and including only SCIT patients, followed 1937 children and adults for a minimum of 3 years and found a nonpersistence rate varying between 12% and 84%, with a mean of 54% [36–38]. Three SLIT studies, published in 2004–2018, studied 2007 patients followed for a minimum of 3 years and reported nonpersistence rates between 15% and 45% [39–41]. However, perhaps the most accurate SLIT nonpersistence rates derive from the sales data of two major SLIT manufacturers, accounting for approximately 60% of the Italian SLIT marketplace from 2006 to 2009 [42]. These data demonstrate 87% nonpersistence over these 3 years [42]. In a U.S. clinical setting without any elements of an observational study, the best data for SCIT persistence, with a 12% nonpersistence rate, were from a region with a homogenous population, served by a large multispecialty medical clinic [38]. Moving away from real life and reviewing two randomized but open-label observation studies, the best overall persistence for SCIT and SLIT is a nonpersistence rate between 11% and 22% [34,39]. Elements incorporated into these observational studies, e.g., intense education, phone support and reminders, diary cards, and quality-of-life measurements, especially during the first 3–12 months of treatment, could dramatically improve persistence in the real-life clinical setting. In summary, outside of controlled studies, there is a wide variation in study size, design, reporting methods, and data elements reported, making it very difficult to predict a realistic persistence rate in the real world. However, it is clear that there is a major problem with attaining the minimum of 3 years of AIT for best long-term outcomes.

The reasons for discontinuation in many of the studies reviewed were not defined, often due to the study design, e.g., pharmacy databases for 6 of the 16 described studies [28,31,33,35–37]. When this information was reported, it was usually based on a random sampling, usually less than 50% of the total patients studied. In three studies, the medical record did not indicate the reason for discontinuation, and/or over 50% of the patients studied were unwilling to state a reason for their discontinuation. Based on limited reporting, reasons given for discontinuation of SCIT (in overall descending order) included inconvenience and excessive time commitment; medical comorbidities, especially psychiatric disorders and pregnancy; financial concerns; relocation of residence; symptom improvement; family problems; and adverse effects. Lack of efficacy was rarely mentioned for SCIT. For SLIT, the reasons for discontinuation (in overall descending order) were lack of efficacy; adverse effects; inability to be compliant; financial concerns; spontaneous symptom improvement; excessive time commitment; and family problems. When comparing dust mite SCIT versus SLIT, most studies showed a higher discontinuation rate for SLIT, with one author commenting on lack of efficacy as the main reason [31]. One 2-year SCIT study that did not qualify for inclusion in the persistence table completed a logistic regression analysis for nonpersistence and found that the absence of allergic conjunctivitis, negative perception of SCIT, nondecrease in use of medication, and missing more than 2 of the 10 previously scheduled injections were all significant at a *p* value .01 or less for discontinuation of SCIT [43]. The U.S. persistence studies were completed before 2011, except for one completed in 2014. Due to the changes in U.S. healthcare delivery over the past 10 years, it is likely that patients' direct financial burden for AIT is currently playing a much larger role in both failure to initiate AIT and nonpersistence of AIT.

Demographic data show children to be the most persistent age group, especially 5–14 years of age, both for SCIT and SLIT. Adolescents and young adults had a high discontinuation rate, while adults over 40 were more persistent. Sex, socioeconomic status, and type of payment for AIT did not seem to be major overall factors in predicting discontinuation of AIT. Most nonpersistence for both SCIT and SLIT occurs during the first year of treatment, especially during the first 3 months. However, SLIT patients tended to discontinue AIT sooner than did SCIT patients. If patients continued into the second year of AIT, they were more likely to complete the third year. Patients prescribed AIT and treated by allergists versus nonallergists had lower discontinuation rates. Patients with more allergies versus those with only a few allergies were more likely to initiate AIT, and often selected SLIT over SCIT. Patients were less likely to initiate and more likely to discontinue AIT if they had multiple medical comorbidities. Failure to initiate AIT, as reported by patients in an internet survey, was due to multiple issues, including financial concerns (34%), practical constraints (31%), insufficient perceived benefit (25%), and fear of adverse events (22%) [13].

31.6 LITERATURE REVIEW FOR CONSISTENCY OF AIT

As with persistence of AIT, when reviewing the literature to compare studies reporting "consistency," exclusion and inclusion criteria were similar to those for "persistence," except that a shorter 2-year period of observation versus 3 years was accepted. Consistency was defined as the percentage of the prescribed doses of SCIT that were actually received as injections or taken in the form of SLIT tablets or liquid. In countries where SLIT and SCIT are dispensed as pharmacy

Table 31.1 Allergen immunotherapy: Persistence and consistency in real life

Author	Study years	Study design	Patients	Dx	Setting	Allergens	Indications for AIT	How nonpersistence determined	Rate of nonpersistence	Consistency	Reason for nonpersistence (or consistency)	Comments
Allam [28]	2006–2014	Retrospective cohort, 3-yr Rx renewal rates	SCIT: 2109 SLIT: 2429 60% adults 40% children (Data available yr 3 for: SCIT 60% of pts. SLIT 61% of pts)	AR, A+ AR (10%)	German IMS Health Dz. Analyzer Extract Rx Database	Grass pollen SCIT: Aqueous SLIT: Tablets	Not stated	<1 Rx filled/ yr for 3 yrs	SCIT: 69% SLIT: 70%	SCIT: 83% SLIT: 81% Defined: persistent pts: % of 1095 days (3 yr) meds were in pt's possession as prescribed. SCIT assumed q 4 wks. Injections; equal across all ages	No info	SLIT pts discontinued sooner than SCIT pts; highest persistence age 4–14; lowest persistence age 15–17; highest persistence: pediatrician Rx vs. nonallergist specialist; consistency equal across all ages
Anolik [29]	2005–2011	Retrospective, randomly selected EMR chart review, followed 3+ yrs	SCIT: 2485 SLIT drops: 701 Children: 1368 (70% SCIT, 30% SLIT) Adults: 1814 (83% SCIT, 16% SLIT)	AR AR + A + AC + CRS (small %)	U.S. outpatient allergy/ asthma practice	Multiple pollen/ perennial allergens; 60% pts had 6–10 allergens		Failure to renew allergen extract when due during 3-yr Tx	Nonpersistent Tx SCIT: 39% SLIT: 43% Completed TX: SCIT: 35% SLIT: 24% Ongoing Tx <3 yrs completed: SCIT: 26% SLIT: 26%	Not reported	SLIT: 69% no reason and 20% "other"; SCIT: 67% no reason and 21% "other"; reasons provided for <10% of pts: inconvenience, lack of efficacy, expense, time-consuming	36% for which AIT recommended started Tx; ↑ allergens = higher % started AIT; ↑ morbidities = ↓ pts on AIT; children with > morbidities chose SLIT vs. SCIT; asthmatics selected SLIT vs. SCIT; SCIT: F > M; children had greater persistence than adults for SCIT and SLIT; SLIT pts discontinued before SCIT pts
Egert-Schmidt [30]	2007–2011	Retrospective	SCIT: 85,241 SLIT: 706 children adolescents, adults	AR	German manufacturer sales data	SLIT: Pollen SCIT: Pollen and D. mite (allergoid and unmodified depot)		Rx refilled to last 3 yrs Preseasonal SCIT: ≥3 Rx; Perennial SCIT: ≥5 Rx; Perennial SLIT: ≥8 Rx	SCIT: 58% pollen SLIT: 55% d. mite SLIT: 84% pollen SCIT: perennial unmodified: 55–58%; SCIT perennial allergoid: 40%; SCIT: preseasonal allergoid: 73%; SLIT: high-dose perennial: 84%	Not reported	No info	Perennial SLIT and preseasonal SCIT had lower persistence than perennial SCIT; children and adolescents more persistent than adults

(Continued)

Table 31.1 (*Continued*) Allergen immunotherapy: Persistence and consistency in real life

Author	Study years	Study design	Patients	Dx	Setting	Allergens	Indications for AIT	How nonpersistence determined	Rate of nonpersistence	Consistency	Reason for nonpersistence (or consistency)	Comments
Hsu and Reisacher [26]	2007–2010	Retrospective	SCIT: 139 SLIT: 78 Children, adults	AR	U.S. ENT clinic Cornell Medical College	Allergen not stated 20 microgram major allergen/ maintenance Tx		<3 yrs of SCIT or SLIT drop vials ordered	SCIT: 45% SLIT: 41%	Not reported	Phone survey 32 SCIT pts: #1 inconvenience; 8 SLIT pts: #1 lack of efficacy, #2 financial	SCIT: F > M; SLIT: M > F; High % SCIT pts discontinued <3 mo; SLIT pts discontinued 2–12 mo
Kiel [31]	1994–2009	Retrospective, Rx database	SCIT: 2796 SLIT: 3690 Adults	AR	Netherlands Community pharmacy database	Grass and Tree Pollen, D. mite; SCIT: 25% >1 allergen SLIT: 37% >1 allergen	+ skin test and/or sIgE; Related symptoms uncontrolled with pharmacotherapy	≥3 mo late for Rx filled during 3 yrs Following 1st Rx	SCIT: 77% SLIT: 93%	Consistent = never late for Rx pickup (persistent pts on one allergen) SCIT: 63% SLIT: 38% inconsistent: Mean 1.4 late Rx pickup (all persistent)	No info	Median duration Tx: SCIT: 1.7 yrs; SLIT: 0.6 yrs; nonpersistence higher in: Single allergen, younger age, lower socioeconomic status, allergist (vs. GP) Rx; 56% persistent pts were never late picking up vials; inconsistency much higher in SCIT vs. SLIT; dust mite allergen highest nonpersistence and SLIT > SCIT; Resource use for persistent/nonpersistent pts included
Leader [32]	2007–2014	Retrospective record review	SCIT: 140 SLIT: 269 Adults	AR	U.S. ENT Clinic Emory University	Not stated		<3 yrs of AIT per chart	SLIT: 95% SCIT: 97% (only 18 pts completed Tx)	SCIT: 62% excellent, 22% good; SLIT: 31% excellent, 35% good; Consistency defined: SCIT: # of 2-wk breaks in Tx schedule/ year 1–2 = excellent 3–4 = good 5–6 = fair ≥7 = poor; SLIT: refill of 3-mo supply (average late days/refill/yr); Late ≤ 10 days = excellent; 11–15 days = good; 16–20 days = fair; ≥ 25 = poor	SCIT: moved, β-blocker use, comorbidities; SLIT: symptom improvement, lack of efficacy, moved, financial concerns (drops were out-of-pocket expense)	Consistency better with SCIT vs. SLIT; Higher rates of consistency for SCIT did not translate into higher persistence

(Continued)

Table 31.1 (*Continued*) Allergen immunotherapy: Persistence and consistency in real life

Author	Study years	Study design	Patients	Dx	Setting	Allergens	Indications for AIT	How nonpersistence determined	Rate of nonpersistence	Consistency	Reason for nonpersistence (or consistency)	Comments
Lemberg [33]	2003–2011	Retrospective, database analysis	SCIT: 207 SLIT: 124 (tablets or drops); Adolescent and Adult patients; SLIT pts younger than SCIT pts	AR	German private allergy clinic with two locations	Grass, tree, d. mites, wasps; 89 different allergen extracts. Pre- and coseasonal; year-round, or both		Completion of 28–36 months AIT	SCIT: 32% SLIT: 39%	Not reported	Only 32 pts willing to say why they discontinued: #1 moved or travel; #2 "noncompliance"; #3 adverse effects; #4 pregnancy	Nonpersistent: M = F; nonpersistent: younger age> older age; most pts discontinued within 1st Tx yr; if continued year 2, more likely to complete year 3; pre- and coseasonal had higher nonpersistence than perennial or perennial + coseasonal; 100% private insurance;
Paino [34]	1998–2003	Prospective, open-label study	SCIT: 1886 SLIT: 806 LNIT: 82 Children	AR, A, or AR + A	Italian hospital setting or private medical office	Type allergen not stated Single allergen/ patient		<3 yrs Tx documented in chart	SCIT: 11% SLIT: 22% LNIT: 73%	Not reported	SCIT: #1 Cost; #2 time-consuming #3 family issues #4 ineffective SLIT: #1 Cost #2 ineffective #3 time-consuming #4 family issues	More of a "study" than "real-life"; pts had scheduled 4-month interval visits with physician for review of consistency; Gov. health services covered allergy extract but pt paid for office services; only 6.4% of SCIT/SLIT discontinued 1st 12 mos.
Sieber [35]	2005–2008	Retrospective chart review	SCIT: 1297 SLIT drops: 112; children, adolescents, and adults	AR	German national Rx database	Grass pollen		No Rx refills in 2nd and 3rd year of 3-yr cycle	SCIT: 64% SLIT: 49%		No info	Nonpersistence: F > M; [pregnancy is contraindication for AIT in Germany]; only study showing higher nonpersistence for SCIT and noted for all 3 yrs
Cohn/Pizzi [24]	1989–1991 (Slightly <3 yrs)	Retrospective, Review of charts	SCIT: 140 SLIT: 269	AR, AR + A	U.S. urban hospital practice	Not stated	Not stated	No vaccine refill in 6 months	50% (Same for AR or AR + A)	50% Same for AR or AR + A	AR pts: #1 Inconvenient (55%) #2 UK AR + A #1 Better with meds (25%) #2 Inconvenient #3 UK #4 other illness	

(Continued)

Table 31.1 (Continued) Allergen immunotherapy: Persistence and consistency in real life

Author	Study years	Study design	Patients	Dx	Setting	Allergens	Indications for AIT	How nonpersistence determined	Rate of nonpersistence	Consistency	Reason for nonpersistence (or consistency)	Comments
Donahue et al. [36]	1988–1992	Retrospective electronic chart review, records available until 1994	SCIT: 384, children and adults; M > F in <10 yrs age	AR, AR + A, A	U.S. HMO database, Harvard Community Health Plan	Pollen, some perennial allergens 84% had multiple inhalant allergens	1. Allergy severe enough to interfere with daily activities 2. Clinical Hx was consistent with long-standing allergic disease 3. Skin test + to clinically relevant antigens 4. Multiple, unsuccessful attempts at allergen avoidance 5. Availability of effective extract 6. Unsuccessful pharmacotherapy	<61 AIT inj. over 3.5 yrs (pts followed last inj. + 1 yr)	SCIT: 67%	Persistent patients were 89%–99% compliant Consistent = completed 50% of recommended Tx in each time intervals (0–3 m, 3–6 m, 6–12 m, 12–24 m; 24–36 m) Note: Study had issues with chart coding errors for compliance <50%; median inj. during year 1–2 was 41% higher for persistent pts; distribution of # Tx/patient was bimodal, peaks at 5 injections and 65 injections	115 surveyed #1 Pt's decision (54%) #2 (30%) Physician's orders (30%) Other reasons (all equal%): Symptoms resolved; Tx completed; lack of efficacy; adverse rxns.; medical complications	2% of pts (122,196) with A or AR Dx started AIT; if A only Dx, 35% had only 1 AIT Tx; 23% discontinued after 3 mo 50% continued into year 3; persistence greater in: M, age 20–40 yrs, Dx. AR + A; persistence lowest in age 10–20 yrs and Dx. A only; adverse reactions captured only if separate encounter; mean post- AIT follow-up only 7 mos; resource utilization included
Hankin [37]	1997–2004	Retrospective database review	SCIT: 520, children	AR	U.S. Medicaid claims database	Not stated		<3 yrs of Medicaid charges for AIT	SCIT: 84%	No info	No info	3% of pts with AR Dx started on AIT; 47% nonpersistent before 12 mos; M>F for AR Dx and SCIT Tx; Hispanics 2× >than African Americans and whites for SCIT Tx (Medicaid population may explain); resource use data included
More and Hagan [67]	June–September 2000	Retrospective chart review	SCIT: 381 Adults and children	AR, AR + A, Fire ant, Hymenoptera	U.S. Military allergy clinic	Not reported	Not reported	N/A	N/A	77.4% consistent Consistency = SCIT: Tx past 3 mos (also included pt who had 5+ yrs of AIT or d/ced by physician)	Reasons for inconsistency: 55 pts surveyed: # 1 inconvenience (35%); #2 other medical conditions (18%); #3 adverse Rxn (18%)	Most consistent: Hymenoptera; least consistent: active servicemen and RUSH (vs. conventional schedule)

(Continued)

Table 31.1 (Continued) Allergen immunotherapy: Persistence and consistency in real life

Author	Study years	Study design	Patients	Dx	Setting	Allergens	Indications for AIT	How nonpersistence determined	Rate of nonpersistence	Consistency	Reason for nonpersistence (or consistency)	Comments
Rhodes [38]	1982–1996	Retrospective chart review	SCIT: 1033 children and adults	AR, A, AR + A (63% had Hx of asthma)	U.S. allergy clinic, academic center	Pollen, mold, dust mite, cat 4–5 allergen types/ patient "High-dose" Tx	2 mo./yr severe symptoms after avoidance and intense multiple meds	<3 yr AIT per chart review	SCIT: 12%	No info	#1A: medical problem (usu. psychiatric) #1B (equal to 1A); #2 moved; #3 inconvenient; # 4 allergic reaction	Discontinuation rate per year very similar, persistence highest: F > M, age > 40; persistence lowest: Age 16–25, pts having a systemic Rxn, inconsistency with prior medication use and allergen avoidance predicted inconsistency with AIT; study had a homogenous population and was a multispecialty clinic; When moved, only 1/3 continued Tx
Klotsiridis [41]	2011–2014 (2015)	Prospective, noninterventional, observational, multicenter, open-label study	SLIT tablets: 399; adults and children	AR and/or AC 100% pts, ±A, AD	50 Sweden and 2 Denmark investigators	Grass, birch pollen; 69% had > 1 allergen	Mod-severe AR	3 years of TX	SLIT: 45% Children: 31% Adults: 55%	Consistency = 6–7 tablets/wk: All patients: 1 mo: 95%; 1 yr: 89%; 3 yrs: 81%; consistency greater in peds. vs. adults; consistency higher in persistent patients (89% reached yr 3)	#1 Adverse events (38%) #2 lost to follow-up (17%) #3 "other" (15%)	Nonpersistent pts usually discontinued 1st year (65%); 67% offered option of a tool for compliance at 1 mo. visit, but only 33%–37% used any tool; Medimemo # 1 tool offered; HRQL improved, greatest in physical functioning; QOL survey, VAS, and compliance evaluated at each visit; consistency did not predict persistence
Lombardi [44]	November 2003 (date of survey)	Multicenter observational study-phone survey	SLIT: 86 Adolescent, Adult	AR, AR + A, A	Italian outpatient clinic	D. mites: 41; pollen: 45	Not reported	N/A	N/A	Dust mites: 97%; pollen: 98%; consistency based on % tablets remaining in supply on day of survey	N/A	National healthcare covered cost of allergy extract

(Continued)

Table 31.1 (*Continued*) Allergen immunotherapy: Persistence and consistency in real life

Author	Study years	Study design	Patients	Dx	Setting	Allergens	Indications for AIT	How nonpersistence determined	Rate of nonpersistence	Consistency	Reason for nonpersistence (or consistency)	Comments
Marogna [39]	Dates not given; 1 yr observation prior to 3-yr study	Randomized, open/ controlled, observational study	SLIT: 319 Age 15–65 Adolescents and adults	R, R + A	Italian outpatients, allergy clinic	Pollen, dust mites		<3 yrs of AIT	SLIT: 15%; control: 12%	Excellent: 72%; Good: 18%; Poor: 10%; compliance defined as % tablets taken over 3 yrs: excellent = 80% good = 60–80% poor = <60%)	#1 UK; #2 lack of efficacy; #3 noncompliant; #4 side effects; discontinuation due to intolerable symptoms: SLIT: 19% control: 64%	More like a research study than "real life"; pt kept diary card for symptoms, meds, adverse reactions, volume of remaining extract
Senna [42]	2006–2009	Retrospective database	SLIT: UK # 60% of Italian immunotherapy market	UK	2 extract Manufacturers' sales figures	UK		Reduced sales over 3 yrs	SLIT: 87% After 3 yrs sales had decreased to 13% compared to star. of year 1	No info	No Info	Identical figures for both allergy extract manufacturers; nonpersistence only marginally dependent upon modality of payment
Trebuchon	2002–2008	Retrospective, observational, multicenter study	SLIT: 1289; children and adults	AR, AR + A	French allergists (139)	D. mite		<3 yr per chart review in 2008	SLIT: 27% (best estimate for 3 yrs) Children: 24%, Adults: 31%	Physician said very good or good: 88% persistent patients said 96%	#1 Poor compliance (32%); #2 poor efficacy (25%)	Study did not provide enough details to accurately determine persistence or consistency

Note: Studies reporting consistency but not reporting persistence: Moore (SCIT) and Lombardi (SLIT). Studies reporting persistence but not reporting persistence: Moore (SCIT) and Lombardi (SLIT). Studies reporting resource use: Kiel (SCIT and SLIT), Donahue (SCIT, and Hankin (SCIT).

Inclusion criteria for persistence:

Real-life practice

3-year minimum study time for persistence of specific immunotherapy (SIT), time must have been specified for some patients had to have completed 3 years of allergen immunotherapy

Stated or implied diagnosis of participants.

Captured but not required: funding source for AIT treatment.

Minimum of 50 patients followed for full 3 years.

If data from insurance claims, had to be enrolled in plan before study started and until end of study.

Desired but not required: date of first AIT, even if prior to onset of study years.

Desired but not required: state indications, e.g., failed pharmacotherapy, for AIT.

Patient has to receive at least one AIT treatment.

Desired but not required: reasons for discontinuation and the number of study participants surveyed.

Exclusion criteria for persistence/consistency:

Controlled research study, e.g., randomized DBPC studies with payment/incentives/research assistants, etc.

Unable to obtain full-text article in English.

Abbreviations: A, asthma diagnosis; AD, atopic dermatitis diagnosis; AIT, allergen immunotherapy; C, conjunctivitis diagnosis; d. mite, dust mite, Dx, diagnosis; dz, disease; HRQL, health-related quality of life; peds, pediatric patients; pt., patient; QOL, quality of life; R, allergic rhinitis diagnosis only; R + A, allergic rhinitis and asthma diagnosis; Rx, prescription; SCIT, subcutaneous immunotherapy; SLIT, sublingual immunotherapy; Tx, treatment; VAS, visual analog scale; wks, weeks; yr, year.

products, the refill records were used to determine consistency. Some studies only reported consistency for the patients who had also been persistent with their AIT. Unfortunately, only three of the nine studies reviewed for persistence also reported on consistency [28,31,32]. These three studies all used different methods to determine consistency. Based on a large German health disease database, of those who were persistent for 3 years, there was 83% and 81% consistency for SCIT and SLIT, respectively, based on the percentage of days for which prescribed doses had been filled at the pharmacy and picked up by the patient [28]. A Netherlands community pharmacy database study defined consistency as not being late for refilling any of the SLIT and SCIT treatment sets [31]. In this study, all nonpersistent patients were considered nonconsistent. Of the persistent patients (23% of all SCIT patients and 7% of all SLIT patients) who were treated with only one allergen (75% and 63% of patients of SCIT and SLIT, respectively), 56% were also consistent (no late pharmacy visits), and 44% had a mean of 1.4 late pharmacy visits [31]. The persistent SLIT group had an odds ratio of 2.8 of being late compared to the persistent SCIT group. Overall, 38% and 62% of the SCIT and SLIT groups, respectively, as defined earlier, were nonconsistent, meaning that they were late for picking up their treatment sets [31]. A U.S. otolaryngology university clinic defined consistency as excellent, good, fair, or poor based on the number of 2-week breaks in scheduled treatments/year [32] (see Table 31.1 for details). Consistency for SCIT patients was excellent or good 62% and 22% of the time, respectively, while for SLIT, the consistency was excellent or good 31% and 35% of the time, respectively [32].

Consistency for studies including only SCIT patients often used the date of last refill of vials or date of last allergy injection to determine consistency. In an urban U.S. hospital allergy practice, based on having no vial refill for 6 months, 50% of patients were found to be inconsistent [24]. Using a large U.S. health maintenance organization database, consistency was defined as completing at least 50% of the scheduled injections within predefined time periods, e.g., 6- to 12-month intervals (see Table 31.1 for details). The study found that 89%–99% of SCIT patients were consistent, although 67% discontinued therapy before the end of 3.5 years [36]. This study suggests that consistence does not necessarily predict persistence. A U.S. military allergy clinic that defined consistency as having received an allergy injection within the previous 3 months demonstrated consistency to be 77.4% [25]. However, this study did not report the persistence of SCIT [25]. It is obvious that consistency for SCIT has many different definitions and that a standardized definition is needed for future studies.

Consistency in studies for SLIT patients is usually based on the number of doses of liquid or tablets taken within a specified time period. While reported as absolute numbers by some, a range of percentage of doses taken is used by others to report consistency. If, by definition, taking six to seven tablets per week is consistence, at the end of a 3-year SLIT study, 89% of patients (all persistent patients) reported consistence [41]. However, there were no objective measurements with the patient self-reporting. While still taking SLIT, at 1 month, 1 year, 2 years, and 3 years, consistency was reported to be 95%, 89%, 91%, and 81%, respectively. However, of the enrolled patients, only 55% completed 3 years of treatment, again demonstrating that consistency does not always translate into persistence [41]. In another study, based on one phone call (at the end of 1 year of dust mite daily treatment or the beginning of pollen season for preseasonal treatment) with patients counting the remaining doses of SLIT, 97% of patients with dust mite allergy

and 98% with pollen allergy reported that they were consistent [44]. Two similar short-term observational, multicenter consistency studies in France involved contacting the patient by phone following 3 and 6 months of SLIT therapy [45,46]. The patients were asked to count their remaining tablets and, based on the expected number that should have been taken, the consistency was calculated. At 3 months, greater than 90% consistency was noted in 76% of adults and 69% of children; at 6 months greater than 90% consistency was described in 75% of adults and 66% of children [45,46]. In a 3-year Italian outpatient, randomized, observational study, patients were described as having excellent, good, or poor consistency if they took 80%, 60%–80%, or less than 60% of the prescribed tablets, respectively [39]. The study reported that 72% and 18% had excellent and good consistency, respectively. In this study, only 15% discontinued SLIT during the 3-year study [39]. In another retrospective, observational French study, physicians rated patients as to their perceived consistency with SLIT, rating 88% of patients either very good or good [40]. However, only 27% of patients completed the prescribed course (3–5 years) of SLIT [40]. Although it should be easier to define consistency in SLIT, which requires one dose per day, than in SCIT, which may be biweekly, weekly, or even every 4 weeks based on the schedule and patients' tolerance of dose escalation, wide variations in the definition of consistency prohibit firm conclusions about degree of consistency or how this impacts persistence. Based on the number of real-life studies reviewed, there is very little correlation of consistency with persistence for either SLIT or SCIT.

Not addressed in the previous studies is the reliability of patient reporting. In a small U.S. otolaryngology clinic setting, using off-label aqueous SLIT liquid therapy, patients' reporting of SLIT use was not reliable as evidenced by 50% claiming never to have missed doses, even among those known to be noncompliant. The most common reason was cost, which is understandable as SLIT liquid (drops or spray) in the United States is not approved by the U.S. Food and Drug Administration and thus is not reimbursed by third-party payors. The second most common reason for discontinuation was minimal effectiveness, which likely results from low-dose SLIT liquid therapy, as administering high-dose liquid therapy using the SCIT aqueous extracts (off-label in the United States) is both impractical and cost prohibitive. However, interestingly, of patients who were noncompliant, 53% reported substantial and 29% reported moderate symptom improvement [47].

31.7 TYPES OF NONADHERENCE

Nonadherence comes in many different forms that can be categorized, in general, as (1) erratic nonadherence, (2) unwitting nonadherence, and (3) intelligent nonadherence [14]. While these terms are often used in conjunction with the management of other chronic diseases, e.g., asthma, they also can be applied to AIT.

31.7.1 Erratic nonadherence

Erratic nonadherence is likely the most common form of nonadherence and the most easily identified by both patients and physicians. It is often due to forgetfulness and complex and/or chaotic lifestyles. In these cases, patients understand the reasons they should be adherent and ideally want to be adherent, but they have not made AIT a high enough priority within their busy schedules. Simplified and convenient treatment regimens, behavior modification, and reminder aids may be helpful for the patient with erratic nonadherence.

31.7.2 Unwitting nonadherence

Unwitting nonadherence is the term used when patients fail to understand fully the specifics of or the necessity for the recommended treatment regimen. With AIT, patients are often unaware or forget that consistency and persistence with AIT are required for immunological changes that provide long-term benefit after cessation of treatment. In other words, patients fail to understand fully that adherence is required even when current symptoms are under excellent control. If at each office visit, including visits for AIT injections only, the physician and staff members recognize the opportunity to engage in ongoing education and discussion of the long-term benefits of AIT, unwitting nonadherence may be diminished.

31.7.3 Intelligent nonadherence

Intelligent nonadherence refers to the patient's completing allergy testing but failing to initiate treatment after having agreed to do so. Additionally, the patient may alter the treatment regimen or even discontinue therapy deliberately and for personal reasons. Patients may reach this decision as they start to feel better and no longer feel the need to take the treatment, dislike or fear short- or long-term side effects of AIT, are encouraged by family members to stop, cannot afford the treatment, are unwilling to devote the time required, or prefer to use pharmacotherapy. The patient has already made, at least informally, a risk-benefit assessment. Many of these patients may be reluctant to provide the reasons that they stopped AIT, if asked. To address this type of nonadherence, the physician must spend time with the patient engaging in an open-ended, nonjudgmental conversation; attempt to provide alternative solutions to the patient's individual barriers and concerns; and be prepared to accept the patient's final decision of continuation or discontinuation of AIT.

31.8 RESEARCH STUDIES ON IMPROVING AIT ADHERENCE

Although much has been written regarding reasons for poor adherence, including both a lack of "persistence" and "consistency," most articles are based on expert opinion and include limited data from clinical research. One common theme with nonadherence, especially with lack of persistence, is that the first 3–12 months are crucial for patient education, engagement, and follow-up, as the number of dropouts peaks during this time [31,33,37,41]. A multinational, online survey of 261 patients from the United States, Russia, Spain, France, and Germany documented the need for better patient education on AIT [13]. In this survey, 28% of patients did not know which allergens were being used for their own AIT, and 27% did not know that allergies are chronic conditions.

Asking the patient about adherence during an interview will likely result in the patient's overestimating his or her degree of consistency with SLIT [47]. Patient's reporting of consistency is likewise overestimated even with SCIT, where office records can easily confirm consistency based on allergy injection administration records. Short-term SLIT studies attempting to obtain a more accurate consistency assessment using an unannounced phone call requesting the patient to count the remaining doses, reported over 90% consistency in 75% of adults and 66% of children at 6 months [45,46]. However, similar long-term (3-year or longer) studies have not been published.

In developing strategies to improve SLIT persistence, Savi employed a combination of education, frequent contact, and strictly scheduled contact involving five office visits or phone contacts and approximately 1 1/2 hours of professional/personnel time over the first year of SLIT treatment. This study reduced the discontinuation rate from 35% (control population) to 12% (intervention group) at the end of the first year of AIT, showing a statistically significant difference ($p < .001$) [48]. Furthermore, this study demonstrated the importance of very close follow-up during the early stages of treatment. Fourteen percent of the control group stopped SLIT during the first 10 days of treatment due to local side effects. Similarly, in the intervention group, 13% had discontinued SLIT due to local side effects during the first 10 days. However, following a supportive phone call from an office nurse at 10 days, only 2% of the study group remained nonpersistent. Similarly, at the 4-month follow-up visit for the intervention group, six additional patients had discontinued SLIT, but two resumed therapy following the visit. Using this approach, 4 months following initiation of treatment, only 5% of the interventional group had discontinued SLIT compared to 17% in the control group [48].

More frequent clinical follow-up visits improve persistence as well. A real life study compared persistence with four visits per year to two visits per year or one visit per year and found that persistence was improved with more frequent visits [49]. Nonpersistence for year 1 was 8.1, 14.7, and 29.3 for four, two, or one visit per year, respectively. Likewise, nonpersistence for year 2 was 10.4, 27.8, and 41.1 for four, two, or one visit per year, respectively [49]. In general, patients attend more clinic visits when reminder phone calls or letters provide information about the reason for the visit [50]. Maintaining good follow-up and consistency can be even more challenging when SCIT allergy extract is administered by another office, e.g., primary care physician (PCP) or college clinic. Communicating with the patient between "refill" appointments is advised.

Factors that interfere with adherence with SCIT are dose reductions for local reactions, symptom peaks associated with specific seasons, or interruptions in treatment. A 2017 review article presented evidence both for and against dose increase (during the buildup phase) and leveling off of dose reductions (maintenance phase) when one of these situations or events occurs [51]. Surveys of U.S. allergists indicate that between 12% and 40% routinely adjust SCIT doses during a patient's peak pollen season [3,52]. Furthermore, data from the American Academy of Allergy, Asthma and Immunology (AAAAI)/American College of Allergy, Asthma, and Immunology (ACAAI) national surveillance studies indicate that lowering or not increasing doses during peak pollen season may lower the risk of a severe systemic reaction [52]. Administration of AIT without dose reduction during the relevant pollen season has been implicated, by some, to be a major factor in both fatal and near-fatal SCIT reactions in the United States [53,54]. However, it may be argued that prospective observational studies have not found any differences in systemic reaction rates during pollen season versus nonpollen season, but these studies are likely confounded by study design [55–57]. One study of SCIT for mountain cedar showed that both the number and the severity of adverse reactions, as well as the treatment outcomes, were the same with or without seasonal dose reductions [58]. If the decision is not to reduce the SCIT dose in all pollen-sensitized patients during pollen season, trying to select which particular patients require dose reduction during peak pollen season has been challenging. The 2012–2013 surveillance study showed that of the various factors studied, only the size of the skin test corresponding to the particular pollen/season was useful for selecting at-risk patients; not escalating doses during the season for these patients resulted in a reduction in systemic reactions of all severity grades [59]. However, caution is advised by others in trying to select at-risk patients, as there is still fear that omitting dose reductions during pollen season will result in an increase in adverse events [60].

With the time commitment for SCIT buildup, alternative, accelerated buildup dosing schedules are being used by some clinicians. Despite the use of premedication (e.g., antihistamines and corticosteroids), accelerated schedules (e.g., ultrarush, rush, and cluster) have been associated with higher rates of systemic reactions when compared to conventional regimens with an escalating rate of systemic reactions inversely related to the number of buildup doses utilized [61]. After disqualifying patients who have poorly controlled asthma, high levels of sensitization by skin testing, comorbid medical conditions (e.g., cardiovascular disease), and young children, the allergist may offer an accelerated AIT schedule, particularly cluster, as an option. Cluster carries somewhat higher but usually acceptable risks [62]. Using more rapid buildup schedules has usually, although not always, been associated with improved adherence due to reduced numbers of injections/visits and lower associated costs [63–67].

Requiring that patients on SCIT refrain from concomitantly taking certain medications, e.g., β-blockers and/or angiotensin-converting enzyme inhibitors or angiotensin receptor blockers, can definitely lead to failure to initiate as well as nonpersistence of SCIT. However, not all studies have shown an increase in the frequency or severity of reactions for SCIT patients who are concomitantly taking these at-risk medications. In a small, prospective observation study, for example, 20 patients were permitted to remain on one of the previously listed medications while on SCIT [68]. They were compared to a matched control group who were on SCIT but not receiving any of these at-risk medications. While the frequency of severe reactions was greater in the study group, the systemic symptoms resolved just as quickly, and the number of doses of epinephrine were not increased for those taking the at-risk medications [68]. Nevertheless, more studies are needed before removing the caution that immunotherapy guidelines recommend [69].

Adverse reactions, both local and systemic, are often stated as the reasons for poor adherence. Most SCIT dosing regimens were initially established for adult patients and have subsequently been used without modification for children. Pediatric AIT schedules may need to be reviewed and possibly revised [70]. One study demonstrated a higher rate of systemic reactions, grades 1 and 2, in children, leading the authors to suggest that a different dosing strategy, e.g., a lower starting dose, a decrease in target maintenance dose, or a slower buildup phase, should be developed for children [71]. Guideline-endorsed strategies (grade A evidence) to reduce local side effects from SLIT include using oral antihistamines prior to SLIT administration [72]. Strategies recommended, but not studied, for SLIT include split tablet administration, moving the tablet to other parts of the vestibulum, and avoiding swallowing the tablet [41].

The use of electronic medication reminder systems, e.g., MEMOZAX or short message service (SMS), may improve adherence. Jansen studied the effects of MEMOZAX, a system that stores and dispenses SLIT tablets, reminds patients to take their medication, and keeps a record of consistency over the previous 7 days [73]. Patients used the reminder system 82% of the time, but only 32% felt that the feedback function of MEMOZAX made them feel motivated to take their SLIT tablets [73]. In another study, when patients were offered an electronic medication reminder system without cost, e.g., MEMOZAX or SMS, only 33%–37% of patients elected to use one [41]. For tablets, pharmaceutical caps, e.g., GlowCaps by Vitality, Inc., incorporate microchips and transmitters that can send information to the physician over the internet via wireless routers [20]. They can be programmed to have the cap blink when it is time to take the tablet, followed by playing a musical jingle if the tablet is not taken, and if still ignored, followed in 1 hour by an automated phone call. Furthermore, when the vial is empty, a new prescription request can be sent to the pharmacy automatically. Not only can the cost for such reminders inhibit their use, but there is also a dearth of real-life clinical studies that demonstrate better consistency or persistence of AIT with the use of these electronic devices.

Patients often say that they forget to use their SLIT on a daily basis. Physicians either recommend morning dosing or allow the patient to decide when to take SLIT during the day. In a randomized, double-blind, placebo-controlled (DBPC) study of adherence to inhaled budesonide in children with asthma, the authors showed adherence rates of 41% in morning and 47% in evening dosages after 27 months, indicating statistically higher adherence to the evening dose [74]. Taking these data into account, consistency might be better if patients are advised to take their daily dose of SLIT in the evening.

One important reason given for discontinuation of AIT is lack of efficacy, especially for SLIT. If a reliable biomarker were available to indicate clinical response, it could potentially be used as an indication of adherence. Limited studies have suggested that measuring increases in specific IgG or IgG4 levels might be effective markers for AIT adherence, but more research is needed [75].

In reviewing multiple studies and recommendations that address adherence to AIT, the 2017 European Academy of Allergy and Clinical Immunology (EAACI) immunotherapy guidelines list the main reasons for poor adherence as side effects, inconvenience, lack of efficacy, and forgetfulness [72]. The use of reminder devices tailored to the patient, patient education, and good physician-patient communication were recommended, but it was acknowledged that these recommendations were based on low-quality (grade C) evidence [72]. The use of frequent, e.g., every 3 months, follow-up visits was recommended based on grade B evidence [72].

Pharmacists are playing an increasing role in education for both disease state management and pharmacologic management of patients with allergic rhinitis and asthma. With the availability of SLIT as a prescription drug, this will extend to immunotherapy. The role of pharmacists in the implementation of care pathways for these diseases is increasing both in Europe and in the United States [76,77]. Allergists and pharmacists ideally should develop and actively participate in a personalized adherence plan for every patient on SLIT.

Pharmaceutical companies are devoting increasing resources to improve adherence, recognizing that they lose billions of dollars in sales when patients do not take their prescribed medications [23]. Recognizing the importance of adherence to their bottom line, pharmaceutical companies increased their budget for adherence by 281% from 2009 to 2012 [20]. The pharmaceutical companies recognize that they cannot directly change patients' beliefs and attitudes about medications, especially those involving nonadherence, but must direct their adherence messages predominantly through nurses, physicians, pharmacists, and other patients, as these are trusted intermediaries who have the largest impact on nonadherent patients. Research shows that nurses, physicians, and pharmacists are the number 1, 2, and 3 most trusted healthcare professionals [78]. Pharmaceutical distribution centers have used behavioral psychologists to train pharmacists in techniques of motivational interviewing to help patients overcome barriers to adherence [20]. While pharmaceutical companies do not dictate what patient ambassadors say, they are very careful about selecting the right patient to tell the desired story. This cherry-picking of patient ambassadors has raised some ethical concerns. With the explosion of expensive designer drugs for orphan diseases, the field has seen huge pharmaceutical investments in conveying marketing information using patient ambassadors. Their methods of reaching patients and healthcare providers is also changing. From 2015 to 2017, the pharmaceutical industry increased its total adherence budget for digital strategies (from 21% to 33% of the total adherence budget) and reduced its budget for adherence strategies that utilized printed material [79].

For SCIT and SLIT to be more widely prescribed and used, it may require that the pharmaceutical manufacturers help the clinician support many of the adherence strategies discussed earlier. A list of obstacles in real life and strategies to improve adherence are summarized in Tables 31.2 and 31.3.

31.9 METHODS OF MEASURING CONSISTENCY OF AIT

31.9.1 Subjective

For the same patient, subjective assessments of adherence are always higher than objective assessments, but subjective measures are low cost, have face validity, and can be applied to both SLIT and SCIT [80]. Maintaining a paper or electronic diary of medication use is a standard method of assessing adherence in controlled trials, and patients in clinical practices who are on SLIT could also be requested to keep such a log or diary. However, keeping a diary is time-consuming for the patient, is influenced by social desirability responding ("faking good"), may be retrospectively completed, and is labor intensive for health professionals to review and to score or to summarize. Both SCIT and SLIT adherence data can be obtained by the patient's verbal report during an office visit. While this method is inexpensive and easy to complete, it is highly influenced by social desirability responding, is limited by the accuracy of the patient's memory, and does not allow for the determination of patterns of nonadherence [81].

Table 31.2 Adherence (persistence and consistency) obstacles in real life

Financial burden of co-pay, high deductibles
Inconvenience of frequent office visits for allergen immunotherapy or daily use of tablets for sublingual immunotherapy (SLIT)
Poor physician/nursing/front office relationship with patients, especially when multiple providers and nursing staff are involved with subcutaneous immunotherapy (SCIT)
Travel and wait time, missing work and school for SCIT
Office locations and hours inconvenient for SCIT
Chastisement when "late" for SCIT
Local reactions from SCIT or SLIT
Stopping treatment when symptoms improve
Perceived ineffectiveness
Symptom control still requires avoidance or pharmacotherapy

Table 31.3 Adherence (persistence and consistency) improvement strategies

Success depends on a multifaceted approach—implementing just one suggestion will not work!
Used to use "shared decision-making" tool before initiating allergen immunotherapy (AIT)
Provide detailed financial cost for AIT prior to initiation and update patient when changes occur, e.g., due to insurance policies
Ask about financial concerns and adverse events at each follow-up visit
Have frequent contact with patient at AIT initiation, e.g., weekly first 3 months
Develop a support line 24/7 for AIT patients
Designate a specific office nurse with a dedicated phone extension for AIT patients
Utilize volunteer patient ambassadors
Use simple and effective electronic tracking of missed SCIT appointments
Send automatic email/SMS messages about upcoming SCIT treatments, SLIT, and follow-up visits for AIT and include reason for visit
Provide verbal and written (pictorial) local reaction explanations for SCIT and SLIT and possible solutions
Provide written directions for when to withhold SCIT or SLIT and when to restart
Obtain pharmacy records for SLIT refill data to discuss during office visits
Use objective measurements for symptom improvement at each visit, e.g., allergy control test (ACT) or rhinitis control assessment test (RCAT)
Complete an "Allergen Immunotherapy Adherence Questionnaire" (a modified Morisky 8 Questionnaire) or similar instrument at each visit and phone call
Use motivational interviewing techniques for each office visit
Develop personalized adherence plan for each patient
Ask patients to complete the Satisfaction Scale for Patients Receiving Allergen Immunotherapy (ESPIA) on an annual basis

It is well established that when patients say that they are nonadherent, this is truly the case. Even when admitting they are nonadherent, they overestimate their adherence by 17% on average [73]. However, when patients report that they are adherent, this is only true about 50% of the time [73]. Perhaps the most inaccurate method of determining patient adherence is "clinical impression." Part of the difficulty of using the clinician's judgment stems from performing an incomplete assessment of adherence during the office visit. The physician may also be unconsciously biased as to the degree of adherence based on patient characteristics such as socioeconomic status or level of education as well as the patient's perceived motivation during the visit [82]. However, even a thorough, informal assessment of adherence is often inaccurate if one considers the improvement or lack thereof in health outcomes, e.g., reduction of allergic symptoms and improvement in quality of life attributed only to AIT. Assuming that a patient who remains symptomatic is nonadherent can be detrimental to the clinician-patient relationship and also may prevent a modification of treatment course that may benefit the patient. Thus, health outcomes can never serve completely as a proxy for a measurement of adherence [80]. Furthermore, only assessing health outcomes offers no insight into patterns of behavior that contribute to nonadherence.

31.9.2 Objective

Direct observation and recording of completed SCIT injections in the office definitely identifies patients who are adherent or nonadherent. Every clinic should have a specific plan for monitoring missed visits and reminding patients of upcoming appointments and allergy injections, using a combination of phone, text, and email reminders. Ideally, a structured provider-patient discussion of completed SCIT treatments, including being consistent with appropriate injection intervals, should be held during all office visits. Unfortunately, it is not standard practice for all office staff to monitor diligently and to complete patient follow-up for missed injections, nor is it typical for physicians to document nonadherence during office visits. Future use of electronic monitors, e.g., flashing red lights on allergy injection vials, could prompt staff that the vial has not been used within the scheduled interval, prompting a patient follow-up phone call.

The most objective method of determining SLIT adherence is through the use of pharmacy and medical claims data. However, this only confirms that the SLIT tablets were picked up and not that they were actually taken. Moreover, it does not indicate whether the SLIT treatment was taken as prescribed. As with oral medications, when patients realize that they are being monitored for adherence and are requested to bring in the remaining tablets, there is often "dumping," i.e., discarding the unused tablets, prior to the office visit. While not yet available for SLIT tablets, a tool incorporating a microchip, e.g., the Medication Event Monitoring System (MEMS) that records the time and date that the tablet is removed from the sealed package or bottle could be a future option [83].

Although not totally objective, the use of standardized, patient-administered questionnaires has been suggested. Unfortunately, those that address global patient characteristics or personality traits are not good predictors of adherence behavior [83]. The eight-item Morisky Medication Adherence Scale (MMAS-8), developed in 2008, is one of the most accepted self-reported measures for adherence to taking prescribed medications for many chronic diseases [84,85]. There are seven questions that are Yes/No and one item that is rated on a five-point Likert scale. For the control of hypertension,

for example, it has a sensitivity of 92% and a specificity of 53% [86]. Although it has not been validated, the authors of this chapter have proposed the use of the "Allergen Immunotherapy Adherence Questionnaire," based on a modification of the Morisky MMAS-8 (see Figure 31.1).

In addition to the use of an adherence questionnaire, including the Rhinitis Control Assessment Test (RCAT) and/or the Allergy Control Test (ACT), both U.S.-validated instruments, can help both the patient and the physician monitor symptom improvement or lack thereof. Patients may fail to realize the degree to which they have improved over a 1- to 2-year time span, as expectations may increase as symptoms improve. Having a record that more objectively documents slow but steady improvement can enhance adherence. Another questionnaire that clinicians may want to consider administering on a yearly basis is the validated (for adults)

Patient answers: Yes or No
Score: Y = 1; N = 0

1. Do you sometimes forget to come in for your allergy injection or to take your SLIT tablet?

2. People sometimes miss their scheduled allergy injection or SLIT tablet for reasons other than forgetting. Thinking over the past 3 months, were there any times when you intentionally did not come in for an allergy injection or failed to take your SLIT tablet?

3. Have you ever cut back or stopped taking your allergy injections or SLIT tablets (without discussing this with your allergist) because you felt worse when you took the allergy treatment?

4. When you travel, do you often skip allergy injections or SLIT tablets?

5. Did you skip or were you late for your last or today's allergy injection or for taking any SLIT tablets this week?

6. When you feel like your symptoms are under control, do you sometimes stop taking your allergy injections or SLIT tablets?

7. Taking allergy injections or SLIT tablets on a regular basis is a real inconvenience for some people. Do you ever feel hassled about sticking to your treatment plan?

8. How often do you have difficulty remembering to come in for your allergy injection or taking your SLIT tablet at home?
   A. Never/rarely
   B. Once in a while
   C. Sometimes
   D. Usually
   E. All the time

A = 0;
B–E = 1

Total score for all 8 questions:
Scores: >2 = low adherence
1 or 2 = medium adherence
0 = high adherence

Morisky DE, Green LW, Levine DM. Concurrent and predictive validity of a self-reported measure of medication adherence. Med Care. 1986;24:67–74.

Figure 31.1 Allergen immunotherapy adherence questionnaire. Adapted from Morisky Medication Adherence Scale [MMAS-8] Morisky DE et al. *Med Care*. 1986;24:67–74.

Satisfaction Scale for Patients Receiving Allergen Immunotherapy (ESPIA) that consists of 16 items with overall satisfaction rated on a 0–100 scale [87].

31.10 WHO IS TO BLAME FOR NONADHERENCE?

If adherence strategies are going to be successful, they must be addressed by the entire healthcare system, in much the same way as medical errors are now handled. Active participants must include the patient and his or her extended family; the physician and related healthcare professionals; all clerical staff within the healthcare setting; third-party payors; and healthcare educators, including professional organizations, researchers, and policy makers. These participants have to consider communication, affordability, simplicity, and convenience, as these are all key to achieving the desired adherence.

All healthcare providers must be sensitive to cultural and ethnic values and beliefs when discussing AIT with the patient and his or her family. Inviting all interested family members to the AIT shared decision-making visit to get "buy-in" is the first step toward adherence. The importance of all staff, from receptionist to nurse to physician, creating a team approach that establishes a caring, friendly, respectful, patient-centered relationship with the entire family cannot be overemphasized. Reprimanding the patient for missed injections or visits, disregarding the patient's concern with minor adverse reactions such as local swelling, and blaming the patient for his or her uncontrolled symptoms can all contribute to nonpersistence and inconsistency of AIT.

In our mobile society and ever-changing provider panels, patients often have to transfer their allergy care and AIT to another allergist. For many patients, this transition is very difficult, even when they desire to continue with AIT. Only about one-third of patients on AIT actually continue AIT when they relocate [38]. Allergists, for the most part, are not using the recommended guidelines regarding (1) format for SCIT allergy extract prescriptions, (2) schedules for AIT administration, (3) ideal maintenance dose, and (4) standardized recording of injections. There remains the unwillingness on the parts of many treating allergists to release detailed allergy extract records, as well as the concern on the part of the new allergist about the accuracy of prior skin testing. Although published studies are not available, it is likely that most SCIT patients are retested and restarted on AIT by the new allergist. All of these issues lead to markedly reduced AIT adherence.

Physicians are under increasing time constraints as fee-for-service and group-contracted reimbursements continued to be reduced each year, making it very difficult to carve out time for shared decision-making and open-ended adherence assessment and problem-solving visits with AIT patients. Patients' perceptions of their physicians' interest in them, as individual patients, is a good predictor of the patients' intentions to adhere to the treatment plan [88]. Whether deciding to initiate or to continue with AIT, patients want to feel that their preferences have been taken into account. Utilizing a standard operating procedure with self-reported questionnaires, short videos, or online educational tools that reinforce shared decision-making [89] and employing a team approach within the clinic may help reduce or eliminate some of these obstacles. Convenience of clinic hours, clinic locations, parking, scheduling of appointments, and waiting times are essential to maintaining patient adherence to AIT.

Many articles have been written on the beneficial effects of shared decision-making and motivational interviewing (MI) [90,91]. MI aims to develop the patient's intrinsic motivation to adhere to the recommended treatment and to resolve any ambivalence about becoming more adherent. The patient must see that following the recommended treatment protocol aligns with his or her own values and goals [92]. Using the four key components of MI, i.e., open-ended questions, affirmations, reflective listening, and summary statements, increases patient satisfaction and treatment adherence [92]. An interview in which the patient is asked yes or no questions leads to limited information being elicited, responses that are more biased, potential damage to the physician-patient relationship, and diminished effect on improving adherence. Expression of empathy, an underlying principle of MI, predicts favorable treatment outcomes.

Some studies demonstrate that using MI actually saves the physician time in the long run. However, most physicians are ill-equipped to engage in MI. Following the MI, the physician is encouraged to use various strategies to enhance the motivation to bring about change, such as allowing the patient to set the agenda, e.g., "Would you rather discuss with me the benefit you are experiencing or not experiencing from your allergy injections, or would you rather discuss any side effects that you are experiencing?" Another strategy is asking the patient to discuss how in a typical day/week/month his or her allergies are impacting his or her life. Asking the patient to rate his or her motivation to adhere to AIT on a 1–10 scale as well as rating his or her confidence in being able to make changes to improve adherence can also be of value. The physician may use the "lower-higher exercise" to have the patient defend his or her number on the scale of confidence in being able to adhere by asking "Why not a lower number?" helping to elicit positive action statements by the patient [92]. Finally, exploring with the patient the costs and benefits of becoming more adherent to AIT would likely conclude the adherence conversation. But for most allergists, following the previous recommendations might seem overwhelming. Proficiency in conducting a shared decision-making conversation, using motivational interviewing, and customizing a personalized adherence plan all in a time-efficient manner are skills that most allergists have not been taught. While the "best approach" to address nonadherence needs additional research, our professional organizations should provide educational tools that present what is currently felt to be the best way to maximize the patient-physician interaction and to achieve better adherence.

In a recent U.S. study that examined reasons for nonadherence to SCIT, inadequate healthcare coverage by a third-party payor was the number one cause for discontinuation for 40% of the 213 patients who were not persistent [93]. In a literature review of 66 articles looking for the relationship between cost-sharing and adherence in multiple disease states, 85% showed that increasing the patient's share of medication costs significantly decreased adherence and negatively impacted disease outcome, irrespective of type of outcome measured or the disease state studied [94]. On average, for a $1 increase in the patient's copay, adherence decreases by 0.4% [94]. One study showed that an increase of $10 for diabetes medications could result in a 19% reduction in adherence [94]. Throughout the course of AIT, the patient will continue to assess if the results, present and future, are worth the out-of-pocket cost and inconvenience of continuing with AIT. It is likely that the cost of AIT in the United States is almost always an underlying consideration, whether deciding to initiate or to continue with AIT, even if other reasons are offered as the principal rationale for nonpersistence. While a zero copay would not provide 100%

adherence, it is unfortunate that third-party payors fail to see that setting unreasonable patient cost for AIT, and thereby encouraging nonadherence, leads to ineffective treatment and worsening of the underlying disease, which can lead to further nonadherence.

Healthcare providers, professional organizations, advocacy groups, and all of our patients need to advocate to policy makers to keep AIT as an affordable option for the treatment of AR and asthma. While research on the efficacy and long-term benefits of SLIT is expanding, mainly smaller and older studies address the efficacy and long-term benefits of SCIT. High-quality research that establishes the long-term benefits of SCIT and SLIT is clearly an unmet need.

31.11 HOW IMPORTANT IS CONSISTENCY FOR SUBCUTANEOUS IMMUNOTHERAPY AND SUBLINGUAL IMMUNOTHERAPY?

The very basic questions of how the varying schedules of pre- and coseasonal versus year-round treatment, as well as the consistency of SCIT or SLIT treatment, correlate with symptom improvement both during and following discontinuation of AIT, remain unanswered. We do not know how consistent the patient must be to increase quality of life and to obtain good, long-term results.

Questions remain regarding recommended duration of AIT for both seasonal and perennial allergens. For year-round SCIT, 3 years is generally accepted as the minimum [95], but the ideal duration of AIT for long-term benefit has not been determined, with longer durations, e.g., 4–5 years versus 3 years, reported to be superior in some studies [96–98]. In a 15-year prospective controlled but nonrandomized study comparing 3, 4, and 5 years of SLIT dust mite year-round treatment, long-term symptom improvement was present during all treatment years and remained statistically reduced (compared to the control group) for 6, 7, and 7 years, respectively, following AIT discontinuation [95,99]. However, symptom scores for the 3-, 4-, and 5-year SLIT groups remained decreased more than 50% of baseline for 7, 8, and 8 years, respectively, after discontinuation of AIT [95]. The researchers, therefore, suggested that 4 years may be the optimal length of SLIT dust-mite treatment [95,100]. Similar data for other perennial allergens have not been published.

Many European studies report excellent results with pre- and coseasonal pollen SCIT [72], although it is rarely used in the United States. These data show that even with long treatment-free intervals (outside of pollen season), there can be long-lasting efficacy following 3 years of treatment. While the two grass SLIT tablets available in the United States have both been approved for pre- and coseasonal use, one grass product (GRASTEK) is also approved for year-round treatment. In controlled trials, following 3 years of year-round treatment with GRASTEK, patients maintained symptom reduction for only 1 year following discontinuation of treatment. In open-label studies, year-round SLIT was not superior to preseasonal treatment [101,102]. But studies showing persistent benefit for 2 years following 3 years of grass pollen SLIT tablets used year-round treatment [100,103]. Even in this study, the 40% improvement in symptoms reported at the end of the 3 years of active treatment had declined to 20% by the end of the second year after treatment was discontinued, losing statistical significance

[100]. Additional studies are needed to firmly establish the long-term benefits of 3 years of pre- and coseasonal treatment. In one large pre- and coseasonal 2-year grass SLIT study, patients reported a persistence of 96.8% and a consistency of 93.3% [104]. If it is established that pre- and coseasonal is just as effective overall as year-round therapy, adherence follow-up could be more intense and, hopefully, result in improved persistence, with reduction in both direct and indirect costs.

Although there are sufficient data to conclude that a minimum of 3–4 years of AIT is needed for the best long-term benefit [2,7,105–108], the data on the effect of missed treatments on short- term symptom control or on the long-term benefit following completion of the ideal 3–5 years of AIT are inconclusive. Is there a threshold, e.g., either a percentage of AIT treatments overall or a certain number within a defined period, below which missed treatments are nonsignificant? Do missed treatments in the first 6–12 months of treatment have a larger impact than missed treatments in the last year of treatment? Do missed treatments have a greater impact with SCIT versus SLIT? As the answers to these questions likely relate to the frequency with which the immune system requires stimulation to bring about the desired immune changes, e.g., tolerance-inducing cells, blocking antibodies, and reduced specific IgE, research is needed that convincingly shows how best to impact the desired immune changes. It is also unknown if the desired immune effects differ among different individuals and with different allergens, especially seasonal versus perennial allergens where, in the latter, stimulation from environmental exposure occurs on a continual basis.

Perhaps a more intriguing question is whether scheduled intermittent administration of SCIT and SLIT for perennial allergens would be effective and safe. One could reason that if intermittent treatment is effective for pollen, it should also be effective for perennial allergens, with similar immunologic responses. Perhaps patients would be willing to take SLIT and SCIT for 2 months on and 2–4 months off, allowing freedom for summer vacations or extended work assignments out of town. With SLIT tablets having no buildup phase, such an intermittent schedule could likely be safely implemented. However, with SCIT, such an approach would probably require having the patient reach the maintenance dose prior to taking an "AIT vacation." When treatment is reinitiated after an AIT vacation, one would likely want to accomplish rapid dose buildup with SCIT in a rush or cluster regimen. In real life, allergists are frequently faced with this dilemma when patients return after a self-imposed break and request to restart AIT. The degree to which the prior dose is reduced likely varies widely from one allergist to another. While most patients seem to tolerate restarting AIT after a prolonged absence and report rapid symptom reduction, the effect of this inconsistency on long-term benefit remains unstudied. One small 12-month randomized, but nonblinded, dust mite SLIT study compared continual versus 2 months of treatment alternating with 2 months of suspension [109]. The continual group administered SLIT 3×/week, while the intermittent group administered SLIT daily, with both groups achieving the same cumulative allergen extract dose at the end of 1 year. There were no intergroup differences in efficacy, side effects, quality of life, or patient satisfaction [109]. While compliance did not differ between the two groups during this short study, one would hope that intermittent treatment might be better accepted by patients, would be easier for physicians to monitor, and could reduce overall costs of AIT. Research data are needed on safety and efficacy for both immediate and long-term symptom reduction with both unintended inconsistency or a planned, intermittent treatment schedule. Furthermore, evidence is needed that an intermittent schedule improves compliance and reduces cost, making quality adjusted life-year (QALY) calculations more favorable.

31.12 COST-EFFECTIVENESS OF AIT

Exploring the literature regarding the pharmacoeconomics of AIT is not an easy task. There are several important issues that add complexity. These include the fact that studies that have examined this question rely on different approaches, with some examining only direct costs, e.g., medicines and medical visits, while others attempt to consider indirect costs, e.g., missed school or work [110]. It must also be noted that beyond AIT's ability to reduce medicine acutely [97], after a 2- to 5-year course, it can provide sustained effect even 12 years after discontinuation [111], can prevent neosensitization to new allergens [112,113], as well as prevent escalation of AR to asthma [112]. Thus, cost reduction could be realized in multiple domains and over an extended time.

There have been many studies exploring the pharmacoeconomics of both SCIT and SLIT in allergic disease, including several recent reviews; but interestingly, very few studies have been performed in the United States [110,114–116]. As noted earlier, determining the cost-effectiveness of AIT is hampered by several impediments, most important being the difficulty in quantifying the long-term efficacy as well as the indirect costs. With that said, these studies almost universally demonstrate the cost savings of AIT, with time to achieve this goal varying from 3 months to several years. In this section, we explore these data in more detail.

One of the first studies to formally consider the economic impact of immunotherapy was performed by Creticos and colleagues [117]. The authors examined the efficacy of SCIT for asthma exacerbated by seasonal ragweed exposure, comparing 2 years of subcutaneous ragweed SCIT to placebo in a double-blind fashion [117]. The authors found a reduction in rhinitis symptoms, skin-test sensitivity, and bronchial hyperresponsiveness, as well as an improvement in peak expiratory flow rates. Although medication scores were lower in the active group at year 1, they were similar at year 2. It should be noted, however, that baseline medication use was higher in the active AIT group. While the retail medication cost was $597 for the placebo group versus $420 for the group randomized to AIT, these cost savings were offset by the charges for SCIT [117].

A series of studies examined resource utilization and costs of SCIT through the examination of a Medicaid population database. The first relied on a retrospective analysis of Florida Medicaid claims data (1997–2004) in children given a new diagnosis of AR, examining characteristics associated with receiving SCIT, patterns of SCIT care, and healthcare use, as well as costs incurred in the 6 months before versus the 6 months after SCIT [37]. They found that despite suboptimal treatment persistence, resource use and costs after treatment were significantly reduced from pre-SCIT levels. Specifically, 47% discontinued SCIT within the first year and only 16% completed 3 years of SCIT. Despite this poor persistence, patients who received SCIT used significantly less pharmacy (12.1 versus 8.9 claims, $P<.0001$), outpatient (30.7 versus 22.9 visits, $P<.0001$), and inpatient (1.2 versus 0.4 admissions, $P<0.02$) resources in the 6 months after compared to the 6 months before SCIT. Pharmacy ($330 versus $60, $P<.0001$), outpatient ($735 versus $270, $P<.0001$), and inpatient ($2441 versus $1, $P<.0001$) costs (including costs for SCIT care) were significantly reduced after

SCIT. It must be kept in mind that this was not a controlled study; therefore, many potential variables unrelated to SCIT could have contributed to the reduced healthcare costs.

The Florida Medicaid database was again utilized to determine whether AIT reduced healthcare utilization and costs in children newly diagnosed as having AR. This second study relied on a retrospective matched cohort design of children with a paid claim between 1997 and 2007 [118]. In the active treatment group, children with newly diagnosed AR and AIT naïve were started on SCIT. The authors looked at the healthcare costs in the active treatment versus the matched controls during the 18 months following the initiation of AIT. The authors found that those children treated with SCIT had significantly lower 18-month median per-patient total healthcare costs ($3247 versus $4872), outpatient costs exclusive of immunotherapy-related care ($1107 versus $2626), and pharmacy costs ($1108 versus $1316) compared with matched controls ($P<.001$ for all). They once again found that a significant difference in total healthcare costs was evident 3 months after initiating AIT and savings increased throughout the study. The authors concluded that the use of SCIT has the potential for early and significant cost savings in children with AR [118]. If these findings can be reproduced in future controlled trials, the use of AIT could significantly reduce AR-related morbidity and its economic burden.

A third study by Hankin and colleagues utilized a similar Florida Medicaid claims database and performed a retrospective analysis in both children and adults who were continuously enrolled, comparing mean 18-month healthcare costs of patients with newly diagnosed AR who began SCIT with matched control subjects not receiving SCIT [119]. The authors found that the group that received SCIT had a 38% ($6637 versus $10,644, $P<.0001$) lower mean 18-month total healthcare cost compared to the matched control subjects, noting significant savings within 3 months of initiating SCIT. Furthermore, they found that the magnitude of 18-month healthcare cost savings seen in AIT-treated adults did not significantly differ from that seen with children ($4397 versus $3965, $P=.435$).

Allen-Ramey and colleagues performed a retrospective cohort study examining the medical and pharmacy claims from the Optum Research Database from January 2009 through February 2014 for adults and pediatric patients with greater than seven (continuers) versus seven or less (discontinuers) injection visits for SCIT, comparing healthcare costs and resource utilization [13,120]. They found that those who continued AIT were less likely to use oral corticosteroids than those who discontinued (27.7% versus 29.6%, $p=.018$). The "continuers" also had fewer respiratory-related emergency room visits (5.4% versus 6.5%, $p=.008$) and hospitalizations (1.1% versus 1.7%; $p=.002$). However, interestingly, the "continuers" were more likely than "discontinuers" to have one or more AR-related office visit (98.8% versus 94.6%, $p<.001$); outpatient hospital visit (2.4% versus 1.7%, $p=.002$), and emergency room visit (3.5% versus 2.7%, $p=.006$). Furthermore, the "continuers" had greater mean total AR-related costs than the "discontinuers" ($1918 versus $646, $p<.001$). Overall, when considering unadjusted mean total respiratory-related costs, the AIT "continuers" were lower than the "discontinuers," but the difference was not statistically significant ($1589 versus $1785, $p=.077$). It should be noted, however, that when adjusted with a generalized linear model, these costs were significantly lower among the "continuers" compared to the "discontinuers" ($p<.001$). The authors concluded that the continued use of SCIT results in lower respiratory-related costs compared to early "discontinuers." These savings are probably a reflection of decrease in overall acute care costs.

It is very difficult to make comparisons due to the different environments and medical systems/payors, as well as disparate pharmacy benefits. However, one German study by Schädlich and Brecht deserves mention, as the authors examined the pharmacoeconomics of SCIT versus pharmacotherapy in patients with seasonal and perennial AR using a model that incorporated a multifaceted assessment of AR with a 10-year follow-up, including the potential impact of AIT on asthma [121]. They found that the breakeven point between AIT with pharmacotherapy versus pharmacotherapy alone was reached between year 6 and year 8, resulting in net savings of between 650 and 1190 deutschmarks (DM) (approximately $380–$693) per patient after 10 years. The authors conclude that SCIT results in net savings for the healthcare system [121].

The SLIT tablet pharmacoeconomic studies have generally demonstrated a pharmacoeconomic advantage with therapy [122–127]. A 2015 German study, which relied upon a Markov model, compared 3 years of AIT with a 5-grass SLIT tablet versus a market mix of injectable allergoids, following outcomes over 9 years [128]. The authors examined several potential cost drivers, including the relative efficacy, expressed as standardized mean difference estimated from an indirect comparison of symptom scores extracted from available clinical trials; the Rhinitis Symptom Utility Index as a proxy to estimate utility values for symptom scores; drug acquisition and other medical costs, derived from published sources; as well as estimates for resource use, immunotherapy persistence, and asthma development. The analysis was executed from the German payor's perspective, which included payments of the Statutory Health Insurance as well as additional payments by insurants. Using this model, the predicted cost-utility ratio of the five-grass tablet versus a market mix of injectable allergoid products was $13,941.90 per QALY in the base case analysis. This suggests that the sublingual native five-grass tablet is cost-effective relative to a mix of SCIT allergoid compounds [128]. There are obvious limitations to this study, including the fact that there are some data that indicate SCIT to be more effective than SLIT. In the United States, most allergists utilize extracts composed of multiple allergenic components versus the European approach of using only one major allergen. Furthermore, this comparison utilized a SCIT extract that is not approved in the United States. Last, all SLIT studies have been performed in Europe, and the results are difficult to generalize to a disparate system such as that in the United States [110].

Overall, studies examining the pharmacoeconomics of AIT demonstrate a cost savings. Studies have varied regarding the breakeven point, with some achieving cost savings in as little as 3 months, while others show 6–8 years are required. It is difficult to truly model all of the possible savings with AIT, as the potential to prevent neosensitization and the development of asthma, as well as the reduction in absenteeism and presenteeism are extremely difficult to quantify as to value. Furthermore, it is even more difficult to compare modes of AIT. Last, further studies are desperately needed regarding the health economics of AIT in the United States. The paucity of patients achieving the recommended 3–5 years of treatment makes it unlikely that the cost-effectiveness of AIT is maximized [128].

31.13 CONCLUSION AND FUTURE NEEDS

Many questions remain unanswered. Perhaps nonadherence itself is a medical condition that needs treatment. It is important to support and not to blame the patient for nonadherence, as it is the joint responsibility of the patient, the physician, and the healthcare system to create an environment to encourage adherence. Nonadherence is multifactorial (see Table 31.2) in most if not all individuals, and the physician must address all of the factors if adherence is to be improved. Perhaps the greatest challenge is taking the time to create an individualized, patient-tailored strategy to improve adherence, as one size does not fit all. Adherence is dynamic, and selecting the best time to start AIT and assuring that there is close follow-up through the years of AIT is essential. The patient who is persistent and consistent in year 1 of AIT may not continue to be so in year 3 without added encouragement and support. As shown in Table 31.1, there are no uniform thresholds for what constitutes good consistency (e.g., efficacy varies between missing just 1 dose, 5 doses, or 10 doses over a specified period of time), and the various methods of defining and documenting persistence (e.g., via tracking lack of pharmacy refills for a specified time prior, no allergy injection documented on the medical record for a specified time period, or some other method) make it impossible to compare studies and determine common factors for nonadherence. Successful strategies to improve adherence require better definition of nonadherence causation. Researchers must agree on clear operational definitions of the terms "compliance," "adherence," "persistence," and "consistency." The percentage and pattern of prescribed doses or SCIT and SLIT that are required for best patient outcomes should be established. Furthermore, the duration of SCIT and SLIT resulting in best or optimal patient outcomes and cost-effectiveness needs to be defined by data.

Healthcare systems and professional organizations need to help empower physicians and their staffs both in utilizing efficient and accurate ways to assess nonadherence and in implementing interventions to optimize adherence. Strategies to improve adherence are summarized in Table 31.3. The multidisciplinary approach to addressing nonadherence will require the involvement of all healthcare professionals, researchers, professional organizations, third-party payors, and policy makers. Ultimately, clinicians need to respect the wishes of our patients and to accept their decisions as to whether to start and to continue with AIT or to discontinue treatment, as long as they are rational, informed decisions based upon the patients' personal experiences and values.

SALIENT POINTS

1. Nonadherence to medicines as a whole is very common, with significant economic consequence, resulting in an estimated cost in the U.S. alone of $100 to $290 billion per year.
2. Only a small proportion of appropriately selected candidates for allergen immunotherapy (AIT) elect to initiate treatment. Of those who begin AIT, a high percentage are nonadherent to the recommended treatment schedule, often discontinuing therapy before completing the optimal length of therapy.
3. In an analysis of nine studies evaluating the 3-year persistence of AIT, the mean nonpersistence rate was 54% for subcutaneous immunotherapy (SCIT) and 58% for sublingual immunotherapy (SLIT). Reported reasons for discontinuation of SCIT included inconvenience and excessive time commitment; medical comorbidities, especially psychiatric disease and pregnancy; financial concerns; relocation of residence; spontaneous symptom improvement; family problems; and adverse effects. Lack of efficacy was rarely

mentioned for SCIT. While for SLIT, the reasons for discontinuation included lack of efficacy; adverse effects; inability to be compliant; financial concerns; spontaneous symptom improvement; excessive time commitment; and family problems.

4. Demographic patterns for nonpersistence of AIT demonstrate children (especially 5–14 years of age) to be the most persistent age group both for SCIT and SLIT. Adolescents and young adults had a high discontinuation rate, while adults over 40 years were more persistent. Sex, socioeconomic status, and type of payment for AIT did not seem to be major factors in predicting discontinuation of AIT. Patients whose AIT was prescribed by allergists demonstrate lower discontinuation rates compared to nonallergists.

5. Shared decision-making and motivational interviewing may be helpful approaches to increase adherence and persistence of AIT.

6. Successful adherence strategies will likely require engagement of the entire healthcare system. Active participants must include the patient and his or her extended family; the physician and related healthcare professionals; all clerical staff within the healthcare setting; third-party payors; healthcare educators, including professional organizations; researchers; and policy makers.

7. Determining the cost-effectiveness of AIT is hampered by several impediments, particularly the difficulty in quantifying the indirect cost and the long-term efficacy, including potential downstream benefits such as prevention of the atopic march or reduction in neosensitization. Studies have, however, demonstrated resource use and costs were improved in as little as 6 months following the initiation of AIT, even despite poor adherence.

8. Additional research is needed for optimal AIT to be attained. Goals include defining the length of time for AIT, further assessment of episodic/coseasonal approaches, tools to identify patients most likely to be adherent with AIT, and strategies to improve adherence.

REFERENCES

1. Bousquet J, Lockey R, Malling HJ et al. Allergen immunotherapy: Therapeutic vaccines for allergic diseases. World Health Organization. American Academy of Allergy, Asthma and Immunology. *Ann Allergy Asthma Immunol* 1998; 81(5): 401–415.

2. Burks AW, Calderon MA, Casale T et al. Update on allergy immunotherapy: American Academy of Allergy, Asthma and Immunology/European Academy of Allergy and Clinical Immunology/PRACTALL consensus report. *J Allergy Clin Immunol* 2013; 131(5): 1288–1296.e3.

3. Ponda P, Mithani S, Kopyltsova Y et al. Allergen immunotherapy practice patterns: A worldwide survey. *Ann Allergy Asthma Immunol* 2012; 108(6): 454–459.e7.

4. Kim JM, Lin SY, Suarez-Cuervo C et al. Allergen-specific immunotherapy for pediatric asthma and rhinoconjunctivitis: A systematic review. *Pediatrics* 2013; 131(6): 1155–1167.

5. Lin SY, Erekosima N, Suarez-Cuervo C et al. *AHRQ Comparative Effectiveness Reviews. Allergen-Specific Immunotherapy for the Treatment of Allergic Rhinoconjunctivitis and/or Asthma: Comparative Effectiveness Review.* Rockville, MD: Agency for Healthcare Research and Quality (US); 2013.

6. Senna G, Ridolo E, Calderon M, Lombardi C, Canonica GW, Passalacqua G. Evidence of adherence to allergen-specific immunotherapy. *Curr Opin Allergy Clin Immunol* 2009; 9(6): 544–548.

7. Canonica GW, Bousquet J, Casale T et al. Sub-lingual immunotherapy: World Allergy Organization Position Paper 2009. *Allergy* 2009; 64(Suppl 91): 1–59.

8. Kristiansen M, Dhami S, Netuveli G et al. Allergen immunotherapy for the prevention of allergy: A systematic review and meta-analysis. *Pediatr Allergy Immunol* 2017; 28(1): 18–29.

9. Incorvaia C, Riario-Sforza GG, Incorvaia S, Frati F. Sublingual immunotherapy in allergic asthma: Current evidence and needs to meet. *Ann Thorac Med* 2010; 5(3): 128–132.

10. Cox L, Cohn JR. Duration of allergen immunotherapy in respiratory allergy: When is enough, enough? *Ann Allergy Asthma Immunol* 2007; 98(5): 416–426.

11. Brehler R, Klimek L, Kopp MV, Christian Virchow J. Specific immunotherapy-indications and mode of action. *Dtsch Arztebl Int* 2013; 110(9): 148–158.

12. Flay BR. Efficacy and effectiveness trials (and other phases of research) in the development of health promotion programs. *Prev Med* 1986; 15(5): 451–474.

13. Calderon MA, Cox L, Casale TB et al. The effect of a new communication template on anticipated willingness to initiate or resume allergen immunotherapy: An internet-based patient survey. *Allergy Asthma Clin Immunol* 2015; 11(1): 17.

14. Sabate E. *Adherence to Long-Term Therapies: Evidence for Action.* Geneva, Switzerland: World Health Organization, 2003.

15. Denford S, Frost J, Dieppe P, Cooper C, Britten N. Individualisation of drug treatments for patients with long-term conditions: A review of concepts. *BMJ Open* 2014; 4(3): e004172.

16. Costa E, Giardini A, Savin M et al. Interventional tools to improve medication adherence: Review of literature. *Patient Prefer Adherence* 2015; 9: 1303–1314.

17. Ho PM, Magid DJ, Masoudi FA, McClure DL, Rumsfeld JS. Adherence to cardioprotective medications and mortality among patients with diabetes and ischemic heart disease. *BMC Cardiovasc Disord* 2006; 6: 48.

18. Krishnan JA, Bender BG, Wamboldt FS et al. Adherence to inhaled corticosteroids: An ancillary study of the Childhood Asthma Management Program clinical trial. *J Allergy Clin Immunol* 2012; 129(1): 112–118.

19. Huetsch JC, Uman JE, Udris EM, Au DH. Predictors of adherence to inhaled medications among veterans with COPD. *J Gen Intern Med* 2012; 27(11): 1506–1512.

20. Lamkin M, Elliott C. Curing the disobedient patient: Medication adherence programs as pharmaceutical marketing tools. 2014. https://digitalcommons.law.utulsa.edu/fac_pub/475

21. New England Healthcare Institute. Thinking outside the pillbox: A system-wide approach to improving patient medication adherence for chronic disease. 2009. https://www.nehi.net/writable/publication_files/file/pa_issue_brief_final.pdf

22. Cutler RL, Fernandez-Llimos F, Frommer M, Benrimoj C, Garcia-Cardenas V. Economic impact of medication non-adherence by disease groups: A systematic review. *BMJ Open* 2018; 8(1): e016982.

23. Lamkin M, Elliott C. Curing the disobedient patient: Medication adherence programs as pharmaceutical marketing tools. *J Law Med Ethics* 2014; 42(4): 492–500.

24. Cohn JR, Pizzi A. Determinants of patient compliance with allergen immunotherapy. *J Allergy Clin Immunol* 1993; 91(3): 734–737.

25. Moore BA, Duffy DJ, Heng HG, Lim CK, Miller MA. What is your diagnosis? *J Am Vet Med Assoc* 2017; 251(11): 1241–1243.

26. Hsu NM, Reisacher WR. A comparison of attrition rates in patients undergoing sublingual immunotherapy vs subcutaneous immunotherapy. *Int Forum Allergy Rhinol* 2012; 2(4): 280–284.

27. Makatsori M, Scadding GW, Lombardo C et al. Dropouts in sublingual allergen immunotherapy trials—A systematic review. *Allergy* 2014; 69(5): 571–580.

28. Allam JP, Andreasen JN, Mette J, Serup-Hansen N, Wustenberg EG. Comparison of allergy immunotherapy medication persistence with a sublingual immunotherapy tablet versus subcutaneous immunotherapy in Germany. *J Allergy Clin Immunol* 2018; 141(5): 1898–1901.e5.

29. Anolik R, Schwartz AM, Sajjan S, Allen-Ramey F. Patient initiation and persistence with allergen immunotherapy. *Ann Allergy Asthma Immunol* 2014; 113(1): 101–107.

30. Egert-Schmidt AM, Kolbe JM, Mussler S, Thum-Oltmer S. Patients' compliance with different administration routes for allergen immunotherapy in Germany. *Patient Prefer Adherence* 2014; 8: 1475–1481.

31. Kiel MA, Roder E, Gerth van Wijk R, Al MJ, Hop WC, Rutten-van Molken MP. Real-life compliance and persistence among users of subcutaneous and sublingual allergen immunotherapy. *J Allergy Clin Immunol* 2013; 132(2): 353–360.e2.

32. Leader BA, Rotella M, Stillman L, DelGaudio JM, Patel ZM, Wise SK. Immunotherapy compliance: Comparison of subcutaneous versus sublingual immunotherapy. *Int Forum Allergy Rhinol* 2016; 6(5): 460–464.

33. Lemberg ML, Berk T, Shah-Hosseini K, Kasche EM, Mosges R. Sublingual versus subcutaneous immunotherapy: Patient adherence at a large German allergy center. *Patient Prefer Adherence* 2017; 11: 63–70.

34. Pajno GB, Vita D, Caminiti L et al. Children's compliance with allergen immunotherapy according to administration routes. *J Allergy Clin Immunol* 2005; 116(6): 1380–1381.

35. Sieber J, De Geest S, Shah-Hosseini K, Mosges R. Medication persistence with long-term, specific grass pollen immunotherapy measured by prescription renewal rates. *Curr Med Res Opin* 2011; 27(4): 855–861.

36. Donahue JG, Greineder DK, Connor-Lacke L, Canning CF, Platt R. Utilization and cost of immunotherapy for allergic asthma and rhinitis. *Ann Allergy Asthma Immunol* 1999; 82(4): 339–347.

37. Hankin CS, Cox L, Lang D et al. Allergy immunotherapy among Medicaid-enrolled children with allergic rhinitis: Patterns of care, resource use, and costs. *J Allergy Clin Immunol* 2008; 121(1): 227–232.

38. Rhodes BJ. Patient dropouts before completion of optimal dose, multiple allergen immunotherapy. *Ann Allergy Asthma Immunol* 1999; 82(3): 281–286.

39. Marogna M, Spadolini I, Massolo A, Canonica GW, Passalacqua G. Randomized controlled open study of sublingual immunotherapy for respiratory allergy in real-life: Clinical efficacy and more. *Allergy* 2004; 59(11): 1205–1210.

40. Trebuchon F, David M, Demoly P. Medical management and sublingual immunotherapy practices in patients with house dust mite-induced respiratory allergy: A retrospective, observational study. *Int J Immunopathol Pharmacol* 2012; 25(1): 193–206.

41. Kiotseridis H, Arvidsson P, Backer V, Braendholt V, Tunsater A. Adherence and quality of life in adults and children during 3-years of SLIT treatment with Grazax—A real life study. *NPJ Prim Care Respir Med* 2018; 28(1): 4.

42. Senna G, Lombardi C, Canonica GW, Passalacqua G. How adherent to sublingual immunotherapy prescriptions are patients? The manufacturers' viewpoint. *J Allergy Clin Immunol* 2010; 126(3): 668–669.

43. Mahesh PA, Vedanthan PK, Amrutha DH, Giridhar BH, Prabhakar AK. Factors associated with non-adherence to specific allergen immunotherapy in management of respiratory allergy. *Indian J Chest Dis Allied Sci* 2010; 52(2): 91–95.

44. Lombardi C, Gani F, Landi M et al. Quantitative assessment of the adherence to sublingual immunotherapy. *J Allergy Clin Immunol* 2004; 113(6): 1219–1220.

45. Passalacqua G, Musarra A, Pecora S et al. Quantitative assessment of the compliance with a once-daily sublingual immunotherapy regimen in real life (EASY Project: Evaluation of a novel SLIT formulation during a Year). *J Allergy Clin Immunol* 2006; 117(4): 946–948.

46. Passalacqua G, Musarra A, Pecora S et al. Quantitative assessment of the compliance with once-daily sublingual immunotherapy in children (EASY project: Evaluation of a novel SLIT formulation during a year). *Pediatr Allergy Immunol* 2007; 18(1): 58–62.

47. Kumar MS, Oh MS, Leader B et al. Perceived compliance and barriers to care in sublingual immunotherapy. *Int Forum Allergy Rhinol* 2017; 7(5): 525–529.

48. Savi E, Peveri S, Senna G, Passalacqua G. Causes of SLIT discontinuation and strategies to improve the adherence: A pragmatic approach. *Allergy* 2013; 68(9): 1193–1195.

49. Vita D, Caminiti L, Ruggeri P, Pajno GB. Sublingual immunotherapy: Adherence based on timing and monitoring control visits. *Allergy* 2010; 65(5): 668–669.

50. Macharia WM, Leon G, Rowe BH, Stephenson BJ, Haynes RB. An overview of interventions to improve compliance with appointment keeping for medical services. *JAMA* 1992; 267(13): 1813–1817.

51. Epstein TE, Tankersley MS. Are allergen immunotherapy dose adjustments needed for local reactions, peaks of season, or gaps in treatment? *J Allergy Clin Immunol Pract* 2017; 5(5): 1227–1233.

52. Epstein TG, Liss GM, Murphy-Berendts K, Bernstein DI. AAAAI and ACAAI surveillance study of subcutaneous immunotherapy, year 3: What practices modify the risk of systemic reactions? *Ann Allergy Asthma Immunol* 2013; 110(4): 274–278.e1.

53. Reid MJ, Lockey RF, Turkeltaub PC, Platts-Mills TA. Survey of fatalities from skin testing and immunotherapy 1985–1989. *J Allergy Clin Immunol* 1993; 92(1 Pt 1): 6–15.

54. Bernstein DI, Wanner M, Borish L, Liss GM, Immunotherapy Committee AAoAA, Immunology. Twelve-year survey of fatal reactions to allergen injections and skin testing: 1990–2001. *J Allergy Clin Immunol* 2004; 113(6): 1129–1136.

55. Tinkelman DG, Cole WQ 3rd, Tunno J. Immunotherapy: A one-year prospective study to evaluate risk factors of systemic reactions. *J Allergy Clin Immunol* 1995; 95(1 Pt 1): 8–14.

56. Lin MS, Tanner E, Lynn J, Friday GA, Jr. Nonfatal systemic allergic reactions induced by skin testing and immunotherapy. *Ann Allergy* 1993; 71(6): 557–562.

57. Moreno C, Cuesta-Herranz J, Fernandez-Tavora L, Alvarez-Cuesta E, Immunotherapy Committee SEdAeIC. Immunotherapy safety: A prospective multi-centric monitoring study of biologically standardized therapeutic vaccines for allergic diseases. *Clin Exp Allergy* 2004; 34(4): 527–531.

58. Wong PH, Quinn JM, Gomez RA, Webb CN. Systemic reactions to immunotherapy during mountain cedar season: Implications for seasonal dose adjustment. *J Allergy Clin Immunol Pract* 2017; 5(5): 1438–1439.e1.

59. Epstein TG, Liss GM, Murphy-Berendts K, Bernstein DI. Risk factors for fatal and nonfatal reactions to subcutaneous immunotherapy: National surveillance study on allergen

immunotherapy (2008–2013). *Ann Allergy Asthma Immunol* 2016; 116(4): 354–359.e2.

60. Leung TF. In-season dosage adjustment for pollen subcutaneous immunotherapy: The controversy continues. *J Allergy Clin Immunol Pract* 2017; 5(5): 1440–1441.

61. Winslow AW, Turbyville JC, Sublett JW, Sublett JL, Pollard SJ. Comparison of systemic reactions in rush, cluster, and standard-build aeroallergen immunotherapy. *Ann Allergy Asthma Immunol* 2016; 117(5): 542–545.

62. Hejjaoui A, Dhivert H, Michel FB, Bousquet J. Immunotherapy with a standardized *Dermatophagoides pteronyssinus* extract. IV. Systemic reactions according to the immunotherapy schedule. *J Allergy Clin Immunol* 1990; 85(2): 473–479.

63. Brehler R, Klimek L, Pfaar O, Hauswald B, Worm M, Bieber T. Safety of a rush immunotherapy build-up schedule with depigmented polymerized allergen extracts. *Allergy Asthma Proc* 2010; 31(3): e31–e38.

64. Cardona R, Lopez E, Beltran J, Sanchez J. Safety of immunotherapy in patients with rhinitis, asthma or atopic dermatitis using an ultra-rush buildup. A retrospective study. *Allergol Immunopathol (Madr)* 2014; 42(2): 90–95.

65. Casanovas M, Martin R, Jimenez C, Caballero R, Fernandez-Caldas E. Safety of an ultra-rush immunotherapy build-up schedule with therapeutic vaccines containing depigmented and polymerized allergen extracts. *Int Arch Allergy Immunol* 2006; 139(2): 153–158.

66. Pfaar O, Mosges R, Hormann K, Klimek L. Safety aspects of cluster immunotherapy with semi-depot allergen extracts in seasonal allergic rhinoconjunctivitis. *Eur Arch Otorhinolaryngol* 2010; 267(2): 245–250.

67. More DR, Hagan LL. Factors affecting compliance with allergen immunotherapy at a military medical center. *Ann Allergy Asthma Immunol* 2002; 88(4): 391–394.

68. Carlson GS, Wong PH, White KM, Quinn JM. Evaluation of angiotensin-converting enzyme inhibitor and angiotensin receptor blocker therapy in immunotherapy-associated systemic reactions. *J Allergy Clin Immunol Pract* 2017; 5(5): 1430–1432.

69. Cox L, Nelson H, Lockey R et al. Allergen immunotherapy: A practice parameter third update. *J Allergy Clin Immunol* 2011; 127(1 Suppl): S1–S55.

70. Comberiati P, Marseglia GL, Barberi S, Passalacqua G, Peroni DG. Allergen-specific immunotherapy for respiratory allergy in children: Unmet needs and future goals. *J Allergy Clin Immunol Pract* 2017; 5(4): 946–950.

71. Lim CE, Sison CP, Ponda P. Comparison of pediatric and adult systemic reactions to subcutaneous immunotherapy. *J Allergy Clin Immunol Pract* 2017; 5(5): 1241–1247.e2.

72. Roberts G, Pfaar O, Akdis CA et al. EAACI guidelines on allergen immunotherapy: Allergic rhinoconjunctivitis. *Allergy* 2018; 73(4): 765–798.

73. Jansen A, Andersen KF, Bruning H. Evaluation of a compliance device in a subgroup of adult patients receiving specific immunotherapy with grass allergen tablets (GRAZAX) in a randomized, open-label, controlled study: An a priori subgroup analysis. *Clin Ther* 2009; 31(2): 321–327.

74. Jonasson G, Carlsen KH, Mowinckel P. Asthma drug adherence in a long term clinical trial. *Arch Dis Child* 2000; 83(4): 330–333.

75. Biomarkers Definitions Working Group. Biomarkers and surrogate endpoints: Preferred definitions and conceptual framework. *Clin Pharmacol Ther* 2001; 69(3): 89–95.

76. Bousquet J, Hellings PW, Agache I et al. ARIA 2016: Care pathways implementing emerging technologies for predictive medicine in rhinitis and asthma across the life cycle. *Clin Transl Allergy* 2016; 6: 47.

77. May JR, Dolen WK. Management of allergic rhinitis: A review for the community pharmacist. *Clin Ther* 2017; 39(12): 2410–2419.

78. Gallup. Honesty/Ethics in Professions 2017. https://news.gallup.com/poll/1654/honesty-eth-ics-professions.aspx

79. Cutting Edge Information. Anticipate Increasing Adherence Budgets for Digital Patient Compliance Activities 2017. http://www.marketwired.com/press-release/anticipate-increasing-adherence-budgets-for-digital-patient-compliance-activities-2216840.htm

80. DiMatteo MR. Variations in patients' adherence to medical recommendations: A quantitative review of 50 years of research. *Med Care* 2004; 42(3): 200–209.

81. Stone A, Turkkan J, Bachrach C, Jobe J, Kurtzmann H, Cain V. *The Science of Self-Report: Implications for Research and Practice.* Mahwah, NJ: Lawrence Erlbaum Associates, 2000.

82. Rand CS, Wise RA. Measuring adherence to asthma medication regimens. *Am J Respir Crit Care Med* 1994; 149(2 Pt 2): S69–S76; discussion S7–8.

83. Farmer KC. Methods for measuring and monitoring medication regimen adherence in clinical trials and clinical practice. *Clin Ther* 1999; 21(6): 1074–1090; discussion 3.

84. Morisky DE, Green LW, Levine DM. Concurrent and predictive validity of a self-reported measure of medication adherence. *Med Care* 1986; 24(1): 67–74.

85. Tan X, Patel I, Chang J. Review of the four item Morisky Medication Adherence Scale (MMAS-4) and eight item Morisky Medication Adherence Scale (MMAS-8). *Innovations in Pharmacy* 2014; 5(3).

86. Morisky DE, Ang A, Krousel-Wood M, Ward HJ. Predictive validity of a medication adherence measure in an outpatient setting. *J Clin Hypertens (Greenwich)* 2008; 10(5): 348–354.

87. Justicia JL, Cardona V, Guardia P et al. Validation of the first treatment-specific questionnaire for the assessment of patient satisfaction with allergen-specific immunotherapy in allergic patients: The ESPIA questionnaire. *J Allergy Clin Immunol* 2013; 131(6): 1539–1546.

88. Martin LR, Williams SL, Haskard KB, Dimatteo MR. The challenge of patient adherence. *Ther Clin Risk Manag* 2005; 1(3): 189–199.

89. American College of Allergy, Ashthma and Immunology. New toolkit helps patients understand immunotherapy choices 2017 [cited August 19, 2018]. https://college.acaai.org/publications/college-insider/new-toolkit-helps-patients-understand-immunotherapy-choices

90. Bender BG. Can health care organizations improve health behavior and treatment adherence? *Popul Health Manag* 2014; 17(2): 71–78.

91. Bender BG, Lockey RF. Solving the problem of nonadherence to immunotherapy. *Immunol Allergy Clin North Am* 2016; 36(1): 205–213.

92. Borrelli B, Riekert KA, Weinstein A, Rathier L. Brief motivational interviewing as a clinical strategy to promote asthma medication adherence. *J Allergy Clin Immunol* 2007; 120(5): 1023–1030.

93. Vaswani R, Garg A, Parikh L, Vaswani S. Non-adherence to subcutaneous allergen immunotherapy: Inadequate health insurance coverage is the leading cause. *Ann Allergy Asthma Immunol* 2015; 115(3): 241–243.

94. Eaddy MT, Cook CL, O'Day K, Burch SP, Cantrell CR. How patient cost-sharing trends affect adherence and outcomes: A literature review. *P T* 2012; 37(1): 45–55.

95. Marogna M, Spadolini I, Massolo A, Canonica GW, Passalacqua G. Long-lasting effects of sublingual immunotherapy according to its duration: A 15-year prospective study. *J Allergy Clin Immunol* 2010; 126(5): 969–975.

96. Frati F, Dell'Albani I, Incorvaia C. Long-term efficacy of allergen immunotherapy: What do we expect? *Immunotherapy* 2013; 5(2): 131–133.

97. Durham SR, Walker SM, Varga EM et al. Long-term clinical efficacy of grass-pollen immunotherapy. *N Engl J Med* 1999; 341(7): 468–475.

98. Des Roches A, Paradis L, Knani J et al. Immunotherapy with a standardized *Dermatophagoides pteronyssinus* extract. V. Duration of the efficacy of immunotherapy after its cessation. *Allergy* 1996; 51(6): 430–433.

99. Durham SR, Emminger W, Kapp A et al. Long-term clinical efficacy in grass pollen-induced rhinoconjunctivitis after treatment with SQ-standardized grass allergy immunotherapy tablet. *J Allergy Clin Immunol* 2010; 125(1): 131–138.e1–7.

100. Durham SR, Emminger W, Kapp A et al. SQ-standardized sublingual grass immunotherapy: Confirmation of disease modification 2 years after 3 years of treatment in a randomized trial. *J Allergy Clin Immunol* 2012; 129(3): 717–725.e5.

101. Pajno GB, Caminiti L, Crisafulli G et al. Direct comparison between continuous and coseasonal regimen for sublingual immunotherapy in children with grass allergy: A randomized controlled study. *Pediatr Allergy Immunol* 2011; 22(8): 803–807.

102. Nakonechna A, Hills J, Moor J, Dore P, Abuzakouk M. Grazax sublingual immunotherapy in pre-co-seasonal and continuous treatment regimens: Is there a difference in clinical efficacy? *Ann Allergy Asthma Immunol* 2015; 114(1): 73–74.

103. Durham SR, investigators GT. Sustained effects of grass pollen AIT. *Allergy* 2011; 66(Suppl 95): 50–52.

104. Antolin-Amerigo D, Tabar IA, Del Mar Fernandez-Nieto M et al. Satisfaction and quality of life of allergic patients following sublingual five-grass pollen tablet immunotherapy in Spain. *Drugs Context* 2017; 6: 212309.

105. Walker SM, Varney VA, Gaga M, Jacobson MR, Durham SR. Grass pollen immunotherapy: Efficacy and safety during a 4-year follow-up study. *Allergy* 1995; 50(5): 405–413.

106. Tabar AI, Arroabarren E, Echechipia S, Garcia BE, Martin S, Alvarez-Puebla MJ. Three years of specific immunotherapy may be sufficient in house dust mite respiratory allergy. *J Allergy Clin Immunol* 2011; 127(1): 57–63.e1–3.

107. Cox L, Calderon MA. Subcutaneous specific immunotherapy for seasonal allergic rhinitis: A review of treatment practices in the US and Europe. *Curr Med Res Opin* 2010; 26(12): 2723–2733.

108. Bousquet J, Lockey R, Malling HJ. Allergen immunotherapy: Therapeutic vaccines for allergic diseases. A WHO position paper. *J Allergy Clin Immunol* 1998; 102(4 Pt 1): 558–562.

109. Cadario G, Ciprandi G, Di Cara G et al. Comparison between continuous or intermittent schedules of sublingual immunotherapy for house dust mites: Effects on compliance, patients satisfaction, quality of life and safety. *Int J Immunopathol Pharmacol* 2008; 21(2): 471–473.

110. Lockey RF, Hankin CS. Health economics of allergen-specific immunotherapy in the United States. *J Allergy Clin Immunol* 2011; 127(1): 39–43.

111. Eng PA, Borer-Reinhold M, Heijnen IA, Gnehm HP. Twelve-year follow-up after discontinuation of preseasonal grass pollen immunotherapy in childhood. *Allergy* 2006; 61(2): 198–201.

112. Marogna M, Falagiani P, Bruno M, Massolo A, Riva G. The allergic march in pollinosis: Natural history and therapeutic implications. *Int Arch Allergy Immunol* 2004; 135(4): 336–342.

113. Des Roches A, Paradis L, Menardo JL, Bouges S, Daures JP, Bousquet J. Immunotherapy with a standardized *Dermatophagoides pteronyssinus* extract. VI. Specific immunotherapy prevents the onset of new sensitizations in children. *J Allergy Clin Immunol* 1997; 99(4): 450–453.

114. Hankin CS, Cox L, Bronstone A. The health economics of allergen immunotherapy. *Immunol Allergy Clin North Am* 2011; 31(2): 325–341, x.

115. Canonica GW, Passalacqua G. Disease-modifying effect and economic implications of sublingual immunotherapy. *J Allergy Clin Immunol* 2011; 127(1): 44–45.

116. Cox LS, Hankin C, Lockey R. Allergy immunotherapy adherence and delivery route: Location does not matter. *J Allergy Clin Immunol Pract* 2014; 2(2): 156–160.

117. Creticos PS, Reed CE, Norman PS et al. Ragweed immunotherapy in adult asthma. *N Engl J Med* 1996; 334(8): 501–506.

118. Hankin CS, Cox L, Lang D et al. Allergen immunotherapy and health care cost benefits for children with allergic rhinitis: A large-scale, retrospective, matched cohort study. *Ann Allergy Asthma Immunol* 2010; 104(1): 79–85.

119. Hankin CS, Cox L, Bronstone A, Wang Z. Allergy immunotherapy: Reduced health care costs in adults and children with allergic rhinitis. *J Allergy Clin Immunol* 2013; 131(4): 1084–1091.

120. CurrAllen-Ramey F, Mao J, Blauer-Peterson C, Rock M, Nathan R, Halpern R. Healthcare costs for allergic rhinitis patients on allergy immunotherapy: A retrospective observational study. *Curr Med Res Opin* 2017; 33(11): 2039–2047.

121. Schadlich PK, Brecht JG. Economic evaluation of specific immunotherapy versus symptomatic treatment of allergic rhinitis in Germany. *Pharmacoeconomics* 2000; 17(1): 37–52.

122. Bériot-Mathiot A, Vestenbæk U, Bo Poulsen P et al. Cost effectiveness of sublingual immunotherapy in children with allergic rhinitis and asthma. *Eur Ann Allergy Clin Immunol* 2005; 37(8): 303–308.

123. Berto P, Passalacqua G, Crimi N et al. Economic evaluation of sublingual immunotherapy vs symptomatic treatment in adults with pollen-induced respiratory allergy: The Sublingual Immunotherapy Pollen Allergy Italy (SPAI) study. *Ann Allergy Asthma Immunol* 2006; 97(5): 615–621.

124. Bachert C, Vestenbaek U, Christensen J, Griffiths UK, Poulsen PB. Cost-effectiveness of grass allergen tablet (GRAZAX) for the prevention of seasonal grass pollen induced rhinoconjunctivitis—A Northern European perspective. *Clin Exp Allergy* 2007; 37(5): 772–779.

125. Canonica GW, Bousquet J, Mullol J, Scadding GK, Virchow JC. A survey of the burden of allergic rhinitis in Europe. *Allergy* 2007; 62(Suppl 85): 17–25.

126. Berto P, Frati F, Incorvaia C et al. Comparison of costs of sublingual immunotherapy and drug treatment in grass-pollen induced allergy: Results from the SIMAP database study. *Curr Med Res Opin* 2008; 24(1): 261–266.

127. Nasser S, Vestenbaek U, Beriot-Mathiot A, Poulsen PB. Cost-effectiveness of specific immunotherapy with Grazax in allergic rhinitis co-existing with asthma. *Allergy* 2008; 63(12): 1624–1629.

128. Verheggen BG, Westerhout KY, Schreder CH, Augustin M. Health economic comparison of SLIT allergen and SCIT allergoid immunotherapy in patients with seasonal grass-allergic rhinoconjunctivitis in Germany. *Clin Transl Allergy* 2015; 5: 1.

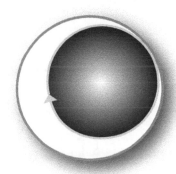

32 Biologics in allergic disease

Tara V. Saco and Farnaz Tabatabaian
University of South Florida Morsani College of Medicine

CONTENTS

32.1 INTRODUCTION

Allergic disease treatment options for respiratory and dermatologic diseases have advanced over the past several years, i.e., targeting the mediators of T2 inflammation, IgE, and interleukins (IL)-5, -4, and -13. It is a challenge for the clinician to choose the appropriate medication for a given subject. Understanding the role of therapeutic agents approved to treat T2 inflammation makes this decision less daunting. This chapter discusses the biologic agents used to treat atopic disease that target T2 inflammation–associated mediators (Table 32.1). First, the central role of T2 inflammation is addressed.

32.2 T2 INFLAMMATION

T2 inflammation in the lungs is associated with elevated bronchial airway eosinophils, basophils, mast cells, and innate lymphoid cell type 2 (ILC2) and Th2 cells (Figure 32.1). Type 2 cytokines, IL-4, -5, and -13 play a key role in the inflammatory process. B cells in the presence of IL-4 further differentiate into plasma cells which produce IgE. The binding of an allergen to IgE located on mast cells, eosinophils, and basophils leads to degranulation and release or production of histamine, prostaglandins, leukotrienes, tumor necrosis factor (TNF)-α, and type 2 cytokines. External stimuli induce epithelial cells lining the lung to produce thymic stromal lymphopoietin (TSLP) and IL-25 and -33 [1–4]. The culmination of this complex pathway of the innate and adaptive immune causes airway inflammation, bronchial hyperresponsiveness, and sometimes airway remodeling.

Skin barrier damage associated with atopic dermatitis contributes to allergen exposure and stimulation of T2 inflammation (Figure 32.2). As allergens traverse the stratum corneum of the skin, they are taken up by Langerhans cells, the local antigen-presenting cells, and presented to naïve T cells. These cells further differentiate into Th2 cells and produce type 2 cytokines, IL-4 and -13, which are central for IgE production, survival of Th2 cells, and to attract eosinophils into the site of inflammation. Both cytokines signal via the IL-4-α receptor. Studies suggest that IL-31, also produced by Th2 cells, causes pruritus. TSLP, IL-25, and IL-33 also play a role in stimulating mast cells and stimulating ILC2 [2,5]. The triggers that cause chronic idiopathic urticaria and angioedema are unknown; however, IgE binding to the FCϵR1 receptor on mast cells and basophils leads to degranulation. Urticaria, associated with auto-inflammatory syndromes, is linked to altered production of IL-1β [6].

Amplification of T2 inflammation in chronic rhinosinusitis with nasal polyps (CRSwNP) is similar to that present in asthma and atopic dermatitis (Figure 32.1). Fungi, *Staphylococcus aureus*, and viruses, for example, induce epithelial cells to produce TLSP and IL-33 and -1,

Table 32.1 Biologic agents used to treat atopic diseases that target T2 inflammation-associated mediators

FDA-Approved Agents (except for nasal polyps)	Mechanism of Action	Black Box Warnings and Important Precautions	Optimal Treatment Duration	Ages Approved	Dosing	Disease State: Asthma				
						Biomarkers	Exacerbation Rate Reduction	Prebronchodilator FEV_1 Improvement	Asthma Symptom Score and Quality of Life Improvements	Corticosteroid-Sparing Effect
Omalizumab (Xolair®)	Binds to IgE (at Fcε3), which prevents IgE binding to the FcεR1 receptor on mast cells and other key inflammatory cells.	*Black Box Warning:* Anaphylaxis (observation for an "appropriate period of time" after injection recommended in package insert, usually 2 hour observation period for first 3 injections) *Precautions:* Possible increased risk of solid tumors (now debunked) *Pregnancy category:* Insufficient data to provide category; monoclonal antibodies are transported across the placenta during the 3rd trimester, thus potential risk is greatest during this time; caution in nursing mothers (unknown if transferred via breast milk)	Unknown	6 years of age and older	Based on IgE and body weight (0.016 mg/kg/IU/mL) SC Q2-4W	IgE 30–700 IU/mL	50%	Minimal or mixed effect	Yes	Data mixed (ICS sparing, PO sparing unclear)
Dupilumab (Dupixent®)	Binds to IL-4Rα, which inhibits both IL-4 and IL-13 signaling.	*Black Box Warning:* None *Precautions:* 1. Hypersensitivity reactions 2. Conjunctivitis in atopic dermatitis subjects *Pregnancy category:* Insufficient data to provide category; monoclonal antibodies are transported across the placenta during the 3rd trimester, thus potential risk is greatest during this time; caution in nursing mothers (unknown if transferred via breast milk)	Unknown	12 years of age and older	Regimens: 1. An initial dose of 400 mg followed by 200 mg SC Q2W OR 2. An initial dose of 600 mg followed by 300 mg SC Q2W 3. For subjects requiring concomitant oral corticosteroids or with comorbid moderate-to-severe atopic dermatitis for which dupilumab is indicated, initial dose of 600 mg SC followed by 300 mg SC Q2W	Blood EOS ≥ 150 cells/µL OR FeNO ≥ 25 ppb	~ 60–80%	~ 0.150–0.160 L	Yes in Phase 2b study	Yes in the VENTURE trial

(Continued)

Table 32.1 (*Continued*) Biologic agents used to treat atopic diseases that target T2 inflammation-associated mediators

FDA-Approved Agents (except for nasal polyps)	Mechanism of Action	Black Box Warnings and Important Precautions	Optimal Treatment Duration	Ages Approved	Dosing	Disease State: Asthma					
						Biomarkers	Exacerbation Rate Reduction	Prebronchodilator FEV$_1$ Improvement	Asthma Symptom Score and Quality of Life Improvements	Corticosteroid-Sparing Effect
Mepolizumab (Nucala®)	Binds to IL-5	*Black Box Warning:* None *Precautions:* 1. Hypersensitivity reactions 2. Increased risk of herpes zoster infections (consider vaccination prior to initiating injections) *Pregnancy category:* Insufficient data to provide category; monoclonal antibodies are transported across the placenta during the 3rd trimester, thus potential risk is greatest during this time; caution in nursing mothers (unknown if transferred via breast milk)	Unknown	12 years of age and older	100 mg (fixed) SC Q4W	Blood eosinophils ≥ 150 cells/μL at initiation OR ≥ 300 cells/μL within the previous year	SC: 53% IV: 47% ≥ 500 eosinophils/ μL: 79%	0.098–0.100 L (based on 1 study after 32 weeks of therapy) ≥ 500 cells/μL: 0.132 L	Varied	Yes
Reslizumab (Cinqair®)	Binds to IL-5	*Black Box Warning:* Anaphylaxis (observation for "an appropriate period of time" recommended in package insert) *Precautions:* Malignancies were observed in clinical trials (6/1028 [0.6%] in treatment group vs 2/730 [0.3%] in placebo group, no predominance of a particular malignancy, most were diagnosed after < 6 months of reslizumab treatment) *Pregnancy category:* Insufficient data to provide category; monoclonal antibodies are transported across the placenta during the 3rd trimester, thus potential risk is greatest during this time; caution in nursing mothers (unknown if transferred via breast milk)	Unknown	18 years of age and older	3.0 mg/kg (weight-based) IV Q4W	Blood eosinophils ≥ 400 cells/ μL	50–60%	0.093–0.160 L (subgroup analysis from 1 study showed 0.270 L improvement)	Varied	Data mixed

(Continued)

Table 32.1 (*Continued*) Biologic agents used to treat atopic diseases that target T2 inflammation-associated mediators

FDA-Approved Agents (except for nasal polyps)	Mechanism of Action	Black Box Warnings and Important Precautions	Optimal Treatment Duration	Ages Approved	Dosing	Biomarkers	Disease State: Asthma			
							Exacerbation Rate Reduction	Prebronchodilator FEV$_1$ Improvement	Asthma Symptom Score and Quality of Life Improvements	Corticosteroid-Sparing Effect
Benralizumab (Fasenra®)	Binds to the IL-5 receptor subunit on eosinophils and basophils. Induces antibody-dependent cell-mediated cytotoxicity of eosinophils and basophils.	*Black Box Warning:* None *Precautions:* Hypersensitivity reactions *Pregnancy category:* Insufficient data to provide category; monoclonal antibodies are transported across the placenta during the 3rd trimester, thus potential risk is greatest during this time; caution in nursing mothers (unknown if transferred via breast milk)	Unknown	12 years of age and older	30 mg (fixed) SC Q8W (first 3 doses Q4W)	Blood eosinophils ≥ 300 cells/ μL	SIROCCO: 45 –51% CALIMA: 28 –36% BISE: Not measured ZONDA: 55 –70%	SIROCCO: • Q4W: ↑ 0.106 L • Q8W: ↑ 0.159 L CALIMA: • Q4W: ↑ 0.125 L • Q8W: ↑ 0.116 L BISE: • Q4W: ↑ 0.070 L (similar in subjects with blood eosinophils ≥ 300 cells/μL and < 300 cells/μL)	Varied	Yes

				Disease State: Atopic Dermatitis			
				Ages Approved	Dosing	Biomarkers	Symptom Score Improvement
Dupilumab (Dupixent®)	Binds to IL-4Rα, which inhibits both IL-4 and IL-13 signaling.	*Black Box Warning:* None *Precautions:* 1. Hypersensitivity reactions 2. Conjunctivitis in atopic dermatitis subjects *Pregnancy category:* Insufficient data to provide category; monoclonal antibodies are transported across the placenta during the 3rd trimester, thus potential risk is greatest during this time; caution in nursing mothers (unknown if transferred via breast milk)	Unknown	18 years of age and older for atopic dermatitis	Initial dose of 600 mg, then 300 mg SC Q2W	None validated	Yes

(*Continued*)

Table 32.1 (Continued) Biologic agents used to treat atopic diseases that target T2 inflammation-associated mediators

FDA-Approved Agents (except for nasal polyps)	Mechanism of Action	Black Box Warnings and Important Precautions	Optimal Treatment Duration	Ages Approved	Disease State: Urticaria — Dosing	Biomarkers	Symptom Score Improvement	Corticosteroid-Sparing Effect
Omalizumab (Xolair®)	Binds to IgE (at Fcε3), which prevents IgE binding to the FcεR1 receptor on mast cells and other key inflammatory cells.	*Black Box Warning:* Anaphylaxis (observation for an "appropriate period of time" after injection recommended in package insert, usually 2 hour observation period for first 3 injections) *Precautions:* Possible increased risk of solid tumors (now debunked) *Pregnancy category:* Insufficient data to provide category; monoclonal antibodies are transported across the placenta during the 3rd trimester, thus potential risk is greatest during this time; caution in nursing mothers (unknown if transferred via breast milk)	Unknown	12 years of age and older for chronic idiopathic urticaria	150 or 300 mg SC Q4W (fixed dose, does not depend on body weight or IgE levels)	None validated	Yes	Yes
Canakinumab (Ilaris®)	Binds to IL-1β	*Black Box Warning:* None *Precautions:* 1. Increased risk of severe infections due to inhibition of IL-1, do not administer during an active infection 2. Should not receive live vaccines during treatment (should receive all recommended vaccines prior to starting canakinumab) *Pregnancy category:* No human data, insufficient data to provide category, caution in nursing mothers (unknown if transferred via breast milk)	Unknown	4 years of age and older for Muckle-Wells Syndrome and Familial Cold Urticaria Syndrome)	Regimens: 1. 150 mg SC Q8W for CAPS subjects with body weight > 40 kg 2. 2 mg/kg SC Q8W for CAPS subjects with body weight ≥ 15 kg and ≤ 40 kg. 3. For children 15–40 kg with inadequate response, dose can be increased to 3 mg/kg SC Q8W	None validated (possibly serum amyloid A and/or CRP)	Yes	Unknown
Anakinra (Kineret®)	Binds to IL-1Rα	*Black Box Warning:* None *Precautions:* 1. Hypersensitivity reactions 2. Increased risk of infections (do not administer during active infection) 3. Should not receive live vaccines during treatment 4. Decrease in neutrophil count (must be assessed prior to initiating and during treatment, monthly for 3 months, and then quarterly for up to 1 year) Pregnancy Category B, caution in nursing mothers (unknown if transferred via breast milk)	Unknown	No official age limit for Neonatal-Onset Multisystem Inflammatory Disease, studied in subjects < 2 years, 2–11 years, and 12–17 years with similar adverse event as subjects ≥ 18 years, with the exception of more frequent infections and related symptoms subjects < 2 years	Starting dose 1–2 mg/kg SC daily, dose can be adjusted to a maximum of 8 mg/kg daily. Consider every other day dosing for subjects with severe renal insufficiency or end stage renal disease (creatinine clearance < 30 mL/min)	None validated (possibly serum amyloid A and/or CRP)	Yes	Unknown

(Continued)

Table 32.1 (Continued) Biologic agents used to treat atopic diseases that target T2 inflammation-associated mediators

Disease State: Urticaria

FDA-Approved Agents (except for nasal polyps)	Mechanism of Action	Black Box Warnings and Important Precautions	Optimal Treatment Duration	Ages Approved	Dosing	Biomarkers	Symptom Score Improvement	Corticosteroid-Sparing Effect
Rilonacept (Arcalyst®)	Soluble decoy receptor that blocks IL-1β	*Black Box Warning:* None *Precautions:* 1. Hypersensitivity reactions 2. Increased risk of infections (do not administer during active infection) 3. Should not receive live vaccines during treatment Pregnancy Category C, caution in nursing mothers (unknown if transferred via breast milk)	Unknown	12 years of age and older for CAPS (including Muckle-Wells Syndrome and Familial Cold Urticaria Syndrome)	Regimens: 18 years and older: 320 mg SC loading dose, then 160 mg Q1W (no more frequently than Q1W) 12 to 17 years: 4.4 mg/kg loading dose up to a maximum of 320 mg, then 2.2 mg/kg up to a maximum of 160 mg Q1W (no more frequently than Q1W)	None validated (possibly serum amyloid A and/or CRP)	Yes	Unknown

Disease State: Nasal Polyps

FDA-Approved Agents (except for nasal polyps)	Mechanism of Action	Black Box Warnings and Important Precautions	Optimal Treatment Duration	Dosing	Biomarkers	Nasal Polyp Score Improvement	Anosmia and Symptom Score Improvement	Sinus Opacification Improvement	Nasal Tissue Inflammation Improvement	Need for Surgery Obviated
Omalizumab (Xolair®)	Binds to IgE (at Fcε3), which prevents IgE binding to the FcεR1 receptor on mast cells and other key inflammatory cells.	*Black Box Warning:* Anaphylaxis (observation for an "appropriate period of time" after injection recommended in package insert, usually 2-hour observation period for first 3 injections) *Precautions:* Possible increased risk of solid tumors (now debunked) *Pregnancy category:* Insufficient data to provide category; monoclonal antibodies are transported across the placenta during the 3rd trimester, thus potential risk is greatest during this time; caution in nursing mothers (unknown if transferred via breast milk)	Unknown	Based on IgE and body weight (0.016 mg/kg/IU/mL) SC Q2-4W studied	None validated	Yes	Yes	Yes	No	Not studied
Dupilumab (Dupixent®)	Binds to IL-4Rα, which inhibits both IL-4 and IL-13 signaling.	*Black Box Warning:* None *Precautions:* 1. Hypersensitivity reactions 2. Conjunctivitis in atopic dermatitis subjects *Pregnancy category:* Insufficient data to provide category; monoclonal antibodies are transported across the placenta during the 3rd trimester, thus potential risk is greatest during this time; caution in nursing mothers (unknown if transferred via breast milk)	Unknown	600-mg loading dose, then 300 mg SC Q1W studied	None validated	Yes	Yes	Yes	Not studied	Not studied

(Continued)

Table 32.1 (Continued) Biologic agents used to treat atopic diseases that target T2 inflammation-associated mediators

FDA-Approved Agents (except for nasal polyps)	Mechanism of Action	Black Box Warnings and Important Precautions	Optimal Treatment Duration	Dosing	Biomarkers	Disease State: Nasal Polyps				
						Nasal Polyp Score Improvement	Anosmia and Symptom Score Improvement	Sinus Opacification Improvement	Nasal Tissue Inflammation Improvement	Need for Surgery Obviated
Mepolizumab (Nucala®)	Binds to IL-5	*Black Box Warning:* **None** *Precautions:* 1. Hypersensitivity reactions 2. Increased risk of herpes zoster infections (consider vaccination prior to initiating injections) *Pregnancy category:* Insufficient data to provide category; monoclonal antibodies are transported across the placenta during the 3rd trimester, thus potential risk is greatest during this time; caution in nursing mothers (unknown if transferred via breast milk)	Unknown	750 mg IV Q4w (6 doses) studied	None validated	Yes	Yes	Not studied	Not studied	Yes

Abbreviations: CRP = C Reactive protein, FcεR1 = High-affinity IgE receptor, FEV$_1$ = Forced expiratory volume in 1 second, ICS = Inhaled corticosteroids. IgE = Immunoglobulin E, IL = Interleukin, LABA = Long-acting β2-agonist, PO = Oral, Q1W = Once weekly, Q2W = Once every other week, Q4W = Once every 4 weeks. Q8W = Once every 8 weeks (first three doses Q4W).; SC = Subcutaneous; IV = Intravenous.

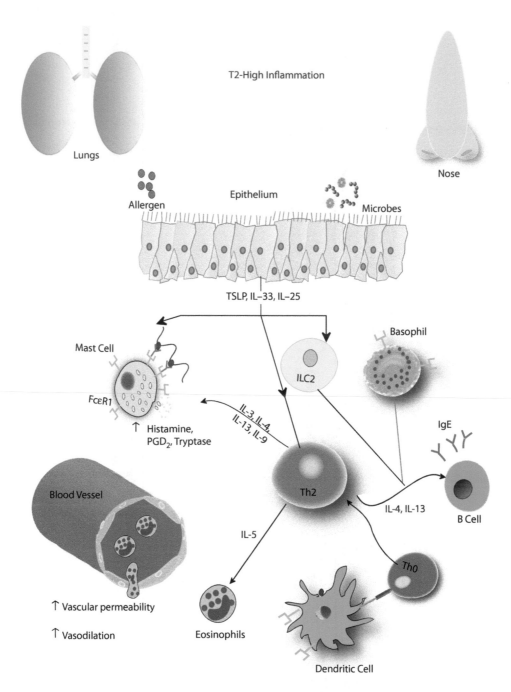

Figure 32.1 The complex interplay of various cytokines and inflammatory cells central in T2 high inflammation in the lungs and nasal cavity. Stimulation via allergens or microbes increases production of TSLP, IL-25, IL-33 from epithelial cells and contributes to the production of type 2 cytokines. Secretion of IL-5 stimulates the migration and stabilization of eosinophils in the area of inflammation. IL-4 contributes to IgE class switching in B cells. (Fc$_\varepsilon$R1, immunoglobulin E receptor; ICL2, innate lymphoid cells type 2; PGD$_2$, prostaglandin D$_2$; TSLP, thymic stromal lymphopoietin.)

important to differentiate naïve T to Th2 cells, upregulate ILC2, and cause mast cell degranulation [7]. IL-13 plays a role in goblet cell hyperplasia and increased mucus production. IL-4, -5, and -13 are central for eosinophil chemotaxis [4].

32.3 BIOLOGIC AGENTS TO TREAT ASTHMA

Th2 asthma is defined by the presence of airway eosinophils and type 2 cytokines. Monoclonal antibodies approved to treat asthma

include omalizumab, mepolizumab, reslizumab, benralizumab, and dupilumab.

32.3.1 Omalizumab

The first monoclonal antibody approved by the U.S. Food and Drug Administration (FDA) for asthma as add-on therapy for moderate to severe persistent asthma for age 6 years and above is omalizumab (Xolair; Genentech USA, Inc. and Novartis Pharmaceuticals

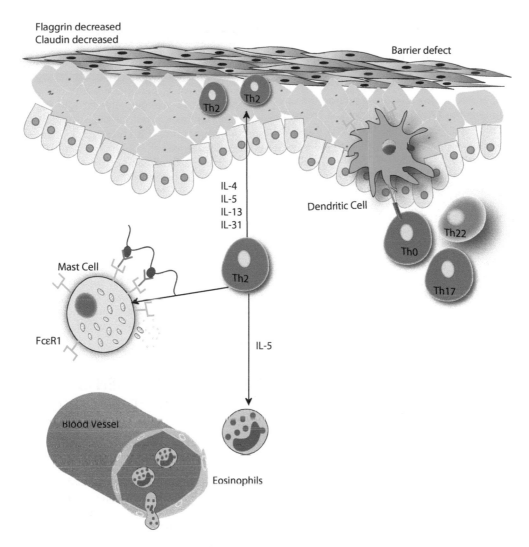

Figure 32.2 T2 inflammation is very important for both acute and chronic atopic dermatitis in the skin. Type 2 cytokines IL-4, IL-5, and IL-13, contribute to IgE class switching and induce the production of both mast cells and peripheral eosinophils. IL-31 plays a role in pruritus. The presence of Th22 cells contributes to IL-33 production, which induces epidermal hyperplasia prominent in this disease.

Corporation, Switzerland) [7]. Omalizumab is a humanized monoclonal antibody with high affinity for the FCε3 section of IgE and prevents the interaction of IgE with the high-affinity IgE receptor (FCεR1) on mast cells, eosinophils, and basophils. Furthermore, increased clearance of IgE associated with omalizumab via the reticuloendothelial system downregulates the FCεR1 on these cells attenuating the allergic response [8]. Omalizumab is administered subcutaneously every 2–4 weeks. Dosing is calculated based on total serum IgE and body weight. Available doses range from 75 to 375 mg given subcutaneously (sub-Q). FDA dosage recommendations for adults are based on IgE levels and range from 30 to 700 IU/mL and in children, age 6–12 years, from 30 to 1300 IU/mL [7]. However, multiple studies show benefit with serum IgE above those limits in both age groups [2,9]. This agent is included as an add-on therapy in step 5 of the Global Initiative for Asthma (GINA) guidelines [10]. Omalizumab decreases asthma exacerbations by 60% in subjects with elevated FeNO and peripheral eosinophil counts of >300 cells/µL [8,11]. Omalizumab decreases inhalation of glucocorticosteroid use but does not consistently decrease oral glucocorticoid use. Furthermore, it did not demonstrate a statistical improvement of the forced expiratory volume in one second

(FEV$_1$) in clinical trials [12,13]. The drug does not immunomodulate; hence, the therapeutic benefit with extended use is not known. Subjects should remain on this medication 16–24 weeks and then be reevaluated to determine whether omalizumab should be continued. Anaphylaxis is listed in a package insert black box warning. Therefore, patients should be monitored for 120 minutes following the first three injections and thereafter, 30 minutes. Pooled analysis from clinical trials fails to support a causal relationship with increased solid tumors, a warning included in the package insert.

32.3.2 Mepolizumab, reslizumab, and benralizumab

Eosinophils are an integral part of Th2 asthma. Elevated sputum and peripheral eosinophils correlate with increased asthma exacerbations and poorly controlled asthma [1,14,15]. IL-5 is necessary for eosinophil growth, differentiation, and migration into the airways [1,16]. Mepolizumab, reslizumab, and benralizumab are three monoclonal antibodies that target IL-5. Mepolizumab and reslizumab directly bind to the IL-5 cytokine and prevent its downstream binding to the IL-5 receptor [14,17–19]. Benralizumab binds to the alpha (α) chain of IL-5 receptor, thus enhancing the antibody-dependent cell-mediated cytotoxicity causing apoptosis of eosinophils, basophils, and eosinophil progenitor cells [20]. Mepolizumab is the first IL-5 inhibitor approved by the FDA as an add-on therapy for severe persistent asthma in the 12 years and older age group. It is administered as a 100 mg subcutaneous injection every 4 weeks [21]. Mepolizumab shows improvement in the quality-of-life scores with decreased emergency room (ER) visits and hospitalizations, a 53% decrease in asthma exacerbation, an improvement of 100 mL in FEV_1, and 50% reduced oral glucocorticoid use in phase 3 studies [22,23]. Subjects with higher levels of peripheral eosinophilia experience greatest benefit. Mepolizumab, 300 mg sub-Q, is FDA approved for eosinophilic granulomatosis with polyangiitis [22].

Reslizumab is also a humanized anti-IL-5 monoclonal antibody approved by the FDA as add-on therapy for patients 18 years or older with severe eosinophilic asthma. It is administered intravenously (IV) at 3 mg/kg over 20–50 minutes every 4 weeks [24]. Castro and colleagues reported a decrease in asthma exacerbations and significant improvement in FEV_1 in subjects with peripheral eosinophil count 400 cell/μL or greater [17]. Reslizumab seems to elicit the greatest improvement in FEV_1 when compared to other IL-5 blocking agents that may be, in part, related to weight dosing.

Benralizumab, a monoclonal antibody that targets the alpha (α) IL-5 receptor, was FDA approved in 2017 as add-on therapy for moderate to severe eosinophilic asthma in the 12 years or older age group. Thirty milligrams sub-Q are injected for the first three doses at 4-week intervals and subsequently, every 8 weeks [20]. Its direct effect on eosinophils is attractive as these cells can subsequently enter the tissue independent of IL-5. Benralizumab does decrease asthma exacerbations, improve the FEV_1, and in asthma improve quality-of-life scores. The greatest effect occurs in subjects with eosinophil count $\geq$300 cells/μL [18,25–27].

The relapse rates of subjects with acute asthma exacerbations presenting to the emergency room (ER) are fairly high in spite of corticosteroid use. The administration of one dose of benralizumab during an acute ER visit decreased exacerbation rates for asthma by 50% over the next 12 weeks [28]. This study has led to the novel concept of using a biologic in the ER to possibly decrease readmission rates as well as cost. In summary, all three biologic agents target IL-5 and decrease asthma exacerbations and improve quality-of-life scores.

32.3.3 Dupilumab

Dupilumab is a fully humanized anti-IL-4 receptor α monoclonal antibody that inhibits both IL-4 and -13 signaling. It is FDA approved as add-on therapy for moderate to severe asthma in ages 12 years and older who have the eosinophilic phenotype or oral corticosteroid dependent asthma [29]. An initial loading dose of 400 mg with subsequent biweekly doses of 200 mg sub-Q decrease asthma exacerbation rates, improve the FEV_1, and improve the quality of life. Greater benefit occurs in patients with higher baseline levels of eosinophils. In glucocorticoid-dependent patients, an initial 600 mg loading dose with a subsequent biweekly dose of 300 mg sub-Q leads to decreased rates of severe exacerbations, reduced oral glucocorticoid use, and improvement in the FEV_1 [30–33]. Hypereosinophilia was observed in some patients and should be monitored if counts get close to or greater than 1500 cells/μL.

32.3.4 What to select?

All monoclonal biologics approved to date target Th2 asthma. Biomarkers used to identify Th2 asthma include fractional exhaled nitric oxide (FeNO), peripheral eosinophilia, blood periostin level, and presence of allergen-specific IgE. Poorly controlled asthma with recurrent exacerbations is associated with increased blood or sputum eosinophils. It is challenging clinically to measure sputum eosinophils. However, obtaining blood eosinophils is relatively simple. Epithelial cells lining the alveoli express high quantity of inducible nitric oxide synthase (iNOS). IL-4 and -13 upregulate the expression of iNOS and hence the production of nitric oxide (NO) [34,35]. Elevated FeNO is a noninvasive biomarker for T2 inflammation. Periostin is increased in the presence of IL-13 [15]. The clinical use of these biomarkers is an indication of upregulation of Th2 inflammatory mediators and possible responsiveness to these biologic agents. There are no head-to-head trials comparing these agents. Factors that may play a role in selecting a biologic agent include ease of therapy, route and frequency of the medication, out-of-pocket cost and confounding atopic comorbidities, such as atopic dermatitis, nasal polyps, food allergy, and allergic rhinoconjunctivitis.

32.4 BIOLOGIC AGENTS USED TO TREAT CHRONIC IDIOPATHIC URTICARIA

The exact stimulus behind mast cell degranulation in chronic idiopathic urticaria (CU) and angioedema is unknown, but presumably IgE plays an etiologic role in this disease. One possible pathogenic mechanism is the development of autoantibodies against the α-chain of the FcϵR1 located on mast cells or against IgE. This can be determined using the chronic urticaria index (CUI), but this has not been validated as a possible marker to predict response to available therapies. The majority ($\sim$50%) of CU subjects are not adequately controlled on high-dose second-generation antihistamines. Previous treatment guidelines recommended consideration of other medications such as tacrolimus, cyclosporine, dapsone, and Plaquenil. In a recent double-blind study, dapsone was shown to be very effective [36]. Guidelines recommend cyclosporine as a third-line agent should patients not respond to omalizumab [37]. However, the overall side-effect profile for glucocorticoids, cyclosporin, tacrolimus, and Plaquenil can limit their use. Monoclonal therapies are effective to treat these subjects with limited associated adverse effects; however, the associated cost is a rate-limiting problem [38]. No validated clinical biomarkers to predict response exist at this time.

Auto-inflammatory syndromes such as Schnitzler syndrome and cryopyrin-associated periodic fever syndromes (CAPSs) are often associated with urticaria. These include Muckle-Wells syndrome, neonatal-onset multisystem inflammatory disease, and familial cold autoinflammatory syndrome. They are believed to be mediated by autosomal dominant mutations in the NLRP3 gene with the subsequent production of altered cryopyrin, which induces constitutive production of IL-1b. Anti-IL-1 monoclonal antibodies are utilized in these subjects to control the urticaria and other associated manifestations of these syndromes [39,40]. The FDA-approved monoclonal options for different types of urticaria include omalizumab, canakinumab, anakinra, and rilonacept.

32.4.1 Omalizumab

Omalizumab is FDA approved for subjects 12 years and older who have uncontrolled chronic urticaria on maximum dose second-generation antihistamines. Omalizumab theoretically binds IgE and thereby increases internalization of FcεR1, thus eliminating targets for autoantibodies. Data from phase 3 studies show a marked improvement in symptom and quality-of-life scores in such subjects. Response to omalizumab is usually dose-dependent with more than half of these subjects achieving complete remission with monthly 300 mg sub-Q injections [41].

It is unknown how long subjects should remain on omalizumab after the desired treatment effect is achieved. "The Xolair Treatment Efficacy of Longer Duration in Chronic Idiopathic Urticaria (XTEND-CIU)" study shows persistent benefit with a 48-week treatment course with reinitiation of omalizumab in subjects who discontinue this drug after 24 weeks and experience a recurrence of symptoms [38]. The European Academy of Allergy and Clinical Immunology (EAACI)/Global Allergy and Asthma European Network (GA2LEN)/European Dermatology Forum (EDF)/World Allergy Organization (WAO) guidelines have been conditionally accepted by the American Academy of Allergy, Asthma and Immunology (AAAAI) and the American College of Allergy, Asthma and Immunology (ACAAI). They list omalizumab as the third step in management of chronic urticaria behind second-generation antihistamine monotherapy or an increase up to four times the recommended dose [37]. The 2014 AAAAI practice parameters do not recommend starting omalizumab until step 4, which also lists cyclosporine as a potential option [42]. The updated practice parameters will likely be more consistent with the EAACI/GA2LEN/EDF/WAO guidelines.

The three FDA-approved IL-1 antagonists for CAPSs-associated urticaria include canakinumab, a humanized anti-IL-1β monoclonal antibody; anakinra, a recombinant human IL-1Rα antagonist; and rilonacept, a soluble decoy receptor that blocks IL-1β. Data from small studies using anakinra and canakinumab in Schnitzler syndrome subjects is favorable. Further studies are underway to examine the utility of using anti-IL-1 monoclonal antibodies for CU.

32.5 BIOLOGIC AGENTS IN ATOPIC DERMATITIS

IL-4, -5, -13, -31 and IgE are involved in the pathogenesis of atopic dermatitis. Although IgE is thought to play a large role, anti-IgE monoclonal antibody therapy has not proven to be successful. The only FDA-approved monoclonal antibody to treat atopic dermatitis is dupilumab, which targets the IL-4 and IL-13.

32.5.1 Dupilumab

Dupilumab is an anti-IL-4Rα humanized monoclonal antibody that blocks IL-4 and IL-13 signaling and is FDA approved for subjects 18 years and older with atopic dermatitis [29]. It also decreases IgE production by almost 40%. It is administered starting with a 600 mg sub-Q dose followed by 300 mg sub-Q every other week [31]. There is no validated biomarker to predict response to dupilumab for atopic dermatitis. Likewise, there are no black box warnings, but an important listed precaution is conjunctivitis. Dupilumab significantly decreases the Eczema Area and Severity Index, Investigator Global Assessment, and pruritus scores. The improvement in pruritus is clinically significant and translates to improvement in quality of life.

32.6 BIOLOGIC AGENTS FOR NASAL POLYPOSIS

Chronic rhinosinusitis with nasal polyposis (CRSwNP) can be refractory to conventional therapy and may require multiple surgical interventions. Mucosal eosinophilia is predictive of increased disease burden with reoccurrence of nasal polyps after surgery [43]. Type 2 cytokines drive mediators of the eosinophilic phenotype. Local IgE production is also linked to disease severity. This raises the question whether biologic agents that target IgE, IL-4, -5, and -13 may be effective to treat this disease. Data indicate omalizumab, mepolizumab, and dupilumab may be useful to treat nasal polyposis, although none are FDA approved as of January 2019. Omalizumab improved sinus opacification and anosmia, and significantly decreased nasal polyp scores in a proof-of-concept study [44]. Data suggest mepolizumab improves nasal symptoms and decreases nasal polyp scores. One randomized double-blind, placebo-controlled trial illustrates that mepolizumab administered over 6 months in subjects with severe nasal polyposis reduces the need for sinus surgery [45]. Several studies suggest that the use of dupilumab in subjects with severe polyposis improves nasal symptoms scores and anosmia [46,47]. While all of these agents are promising, none are FDA approved, and further studies are needed to prove dose-related efficacy.

32.7 CONCLUSION

Asthma, urticaria, atopic dermatitis, CAPs, and CRSwNP can be chronic and debilitating diseases. The development of biologic agents to target underlying mechanisms associated with these diseases is innovative, leading to the use of more precision medicine. However, uncertainties exist with the growing repertoire of biologics in that none of the existing biologics are immunomodulating. Therefore, it is unknown how long they should be utilized and if they will lead to disease remission, at least in some subjects. This presents a dilemma with regard to the cost attributed to the utilization of biologics. These drugs on average cost between $2000 and $4000 per month depending on the dose and the medication. The biologics to treat moderate to severe asthma all target Th2 inflammation. Choosing the right one is challenging; however, biomarkers, such as FeNO, blood and sputum eosinophils, specific IgE, and periostin are consistent with Th2-mediated inflammation and can be helpful to the clinician. The one chosen depends on the severity of disease, biomarkers, comorbid conditions, efficacy, convenience, and cost.

SALIENT POINTS

1. Type 2 cytokines (IL-4, IL-5, IL-13) and IgE all play an important role in T2 inflammation.
2. Biologic agents that target type 2 cytokines and IgE provide an avenue to treat patients with asthma, chronic idiopathic urticaria, and atopic dermatitis not controlled by more conventional therapy.

3. FDA-approved medications to treat moderate to severe asthma include dupilumab, omalizumab, resilizumab, mepolizumab, and benralizumab. They primarily decrease the exacerbation rate of asthma. None are immunomodulatory or result in remission of the disease. Baseline measurement of peripheral eosinophils is needed with counts greater than 150–300 cells/μL for approval of medication depending on the agent.
4. Dupilumab is approved for moderate to severe atopic dermatitis.
5. Omalizumab is recommended as a second-line agent in chronic idiopathic urticaria.
6. The lack of major side effects of these biologics makes them attractive to use to treat these diseases. However, their excessive cost is of concern, in particular, since none are immunomodulatory or seem to remit the disease.

REFERENCES

1. Tabatabaian F, Ledford DK, Casale TB. Biologic and new therapies in asthma. *Immunol Allergy Clinics North Am* 2017; 37(2): 329–343.
2. Casale TB. Biologics and biomarkers for asthma, urticaria, and nasal polyposis. *J Allergy Clin Immunol* 2017; 139(5): 1411–1421.
3. Sonnenberg GF, Artis D. Innate lymphoid cells in the initiation, regulation and resolution of inflammation. *Nat Med* 2015; 21(7): 698–708.
4. Fahy JV. Type 2 inflammation in asthma—Present in most, absent in many. *Nat Rev Immunol* 2015; 15(1): 57–65.
5. Werfel T, Allam JP, Biedermann T et al. Cellular and molecular immunologic mechanisms in patients with atopic dermatitis. *J Allergy Clin Immunol* 2016; 138(2): 336–349.
6. Kuemmerle-Deschner JB. CAPS—Pathogenesis, presentation and treatment of an autoinflammatory disease. *Sem Immunopathol* 2015; 37(4): 377–385.
7. XOLAIR (omalizumab) prescribing information. http://www.xolair.com/allergic-asthma/hcp/
8. Hanania NA, Wenzel S, Rosen K et al. Exploring the effects of omalizumab in allergic asthma: An analysis of biomarkers in the EXTRA study. *Am J Respiratory Crit Care Med* 2013; 187(8): 804–811.
9. Cardet JC, Casale TB. New insights into the utility of omalizumab. *J Allergy Clin Immunol* 2019; 143(3): 923–926.e1
10. Becker AB, Abrams EM. Asthma guidelines: The Global Initiative for Asthma in relation to national guidelines. *Curr Opin Allergy Clin Immunol* 2017; 17(2): 99–103.
11. Busse W, Spector S, Rosen K et al. High eosinophil count: A potential biomarker for assessing successful omalizumab treatment effects. *J Allergy Clin Immunol* 2013; 132(2): 485–486.e11.
12. Normansell R, Walker S, Milan SJ et al. Omalizumab for asthma in adults and children. *Cochrane Database Syst Rev* 2014; (1): Cd003559.
13. Busse WW, Morgan WJ, Gergen PJ et al. Randomized trial of omalizumab (anti-IgE) for asthma in inner-city children. *N Engl J Med* 2011; 364(11): 1005–1015.
14. Pavord ID, Korn S, Howarth P et al. Mepolizumab for severe eosinophilic asthma (DREAM): A multicentre, double-blind, placebo-controlled trial. *Lancet (London, England)* 2012; 380 (9842): 651–659.
15. Berry A, Busse WW Biomarkers in asthmatic patients: Has their time come to direct treatment? *J Allergy Clin Immunol* 2016; 137(5): 1317–1324.
16. Fajt ML, Wenzel SE. Asthma phenotypes and the use of biologic medications in asthma and allergic disease: The next steps toward personalized care. *J Allergy Clin Immunol* 2015; 135(2): 299–310, quiz 1.
17. Castro M, Zangrilli J, Wechsler ME et al. Reslizumab for inadequately controlled asthma with elevated blood eosinophil counts: Results from two multicentre, parallel, double-blind, randomised, placebo-controlled, phase 3 trials. *Lancet Respir Med* 2015; 3(5): 355–366.
18. Laviolette M, Gossage DL, Gauvreau G et al. Effects of benralizumab on airway eosinophils in asthmatic patients with sputum eosinophilia. *J Allergy Clin Immunol* 2013; 132(5): 1086–1096.e5.
19. Cabon Y, Molinari N, Marin G et al. Comparison of anti-interleukin-5 therapies in patients with severe asthma: Global and indirect meta-analyses of randomized placebo-controlled trials. *Clin Exp Allergy* 2017; 47(1): 129–138.
20. Fasenra (benralizumab) prescribing information. https://www.fasenrahcp.com
21. NUCALA (mepolizumab). https://www.gsksource.com/pharma/content/gsk/source/us/en/brands/nucala/pi.html?cc=F736CF99B6F1&pid=
22. Bel EH, Wenzel SE, Thompson PJ et al. Oral glucocorticoid-sparing effect of mepolizumab in eosinophilic asthma. *N Engl J Med* 2014; 371(13): 1189–1197.
23. Nair P, Pizzichini MM, Kjarsgaard M et al. Mepolizumab for prednisone-dependent asthma with sputum eosinophilia. *N Engl J Med* 2009; 360(10): 985–993.
24. CINQAIR (reslizumab) prescribing information. http://www.cinqair.com
25. Castro M, Wenzel SE, Bleecker ER et al. Benralizumab, an anti-interleukin 5 receptor α monoclonal antibody, versus placebo for uncontrolled eosinophilic asthma: A phase 2b randomised dose-ranging study. *Lancet Respir Med* 2014; 2(11): 879–890.
26. Nair P, Barker P, Goldman M. Glucocorticoid sparing of Benralizumab in asthma. *N Engl J Med* 2017; 377(12): 1205.
27. FitzGerald JM, Bleecker ER, Nair P et al. Benralizumab, an anti-interleukin-5 receptor α monoclonal antibody, as add-on treatment for patients with severe, uncontrolled, eosinophilic asthma (CALIMA): A randomised, double-blind, placebo-controlled phase 3 trial. *Lancet (London, England)* 2016; 388(10056): 2128–2141.
28. Nowak RM, Parker JM, Silverman RA et al. A randomized trial of benralizumab, an anti-interleukin 5 receptor α monoclonal antibody, after acute asthma. *Am J Emerg Med* 2015; 33(1): 14–20.
29. DUPIXENT. Dupilumab prescribing information. https://www.dupixent.com
30. Busse WW, Maspero JF, Rabe KF et al. Liberty asthma QUEST: Phase 3 randomized, double-blind, placebo-controlled, parallel-group study to evaluate dupilumab efficacy/safety in patients with uncontrolled, moderate-to-severe asthma. *Adv Ther* 2018; 35(5): 737–748.
31. Beck LA, Thaci D, Hamilton JD et al. Dupilumab treatment in adults with moderate-to-severe atopic dermatitis. *N Engl J Med* 2014; 371(2): 130–139.
32. Castro M, Corren J, Pavord ID et al. Dupilumab efficacy and safety in moderate-to-severe uncontrolled asthma. *N Engl J Med* 2018; 378(26): 2486–2496.
33. Rabe KF, Nair P, Brusselle G et al. Efficacy and safety of dupilumab in glucocorticoid-dependent severe asthma. *N Engl J Med* 2018; 378(26): 2475–2485.

34. Petsky HL, Kew KM, Turner C et al. Exhaled nitric oxide levels to guide treatment for adults with asthma. *Cochrane Database Syst Rev* 2016; 9: Cd011440.

35. Pijnenburg MW, Bakker EM, Lever S et al. High fractional concentration of nitric oxide in exhaled air despite steroid treatment in asthmatic children. *Clin Exp Allergy* 2005; 35(7): 920–925.

36. Liang SE, Hoffmann R, Peterson E et al. Use of dapsone in the treatment of chronic idiopathic and autoimmune urticaria. *JAMA Dermatol* 2019; 155(1): 90–95.

37. Shahzad Mustafa S, Sanchez-Borges M. Chronic urticaria: Comparisons of US, European, and Asian guidelines. *Curr Allergy Asthma Rep* 2018; 18(7): 36.

38. Maurer M, Kaplan A, Rosen K et al. The XTEND-CIU study: Long-term use of omalizumab in chronic idiopathic urticaria. *J Allergy Clin Immunol* 2018; 141(3): 1138–1139.e7.

39. Hausmann JS. Targeting cytokines to treat autoinflammatory diseases. *Clin Immunol.* 2019; 206: 23–32.

40. Davis MDP, van der Hilst JCH. Mimickers of urticaria: Urticarial vasculitis and autoinflammatory diseases. *J Allergy Clin Immunol Pract* 2018; 6(4): 1162–1170.

41. Altman MC, Naimi DR. Omalizumab for chronic urticaria. *N Engl J Med* 2013; 368(26): 2528–2530.

42. Bernstein JA, Lang DM, Khan DA et al. The diagnosis and management of acute and chronic urticaria: 2014 update. *J Allergy Clin Immunol* 2014; 133(5): 1270–1277.

43. Kato A. Immunopathology of chronic rhinosinusitis. *Allergol Int* 2015; 64(2): 121–130.

44. Gevaert P, Calus L, Van Zele T et al. Omalizumab is effective in allergic and nonallergic patients with nasal polyps and asthma. *J Allergy Clin Immunol* 2013; 131(1): 110–116.e1.

45. Bachert C, Sousa AR, Lund VJ et al. Reduced need for surgery in severe nasal polyposis with mepolizumab: Randomized trial. *J Allergy ClinImmunol* 2017; 140(4): 1024–1031.e14.

46. Bachert C, Mannent L, Naclerio RM et al. Effect of subcutaneous dupilumab on nasal polyp burden in patients with chronic sinusitis and nasal polyposis: A randomized clinical trial. *JAMA* 2016; 315(5): 469–479.

47. Shirley M. Dupilumab: First global approval. *Drugs* 2017; 77(10): 1115–1121.

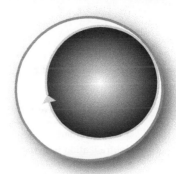

33 Unproven and epicutaneous and other investigational forms of immunotherapy

Haig Tcheurekdjian

Allergy/Immunology Associates, Inc.
Case Western Reserve University

Abba I. Terr

University of California San Francisco Medical Center

CONTENTS

33.1 INTRODUCTION

Specific subcutaneous allergen immunotherapy is the accepted practice throughout the world for the treatment of selected patients with respiratory allergy or Hymenoptera venom anaphylaxis. Numerous placebo-controlled clinical trials document its efficacy and therefore support its use. The precise mechanism by which allergen immunotherapy renders the allergic patient clinically tolerant to ambient allergen exposure remains elusive.

This treatment evolved from the preseasonal grass pollen injections recommended empirically by Noon and Freeman in 1910. Efforts to improve allergen immunotherapy, because it is time consuming, costly, and prone to serious adverse effects, include chemical alterations of the allergen, the use of immunologic adjuvants, and different routes of administration.

The purpose of this chapter is twofold. The first intent is to describe certain unproven and unconventional ("alternative") methods of allergen immunotherapy that have been tried but cannot be recommended because they are unsubstantiated, unscientific in concept, and/or have an unfavorable risk/benefit ratio (Table 33.1). The second is to describe investigational methods of inhalant allergen immunotherapy that are grounded in sound scientific principles but have not yet undergone enough investigation to warrant their use in clinical practice (Table 33.2). Investigational methods of allergen administration are discussed in this chapter, while experimental modification of allergen structure for immunotherapy is discussed

Table 33.1 Unconventional forms of immunotherapy

Serial endpoint titration

Neutralization or symptom-relieving therapy

Enzyme-potentiated desensitization

Autogenous urine injections

Table 33.2 Investigational forms of aeroallergen immunotherapy

Intralymphatic

Epicutaneous

Intradermal

in Chapter 30. In the past, sublingual immunotherapy (SLIT) for respiratory allergy using inhalant allergens and oral immunotherapy (OIT) for food allergy have been considered controversial. Based on scientifically valid ongoing studies, SLIT is now an accepted form of therapy for respiratory allergy, and both SLIT and OIT are recognized as promising approaches for food allergy.

33.2 UNPROVEN FORMS OF IMMUNOTHERAPY

33.2.1 Immunotherapy based on serial endpoint titration

Serial endpoint titration utilizes semiquantitative skin testing to establish the dose of allergen for initiating and optimizing injection treatment of allergic disease. Rinkel, whose name is typically associated with this method of immunotherapy, developed this technique, which others modified. The "Rinkel" method was used for treatment of respiratory diseases caused by the common inhalant allergens (pollens, molds, dust) and, subsequently, for the treatment of food allergy [1–4]. It is currently favored by some otolaryngologists in the United States who include allergy practice in their specialty.

Rinkel's method of testing uses serial fivefold decreasing dilutions (i.e., increasing concentrations) of allergen. Allergen extracts are injected intradermally in a volume of 0.01 mL until an "endpoint is achieved." The wheal diameter is recorded 10 minutes after injection [5,6]. The "endpoint" of the test (i.e., a "positive" test) for each allergen is the lowest concentration that results in a 2 mm or greater increase in wheal diameter compared to the prior fivefold dilution. As many as nine serial intradermal injections can be administered. The initial test dose is very low, generally 1:1,953,125 of the concentrated allergen.

Certain features of this testing protocol must be considered in assessing its relationship to treatment. The presence or absence of erythema accompanying the wheal is ignored [7], which could lead to a false-positive test result. The use of a latent period of only 10 minutes could result in a false-negative interpretation for an IgE-mediated allergic skin test reaction. In some cases, this testing method does not produce the expected progressive increase in wheal diameters. These variations are referred to as "bizarre responses" and are categorized as "hour-glass, plateau, and flash responses" [7]. In the hour-glass response, escalating

allergen concentrations initially lead to decreasing wheal sizes on skin testing followed by an increasing diameter. Plateau responses are characterized as sequential escalating allergen concentrations that result in no change in wheal sizes. The flash response is a large wheal size that on repeat testing with the same allergen concentration leads to a much smaller reaction. Proponents of the Rinkel method attribute these variations to extraneous factors such as concurrent infection, airborne allergen exposure, or incidental food allergy, for which proof is lacking.

The "endpoint," as defined earlier, is considered to be a safe dose to initiate immunotherapy for that particular allergen and patient. This procedure is a safe method for preventing a systemic reaction to the first subcutaneous treatment dose, although the dose is almost always too conservative (i.e., the allergen solution is excessively dilute). The low, initial dose unnecessarily prolongs the course of treatment [8–11].

In addition to establishing the initial dose of immunotherapy, an "optimal" dose is calculated as certain arbitrary multiples of the endpoint, usually between 25 and 50 times the quantity of allergen producing the endpoint. Practitioners of this procedure may vary these multiples empirically, depending on the allergen.

The "optimal dose," as determined by this protocol, is claimed to be the dose at which symptoms will be controlled during immunotherapy. Clinical trials, however, show that such a calculated "optimal" immunotherapy dose is almost always too low so that treatment based on the endpoint procedure leads to therapy that is ultimately no more effective than placebo [12].

Proponents of the Rinkel method recommend retesting during the course of immunotherapy to establish a new "endpoint" if the patient fails to improve as expected. There are no clinical studies to validate this recommendation.

33.2.2 Provocation-neutralization

"Neutralization" (also called "symptom-relieving" or "tolerance" therapy) is also based on a testing procedure related to the method of treatment. "Provocation-neutralization," which evolved from serial endpoint titration described earlier, is based on the concept that an extremely small quantity of allergen ("provocation") can cause the immediate appearance of a symptomatic allergic reaction with the prompt disappearance ("neutralization") of these symptoms with further administration of the allergen. In actual practice, the symptoms that are provoked and cleared in this way are subjective, nonspecific, and not consistent with those symptoms widely recognized as indicative of allergic disease [13–18]. Objective physical signs are ignored.

Provocation-neutralization testing is performed in a manner similar to skin endpoint titration with increasing or decreasing fivefold serial dilutions of the allergen [4]. Many practitioners of this procedure use skin-test extracts that include not only the usual inhalant and food allergens but also solutions of environmental chemicals, drugs, hormones, and many other items that are unlikely to cause atopic disease. Testing is performed by exposing the patient to the allergen via the intracutaneous, subcutaneous, or sublingual route. There is no rational explanation for selecting the route of administration. The sublingual route is used especially, although not exclusively, to diagnose food allergy. Injections are given in the arm. Intracutaneous testing volumes are 0.01, 0.02, or 0.05 mL. The patient keeps a written record of all "sensations" (i.e., any symptom) experienced over a 10-minute period following each injection or sublingual drop. There is no standardized protocol for grading the subjective response, so any symptom or sensation reported by the patient constitutes a positive test result. If the patient reports no symptoms, higher doses are administered in a serial fashion until symptoms are reported. Once a test result is considered positive, further testing proceeds by progressively lowering concentrations until a dose is reached at which the patient reports no sensations. This particular dose is considered to be the "neutralizing dose," which is then used for subsequent treatment.

Each allergen or other test substance must be given separately in a serial fashion, so complete testing can require many days, weeks, or months. No negative controls are included, and there is no provision to account for spontaneous symptoms.

There are variations on this basic protocol. Wheal diameter may be used in addition to subjective symptoms in determining a positive response, but there are no published criteria for wheal sizes indicating a positive or negative result [14]. Some practitioners of provocation-neutralization use the *absence* of symptoms as a positive test [14,16]. In this scheme, a negative test is followed by a serial decrease in subsequent doses; after a positive test the dosages are increased until a negative ("neutralizing") dose is achieved.

The "neutralizing" doses of one or more test substances are then self-administered by the patient as treatment. Where more than one substance is required for treatment, they can be used separately or combined. Treatment can be administered intracutaneously, subcutaneously, or sublingually. The choice is arbitrary, because there are no established protocols and published clinical trials. The patient is advised to administer the neutralizing solution either after symptoms appear or before anticipated exposure to a substance that the patient believes is the cause of the illness. Treatment can also be given on a regular maintenance schedule, usually daily or twice weekly.

Historically, this procedure evolved from the serial intradermal endpoint technique, and certain theories have been offered to justify the results. It is claimed that allergen is present in the injected wheal and released into the systemic circulation from which it elicits symptoms [13]. However, the minute quantity of allergen and the nonallergic nature of induced symptoms make this theory unlikely. Another hypothesis states that allergen introduced into the skin or under the tongue induces antibody formation with the development of circulating immune complexes, but this an untenable scenario, based on the kinetics and time required for these events. Other theories postulate antigen stimulation, suppression of lymphocyte function, and/or induction of immunologic tolerance. Sublingual "desensitization" of lymphocytes also has been postulated as a consequence of antigen absorption from the sublingual route. There are no published results of experimental proof for any of these theories.

Neutralizing therapy is recommended to treat a wide variety of conditions, including atopic asthma, rheumatic diseases, premenstrual syndrome, viral infections, headache, musculoskeletal complaints, attention deficit disorder in children, and others. Neutralizing "antigens" include extracts of known allergens, environmental chemicals, hormones, viral vaccines, foods, histamine, serotonin, saline, and even distilled water.

Published clinical trials of "neutralization" therapy are few in number [17–21,23–25]. One preliminary report of a double-blind, placebo-controlled crossover study of subcutaneous injections of foods administered daily to eight patients revealed improvement with both placebo and active vaccines, but the results from the latter were said to be superior [21]. Another report claims both

subjective and objective improvement in 20 patients with perennial rhinitis treated with sublingual dust vaccine. These results are of questionable significance since the duration of the study period was only 2 weeks, and five of the subjects were not, in fact, allergic to the house dust mite as determined by the investigators reporting the study [25]. A well-conducted, double-blind, placebo-controlled study investigated provocation-neutralization for food-sensitivity in subjects who had consistent, reproducible symptoms on unblinded provocation testing. There was no difference in provocation of symptoms between injections containing allergen and those containing placebo. Furthermore, neutralizing doses were equally efficacious whether allergen or placebo was administered [26].

33.2.3 Enzyme-potentiated desensitization

In 1973, McEwen reported that the enzyme β-glucuronidase acts as an adjuvant or promoter of an immune response when added to the antigen immediately before injection [27]. Since then, a small number of allergists have recommended a procedure known as enzyme-potentiated desensitization (EPD) as an improvement over conventional immunotherapy, claiming that it requires many fewer injections compared to conventional immunotherapy and has an 80% effectiveness rate.

A very low dose of allergen (1–2.5 Noon units, approximately the amount delivered into the skin in a standard prick test) is mixed with a partially purified enzyme, β-glucuronidase, in a dose (100 Fishman units, <40 mg) equivalent to the amount of enzyme normally present in 4 mL of human blood. The mixture is immediately injected intradermally in a volume of approximately 0.125 mL. This is considered sufficient immunization to produce a therapeutic effect for an entire pollen season when given as a single dose preseasonally. For perennial allergy, the intradermal injections are given every 2–6 months. Both inhalant and food allergens have been used in this fashion. A single intradermal injection may contain as many as 150 allergens, typically including inhalants, foods, and certain food additives.

Proponents of this form of treatment claim success in treating not only allergic rhinitis, asthma, and eczema, but also sinusitis, nasal polyposis, urticaria, migraine headaches, ulcerative colitis, irritable bowel syndrome, chronic fatigue syndrome, "immune dysfunction," attention deficit hyperactivity disorder, anxiety, rheumatoid arthritis, grand mal and petit mal seizures, and anaphylaxis from food allergy.

None of the published research findings in patients treated by enzyme-potentiated desensitization substantiate this theory. The effectiveness of this method and the presumed pharmacologic property of β-glucuronidase on the immune system are based on anecdotal evidence or clinical trials of generally inferior quality. Several published double-blind reports claim symptomatic improvements in adults or children with allergic rhinoconjunctivitis or asthma along with conflicting results of immunologic changes [28–36]. These studies suffer from a number of limitations including small sample sizes, brief follow-up periods, and/or lack of objective measures of disease activity. A double-blind, placebo-controlled trial of enzyme-potentiated desensitization for large local reactions to mosquito bites, conducted by investigators who had identified this therapy as being effective in a retrospective analysis, showed no difference between active treatment and placebo [36]. The most rigorously performed double-blind study, which included 183 subjects and objective outcome measures, showed no benefit to enzyme-potentiated desensitization in comparison to placebo for children with allergic rhinitis [35]. Furthermore, the U.S. Food and Drug Administration has banned the import of enzyme-potentiated desensitization products prepared by the primary manufacturer because these allergens are unlicensed in the United States and have previously been imported illegally [37].

The proponents of enzyme-potentiated desensitization hypothesize that the enzyme recruits and activates a new population of CD8+ lymphocytes that downregulates the response to the injected antigens, thereby suppressing the immune response. The claim that this method of treatment requires infrequent injections of allergen is based on the supposition that specific "suppressor" CD8+ T cells persist for up to 2 years. When prescribed for perennial allergies, the first few injections are given every 2 months, after which they are as infrequent as once or twice yearly. For treatment of seasonal pollen allergy, a single dose is given no longer than 4 months before the expected season. Booster doses are given "as required." The effectiveness for house dust allergy is said to be evident almost immediately, for hay fever after 3–4 weeks and for food allergy after 6–9 months.

Advocates of this treatment frequently require their patients to follow certain rules to avoid treatment failure. The patients must not be exposed to allergens for which they are being treated for a period of 24 hours before and 48 hours after the injection. They must consume a special "EPD diet" of lamb, sweet potatoes, carrots, celery, lettuce, sago, tapioca, rhubarb, sea salt, and bottled water for 24 hours before and 48 hours after the injection. They are prescribed specific vitamins and minerals. The injection is given only during the first 2 weeks of the menstrual cycle, and a number of specified medications must be avoided. It is not to be used during pregnancy or within 5 days of an upper respiratory infection. The patient must not use scented products or ointments on the skin near the injection site. Exposure to heat, stress, environmental chemicals, smoke, air-conditioning, newsprint, and photocopiers must be avoided. Efficacy also is believed to be enhanced by taking zinc, folic acid, vitamin A, pyridoxine, and magnesium orally or intravenously for several days before the injection. Delayed reactions, described as a temporary return of the allergic symptoms for which the patient is being treated, are considered a favorable sign that the treatment will be effective.

33.2.4 Autogenous urine immunotherapy

In the early 1930s, several medical publications appeared claiming that a specific substance, called "proteose," is present in the urine during the course of allergic disease [38,39]. Urinary proteose refers to a mixture of partially to completely hydrolyzed protein from the glomerular filtrate. It is therefore postulated to contain allergen peptide fragments, and in particular, those peptides that are "specific" or most allergenic for each individual allergic person. This substance was believed to be a source of allergen for therapy superior to the usual allergen vaccines used in immunotherapy.

Several chemical extraction procedures were recommended to obtain "proteose" from the urine of allergic patients. The extract was suspended in a buffered solution and then used for intradermal testing and for subcutaneous therapeutic injections. This practice seemed to thrive briefly in the mid-1900s, subsided after several years, and then resurfaced in the latter half of the twentieth century.

The published reports consist of uncontrolled, anecdotal histories of apparently successful treatment of a variety of allergic conditions, including asthma, rhinitis, anaphylaxis, urticaria, angioedema, and

serum sickness [40–42]. None of these studies used proper controls; therefore, they cannot be used to show efficacy.

There is no investigation of long-term safety. This is a critical issue, since small quantities of glomerular basement membrane antigens are found in normal urine. It is not unreasonable to assume that alteration by chemical treatment during the extraction process could lead to the production of altered renal proteins that might prove to be antigenic and induce autoantibodies, potentially resulting in autoimmune nephropathy.

33.2.5 Scope of the problem

Some of the unproven treatment methods discussed previously, such as autogenous urine immunotherapy, are rarely utilized today. Others such as provocation-neutralization, however, persist [43]. In particular, neutralization therapy using either the injection or sublingual route and enzyme-potentiated desensitization form an important part of the practice of those who subscribe to theories whereby certain people are believed to react to ordinary or even exceedingly minute exposures to common environmental items that can be detected by odor, such as perfumes, organic solvents, and other ubiquitous chemicals. The clinical manifestations of this condition are numerous but entirely subjective [44]. Extracts of chemicals and foods are typically included in the "neutralizing" or "enzyme potentiating" treatment. This "condition" has not been shown to be caused by chemicals or to involve a physical sensitivity [45], and evidence abounds that psychological factors are important in these beliefs [44].

33.2.6 Costs to the healthcare system

There is no reliable method to assess or even estimate the cost of these unproven immunotherapy methods in either absolute amounts or as a percentage of the total healthcare expenditure. Since they are controversial and not considered standard forms of medical practice, they are not listed or codified in the Common Procedural Terminology publication [46]. Nonetheless, it is likely that the costs are substantial considering that, in the United States, out-of-pocket annual expenditures for alternative therapies such as these are estimated to be approximately $34 billion, and rhinosinusitis and asthma are two of the most common conditions for which alternative therapies are sought [47]. Furthermore, in most instances, payment for these services in the United States is made by the patient directly to the practitioner and not by third-party payors, limiting the available data as to the total expenditure for unproven immunotherapy.

33.3 INVESTIGATIONAL FORMS OF IMMUNOTHERAPY

33.3.1 Intralymphatic immunotherapy

The scientific principle behind intralymphatic immunotherapy is to deliver allergen directly to the immune cells involved in generating tolerance during immunotherapy [48]. The hypothesis is that this mode of administration will induce a tolerogenic immune response in a shorter period of time and with fewer doses than the subcutaneous or sublingual routes. In this form of immunotherapy, a superficial inguinal lymph node is injected with allergen under ultrasound guidance, thus introducing the allergen directly into an environment rich with antigen-presenting cells, T cells, and B cells. Furthermore, there is a paucity of mast cells in lymph nodes which may decrease the rate and severity of adverse reactions. Generally, patients receive three allergen injections over 12 weeks. The immune cells in the lymph node are exposed to approximately 100 times the allergen amount per injection when compared to allergen delivered by other routes of immunotherapy [49], but the cumulative amount of allergen administered over the course of therapy is eight times less [50].

Intralymphatic immunotherapy is effective in double-blind placebo-controlled trials with tree pollen [51,52], grass pollen [51–53], and a modified cat dander protein [54]. In general, symptom scores during the pollen season and following intranasal allergen challenges are improved compared to placebo, but medication usage is not necessarily decreased with intralymphatic immunotherapy [51]. The benefits achieved from three intralymphatic immunotherapy injections appear to be long lived. In a randomized, open-label study of grass pollen immunotherapy, clinical benefits of three injections of intralymphatic immunotherapy were similar to that achieved by standard subcutaneous immunotherapy 3 years after treatment [50]. Systemic adverse reactions are rarely reported, although localized lymph node swelling occurs in 33% of injections as compared to 4% in placebo-treated subjects [51]. The injections themselves are well tolerated [55].

A well-designed study showed no benefit to grass pollen intralymphatic immunotherapy as assessed by symptom score and medication use during pollen season [55]. The primary difference in this study as compared to the studies showing clinical benefit is that the time interval between injections was decreased to 2 weeks from 4 weeks. The authors of the studies showing benefit suggest that this shortened time-frame does not allow for appropriate memory B-cell formation and affinity maturation, and selectively generates T cells with low allergen affinity, thereby adversely affecting clinical outcomes [56].

Intralymphatic immunotherapy is a promising treatment modality that can decrease the number of injections administered, decrease the cumulative amount of allergen administered, and potentially provide clinical benefits similar to that of subcutaneous immunotherapy for respiratory allergic disease. Studies to date have generally recruited small numbers of subjects, have not consistently shown clinical benefit, and medication usage has not necessarily decreased with the use of intralymphatic immunotherapy. Furthermore, specific resources are required for injections, such as ultrasonography, which may not be available in many locations. Large and well-conducted studies are still required to determine whether intralymphatic immunotherapy is an effective modality of allergen immunotherapy.

33.3.2 Epicutaneous immunotherapy

Epicutaneous allergen immunotherapy has been used as a treatment modality for respiratory allergic disease since the early 1900s and has been investigated in a number of studies over the following decades [48]. The technique generally involved scratching the patient's skin in a checkerboard pattern to disrupt the epidermis followed by application of allergen to the disrupted skin. The strategy is to allow allergen to diffuse from the scarified epidermis to the immune cells in the dermis while simultaneously avoiding allergen administration directly to the highly vascularized dermis, which could increase the risk of adverse events. Because allergen is being exposed to both the epidermis and the dermis, it is likely that immune cells in both areas are involved in development of tolerance to the allergen. Furthermore, once the allergen diffuses to the dermis, the allergen and locally activated immune cells can be more efficiently drained to the lymph nodes, potentially allowing for an enhanced immunologic response. More recently, repeated tape stripping has been used as a modality to replace skin scarification in order to improve patient comfort while still allowing for allergen administration epicutaneously. This also induces the localized production of cytokines that may enhance the efficacy of the immunotherapy [57].

Three double-blind, placebo-controlled trials from the same research group demonstrated improvement in grass pollen–induced rhinoconjunctivitis symptoms after treatment with epicutaneous allergen immunotherapy [58–60]. The general process involves the administration of a patch loaded with grass pollen to tape-stripped skin on the upper arm. Patches are applied weekly for 6 weeks with patches kept on the skin for 8 hours. Therapy is started prior to the beginning of the grass pollen season. In the latest study [60], subjects treated with grass pollen patches reported 48% improvement in symptoms compared to a 10% improvement in the placebo arm. One year after therapy, the benefits were lost, although this is in contrast to a prior study showing sustained improvement 1 year after therapy [58]. Importantly, a combined endpoint measuring improvement in both symptoms and medication use showed no improvement with grass pollen patch treatment. Likewise, nasal provocation test scores were unchanged in one study [59]. Systemic reactions can occur, especially if the skin is aggressively abraded with a file instead of tape stripping prior to application of patches [61]. Localized reactions, such as eczema at the site of patch placement, are common and occur in most individuals if patches are left in place for 48 hours instead of the shorter 8-hour protocol.

Although epicutaneous allergen immunotherapy is a potential future treatment modality for allergic rhinoconjunctivitis, many of the same limitations seen with intralymphatic immunotherapy are present, such as inconsistent reports of efficacy, unchanged medication usage with therapy, and small study sizes. If further studies show promising results, epicutaneous allergen immunotherapy may allow for easily administered treatment of allergic rhinoconjunctivitis that can be achieved with a short course of therapy. Epicutaneous food immunotherapy currently is more promising than aeroallergen treatment. This is discussed in Chapter 8.

33.3.3 Intradermal immunotherapy

Data regarding intradermal immunotherapy for rhinoconjunctivitis are limited, and further investigation is required. A study assessing cutaneous late response (wheal size 24 hours after intradermal injection of grass pollen) demonstrated a decrease in this response after 6 every other week intradermal grass pollen injections [62]. A subsequent double-blind, placebo-controlled study confirmed that intradermal grass pollen immunotherapy suppresses the cutaneous late response, but it does not lead to improvement in a combined symptom-medication score and is actually associated worse rhinitis and asthma symptom control [22]. At present, there are no data suggesting that intradermal immunotherapy has a role in the treatment of allergic rhinoconjunctivitis.

SALIENT POINTS

Unproven forms of immunotherapy

1. The same controversial treatment is often claimed to be efficacious for a variety of unrelated illnesses.
2. Theories in support of controversial allergy procedures frequently change.
3. Controversial allergy treatments are often linked to unproven forms of allergy diagnostic testing.
4. Clinicians should be familiar with unproven and controversial treatments and their pitfalls to properly advise their patients.
5. Unproven treatments flourish, in part, because of the placebo effect inherent in every form of treatment.

Investigational forms of immunotherapy

1. Different routes of immunotherapy administration may decrease the number of doses of immunotherapy and the time required to complete therapy.
2. Intralymphatic, epicutaneous, and intradermal routes of administration seek to administer allergen to immune cells more effectively than current forms of immunotherapy.
3. Larger studies are needed to confirm efficacy and determine optimal dosing regimens.

REFERENCES

1. Rinkel HJ. The management of clinical allergy, part ll, etiologic factors and skin titration. *Arch Otolaryngol* 1963; 77: 42.
2. Rinkel HJ. The management of clinical allergy, Pt ill: Inhalation allergy therapy. *Arch Otolaryngol* 1963; 77: 205.
3. Rinkel HJ. The management of clinical allergy, Pt IV: Food and mold allergy. *Arch Otolaryngol* 1963; 77: 302.
4. Rinkel HJ, Lee CH, Crown DW Jr et al. The diagnosis of food allergy. *Arch Otolaryngol* 1964; 79: 71.
5. Williams RI. Skin titration; testing and treatment. *Otolaryngol Clin North Am* 1971; 3: 507.
6. Richardson AS. Titration; evaluation of an office system of allergy diagnosis and treatment: Its use in otolaryngology. *Ann Otol Rhinol Laryngol* 1961; 70: 344.
7. Willoughby JW. Serial dilution titration skin tests in inhalant allergy; a clinical quantitative assessment of biologic skin reactivity to allergenic extracts. *Otolaryngol Clin North Am* 1974; 7: 579.
8. Hirsch S, Kalbfleisch JH, Golbert TM et al. Rinkel method; a controlled study. Second report. *J Allergy Clin Immunol* 1980; 65: 192.
9. Hirsch S, Kalbfleisch JH, Golbert TM et al. Rinkel injection therapy; a multicenter controlled study. *J Allergy Clin Immunol* 1981; 68: 133.
10. Van Metre TE, Adkinson NF, Amodio FJ et al. A comparative study of the effectiveness of the Rinkel method and the current standard method of immunotherapy for ragweed pollen hay fever. *J Allergy Clin Immunol* 1980; 66: 500.
11. Van Metre TE, Adkinson NF, Lichtenstein LM et al. A controlled study of the effectiveness of the Rinkel method of immunotherapy for ragweed pollen hay fever. *J Allergy Clin Immunol* 1980; 65: 288.
12. Van Metre TE. Critique of controversial and unproven procedures for diagnosis and therapy of allergy disorders. *Ped Clin North Am* 1983; 30: 807.
13. Morris DL. Use of sublingual antigen in diagnosis and treatment of food allergy. *Ann Allergy* 1971; 27: 289.
14. Lee CH, Williams RT, Binkley EL. Provocative testing and treatment for foods. *Arch Otolaryngol* 1969; 90: 87.
15. Breneman JC, Crook WC, Deamer W et al. Report of the Food Allergy Committee on the sublingual method of provocation testing for food allergy. *Ann Allergy* 1973; 31: 382.
16. Willoughby JW. Provocative food test technique. *Ann Allergy* 1965; 23: 543.
17. Lee CH, Williams RT, Binkley EL. Provocative inhalation testing and treatment. *Arch Otolaryngol* 1969; 90: 173.
18. Kailin EW, Collier R. "Relieving" therapy for antigen exposure. *JAMA* 1971; 217: 78.
19. Dickey LD, Pfeiffer G. Sublingual therapy in allergy. *Trans Am Soc Ophthal Otolaryngol Allergy* 1964; 5: 37.
20. Warren CM. Inhalant allergy: Diagnosis and treatment by provocation intracutaneous method. *Med Dig* 1978; 33.
21. Miller JB. A double-blind study of food extract injection therapy: A preliminary report. *Ann Allergy* 1977; 38: 185.
22. Slovick A, Douiri A, Muir R et al. Intradermal grass pollen immunotherapy increases Th2 and IgE responses and worsens respiratory allergic symptoms. *J Allergy Clin Immunol* 2017; 139: 1830–1839.
23. Morris DL. Treatment of respiratory disease with ultra-small doses of antigen. *Ann Allergy* 1970; 28: 494.
24. Morris DL. Treatment of atopic dermatitis with tolerogenic doses of antigen. *Acta Dermatovenerol* 1980; 92(suppl): 97.
25. Scadding GK, Brostoff J. Low dose sublingual therapy in patients with allergic rhinitis due to house dust mite. *Clin Allergy* 1986; 16: 483.
26. Jewett DL, Fein G, Greenberg MH. A double-blind study of symptom provocation to determine food sensitivity. *N Engl J Med* 1990; 323: 429.
27. McEwen LM, Nicholson M, Kitchen I, White S. Enzyme potentiated desensitization. III. Control by sugars and diols of the immunological effect of glucuronidase in mice and patients with hay fever. *Ann Allergy* 1973; 31: 543.
28. Fell P, Brostoff J. A single dose desensitization for summer hay fever. Results of a double blind study-1988. *Eur J Clin Pharmacol* 1990; 38: 77.
29. Cantani A, Ragno V, Monteleone MA, Lucenti P, Businco L. Enzyme-potentiated desensitization in children with asthma and mite allergy: A double-blind study. *J Invest Allergol Clin Immunol* 1996; 6: 270.
30. Astarita C, Scala G, Sproviero S, Franzese A. Effects of enzyme-potentiated desensitization in the treatment of pollinosis: A double-blind placebo-controlled trial. *J Invest Allergol Immunol* 1996; 6: 248.
31. Di Stanisloa C, Di Berardino L, Bianchi I, Bologna G. A double-blind, placebo controlled study of preventive immunotherapy with E.P.D., in the treatment of seasonal allergic disease. *Allerg Immunol (Paris)* 1997; 29: 39–42.
32. Caramia G, Franceschini F, Cimarelli ZA, Ciucchi MS, Gagliardini R, Ruffini E. The efficacy of E.P.D., a new immunotherapy, in the treatment of allergic diseases in children. *Allerg Immunol (Paris)* 1996; 28: 308–310.
33. Di Stanislao C, Angelini F, Gagliardi MC et al. β-Glucuronidase short-term immunotherapy. *Allergy* 2003; 58: 459.
34. Galli E, Bassi MS, Mora E et al. A double-blind randomized placebo-controlled trial with short-term β-glucuronidase

therapy in children with chronic rhinoconjunctivitis and/or asthma due to dust mite allergy. *J Investig Allergol Clin Immunol* 2006; 16: 345–350.

35. Radcliffe MJ, Lewith GT, Turner RG, Prescott P, Church MK, Holgate ST. Enzyme potentiated desensitization in treatment of seasonal allergic rhinitis: Double blind randomized controlled study. *BMJ* 2003; 327: 251–254.

36. Berkovitz S, Hill N, Radcliffe M, Ambler G. A randomised, double-blind pilot study of enzyme-potentiated desensitisation for prophylaxis of large local reactions to mosquito bites. *J Allergy (Cairo)* 2012; 2012: 106069.

37. U.S. Food and Drug Administration. 2016 January 14 [cited 2018 March 10]. FDA Import Alert 57–15. Detention Without Physical Examination of Allergens And/Or Allergenic Products. http://www.accessdata.fda.gov/cms_ia/importalert_154.html

38. Steel RS. The specificity of urinary proteose. *Med J Aust* 1932; 2: 800.

39. Oriel OH, Barber HW. Proteose in urine excreted in anaphylactic and allergic conditions. *Lancet* 1930; 2: 1304.

40. Whitehead RW, Darley W, Dickman PA. Therapeutic use of urinary proteose. *Colorado Med* 1934; 56.

41. Liberman I, Bigland AD. Autogenous urinary proteose in asthma and other allergic conditions. *Br Med J* 1937; 1: 62.

42. Plesch J. Urine therapy. *Med. Press* 1947; 218: 128.

43. Kelso JM. Unproven diagnostic tests for adverse reactions to foods. *J Allergy Clin Immunol Pract* 2018; 6: 362–365.

44. Bielory L, Terr AI. Unconventional theories and unproven methods in allergy. Ch. 101. In: Adkinson Jr NF et al., editor. *Middleton's Allergy; Principles and Practice*, 8th ed. Philadelphia, PA: Elsevier, 2014: 1616–1635.

45. UNEP-ILO-WHO et al. Conclusions and recommendations of a workshop on multiple chemical sensitivities (MCS). *Reg Toxicol Pharmacol* 1996; 24: S188–S189.

46. American Medical Association. *Current Procedural Terminology 2018*. Chicago, IL: American Medical Association, 2017.

47. Nahin RL, Barnes PM, Stussman BJ, Bloom B. Costs of complementary and alternative medicine (CAM) and frequency of visits to CAM practitioners: United States, 2007. *Natl Health Stat Report* 2009; 30: 1–14.

48. Senti G, Kundig TM. Novel delivery routes for allergen immunotherapy: Intralymphatic, epicutaneous, and intradermal. *Immunol Allergy Clin N Am* 2016; 36: 25–37.

49. Senti G, Johansen P, Kundig TM. Intralymphatic immunotherapy: From the rationale to human applications. *Curr Top Microbiol Immunol* 2011; 352: 71–84.

50. Senti G, Vavricka BMP, Erdmann I et al. Intralymphatic allergen administration renders specific immunotherapy faster and

safer: A randomized controlled trial. *PNAS* 2008; 105: 17908–17912.

51. Hylander T, Larsson O, Petersson-Westin U et al. Intralymphatic immunotherapy of pollen-induced rhinoconjunctivitis: A double-blind placebo-controlled trial. *Respiratory Research* 2016; 17: 10–18.

52. Hylander T, Latif L, Petersson-Westin U, Cardell, LO. Intralymphatic allergen-specific immunotherapy: An effective and safe alternative treatment route for pollen-induced allergic rhinitis. *J Allergy Clin Immunol* 2013; 131: 412–420.

53. Patterson AM, Bonny AE, Shiels WE, Erwin EA. Three injection intralymphatic immunotherapy in adolescents and young adults with grass pollen rhinoconjunctivitis. *Annals Allergy Asthma Immunol* 2016; 116: 168–170.

54. Senti G, Crameri R, Kuster D et al. Intralymphatic immunotherapy for cat allergy induces tolerance after only three injections. *J Allergy Clin Immunol* 2012; 129: 1290–1296.

55. Witten M, Malling H-J, Blom L, Poulsen BC, Poulsen, LK. Is intralymphatic immunotherapy ready for clinical use in patients with grass pollen allergy? *J Allergy Clin Immunol* 2013; 132: 1248–1252.

56. Kundig TM, Johansen P, Bachmann MF, Cardell LO, Senti G. Intralymphatic immunotherapy: Time interval between injections is essential. *J Allergy Clin Immunol* 2014; 133: 930–931.

57. Nickoloff B, Naidu Y. Perturbation of epidermal barrier function correlates with initiation of cytokine cascade in human skin. *J Am Acad Dermatol* 1994; 30: 535–546.

58. Senti G, Graf N, Haug S et al. Epicutaneous allergen administration as a novel method of allergen-specific immunotherapy. *J Allergy Clin Immunol* 2009; 124: 997–1002.

59. Senti G, von Moos S, Tay F et al. Epicutaneous allergen-specific immunotherapy ameliorates grass pollen-induced rhinoconjunctivitis: A double-blind, placebo-controlled dose escalation study. *J Allergy Clin Immunol* 2012; 129: 128–135.

60. Senti G, von Moos S, Tay F, Graf N, Johansen P, Kundig TM. Determinants of efficacy and safety in epicutaneous allergen immunotherapy: Summary of three clinical trials. *Allergy* 2015; 70: 707–710.

61. von Moos S, Johansen P, Tay F, Graf N, Kundig TM, Senti G. Comparing safety of abrasion and tape-stripping as skin preparation in allergen-specific epicutaneous immunotherapy. *J Allergy Clin Immunol* 2014; 134: 965–967.

62. Rotiroti G, Shamji M, Durham SR, Till SJ. Repeated low-dose intradermal allergen injection suppresses allergen-induced cutaneous late responses. *J Allergy Clin Immmunol* 2012; 130: 918–924.

SECTION V

Recognition, management, and prevention of adverse effects of allergen immunotherapy

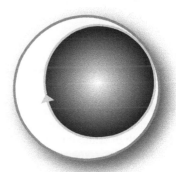

34 Adverse effects and fatalities associated with allergen skin testing and subcutaneous allergen immunotherapy*

Andrew S. Bagg
University of Central Florida College of Medicine

Richard F. Lockey
University of South Florida Morsani College of Medicine

CONTENTS

34.1 INTRODUCTION

Most local and systemic reactions that develop during subcutaneous allergen immunotherapy (SCIT) occur within 20–30 minutes of injection but can occur later than 30 minutes. Subcutaneous nodules at the site of injection are more common with aluminum-adsorbed vaccines, may persist, but usually disappear and do not necessitate an adjustment in the SCIT dose. Patients who develop nodules that persist should be injected with aqueous preparations.

Van Arsdel's and Sherman's [1] comprehensive review in 1957 analyzed retrospectively the incidence of constitutional reactions in a population of 8706 patients who had received a total of 1,250,000 allergen injections during the 21 years between 1935 and 1955. Their patients experienced a total of 1774 constitutional reactions, about 1 in 700 of the 1,250,000 injections given. The

reactions occurred in 663 patients, an incidence of 1.9% (versus the 3.5% reported in 1916 by Cooke and Vanderveer) [2]. Of the 663 reacting patients, 635 were pollen sensitive, representing about 15% of the 4215 pollen-sensitive patients, contrasted with a 0.6% incidence in the remaining 4491 patients. Most of the studies on adverse reactions to SCIT have been concerned with reactions resulting from the injection itself.

Reports of adverse effects from prick-puncture skin tests prompted an analysis of data derived from the Second National Health and Nutrition Examination Survey (NHANES II) [3]. This study revealed that the risk of prick-puncture allergy skin testing was low when carried out with eight extracts licensed by the U.S. Food and Drug Administration (FDA) on a randomly selected population.

The incidence of adverse reactions during SCIT reported in retrospective and prospective studies has varied considerably, depending

---

* In earlier editions, this chapter was co-authored by our dear friend and colleague, the late Samuel C. Bukantz, MD.

on several factors, including the type of allergen vaccine preparation, the patients selected, route of administration, and treatment schedule used, with or without pretreatment and/or preventive procedures [4–12]. All studies carried out between 1980 and 1989 established the safety of SCIT when performed on selected patients by experienced physicians who exercised caution and provided adequate monitoring and appropriate treatment, when anaphylaxis does occur. The nonfatal adverse reaction rate ran from less than 1% of patients on regular SCIT to 36.2% on rush SCIT, without pretherapy.

These data have been obtained in studies utilizing the subcutaneous route of injection of allergen vaccines obtained by aqueous extraction of allergens. An "Immunotherapy Coalition" consisting of the American Academy of Allergy, Asthma and Immunology (AAAAI), the American College of Allergy, Asthma, and Immunology (ACAAI), and allergy extract manufacturers supported the benefits of SCIT and pretreatment to reduce adverse effects associated with the therapy [13–24].

Other allergen molecules and techniques of AIT have also been explored to decrease the potential for adverse reactions and to increase efficacy [25–33]. These have included oral administration [34,35], nasal administration [36,37], and sublingual-swallow immunotherapy (SLIT) [38–42]. A review of the available literature by the World Health Organization (WHO) in 1998 concluded that oral immunotherapy was ineffective, whereas SLIT is a viable alternative to the subcutaneous injection route (see Chapter 35). These conclusions were also made in a position paper of the European Academy of Allergy and Clinical Immunology. This is reviewed in the paper by Passalacqua et al. [42]. Cox et al. have reviewed the literature regarding SLIT from the AAAAI and ACAAI Task Force and report evidence of clinical efficacy and a favorable safety profile [43]. A Cochrane database systematic review and review of meta-analyses also support this [118,120]. SLIT is also well tolerated in children as young as 2 years [44,119]. The adverse effects associated with SLIT are covered in Chapter 35. Alternative methods for AIT are covered in Chapters 30 and 33.

34.2 FREQUENCY OF IgE SYSTEMIC REACTIONS

The risk of death after the injection of a foreign substance has been known since Lamson's report in 1924 [45]. No other cited studies had reported fatalities; however, in 1942, Vance and Strassman [46] reported seven cases of sudden death following injection of foreign protein, and James and Austin [47] published an analysis of six instances of fatal anaphylaxis in humans following parenteral administration of antigen (penicillin, guinea pig hemoglobin, bee venom, and ragweed vaccine), citing several single case reports by Sheppe [48] and Blanton and Sutphin [49], as well as the seven cases of Vance and Strassman by Rosenthal [50] following penicillin injection.

Rands, a general practitioner in the United Kingdom, published a report of a single fatality of a 19-year-old female due to nonresponsive bronchoconstriction developing within 5 minutes following the injection of her usual maintenance dose of Pollinex (a commercial pollen vaccine manufactured in Toronto, Canada) given 5 weeks after the same dose had been administered without effect [51]. In 1985, 13 fatalities from SCIT were reported at the annual meeting of the AAAAI [10]. Stemming from the findings published in this abstract, concerns over the safety of SCIT began to build in North America and Great Britain because of two almost simultaneously

published reports describing 40 and 26 fatalities associated with SCIT in the United States and Great Britain, respectively [11,12]. Based on these reports, changes took place in the United States, with the institution of SCIT practice parameters leading to a sharp decline in fatalities secondary to this form of therapy. Similarly, in Europe, restrictions on the administration of SCIT were levied by the British Committee for the Safety of Medicines resulting in a sharp decline in SCIT given in the United Kingdom over subsequent years.

A major objective of this chapter is to compare the retrospective reviews of fatalities occurring during skin testing and immunotherapy made by the Committee on Allergen Standardization of the AAAAI [82] and by the Paul Ehrlich Institute, the German Federal Agency for Sera and Vaccines [53]. These studies analyzed the factors contributing to fatalities occurring during skin tests or immunotherapy with a view to diminishing and, hopefully, eliminating them.

34.3 NON-IgE-MEDIATED ADVERSE REACTIONS

It is appropriate to review reports of some aspects of adverse reactions to SCIT that are controversial. The possible role of precipitins as responsible for adverse reactions was addressed by Busse et al. in a study correlating *Alternaria* IgG precipitins and adverse reactions [54]. Their prospective study revealed that 5 of 23 *Aternaria*-sensitive persons had IgG precipitins before SCIT and another six developed precipitins during therapy. Only one of the 23 experienced a reaction to *Alternaria* 4–6 hours after an injection of *Alternaria* vaccine. They conclude that precipitins to *Alternaria* are common and do not seem to be the basis for late reactions, and their presence is not a contraindication to AIT. A contrasting report by Kaad and Ostergaard suggests that SCIT of asthmatic children with mold vaccines might be hazardous by provoking immune complex reactions [55]. Of 38 children with bronchial asthma who were immunized with mold vaccines, seven (19%) were withdrawn due to "serious" side effects that were considered clinically consistent with an immune complex reaction. These seven children exhibited a two- to fourfold increase in circulating precipitating antibodies to the injected vaccines. Of the remaining 31 patients also treated with mold vaccines, 14, who were without side effects, did not develop precipitating antibodies. The sera of these patients were not examined for immune complexes, and the authors quote the contradictory findings of the Kemler and Stein [56,57] groups as well as apparently supportive reports by Stendardi et al., Cano et al., El-Hefny et al., Moore and Fink, and Kuukiala et al. [58–62].

Relevant to these studies is the report by Clausen and Yanari that immune complex–mediated disease is not a factor in patients on maintenance venom immunotherapy [63]. They evaluated the problem in 30 adults and 15 pediatric patients receiving regular monthly doses of venom (100 μg of antigen), all between 12 and 9 months. A serum sickness–like presentation had been reported as a sequela of Hymenoptera stings, but the possible role of immune complexes had not been addressed.

No patients developed clinical manifestations suggestive of immune complex pathology: all urinalyses were negative for gross and microscopic hematuria, no sera showed an elevation of Clq, and only 4 of the 45 patients had significantly elevated Raji cell assays. Prospective reevaluation showed the presence of immune complexes before venom administration with no change in acute-phase reactants or Raji cell titers 12 hours later. The authors conclude that monthly administration of Hymenoptera venom does not appear to be associated with immune complex disease by either clinical or immunologic parameters. A further relevant article was contributed by Umetsu et al. who described an 8-year-old male child with rhinitis and asthma who developed serum sickness triggered by anaphylaxis complicating SCIT with multiple inhalant allergens (ragweed, grass, and tree pollens; mold spores; and dust) [64]. This child developed puffy eyelids 1 hour following a half-dose of his vaccine and progressed thereafter to an impressive serum sickness syndrome characterized by severe generalized raised annular urticaria, severe asthma, angioedema, severe arthralgias, fever, and episodes of confusion and disorientation. The authors hypothesized that the enhanced vascular permeability that accompanied the anaphylaxis allowed immune complexes that may have persisted in the circulation to deposit in the blood vessels of the patient. The immune complexes may or may not have been related to the SCIT itself; tests for these complexes, however, were negative. Clemmensen and Knudsen reported a patient with eczema who apparently developed contact sensitivity to aluminum while receiving SCIT for hay fever with an aluminum-precipitated allergen [65]. Standard patch testing was positive to the aluminum discs used for testing and negative in 53 controls; the eczema disappeared when therapy was discontinued.

An association between brachial plexus neuropathy and AIT was reported by Wolpow [66]. Two patients were described who developed acute, self-limiting, unilateral brachial plexus neuropathy in association with SCIT of dust and molds. Previous reports of this neurologic illness had "in many cases followed injection of foreign substances, but usually of animal rather than vegetable origin."

Schatz et al. call attention to what they termed *nonorganic adverse reactions* to AIT [67]. They described 10 patients who presented adverse reactions to SCIT that mimicked immunologically mediated reactions but were believed to be "nonorganic" in etiology—with a high incidence of coexisting or contributory psychiatric problems.

34.4 LONG-TERM SEQUELAE

The possibility that chronic injection of foreign proteins might induce long-term sequelae had been addressed by both experimental animal studies and anecdotal reports in humans. Rabbits hyperimmunized with various vaccines make cryoprecipitating proteins, monoclonal antibody, rheumatoid factor, and anti-DNA antibodies [68–70], and such, hyperimmunized animals may develop amyloidosis and myeloma [71,72]. There are anecdotal reports of multiple myeloma and Waldenström's macroglobulinemia in patients on long-term SCIT [73] and a report of a striking incidence of positive rheumatoid factors in atopic children on such therapy [74].

Levinson et al. undertook to determine if long-term AIT caused late sequelae, particularly those reflecting abnormal immunologic responses [75]. Their study, the first systematic investigation of potential adverse effects of long-term SCIT, examined 41 patients between 18 and 50 years of age who had received such therapy with three or more allergen vaccines for 5 or more years at the Walter Reed Army Medical Center Allergy Clinic. Twenty-one age- and gender-matched atopic individuals served as controls prior to initiating such therapy. The treated individuals showed no increased autoimmune, collagen, vascular, or lymphoproliferative disease. Furthermore, long-term allergen immunotherapy had no adverse effects on immunologic reactivity as assessed by a number of immunologic parameters—with a particularly noteworthy absence

of immune complexes in the serum of patients undergoing long-term AIT. It is true for at least this study of 41 patients, mostly Caucasian females, of an average age of 30 years, treated for allergic rhinitis and asthma for 5 or more years in the U.S. Army Allergy Clinic.

Phanuphak and Kohler [76] described in 6 of 20 consecutive patients the onset of polyarteritis nodosa, of vasculitic symptoms that coincided with SCIT for presumptive atopic (IgE-mediated) respiratory disease. Compared with 14 other patients with polyarteritis nodosa, the six on AIT had significantly greater skin involvement and peripheral blood eosinophils. There was evidence for circulatory complexes with decreased hemolytic complement, increased cryoglobulins, or increased C1q binding in both groups but no allergen-precipitating antibodies.

A possible association between pemphigus vulgaris and allergen injections with cat pelt vaccine was raised by McCombs et al. [77]. Although intriguing, it seems irrelevant since such therapy today is performed with purified cat allergens.

The conflicting results of studies in patients receiving long-term SCIT might be explained by a nonuniformity of detection methods used. This prompted a group of Australian investigators to examine a population of older patients with documented prolonged AIT extending over many years. They examined 35 older patients (mean age 62 years, range 53–85 years) who received injections of allergen vaccines for between 2 and 30 years (mean of 13 years) and compared them with an age-matched control group (mean age 64.7, range 42–87 years). Treated patients had significantly higher IgG and lower total IgE than controls but no increased incidence of paraproteins or evidence of immune complex disease such as urinary abnormalities, increased C1q binding levels, cryoglobulins, or rheumatoid fever [78].

34.5 FATALITIES

Fatalities, carefully documented, constitute a less controversial measure of adverse effects related to either skin testing or allergen immunotherapy. Since Lamson's first description of death from anaphylaxis associated with SCIT [45], six fatalities have been reported related to or associated with SCIT [46,47,51,79–81]. More than 70 deaths (between 1895 and 1964) have been reported after skin testing, the majority of these associated with antigens such as horse serum–derived tetanus or diphtheria antitoxins and pneumococcus antiserum, none of which is currently in use. Nine of these 70 deaths from skin testing were associated with allergens similar to allergens used today. No articles on fatalities associated with SCIT or skin testing have been published in the United States between 1980 and 1987.

A project defining risk factors for fatalities from skin testing and SCIT was instituted as a retrospective study by the Committee on Allergen Standardization of the AAAAI in 1983. For this project, Lockey and his coworkers composed a 64-item questionnaire designed to obtain data on fatalities from skin testing and SCIT. The questionnaire was mailed to the then 3400 members and fellows of the AAAAI. In 1985, 13 fatalities from SCIT were reported at the annual meeting of the AAAAI. An extensive analysis was published in the *Journal of Allergy and Clinical Immunology* in April 1987 [82]. Although 46 fatalities had been reported from 1945 to 1984, 30 (6 fatalities from skin testing and 24 from SCIT) had sufficient data for analysis. Tables 34.1 and 34.2 (modified from [82]) summarize the data on fatalities associated with skin testing and SCIT, respectively.

Table 34.1 Case reports from the literature—Fatalities from skin tests

Author/year	Age/medical disease	Injected vaccine	Onset of symptoms	Initial symptoms	Cause of death
Baagoe, 1928	Unknown	Egg white, 0.1 cc	Sudden	Dyspnea	Unknown
Lamson, 1929	5 mo, eczema	Ovomucoid, 0.05 cc	2 min	Cyanosis	Respiratory arrest
Lamson, 1929	34 yr, asthma	Buckwheat 1:500, ID	2–3 min	Lacrimation, cyanosis, respiratory difficulty	Anaphylactic shock
Vance and Strassman, 1942	4 yr	Silkworm, sheep's wool, kapok extracts, IC	5 min	Shock/unconscious	Anaphylactic shock[a]
Wiseman and McCarthy-Brough, 1945	78 yr, asthma	17 environmental allergens, 0.01 cc, IC	5 min	Cough, asthma	Anaphylactic arrest
Swineford, 1946	49 yr, asthma	56 food extracts, 8–9 inhalant extracts, IC	3 min	"Not feeling well," dyspnea	Cardiovascular collapse
Blantin and Sutphin, 1949	57 yr, asthma	56 skin tests, scratch and IC	Sudden	Air hunger	Anaphylactic shock[a]
Harris and Shure, 1950	25 yr, asthma	Environmental substances, ID	1 min	Dyspnea	Respiratory arrest[a]
Dogliotti, 1968	35 yr	Penicillin scratch	4–5 min	Flush, abdominal Pain	Anaphylactic shock
Lockey et al., 1987	6 subjects, 10–50 yrs	Variable	3–20 min	Variable	Asthma, anaphylactic shock, others
Reid et al., 1995	1 subject	Unknown	Unknown	Unknown	Unknown
Bernstein et al., 2004	1 young subject, asthma, food allergy	90 food scratch tests	Unknown	Bronchospasm	Respiratory arrest

Source: Adapted from Lockey RF et al. *J Allergy Clin Immunol* 1987; 79(4): 660–677.
Note: No new skin test deaths from my research—AB.
[a] Autopsy confirmed anaphylactic shock.

Although all ages were affected (range 7–70 years), the mean ages of the fatalities following skin testing or SCIT were 30 and 34 years, respectively. There was no gender predilection. Errors of administration appeared to be responsible for three fatalities and questionable for an additional three. Ten patients had died after skin tests or SCIT during a seasonal exacerbation of the patients' allergic disease, four in patients who had been symptomatic at the time of injection, two of whom had been receiving β-adrenergic blockers. Of the 24 fatalities associated with SCIT, 4 had experienced previous reactions, 11 had a high degree of sensitivity, and 4 had been injected with newly prepared vaccines. Fifteen of the total of 30 fatalities had received a pollen vaccine as part of the fatal injection. Five of the six fatalities associated with skin testing had occurred without prior prick-puncture testing. Signs and symptoms of systemic reactions were not reliable predictors of death. The onset of systemic reactions was 30 minutes or less after injection in 23 of 30 patients, more than 30 minutes after injection in two, and had not been reported on five. The cause of death in 14 of 16 patients with asthma was respiratory. Epinephrine had been administered to 18 patients, not given to 3, and was either not recorded or unknown in 9 patients.

A later supplemental survey conducted by Reid, Lockey, Turkeltaub, and Platts-Mills on deaths in the United States from SCIT between 1985 and 1989 was reported at the 1990 AAAAI meeting in Baltimore, Maryland [83]. There were no deaths from skin testing reported; however, 16 deaths were reported from SCIT.

These deaths were reported in the *Journal of Allergy and Clinical Immunology* and included one additional death for a total of 17 [84]. The mean age was 36 years (range 10–77), and there were 5 males and 11 females (gender of one subject not reported) versus 11 males and 13 females in the earlier study. Eighty-seven percent of the subjects had asthma, 1 was on β-blocker therapy, and 10 of 17 were "highly sensitive" by skin testing or the radioallergosorbent test (RAST). Fourteen of 17 were on aqueous vaccines, 10 of 17 on increasing doses, and 9 of 17 received epinephrine. The results obtained in this study are similar to those reported previously.

Reid and Gurka presented an abstract at the 1996 Academy of Allergy, Asthma and Immunology meeting about the continuation of the above-mentioned study that covered events from January 1990 to June 1995 [85]. They reported 28 deaths during this time, with an average of five deaths per year with incomplete data for 19 of the 28 reports. One of the 28 deaths was associated with intradermal skin testing and 27 with SCIT. Four of the SCIT deaths occurred following home injections or injections given with no physician present, 3 were associated with an incorrect dose, 19 occurred in individuals with atopic asthma, and 5 deaths occurred despite postreaction intervention. The age range at the time of death was 12–73 years, and there was no gender predilection. Data in this study are similar to previous reports of fatalities.

The Committee on the Safety of Medicine of the United Kingdom reported in 1986 that 26 deaths from anaphylaxis due to SCIT had occurred in the United Kingdom since 1957. All died

Table 34.2 Case reports from the literature—Fatalities from subcutaneous immunotherapy

Author	Gender	Age (yr)	Medical disease	Allergen	Status of immunotherapy	Onset of symptoms	Symptoms	Cause of death
Lamson, 1929	M	34	Asthma	Bermuda grass pollen, 0.05 cc, 1:100	(Because of "nervousness" with preceding reaction)	<3 min	Flushing, athetoid movements, dyspnea	Anaphylactic shock[a]
Waldbott, 1932	F	40		Ragweed vaccine, 1400 units	Unk	<3 min	Dyspnea, urticaria	Anaphylactic shock
Vaughn, Black 1939	Unk	Unk	Unk	Unk	Unk	Unk	Unk	Unk
Vance, Strassman, 1964	M	35	Asthma	Ragweed vaccine	Unk	1 hr	Unk	Anaphylactic shock[a]
James, Austen, 1964	M	56		Hay fever desensitization	Unk (11 of 21)	<45 min	Dyspnea	Anaphylactic shock[a]
Rands, 1980	F	19	Asthma	Pollinex, Migen[b]	Maintenance	3–10 min	Rushing, tachycardia	Anaphylactic shock[a]
Pollard, 1980	M	24	Asthma	Bencard Product[c]	Unk (15th injection)	25 min	Unk	Status asthmaticus
CSM Update, 1986	F, 13 M, 12 Unk, 1	11–57 x, 01	Asthma, hay fever, Unk	Varied, mite	Normal course, 16[d] Maintenance, 4 Unk, 6	<10 min, 14 <30 min, 4 <90 min, 2 Unk, 6	Asthma and anaphylaxis	Asthma and anaphylaxis
Lockey et al., 1987	F, 13 M, 11	7–70 x, 34	Unk[e]	Varied pollens, Molds	Maintenance, 7 Increasing, 9 Decreasing, 1 1st injection, 1 NA, 6	<20 min, 15 20–30 min, 3 >30 min, 2 Unk, 4	Pruritus, 3 Angioedema, 0 UAO/LAO and/or asthma, 12 Shock, 4 Coma, 9 Hypotension, 6 Myocardial infarction, 1 NA or unk, 6	UAO/LAO and/or asthma, 13 Cardiovascular, 6 Anaphylactic shock, 13 Others, 4 NA or unk, 3
Reid, Lockey et al., 1989	F, 11 M, 5 Unk, 1	10–77 x, 36	Asthma, 13 AR, 7 CV, 3 DM, 1 HtD, 1 Unk, 1	Aqueous, 14 Unk, 2	Maintenance, 3 Increasing, 9 Decreasing, 1 Unk, 3	<20 min, 8 20–30 min, 3 >30 min, 1[f] Unk, 4	U and A, 1 LAO, 5 UAO and LAO, 4 UAO, 1 Shock 4 Unk, 5	Resp, 8 Shock, 0 Both, 4 Other, 1 Unk, 3
Reid et al., 1995	Unk	12–73	Asthma, 19	Unk	Unk	Unk	Unk	Unk
Lüderitz-Puchel et al., 1996	Unk, 40 28 analyzed	Unk	Aqueous, 6 Semidepot, 22	Unk	Unk	Unk	Shock, 7 Unk, 21	

(Continued)

Table 34.2 (Continued) Case reports from the literature—Fatalities from subcutaneous immunotherapy

Author	Gender	Age (yr)	Medical disease	Allergen	Status of immunotherapy	Onset of symptoms	Symptoms	Cause of death
Bernstein et al., 2004	F, 6 M, 11	5–81 x, 39	Asthma, 15 AR, 2	Mix 14, mite 3	Maintenance 10, Increasing 7	<30 min, 10 >30 min, 3 Unk, 4	LOA 8, UAO 2, UAO and-LAO 6, Shock 13, Pruritus 3, A 3	Upper airway edema, 5 asthma, 6 shock, 6
Bernstein et al., 2010			6 fatal reactions to SCIT were reported retrospectively from 2001 to 2007 (further details not available)					
Bernstein et al., 2009	M	43	Asthma, DM, HTN, obese	Grass, weeds, cat, dog	0.2mL 1:10 increasing	3-10 minutes	U, A, LAO, UAO, shock	Anaphylactic shock
Bernstein et al., 2014	Unk	Unk	Unk	11th injection from same vial (unknown if buildup or maintenance)		Unk	Unk, No dosing error	Unk
Bernstein et al., 2015	M	33	Asthma (Advair 500)	0.1 mL of 1:1 vial, just finished cluster buildup		Unk	Asthma symptoms	Anaphylaxis
Bernstein et al., 2015	Unk	Adult	Severe Asthma	On maintenance dosing after standard buildup		Unk	Unk	Unk
Bernstein et al., 2016	M	Adult	Unk	Shots given at local healthcare clinic by nurse practitioner who did not recognize anaphylaxis		Unk	Unk	Anaphylaxis confirmed by autopsy
Bernstein et al., 2017	M	13	Asthma, most recent FEV$_1$ >80%	0.15 mL of 1:1 (maintenance) vial; no dosing error		Waited less than 20 minutes; he was wheezing when parent arrived home 1.5 hours later	Wheezing; administered epinephrine and called EMS; EMT intubated; pronounced dead in ED	Anaphylaxis confirmed by autopsy
Bernstein et al., 2017	Unk	Unk	Unk	Unk		Unk	Unk	Unk

Source: Adapted from Lockey RF et al. *J Allergy Clin Immunol* 1987; 79(4): 660–677.
Abbreviations: A, angioedema; AR, allergic rhinitis; CV, cardiovascular; DM, diabetes mellitus; HtD, heart disease; LAO, lower airway obstruction; NA, not available; U, urticaria; UAO, upper airway obstruction; Unk, unknown.
[a] Autopsy confirmed.
[b] Not in article, listed only as Pollinex, pollen vaccine; Migen, house dust mite vaccine.
[c] Bencard Allergy Unit, Brentford, Middlesex, United Kingdom.
[d] ? meaning of normal course.
[e] Not requested.
[f] Not witnessed.

from AIT-induced bronchospasm and/or anaphylaxis, 11 of these since 1980 and 5 during the preceding 18 months. In most of the cases, adequate facilities for cardiorespiratory resuscitation were not available. Asthma was the indication for treatment in 16 of the 26, allergic rhinitis in 1, and the indicator was unknown in 9. In two patients, the ultimately fatal systemic reaction allegedly began more than 30 minutes after injection, resulting in a recommendation that patients remain in a medical facility for 2 hours after their injection [52]. Currently, 26 centers throughout the United Kingdom are equipped to perform SCIT in specialist hospital settings. About 500 courses of SCIT are initiated annually, and the minimum waiting period is now 60 minutes [86,87].

In Sweden, introduction of potent mite, mold, and animal dander vaccines was accompanied by some anaphylactic deaths that prompted the regulatory agency to restrict the use of these vaccines to physicians and clinics specializing in this issue [88].

The Paul Ehrlich Institute in Germany reported 40 fatalities between 1977 and 1994, with complete data available for 20 reports in Germany and 8 reports elsewhere in Europe. For 23 of the 28 reports analyzed, it was not possible to rule out error on the part of the physician and/or inadequate information given to the patient as factors contributory to the fatal outcomes [53]. Three cases with permanent hypoxic brain damage as a result of anaphylactic shock were also reported. Semidepot preparations, which are not used in the United States, were involved in most of the adverse and fatal reactions. Mite allergen vaccines were used in 18 of the cases reported.

There are 41 fatalities identified from SCIT in Bernstein et al. from the AAAAI physician member survey of fatal reactions and near-fatal reactions (NFRs) from 1990 to 2001 [89]. The estimated fatality rate is 1 per 2.5 million injections (average of 3.4 deaths per year), similar to the results in the previous AAAAI physician member surveys [82,84,85]. One skin test fatality was confirmed in a young woman with allergic rhinitis, moderate persistent asthma, and food allergy who had a fatal anaphylactic reaction after application of prick-puncture tests to 90 food antigens [89].

A Danish 10-year prospective study from 2004 to 2013 of 102,274 allergy injections showed no reported fatalities [122].

In 2008, physicians were asked to complete a web-based survey reporting allergy injection and skin test–related fatal and nonfatal reactions during their clinical practices for the prior 12 months. No fatal reactions to SCIT were identified. However, six fatal reactions to SCIT were reported retrospectively from 2001 to 2007 [114]. In 2009, year 2 of this survey, again no fatal reactions were reported [115]. From 2010 to 2011, year 3 of the study, no fatal reactions were directly or indirectly reported [121]. In this same study at year 4, there was one confirmed fatality in 2009 [123]. This study was continued from 2008 to 2012. There was one reported fatality during that time. Bernstein et al. confirmed one fatality in 2014 and an additional five fatalities between 2016 and 2017 (see Table 34.2) [133,134].

34.6 ANAPHYLAXIS ASSOCIATED WITH SKIN TESTING AND SUBCUTANEOUS IMMUNOTHERAPY

The study by Van Arsdel and Sherman [1] supports the general safety of SCIT for the control of IgE-mediated allergic diseases in that over one million allergen vaccine injections given to 8700 patients from 1935 to 1955 had been administered without a fatality. In a prospective study on AIT, Hepner et al. reported in 1987 that 25 out of 2989 patients, over a 7-month period, experienced systemic reactions, and there were no fatalities [6]. Based on annual studies from a panel of 2000 physicians in the United States, the National Disease and Therapeutic Index indicated that in each of the five previous years, 7–10 million allergen injections had been given [90]. Since so many injections are administered yearly, the risk of a fatal reaction is low. Lockey et al. reported that 45 (1.4%) of 3236 patients who had a clinical history of Hymenoptera hypersensitivity and were skin tested had systemic hypersensitivity reactions during skin testing, and eight of these (0.25% of the subjects tested) were severe [91]. Of 1410 patients placed on SCIT, 171 experienced 327 systemic reactions, of which 28 reactions (9%) were severe but not fatal [92]. These studies illustrate that SCIT with a standardized vaccine, used as indicated, in individuals with an allergic disease that may be life threatening, induces a low incidence of adverse reactions, most of which are mild to moderate.

The systemic reaction rate to skin testing is significantly lower than the rate of reactions to SCIT, but it is not negligible. Lin et al. reported only two patients with systemic allergic reactions to skin testing in 10,400 patients tested [93]. The overall risk of inducing anaphylaxis by skin testing was 0.02%, and other studies have produced similar results [93–95]. The rate of systemic reactions to skin testing is likely underreported. Thompson et al. reported a systemic reaction rate of 6% of patients receiving skin testing [96]. Bagg reported a 3.5% systemic reaction rate of 1456 patients receiving skin testing in a retrospective review over 1 year [97]. All patients were given epinephrine for any systemic symptoms that occurred during skin testing, and all readily responded to early intervention with epinephrine [97]. It is important to recognize the risk of systemic reactions from skin testing as well as the treatment for these reactions in order to prevent progression. The early administration of epinephrine appears to prevent more serious and late-phase reactions.

The incidence of unconfirmed NFRs from 1990 to 2001 was 23 per year (5.4 events per million injections) in the latest mentioned AAAAI survey of fatal and NFRs from SCIT [98]. There were 115 systemic reactions (5.2% of patients and 0.06% of injections) from 1981 to 1990 [99] and 26 systemic reactions (1.08% of patients and 0.01% of injections) from 1991 to 2000 [100] in another retrospective analysis of nonfatal systemic reactions to SCIT. Based on the AAAAI/ACAAI collaborative surveillance study (2008–2011), in year 1 there were 10.2 systemic reactions per 10,000 injection visits or 0.1% of allergy injection visits [114]. Most were mild reactions; however, 3% were severe anaphylactic events (3 severe reactions for every 100,000 injection visits) [114]. Between 2008 and 2012, data were gathered on 23.3 million injection visits. Overall systemic reaction rates remained stable at 0.1%. The rate of very severe, World Allergy Organization (WAO) grade 4, systemic reactions was similar to previously reported rates of near-fatal reactions (1 in 1 million injections) [123]. A 10-year retrospective study from Denmark of 102,274 injections during 7218 patient-years of treatment observed only three severe (WAO grade 4) reactions. These are three severe reactions per 102,274 injections (0.0029%) [122,128].

In a 1-year retrospective study of 773 subjects, Phillips reports that systemic reactions occurred in 4% of patients receiving SCIT, and all received early intervention with epinephrine and responded successfully [117]. There were no late-phase or protracted-phase reactions.

A review by Stewart and Lockey [101] in 1992, which examined the incidence of systemic reactions to SCIT, concluded that the percentage of subjects experiencing a systemic reaction is small but will probably increase as the AIT schedule is accelerated and when or if high-dose regimens are required in highly sensitive subjects. In addition, maintenance AIT is associated with fewer systemic reactions than the buildup period of rush and accelerated schedules. In 2007, a case series of biphasic anaphylaxis revealed that in patients who received treatment with epinephrine within 30 minutes of symptom onset, the incidence of biphasic response was zero compared with the overall mean of 19% [116].

Premedication with a combination of methylprednisolone, ketotifen (a mast-cell stabilizer not available in the United States), and long-acting theophylline may decrease the incidence of systemic reactions associated with rush protocols. Concern was voiced over masking a mild reaction by using premedication, which might therefore be followed by a later, more serious, reaction or delay the onset of a reaction beyond the waiting period. However, premedication with antihistamine reduced the frequency of severe systemic reactions caused by conventional SCIT and increased the proportion of patients who achieved the target maintenance dose in one randomized controlled study [102]. In other studies, premedication with antihistamines significantly reduced the incidence of systemic reactions during rush AIT or specific cluster AIT [103–105,125,130]. There was no evidence that antihistamines masked the early warning signs or delayed the onset of systemic reactions. In the Casale et al. study, pretreatment with omalizumab resulted in a fivefold decrease in risk of anaphylaxis caused by a ragweed rush protocol [106]. Further studies involving larger groups of patients and different dosage regimens are necessary to define the future role of antihistamine and other pharmacologic pretreatment in SCIT. Dose adjustment during peak pollen season was associated with fewer WAO grade 3 or 4 systemic reactions [123]. Finally, a minimum of a 30-minute waiting period, as recommended by the AAAAI and the ACAAI "Allergen Immunotherapy: A Practice Parameter Third Update," was deemed appropriate with a longer waiting period for high-risk patients [13,127].

34.7 RISK FACTORS FOR SKIN TESTING AND IMMUNOTHERAPY

It is essential that strict attention be paid to risk factors for systemic reactions and that techniques of management are initiated both before and after skin testing or SCIT to minimize these risks. Several guidelines have been suggested that emphasize thorough training of all personnel involved in these procedures as well as the prompt treatment of systemic reactions [82,88]. These have encouraged the development and use of standardized vaccines and emphasize certain risk factors, including the following:

1. Patients, particularly asthmatics, suffering a seasonal exacerbation of their symptoms [124]
2. Patients who demonstrate exquisite sensitivity to particular allergen(s) [107]
3. Patients on β-blockers [107,108]
4. Patients with asthma, especially when their asthma is unstable [109,126,132]
5. Patients in whom rush SCIT is used (both venoms and inhalant allergens) [101,103,105,107,129]
6. Patients in whom high doses of potent standardized allergen vaccines are utilized
7. Injections from new vials [107]
8. Dosing errors [107]

34.8 PRECAUTIONS FOR SKIN TESTING AND IMMUNOTHERAPY

The following guidelines are suggested:
1. Always begin with a percutaneous procedure for skin testing (i.e., prick-puncture).
2. When possible, do not use β-adrenergic blocking agents concomitantly during skin testing or immunotherapy.
3. Keep patients under observation for at least 30 minutes or even longer for those at greatest risk since most fatal systemic reactions begin within that time [13].
4. When SCIT is prescribed, give the patient written and/or verbal guidelines outlining methods of AIT and the importance of adherence to these guidelines to prevent an adverse reaction (see Chapter 37).

5. Inform patients receiving AIT of its potential risk and obtain informed consent.
6. Administer SCIT in an office or clinical setting with a physician present and with optimal care available for the treatment of a systemic reaction.
7. Monitor patients to assure they are waiting a proper time in the facility where they receive their AIT injections.
8. Provide adequate instructions to another physician who may give the injections elsewhere from vials of vaccine taken from the prescribing physician's office or clinic (see Chapter 37).

The safety of SCIT has been reviewed in detail by Norman and Van Metre [110].

34.9 EQUIPMENT RECOMMENDED FOR SETTINGS WHERE ALLERGEN IMMUNOTHERAPY IS ADMINISTERED

The following equipment is recommended by the Joint Task Force on Practice Parameters [13]:
1. Stethoscope and sphygmomanometer
2. Tourniquets, syringes, hypodermic needles, large-bore needles (14 gauge)
3. Aqueous epinephrine HCL 1:1000 wt/vol
4. Equipment to administer oxygen by mask
5. Equipment to administer intravenous fluids
6. Antihistamines for injection (second-line agents for anaphylaxis, but H1 and H2 antihistamines work better together than either one alone)
7. Corticosteroids for intramuscular or intravenous injection (second-line agents for anaphylaxis)
8. Equipment to maintain an airway appropriate for the supervising physician's expertise and skill
9. Glucagon kit available for patients receiving β-blockers

The prompt recognition of systemic reactions and the immediate use of epinephrine are the mainstays of therapy [111–113].

SALIENT POINTS

1. Physicians who administer subcutaneous allergen immunotherapy (SCIT) should have the appropriate equipment and personnel to treat a systemic reaction.
2. No allergen vaccine can be considered completely safe for a given patient allergic to that vaccine.
3. The risk of a fatal reaction can be reduced and even eliminated by the careful selection and monitoring of allergic patients on SCIT, by using improved biologically standardized vaccines and by skilled and timely treatment of systemic reactions.
4. The wait period of 30 minutes is adequate for most patients but should be extended for high-risk patients.
5. Patients at highest risk for allergen immunotherapy (AIT) are patients with asthma, especially unstable asthma.
6. Other high-risk patients include those with a seasonal exacerbation and exquisite sensitivity, and those on β-blockers and rush schedules.
7. Fatal reactions (one reported 2008–2012) to SCIT appear to be declining, possibly related to universal screening of asthmatic patients prior to injection and to adjusting doses during the pollen season [123,131].

REFERENCES

1. Vanarsdel PP, Sherman WB. Risk of inducing constitutional reactions in allergic patients. *J Allergy* 1957; 28(3): 251–261.
2. Cooke RA, Veer AV. Human sensitization. *J Immunol* 1916; 1(3): 201–305.
3. Turkeltaub PC, Gergen PJ. The risk of adverse reactions from percutaneous prick-puncture allergen skin testing, venipuncture, and body measurements: Data from the second National Health and Nutrition Examination Survey 1976–1980 (NHANES II). *J Allergy Clin Immunol* 1989; 84(6 Pt 1): 886–890.
4. Greenberg MA et al. Late and immediate systemic-allergic reactions to inhalant allergen immunotherapy. *J Allergy Clin Immunol* 1986; 77(6): 865–870.
5. Hejjaoui A et al. Immunotherapy with a standardized *Dermatophagoides pteronyssinus* extract. IV. Systemic reactions according to the immunotherapy schedule. *J Allergy Clin Immunol* 1990; 85(2): 473–479.
6. Hepner M OD, MacKechnie H, Rowe M, Anderson J. The safety of immunotherapy—A prospective study. *J Allergy Clin Immunol* 1987; 79(133).
7. Levine MI. Systemic reactions to immunotherapy. *J Allergy Clin Immunol* 1979; 63(3): 209.
8. Nelson BL, Dupont LA, Reid MJ. Prospective survey of local and systemic reactions to immunotherapy with pollen extracts. *Ann Allergy* 1986; 56(4): 331–334.
9. Osterballe O. Side effects during immunotherapy with purified grass pollen extracts. *Allergy* 1982; 37(8): 553–562.
10. Rawlins MD, Wood SM, Mann RD. Hazards with desensitising vaccines. *Arb Paul Ehrlich Inst Bundesamt Sera Impfstoffe Frankf A M* 1988; (82): 147–151.
11. Rieckenberg MR, Khan RH, Day JH. Physician reported patient response to immunotherapy: A retrospective study of factors affecting the response. *Ann Allergy* 1990; 64(4): 364–367.
12. Vervloet D et al. A prospective national study of the safety of immunotherapy. *Clin Allergy* 1980; 10(1): 59–64.
13. Cox L, Nelson H, Lockey RF. Allergen immunotherapy: A practice parameter third update. *J Allergy Clin Immunol* 2011; 127(1): S1–S55.
14. Akcakaya N et al. Local and systemic reactions during immunotherapy with adsorbed extracts of house dust mite in children. *Ann Allergy Asthma Immunol* 2000; 85(4): 317–321.
15. Brockow K et al. Efficacy of antihistamine pretreatment in the prevention of adverse reactions to Hymenoptera immunotherapy: A prospective, randomized, placebo-controlled trial. *J Allergy Clin Immunol* 1997; 100(4): 458–463.
16. Karaayvaz M et al. Systemic reactions due to allergen immunotherapy. *J Investig Allergol Clin Immunol* 1999; 9(1): 39–44.
17. Lockey RF et al. Systemic reactions and fatalities associated with allergen immunotherapy. *Ann Allergy Asthma Immunol* 2001; 87(1 Suppl 1): 47–55.
18. Machin IS et al. Immunotherapy units: A follow-up study. *J Investig Allergol Clin Immunol* 2001; 11(3): 167–171.
19. Malling HJ. Minimising the risks of allergen-specific injection immunotherapy. *Drug Saf* 2000; 23(4): 323–332.
20. Mellerup MT et al. Safety of allergen-specific immunotherapy. Relation between dosage regimen, allergen extract, disease and systemic side-effects during induction treatment. *Clin Exp Allergy* 2000; 30(10): 1423–1429.
21. Nettis E et al. Safety of inhalant allergen immunotherapy with mass units-standardized extracts. *Clin Exp Allergy* 2002; 32(12): 1745–1749.
22. Tankersley MS et al. Local reactions during allergen immunotherapy do not require dose adjustment. *J Allergy Clin Immunol* 2000; 106(5): 840–843.
23. Winther L, Malling HJ, Mosbech H. Allergen-specific immunotherapy in birch- and grass-pollen-allergic rhinitis. II. Side-effects. *Allergy* 2000; 55(9): 827–835.
24. Wuthrich B et al. Safety and efficacy of specific immunotherapy with standardized allergenic extracts adsorbed on aluminium hydroxide. *J Investig Allergol Clin Immunol* 2001; 11(3): 149–156.
25. Bhalla PL. Genetic engineering of pollen allergens for hayfever immunotherapy. *Expert Rev Vaccines* 2003; 2(1): 75–84.
26. Chen D, Maa YF, Haynes JR. Needle-free epidermal powder immunization. *Expert Rev Vaccines* 2002; 1(3): 265–276.
27. Di Gioacchino M et al. Allergen immunotherapy: an effective immune-modifier. *Int J Immunopathol Pharmacol* 1999; 12(1): 1–5.
28. Holt PG et al. Developmental factors associated with risk for atopic disease: Implications for vaccine strategies in early childhood. *Vaccine* 2003; 21(24): 3432–3435.
29. Koh YY, Kim CK. The development of asthma in patients with allergic rhinitis. *Curr Opin Allergy Clin Immunol* 2003; 3(3): 159–164.
30. Reyes Moreno A, Castrejon Vazquez MI, Miranda Feria AJ. Failure of allergen-based immunotherapy in adults with allergic asthma. *Rev Alerg Mex* 2003; 50(1): 8–12.
31. Spiegelberg HL et al. DNA-based vaccines for allergic disease. *Expert Rev Vaccines* 2002; 1(2): 169–177.
32. Tarzi M, Larche M. Peptide immunotherapy for allergic disease. *Expert Opin Biol Ther* 2003; 3(4): 617–626.
33. Tella R et al. Effects of specific immunotherapy on the development of new sensitisations in monosensitised patients. *Allergol Immunopathol (Madr)* 2003; 31(4): 221–225.
34. Criado Molina A et al. Immunotherapy with an oral *Alternaria* extract in childhood asthma. Clinical safety and efficacy and effects on *in vivo* and *in vitro* parameters. *Allergol Immunopathol (Madr)* 2002; 30(6): 319–330.
35. Litwin A et al. Oral immunotherapy with short ragweed extract in a novel encapsulated preparation: A double-blind study. *J Allergy Clin Immunol* 1997; 100(1): 30–38.
36. Liu YH et al. Efficacy of local nasal immunotherapy for Dp2-induced airway inflammation in mice: Using Dp2 peptide and fungal immunomodulatory peptide. *J Allergy Clin Immunol* 2003; 112(2): 301–310.
37. Passali D et al. Nasal immunotherapy is effective in the treatment of rhinitis due to mite allergy. A double-blind, placebo-controlled study with rhinological evaluation. *Int J Immunopathol Pharmacol* 2002; 15(2): 141–147.
38. Andre C et al. A double-blind placebo-controlled evaluation of sublingual immunotherapy with a standardized ragweed extract in patients with seasonal rhinitis. Evidence for a dose-response relationship. *Int Arch Allergy Immunol* 2003; 131(2): 111–118.
39. Cirla AM et al. A pre-seasonal birch/hazel sublingual immunotherapy can improve the outcome of grass pollen injective treatment in bisensitized individuals. A case-referent, two-year controlled study. *Allergol Immunopathol (Madr)* 2003; 31(1): 31–43.

40. Di Rienzo V et al. Long-lasting effect of sublingual immunotherapy in children with asthma due to house dust mite: A 10-year prospective study. *Clin Exp Allergy* 2003; 33(2): 206–210.

41. Grosclaude M et al. Safety of various dosage regimens during induction of sublingual immunotherapy. A preliminary study. *Int Arch Allergy Immunol* 2002; 129(3): 248–253.

42. Passalacqua G et al. Oral and sublingual immunotherapy in paediatric patients. *Curr Opin Allergy Clin Immunol* 2003; 3(2): 139–145.

43. Cox LS et al. Sublingual immunotherapy: A comprehensive review. *J Allergy Clin Immunol* 2006; 117(5): 1021–1035.

44. Cox L. Sublingual immunotherapy in pediatric allergic rhinitis and asthma: Efficacy, safety, and practical considerations. *Curr Allergy Asthma Rep* 2007; 7(6): 410–420.

45. Lamson R. Death associated with injection of foreign substances. *JAMA* 1924; 82(1090).

46. Vance BM, Strassman G. Sudden death following injection of foreign protein. *Arch Pathol* 1942; 34(849).

47. James LP Jr, Austen KF. Fatal systemic anaphylaxis in man. *N Engl J Med* 1964; 270: 597–603.

48. Sheppe WM. Fatal anaphylaxis in man. *J Lab Clin Med* 1930; 16(372).

49. Blanton WV, Sutphin AK. Death during skin testing. *Am J M Sci* 1949; 217(169).

50. Rosenthal A. Fatal anaphylactic reactions to penicillin. *NY State J Med* 1954; 54(1485).

51. Rands DA. Anaphylactic reaction to desensitisation for allergic rhinitis and asthma. *Br Med J* 1980; 281(6244): 854.

52. Committee, Update: Desensitization vaccines. *Br Med J* 1986; 293(948).

53. Lüderitz-Puchel U, May S, Haustein D. Incidents following hyposensitization. *Münch med Wschr* 1996; 138: 1–7.

54. Busse WW, Storms WW, Flaherty DK, Crandall M, Reed CE. *Alternaria* IgG precipitins and adverse reactions. *J Allergy Clin Immunol* 1976; 57(367).

55. Kaad PH, Ostergaard PA. The hazard of mould hyposensitization in children with asthma. *Clin Allergy* 1982; 12(3): 317–320.

56. Kemler BJ et al. Failure to detect circulating immune complexes in allergic patients on injection therapy. *Clin Allergy* 1979; 9(5): 473–478.

57. Stein MR et al. A laboratory evaluation of immune complexes in patients on inhalant immunotherapy. *J Allergy Clin Immunol* 1978; 62(4): 211–216.

58. Cano PO et al. Circulating immune complexes in patients with atopic allergy. *Clin Allergy* 1977; 7(2): 167–171.

59. El-Hefny A et al. Extrinsic allergic bronchiolo-alveolitis in children. *Clin Allergy* 1980; 10(6): 651–658.

60. Kuuliala O et al. Haemagglutinating antibodies to cat dander in relation to exposure and respiratory allergy. *Clin Allergy* 1979; 9(4): 391–395.

61. Moore VL, Fink JN. Immunologic studies in hypersensitivity pneumonitis—Quantitative precipitins and complement-fixing antibodies in symptomatic and asymptomatic pigeon breeders. *J Lab Clin Med* 1975; 85(4): 540–545.

62. Stendardi L, Delespesse G, Debisschop MJ. Circulating immune complexes in bronchial asthma. *Clin Allergy* 1980; 10(4): 405–411.

63. Clausen RW, Yanari SS. Immune complex-mediated disease not a factor in patients on maintenance venom immunotherapy. *J Allergy Clin Immunol* 1983; 72(2): 199–203.

64. Umetsu DT et al. Serum sickness triggered by anaphylaxis: A complication of immunotherapy. *J Allergy Clin Immunol* 1985; 76(5): 713–718.

65. Clemmensen O, Knudsen HE. Contact sensitivity to aluminium in a patient hyposensitized with aluminium precipitated grass pollen. *Contact Dermatitis* 1980; 6(5): 305–308.

66. Wolpow ER. Brachial plexus neuropathy. Association with desensitizing antiallergy injections. *JAMA* 1975; 234(6): 620–621.

67. Schatz M, Patterson R, DeSwarte R. Nonorganic adverse reactions to aeroallergen immunotherapy. *J Allergy Clin Immunol* 1976; 58(1 Pt. 2): 198–203.

68. Bokisch VA, Bernstein D, Krause RM. Occurrence of 19S and 7S anti-IgGs during hyperimmunization of rabbits with streptococci. *J Exp Med* 1972; 136(4): 799–815.

69. Christian CL, Desimone AR, Abruzzo JL. Anti-DNA antibodies in hyperimmunized rabbits. *J Exp Med* 1965; 121: 309–321.

70. Eichmann K, Braun DG, Krause RM. Influence of genetic factors on the magnitude and the heterogeneity of the immune response in the rabbit. *J Exp Med* 1971; 134(1): 48–65.

71. Potter M. Myeloma proteins (M-components) with antibody-like activity. *N Engl J Med* 1971; 284(15): 831–838.

72. Riesen W, Rudikoff S, Oriol R, Potter M. An IgM Waldenstrom with specificity against phosphorylcholine. *Biochemistry* 1975; 14(5): 1052–1057.

73. Penny R, Hughes S. Repeated stimulation of the reticuloendothelial system and the development of plasma-cell dyscrasias. *Lancet* 1970; 1(7637): 77–78.

74. Raphael SA, Nell PA, Hymchuk Lischner HW. Positive late antiglobulin test in atopic pediatric subjects receiving hyposensitization therapy. *J Allergy Clin Immunol* 1976; 57(103).

75. Levinson AI et al. Evaluation of the adverse effects of long-term hyposensitization. *J Allergy Clin Immunol* 1978; 62(2): 109–114.

76. Phanuphak P, Kohler PF. Onset of polyarteritis nodosa during allergic hyposensitization treatment. *Am J Med* 1980; 68(4): 479–485.

77. McCombs CC, Michalski JP, Jerome DC. Case 26-1980: *Pemphigus vulgaris* after hyposensitization injections. *N Engl J Med* 1980; 303(20): 1179.

78. Katelaris CH, Walls RS. A study of possible ill effects from prolonged immunotherapy in treatment of allergic diseases. *Ann Allergy* 1984; 53(3): 257–261.

79. Waldbatt GL. The prevention of anaphylactic shock. *JAMA* 1932; 98(446).

80. Vaughan VA, Black JR. *Practice of Allergy*. St. Louis, MO: C.V. Mosby, 1939.

81. Pollard RCH. Anaphylactic reaction to desensitization. *Br Med J* 1980; 281(1429): 481.

82. Lockey RF et al. Fatalities from immunotherapy (IT) and skin testing (ST). *J Allergy Clin Immunol* 1987; 79(4): 660–677.

83. Reid MJ, Lockey RF, Turkeltaub PC, Platts-Mills TA. Fatalities (F) from immunotherapy (IT) and skin testing (ST). *J Allergy Clin Immunol* 1990; 85(180).

84. Reid MJ et al. Survey of fatalities from skin testing and immunotherapy 1985–1989. *J Allergy Clin Immunol* 1993; 92(1 Pt 1): 6–15.

85. Reid M, Gurka G. Deaths associated with skin testing and immunotherapy. *J Allergy Clin Immunol* 1996; 97(231).

86. Durham SR. Personal Communication. 2007 November: Allergy and Clinical Immunology, National Heart and Lung Institute, Imperial College. London, United Kingdom.

87. Andersen P. Personal Communication. 2007 November: General Manager, ALK-Abelló UK.

88. Norman PS. Fatal misadventures. *J Allergy Clin Immunol* 1987; 79(572).

89. Bernstein DI, Wanner M, Borish L, Liss GM. Twelve-year survey of fatal reactions to allergen injections and skin testing: 1990–2001. *J Allergy Clin Immunol* 2004; (113): 1129–1136.

90. National Disease and Therapeutic Index. IMS America, L.

91. Lockey RF, Turkeltaub PC, Olive CA, Baird-Warren LA, Olive ES, Bukantz SC. The Hymenoptera venom study II: Skin test results and safety of venom skin testing. *J Allergy Clin Immunol* 1989; 84(967).

92. Lockey RF, Turkeltaub PC, Olive ES, Hubbard JM, Baird-Warren IA, Bukantz SC. The Hymenoptera venom study, III, safety of venom immunotherapy. *J Allergy Clin Immunol* 1990; 86(775).

93. Lin MS et al. Nonfatal systemic allergic reactions induced by skin testing and immunotherapy. *Ann Allergy* 1993; 71(6): 557–562.

94. Liccardi G et al. Anaphylaxis caused by skin prick testing with aeroallergens: Case report and evaluation of the risk in Italian allergy services. *J Allergy Clin Immunol* 2003; 111(6): 1410–1412.

95. Valyasevi MA, Maddox DE, Li JT. Systemic reactions to allergy skin tests. *Ann Allergy Asthma Immunol* 1999; 83(2): 132–136.

96. Thompson M, Shearer D, Lockey R, Fox R, Ledford D. Systemic reactions to percutaneous (P) and intradermal (ID) skin tests (ST). *J Allergy Clin Immunol* 1998; (101): S30.

97. Bagg A, Chacko T, Lockey RF. Reactions to prick and intradermal skin tests. *Ann Allergy Asthma Immunol* 2009; 102: 400–402.

98. Amin HS, Liss GM, Bernstein DI. Evaluation of near-fatal reactions to allergen immunotherapy injections. *J Allergy Clin Immunol* 2006; 117(1): 169–175.

99. Ragusa FV et al. Nonfatal systemic reactions to subcutaneous immunotherapy: A 10-year experience. *J Investig Allergol Clin Immunol* 1997; 7(3): 151–154.

100. Ragusa VF, Massolo A. Non fatal systemic reactions to subcutaneous immunotherapy: A 20-year experience comparison of two 10-year periods. *Allerg Immunol (Paris)* 2004; 36(2): 52–55.

101. Stewart E, Lockey RF. Systemic reactions from allergen immunotherapy. *J Allergy Clin Immunol* 1992; 90(4 pt 1): 567–578.

102. Ohashi Y., Nakai Y., Murata K. Effect of pretreatment with fexofenadine on the safety of immunotherapy in patients with allergic rhinitis. *Ann Allergy Asthma Immunol* 2006; 96: 600–605.

103. Berchtold E, Maibach R, Muller U. Reduction of side effects from rush-immunotherapy with honey bee venom by pretreatment with terfenadine. *Clin Exp Allergy* 1992; 22(1): 59–65.

104. Nielsen L et al. Antihistamine premedication in specific cluster immunotherapy: A double-blind, placebo-controlled study. *J Allergy Clin Immunol* 1996; 97(6): 1207–1213.

105. Portnoy J et al. Premedication reduces the incidence of systemic reactions during inhalant rush immunotherapy with mixtures of allergenic extracts. *Ann Allergy* 1994; 73(5): 409–418.

106. Casale TB et al. Omalizumab pretreatment decreases acute reactions after rush immunotherapy for ragweed-induced seasonal allergic rhinitis. *J Allergy Clin Immunol* 2006; 117(1): 134–140.

107. Allergen immunotherapy: Therapeutic vaccines for allergic diseases. Geneva: January 27–29 1997. *Allergy* 1998; 53(44 Suppl): 1–42.

108. Kaplan AP et al. β-Adrenergic blockers, immunotherapy, and skin testing. American Academy of Allergy and Immunology. *J Allergy Clin Immunol* 1989; 84(1): 129–130.

109. Bousquet J et al. Immunotherapy with a standardized *Dermatophagoides pteronyssinus* extract. Systemic reactions during the rush protocol in patients suffering from asthma. *J Allergy Clin Immunol* 1989; 83(4): 797–802.

110. Norman PS, Van Metre TE Jr. The safety of allergenic immunotherapy. *J Allergy Clin Immunol* 1990; 85(2): 522–525.

111. Personnel and equipment to treat systemic reactions caused by immunotherapy with allergenic extracts. American Academy of Allergy and Immunology. *J Allergy Clin Immunol* 1986; 77(2): 271–273.

112. Bousquet J et al. Allergen immunotherapy: Therapeutic vaccines for allergic diseases. World Health Organization. American Academy of Allergy, Asthma and Immunology. *Ann Allergy Asthma Immunol* 1998; 81(5 Pt 1): 401–405.

113. Kemp SF, Lockey RF. Anaphylaxis: A review of causes and mechanisms. *J Allergy Clin Immunol* 2002; 110(3): 341–348.

114. Bernstein DI et al. Surveillance of systemic reactions to subcutaneous immunotherapy injections: Year 1 outcomes of the ACAAI and AAAAI collaborative study. *Ann Allergy Asthma Immunol* 2010; 104: 530–535.

115. Epstein TG et al. Immediate and delayed-onset systemic reactions after subcutaneous immunotherapy injections: ACAAI/AAAAI surveillance study of subcutaneous immunotherapy—Year 2. *Ann Allergy Asthma Immunol* 2011; 107: 426–431.

116. Ellis A, Day J. Incidence and characteristics of biphasic anaphylaxis: A prospective evaluation of 103 patients. *Ann Allergy Asthma Immunol* 2007, 98: 64–69.

117. Phillips JF et al. Systemic reactions to subcutaneous allergen immunotherapy and the response to epinephrine. *Allergy Asthma Proc* 2011; 32: 288–294.

118. Radulovic S, Wilson D, Calderon M, Durham S. Systematic reviews of sublingual immunotherapy (SLIT). *Allergy* 2011; 66: 740–752.

119. Penagos M et al. Metaanalysis of the efficacy of sublingual immunotherapy in the treatment of allergic asthma in pediatric patients, 3 to 18 years of age. *Chest* 2008; 133: 599–609, Ia.

120. Nieto A, Mazon A, Pamies R, Bruno L, Navarro M, Montanes A. Sublingual immunotherapy for allergic respiratory diseases: An evaluation of meta-analyses. *J Allergy Clin Immunol* 2009; 124: 157–161, e1–32. IV.

121. Epstein TG, Liss GM, Murphy-Berendts K, Bernstein DI. AAAAI and ACAAI surveillance study of subcutaneous immunotherapy, Year 3: what practices modify the risk of systemic reactions? *Ann Allergy Athma Immunol* 2013; 110: 274–278.

122. Madsen F, Sidenius K, Enevoldsen H, Frølund L, Guul S-J, Søes-Petersen U. Safety of allergen immunotherapy: A 10-year prospective study. *J Allergy Clin Immunol* 2016; 138(5).

123. Epstein TG et al. AAAAI/ACAAI Surveillance Study of Subcutaneous Immunotherapy, Years 2008–2012: An update on fatal and nonfatal systemic allergic reactions. *J Allergy Clin Immunol: In Practice* 2014; 2(2): 161–167.

124. Epstein TG et al. Risk factors for fatal and nonfatal reactions to subcutaneous immunotherapy National surveillance study on allergen immunotherapy. *Ann Allergy Asthma Immunol* 2016; 116: 354–359.

125. Winslow AW et al. Comparison of systemic reactions in rush, cluster, and standard-build aeroallergen immunotherapy. *Ann Allergy Asthma Immunol* 2016; 117: 542.

126. Matloff SM, Bailit IW, Parks P, Madden N, Greineder DK. Systemic reactions to immunotherapy. *Allergy Proc* 1993; 14: 347–350.

127. Rank MA, Oslie CL, Krogman JL, Park MA, Li JT. Allergen immunotherapy safety: Characterizing systemic reactions and identifying risk factors. *Allergy Asthma Proc* 2008; 29: 400–405.

128. Cox L et al. Speaking the same language: The World Allergy Organization Subcutaneous Immunotherapy Systemic Reaction Grading System. *J Allergy Clin Immunol* 2010; 125(3): 569–574.

129. Copenhaver C et al. Systemic reactions with aeroallergen cluster immunotherapy in a clinical practice. *Ann Allergy Asthma Immunol* 2011; 107(5): 441–447.

130. Calabria C et al. Accelerated immunotherapy schedules and premedication. *Immunol Allergy Clin North Am* 2011; 31(2): 251–263.

131. Liss GM, Murphy-Berendts K, Epstein T, Bernstein DI. Factors associated with severe versus mild immunotherapy-related systemic reactions: A case-reference study. *J Allergy Clin Immunol* 2011; 127: 1298–1300.

132. Kannan J, Epstein T. Immunotherapy safety: What have we learned from surveillance surveys? *Curr Allergy Asthma Rep* 2013; 13(4): 381–388.

133. Epstein T et al. Recent trends in fatalities, waiting times, and use of epinephrine auto-injectors for subcutaneous allergen immunotherapy (SCIT): AAAAI/ACAAI National Surveillance Study 2008–2016. *JACI* 2018; 141.

134. Bernstein D et al. Fatalities from Subcutaneous Allergen Immunotherapy (SCIT) occurring under the care of allergists from 2009–2017. Personal Communication. November 6, 2018.

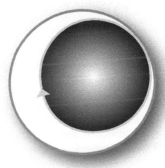

35 Recognition, prevention, and treatment of adverse effects associated with sublingual immunotherapy

Giovanni Passalacqua and Diego Bagnasco
University of Genoa

Giorgio Walter Canonica
University of Genoa
Humanitas University

CONTENTS

35.1 HISTORICAL PERSPECTIVE

Allergen-specific immunotherapy (AIT) is a biological form of therapy that can redirect and modify the abnormal response to allergens that occurs in allergic individuals. It is considered one of the cornerstones in the management of allergic respiratory diseases and Hymenoptera venom allergy. Subcutaneous immunotherapy (SCIT) has been utilized to treat allergic diseases since the beginning of the twentieth century. Favorable results obtained by empirical methods resulted in its widespread use, but it has remained unchanged for decades until the latter years of the twentieth century. Attempts were made by several clinicians to use other forms of such therapy [1–3], but SCIT was well established, and alternative forms of administration remained of limited interest [4]. Following early reports [5], in 1986 the British Committee for the Safety of Medicines [6] and Lockey et al. [7] reported multiple deaths from SCIT. As a consequence, there were recommendations and implementation of additional safety measures made throughout the world for SCIT; in the United Kingdom, SCIT use was made impractical because

of a mandatory 2-hour wait in a medical facility after an injection. The safety concerns with SCIT stimulated other AIT modalities, and noninjection routes gained new interest. Although some systemic adverse events (SAEs) of SCIT are avoidable, others occur unpredictably [7,8], thus contributing to the growth of interest in safer noninjection routes. Sublingual immunotherapy (SLIT) was used in the United States early in the first half of the twentieth century [9]. However, the first controlled trial with positive results with SLIT was published in 1986 [10].

With time, an increased number of positive studies were published in the literature. The 2009 and 2013 World Allergy Organization position papers listed 60 and 77 randomized clinical trials, respectively [11,12], and currently the number reaches about 90 trials. Several meta-analyses were published [13,14] and conclude that SLIT and SCIT are effective. Approximately 10 years prior to that time, the use of SLIT was mentioned in the World Health Organization position paper on AIT [15]. Such therapy also has been highlighted in subsequent guidelines [16], until 2017 when SLIT was finally accepted as an add-on option also to treat asthma [17]. In all cases, SLIT is categorized as a reasonable alternative to SCIT, and SLIT is routinely used in several European countries where standardized extracts for relevant allergens are available. Currently, some standardized SLIT products (ragweed, grass, mite) are also approved by the U.S. Food and Drug Administration (FDA) [18]. Finally, over the last 10 years, oral and sublingual administration AIT has been intensively studied in the field of food allergy (milk, egg, peanut) with favorable results, although in this latter case, safety aspects remain a problem [19,20].

35.2 SAFETY OF ALLERGEN IMMUNOTHERAPY: GENERAL ASPECTS

A detailed description of the adverse events (AEs) that are possibly, probably, or likely related to treatment can be provided by the careful reporting of such events during clinical trials or collection of such data after medications are introduced onto the market. SCIT causes a wide variety of AEs, ranging from local wheal-and-flare reactions at the site of the injection to systemic allergic reactions (SARs). The majority of SAEs occur within 30 minutes and therefore are presumed to be secondary to specific IgE reactions. Delayed reactions also occur and are probably most likely IgE-mediated late-phase responses. SAEs due to SCIT are classified according to a system introduced in 1993 [21] and updated in 2010 by the World Allergy Organization, a modification of which was proposed by Cox et al. in 2017 [22]. With SCIT, the rate of SAEs depends on the schedule used to administer the allergen extract, the type of allergen utilized, and survey methods. SAEs with SCIT occur at approximately 0.05%–0.6% of doses administered [23,24]. The risk of severe SARs leading to fatalities is approximately 1 per 2.5 million injections. Although six fatalities from SCIT were documented in the United States between 2001 and 2007, no fatalities have been directly or indirectly reported from SCIT during the first 2 years of a surveillance project by the American specialty organizations 2008–2010 [24]. However, in an abstract presented at the 2019 American Academy of Allergy, Asthma and Immunology (AAAAI) meeting, five additional deaths were reported between 2009 and 2016.

AE reports associated with SCIT are often incomplete, for example, no information is provided in approximately 20% of published SCIT clinical trials [25]. In studies where such data are reported, SARs occurred on average in 14% of subjects. In a 2004 survey, human error remained a major cause of SARs, but the cause of many serious SCIT reactions are still unclear [26].

AEs are carefully reported in the majority of the SLIT "big trial" studies, since the treatment was specifically developed to minimize them. Concerning the classification and grading of systemic AEs from SLIT, the method proposed recently is shared with SCIT [22]. Nonetheless, since the vast majority of the AEs with SLIT involve the digestive system, that is the specific site of administration, a dedicated grading of local side effects has been developed [27]. For practical reasons, in addition to AEs strictly localized in the upper digestive system (itching/swelling/burning of the lips or mouth), also nausea, diarrhea, and abdominal pain are considered "local" [27] (Figure 35.1, Table 35.1).

Most studies report that up to 50% of treated subjects experience oral or gastrointestinal reactions. The mechanisms of AEs with SLIT are not understood, but the amount of allergen (and possibly the number of allergens administered) plays an important role. When the allergen extract is immediately swallowed, i.e., oral

SLIT: KNOWN SIDE EFFECTS

Figure 35.1 Description of the possible side effects of SLIT and the actions to be taken.

swallow route, there are few side effects involving the oral cavity, whereas abdominal pain and nausea occur more frequently. When the dose is held under the tongue, then spat, oral reactions are more common and abdominal symptoms less frequent. Reactions involving the lower digestive tract, e.g., diarrhea or abdominal discomfort, could, in principle, be classified as a "systemic" reaction but, in general, such reactions are classified as local in nature when they are not accompanied by other systemic signs and symptoms of a SAR [27]. The relationship between allergen dose and side effects is unclear, although a certain dose-dependency is described, at least for local AEs [28]. Many local AEs, especially those involving the oral pharynx, tend to disappear with subsequent treatment [29,30]. The severity of AEs is usually mild; therefore, the frequency of SLIT AEs is probably underestimated. Finally, in many studies there is no updosing phase, thus treatment is started with the maintenance dose. The lack of updosing and beginning with maintenance treatment does not seem to increase the incidence of AEs [31,32]. SLIT is administered at home by the patient; however, it is suggested that the first dose be given in a clinic under the supervision of a physician [12,18].

35.3 DATA FROM RANDOMIZED DOUBLE-BLIND CLINICAL TRIALS

There are now more than 90 randomized double-blind, controlled clinical trials with SLIT. No fatality or life-threatening reactions are described, although exceptional cases of "anaphylaxis" are reported (see Table 35.2). Fifteen published trials report no AEs.

The most frequently described AEs in children and adults are the immediate onset of oral/sublingual pruritus after dosing, ranging from 0% to 50%, followed in frequency by abdominal pain, nausea, and/or diarrhea. These AEs are usually, but not always, described as mild and self-limited and do not require dose adjustment or medical treatment [22]. SARs, e.g., asthma, rhinitis, urticaria, angioedema, or severe abdominal complaints are reported in less than 0.3% of patients [27]. In the largest published SLIT trials, involving hundreds of subjects [33–45] utilizing various allergen doses, AEs were reported by 50%–60% of patients. Almost all were mild to moderate, and self-limited, but one involved uvular edema and was judged as being a serious AE. Overall, only about 2%–5% of the participants withdrew for AEs, probably or possibly related to

Table 35.1 Grading system for sublingual immunotherapy (SLIT) local adverse events (AEs) [27]: MedDRA description of adverse events

	Local side effect	MedDRA preferred term	MedDRA code	MedDRA low-level term
Mouth/ear	Altered taste perception	Dysgeusia	10013911	Taste alteration
	Itching of lips	Oral pruritus	10052894	Itching of mouth
	Swelling of lips	Swelling of lips	10024570	Swelling of lips
	Itching of oral mucosa	Oral pruritus	10052894	Itching of mouth
	Swelling of oral mucosa	Mucosal edema	10030111	Mucosal swelling
	Itching of ears	Ear pruritus	10052138	Ear pruritus
	Swelling of tongue	Swollen tongue	10042727	Swelling of tongue, nonspecific
	Glossodynia	Glossodynia	10018388	Glossodynia
	Mouth ulcer	Mouth ulceration	10028034	Mouth ulcer
	Tongue ulcer	Tongue ulceration	10043991	Tongue ulceration
	Throat irritation	Throat irritation	10043521	Throat irritation
	Uvular edema	Pharyngeal edema	10034829	Pharyngeal edema
Upper	Nausea	Nausea	10028813	Nausea
gastrointestinal	Stomachache	Abdominal pain, upper	10000087	Stomachache
	Vomiting	Vomiting	10047700	Vomiting
Lower	Abdominal pain	Abdominal pain	10000081	Abdominal pain
gastrointestinal	Diarrhea	Diarrhea	10012735	Diarrhea

Proposed World Allergy Organization grading

Symptom/sign	Grade 1: Mild	Grade 2: Moderate	Grade 3: Severe	Unknown severity
Pruritus/swelling of mouth, tongue, or lip; throat irritation, nausea, abdominal pain, vomiting, diarrhea, heartburn, or uvular edema	• Not troublesome AND • No symptomatic treatment required AND • No discontinuation of SLIT because of local side effects	• Troublesome OR • Requires symptomatic treatment AND • No discontinuation of SLIT because of local side effects	• Grade 2 AND • SLIT discontinued because of local side effects	Treatment is discontinued, there is no subjective, objective, or both description of severity from the patient/physician

SLIT treatment. In some studies, local side effects were reported frequently (50%–80% of patients), but severe AEs occurred in less than 2% [33–45].

SLIT has been utilized in numerous pediatric studies, including children from ages 3 to 17 years. All report an acceptable safety profile, and four report no side effects. Local oral side effects are most frequently reported in children [31,38,40,41] but are mild in the majority of patients.

35.4 SAFETY IN ASTHMA

Symptomatic and severe asthma is considered a contraindication to AIT, as reported in guidelines [15]. This was deduced by the historical evidence that most fatal or near-fatal adverse events occurred in asthmatic patients [5,6,8], always with SCIT. Indeed, SLIT has an overall more favorable safety profile in asthma. A 2006 randomized, controlled trial was designed specifically to assess the safety and efficacy of SLIT in asthmatic subjects [46]. The occurrence of asthma was not different in SLIT compared to placebo treatment in 114 subjects. Mild, local discomfort (oral itching/swelling/burning) occurred in 53% of the SLIT subjects and none in the placebo-treated subjects. No severe AEs occurred. Another controlled trial on safety [28] was conducted in 48 grass-allergic patients outside the pollen season with progressively increasing doses, up to 200 mcg Phl p 5. The overall incidence of all AEs was 74%, all of mild or moderate intensity (oral itching and irritation of mouth/throat).

Table 35.2 Case reports of suspected anaphylaxis with sublingual immunotherapy

Author (Reference)	Sex (age)	Allergen	Onset	Description	Epinephrine
Dunsky et al. [70]	F (31)	*Alternaria*, cat, dog, grass, ragweed	5 min	Angioedema, dizziness, dyspnea, generalized itching	NO
Antico et al. [71]	F (36)	Latex	10 min	Asthma, generalized urticaria	Not specified
Eifan et al. [72]	F (11)	Dust mite + grass pollen	3 min	Abdominal pain, chest pain, fever, nausea	Not specified
Rodnguez-Perez et al. [73]	F (7) 11 (M)	Mite	20 min 30 min	Wheezing, dyspnea Wheezing, dyspnea, urticaria	YES YES
Blazowski [74]	F (16)	Mite (Overdose)	10 min	Collapse, flushing, urticaria	YES
De Groot and Bijl [75]	M (13) F (27)	Grass	15 min Not spec	Generalized urticaria, swelling of tongue	NO YES
Hsiao and Smart [76]	F (7)	Grass	10 min	Laryngeal edema, asthma	YES
Van Dyken et al. [77]	F (15)	Mite	30 min	Asthma, urticaria	YES
Wasan and Nanda [78]	M (35)	Grass	30 min	Asthma	YES

Two large trials specifically designed to assess the efficacy and safety of SLIT in allergic asthma were conducted [33,34]. In the first one [34] involving 604 patients, the occurrence of all AEs was 54% and 64% in the placebo and active groups, respectively, with asthma exacerbations in 5% of placebo and 8% of active patients. The other study [33] involved 834 asthmatic patients (277 placebo) and demonstrated an overall occurrence of AE in 17% of placebo and 42% of active (mostly local) group, but a significant difference was seen in asthma exacerbation rate in favor of the active groups. Thus, considering these studies, asthma does not represent an absolute contraindication to SLIT if it is well controlled by standard therapy. Also, based on an extensive literature review, only uncontrolled asthma remains an absolute contraindication to SLIT [47]. From the available data, it appears that an optimal control of asthma (i.e., no symptoms) is required as a mandatory limitation for the prescription of SLIT and of AIT in general.

35.5 SPECIFIC CLINICAL PROBLEMS ABOUT SAFETY OF SUBLINGUAL IMMUNOTHERAPY

SLIT, in general, is safer than SCIT; although the local side effects are frequent, they are easily manageable and rarely place the person at risk. There are specific problems about the safety of SLIT: the use of multiple allergens, the lower age limit of initiation, and the possibility of causing or exacerbating eosinophilic esophagitis.

SCIT is not usually recommended for children younger than 5 years of age because potential systemic side effects may be more difficult to recognize or treat. There are two postmarketing surveys of SLIT performed in children between ages 3 and 5 years. The first [48] reported AEs in 5% of 36 subjects with an incidence rate of 0.071 per 1000 doses. The symptoms were gastrointestinal and mild. Another survey [49] involved 128 children and reported AEs in 5.6% or 0.2 per 1000 doses. Two AEs were local and mild, and the

remaining were moderate and consisted of nausea and diarrhea. The use of multiple extracts (different class allergens) for SLIT did not increase the occurrence of adverse events in adults and children [50,51]. According to the literature, the compliance with SLIT in very young children is low under the age of 4 years [52]. Of note, in a retrospective study [53] involving about 5000 children treated with SCIT or SLIT, 8.3% of the SCIT group were shifted to SLIT due to adverse effects.

There are also case reports of anaphylaxis [54–56] probably related to SLIT (summarized in Table 35.2). In some of the reports, the diagnosis of anaphylaxis remains unclear, and the use of intramuscular epinephrine is not always reported [54]. Nonetheless, the administration of an allergen to which the patient is clearly sensitized is a possible risk factor. Therefore, the first dose of SLIT should be done under medical supervision [22,27]. Likewise, it is important to know whether previous SARs occurred to SCIT in patients prescribed SLIT. They may be at higher risk for AEs, although case reports are too few to provide definitive recommendations. Finally, it is necessary to instruct patients in the use of SLIT, as for any medication, in order to avoid accidental overdose and secondary side effects.

Some cases of esophagitis have been associated with SLIT [57–60], but such an association has not been documented [61]. It remains unclear if SLIT can exacerbate preexistent eosinophilic esophagitis or if SLIT can cause it. From a clinical point of view, and considering safety considerations, SLIT for aero-allergens should not be prescribed in subjects with eosinophilic esophagitis.

Sublingual (and oral) AIT is under investigation, with very promising results to treat food allergy. About 75% of children can be desensitized, but at least one-quarter of this selected population can experience SARs [62–64]. Thus, oral or sublingual desensitization for food allergy is primarily considered experimental, although there are some practitioners in the United States who actively practice oral immunotherapy (OIT) in their clinics [65]. In addition, it is important to remind that the efficacy of SLIT is not a "class effect," but it should be documented for each specific product [66,67].

SALIENT POINTS

1. The overall safety of sublingual immunotherapy (SLIT) is confirmed by clinical trials, postmarketing surveillance, and more than 20 years of clinical use [68,69].
2. The occurrence and severity of adverse events (AEs) does not differ between children, even those younger than 5 years of age, and adults.
3. No fatalities due to SLIT are reported.
4. Anaphylaxis with SLIT is rare and remains unpredictable. If anaphylaxis occurs, SLIT should be discontinued since it is administered at home without immediate access to optimal medical treatment.
5. The first dose of SLIT should be administered under medical supervision with appropriate education/information on its use and expected results.
6. Severe uncontrolled asthma remains an absolute contraindication for SLIT as with subcutaneous immunotherapy (SCIT).
7. The severity of the large majority of the AEs reported is mild. Most AEs involve the mouth (burning or itching) or the gastrointestinal tract (abdominal pain, nausea) and usually resolve within a few days of continuation of therapy.
8. A temporary dose-reduction and concomitant antihistamine therapy are considerations in cases of persisting or moderate severe local AEs. If an AE persists and remains troublesome, SLIT should be discontinued.
9. Systemic allergic reactions (SARs), such as urticaria, rhinitis, or asthma, require treatment and temporary dose reduction and may indicate that such therapy should be discontinued.
10. Excluding updosing regimens versus beginning with the therapeutic dose, in general, does not increase the occurrence of AEs.
11. A grading system for the local side effects of sublingual immunotherapy for respiratory diseases is now available to improve and harmonize surveillance as well as the universal reporting of ARs associated with SLIT.
12. SLIT is marketed and used in clinical practice in many European countries and the United States. Detailed data on its safety are available in clinical trials and postmarketing surveys.
13. The literature consistently shows that the side effects of SLIT are mostly local, mild, and consist of oral itching/burning and stomachache. These very rarely lead to discontinuation of therapy.

REFERENCES

1. Herxeimer H. Bronchial hypersensitization and hyposensitization in man. *Int Arch Allergy Appl Immunol* 1951; 40: 40–57.
2. Taylor G, Shivalkar PR. Local nasal desensitization in allergic rhinitis. *Clin Allergy* 1972; 2: 125–126.
3. Taudorf E, Weeke B. Orally administered grass pollen. *Allergy* 1983; 38: 561–564.
4. Canonica GW, Passalacqua G. Non-injection routes for immunotherapy. *J Allergy Clin Immunol* 2003; 111: 437–448.
5. Lockey RF, Benedict LM, Turkeltaub PC, Bukantz SC. Fatalities associated with immunotherapy and skin testing. *J Allergy Clin Immunol* 1987; 79: 660–677.
6. Committee on the Safety of Medicines. CSM update. Desensitizing vaccines. *Br Med J* 1986; 293: 948.
7. Lockey RF, Benedict LM, Turkeltaub PC, Bukantz SC. Fatalities from immunotherapy and skin testing. *J Allergy Clin Immunol* 1987; 79: 660–677.
8. Reid MJ, Lockey RF, Turkeltaub PC, Platt-Mills TAE. Survey of fatalities from skin testing and immunotherapy. *J Allergy Clin Immunol* 1993; 92: 6–15.
9. Hansel FK. Treatment of allergic manifestations by immunologic methods. In: Hansel FK, editor. *Clinical Allergy*. Chapter 39. St. Louis, MO: C.V. Mosby, 1953: 745–765.
10. Scadding K, Brostoff J. Low dose sublingual therapy in patients with allergic rhinitis due to dust mite. *Clin Allergy* 1986; 16: 483–491.
11. Bousquet PJ, Durham SR, Cox L et al. Sublingual immunotherapy: WAO Position Paper 2009. Canonica GW et al. editors. *Allergy* 2009; 64(Suppl 91): 3–45.
12. Canonica GW, Cox L, Pawankar R et al. Sublingual immunotherapy: World Allergy Organization position paper 2013 update. *World Allergy Organ J* 2014; 7(1): 6.
13. Dhami S, Nurmatov U, Arasi S et al. Allergen immunotherapy for allergic rhinoconjunctivitis: A systematic review and meta-analysis. *Allergy* 2017; 72: 1597–1631.
14. Durham SR, Penagos M. Sublingual or subcutaneous immunotherapy for allergic rhinitis? *J Allergy Clin Immunol* 2016; 137: 339–349.
15. Bousquet J, Lockey RF, Malling HJ, editors. WHO Position Paper. Allergen immunotherapy: Therapeutic vaccines for allergic diseases. *Allergy* 1998; 53: 1069–1088.
16. Brożek JL, Bousquet J, Agache I et al. Allergic Rhinitis and its Impact on Asthma (ARIA) guidelines, 2016 revision. *J Allergy Clin Immunol* 2017; 140: 950–958.
17. Global Initiative on the Management of Asthma (GINA). 2017 update. https://ginasthma.org. Accessed October 2018.
18. Li JT, Bernstein DI, Calderon MA et al. Sublingual grass and ragweed immunotherapy: Clinical considerations— A PRACTALL consensus report. *J Allergy Clin Immunol* 2016; 137: 369–376.
19. Passalacqua G, Canonica GW. Allergen immunotherapy: History and future developments. *Immunol Allergy Clin North Am* 2016; 36: 1–12.
20. Pajno GB, Bernardini R, Peroni D et al. Allergen-specific Immunotherapy panel of the Italian Society of Pediatric Allergy and Immunology (SIAIP). Clinical practice recommendations for allergen-specific immunotherapy in children: The Italian consensus report. *Ital J Pediatr* 2017; 43: 13.
21. Stewart GE, Lockey RF. Systemic reactions from allergen immunotherapy. *J Allergy Clin Immunol* 1992; 90: 567–578.
22. Cox L, Larenas-Linnemann D, Lockey RF, Passalacqua G. Speaking the same language: The World Allergy Organization subcutaneous immunotherapy systemic reaction grading system. *J Allergy Clin Immunol* 2010; 125: 569–574.
23. Lockey RF, Nikoara-Kasti GL, Theodoropoulos DS, Bukantz SC. Systemic reactions and fatalities associated with allergen immunotherapy. *Ann Allergy Asthma Immunol* 2001; 87(1 Suppl 1): 47–55.
24. Bernstein DI, Epstein T, Murphy-Berendts K, Liss GM. Surveillance of systemic reactions to subcutaneous immunotherapy injections: Year 1 outcomes of the ACAAI and AAAAI collaborative study. *Ann Allergy Asthma Immunol* 2010; 104: 530–535.
25. Malling HJ. Immunotherapy as an effective tool in allergy treatment. *Allergy* 1998; 53: 461–472.
26. Aaronson DW, Gandhi TK. Incorrect allergy injections: Allergists' experiences and recommendations for prevention. *J Allergy Clin Immunol* 2004; 113: 1117–1121.

27. Passalacqua G, Baena-Cagnani CE, Bousquet J et al. Grading local side effects of sublingual immunotherapy for respiratory allergy: Speaking the same language. *J Allergy Clin Immunol* 2013; 132: 93–98.

28. Kleine-Tebbe J, Ribel M, Herold DA. Safety of a SQ-standardised grass allergen tablet for sublingual immunotherapy: A randomized, placebo-controlled trial. *Allergy* 2006; 61:181–184.

29. Didier A, Worm M, Horak F et al. Sustained 3-year efficacy of pre- and coseasonal 5-grass-pollen sublingual immunotherapy tablets in patients with grass pollen-induced rhinoconjunctivitis. *J Allergy Clin Immunol* 2011; 128: 559–566.

30. Durham SR, Emminger W, Kapp A, de Monchy JG, Rak S, Scadding GK. SQ-standardized sublingual grass immunotherapy: Confirmation of disease modification 2 years after 3 years of treatment in a randomized trial. *J Allergy Clin Immunol* 2012; 129: 717–725.

31. Ibanez MD, Kaiser F, Knecht R et al. Safety of specific sublingual immunotherapy with SQ standardized grass allergen tablets in children. *Pediatr Allergy Immunol* 2007; 18: 516–522.

32. Rodriguez F, Boquete M, Ibanez MD, de la Torre-Martinez F, Tabar AI. Once daily sublingual immunotherapy without updosing—A new treatment schedule. *Int Arch Allergy Immunol* 2006; 140: 321–326.

33. Virchow JC, Backer V, Kuna P et al. Efficacy of a house dust mite sublingual allergen immunotherapy tablet in adults with allergic asthma: A randomized clinical trial. *JAMA* 2016; 315: 1715–1725.

34. Mosbech H, Deckelmann R, de Blay F et al. Standardized quality (SQ) house dust mite sublingual immunotherapy tablet (ALK) reduces inhaled corticosteroid use while maintaining asthma control: A randomized, double-blind, placebo-controlled trial. *J Allergy Clin Immunol* 2014; 134: 568–575.

35. Durham SR, Yang WH, Pedersen MR, Johansen N, Rak S. Sublingual immunotherapy with once-daily grass-allergen tablets: A randomised controlled trial in seasonal allergic rhinoconjunctivitis. *J Allergy Clin Immunol* 2006; 117: 802–809.

36. Dahl R, Kapp A, Colombo G et al. Efficacy and safety of sublingual immunotherapy with grass allergen tablets for seasonal allergic rhinoconjunctivitis. *J Allergy Clin Immunol* 2006; 118: 434–440.

37. Didier A, Malling HJ, Worm M et al. Optimal dose, efficacy, and safety of once-daily sublingual immunotherapy with a 5-grass pollen tablet for seasonal allergic rhinitis. *J Allergy Clin Immunol* 2007; 120: 1338–1345.

38. Wahn U, Tabar A, Kuna P et al. Efficacy and safety of 5 grass pollen sublingual immunotherapy in pediatric allergic rhinoconjunctivitis. *J Allergy Clin Immunol* 2009; 123: 160–166.

39. Ott H, Sieber J, Brehler R et al. Efficacy of grass pollen sublingual immunotherapy for three consecutive seasons and after cessation of treatment: The ECRIT study. *Allergy* 2009; 64: 179–186.

40. Bufe A, Eberle P, Franke-Beckmann E et al. Safety and efficacy in children of an SQ-standardized grass allergen tablet for sublingual immunotherapy. *J Allergy Clin Immunol* 2009; 123: 167–173.

41. Blaiss M, Maloney J, Nolte H, Gawchik S, Yao R, Skoner DP. Efficacy and safety of timothy grass allergy immunotherapy tablets in North American children and adolescents. *J Allergy Clin Immunol* 2011; 127: 64–71.

42. Nelson HS, Nolte H, Creticos P, Maloney J, Wu J, Bernstein DI. Efficacy and safety of timothy grass allergy immunotherapy tablet treatment in North American adults. *J Allergy Clin Immunol* 2011; 127: 72–80.

43. Maloney J, Bernstein DI, Nelson H et al. Efficacy and safety of grass sublingual immunotherapy tablet, MK-7243: A large randomized controlled trial. *Ann Allergy Asthma Immunol* 2014; 112: 146–153.

44. Creticos PS, Esch RE, Couroux P et al. Randomized, double-blind, placebo-controlled trial of standardized ragweed sublingual-liquid immunotherapy for allergic rhinoconjunctivitis. *J Allergy Clin Immunol* 2014; 133: 751–758.

45. Cox LS, Casale TB, Nayak AS et al. Clinical efficacy of 300IR 5-grass pollen sublingual tablet in a US study: The importance of allergen-specific serum IgE. *J Allergy Clin Immunol* 2012; 130: 1327–1334.

46. Dahl R, Stender A, Rak S. Specific immunotherapy with SQ standardized grass allergen tablets in asthmatics with rhinoconjunctivitis. *Allergy* 2006; 61: 185–190.

47. Pitsios C, Demoly P, Bilò MB et al. Clinical contraindications to allergen immunotherapy: An EAACI position paper. *Allergy* 2015; 70: 897–909.

48. Agostinis F, Tellarini L, Falagiani P, Canonica GW, Passalacqua G. Safety of SLIT in very young children. *Allergy* 2005; 60: 133.

49. Di Rienzo V, Minelli M, Musarra A et al. Post-marketing survey on the safety of sublingual immunotherapy in children below the age of 5 years. *Clin Exp Allergy* 2005; 35: 560–564.

50. Lombardi C, Gargioni S, Cottini M, Canonica GW, Passalacqua G. The safety of sublingual immunotherapy with one or more allergens in adults. *Allergy* 2008; 63: 375–376.

51. Agostinis F, Foglia C, Landi M et al. The safety of sublingual immunotherapy with one or multiple pollen allergens in children. *Allergy* 2008; 63: 1637–1639.

52. Pajno GB, Caminiti L, Crisafulli G et al. Adherence to sublingual immunotherapy in preschool children. *Pediatr Allergy Immunol* 2012; 23: 688–689.

53. Pajno GB, Caminiti L, Passalacqua G. Changing the route of immunotherapy administration: An 18-year survey in pediatric patients with allergic rhinitis and asthma. *Allergy Asthma Proc* 2013; 34: 523–526.

54. Calderón MA, Simons FE, Malling HJ, Lockey RF, Moingeon P, Demoly P. Sublingual allergen immunotherapy: Mode of action and its relationship with the safety profile. *Allergy* 2012; 67: 302–311.

55. Nolte H, Casale TB, Lockey RF et al. Epinephrine use in clinical trials of sublingual immunotherapy tablets. *J Allergy Clin Immunol Pract* 2017; 5: 84–89.

56. Makatsori M, Calderon MA. Anaphylaxis: Still a ghost behind allergen immunotherapy. *Curr Opin Allergy Clin Immunol* 2014; 14: 316–322.

57. Kawashima K, Ishihara S, Masuhara M et al. Development of eosinophilic esophagitis following sublingual immunotherapy with cedar pollen extract: A case report. *Allergol Int* 2018; 67: 515–517.

58. Béné J, Ley D, Roboubi R, Gottrand F, Gautier S. Eosinophilic esophagitis after desensitization to dust mites with sublingual immunotherapy. *Ann Allergy Asthma Immunol* 2016; 116: 583–584.

59. Miehlke S, Alpan O, Schröder S, Straumann A. Induction of eosinophilic esophagitis by sublingual pollen immunotherapy. *Case Rep Gastroenterol* 2013; 7: 363–368.

60. Rokosz M, Bauer C, Schroeder S. Eosinophilic esophagitis induced by aeroallergen sublingual immunotherapy in an enteral feeding tube-dependent pediatric patient. *Ann Allergy Asthma Immunol* 2017; 119: 88–89.

61. Egan M, Atkins D. What is the relationship between eosinophilic esophagitis (EoE) and aeroallergens? Implications for allergen immunotherapy. *Curr Allergy Asthma Rep* 2018; 18: 43.

62. Passalacqua G, Nowak-Węgrzyn A, Canonica GW. Local side effects of sublingual and oral immunotherapy. *J Allergy Clin Immunol Pract* 2017; 5(1): 13–21.

63. Arasi S, Passalacqua G, Caminiti L, Crisafulli G, Fiamingo C, Pajno GB. Efficacy and safety of sublingual immunotherapy in children. *Expert Rev Clin Immunol* 2016; 12: 49–56.

64. Pajno GB, Bernardini R, Peroni D et al. Clinical practice recommendations for allergen-specific immunotherapy in children: The Italian consensus report. *Ital J Pediatr* 2017; 43: 13.

65. Wasserman RL, Jones DH, Windom HH et al. Oral immunotherapy for food allergens: The FAST perspective. *Ann Allergy Asthma Immunol* 2018; 121(3): 272–275.

66. Bachert C, Larché M, Bonini S et al. Allergen immunotherapy on the way to product-based evaluation—A WAO statement. *World Allergy Organ J* 2015; 8: 29.

67. Passalacqua G, Bagnasco D, Ferrando M et al. Current insights in allergen immunotherapy. *Ann Allergy Asthma Immunol* 2018; 120: 152–154.

68. Muraro A, Roberts G, Halken S et al. EAACI guidelines on allergen immunotherapy: Executive statement. *Allergy* 2018; 73: 739–743.

69. Pfaar O, Alvaro M, Cardona V et al. Clinical trials in allergen immunotherapy: Current concepts and future needs. *Allergy* 2018; 73: 1775–1783.

70. Dunsky EH, Goldstein MF, Dvorin DJ, Belecanech GA. Anaphylaxis to sublingual immunotherapy. *Allergy* 2006; 61(10): 1235.71.

71. Antico A, Pagani M, Crema A. Anaphylaxis by latex sublingual immunotherapy. *Allergy* 2006; 61(10): 1236–1237.

72. Eifan AO, Keles S, Bahceciler NN, Barlan IB. Anaphylaxis to multiple pollen allergen sublingual immunotherapy. *Allergy* 2007; 62(5): 567–568.

73. Rodriguez-Perez N, Ambriz-Moreno MDJ, Canonica GW, Penagos M. Frequency of acute systemic reactions in patients with allergic rhinitis and asthma treated with sublingual immunotherapy. *Ann Allergy Asthma Immunol* 2008; 101(3): 304–310.

74. Blazowski L. ALLERGY net: Anaphylactic shock because of sublingual immunotherapy overdose during third year of maintenance dose. *Allergy* 2008; 63(3): 374.

75. De Groot HD, Bijl A. Anaphylactic reaction after the first dose of sublingual immunotherapy with grass pollen tablet. Allergy 2009; 64(6): 963–964.

76. Hsiao KC, Smart J. Anaphylaxis caused by in-season switchover of sublingual immunotherapy formulation. *Pediatr Allergy Immunol* 2014; 25(7): 714–715.

77. Van Dyken AM, Smith PK, Fox TL. Clinical case of anaphylaxis with sublingual immunotherapy: House dust mite allergen. *J Allergy Clin Immunol Pract* 2014; 2(4): 485–486.

78. Wasan A, Nanda A. Systemic reaction to timothy grass pollen sublingual immunotherapy. *Allergy Asthma Immunol* 2017; 118(6): 732–733.

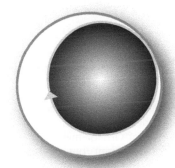

36 Recognition, prevention, and treatment of adverse effects associated with oral allergen immunotherapy

Jennifer A. Dantzer and Robert A. Wood
Johns Hopkins University School of Medicine

CONTENTS

36.1 INTRODUCTION

Oral immunotherapy (OIT) refers to the ingestion of an allergen, usually in a powdered form, in an effort to desensitize or induce long-term tolerance to that allergen. It has been studied experimentally for both food and inhalant allergens, although limited inhalant allergen OIT studies are not encouraging; therefore, OIT is not currently considered to be a likely alternative to subcutaneous or sublingual immunotherapy (SCIT/SLIT). Over the past several decades, multiple routes of immunotherapy have been investigated for food allergy, including oral (OIT), subcutaneous (SCIT), sublingual (SLIT), and epicutaneous (EPIT) [1–3]. For food allergy, OIT shows more promise, with preliminary studies suggesting that it is likely to be more effective at desensitizing to foods than SLIT or EPIT and far safer than SCIT. It is therefore under active investigation for the treatment of food allergy and appears to be the most attractive option at this time, for said purpose [1–8]. OIT is currently practiced in Japan, Europe, and by some physicians and clinics in North America. However, its safety remains a major concern and therefore is considered experimental and currently not recommended for clinical use by the authors [2]. This chapter

reviews the adverse effects associated with food OIT. However, it is important to recognize that data on this subject are relatively limited due to the small number of studies conducted, as well as the fact that the sample sizes of all the studies to date are small, that very few studies are placebo-controlled, that dosing regimens are highly variable, and that the adverse effects associated with treatment are not always described and there is a paucity of long-term data [1,9]. There are a number of larger, placebo-controlled studies that are ongoing and will provide new and more extensive information about OIT in the future.

36.2 RATIONALE AND GENERAL APPROACH

The rationale for using the oral route for food immunotherapy is that ingestion of a food antigen preferentially results in an active immune system response, one that does not trigger an allergic reaction toward the punitive antigen, akin to the natural development of oral tolerance [10]. OIT has been studied most extensively for cow's milk, egg, and peanut, but protocols have also been reported for several other single foods and recently, for multiple foods simultaneously. A high rate of desensitization has been demonstrated in both randomized trials and observational studies of OIT for milk, egg, and peanut. Fewer treated patients become tolerant, but the rate of acquisition of tolerance is likely to be higher than that seen in patients who completely avoid the allergen. OIT is likely to cause more adverse reactions than SLIT or EPIT, given the fact that much higher doses are used in OIT. Preliminary studies suggest that OIT is more effective than SLIT or EPIT to treat milk and peanut allergy [1,11–13]. Selected studies with specific emphasis on dose and reported adverse reactions with OIT for food allergy are summarized in Table 36.1.

Although published protocols vary widely, the general approach to OIT is to start patients on a very low dose of the relevant allergen, for example, 0.01 mg of peanut protein or four drops per day of a solution of 10 drops of cow's milk in 10 mL of water, and advance to a maintenance dose, e.g., 300–4000 mg of milk, egg, or peanut protein, over several months. In most protocols, dose escalation is accomplished by providing 25%–50% dose increases every 1–2 weeks, while the patient is under observation, with daily home administration of that same dose until the next observed dose increase. Maintenance dosing may then last for months to years; however, it is still not clear what period of maintenance dosing is needed for optimal outcomes. A repeat open food challenge (OFC) is then performed, and many studies also include a final challenge after a period of time off therapy to determine sustained unresponsiveness, or "lack of a clinical reaction to a food allergen after active therapy has been stopped" (quote from [1]) [6]. While protocols provide a single dosing strategy for all subjects, it is critical that each subject be monitored individually and that dose adjustments be considered following adverse reactions. Hopefully, in the future, individualized therapy based on one or more specific biomarkers will lead to better results.

OIT studies to date have shown high rates of adverse reactions, affecting virtually all treated patients, ranging from mild, local symptoms, such as oral pruritus, to severe systemic reactions [1,6]. Approximately 10%–25% of subjects have dropped out of OIT trials due to adverse reactions, most commonly gastrointestinal (GI) symptoms, with an estimated risk of eosinophilic esophagitis (EoE) of 2%–5% [1,6,8].

A possible alternative approach is to combine OIT with anti-IgE therapy as with omalizumab [1,6,14]. Anti-IgE therapy with omalizumab has been studied as an adjunct to milk, peanut, egg, and multifood OIT [15–21]. Studies indicate that omalizumab in addition to OIT can decrease, but not eliminate, the risk for adverse reactions and can reduce the time required to reach maintenance dosing [14]. To date, there have been small pilot studies, case reports, and two small double-blind placebo-controlled trials, and additional studies are underway exploring this approach, and others may evolve as newer, higher-affinity anti-IgE molecules are introduced.

The following sections of this chapter are divided into reviews of specific studies on milk, egg, peanut, wheat, and multifood OIT. Again, the focus is on adverse reactions, with data on efficacy found in Chapter 28 and immunologic response in Chapter 5.

36.2.1 Milk oral immunotherapy

Two different systematic reviews and meta-analyses of milk OIT trials found that the relative risk of developing full tolerance to cow's milk was 10-fold higher in children treated with milk OIT versus avoidance of milk [22,23]. In addition, similar results are reported in observational studies. However, the risk of an adverse reaction is 34-fold higher (95% CI: 4.8–244.7) in children receiving OIT compared with those on an elimination diet, with reactions occurring with 16% of doses [23]. Lip/mouth pruritus is the most common symptom, but rates of systemic reactions and use of epinephrine also are greater with OIT than with avoidance [22,23].

A few key studies are informative regarding adverse reactions with milk OIT, especially those that are randomized to treated and untreated groups and/or a true placebo group. Nine subjects (36%), in a randomized trial by Staden et al. that included OIT to egg and milk, were not able to tolerate OIT due to flares of atopic dermatitis or recurrent acute adverse effects, e.g., urticaria, abdominal pain, and emesis [24]. In addition, all subjects experienced some adverse reactions, and many children had significant reactions even while on a stable dosing regimen. Many of these adverse reactions occurred in the setting of what the authors describe as augmentation factors, most notably exercise or febrile illnesses, as is the case in most other studies. Also of note in this trial is that the control group, who maintained an avoidance diet, had far fewer reactions during the study period. Somewhat surprisingly, spontaneous resolution rates of milk or egg allergy were comparable, 7 of 20 (35%), to that seen in the treatment group.

In another randomized study of milk OIT, published by Longo et al., 3 of the 30 treated children discontinued the study because of significant respiratory or abdominal side effects [25]. All experienced one or more adverse reactions, mainly urticaria and angioedema or abdominal discomfort, but no child had severe anaphylaxis. During the in-hospital rush escalation, intramuscular epinephrine was administered 4 times in 4 children, whereas nebulized epinephrine was used in 18 children and more than one in 7 because of recurring respiratory symptoms. Two children required treatment in the emergency department during home dosing. They were initially treated by their parents in accordance with the protocol for adverse events and then received further treatment in the hospital with a glucocorticosteroid, antihistamine, and intramuscular epinephrine. In the untreated control group, six children (20%) had mild reactions caused by accidental exposure to milk during the study period.

Adverse reaction rates, as well as rescue medication use, were reported in greater detail, as displayed in Table 36.2 in the first double-blind, placebo-controlled trial of milk OIT published by Skripak et al. [26]. The median frequency for total reactions per participant was 35%, with a wide range from 1% to 95% in the active versus 1% in the placebo group, range, 0 to 53%; $P = .02$. The most common reactions in the active group were local, mostly oral pruritus, and gastrointestinal, mainly abdominal pain, with a median frequency of 16% and 2% of active doses, respectively. Reactions involving multiple systems were uncommon, occurring with a median frequency of 1% of active doses versus none in the placebo-treated group ($P = .01$).

Data on treatment of reactions in this study reveal that diphenhydramine was given with a median frequency of 10% of active doses compared with 1% of placebo doses. As with the symptom data, the frequency of diphenhydramine use varied widely in the active group, from never to 58% of OIT doses. Four doses of epinephrine were utilized to treat reactions in four different participants in the active group; two of these occurred with the initial in-hospital buildup doses and the other two occurred with home doses.

There was one participant in each treatment group who experienced a significant eczema flare. The placebo group

Table 36.1 Oral immunotherapy studies and reported adverse events

Author (reference number)	Food(s) (N)	Subjects	Starting dose	Time to maintenance/ maintenance dose	Adverse reactions/other comments
Patriarca et al. 1984 [53]	Milk (8)	n = 19 Age: 5–55 years	10 drops of CM in 10 mL of water, four drops/day	100 mL of undiluted CM/day in 104 days.	Side effects in 11 of 19 patients: urticaria, pruritus, emesis, angioedema, abdominal pain, rhinitis, dyspnea.
	Egg (8)		10 drops of beaten egg in 100 mL of water, four drops/day	120 drops of pure beaten egg/day in 90 days.	
	Fish (2)		10 mL of mixed fish commercial extract (eel, sardine, codfish, anchovy) in 90 mL of water, four drops/day	200 g of cooked fish/day in 120 days.	
	Orange (1)		Unspecified	3 months.	
Patriarca et al. 1998 [54]	CM (6), egg (5), fish (2), apple (1)	n = 14 Age: 4–14 years	Modification of previously published protocol	Modification of previously published protocol.	All of the children who achieved maintenance continued to tolerate the foods at least two to three times per week for 3–6 years. 10 of 14 patients experienced side effects during treatment.
Patriarca et al. 2003 [55]	CM (29), egg (15), fish (11), orange (2), and other	n = 59 Age: 3–55 years	Modification of previously published protocol	Modification of previously published protocol.	51% of patients experienced urticaria, emesis, diarrhea, or abdominal pain. In 9 patients (16.7%), protocol was stopped due to side effects. No differences between children and adults. SPT became negative after 18 months in 78%; Food-IgE decreased and food-IgG4 increased after 18 months.
Meglio et al. 2004 [56]	Milk (19)	n = 21 Age: 5–10 years	One drop of milk diluted 1:25 in water	200 mL undiluted CM per day over 180 days.	Three of 21 reacted to minimal dose of diluted CM; 3 of 21 tolerated only 40–80 CM/day; 15 of 21 tolerated 200 mL CM/day for 6 months. Side effect rate 13 of 21. SPT to BLG and CS significantly decreased at 6 months ($p < .001$); CM-IgE levels not significantly different.

(Continued)

Table 36.1 (*Continued*) Oral immunotherapy studies and reported adverse events

Author (reference number)	Food(s) (N)	Subjects	Starting dose	Time to maintenance/ maintenance dose	Adverse reactions/other comments
	Egg (2)		0.01 mg egg per day at home	2.5 g egg per day (1/2 egg) over 41–52 weeks.	
Buchanan et al. 2007 [46]	Egg	n = 7 Mean age: 4 years (subjects with history of egg-induced anaphylaxis were excluded)	0.1 mg of powdered egg white followed by doubling doses every 30 minutes until the highest tolerated dose was determined	Modified rush and buildup phase in the hospital, maintenance dosing once a day at home. Increases by 25 mg every 2 weeks until 150 mg, then by 50 mg until reaching maintenance of 300 mg.	Four subjects tolerated egg challenge at the end of 24 months. Two of them reacted to a subsequent egg challenge done 3 months after treatment was stopped. Egg-specific IgG increased significantly from baseline to 24 months ($p = .002$). Five subjects showed an overall decrease in egg-specific IgE.
Morisset et al. 2007 [57]	Milk (57)	n = 141 Mean age: 2.2 years	1 mL/day	Home buildup over 6 weeks, up to a dose of 250 mL/ day.	Only children tolerating at least 60 mL of milk or 965 mg of raw egg white on a baseline food challenge were included. SPT sizes and specific IgE levels were significantly decreased in children who developed tolerance to milk or egg.
	Egg (84)	n = 141 Mean age: 3.5 years	1 g of hard-boiled egg yolk	Home buildup over 4 weeks to 4 g of yolk and 4 g of egg white once a day, every other day.	
Staden et al. 2007 [24]	Milk (14) Egg (11)	Total N = 45: 14 Milk 11 Egg 20 Untreated controls Age: 0.6–12.5 years (median 2.5 years)	Milk 0.02 mg protein, egg 0.006 mg protein	Slow induction phase at home, median duration 7 months, followed by a maintenance phase of milk 3300 mg (100 mL) and egg 2800 mg (1/2 egg); median duration 9 months.	Nine subjects (36%) were not able to tolerate OIT due to flares of atopic dermatitis or recurrent acute adverse effects (e.g., urticaria, abdominal pain, emesis).
Longo et al. 2008 [25]	Milk	n = 60 Mean age: 7.9 years (5–17)	Five drops of one drop of milk in 10 mL of water	10 day rush phase in the hospital, followed by home dosing, goal of minimum 150 mL milk/day for 1 year.	Three children discontinued the study due to significant respiratory or abdominal side effects. At home, 17 of 30 children reported side effects: 17 children received oral steroids, 6 received nebulized epinephrine, and 2 received intramuscular epinephrine.

(*Continued*)

Table 36.1 (*Continued*) Oral immunotherapy studies and reported adverse events

Author (reference number)	Food(s) (N)	Subjects	Starting dose	Time to maintenance/ maintenance dose	Adverse reactions/other comments
Skripak et al. 2008 [26]	Milk	*n* = 20; active to placebo 2:1 ratio	0.4 mg milk protein	Dose increase every 1–2 weeks, 12 mg minimum tolerated dose to proceed to home dosing; maximum dose 500 mg.	The median frequency of side effects was 35% in the active group compared with 1% in the placebo group.
Narisety et al. 2009 [27]	Milk	*n* = 15 Age: 6–16 years (follow-up of the Skripak study)	500 mg milk (median)	Dose increase by ≤50% every 2 weeks.	Adverse reactions were common and largely unpredictable, with several systemic reactions occurring at previously tolerated doses, often in the setting of exercise or viral illness. However, the overall rate of reactions decreased over time, even as milk doses increased.
Jones et al. 2009 [58]	Peanut	*n* = 29	0.1 mg peanut protein	Initial day escalation phase 0.1 mg peanut protein doubled every 30 minutes, up to 50 mg. Buildup phase: increase by 25 mg every 2 weeks, up to 300 mg.	Open-label study. Most symptoms noted during OIT resolved spontaneously or with antihistamines.
Hofmann et al. 2009 [66]	Peanut	*n* = 20			The probability of having any symptoms after a buildup phase dose was 46%, with a risk of 29% for skin symptoms. The risk of reaction with any home dose was 3.5%. Treatment was given for 0.7% of home doses. Two subjects received epinephrine after one home dose each.
Blumchen et al. 2010 [59]	Peanut	*n* = 23	OIT was started with approximately 1/100 of the eliciting reaction dose during the baseline DBPCFC; range 0.8–24 mg	14 patients required a median of 7 months (range 0–560 days) to reach their individual stable maintenance dose (0.5–2 g peanut) after the rush phase.	In 2.6% of 6137 total daily doses, mild to moderate side effects were observed; in 1.3%, lower respiratory symptoms occurred. OIT was discontinued in 4 of 22 (18%) patients because of adverse events. No epinephrine was used for treatment of adverse reactions.

(Continued)

Table 36.1 (*Continued*) Oral immunotherapy studies and reported adverse events

Author (reference number)	Food(s) (N)	Subjects	Starting dose	Time to maintenance/ maintenance dose	Adverse reactions/other comments
Varshney et al. 2011 [62]	Peanut	*n* = 28	0.1 mg peanut protein	Initial escalation day: 0.1–6 mg, subjects not tolerating 1.5 mg were withdrawn from the study; dose escalation lasted 44 weeks, maintenance phase lasted 1 month; the oral food challenge was done at 48 weeks.	During the initial escalation day, 9 (47%) of 19 peanut OIT subjects experienced clinically relevant side effects requiring antihistamine treatment. Of these, two were treated with epinephrine. One peanut OIT subject withdrew from the study after the first dose escalation because of mild gastrointestinal symptoms. No peanut OIT subjects needed epinephrine with home doses.
Anagnostou et al. 2011 [60]	Peanut	*n* = 22 (median age 11 years)		800 mg	Reactions, mostly mild, occurred in 86% during immunotherapy, adrenaline was not required. 12/22 (54%) required a transient dose reduction because of reactions possibly related to extrinsic factors: tiredness, infection, and exercise.
Keet et al. 2012 [11]	Milk	*n* = 30 Age: 6–17 years	0.0000017 mg	Children with CM allergy were randomized to SLIT alone or SLIT followed by OIT. SLIT initial escalation day: 0.0000017–0.07 mg. SLIT buildup phase: dose increased every 1–2 weeks up to 3.73 mg. SLIT/SLIT advanced to 7 g in two dose increases. SLIT/OIT advanced to 985 (OITB) or 1969 (OITA) in 14 dose increases.	The overall reaction rate was similar, but systemic reactions were more common during OIT than during SLIT. Six of 15 subjects who passed a full milk challenge after 60 weeks of maintenance lost desensitization within 6 weeks.

(Continued)

Table 36.1 (*Continued*) Oral immunotherapy studies and reported adverse events

Author (reference number)	Food(s) (N)	Subjects	Starting dose	Time to maintenance/maintenance dose	Adverse reactions/other comments
Burks et al. 2012 [42]	Egg	$n = 55$ Age: 5–11 years	0.1 mg raw egg white powder	Double-blind, randomized, placebo-controlled study, 40 children received OIT (maximum dose 2000 mg egg protein over 8–9 months) and 15 received placebo.	The rates of adverse events were highest during the first 10 months of oral immunotherapy. Adverse events, most of which were oral or pharyngeal, were associated with 25% of 11,860 doses of oral immunotherapy with egg and 3.9% of 4018 doses of placebo. After 10 months, the rate of symptoms in the oral-immunotherapy group decreased to 8.3% of 15,815 doses.
Vazquez-Ortiz et al. [29]	Milk	$n = 81$ Age: 5–18 years	1 mL of CM diluted 1/100 with water	Subjects were admitted to the hospital for 2–4 days for IDE. They then increased weekly to a maximum of 200 mL of CM.	Dose-related reactions occurred in 95% of children. 7.5% withdrew due to AEs. Salbutamol was administered in 54 children and epinephrine in 9. 12% of reactions occurred in the setting of cofactors. One patient was diagnosed with EoE after 3 weeks of OIT.
Anagnostou et al. 2014 [61]	Peanut	$n = 99$ (49 active, 50 control) Age: 7–16 years	2 mg of peanut protein	Randomized, placebo-controlled crossover trial. Maintenance goal of 800 mg/day.	During the first phase, 1 subject discontinued and 5 withdrew in the active group and 1 discontinued and 4 withdrew from the control group. Most side effects were mild (81% had oral pruritus, 57% abdominal pain, 33% nausea, 33% vomiting, 22% wheeze). One participant received epinephrine at home on two occasions and 18 (19%) were treated with an inhaled B2 agonist.
Vickery et al. 2014 [67]	Peanut	$n = 24$ Age: 1–16 years	Initial dose escalation dosing began at 0.1 mg and increased up to 50 mg	Open-label OIT, Up to 4000 mg for a maximum of 5 years.	Safety data not provided.

(Continued)

Table 36.1 (*Continued*) Oral immunotherapy studies and reported adverse events

Author (reference number)	Food(s) (N)	Subjects	Starting dose	Time to maintenance/maintenance dose	Adverse reactions/other comments
Narisety et al. 2014 [64]	Peanut	n = 20	SLIT: 0.000165 μg escalated on IDE to 0.066 μg OIT: 0.1 mg escalated on IDE to 6 mg	DBPC SLIT versus OIT; Goal maintenance of 3.7 mg/day (SLIT) and 2000 mg/day (OIT) of peanut protein.	Significantly more dosing-related adverse reactions in the OIT compared to the SLIT group (43% of doses compared to 9%). Most reactions were mild. All but one subject had at least one dosing-related AE. Antihistamines were used to treat symptoms in 40.9% of OIT doses and 23.1% of SLIT doses. Four subjects in the active OIT group required a total of five doses of epinephrine (one during buildup and four during maintenance).
Begin et al. 2014 [75]	Multifood versus peanut single food OIT	n = 40 (n = 25: multiple food OIT, median age 8) (n = 15: peanut OIT, median age 10)	0.1 mg	4000 mg per allergen.	Similar reaction rates between groups, which were mostly mild. Both groups had two severe reactions requiring epinephrine.
Begin et al. 2014 [20]	Multifood + omalizumab	n = 25 (median age 7 years)	On IDE, dosing began at 5 mg total food allergen divided equally between the included foods. On IDE, dosing then increased up to 1250 mg total protein	After 8 weeks' pretreatment with omalizumab, rush OIT for up to five allergens simultaneously. Subjects reached maintenance dose of 4000 mg protein per allergen at median of 18 weeks.	52% of subjects had symptoms during the IDE. All were mild. Reactions occurred with 5.3% of doses. 94% of reactions were mild. There was one severe reaction that required epinephrine (during home dosing).
Wood et al. 2015 [30]	Milk	n = 57 Age: 7–32 years Randomized 1:1 to omalizumab or placebo, plus open label milk OIT	0.07 mg milk Required to tolerate 2.1 mg at dosing visit #1	After 4 months of omalizumab/placebo, milk OIT was started with initial dose escalation up to 2.1 mg, followed by dose buildup over 22–40 weeks and then maintenance dosing through month 28 (minimum dose of 520 mg of milk protein, goal dose of 3300 mg).	Compared to the placebo group, the omalizumab group had decreased (1) adverse reactions, (2) doses with symptoms, and (3) dose-related reactions requiring treatment.

(Continued)

Table 36.1 (*Continued*) Oral immunotherapy studies and reported adverse events

Author (reference number)	Food(s) (N)	Subjects	Starting dose	Time to maintenance/maintenance dose	Adverse reactions/other comments
Jones et al. 2016 [43]	Egg	*n* = 40 Age: 5–18 years 22 subjects were on eOIT in years 3 and 4	Follow-up study to Burks et al. 2012 [42]	Maintenance dose of 2 g of egg protein continued for 4 years.	In years 3–4, 12/22 (54.5%) had symptoms with dosing (all mild). Subjects had a reduction in dosing symptoms after year 2 (median percent of doses per subject was 8% prior to year 2 and 0.2% after year 2). The most common symptoms were respiratory, skin, or GI. 1.9% of doses caused symptoms lasting >30 minutes during home dosing. No dosing-related symptoms required epinephrine.
Vickery et al. 2017 [38]	Peanut	*n* = 40 Age: 9–36 months		Double-blind two-dose trial. Subjects were randomized 1:1 to low dose (target maintenance dose of 300 mg peanut protein) or high dose (3000 mg peanut protein). The median duration of treatment was 29.1 months.	95% of subjects had at least one AE, of which 85% of these AEs were mild, 15% moderate, and none severe. Moderate AEs were more likely during buildup and in the low-dose group compared to the high-dose group. Two subjects withdrew due to persist GI AEs. One had resolution of abdominal pain after stopping OIT. The second who had "gastroesophageal reflux" before starting OIT, underwent an EGD that showed esophageal eosinophils that persisted even after stopping OIT. Epinephrine was administered once (at home).

(Continued)

Table 36.1 (*Continued*) Oral immunotherapy studies and reported adverse events

Author (reference number)	Food(s) (N)	Subjects	Starting dose	Time to maintenance/ maintenance dose	Adverse reactions/other comments
Bird et al. 2018 [39]	Peanut	n = 55 AR101 peanut powder = 29; Placebo = 26; Age: 4–26 years	0.5 mg	Randomized, DBPC phase 2 trial; maintenance dose: 300 mg/day.	Reactions were common, but 94% were mild. There was one treatment-related SAE treated with epinephrine. The most common dosing-related AE in both groups was GI symptoms. Six patients on peanut OIT (21%) withdrew, four due to recurrent GI symptoms. In one case, biopsies showed eosinophilic esophagitis. In all cases, GI symptoms resolved within 3 weeks of stopping OIT.
Andorf et al. 2018 [21]	Multifood (up to five foods)	n = 48 Age: 4–15 (n = 36: omalizumab arm) (n = 12: placebo arm)	5 mg food protein (1 mg of each food)	Randomized, DBPC phase 2 clinical trial; Randomized 3:1 to received omalizumab or placebo for 16 weeks. Multifood OIT weeks 8–36, with updosing to 2 g per food. Maintenance was reached as early as 12 weeks in the omalizumab group and 20 weeks in the placebo group.	All participants experienced at least one adverse event, but the per-participant percentage of OIT-associated AEs was significantly lower in the omalizumab group (27% versus 68%). No serious adverse events.

Note: Missing data not provided in that specific manuscript.
Abbreviations: AE, adverse event; BLG, beta-lactoglobulin; CM, cow's milk; CS, casein; DBPC, double blind, placebo controlled; DBPCFC, double-blind, placebo-controlled food challenge; EGD, esophagogastroduodenoscopy; GI, gastrointestinal; IDE, initial dose escalation; OIT, oral immunotherapy; SAE, serious adverse event; SLIT, sublingual immunotherapy; SPT, skin prick test.

Table 36.2 Safety data from milk oral immunotherapy trial of Skripak et al. [26]

	Active (*n* = 13)		Placebo (*n* = 7)		*p*-value
Doses per child, median (range)	177 (155–242)		171 (152–199)		0.05
Total doses	2437		1193		N/a
Symptom/treatment	Number (%) of total doses	% of doses with reaction/treatment per child, median (range)	Number (% of total doses)	% of doses with reaction/ treatment per child, median (range)	
Total reactions	1107 (45.4)	35 (1–95)	134 (11.2)	1 (0–53)	0.02
Local symptoms	870 (35.7)	16 (1–90)	104 (8.7)	1 (0–53)	0.006
Gastrointestinal	458 (18.7)	2 (0–93)	16 (1.3)	0 (0–3)	0.02
Lower respiratory	198 (8.1)	1 (0–82)	28 (2.3)	1 (0–12)	0.3
Skin	22 (0.9)	0 (0–8)	1 (0.1)	0 (0–1)	0.1
Multiple systems	29 (1.2)	1 (0–7)	0	0	0.01
Eczema flare	1 patient	n/a	1 patient	n/a	ns
Diphenhydramine	249 (10.2)	1 (0–58)	14 (1.1)	1 (0–6)	0.3
Albuterol	21 (0.9)	0 (0–4)	2 (0.2)	0 (0–1)	0.2
Epinephrine	4 (0.2)	0 (0–1)	0	0	0.1

participant's flare was managed with topical medications and oral antibiotics for a skin infection. The active group participant continued to have significant eczema despite aggressive management, which resulted in her early withdrawal from the study. In general, although reactions were common and all active-treated patients experienced at least one adverse event, nearly 90% of all acute reactions were transient and required no treatment. It is also important to note that reactions occurred sporadically at all dose levels, including during maintenance therapy at previously tolerated doses.

An open-label follow-up of the Skripak study was published by Narisety et al. [27]. Of note, all patients had reactions to at least some home doses, 17% of which (*N* = 2465, median 157 per subject) were associated with local reactions. Other reactions included gastrointestinal, 3.7%; respiratory, 0.9%; cutaneous, 8%; and multisystem, 5.8%. Treatment included diphenhydramine for 93 (3.8%), albuterol for 12 (0.5%), prednisone for 3 (0.1%), and epinephrine for 6 (0.2%; 4 subjects). The authors concluded that while the rate of reactions appeared to decrease over time for most subjects, reactions were common and largely unpredictable, with several systemic reactions occurring at previously tolerated doses, often with exercise or a viral illness. In addition, in one subject, apparent clinical reactivity to milk recurred, primarily manifesting as GI symptoms, suggesting the possibility of EoE that resolved with resumption of a strict milk avoidance diet.

Keet et al. performed the first direct comparison of milk OIT and milk SLIT in a randomized unblinded trial [11]. While OIT was more efficacious than SLIT in inducing milk desensitization, it was accompanied by more systemic side effects. Overall, reaction rates were similar, occurring with 29% of SLIT and 23% of OIT doses. However, compared with SLIT, OIT reactions were significantly more multisystem, involving the upper and lower respiratory and GI tracts, and required more rescue medication with β-agonists and antihistamines.

While not a direct adverse effect, it is important to note that desensitization with OIT is transient in many patients, especially after a period of avoidance. This was highlighted in a study by Keet illustrating that some subjects begin to lose protection within 1 week of discontinuing treatment [11]. This was confirmed by a longer-term follow-up study of participants from both the Skripak and Keet OIT trials [28]. In this study, 3–5 years after completing treatment, only 19% of subjects were consuming milk in an unrestricted fashion, 31% were consuming at least one serving/day but still were restricted, 28% consumed some uncooked milk but less than a serving/day, 6% had minimal milk or milk in a baked food only, and 16% were strictly avoiding milk. Twenty-two percent limited their consumption because of symptoms, and an additional 25% limited milk while exercising and 6% limited milk with an illness. Notably, some subjects who initially did well subsequently had increased symptoms that led to resumption of a strict milk avoidance diet. Several experienced repeated episodes of anaphylaxis after periods of apparent tolerance.

Vazquez-Ortiz et al. performed a prospective longitudinal study of cow's milk OIT in 81 children, age 5–18 years [29]. This study found that 95% of children experienced at least one dose-related reaction; 91% of reactions affected a single organ; 14 children (17.5%) had persistent reactions; and 6 children (7.5%) withdrew due to adverse events. These 20 children accounted for 78% of all reactions detected. Salbutamol was administered in 54 children and epinephrine in 9. Twelve percent of reactions occurred in the setting of cofactors, such as exercise, infection, emotional stress, asthma exacerbation, fasting, lying down, and tiredness. One patient was diagnosed with EoE by biopsy after 3 weeks of cow's milk OIT.

Wood et al. conducted the first double-blind, placebo-controlled trial of milk OIT with omalizumab or placebo [30]. There were no significant differences between the groups in regard to OIT efficacy (*p* = .18). However, the omalizumab group had significantly fewer doses with symptoms (2.1% versus 16.1%, $p = .005$) and dosing-related reactions that required treatment (0% versus 3.8%, $p = .0008$).

While severe reactions to milk OIT, as well as to other foods, are relatively uncommon, they can occur. While these reactions can occur in an unpredictable fashion and are not all preventable, some may be preventable by taking care to always exercise extreme caution in dose administration, especially during dose escalation. This is evidenced by one case report of life-threatening anaphylaxis in a patient during the dose-escalation phase of milk OIT, when dose escalation was continued despite a serious reaction that occurred earlier on the same day [31].

In all OIT studies to date, GI side effects occur in approximately 20% of participants on active therapy, and this is the most common reason for withdrawal from treatment [6,8]. The potential to induce, or possibly unmask, EoE via OIT is documented in studies for milk, egg, and peanut [26,29,32–40]. A 2014 systematic review reported the prevalence of biopsy-proven EoE after OIT was 2.7% (CI: 1.7 to 4%) [34]. In a prospective study of 128 children undergoing milk and/or egg OIT, primary eosinophilic GI disease was diagnosed in 8/128 children (6.25%), of which 6 had EoE, 1 had esophageal and duodenal disease, and 1 had esophageal and colon involvement [35]. Burk et al. reported two cases of EoE during peanut OIT despite treatment with omalizumab [33]. In an egg OIT study, one patient was diagnosed with EoE after developing acute symptoms of dyspepsia and solid food dysphagia 5 months after completing egg OIT [40]. In 2017, a literature review of 110 OIT studies of patients' milk, egg, or peanut allergy reported an overall rate of biopsy-proven EoE in 5.3% (egg, 4.2%; milk, 5.4%; and peanut, 5.2%) [37]. There were much higher rates of reported GI symptoms. It is important to recognize that chronic abdominal symptoms are common in patients undergoing OIT to egg, peanut, and milk and are overall the most common cause of treatment discontinuation. Furthermore, since most of these symptoms resolve with discontinuation of the OIT, endoscopies are usually not performed, and the true risk of EoE remains unknown.

36.2.2 Egg OIT

Egg OIT, as with milk OIT, appears to be effective in desensitizing most patients. Permanent tolerance occurs less frequently than desensitization but likely occurs at a higher rate in OIT-treated patients than in those who follow a strict elimination diet. A 2014 Cochrane database systematic review and meta-analysis analyzed four randomized, controlled trials of egg OIT in children [41]. Three studies used avoidance diet as a control, and one study used a placebo group. In the egg OIT groups ($n = 100$), 39% tolerated a full serving of egg compared to 11% of controls ($n = 67$) (RR 3.39, 95% CI: 1.74–6.62). During egg OIT, 69% of subjects reported mild to severe adverse events, and 5/100 (5%) required epinephrine.

These findings are best illustrated in a randomized trial of 55 children, aged 5–11 years (median age 7 years), who received either egg-white powder OIT with a maintenance dose goal of 2 g ($n = 40$) or placebo ($n = 15$) [42]. OIT was discontinued for 2 months in the children who passed the 22-month OFC. Eleven of 29 patients, or 27.5% of the original 40 on OIT, who underwent the OFC at 24 months passed, demonstrating sustained unresponsiveness. An open label long-term follow-up period of this cohort showed a benefit of longer therapy with 20/40 (50%) achieving sustaining unresponsiveness by year 4 [43].

Reports of adverse events in this important study reveal that no severe reactions were reported but that mild oropharyngeal symptoms were common, particularly during the first 10 months of escalating dosing (Table 36.3) [42]. Of the five children in the oral-immunotherapy group who withdrew within 5.5 months after beginning therapy, four did so because of chronic abdominal complaints and one because of an anxiety reaction. One additional child in the oral immunotherapy group withdrew secondary to an allergic reaction associated with dosing after the oral food challenge at 10 months but before the challenge at 22 months. The rates of all adverse events were highest during the first 10 months of OIT. Adverse events were associated with 25% of 11,860 doses of OIT with egg and 3.9% of 4018 doses of placebo. In the OIT group, 78%

Table 36.3 Symptoms with egg oral immunotherapy in the first 10 months of treatment [42]

| Visit type | Number of doses | Any symptom | Symptom type | | | | | | | Symptom severity | | |
			Oral/phary Only	Skin	Resp.	GI	Other	Persist >30 minutes	Treated	Mild	Moderate	Severe
Placebo												
Escalation	150	4.0	1.3	0.7	2.0	1.3	0.7	1.3	1.3	2.0	0.7	0.0
Clinic	235	6.0	0.4	1.3	3.8	0.4	0.9	0.0	0.0	5.5	0.0	0.0
Home	3633	3.7	0.2	0.7	2.4	0.3	0.8	1.4	0.5	3.6	0.0	0.0
All	4018	3.9	0.2	0.8	2.4	0.3	0.8	1.3	0.5	3.7	0.1	0.0
Egg OIT												
Escalation	347	27.4	13.8	8.1	9.8	9.5	3.5	8.4	7.2	16.7	3.7	0.0
Clinic	730	35.9	19.7	5.8	13.4	8.8	3.2	4.5	3.7	22.1	1.9	0.0
Home	10783	24.2	15.1	4.2	7.4	5.1	2.1	4.7	3.5	13.7	0.6	0.0
All	11860	25.0	15.4	4.4	7.8	5.5	2.2	4.8	3.6	14.3	0.7	0.0

Abbreviations: GI, gastrointesitnal; phary., pharyngeal; Resp, respiratory.

of children had oral or pharyngeal adverse events, compared with 20% of those in the placebo group ($p < .001$). After 10 months, the rate of adverse effects in the OIT group decreased to 8.3% of the 15,815 doses provided in this phase of the trial.

During the open-label follow-up study, 12/22 subjects (54.5%) receiving OIT in years 3 to 4 had symptoms with dosing, but all were classified as mild [43]. In these 22 subjects, the median percentage of doses per subject with any symptoms decreased after year 2 compared to before year 2 (0.2% versus 8%); 95% of doses were symptom-free. During years 3 and 4, no one required epinephrine for dosing-related symptoms; 1.6% of doses required treatment with antihistamines.

Another double-blind, placebo-controlled study randomized egg allergic children to OIT ($n = 17$) or placebo ($n = 14$) for 4 months [44]. In the egg OIT group, 16 achieved desensitization at 4 months compared to none in the placebo group. After a 3-month avoidance period, 5 of 16 (31%) in the egg OIT group achieved tolerance. Adverse events were reported in three subjects during the desensitization period, and one of these subjects discontinued. During the maintenance period, two subjects reported adverse events.

Similar findings are reported in several other studies, although most are just observational in nature [45–57]. In addition, in a randomized but open-label trial by Staden et al., egg OIT did not expedite the natural acquisition of tolerance [24]. Adverse events from these studies are summarized in Table 36.1.

36.2.3 Peanut OIT

Studies of OIT for peanut allergy demonstrate successful desensitization to peanut in most patients [38,39,58–64]. In one randomized trial, 28 children aged 1–16 years, received OIT with peanut flour ($n = 19$) or placebo ($n = 9$) [62]. Three in the treatment group dropped out due to allergic side effects. Double-blind, placebo-controlled food challenges (DBPCFCs) were performed approximately 1 year after the onset of treatment and 4 weeks after reaching maintenance therapy. All 16 subjects on peanut OIT tolerated the maximum total dose of 5000 mg of peanut protein, whereas the median dose reached by the placebo subjects was 280 mg.

Varshney et al. did a detailed analysis of adverse events associated with peanut OIT at Duke University and Arkansas Children's Hospital [65]. Adverse reactions were categorized as those occurring during the initial escalation day, the buildup phase, and the home dosing phase. Twenty of 28 patients between the ages of one and 16 years, who completed all phases of the study, were included. This study used a maintenance dose of just 300 mg of peanut protein, far lower than the 1000–2000 mg doses used in many subsequent studies. As summarized in Table 36.4, during the initial escalation day, upper respiratory (79%) and abdominal (68%) symptoms were most commonly experienced. The risk of mild wheezing during the initial escalation day was 18%. The probability of having any symptoms after a buildup phase dose was 46%, with a risk of 29% for upper respiratory and 24% for cutaneous symptoms. The risk of a reaction with any home dose was 3.5%, with upper respiratory (1.2%) and cutaneous (1.1%) symptoms being most common. Treatment was given with 0.7% of home doses, two of which included epinephrine. The authors conclude that subjects were more likely to have significant allergic symptoms during the initial escalation day when they were under close supervision rather than during other phases of the study and that allergic reactions with home doses are rare.

Table 36.4 Risk of symptom occurrence with peanut oral immunotherapy (with 95% confidence intervals) [62]

	Initial escalation day	Buildup phase	Home dosing
Any symptom	93% (77%, 99%)	46% (37%, 56%)	3.5% (2.3%, 5.1%)
Upper respiratory	79% (59%, 92%)	29% (20%, 41%)	1.2% (0.6%, 2.5%)
Skin	61% (41%, 79%)	24% (17%, 32%)	1.1% (0.7%, 1.8%)
Abdominal	68% (48%, 84%)	5.5% (3.2%, 9.2%)	0.9% (0.6%, 1.4%)
Chest	18% (6%, 37%)	1.7% (0.6%, 5.1%)	0.3% (0.1%, 0.4%)

An additional publication from the investigators at Duke and Arkansas also focused on adverse reactions to peanut OIT, using specific examples to highlight potential risk factors for adverse reactions and possible preventative strategies [66]. Five risk factors are described for patients who previously tolerated peanut OIT. These include (1) concurrent illness, (2) suboptimally controlled asthma, (3) timing of dose administration after food ingestion (fewer reactions when doses taken with food), (4) physical activity following dosing, and (5) dosing during menses. Based on these observations, they recommend (1) withholding OIT during acute illnesses and advising subjects to resume dosing at home only if fewer than three doses are missed. Otherwise, reinstitution of dosing should occur under observation. (2) They also recommend close monitoring of asthma with the regular use of peak flow and pulmonary function testing. (3) Because reactions were more common on an empty stomach, doses should be taken with food. (4) Exercise should be avoided for 2 hours following dosing, especially in children who have experienced such a reaction. (5) Although an association with menses was reported only in one subject, the severity of her reaction led to her withdrawal from the study, thus the admonition that concurrent menses is a possible risk factor.

Vickery et al. performed the first study to examine sustained unresponsiveness following peanut OIT [67]. This study included 24 patients aged 1–16 years who completed peanut OIT with a maintenance dose of 4000 mg for up to 5 years. Fifty percent of subjects demonstrated sustained unresponsiveness at a 5000 mg OFC 1 month after stopping OIT. Six of 39 subjects originally enrolled withdrew due to allergic side effects. More detailed adverse event data were not provided.

A more recent open-label study of peanut OIT randomized 40 children, aged 9–36 months, to low-dose (300 mg/day) or high-dose (3000 mg/day) peanut protein [38]. In the intent to treat analysis, 29 of 37 (78%) had sustained unresponsiveness 4 weeks after stopping treatment (300 mg arm: 17/20 [85%]; 3000 mg arm: 12/17 [71%]). AEs occurred in 95% of subjects at an average per-dose rate of 0.8%. AEs were more common during buildup, and symptoms mainly involved the upper airway and the GI tract. AEs were mild in 85%, moderate in 15%, and severe in 0%. Treatment was required in 25% of events, with most requiring only antihistamines and only one reaction requiring epinephrine. Two subjects withdrew due to persistent GI symptoms. In one subject, symptoms resolved with stopping OIT. In the second subject, symptoms persisted, and he was found to have more than 30 eos/hpf in the esophagus, which persisted on repeat endoscopy 3 months after stopping OIT.

The first phase 2, multicentered, randomized, double-blind, placebo-controlled trial of peanut oral immunotherapy was published in 2018 [39]. Subjects were randomized 1:1 to daily peanut OIT (AR101) or placebo and slowly upposed to a goal of 300 mg/day. At the exit DBPCFC, 79% of AR101 subjects tolerated ≥443 mg of peanut protein and 62% tolerated 1043 mg compared to 19% and 0% in the placebo group (both $p < .0001$). AEs that were possibly, probably, or definitely related to study product occurred in 93% (27/29) of peanut OIT subjects and 46% (12/26) of placebo subjects. In both groups, 94% or more of treatment-related AEs were graded as mild, and the most common AE was GI symptoms (AR101: 66%, placebo: 27%). One subject had anaphylaxis requiring epinephrine at home that occurred while playing basketball 16 hours after the dose. Six of the 29 (21%) AR101 subjects withdrew, primarily due to GI symptoms, and one of these subjects had biopsy-proven EoE that resolved with stopping OIT.

Two meta-analyses specifically addressing peanut OIT were published in 2012 (Table 36.5) [63,68]. Adverse reactions occur in all subjects treated with OIT, but most reactions are mild. In the intervention arm, 47% ($n = 9$) of subjects experienced clinically relevant adverse reactions during the initial-day escalation (none in the placebo arm), and clinically relevant symptoms occurred during the buildup phase after 1.2% of 407 buildup doses. Nine children (47%) receiving peanut OIT were treated with antihistamines during the initial-day escalation, and two required epinephrine, but no medication use was reported during the buildup dosing. None of the placebo subjects required treatment during initial-day escalation or buildup dosing. The investigators of the Cochrane report concluded that larger studies are needed prior to recommending the routine use of peanut OIT for people with peanut allergy [63].

In 2017, Virkud et al. performed a retrospective analysis of three peanut OIT studies, which included 104 children with peanut allergy [69]. At least one likely related AE occurred in 80% of subjects with a mean AE rate of 1.7% of dosing days. The rate of AEs and number of subjects affected by AEs decreased from buildup to maintenance. They found that 93% of all likely related AEs occurred at home. Overall, 85% of reactions were mild, 15% moderate, and 0% severe. There were 113 systemic reactions (10%). Fifty-one of the 104 children (49%) had GI symptoms at some point during treatment. The most common treatment was antihistamines, but 18 events required epinephrine administration (all occurred at home). They found that the presence of allergic rhinitis and the wheal size of the peanut skin prick test were the only significant predictors of AEs.

36.2.4 Wheat OIT

Compared to milk, egg, and peanut, there have only been a few clinical trials of wheat OIT. In 2005, Nucera et al. published the first successful OIT protocol in a 7-year-old female with a wheat allergy [70]. The subject underwent OIT up to 1.5 g of semolina three times per day, and then the protocol switched to pasta (1.2 g up to 49 g) three times per day. They report that she did not have any adverse reaction during either stage of the desensitization.

In 2014, Kusunoki published a case report of a 7-year-old boy who had two episodes of wheat-dependent exercise-induced anaphylaxis after successful treatment with OIT [71]. The child underwent desensitization during a 4-month hospital stay. He started with a dose of 1 g of noodles that was then increased 1.5-fold twice a week until he reached 100 g of noodles. He developed localized hives after the 2.7 and 22 g doses. He was discharged

Table 36.5 Examples of reactions during peanut oral immunotherapy (OIT) home dosing [63]

Subject	Age at reaction (months)	Pattern	Reaction	Dose	Length of time on OIT (months)	Length of time on dose	Baseline IgE (kU/L)	IgE at time of reaction	Treatment	Recommendations to subject
1	70	Fever	AE, LR	300 mg	12	5 months	23.6	13.9	H1, E, A	Hold dose if ill
2	131	Fever	AE, U, LR	1200 mg	19	3 months	>100	136.5	H1, E, CS, A	Hold dose if ill
3	38	Asthma	LR	300 mg	10	4 months	22.7	9.3	H1, A	Start inhaled CS
4	83	Empty stomach	U, LR, G	1800 mg	27	7 months	>100	115	H1, A	Take all doses with meal
5	102	Exertion	LR	2400 mg	49	2 months	58.3	4.7	H1, A	Avoid exercise for 2 hours after dose
6	99	Exertion	U, LR	3000 mg	47	2 days	73.1	7.3	H1, CS	Avoid exercise for 2 hours after dose; decrease dose to 2400 mg
7	145	Menses and exertion	AE, U, UR, LR, G	4000 mg	20	9 months	85.1	59.5	H1, E, CS	Discontinued participation in study after second occurrence

Abbreviations: A, albuterol; AE, angioedema; CS, corticosteroids; E, epinephrine; G, gastrointestinal; H1, antagonist; IgE, immunoglobulin E; LR, lower respiratory; U, urticaria; UR, upper respiratory.

home consuming regular intake of wheat-containing products. Two months later, he developed cough, wheezing, breathing difficulty, and hives while playing soccer after eating wheat. He was treated with epinephrine. He was advised to avoid exercise after eating wheat-containing foods; however, he had a similar reaction while running around at home after eating wheat bread for breakfast. He again received epinephrine. He was again advised to avoid eating wheat prior to exercise, and no further episodes were reported.

Rodríguez del Río et al. studied the safety and efficacy of wheat OIT and the impact of wheat OIT in the treatment of allergy to other gluten-containing cereals [72]. The protocol included an updosing phase that started with semolina porridge (0.0005 g up to 4 g) and then semolina pasta (8 g up to 100 g = 13 g of wheat protein), followed by maintenance phase. Seven children were enrolled (median age of 5.5 years). During updosing, adverse reactions occurred with 6.25% of doses. One patient discontinued the study and had recurrent abdominal pain. One patient had a reaction during maintenance, which was felt to be related to exercise and was treated with antihistamines and corticosteroids.

In 2015, Sato et al. investigated the efficacy of open-label wheat OIT in 18 subjects (median age of 9 years) with a history of wheat-induced anaphylaxis [73]. Eleven subjects (median age of 7 years) were selected as historical controls. The study had four phases: rush (5 days in the hospital), long-term buildup, maintenance, and 2 weeks of complete avoidance. During the rush phase, adverse reactions occurred with 42/143 (26.4%) of total doses, but none required epinephrine. Two subjects dropped out. Adverse events occurred after 486 of the 5778 (6.8%) total doses, and one reaction required epinephrine.

A more recent study was published in 2018 by Kulmala et al. [74]. One hundred wheat-allergic children aged 6–18 years were treated with OIT using well-cooked wheat spaghetti. Buildup occurred over 4 months with a goal maintenance dose of 2000 mg of wheat protein. All subjects were treated with daily antihistamines during the buildup phase. Subjects continued their wheat dose for 3 months (maintenance phase 1) and were then advised to eat wheat daily with no restrictions (maintenance phase 2). Of the 100 patients enrolled, 43% of subjects discontinued therapy at some point during the study. The majority of patients (94/100) had a reaction at some phase of the study. Overall, 34% were mild, 36% moderate, and 24% severe. The most common symptoms were oral itching, wheezing, and abdominal pain. The proportion of participants with symptoms was similar during all three phases of the study (buildup: 70% [43% were moderate or severe], maintenance phase 1: 78% [35% were moderate or severe], maintenance phase 2: 72% [24% were moderate or severe]). Physical activity 1–4 hours after dosing was a cofactor in 11 reactions. Epinephrine was used by 12 subjects a total of 13 times during the study.

36.2.5 Multifood OIT

In 2014, Begin et al. published a phase 1 study to evaluate the safety of a modified OIT to multiple allergens [75]. Twenty-five subjects (4–25 years) were treated with multiple food OIT, and 15 subjects (5–46 years) were treated with single food OIT. All subjects underwent (1) initial dose escalation (IDE), (2) home dosing with biweekly updosing, and (3) maintenance phase. There was no significant difference in reaction rate between those on multiple-food OIT compared to single-food OIT. During IDE, 60% of subjects in the multiple food OIT group had reactions compared to 40% in

the single-food OIT group (p = .22). Similarly, the median reaction rate during dose escalation and home dosing was 3.4% and 3.1% in the multiple-food OIT group compared to 3.7% and 2.9% in the single-food OIT group (p = .31 and .65, respectively). Most reactions in both groups were mild. Both groups had two severe reactions after home dosing that required epinephrine. All participants were advised to take cetirizine 1 hour prior to each dose.

The same group conducted a phase 1 trial of the safety of dose tolerability of rush OIT to multiple foods using omalizumab [20]. Subjects received omalizumab for 8 weeks, followed by rush OIT to up to five foods simultaneously. On IDE, the dosing scheduled was 5, 50, 150, 300, 625, 1250 mg total protein (250 mg/food for five allergens). Omalizumab was then continued for an additional 8 weeks following initial dose escalation. Subjects reached maintenance dose of 4000 mg protein per allergen at median of 18 weeks. Fifty-two percent of subjects had symptoms during the IDE. All were mild. Reactions occurred with 5.3% of doses (401/7530). Ninety-four percent of reactions were mild. There was one severe reaction that required epinephrine (during home maintenance dosing). Authors concluded that patients with multiple-food allergies could be safely and rapidly desensitized to multiple foods during 16 weeks of treatment with omalizumab plus rush OIT.

In 2018, Andorf et al. published a phase 2 DBPC trial of multiple-food OIT plus omalizumab or placebo [21]. Forty-eight patients were enrolled, 36 were randomized to omalizumab and 12 received placebo for 16 weeks. All subjects received multifood OIT with two to five foods starting at week 8. The omalizumab group had tolerated a significantly higher dose on IDE compared to the placebo group (250 mg per food versus 11 mg per food, p < .001). Similarly, maintenance was reached as early as 12 weeks in the omalizumab group and 20 weeks in the placebo group. A greater proportion of participants in the omalizumab group passed the 36 weeks DBPCFC to 2 g protein for two to five foods compared with the placebo group. All participants experienced at least one adverse event, but the per-participant percentage of OIT-associated AEs was significantly lower in the omalizumab group (27% versus 68%). No serious adverse events were reported.

36.3 CONCLUSION

Progress has been made in the area of food OIT. This fact does provide considerable optimism about its potential role for its routine use in clinical practice in the future. However, given the profile of adverse events outlined in this chapter, it is clear that the picture is not universally positive. Adverse events are common, sometimes severe, and certainly occur with greater frequency than in patients who simply follow a strict avoidance diet.

SALIENT POINTS

1. The rate and severity of adverse reactions with food oral immunotherapy (OIT) appear similar for the three main foods thus far studied, milk, egg, and peanut.
2. While acute severe reactions certainly draw the most obvious attention, the reader should recognize that the most common reasons that indicate the discontinuation of OIT are "chronic" side effects, most commonly abdominal pain, and the true risk of eosinophilic GI disease is still unknown.

3. No specific biomarkers—for example, baseline challenge results, specific IgE or IgG4 levels, or skin test size—can accurately predict adverse events or response to therapy.

4. The long-term outcomes of food OIT need careful, ongoing study. While many studies demonstrate loss of protection over a period of weeks upon completion of OIT, at least one study now demonstrates that even some patients who appeared to do well during and shortly after treatment regain considerable, sometimes anaphylactic, reactivity over the next several years. These patients may be at greatest risk in that they have a false sense of security about future reactions. All investigators remain hopeful that adverse events can be significantly reduced in the future with newer techniques and the coadministration of immunomodulators, such as anti-IgE.

5. In the end, a balance between risk/benefit will become clearer, primarily based on long-term outcomes. If long-term tolerance is achievable in a large number of patients, some adverse events may be justifiable. However, if reactions continue to occur after years of therapy, and the transient nature of the desensitization makes lifetime treatment necessary, the balance between risk/benefit becomes far less clear.

REFERENCES

1. Burks AW, Sampson HA, Plaut M, Lack G, Akdis CA. Treatment for food allergy. *J Allergy Clin Immunol* 2018; 141(1): 1–9.
2. Rachid R, Keet CA. Current status and unanswered questions for food allergy treatments. *J Allergy Clin Immunol Pract* 2018; 6(2): 377–382.
3. Cox L, Compalati E, Kundig T, Larche M. New directions in immunotherapy. *Curr Allergy Asthma Rep* 2013; 13(2): 178–195.
4. Burbank AJ, Sood P, Vickery BP, Wood RA. Oral immunotherapy for food allergy. *Immunol Allergy Clin North Am* 2016; 36(1): 55–69.
5. Wood RA. Food allergen immunotherapy: Current status and prospects for the future. *J Allergy Clin Immunol* 2016; 137(4): 973–982.
6. Wood RA. Oral immunotherapy for food allergy. *J Investig Allergol Clin Immunol* 2017; 27(3): 151–159.
7. Parrish CP, Har D, Andrew Bird J. Current status of potential therapies for IgE-mediated food allergy. *Curr Allergy Asthma Rep* 2018; 18(3): 18.
8. Scurlock AM, Jones SM. Advances in the approach to the patient with food allergy. *J Allergy Clin Immunol* 2018; 141(6): 2002–2014.
9. Nurmatov U, Dhami S, Arasi S et al. Allergen immunotherapy for IgE-mediated food allergy: A systematic review and meta-analysis. *Allergy* 2017; 72(8): 1133–1147.
10. Burks AW, Laubach S, Jones SM. Oral tolerance, food allergy, and immunotherapy: Implications for future treatment. *J Allergy Clin Immunol* 2008; 121(6): 1344–1350.
11. Keet CA, Frischmeyer-Guerrerio PA, Thyagarajan A et al. The safety and efficacy of sublingual and oral immunotherapy for milk allergy. *J Allergy Clin Immunol* 2012; 129(2): 448–455, 455.e1–5.
12. Kim EH, Bird JA, Kulis M et al. Sublingual immunotherapy for peanut allergy: Clinical and immunologic evidence of desensitization. *J Allergy Clin Immunol* 2011; 127(3): 640–646.e1.
13. Fleischer DM, Burks AW, Vickery BP et al. Sublingual immunotherapy for peanut allergy: A randomized, double-blind, placebo-controlled multicenter trial. *J Allergy Clin Immunol* 2013; 131(1): 119–127.e1–7.
14. Dantzer JA, Wood RA. The use of omalizumab in allergen immunotherapy. *Clin Exp Allergy* 2018; 48(3): 232–240.
15. Nadeau KC, Schneider LC, Hoyte L, Borras I, Umetsu DT. Rapid oral desensitization in combination with omalizumab therapy in patients with cow's milk allergy. *J Allergy Clin Immunol* 2011; 127(6): 1622–1624.
16. Wood RA, Kim JS, Lindblad R et al. A randomized, double-blind, placebo-controlled study of omalizumab combined with oral immunotherapy for the treatment of cow's milk allergy. *J Allergy Clin Immunol* 2016; 137(4): 1103–1110.e1–11.
17. Schneider LC, Rachid R, LeBovidge J, Blood E, Mittal M, Umetsu DT. A pilot study of omalizumab to facilitate rapid oral desensitization in high-risk peanut-allergic patients. *J Allergy Clin Immunol* 2013; 132(6): 1368–1374.
18. MacGinnitie AJ, Rachid R, Gragg H et al. Omalizumab facilitates rapid oral desensitization for peanut allergy. *J Allergy Clin Immunol* 2017; 139(3): 873–881.e8.
19. Lafuente I, Mazon A, Nieto M, Uixera S, Pina R, Nieto A. Possible recurrence of symptoms after discontinuation of omalizumab in anti-IgE-assisted desensitization to egg. *Pediatr Allergy Immunol* 2014; 25(7): 717–719.
20. Begin P, Dominguez T, Wilson SP et al. Phase 1 results of safety and tolerability in a rush oral immunotherapy protocol to multiple foods using Omalizumab. *Allergy Asthma Clin Immunol* 2014; 10(1): 7.
21. Andorf S, Purington N, Block WM et al. Anti-IgE treatment with oral immunotherapy in multifood allergic participants: A double-blind, randomised, controlled trial. *Lancet Gastroenterol Hepatol* 2018; 3(2): 85–94.
22. Martorell Calatayud C, Muriel Garcia A, Martorell Aragones A, De La Hoz Caballer B. Safety and efficacy profile and immunological changes associated with oral immunotherapy for IgE-mediated cow's milk allergy in children: Systematic review and meta-analysis. *J Investig Allergol Clin Immunol* 2014; 24(5): 298–307.
23. Brozek JL, Terracciano L, Hsu J et al. Oral immunotherapy for IgE-mediated cow's milk allergy: A systematic review and meta-analysis. *Clin Exp Allergy* 2012; 42(3): 363–374.
24. Staden U, Rolinck-Werninghaus C, Brewe F, Wahn U, Niggemann B, Beyer K. Specific oral tolerance induction in food allergy in children: Efficacy and clinical patterns of reaction. *Allergy* 2007; 62(11): 1261–1269.
25. Longo G, Barbi E, Berti I et al. Specific oral tolerance induction in children with very severe cow's milk-induced reactions. *J Allergy Clin Immunol* 2008; 121(2): 343–347.
26. Skripak JM, Nash SD, Rowley H et al. A randomized, double-blind, placebo-controlled study of milk oral immunotherapy for cow's milk allergy. *J Allergy Clin Immunol* 2008; 122(6): 1154–1160.
27. Narisety SD, Skripak JM, Steele P et al. Open-label maintenance after milk oral immunotherapy for IgE-mediated cow's milk allergy. *J Allergy Clin Immunol* 2009; 124(3): 610–612.
28. Keet CA, Seopaul S, Knorr S, Narisety S, Skripak J, Wood RA. Long-term follow-up of oral immunotherapy for cow's milk allergy. *J Allergy Clin Immunol* 2013; 132(3): 737–739.e6.
29. Vazquez-Ortiz M, Alvaro-Lozano M, Alsina L et al. Safety and predictors of adverse events during oral immunotherapy for milk allergy: Severity of reaction at oral challenge, specific IgE and prick test. *Clin Exp Allergy* 2013; 43(1): 92–102.
30. Wood RA, Kim JS, Lindblad R et al. A randomized, double-blind, placebo-controlled study of omalizumab combined with oral immunotherapy for the treatment of cow's milk allergy. *J Allergy Clin Immunol* 2016; 137(4): 1103–1110.

31. Nieto A, Fernandez-Silveira L, Mazon A, Caballero L. Life-threatening asthma reaction caused by desensitization to milk. *Allergy* 2010; 65(10): 1342–1343.

32. Sanchez-Garcia S, Rodriguez Del Rio P, Escudero C, Martinez-Gomez MJ, Ibanez MD. Possible eosinophilic esophagitis induced by milk oral immunotherapy. *J Allergy Clin Immunol* 2012; 129(4): 1155–1157.

33. Burk CM, Dellon ES, Steele PH et al. Eosinophilic esophagitis during peanut oral immunotherapy with omalizumab. *J Allergy Clin Immunol Pract* 2017; 5(2): 498–501.

34. Lucendo AJ, Arias A, Tenias JM. Relation between eosinophilic esophagitis and oral immunotherapy for food allergy: A systematic review with meta-analysis. *Ann Allergy Asthma Immunol* 2014; 113(6): 624–629.

35. Echeverria-Zudaire LA, Fernandez-Fernandez S, Rayo-Fernandez A, Munoz-Archidona C, Checa-Rodriguez R. Primary eosinophilic gastrointestinal disorders in children who have received food oral immunotherapy. *Allergol Immunopathol (Madr)* 2016; 44(6): 531–536.

36. Garcia Rodriguez R, Mendez Diaz Y, Moreno Lozano L, Extremera Ortega A, Gomez Torrijos E. Eosinophilic esophagitis after egg oral immunotherapy in an adult with egg-allergy and egg-bird syndrome. *J Investig Allergol Clin Immunol* 2017; 27(4): 266–267.

37. Petroni D, Spergel JM. Eosinophilic esophagitis and symptoms possibly related to eosinophilic esophagitis in oral immunotherapy. *Ann Allergy Asthma Immunol* 2018; 120(3): 237–240.e4.

38. Vickery BP, Berglund JP, Burk CM et al. Early oral immunotherapy in peanut-allergic preschool children is safe and highly effective. *J Allergy Clin Immunol* 2017; 139(1): 173–181.e8.

39. Bird JA, Spergel JM, Jones SM et al. Efficacy and safety of AR101 in oral immunotherapy for peanut allergy: Results of ARC001, a randomized, double-blind, placebo-controlled phase 2 clinical trial. *J Allergy Clin Immunol Pract* 2018; 6(2):476–485.e3.

40. Ridolo E, De Angelis GL, Dall'aglio P. Eosinophilic esophagitis after specific oral tolerance induction for egg protein. *Ann Allergy Asthma Immunol* 2011; 106(1): 73–74.

41. Romantsik O, Bruschettini M, Tosca MA, Zappettini S, Della Casa Alberighi O, Calevo MG. Oral and sublingual immunotherapy for egg allergy. *Cochrane Database Syst Rev* 2014; (11): CD010638.

42. Burks AW, Jones SM, Wood RA et al. Oral immunotherapy for treatment of egg allergy in children. *N Engl J Med* 2012; 367(3): 233–243.

43. Jones SM, Burks AW, Keet C et al. Long-term treatment with egg oral immunotherapy enhances sustained unresponsiveness that persists after cessation of therapy. *J Allergy Clin Immunol* 2016; 137(4): 1117–1127.e10.

44. Caminiti L, Pajno GB, Crisafulli G et al. Oral immunotherapy for egg allergy: A double-blind placebo-controlled study, with postdesensitization follow-up. *J Allergy Clin Immunol Pract* 2015; 3(4): 532–539.

45. Burks AW, Jones SM. Egg oral immunotherapy in non-anaphylactic children with egg allergy: Follow-up. *J Allergy Clin Immunol* 2008; 121(1): 270–271.

46. Buchanan AD, Green TD, Jones SM et al. Egg oral immunotherapy in nonanaphylactic children with egg allergy. *J Allergy Clin Immunol* 2007; 119(1): 199–205.

47. Vickery BP, Pons L, Kulis M, Steele P, Jones SM, Burks AW. Individualized IgE-based dosing of egg oral immunotherapy and the development of tolerance. *Ann Allergy Asthma Immunol* 2010; 105(6): 444–450.

48. Garcia Rodriguez R, Urra JM, Feo-Brito F et al. Oral rush desensitization to egg: Efficacy and safety. *Clin Exp Allergy* 2011; 41(9): 1289–1296.

49. Maeta A, Matsushima M, Muraki N et al. Low-dose oral immunotherapy using low-egg-allergen cookies for severe egg-allergic children reduces allergy severity and affects allergen-specific antibodies in serum. *Int Arch Allergy Immunol* 2018; 175(1–2): 70–76.

50. Dello Iacono I, Tripodi S, Calvani M, Panetta V, Verga MC, Miceli Sopo S. Specific oral tolerance induction with raw hen's egg in children with very severe egg allergy: A randomized controlled trial. *Pediatr Allergy Immunol* 2013; 24(1): 66–74.

51. Meglio P, Giampietro PG, Carello R, Gabriele I, Avitabile S, Galli E. Oral food desensitization in children with IgE-mediated hen's egg allergy: A new protocol with raw hen's egg. *Pediatr Allergy Immunol* 2013; 24(1): 75–83.

52. Fuentes-Aparicio V, Alvarez-Perea A, Infante S, Zapatero L, D'Oleo A, Alonso-Lebrero E. Specific oral tolerance induction in paediatric patients with persistent egg allergy. *Allergol Immunopathol (Madr)* 2013; 41(3): 143–150.

53. Patriarca C, Romano A, Venuti A et al. Oral specific hyposensitization in the management of patients allergic to food. *Allergol Immunopathol (Madr)* 1984; 12(4): 275–281.

54. Patriarca G, Schiavino D, Nucera E, Schinco G, Milani A, Gasbarrini GB. Food allergy in children: Results of a standardized protocol for oral desensitization. *Hepatogastroenterology* 1998; 45(19): 52–58.

55. Patriarca G, Nucera E, Roncallo C et al. Oral desensitizing treatment in food allergy: Clinical and immunological results. *Aliment Pharmacol Ther* 2003; 17(3): 459–465.

56. Meglio P, Bartone E, Plantamura M, Arabito E, Giampietro PG. A protocol for oral desensitization in children with IgE-mediated cow's milk allergy. *Allergy* 2004; 59(9): 980–987.

57. Morisset M, Moneret-Vautrin DA, Guenard L et al. Oral desensitization in children with milk and egg allergies obtains recovery in a significant proportion of cases. A randomized study in 60 children with cow's milk allergy and 90 children with egg allergy. *Eur Ann Allergy Clin Immunol* 2007; 39(1): 12–19.

58. Jones SM, Pons L, Roberts JL et al. Clinical efficacy and immune regulation with peanut oral immunotherapy. *J Allergy Clin Immunol* 2009; 124(2): 292–300, 300.e1–97.

59. Blumchen K, Ulbricht H, Staden U et al. Oral peanut immunotherapy in children with peanut anaphylaxis. *J Allergy Clin Immunol* 2010; 126(1): 83–91.e1.

60. Anagnostou K, Clark A, King Y, Islam S, Deighton J, Ewan P. Efficacy and safety of high-dose peanut oral immunotherapy with factors predicting outcome. *Clin Exp Allergy* 2011; 41(9): 1273–1281.

61. Anagnostou K, Islam S, King Y et al. Assessing the efficacy of oral immunotherapy for the desensitisation of peanut allergy in children (STOP II): A phase 2 randomised controlled trial. *Lancet* 2014; 383(9925): 1297–1304.

62. Varshney P, Jones SM, Scurlock AM et al. A randomized controlled study of peanut oral immunotherapy: Clinical desensitization and modulation of the allergic response. *J Allergy Clin Immunol* 2011; 127(3): 654–660.

63. Nurmatov U, Venderbosch I, Devereux G, Simons FE, Sheikh A. Allergen-specific oral immunotherapy for peanut allergy. *Cochrane Database Syst Rev* 2012; (9):CD009014.

64. Narisety SD, Frischmeyer-Guerrerio PA, Keet CA et al. A randomized, double-blind, placebo-controlled pilot study of sublingual versus oral immunotherapy for the treatment of peanut allergy. *J Allergy Clin Immunol* 2015;135(5):1275–1282.e1–6.

65. Varshney P, Steele PH, Vickery BP et al. Adverse reactions during peanut oral immunotherapy home dosing. *J Allergy Clin Immunol* 2009; 124(6): 1351–1352.

66. Hofmann AM, Scurlock AM, Jones SM et al. Safety of a peanut oral immunotherapy protocol in children with peanut allergy. *J Allergy Clin Immunol* 2009; 124(2): 286–291, 291.e1–6.

67. Vickery BP, Scurlock AM, Kulis M et al. Sustained unresponsiveness to peanut in subjects who have completed peanut oral immunotherapy. *J Allergy Clin Immunol* 2014; 133(2): 468–475.

68. Sheikh A, Nurmatov U, Venderbosch I, Bischoff E. Oral immunotherapy for the treatment of peanut allergy: systematic review of six case series studies. *Prim Care Respir J* 2012; 21(1): 41–49.

69. Virkud YV, Burks AW, Steele PH et al. Novel baseline predictors of adverse events during oral immunotherapy in children with peanut allergy. *J Allergy Clin Immunol* 2017; 139(3): 882–888.e5.

70. Nucera E, Pollastrini E, De Pasquale T et al. New protocol for desensitization to wheat allergy in a single case. *Dig Dis Sci* 2005; 50(9): 1708–1709.

71. Kusunoki T, Mukaida K, Hayashi A et al. A case of wheat-dependent exercise-induced anaphylaxis after specific oral immunotherapy. *J Investig Allergol Clin Immunol* 2014; 24(5): 358–359.

72. Rodriguez del Rio P, Diaz-Perales A, Sanchez-Garcia S et al. Oral immunotherapy in children with IgE-mediated wheat allergy: Outcome and molecular changes. *J Investig Allergol Clin Immunol* 2014; 24(4): 240–248.

73. Sato S, Utsunomiya T, Imai T et al. Wheat oral immunotherapy for wheat-induced anaphylaxis. *J Allergy Clin Immunol* 2015;136(4):1131–1133.e7.

74. Kulmala P, Pelkonen AS, Kuitunen M et al. Wheat oral immunotherapy was moderately successful but was associated with very frequent adverse events in children aged 6–18 years. *Acta Paediatr* 2018; 107(5): 861–870.

75. Begin P, Winterroth LC, Dominguez T et al. Safety and feasibility of oral immunotherapy to multiple allergens for food allergy. *Allergy Asthma Clin Immunol* 2014; 10(1): 1.

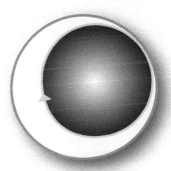

37 Instructions and consent forms for subcutaneous allergen immunotherapy

Shiven S. Patel
University of South Florida Morsani College of Medicine

Linda Cox
Nova Southeastern University

Richard F. Lockey
University of South Florida Morsani College of Medicine

CONTENTS

37.1 INTRODUCTION

The primary objective of allergy skin test and allergen immunotherapy (AIT) forms is to provide sufficient information to be universally interpreted by physicians and other healthcare professionals, regardless of their practice location or training program. The immunotherapy and allergy skin test forms also should be sufficiently detailed to enable all physicians to make treatment decisions.

The recommended information to be included on the forms is outlined in the American Academy of Allergy, Asthma and Immunology (AAAAI) and the American College of Allergy, Asthma, and Immunology (ACAAI) Joint Task Force on Practice Parameters (JTPP): "Allergen Immunotherapy: A Practice Parameter Third Update" (JAIPP). The purpose of these guidelines is to optimize the practice of clinical allergy through objective, scientific, and reproducible documentation and standardization of skin testing and immunotherapy procedures. The intended outcome is enhanced safety, accuracy, and efficacy of allergy diagnostic testing and allergy immunotherapy treatment.

This chapter reviews these guidelines and recommendations and includes examples of the standardized immunotherapy and allergy skin test forms developed by the AAAAI's Immunotherapy, Allergen Standardization and Allergy Diagnostic Testing Committee (ICOM) and the JTPP. The immunotherapy forms are provided as a courtesy of the AAAAI/ACAAI JTPP and are included in the JAIPP [1]. They can be downloaded from the AAAAI's website (http://www.aaaai.org/practice-resources/tools-and-technology/immunotherapy-forms.aspx). Examples of consent and instruction forms are also included on the AAAAI's website (https://www.aaaai.org). Patient instruction and consent forms are also available in Spanish.

The forms integrate the guidelines into editable documents. Physicians may use these forms as a template and customize them for their practice, while maintaining the basic information recommended in the published guidelines. Utilization of these forms will encourage uniformity of allergy skin testing and immunotherapy procedures and improve the safety and accuracy of allergy care. This will help facilitate continuity of patient care if there is a transfer or change that could potentially affect allergy services, such as a move to a new location, a new physician, or new nursing staff.

37.2 ALLERGY SKIN TEST FORMS

The use of immediate hypersensitivity (allergy) skin testing as a diagnostic tool in clinical allergy dates to the late 1800s with the work of Charles Blakely (1820–1900), an English physician and "hay fever" sufferer, who discovered that he could elicit a skin test response if he rubbed the pollen into his scratched skin [2]. Allergy skin testing continues to be the primary diagnostic tool for subjects with allergic diseases in most clinical practices. In AIT clinical trials, it is used both as a patient selection criteria and outcome assessment parameter. There is considerable variability in how allergy skin test results are performed and recorded [3]. This is likely because there have been, until recently, few guidelines aimed at ensuring that the clinical practice of allergy skin testing is uniform and consistent [4,5]. This variability in allergy skin test practices can adversely impact patient care, particularly individuals who may require a transfer of their allergy care. Physicians may have difficulty interpreting allergy skin test results performed in another facility and recommend the transferring patient undergo a repeat allergy evaluation. Guidelines to ensure a more uniform practice for allergy skin reporting were first developed by AAAAI's ICOM in 1999 [6]. Similar guidance was provided 14 years later in a position paper statement on skin prick tests developed as a collaborative effort of two international organizations, the Global Allergy and Asthma European Network (GA²LEN) and the Allergic Rhinitis and its Impact on Asthma (ARIA) [5]. The goal of both guidelines is to improve the quality of allergy skin testing and reduce undesirable variation by documenting the results in an objective, scientific, and reproducible manner.

The completed allergy skin test form should provide enough information to allow other physicians to understand the type of test and the manner in which it was performed. Many variables can potentially affect allergy skin test results and are included in the skin test form developed by the AAAAI's ICOM. These variables include location of the testing site [7], skin test device [8–10], combination of testing device and location [11], testing technician, patient's age [12], sun damage of the skin [12]. and medications [4,13]. These variables can influence the interpretation of the allergy skin test results. Therefore, it is important to include details about these variables on the allergy skin test form.

The key purpose of the allergy skin test report is to convey information about the test results. The skin test results should be recorded in a manner permitting other physicians to readily interpret the patient's positive and negative allergy skin test profile. The two most commonly used methods of reporting allergy skin test results are as follows:

Quantitative results are reported as measurement of the longest diameter of wheal and diameter of erythema/flare *or* the longest diameter and the widest perpendicular diameter (orthogonal) in millimeters. The mean wheal diameter and actual area can be calculated from these measurements. Studies demonstrate that both correlate with the longest diameter. The latter are not generally used in clinical practice, primarily because the calculation requires more time than simply recording a measurement.

Semiquantitative scoring is reported on a scale of 0 to 4+. The key to scoring must be included and must be based on measurement of wheal and flare.

One of the limitations of the semiquantitative scoring method is that it fails to provide specific information about the degree of skin test reactivity (i.e., a 4+ could represent a wide range of wheal sizes in many of the scoring systems). Reporting the skin test response in millimeters of the longest diameters of the wheal and erythema/flare may provide more specific information. The longest diameter of the skin test response correlated with the actual area in a study that compared computer-determined areas of 50 skin test responses with measured skin test responses [14]. The sums and products of orthogonal diameters also highly correlated with the actual areas but added little to the correlation of the longest diameter. This study also compared area and longest diameter measurements of prick skin test responses applied by different persons and found significant differences in the area measurements between testers, which were not found when longest diameter measurements were compared. Another study, comparing the mean and longest wheal diameters, determined that the longest wheal diameter was the optimal measurement for the evaluation of skin prick tests because it was a better surrogate marker of the wheal surface area in addition to being easier and faster to measure [15]. The AAAAI ICOM form recommends recording results as either the longest diameter or the longest diameter and its widest perpendicular diameter. Although the latter method is not superior to measuring the longest diameter alone, some prefer this additional measurement, because it may possibly identify an unusual response related to technique variation (e.g., a wheal of 10 mm by 2 mm caused by stroking the device along the skin instead downward prick/puncture).

There are some clinical implications associated with the degree of skin test reactivity that are pertinent to patients on AIT:

- High degree of skin test reactivity associated with greater risk during AIT [16,17]
- Starting dose of AIT may be based on skin test reactivity [1]
- Change in skin test reactivity with AIT may predict who is less likely to experience clinical relapse after discontinuing AIT, although this is controversial [18]

Recording the allergy skin test results as measurements of the wheal and erythema in millimeters will provide the physician with precise, reproducible information about the patient's degree of allergen sensitivity.

An objective test protocol for quality assurance should be used to assess the allergy skin test technician's testing proficiency. One suggested protocol for quality assurance and proficiency testing is to have the skin testing technician test 20 alternating positive and negative controls on the back (Figure 37.1a and b) [19]. The longest diameters of the wheal and the longest diameters of the erythema/flare should be measured and recorded in millimeters. The coefficient of variation, which is a measure of skin test reproducibility, can be calculated with the following formula: standard deviation of wheal divided by mean wheal diameter. Ideally, the coefficient of variation should be less than 30%.

The skin testing form should contain the information listed in the following sections.

37.2.1 Patient and prescribing physician information

1. Patient name, date of birth, and identifying number (if applicable)
2. Prescribing physician name, address, and telephone number
3. Testing date
4. Last time of administration of medications, which may affect the skin test response (e.g., antihistamines, psychotropic medications)

37.2.2 Allergy skin test methods

1. Skin test technician (the clinic should have documentation of the quality assurance evaluation of the skin test technician's proficiency with the device used for skin testing)
2. Location of test (e.g., back or arm)
3. Type of test (e.g., percutaneous and/or intradermal)
4. Instrument used (e.g., testing device, needle size, commercial kit)
5. Elapsed time between application and reading of tests
6. Amount injected with intradermal technique

37.2.3 Testing materials

1. Positive and negative controls
2. Manufacturing company or source of reagents
3. Common name (scientific name optional) of allergens
4. Concentration used in testing
5. Dilution and diluent where applicable
6. Contents, concentrations, and diluents of any mixtures

(a) **Suggested Proficiency Testing/Quality Assurance Technique for Skin Prick Testing**

- Using desired skin test device, perform skin testing with positive and negative controls in an alternate pattern on a subject's back (histamine 1–10 [10 mg/mL] and saline 1–10)

- Record histamine results at 8 minutes by outlining wheals with a felt-tip pen and transferring with transparent tape to a blank sheet of paper

- Record saline results at 15 minutes by outlining wheal and flares with a felt-tip pen and transferring results with transparent tape to a blank sheet of paper

- Calculate the mean diameter $X = (D + d)/2$; D = largest diameter and d = *perpendicular at midpoint of D*

- **Histamine**
  Calculate the mean and standard deviations of each mean wheal diameter
  Determine coefficient of variation = standard deviation/mean
  Quality standard should be less than 30%

- **Saline**
  All negative controls should be <3-mm wheals and <10-mm flares

(b)

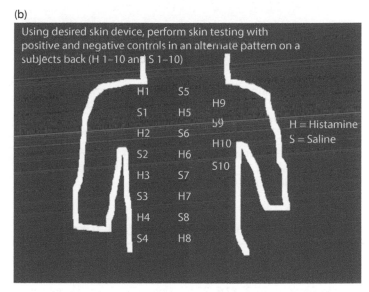

Figure 37.1 (a) Skin Test Proficiency Test. (b) Diagram of the layout of a skin test proficiency test. (From Oppenheimer J, Nelson HS. *Ann Allergy Asthma Immunol* 2006; 96: 19–23. With permission.)

37.2.4 Recording of results

The Joint Task Force's Allergy Diagnostics: A Practice Parameter summary statement addressing recording of skin test results states that "The peak reactivity of prick/puncture tests is 15 to 20 minutes at which time both wheal and erythema diameters (or areas) should be recorded in millimeters and compared with positive and negative controls" [4].

The AAAAI's ICOM skin test reporting guidelines, which were originally published in the *Academy News* [6] and currently are available on the AAAAI's website (https:// www.aaaai.org), also recommend recording results as the longest diameters of wheal and erythema/flare in millimeters or the longest diameter and its widest perpendicular diameter (e.g., longest diameter; wheal 5 mm erythema 10 mm, or longest diameter and widest perpendicular;

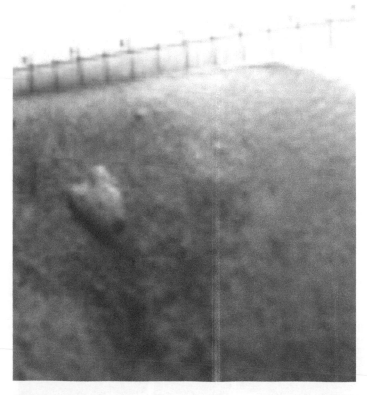

Figure 37.2 Recording skin test results by measuring the longest diameter wheal and surrounding erythema. (Provided with the permission of Linda Cox, MD.)

wheal 5/8 and erythema 10/10 mm). The GA²LEN-ARIA position statement on skin prick tests also recommends recording the longest wheal diameter (Figure 37.2).

37.2.5 Example of allergy skin test form

The following forms were developed by the AAAAI's ICOM and include the information recommended by its earlier published guidelines (see Sections 37.3, 37.6–37.10). Figure 37.3 is an example of a blank allergy skin test form.

37.3 ALLERGEN IMMUNOTHERAPY PRESCRIPTION FORMS

The AIT prescription form should provide specific information about the contents of the vaccine. Precise details are necessary for any other physician or healthcare professional to replicate the prescription without significant variation from the previous formulation, aside from known differences of lots and manufacturers. AIT vaccines differ when there are changes in the constituents of the mixture, including the diluent, manufacturer, and vaccine type (aqueous versus glycerinated) [1]. The AIT vaccine label is important and should contain sufficient details to allow physicians, other healthcare professionals, and the patient to recognize for whom the AIT vaccine is indicated as well as pertinent information about its content. The JAIPP has proposed a nomenclature system for labeling allergen

vaccine dilutions (Table 37.1; see Figures 37.4 and 37.5 that present examples of color-coded allergy immunotherapy vaccine vials and labels). Uniform adoption of this system should reduce errors in administration of AIT, particularly when administered outside of the prescribing physician's office.

Allergy immunotherapy prescription forms should contain the information that follows.

37.3.1 Patient information

1. Patient name and number (if applicable), birth date, telephone number, and picture (optional but helpful).

37.3.2 Preparation information

1. Name and signature of person preparing the vaccine
2. Date of preparation
3. Vial name

For example, a name could be "Trees and Grasses." If abbreviations are used, a legend should be included to describe the meanings of the abbreviations.

37.3.3 Allergen immunotherapy content information (information for each allergen should be included on the form in a separate column)

1. Content of the allergen extract including common name or genus and species of individual allergens and detail of all mixes
2. Concentration of manufacturer's extract
3. Volume of manufacturer's extract to add to achieve a selected volume of the projected effective concentration

This can be calculated by dividing the projected effective concentration by the concentration of the available manufacturer's extract and multiplying by the selected volume. For example, the effective dosing range for cat is between 1000 and 4000 BAU (bioequivalent allergen unit). To deliver 2000 BAU in a 0.5 mL maintenance injection, the following formula $V1 \times C1 = V2 \times C2$, is used, where

V1 = 5 mL	Final volume you want to prepare
C1 = 4000 BAU/mL	Concentration you want to prepare
V2 = Unknown	Volume of extract you will need for dilution
C2 = 10,000 BAU	Concentration of extract you will use
Add values into formula:	
V1 × C1 = V2 × C2	5 × 4000 = V2 × 10,000
V2 = (V1 × C1)/C2	V2 = 20,000/10,000 = 2 mL cat extract
To determine amount of diluent needed:	
V1–V2	5–2 = 3 mL of diluent

Source: Adapted from Table II in Cox L et al. *J Allergy Clin Immunol* 2011; 127: S1–55.

(a)
Allergy Skin Test Report Form

Practice name:	Ordering physician:		
Street address	City	State	Zip
Telephone	Fax		

Patient name: _____ Date of birth: __/__/__ Patient number: _____

Testing Technician: _____

Last use of antihistamine (or other med affecting response to histamine): ___ days

Were any medications known to interfere with test? Yes or No   List if necessary: _____

Testing Date (s) and Time: Percutaneous   /   /   AM PM Intradermal   /   /   AM PM

1) **General information about skin test protocol**
   - ☐ **Percutaneous** reported as: **Allergen: Testing concentration: Extract company** (*see below)
     - o **Location**: back___ arm___ **Device**: _____
   - ☐ **Intradermal**: 0.__ml injected, **Testing concentration**: _____ w/v, BAU, AU/ml, PNU (circle one)
2) **Results:** record longest diameter **or** longest diameter and orthogonal diameter (perpendicular diameters) of wheal (W) and erythema (flare) (F) measured in millimeters at 15-20 minutes
   ND or blank in results column indicates test was not performed, 0=negative

* Extract manufacturer abbreviations: G=Greer, AL=Allergy Labs, Ohio, LO Allergy Labs, Oklahoma, AK=ALK, HS=Hollister–Stier, , NE=Nelco, AM=Allermed, AT=Antigen Labs

Allergen: Concentration: Extract Manufacturer. *	Percutaneous W (mm) F	Intradermal W (mm) F	Allergen: Concentration: Extract Manufacturer. *	Percutaneous W (mm) F	Intradermal W (mm) F
			Controls		
			Percutaneous		
			Negative:		
			Positive:		
			Intradermal		
			Negative		
			Positive:		

Interpretation:

Figure 37.3 (a and b) An example of an allergy skin test form. (Reprinted with permission from the American Academy of Allergy, Asthma & Immunology. Visit https://www.AAAAI.org for additional information and updates.) *(Continued)*

(b)

> **Dr. Ah Choo, M.D.**
> **Address: 665 Rosebud Lane**
> **Hollywood, Fl. 33424**
> **Telephone: 645-123-4444 Fax: 645-123-4567**

Patient name: Jerry Cleanex   **Date of birth:** 05/05/90   **Patient number:** 23456
Testing Technician: Mary Lancet
Last use of antihistamine (or other med affecting response to histamine): 10 days ago **Medication**: cetirizine
Testing Date (s) and Time: Percutaneous 5/30/10_ 10:30_AM   **Intradermal** 6/2/02 11:15 AM

3) **General information about skin test protocol**
   - ☐ **Percutaneous** reported as: **Allergen: Testing concentration: Extract compan**y (*see below)
     - o **Location**: back_x__arm___   **Device**: Quintip
   - ☐ **Intradermal**: 0.2_ml injected, **Testing concentration**: 1:1000_w/v or 100 BAU or AU/ml, PNU
4) **Results:** record longest diameter **or** longest diameter and orthogonal diameter (perpendicular diameters) of wheal (W) and erythema (flare) (F) measured in millimeters at 15 minutes
   ND or blank in results column indicates test was not performed, 0=negative
* Extract manufacturer abbreviations: G=Greer, AL=Allergy Labs, Ohio, LO Allergy Labs, Oklahoma, AK=ALK, HS=Hollister–Stier, , N=Nelco, AM=Allermed, AT=Antigen Labs

Allergen: Concentration: Extract Manufacturer. *	Percutaneous W (mm) F		Intradermal W (mm) F		Allergen: Concentration: Extract Manufacturer. *	Percutaneous W (mm) F		Intradermal W (mm) F	
Trees					**Weeds**				
Ulmaceae					*Composite family*				
1. American Elm 1:20 G	0	0			20. Mugwort 10,000 PNU AD	4/6	18/15		
Cupressaceae					21. Short Ragweed 1:10 H	10/6	20/20		
2. Mountain Cedar 1:10 AL	0	0			*Chenopod*				
Betulaceae					22. Russian Thistle 1:20 AG	3/7	10/15		
3. Paper Birch 1:20 AK	3	15			23. Burning Bush 20,000 PNU N	4/6	15/20		
4. Red Alder 1:20 AD	3	10			24. Lamb's Quarter 1:40 AM	6/10	15/20		
Fagaceae					*Amaranth*				
5. Red oak 1:10 H	0	0	10	20	25. Red Root Pigweed G	8/10	20/30		
Aceraceae					*Plantaginaceae*				
6. Box Elder 1:20 N	0	0			26. English Plantain AK	10/9	20/18		
Oleaceae					**Molds/Fungi**				
7. White Ash 1:20 AM	0	0			27. Alternaria alternata AD	10/9	20/18		
8. Olive 1:20 G	5	20			28. Cladosporium herbarum H	0	0	15/18	25/20
Salicaciae					29. Penicillium chrysogenum N	4/5	15/10		
9. Cottonwood Eastern 1:40 AL	6	25			30. Aspergillus fumigatus AM	5/7	20/16		
Moraceae					31. Epicoccum nigrum G	0	0		
10. Mulberry 1:20 AK	7	30			32. Helminthosporium solani AL	0	0		
Juglandaceae					33. Penicillium chrysogenum N	4/5	15/10		
11. Pecan 1:20 AD	0	0							
12. Black Walnut 1:20 H	0	0			**Animals/Mites /Cockroach/Others**				
Plantaceae					34. D. Pteronyssinus AK	20/30	40/30		
13. Sycamore 1:40 AG	0	0			35. D. Farinae AD	15/9	32/40		
Aceraceae					36. American Cockroach H	5/6	12/10		
					37. German Cockroach AG	7	18		
Grasses					38. Cat hair G	15	30		
14. Bahia 1:20 N	20	40			39. AP Dog hair &dander 1:100 HS	5	20		
15. Bermuda 10,000 BAU/ml AM	15	35			**Controls**				
16. Sweet Vernal 1:20 G	25	40			**Percutaneous**				
17. Timothy 100,000BAU/ml AL	30	45			**Negative:** 50% glycerine-saline G	0	0		
18. Johnson 1:10 AK	15	30			**Positive:** Histamine 10mg/ml HS	5/7	20/15		
Weeds					*Intradermal*				
Polygonaceae					**Negative:** 0.05 % glycerine-saline AK			0	7/8
19. Sheep sorrel H	4/9	15/12			**Positive:** Histamine 0.1mg/ml AK			15/20	25/15
Interpretation:									

Figure 37.3 (Continued) (a and b) An example of an allergy skin test form. (Reprinted with permission from the American Academy of Allergy, Asthma & Immunology. Visit https://www.AAAAI.org for additional information and updates.)

Table 37.1 Suggested nomenclature for labeling AIT extract dilutions

Dilution from maintenance concentrate	V/V[a] label	Number[b]	Color
Maintenance concentrate	1:1	1	Red
10-fold	1:10	2	Yellow
100-fold	1:100	3	Blue
1000-fold	1:1000	4	Green
10,000-fold	1:10,000	5	Silver

Source: Based on the system proposed by the JAIPP.

[a] V/V refers to volume per volume dilution with 1:1 being the maintenance concentrate and subsequent dilutions based on the maintenance concentrate.

[b] It is recommended that the numbering system begin with the highest concentration, the maintenance concentrate. This will provide consistency in labeling in the event a greater number of dilutions are needed.

4. The type of diluent (if used)
5. Extract/vaccine manufacturer
6. Lot number
7. Expiration date (This date should not be later than the expiration date of any of the individual components.)

37.3.4 Example of an allergen immunotherapy prescription form

The AAAAI's ICOM developed standardized forms for AIT prescription writing. These forms are included in the JAIPP third update and can be found on the AAAAI website (https://www.aaaai.org). The different forms included can be used for buildup and maintenance phases of immunotherapy and to document the components of any mixes used in the vaccine and would accompany the primary AIT prescription (Figure 37.6). The latter includes a section to document subsequent dilutions from the maintenance concentration.

37.4 ALLERGEN IMMUNOTHERAPY ADMINISTRATION FORMS

The fundamental purpose of the AIT administration form is to provide enough information to enable physicians and other healthcare personnel to know precisely the prior dosing and to furnish a detailed record of the patient's AIT history to include the following:

- A record of any systemic allergic reactions (SARs) and treatment administered
- Other adverse reactions encountered during AIT such as large local reactions

Several risk factors for AIT have been identified and include symptomatic asthma [20], high degree of hypersensitivity [16,17,21], use of β-blockers, dosing errors, and injections given during periods of symptom exacerbation [21–23]. With the exception of dosing errors and high degree of hypersensitivity, these risk factors can be minimized with a preinjection health screen prior to the administration of the allergy vaccine [23]. This preinjection evaluation may include a peak flow measurement for asthmatic patients and a health inquiry administered verbally or as a written questionnaire. The health inquiry is to determine if there were any recent health changes that may require modifying or withholding that patient's AIT (e.g., the addition of a β-blocker medication to treat hypertension). Although a possible risk factor, β-blocker use may not require increased doses of epinephrine for anaphylaxis [24]. The AIT administration form is used to document an evaluation of the patient's health status prior to administering the allergy injection. The form was created by the AAAAI's ICOM and is based on the recommendations of the JAIPP. The information recommended on an AIT administration form is summarized in the next sections.

37.5 SUMMARY POINTS OF ALLERGEN IMMUNOTHERAPY ADMINISTRATION FORMS

37.5.1 Patient information

1. Patient name, date of birth, telephone number, patient picture (optional but helpful)

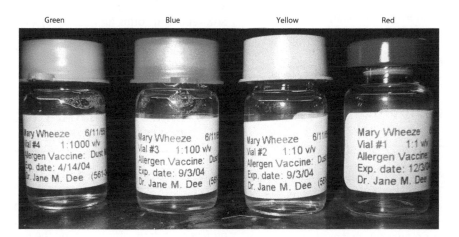

Figure 37.4 Color-coded labeled allergen immunotherapy vaccines with dilutions from maintenance concentrates.

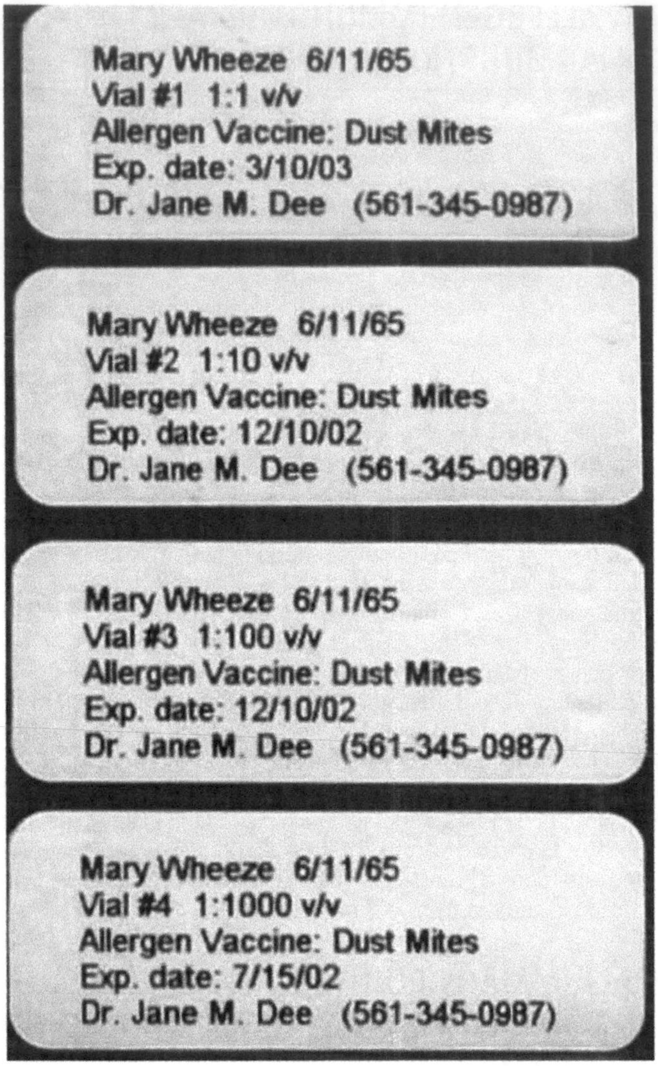

Mary Wheeze 6/11/65
Vial #1 1:1 v/v
Allergen Vaccine: Dust Mites
Exp. date: 3/10/03
Dr. Jane M. Dee   (561-345-0987)

Mary Wheeze 6/11/65
Vial #2 1:10 v/v
Allergen Vaccine: Dust Mites
Exp. date: 12/10/02
Dr. Jane M. Dee   (561-345-0987)

Mary Wheeze 6/11/65
Vial #3 1:100 v/v
Allergen Vaccine: Dust Mites
Exp. date: 12/10/02
Dr. Jane M. Dee   (561-345-0987)

Mary Wheeze 6/11/65
Vial #4 1:1000 v/v
Allergen Vaccine: Dust Mites
Exp. date: 7/15/02
Dr. Jane M. Dee   (561-345-0987)

Figure 37.5 Example of a completed allergen extract label.

37.5.2 Allergy immunotherapy extract information

1. AIT vaccine name and dilution from maintenance concentrate in volume per volume (Table 37.1), vial letter (e.g., A, B), color, or number if used
2. Expiration date of all dilutions

37.5.3 Administration information in separate columns

1. Date of injection.
2. Patient's health prior to injection. This is obtained via a verbal or written interview of the patient prior to administering the AIT injection. Among other issues, the patient is questioned about increased asthma or allergy symptoms, β-blocker use, change in health status (including pregnancy), or an adverse reaction to previous injection (including delayed large local reactions).

Patients with a significant systemic illness, such as influenza, usually should not receive an allergy injection.
3. Antihistamine use. There have been very few studies that have investigated the effect of premedication on conventional AIT buildup schedules. One concern is that antihistamines taken prior to each injection during a conventional AIT buildup might mask a minor reaction that would otherwise alert a physician to an impending SAR. However, one randomized-controlled study demonstrated that premedication with fexofenadine reduced the frequency of severe SARs during a conventional AIT buildup as well as increased the proportion of patients who achieved the target maintenance dose [25].

The JAIPP suggests noting if the patient is taking an antihistamine in order to consistently interpret reactions. It may also be desirable for a patient to be consistent and either take or not take an antihistamine on the day the patient receives his or her injection. The AIT administration form is a means by which antihistamine use is documented and reflects specific instructions from the treating physician about an antihistamine on injection days.
4. Peak flow reading. Symptomatic asthma is a risk factor for AIT [16,21,22]. Obtaining a peak flow measurement prior to the AIT injection may help screen patients with active asthma who should not receive their AIT injection on that day. The form should provide the patient's best peak flow baseline as a reference, and the healthcare professional giving the injection should be provided with specific guidelines about the degree of diminished peak flow for which an injection should be withheld.
5. Baseline blood pressure. It is desirable to record the patient's baseline blood pressure for future reference.
6. Arm administered. Noting into which arm each vaccine is injected facilitates identification of the cause of a large local reaction.
7. Projected buildup schedule
8. Delivered volume reported in milliliters
9. Injection reaction. The details of any treatment given in response to either an SAR or large local reaction should be documented on the health screen (second page of the administration form) or elsewhere in the medical record and referenced on the administration form.

The initials of the individual who gives the injection should be included. The AIT administration forms were developed as two-part forms (Figures 37.7 and 37.8) and are included in the JAIPP. Figures 37.9 and 37.10 present the pre-AIT injection questionnaire and the SAR reporting forms (developed by the AAAAI's Immunotherapy and Anaphylaxis Committee). The SAR reporting form uses the World Allergy Organization Grading System for classifying systemic reactions (Figure 37.11) [6].

37.6 IMMUNOTHERAPY INSTRUCTION AND CONSENT FORMS

37.6.1 Instruction forms

There are two types of instruction forms pertinent to AIT treatment. One form is designed to instruct physicians and other healthcare professionals from offices outside the prescribing allergist's office if the patient transfers his or her AIT treatment. The other is directed

Patient Name:
Patient Number:
Birth Date:
Telephone:

Prescribing physician:
Address:

Telephone:
Fax:

Allergen Extract Content:

Maintenance Concentrate Prescription Form

Bottle Name Abbreviations

Tree: T	Mold: M
Grass: G	Cat: C
Weed: W	Dog: D
Ragweed: R	Cockroach: Cr
Mixture: Mx	Dust Mite: Dm

* Components of mixes listed on a separate sheet

Antigen Number	Extract Name Allergen or Diluent (Common name or *Genus ,species*)*	Concentration and Type of Manufacturer's Extract (AU, BAU, W/V, PNU)/ (50% G, Aq, Ly, AP, AL)	Volume of Manufacturer's Extract to Add	Extract Manufacturer	Lot Number	Expiration Date
1						
2						
3						
4						
5						
6						
7						
8						
9						
10						
Diluent						
Total Volume						

Specific Instructions:

_____

_____

_____

$$\text{Volume to add} = \frac{\text{Maintenance Concentration}}{\text{Conc. of Manufacturer's Extract}} \times \text{Total volume volume*}$$

Maintenance concentration and subsequent dilutions reported as volume/volume (v/v) dilutions with maintenance concentration=1:1 v/v

BAU = Bioeqivalent Allergy Unit, AU =Allergy Unit
PNU=Protein Nitrogen Unit
W/V=Weight per Volume Ratio
G= 50 % Glycerinated
Aq=Aqueous, Ly=Lyophilized
AL= Alum precipitated, AP= Acetone precipitated

Prepared by:_____ **Date Prepared:**_____/_____/_____

Figure 37.6 Example of a completed allergen immunotherapy prescription. (Reprinted with permission from the American Academy of Allergy, Asthma & Immunology. Visit https://www.AAAAI.org for additional information and updates.)

Allergen Immunotherapy Administration Form

Patient Name:	Date of Birth:	Prescribing Physician:
Patient Number:		Address:
Telephone Number:	Diagnosis:	Telephone: Fax:

Dilution	1:10,000 (v/v)	1:1000 (v/v)	1:100 (v/v)	1:10 (v/v)	Maintenance	Immunotherapy A B
Color	Silver	Green	Blue	Yellow	1:1 (v/v) Red	Date started
Vial number	5	4	3	2	1	Date maintenance
Expiration date(s)	__/__/__	__/__/__	__/__/__	__/__/__	__/__/__	dose reached
						Maintenance dose
						Maintenance interval

Best Baseline Peak Flow: _____
Baseline Blood pressure: _____

Allergen extract: _contents_

	Date	Time	Health screen abnormal[1]	Anti-histamine taken?[2] or premedication	Peak Flow	Arm	Vial Number or Dilution	Delivered Volume	Reaction [3]	Injector Initials
1.	/ /		Y N	Y N	____	R L	_____	_____	_____	_____
2.	/ /		Y N	Y N	____	R L	_____	_____	_____	_____
3.	/ /		Y N	Y N	____	R L	_____	_____	_____	_____
4.	/ /		Y N	Y N	____	R L	_____	_____	_____	_____
5.	/ /		Y N	Y N	____	R L	_____	_____	_____	_____
6.	/ /		Y N	Y N	____	R L	_____	_____	_____	_____
7.	/ /		Y N	Y N	____	R L	_____	_____	_____	_____
8.	/ /		Y N	Y N	____	R L	_____	_____	_____	_____
9.	/ /		Y N	Y N	____	R L	_____	_____	_____	_____
10.	/ /		Y N	Y N	____	R L	_____	_____	_____	_____
11.	/ /		Y N	Y N	____	R L	_____	_____	_____	_____
12.	/ /		Y N	Y N	____	R L	_____	_____	_____	_____
13.	/ /		Y N	Y N	____	R L	_____	_____	_____	_____
14.	/ /		Y N	Y N	____	R L	_____	_____	_____	_____
15.	/ /		Y N	Y N	____	R L	_____	_____	_____	_____
16.	/ /		Y N	Y N	____	R L	_____	_____	_____	_____
17.	/ /		Y N	Y N	____	R L	_____	_____	_____	_____
18.	/ /		Y N	Y N	____	R L	_____	_____	_____	_____
19.	/ /		Y N	Y N	____	R L	_____	_____	_____	_____
20.	/ /		Y N	Y N	____	R L	_____	_____	_____	_____
21.	/ /		Y N	Y N	____	R L	_____	_____	_____	_____
22.	/ /		Y N	Y N	____	R L	_____	_____	_____	_____
23.	/ /		Y N	Y N	____	R L	_____	_____	_____	_____
24.	/ /		Y N	Y N	____	R L	_____	_____	_____	_____

1. Health screen refers to either a written or verbal interview of the patient prior to the administration of the allergy injection regarding: the presence of increased asthma symptoms or symptoms of respiratory tract infection, beta-blocker use, change in health status (including pregnancy) or adverse reaction to previous injection. A yes answer to this health screen may require further evaluation (see health screen record on back page).

2. Antihistamine use: to improve consistency in interpretation of reactions it should be noted if the patient has taken an antihistamine on injection days. Physician may also request that antihistamines be taken consistently on injection days: recommended: Y N

3. Reaction: refers to either immediate or delayed systemic or local reactions. Local reactions (noted as LR) can be reported in millimeters as the longest diameter of wheal and erythema. The details of the symptoms and treatment of a systemic reaction (noted as SR) would be recorded elsewhere in the medical record.

Injector signature	Initials	Projected Buildup Schedule				
		Vial 5	Vial 4	Vial 3	Vial 2	Vial 1

Date to reorder: __/__/____

Figure 37.7 Allergen immunotherapy administration. (Reprinted with permission from the American Academy of Allergy, Asthma & Immunology. Visit https://www.AAAAI.org for additional information and updates.)

Health Screen Record

Patient name:_____ Date of birth:_____ Patient number:_____

Health Screen Record

1. Date of immunotherapy injection visit: __/__/___
Patient's response to pre-injection screening questions: _____

Staff action taken (if any): _____

2. Date of immunotherapy injection visit: __/__/___
Patient's response to pre-injection screening questions: _____

Staff action taken (if any): _____

3. Date of immunotherapy injection visit: __/__/___
Patient's response to pre-injection screening questions: _____

Staff action taken (if any): _____

4. Date of immunotherapy injection visit: __/__/___
Patient's response to pre-injection screening questions: _____

Staff action taken (if any): _____

5. Date of immunotherapy injection visit: __/__/___
Patient's response to pre-injection screening questions: _____

Staff action taken (if any): _____

6. Date of immunotherapy injection visit: __/__/___
Patient's response to pre-injection screening questions: _____

Staff action taken (if any): _____

7. Date of immunotherapy injection visit: __/__/___
Patient's response to pre-injection screening questions: _____

Staff action taken (if any): _____

8. Date of immunotherapy injection visit: __/__/___
Patient's response to pre-injection screening questions: _____

Staff action taken (if any): _____

9. Date of immunotherapy injection visit: __/__/___
Patient's response to pre-injection screening questions: _____

Staff action taken (if any) : _____

10. Date of immunotherapy injection visit: __/__/___
Patient's response to pre-injection screening questions: _____

Staff action taken (if any): _____

11. Date of immunotherapy injection visit: __/__/___
Patient's response to pre-injection screening questions: _____

Staff action taken (if any): _____

12. Date of immunotherapy injection visit: __/__/___
Patient's response to pre-injection screening questions: _____

Staff action taken (if any): _____

Figure 37.8 Example of a health screen record. (Reprinted with permission from the American Academy of Allergy, Asthma & Immunology. Visit https://www.AAAAI.org for additional information and updates.)

Immunotherapy Pre-Injection Questionnaire

Patient Name:_____ Date:_____

This questionnaire is designed to optimize safety precautions already in place for your allergen immunotherapy injection (s) (allergy shot). Please review and answer the following questions. The nursing staff will review your responses and notify your physician if they have any questions or concerns about whether you should receive your injection(s) today. **If you are pregnant or have been diagnosed with a new medical condition, please notify the staff.** (Please circle the appropriate answer.)

I have confirmed that the name and birth date on my immunotherapy vial(s) are correct **yes no**

1. Have you had increased asthma symptoms (chest tightness, increased cough, wheezing, or

   shortness of breath) in the past week?   **Yes   No**

2. Have you had increased allergy symptoms (itching eyes or nose, sneezing, runny nose,

   post-nasal drip, or throat-clearing) in the past week?   **Yes   No**

3. Have you had a cold, respiratory tract infection, or flu-like symptoms

   in the past two weeks?   **Yes   No**

4. Did you have any problems such as increased allergy or asthma symptoms, hives, or

   generalized itching within 12 hours of receiving your last injection?

                                                             Yes   No

5. Are you on any new medications? Any new eye drops? Please specify._____

Staff intervention/office visit:

_____

_____

_____

Staff Signature:_____

Figure 37.9 Immunotherapy preinjection questionnaire. (Reprinted with permission from the American Academy of Allergy, Asthma & Immunology. Visit https://www.AAAAI.org for additional information and updates.)

at the patient or patient's guardian. If a patient's AIT treatment is transferred from one physician to another, there is an added risk for a SAR because of the multiple variables that may change with the transfer of care. Changes in the allergen vaccine components, such as the extract manufacturer, may be one of the reasons for the added risk following transfer of AIT treatment. Additional risk may come from staff unfamiliar with the prescribing allergist's AIT schedule, vial color-coding, and nomenclature system. Therefore, it is important that AIT transfer forms provide clear, specific instructions and information. When such documentation is provided and there is no change in the allergy vaccine components or AIT schedule, the risk of a systemic reaction from transferring care is minimized.

It is important to provide patients with information about AIT prior to starting treatment. Compliance with AIT is historically poor [27,28], which should improve by enhancing a patient's understanding of the AIT process. A study of patients receiving AIT demonstrated that a

Allergen Immunotherapy Systemic Reaction/Anaphylaxis Treatment Record

Name:_____Date:_____

Date of Birth:_____Prescribing Physician:_____

Allergens: Tree-Grass-Weed-Mites-Cockroach-Animal Dander-Mold-Hymenoptera

Prior systemic rxn:_____Hx of asthma?_____

Date/time of injection:_____Date/time of rxn:_____

Dilution (Vial #):_____New? Yes No

History of the systemic reaction (SR):

Immediate measures:
__Assess airway, breathing, circulation, and orientation
__Epinephrine IM into arm or when possible anterolateral thigh
__Activate EMS (call 911 or local rescue squad) Y/N Time called:_____AM/PM
__Management algorithm reviewed (as needed)

Signs and Symptoms

Respiratory:	Skin:	Eye/Nasal:	Vascular:	Other:
Shortness of Breath	Hives	Runny Nose	Hypotension	Difficulty Swallowing
Wheezing	Angioedema	Red Eyes	Chest Discomfort	Abdominal pain, nausea, diarrhea
Cough	Generalized Itch	Congestion	Dizziness	Diaphoresis
Stridor	Flushing	Sneezing		Headache
				Uterine cramps
				Impending doom

Time	Resp. rate/ PEFR	Pulse/ O2 Saturation	BP	Intervention, Medications, Exam Comments

Time of discharge from the office:_____Condition upon release: _____
Patient instructions:
_____
Follow-up call to patient: Date/Time_____

Comments:
_____ _
_____ _
_____ _

WAO Subcutaneous Immunotherapy Systemic Reaction Grading System Final Report:

Grade a-d,or z_____First symptom_____Time of onset of first symptom _____

Dosage adjustment? _____

Signatures_____RN_____ARNP/PA_____MD/DO

Figure 37.10 Allergen immunotherapy systemic reaction/anaphylaxis treatment record. (Reprinted with permission from the American Academy of Allergy, Asthma & Immunology. Visit https://www.AAAAI.org for additional information and updates.)

World Allergy Organization Subcutaneous Immunotherapy Systemic Reaction Grading System (see text)				
Grade 1	Grade 2	Grade 3	Grade 4	Grade 5
Symptom(s)/ sign(s) of one organ system present [i] **Cutaneous** Generalized pruritus, urticaria, flushing or sensation of heat or warmth[ii] or Angioedema (not laryngeal, tongue or uvular) or **Upper** **respiratory** Rhinitis (e.g., sneezing, rhinorrhea, nasal pruritus and/or nasal congestion) or Throat-clearing (itchy throat) or Cough perceived to come from the upper airway, not the lung, larynx, or trachea or **Conjunctival** Conjunctival erythema, pruritus or tearing **Other** Nausea, metallic taste, or headache	*Symptom(s)/ sign(s) of more than one organ system present* or **Lower respiratory** Asthma: cough, wheezing, shortness of breath (e.g., less than 40% PEF or FEV1 drop, responding to an inhaled bronchodilator) or **Gastrointestinal** Abdominal cramps, vomiting, or diarrhea or **Other** Uterine cramps	**Lower respiratory** Asthma (e.g., 40% PEF or FEV1 drop, NOT responding to an inhaled bronchodilator) or **Upper respiratory** Laryngeal, uvula or tongue edema with or without stridor	**Lower or Upper respiratory** Respiratory failure with or without loss of consciousness or **Cardiovascular** Hypotension with or without loss of consciousness	Death

Patients may also have a feeling of impending doom, especially in grades 2, 3, or 4.

Note: children with anaphylaxis seldom convey a sense of impending doom and their behavior changes may be a sign of anaphylaxis, e.g., becoming very quiet or irritable and cranky.

Scoring includes a suffix that denotes if and when epinephrine is or is not administered in relationship to symptom(s)/sign(s) of the SR: a, ≤ 5 minutes; b, >5 minutes to ≤10 minutes; c, >10 to ≤ 20 minutes; d, >20 minutes; z, epinephrine not administered.

The final grade of the reaction will not be determined until the event is over, regardless of the medication administered. The final report should include the first symptom(s)/sign(s) and the time of onset after the subcutaneous allergen immunotherapy injection [iii] and a suffix reflecting if and when epinephrine was or was not administered, e.g., Grade 2a; rhinitis:10 minutes.

Final report: Grade a-d,or z_____First symptom_____Time of onset of first symptom _____

Comments[iv]

i. Each Grade is based on organ system involved and severity. Organ systems are defined as: cutaneous, conjunctival, upper respiratory, lower respiratory, gastrointestinal, cardiovascular and other. A reaction from a single organ system such as cutaneous, conjunctival, or upper respiratory, but not asthma, gastrointestinal, or cardiovascular is classified as a Grade 1. Symptom(s)/sign(s) from more than one organ system or asthma, gastrointestinal, or cardiovascular are classified as Grades 2 or 3. Respiratory failure or hypotension, with or without loss of consciousness, defines Grade 4 and death Grade 5. The Grade is determined by the physician's clinical judgment.

ii. This constellation of symptoms may rapidly progress to a more severe reaction.

iii. Symptoms occurring within the first minutes after the injection may be a sign of severe anaphylaxis. Mild symptoms may progress rapidly to severe anaphylaxis and death.

iv. If signs or symptoms are not included in the Table or the differentiation between an SR and vasovagal (vasodepressor) reaction, which may occur with any medical intervention, is difficult, please include comment, as appropriate.

Figure 37.11 World Allergy Organization subcutaneous immunotherapy systemic reaction grading system. (From Cox et al. *J Allergy Clin Immunol* 2010; 125: 569–574, 74.e1–74.e7.)

substantial number of patients have poor knowledge, many misconceptions, and unfounded expectations of various important aspects of such therapy [29]. In outpatient practices, informed decision-making is often incomplete and inadequate [30,31]. AIT patients should be familiar with the potential risks involved and the time commitment necessary to receive such therapy. They should also understand the time necessary before they will begin to improve.

37.6.2 AIT instruction forms for physicians supervising AIT prescribed by another physician

Instruction forms for patients transferring from one physician to another should provide the following:

1. Detailed documentation of the patient's previous AIT treatment, which should include specific information about the components of the AIT vaccine, details of any adverse allergic reaction to AIT, schedule and allergy skin test results
2. Specific instructions for administering AIT and treatment of AIT large local reactions and SARs
3. Guidelines for dosage adjustments for unexpected interruptions in AIT injections and systemic reactions

37.6.3 Patient immunotherapy instruction forms

Instructions for patients beginning AIT should provide the following information:

1. Description of what AIT treatment involves and what alternative treatments are available
2. Potential benefits to be expected from the treatment and the expected timing of these benefits
3. Potential risk of AIT, including the remote possibility of death
4. Costs and who pays these costs
5. Anticipated duration of treatment
6. Any specific office policies regarding AIT, such as deferment of AIT injections with acute illness

Examples of consent and instruction forms, allergy skin test forms, AIT and administration forms can be downloaded from the AAAAI website (https:// www.aaaai.org).

SALIENT POINTS

1. Allergen immunotherapy (AIT) administration forms should include patient information, allergen vaccine information, and administration information.
2. Patient information on AIT forms should include the patient's name and sufficient data to allow identification of the patient. These data include date of birth, telephone number, record number, or patient picture.
3. Allergy vaccine information on AIT forms should convey the contents of the maintenance vaccine with sources of components, the expiration date, and the dilution from maintenance in volume per volume of each vial. The dilutions may be designated with numbers (e.g., 1:1 v/v, 1:10 v/v, etc.), letters (e.g., A, B, etc.), or color (e.g., red, yellow, etc.). A combination of two is desirable.

4. Administration information on an AIT form should include date, dose, arm in which dose was administered, side effects, and initials of professional administering the injection. Additional information desirable in select cases includes blood pressure, peak flow, premedication, current health status, and use of other medications. Subsequent doses and dosing interval should be clearly displayed.
5. Forms for administration of AIT by another, nonprescribing physician should include vaccine contents, schedule and dose of AIT, history of significant prior reactions, and guidelines for change following local reactions or SARs or following interruptions in treatment schedule. Contact information for the prescribing physician also should be clearly displayed. Recommendations for required observation time after treatment and equipment and medication recommended on site should be considered.
6. Patient instruction forms for AIT should include a simple description of treatment, treatment options other than AIT, potential benefits and risks, required waiting time after injections, estimated cost, estimated duration of treatment, and specific office/clinic policies related to deferment of treatment for illness.

REFERENCES

1. Cox L, Nelson H, Lockey R et al. Allergen immunotherapy: A practice parameter third update. *J Allergy Clin Immunol* 2011; 127: S1–S55.
2. Simons EF. *Ancestors of Allergy*. New York, NY: New York Global Medical Communications Ltd., 1994.
3. Coifman R, Cox L. 2006 American Academy of Allergy, Asthma & Immunology member immunotherapy practice patterns and concerns. *J Allergy Clin Immunol* 2007; 119: 1012–1013.
4. Bernstein IL, Li JT, Bernstein DI et al. Allergy diagnostic testing: An updated practice parameter. *Ann Allergy Asthma Immunol* 2008; 100: S1–S148.
5. Bousquet J, Heinzerling L, Bachert C et al. Practical guide to skin prick tests in allergy to aeroallergens. *Allergy* 2012; 67: 18–24.
6. American Academy of Allergy, Asthma and Immunology's Immunotherapy Committee's Guidelines for Reporting Immediate Allergy Skin Test Results. Academy News 1999.
7. Carr WW, Martin B, Howard RS, Cox L, Borish L. Comparison of test devices for skin prick testing. *J Allergy Clin Immunol* 2005; 116: 341–346.
8. Nelson HS, Lahr J, Buchmeier A, McCormick D. Evaluation of devices for skin prick testing. *J Allergy Clin Immunol* 1998; 101: 153–156.
9. Nelson HS, Rosloniec DM, McCall LI, Ikle D. Comparative performance of five commercial prick skin test devices. *J Allergy Clin Immunol* 1993; 92: 750–756.
10. Dykewicz MS, Dooms KT, Chassaing DL. Comparison of the Multi-Test II and ComforTen allergy skin test devices. *Allergy Asthma Proc* 2011; 32: 198–202.
11. Nelson HS, Kolehmainen C, Lahr J, Murphy J, Buchmeier A. A comparison of multiheaded devices for allergy skin testing. *J Allergy Clin Immunol* 2004; 113: 1218–1219.
12. King MJ, Lockey RF. Allergen prick-puncture skin testing in the elderly. *Drugs Aging* 2003; 20: 1011–1017.
13. Shah KM, Rank MA, Davé SA, Oslie CL, Butterfield JH. Predicting which medication classes interfere with allergy skin testing. *Allergy Asthma Proc* 2010; 31: 477–482.

14. Ownby DR. Computerized measurement of allergen-induced skin reactions. *J Allergy Clin Immunol* 1982; 69: 536–538.

15. Konstantinou GN, Bousquet PJ, Zuberbier T, Papadopoulos NG. The longest wheal diameter is the optimal measurement for the evaluation of skin prick tests. *Int Arch Allergy Immunol* 2010; 151: 343–345.

16. Bousquet J, Lockey R, Malling HJ. Allergen immunotherapy: Therapeutic vaccines for allergic diseases. A WHO position paper. *J Allergy Clin Immunol* 1998; 102:558–562.

17. DaVeiga SP, Liu X, Caruso K, Golubski S, Xu M, Lang DM. Systemic reactions associated with subcutaneous allergen immunotherapy: Timing and risk assessment. *Ann Allergy Asthma Immunol* 2011; 106: 533–537.e2.

18. Des Roches A, Paradis L, Knani J et al. Immunotherapy with a standardized *Dermatophagoides pteronyssinus* extract. V. Duration of the efficacy of immunotherapy after its cessation. *Allergy* 1996; 51: 430–433.

19. Oppenheimer J, Nelson HS. Skin testing: A survey of allergists. *Ann Allergy Asthma Immunol* 2006; 96: 19–23.

20. Bernstein DI, Wanner M, Borish L, Liss GM. Twelve-year survey of fatal reactions to allergen injections and skin testing: 1990–2001. *J Allergy Clin Immunol* 2004; 113: 1129–1136.

21. Lockey RF, Benedict LM, Turkeltaub PC, Bukantz SC. Fatalities from immunotherapy (IT) and skin testing (ST). *J Allergy Clin Immunol* 1987; 79(4): 660–667.

22. Amin HS, Liss GM, Bernstein DI. Evaluation of near-fatal reactions to allergen immunotherapy injections. *J Allergy Clin Immunol* 2006; 117: 169–175.

23. Epstein T, Liss G, Murphy-Berendts K, Bernstein D. AAAAI/ACAAI Surveillance Study of Subcutaneous Immunotherapy—Year 3: What practices modify the risk of systemic reactions? *Ann Allergy Asthma Immunol* 2013; 110: 274–278.

24. White J, Gregor K, Lee S et al. Patients taking β-blockers do not require increased doses of epinephrine for anaphylaxis. *J Allergy Clin Immunol Pract* 2018; 6(5): 1553–1558.e1.

25. Ohashi Y, Nakai Y, Murata K. Effect of pretreatment with fexofenadine on the safety of immunotherapy in patients with allergic rhinitis. *Ann Allergy Asthma Immunol* 2006; 96(4): 600–605.

26. Cox LS, Sanchez-Borges M, Lockey RF. World Allergy Organization systemic allergic reaction grading system: Is a modification needed? *J Allergy Clin Immunol Pract* 2017; 5(1): 58–62.e5.

27. Hankin CS, Lockey RF. Patient characteristics associated with allergen immunotherapy initiation and adherence. *J Allergy Clin Immunol* 2011; 127: 46–48.e1–3.

28. Hankin CS, Cox L, Lang D et al. Allergy immunotherapy among Medicaid-enrolled children with allergic rhinitis: Patterns of care, resource use, and costs. *J Allergy Clin Immunol* 2008; 121: 227–232.

29. Sade K, Berkun Y, Dolev Z, Shalit M, Kivity S. Knowledge and expectations of patients receiving aeroallergen immunotherapy. *Ann Allergy Asthma Immunol* 2003; 91: 444–448.

30. Braddock CH III, Edwards KA, Hasenberg NM et al. Informed decision making in outpatient practice: Time to get back to the basics. *JAMA* 1999; 282(24): 2313–2320.

31. Fernandez Lynch H, Joffe S, Feldman EA. Informed consent and the role of the treating physician. *N Engl J Med* 2018; 378(25): 2433–2438.

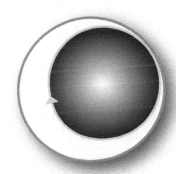

38 Recognition, treatment, and prevention of systemic allergic reactions and anaphylaxis*

Emma Westermann-Clark
University of South Florida Morsani College of Medicine

Stephen F. Kemp and Richard D. deShazo
University of Mississippi Medical Center

CONTENTS

---

* This chapter updates and extends the chapter from the 5th edition. Kemp SF, deShazo RD. Prevention and treatment of anaphylaxis. In: Lockey RF, Ledford DK (eds.). *Allergens and Allergen Immunotherapy*, 5th edition. New York: Informa Healthcare, 2013.

38.1 ANAPHYLAXIS AND ALLERGEN IMMUNOTHERAPY

38.1.1 Introduction

Systemic allergic reactions (SARs), including anaphylaxis, are not required to be reported to public health authorities. Therefore, both morbidity and mortality of SARs are probably underestimated. Tanno et al. call for a revision of the World Health Organization *International Classification of Diseases* (*ICD*) system to include anaphylaxis as a cause of death that may be included on death certificates [1]. Debate surrounding terminology used to describe allergic reactions is summarized in the 2015 American Academy of Allergy, Asthma and Immunology/American College of Allergy, Asthma, and Immunology/Joint Council of Allergy, Asthma and Immunology (AAAAI/ACAAI/JCAAI) Practice Parameter Update on Anaphylaxis [2]. The 2014 International Consensus on Anaphylaxis described anaphylaxis as "a serious, generalized or systemic, allergic or hypersensitivity reaction that can be life threatening or fatal" [3]. The term *systemic allergic reaction* (SAR) is preferred by some to *anaphylaxis* because the term *anaphylaxis* conveys a severity that belies the clinical subtlety of some SARs. A SAR, if not recognized and treated early, can progress to a level of severity termed *anaphylaxis*, which indicates respiratory and/or circulatory deterioration/collapse. The World Allergy Organization (WAO), an international umbrella organization whose members represent 99 national and regional professional societies dedicated to allergy and clinical immunology, created a grading system in 2010 applicable to reactions to subcutaneous allergen immunotherapy (SCIT) [4]. A 2017 rostrum called for expansion of the WAO SAR grading system to apply to all allergens [5]. In this grading system, the term *anaphylaxis* applies to grade 4 or 5 SARs. There is no universally accepted clinical definition of anaphylaxis or SAR [6,7]. In this chapter, the term *anaphylaxis* is used because it is more widely accepted, but the term *SAR* is more inclusive. The terms SAR and anaphylaxis are sometimes used interchangeably. The traditional nomenclature for anaphylaxis reserves the term *anaphylaxis* for IgE-dependent reactions and the term *anaphylactoid* for IgE-independent events, which are often clinically indistinguishable. The term *anaphylactoid* has fallen out of favor; some experts recommend the replacement of this terminology with *immunologic* (IgE-mediated and non-IgE-mediated [e.g., IgG and immune complex/complement-mediated]) and *nonimmunologic* anaphylaxis [2,6,8].

Anaphylaxis is considered likely if any one of three criteria is satisfied within minutes to hours: (1) acute onset of illness with involvement of skin, mucosal surface, or both, and at least one of the following: respiratory compromise, hypotension, or end-organ dysfunction; (2) two or more of the following occur rapidly after exposure to a likely allergen: involvement of skin or mucosal surface, respiratory compromise, hypotension, or persistent gastrointestinal symptoms; and (3) hypotension develops after exposure to a known allergen for that patient: age-specific low blood pressure or decline of systolic blood pressure of greater than 30% compared to baseline [9]. In clinical practice, however, waiting until the development of multiorgan symptoms is imprudent since the ultimate severity of anaphylaxis is difficult to predict from the outset. As previously mentioned, the WAO has developed clinical criteria for immunotherapy-associated anaphylaxis, which generally agree with the NIAID/FAAN criteria but also permit diagnosis of SAR as the sudden onset of symptoms in one body organ

Table 38.1 Epidemiology of anaphylaxis

Statistic	Value	Reference
Incidence/person-years	80–210/1,000,000	[14–16]
Risk/person in United States	0.05%–2.0%	[14,156]
U.S. persons at increased risk	1.24%–16.74%	[18]
Risk in hospitalized subjects	1/2700	[19]
Hospital fatalities/number of subjects	$154/10^6$	[99]
Mortality rate/year	<1% or 1–5.5/1,000,000	[15]
Food anaphylaxis fatalities/year	150	[20]
Peanuts or tree nuts	88% based on registry data	[21,22]
Fatal reactions to β-lactam antibiotics/year	400–800	[19]
Fatalities from subcutaneous immunotherapy/injection visit	1/9,100,000 injections	[35]
Anaphylaxis to Hymenoptera stings	0.4%–4%	[25]
Prevalence of idiopathic anaphylaxis	34,000 subjects	[26]

system after administration of a known allergen for that subject [4,5,10].

Signs and symptoms of anaphylaxis vary, but cutaneous features (urticaria, angioedema, erythema) are the most common overall [11]. Reactions may be immediate and uniphasic, or they may be delayed in onset, biphasic (recurrent), or protracted (discussed later). Respiratory compromise and cardiovascular collapse cause most fatalities [12,13]. An analysis of 202 anaphylaxis fatalities from 1992 to 2001 in the United Kingdom concluded that the interval between initial onset of food anaphylaxis symptoms and fatal cardiopulmonary arrest averaged 25–35 minutes, which was longer than for insect stings (10–15 minutes) or for drugs (mean, 5 minutes in hospital; 10–20 minutes prehospital) [13]. A variety of statistics on the epidemiology of anaphylaxis are published ([14–30]; Table 38.1). Challenges in diagnosing anaphylaxis and the various biomarkers and endotypes of anaphylaxis are reviewed by Castells [31].

38.1.1.1 SUBCUTANEOUS ALLERGEN IMMUNOTHERAPY AND ANAPHYLAXIS

Fatalities from SCIT occur at a rate of approximately 1 per 9.1 million injection visits, a decrease from 1 per 2,500,000 injections prior to year 2001 (see Chapter 34) [32–35]. A surveillance study sponsored by the AAAAI/ACAAI from 2013 to 2017 found that the fatality rate from SCIT had decreased to 0.8 SCIT-related fatalities annually compared to 3.4 SCIT-related fatalities annually in a 1990–2001 surveillance study [35,36]. In the intervening years, six fatal SCIT reactions were identified from 2001 to 2007, but no fatalities were reported from 2008 to 2010 [23,24].The physicians in these surveys included only members of the AAAAI. Therefore, the prevalence of fatalities resulting from SCIT administered by physicians who are not specifically trained to practice allergy and immunology remains unknown. Most SCIT-related fatalities occurred from reactions that took place within 30 minutes of the injection. Asthma is a risk factor for fatal anaphylaxis. Subjects who were symptomatic, especially with asthma, at the time of the injection or who were in their "allergy season" were also at increased risk. Errors in vial selection, especially when advancing to the next vial, and mistakes in dosage or administration also were important in some deaths. Increased subcutaneous tissue may preclude effective delivery of intramuscular (IM) epinephrine; therefore, obesity has been proposed as a risk factor for fatal anaphylaxis. Obesity is thought to have impacted at least one case of fatal anaphylaxis in the United States since 2008 [35]. In a study of 28 adults who had been prescribed epinephrine auto-injectors, needle length was insufficient in 68% of subjects due to increased subcutaneous tissue [37].

Near-fatal reactions (NFRs) to SCIT also have been examined retrospectively. Of 646 survey allergist-immunologist respondents, 273 reported NFRs. The investigators defined NFRs as respiratory compromise, hypotension, or both, requiring emergency epinephrine. Hypotension was reported in 80%, and respiratory failure occurred in 10% of NFRs, exclusively in asthmatic subjects. Epinephrine was delayed or not administered in 6% of these cases [38]. Grade 4 SARs occurred in 1/20,000 patients receiving SCIT in years 2013–2016 [35].

Stewart and Lockey reviewed 38 studies for SARs associated with SCIT [39]. The percentage of subjects experiencing one or more SARs ranged from 0.8% to 46.7% for conventional dose schedules (mean 12.92%, SD 10.8%). Rate of SARs per injection ranged from 0.05% to 3.2% (mean 0.5%, SD 0.87%). All but one study reported rates per injection of 0.6% or less. The 23 studies in which rush or accelerated schedules were used also were reviewed. The percentage of subjects experiencing one or more SARs during the maintenance phase of rush or accelerated SCIT ranged from 0 to 21.1% (mean 4.77%, SD 6.47%). However, the number of SARs was higher during buildup when the interval between injections was reduced ("rush" or "semirush" protocols). Subjects experiencing one or more SAR ranged from 0 to 66.7% with these accelerated schedules (mean 21.33%, SD 17.86%). Accelerated protocols were associated with rates of SARs per injection ranging from 0 to 6.4% (mean 2.36%, SD 1.7%).

38.1.1.2 SUBLINGUAL ALLERGEN IMMUNOTHERAPY AND ANAPHYLAXIS

Nolte and colleagues reviewed epinephrine administration for 29 sublingual immunotherapy (SLIT) clinical trials ($n = 8152$ SLIT, $n = 5155$ placebo) and found that the rate of anaphylaxis on SLIT was very low (see also Chapter 35). Among 8152 subjects on SLIT, epinephrine was administered 25 times, and 16 of these 25 administrations were related to SLIT, resulting in an event rate of 0.2% (16/8152 subjects). The remaining 9 of 25 epinephrine administrations in the SLIT group were for reasons unrelated to SLIT.

Among 5155 subjects on placebo, epinephrine was administered 10 times, resulting in an event rate of 0.2%, identical to the SLIT-treated group event rate [40]. Calderon and colleagues reviewed 11 published case reports of anaphylaxis (all nonfatal) diagnosed according to WAO anaphylaxis criteria following SLIT and calculated an approximate incidence of one case of anaphylaxis per 100 million SLIT administrations. All 11 subjects had skin/mucosal symptoms, which typically predominate in anaphylaxis from any cause. Six of 11 "probably had hypotension and shock," two had abdominal pain, and two others reported chest pain. The investigators noted that the 11 cases did not typify standard SLIT practice since they variously involved rush protocols, overdosage, allergen mixtures, nonstandardized extracts, and subjects who had previously experienced severe adverse reactions from SCIT. Compared with SCIT, SLIT has a better safety profile, although the investigators caution that anaphylaxis risk factors associated with both routes of administration should be characterized further [41].

38.2 MECHANISMS OF ANAPHYLAXIS

38.2.1 Chemical mediators of anaphylaxis

The chemical mediators associated with anaphylaxis are pre-formed and released from granules (histamine, tryptase, chymase, heparin, and carboxypeptidase A_3) or are generated from membrane lipids (prostaglandin D_2, leukotrienes, and platelet-activating factor [PAF]) by the activated mast cell and basophil [12]. The specific roles of individual mediators and their combinations in clinical reactions are hypothetical in most instances and based on animal studies. The development and severity of anaphylaxis appear to depend on the responsiveness of cells targeted by these mediators. Interleukin (IL)-4 and IL-13 are cytokines important in the initial generation of antibody and inflammatory cell responses during anaphylaxis. No comparable studies have been conducted in humans, but anaphylactic effects in the mouse depend on IL-4Rα-dependent IL-4/IL-13 activation of a transcription factor: signal transducer and activator of transcription 6 (STAT-6) [42].

The roles of *PAF* and *PAF acetylhydrolase*, the enzyme that inactivates PAF, appear to be important in human anaphylaxis. In a prospective controlled study, serum PAF levels directly correlated and PAF acetylhydrolase levels inversely correlated with anaphylaxis severity [43]. Retrospective analysis demonstrates that PAF acetylhydrolase activity is significantly lower in subjects experiencing fatal peanut anaphylaxis than for five control groups. Similarly, PAF levels correlated with the severity of acute allergic reactions in 41 patients who presented to an emergency room for treatment, more so than blood levels of histamine or tryptase [44].

Eosinophils appear to exert both pro-inflammatory (e.g., release of cytotoxic granule-associated proteins) or anti-inflammatory (e.g., metabolism of vasoactive mediators) effects [12]. A guinea pig anaphylaxis model suggests that eosinophils already present in chronically inflamed airways may participate in the immediate-phase response to allergen exposure, as well as their traditional roles in the late-phase allergic response [45]. Potential implications for human anaphylaxis have not been determined.

Histamine is only one of the mast cell mediators released in anaphylaxis, but its systemic effects have been studied more than other mediators. In one study, investigators infused histamine into normal volunteers at doses ranging from 0.05 to 1.0 μg/kg/min over 30 minutes to determine the plasma levels required to elicit symptoms of anaphylaxis [46]. A mean plasma level of 1.61 ± 0.30 ng/mL induced a 30% increase in heart rate; a level of 2.39 ± 0.52 ng/mL induced flushing and headache; and a level of 2.45 ± 0.13 ng/mL induced a 30% increase in pulse pressure. Pretreatment with an H_2-antagonist (cimetidine) did not alter these reactions. However, pretreatment with the H_1-antagonist, hydroxyzine hydrochloride, increased the level of histamine necessary to increase the heart rate by 30%. Combining the H_1 and H_2 antihistamines significantly raised the level at which histamine elicited all responses. On the basis of these results, the authors concluded that flushing, hypotension, and headache associated with histamine infusion are mediated by both H_1 and H_2 receptors, whereas tachycardia, pruritus, rhinorrhea, and bronchospasm are associated only with H_1 receptors.

Canine models suggest H_3 receptors modulate cardiovascular responses to norepinephrine in anaphylaxis, whereas mouse models suggest H_4 receptors might be involved in chemotaxis and mast cell cytokine release and might also factor in pruritus [47,48]. Potential implications for human subjects have not been studied.

Tryptase is concentrated selectively in the secretory granules of human mast cells and released when these cells degranulate. It can activate complement, coagulation pathways, and the kallikrein-kinin contact system with the potential clinical consequences of hypotension, angioedema, clotting, and clot lysis (disseminated intravascular coagulation) [11]. Release of β-tryptase (mature tryptase) stored in mast cell secretory granules is more specific for activation than α-protryptase, which is an inactive monomer that is secreted constitutively without stimulation. Tryptase levels generally correlate with the clinical severity of anaphylaxis [12]. However, a dichotomy may exist in the magnitude of tryptase elevations for those individuals experiencing anaphylaxis after parenteral exposure (e.g., injection, insect sting) versus oral exposure (e.g., food ingestion). Clinicians should be aware that the commercial tryptase assay does not measure beta-tryptase but total tryptase. In an analysis of anaphylaxis fatalities, the parenterally exposed subjects had higher serum levels of tryptase and lower levels of antigen-specific IgE, whereas those who succumbed after oral exposure had low tryptase levels and comparatively higher levels of antigen-specific IgE [49]. This difference may be related to the mast cell phenotype first encountered by the culprit antigen. Tryptase- and chymase-containing mast cells (MC_{TC}) are threefold more common in connective tissue than tryptase-containing mast cells (MC_T). The latter predominate in the mucosa of the lung and small intestine [49].

Levels of total tryptase peak 60–90 minutes after the onset of anaphylaxis and can persist as long as 5 hours after the onset of symptoms [11]. The estimated positive predictive value of tryptase elevations in 259 subjects with anesthesia-associated anaphylaxis is 92.6%, and the estimated negative predictive value of normal tryptase levels is 54.3% [50]. Serial tryptase measurements might improve diagnostic sensitivity, but further investigation is needed [7]. Tryptase levels should be checked in subjects who experience anaphylaxis after an insect sting, and these patients should be evaluated for mast cell disorders. A baseline elevation of serum tryptase can indicate an increased risk for insect sting anaphylaxis. It is generally accepted that an increase in serum tryptase of ($1.2\times$ baseline tryptase levels $+2$ [ng/mL]) is a clinically relevant elevation in tryptase and can indicate a mast cell activation–related

event [51,52]. Although an elevation in tryptase can support a diagnosis of anaphylaxis, there is no consensus regarding tryptase as a biomarker for anaphylaxis. Reactions to foods are less likely to be associated with tryptase elevation, but a 2018 prospective study of 160 adult peanut challenges, which analyzed subjects for potential increases in tryptase levels from baseline postchallenge, demonstrated an increase in 100 (62.5%) of 160 subjects with food-allergic reactions of any type, and four (100%) of four who experienced "severe anaphylaxis." A 30% elevation in tryptase compared to baseline was suggested by the authors to be the optimal cutoff to identify a reaction to food challenge, peaking at 2 hours postreaction [53].

Elevations of histamine and tryptase may not correlate clinically. In an emergency department study evaluating subjects who presented with acute allergic reactions, elevated histamine was observed in 42 of 97 subjects, but only 20 exhibited increased tryptase levels [54]. Serum histamine levels also correlate with the severity and persistence of cardiopulmonary manifestations but not with urticaria [54,55].

Nitric oxide (NO), a potent autacoid vasodilator formerly known as endothelium-derived relaxing factor, appears to be involved in the complex interaction of regulatory and counter-regulatory mediators in mast cell activation, including anaphylaxis [12]. Nitric oxide is derived from L-arginine through the activity of various isoforms of nitric oxide synthase as histamine binds to H_1-receptors during phospholipase-C-dependent calcium mobilization. Physiologically, NO participates in the homeostatic control of vascular tone and regional blood pressure. Experiments with NO inhibitors in mice, rabbits, and dogs demonstrate that NO promotes bronchodilation, promotes coronary artery vasodilation, and decreases histamine release. However, its net effects in anaphylaxis appear to enhance vascular smooth muscle relaxation and vascular permeability [12,56]. Several studies have demonstrated that NO is also increased in exhaled air during human anaphylaxis [57,58].

Metabolites of arachidonic acid include products of lipoxygenase and cyclooxygenase pathways. Of note, leukotriene B_4 is a chemotactic agent and thus can solicit other cells to participate in anaphylaxis. These cells theoretically contribute to biphasic (recurrent) anaphylaxis and to protracted reactions. Other effects of arachidonic acid metabolites associated with mast cell activation, including elevations in platelet-activating factor, tryptase, and histamine, contribute to the clinical manifestations of anaphylaxis in relative proportions that are still unclear [11].

Inflammatory mediators also activate the contact system. These consist of kininogen, kallikrein, and tryptase. Release of these mediators may induce formation of bradykinin as well as the activation of factor XII. This, in turn, may produce clotting, clot lysis, and subsequent activation of complement. In contrast, some mediators may have a salubrious effect that limits anaphylaxis. For example, chymase may activate angiotensin II, which can modulate hypotension. Heparin inhibits clotting, kallikrein, and plasmin, opposes complement formation, and modulates tryptase activity [11].

There are *other inflammatory pathways* that participate in anaphylaxis. These may be extremely important in the prolongation and amplification of anaphylaxis. Much of the supporting evidence derives from data obtained during experimental insect sting challenges. During severe anaphylaxis, there is concomitant activation of complement, coagulation pathways, and the contact (kallikrein-kinin) system. Decreases in C4 and C3, as well as the formation of C3a, have been observed in anaphylaxis. Demonstrable evidence for coagulation pathway activation during severe anaphylaxis includes decreases in factor V, factor VIII, and fibrinogen, and fatal disseminated intravascular coagulation in some instances [12,13]. Of 202 anaphylaxis fatalities analyzed retrospectively over a 10-year period in the United Kingdom, 7 (8%) were attributable to disseminated intravascular coagulation [13]. Successful treatment with tranexamic acid is reported [59]. Contact system activation is indicated by decreased high molecular weight kininogen and the formation of kallikrein-C1 inhibitor and factor XIIa-C1 inhibitor complexes. Kallikrein activation not only results in the formation of bradykinin but also activates factor XII. Factor XII alone can lead to clotting and clot lysis via plasmin formation, and plasmin can also activate complement [18]. Finkelman review the evidence in murine models and in humans for immunologic non-IgE-mediated anaphylaxis and conclude that evidence is emerging to support a role for IgG-mediated, complement-mediated anaphylaxis as well as direct basophil and mast cell activation [42]. Reber et al. provide a general up-to-date review of the pathophysiologic mechanisms of anaphylaxis [60].

38.2.2 Effects on the cardiovascular system

Anaphylaxis can be associated with *myocardial effects* including myocardial ischemia, conduction defects, atrial and ventricular arrhythmias, and T-wave abnormalities [61]. Whether such changes are related to direct mediator effects on the myocardium, exacerbation of preexisting myocardial insufficiency by the hemodynamic stress of anaphylaxis, endogenous release of epinephrine as a stress response, or therapeutically administered epinephrine is unclear [12,61–63].

Histamine exerts its pathophysiologic effects during anaphylaxis via both H_1 and H_2 receptors. H_1 receptors mediate coronary artery vasoconstriction and increased vascular permeability, whereas H_2 receptors increase atrial and ventricular inotropy, atrial chronotropy, and coronary artery vasodilation. The interaction of H_1 and H_2 receptor stimulation appears to mediate decreased diastolic pressure and increased pulse pressure [64]. Animal studies suggest a possible modulatory role for H_3 receptors [47]. PAF also decreases coronary blood flow, delays atrioventricular conduction, and has negative inotropic effects on the heart [61].

Raper and Fisher describe two previously healthy subjects who developed profound myocardial depression during anaphylaxis [62]. Echocardiography, nuclear imaging, and hemodynamic measurements confirmed the presence of myocardial dysfunction. Intra-aortic balloon counterpulsation provided hemodynamic support to supplement anaphylaxis treatment. Balloon counterpulsation was required for up to 72 hours because of persistent myocardial depression, even though other clinical signs of anaphylaxis had resolved. Both subjects recovered with no subsequent evidence of myocardial dysfunction. Thus, the heart may be a primary target for anaphylaxis, even in subjects with no preexisting cardiovascular disease.

Increased vascular permeability during anaphylaxis can shift up to 35% of intravascular volume to the extravascular space within 10 minutes [65]. Intrinsic compensatory responses to anaphylaxis include endogenous catecholamines, angiotensin II, and endothelins. These compensatory responses, however, produce variable effects on peripheral vascular resistance. Some subjects experience abnormal elevation of the peripheral vascular resistance (maximal vasoconstriction), yet shock persists due to reduced intravascular volume, while others have decreased systemic vascular resistance despite elevated levels of catecholamines [12]. These differences have important clinical implications since the latter scenario may respond favorably to therapeutic doses of vasoconstrictor agents while the former is vasoconstrictor-unresponsive and requires large-volume fluid resuscitation.

In a retrospective review of prehospital anaphylactic fatalities in the United Kingdom, the posture during the episode was known in 10 individuals [66]. Four of the 10 fatalities were associated with the upright or sitting posture. Postmortem findings were consistent with pulseless electrical activity and an "empty heart" attributed to reduced venous return from vasodilation and concomitant volume redistribution.

Since IgE attached to mast cells can trigger mast cell degranulation, and mast cells accumulate at sites of coronary atherosclerotic plaques, some investigators suggest that anaphylaxis promotes *plaque rupture*, thus risking myocardial ischemia [67–69]. Stimulation of the H_1 histamine receptor may also produce coronary artery *vasospasm* [68,70,71]. *Calcitonin gene-related peptide* (CGRP) released during anaphylaxis may help to counteract coronary artery vasoconstriction during anaphylaxis [72]. CGRP, a sensory neurotransmitter widely distributed in cardiovascular tissues, relaxes vascular smooth muscle and has cardioprotective effects in animal models of anaphylaxis [73].

While tachycardia is the rule, bradycardia may occur during anaphylaxis, so bradycardia may not be as useful to separate anaphylaxis from a vasodepressor reaction as previously thought. *Relative bradycardia*, initial tachycardia followed by a reduction in heart rate despite worsening hypotension, is reported in experimentally induced insect sting anaphylaxis, as well as in trauma victims [55,74–77].

Two distinct phases of physiologic response occur in mammals subjected to hypovolemia. The initial response is a baroreceptor-mediated sympathoexcitatory phase composed of an overall increase in cardiac sympathetic drive and concomitant withdrawal of resting vagal drive, which together produce tachycardia and peripheral vasoconstriction [76]. When the effective blood volume falls by 20%–30%, a second phase follows characterized by withdrawal of the vasoconstrictor drive, relative or absolute bradycardia, increased vasopressin, further catecholamine release as the adrenal axis becomes more active, and hypotension [76,77]. Hypotension in this hypovolemic scenario is independent of the bradycardia, since it persists after atropine reverses bradycardia. The acute vascular effects that occur in anaphylaxis may explain why hemodynamic collapse may occur immediately with no cutaneous or respiratory symptoms [78,79].

The clinical implications of bradycardia in human anaphylactic shock have not been studied. However, one retrospective review of approximately 11,000 trauma subjects observed that mortality was lower with the 29% of hypotensive subjects who were bradycardic when they were compared to the group of hypotensive subjects who were tachycardic, after adjustment for other mortality factors [77]. Thus, bradycardia may have a compensatory role in these hypovolemic settings.

Conduction defects and sympatholytic medications may also produce bradycardia [12]. Excessive venous pooling with decreased venous return, also present in vasodepressor reactions, may activate tension-sensitive sensory receptors in the inferoposterior portions of the left ventricle, resulting in a cardioinhibitory (Bezold-Jarisch) reflex that stimulates the vagus nerve and causes bradycardia [11].

38.3 AGENTS OF ANAPHYLAXIS

No evaluation can conclusively prove causation of anaphylaxis without directly challenging the subject with the suspected agent. Direct challenge is generally contraindicated due to safety concerns in subjects who have experienced potentially life-threatening anaphylaxis. Cause-and-effect may often be demonstrated historically in subjects who experience recurrent, objective findings of anaphylaxis upon inadvertent reexposure to the offending agent. Specific diagnostic testing, where appropriate, may confirm the presence of specific IgE and/or the degranulation of mast cells and basophils.

Virtually any agent capable of activating mast cells or basophils may potentially precipitate anaphylaxis. Table 38.2 lists common causes of anaphylaxis classified by pathophysiologic mechanism. Idiopathic anaphylaxis may be one of the most common, since this diagnosis accounts for approximately one-third of cases in most retrospective studies of anaphylaxis [11,14,80]. Of 601 subjects evaluated over two decades in a university-affiliated practice,

Table 38.2 Representative agents that cause anaphylaxis and their putative mechanisms

IgE-dependent
Foods
Medications
Insect venoms
Allergen immunotherapy
IgE-independent
Nonspecific degranulation of mast cells and basophils
Radiocontrast media (due to osmolarity of media)
Opioids
Muscle paralytics[a]
Idiopathic
Exercise
Cold, heat
Disturbance of arachidonic acid metabolism
Nonsteroidal anti-inflammatory drugs
Complement activation/activation of contact system
Radiocontrast media
Angiotensin-converting enzyme inhibitors
Other
c-kit mutation (D816V)—persons with this mutation are at increased risk for anaphylaxis
Protamine reactions can be IgE, IgG, or complement mediated [32]

[a] Can also be IgE-mediated.

Source: Modified from Kemp SF, Lockey RF. *J Allergy Clin Immunol* 2002; 110: 341–348.

356 (59%) were thought to have idiopathic anaphylaxis [81]. This series excluded anaphylaxis due to SCIT and insect stings. Idiopathic anaphylaxis remains a diagnosis of exclusion.

The most common identifiable causes of anaphylaxis are foods, medications, insect stings, and allergen immunotherapy injections [11,14,30,39,80] (Figure 38.1). Anaphylaxis to peanuts and/or tree nuts causes the greatest concern because it is potentially life-threatening, especially in subjects with asthma, and because of the propensity for life-long allergic sensitivity to these foods.

Anaphylaxis following ingestion of mammalian meat, termed "α-gal" allergy, is attributed to preexisting IgE antibodies specific for the glycosylation product galactose-α-1,3-galactose ("α-gal"). The same glycosylation product is present in and responsible for anaphylaxis secondary to a monoclonal antibody, cetuximab, in sensitized subjects. Certain species of ticks inhabit the Southeastern United States, where reactions to cetuximab were noted in clinical trials. There is some evidence to support tick bites as a sensitizing event leading to IgE-antibodies to α-gal and subsequent mammalian meat and cetuximab allergy. Unlike anaphylaxis to most food allergens, which tend to occur within 30 minutes of ingestion, anaphylaxis to α-gal usually occurs 4–6 hours or more after ingestion of mammalian meat [82].

Individuals rarely have experienced have experienced anaphylaxis after receiving therapeutic preparations of monoclonal IgG antibody to IgE (omalizumab) [83,84]. Reactions to other monoclonal antibodies also occur, the mechanism for which is unclear [85–87].

38.4 MANIFESTATIONS AND DIFFERENTIAL DIAGNOSIS

38.4.1 Clinical manifestations of anaphylaxis

The spectrum of clinical presentations may complicate the diagnosis. Regardless, when the diagnosis is suspected, special attention should be directed toward assessment of both upper and lower airways, respiratory and pulse rates, blood pressure, tissue perfusion, and appearance of the skin. Measurement of peak expiratory flow rate and pulse oximetry may also be useful, where appropriate.

Anaphylaxis is associated with the following signs and symptoms, alone or in combination: diffuse erythema, pruritus, and urticaria; angioedema; bronchospasm; laryngeal edema; hyperperistalsis (e.g., abdominal cramps, emesis, diarrhea); uterine cramps; hypotension; or cardiac arrhythmias. Urticaria and angioedema are the most common manifestations [81,88]. Anaphylaxis (grade 4/5 SAR) occurs as part of a clinical continuum. It can begin with relatively minor symptoms such as itchy palms, eyes, nose, or skin and rapidly progress to a life-threatening respiratory and cardiovascular reaction. Cutaneous findings may be delayed or absent in rapidly progressive anaphylaxis. The next most common manifestations of anaphylaxis are respiratory symptoms, followed by dizziness, syncope, and gastrointestinal symptoms. The more rapidly anaphylaxis occurs after exposure to an offending stimulus, the more likely the reaction is to be severe and potentially life-threatening [33,89].

38.4.2 Differential diagnosis for anaphylaxis

Several systemic disorders share clinical features with anaphylaxis, with the vasodepressor (vasovagal) reaction probably the condition

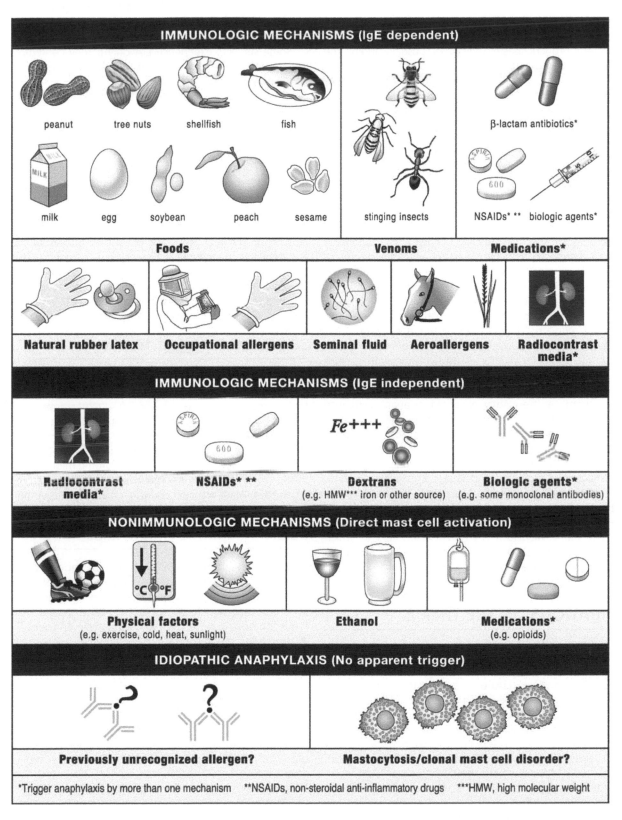

Figure 38.1 Anaphylaxis mechanisms and triggers. Anaphylaxis typically occurs through an IgE-dependent immunologic mechanism. Foods, stinging insect venoms, or medications are common triggers. Medications can also lead to anaphylaxis through an IgE-independent immunologic mechanism or through direct mast cell activation. Radiocontrast media is thought to instigate anaphylaxis through both IgE-dependent and IgE-independent mechanisms. Rarely, inhalant allergens can trigger anaphylaxis. In cases of idiopathic anaphylaxis, clinicians should consider a novel allergen trigger, underlying mastocytosis or a clonal mast cell disorder. *Abbreviations:* NSAID, nonsteroidal anti-inflammatory drug; HMW, high molecular weight. (Used with permission, Simons FER et al. *World Allergy Organization Journal* 2011; 4(2): 13–37. https://doi.org/10.1097/WOX.0b013e318211496c.)

most commonly confused with it. In vasodepressor reactions, however, urticaria is absent, diaphoresis is often present, bradycardia is typically present, bronchospasm or dyspnea is usually absent, the blood pressure may be normal or depressed, and the skin is usually cool and pale. Tachycardia is the rule in anaphylaxis, but it may be absent in subjects with hypovolemia (after initial tachycardia), conduction defects, increased vagal tone due to a cardioinhibitory (Bezold-Jarisch) reflex, or in those who take sympatholytic (e.g. β-blockers) medications. Myocardial dysfunction may cause sudden hemodynamic collapse with or without an arrhythmia. A pulmonary embolism may produce tachycardia, dyspnea, tachypnea, and chest discomfort that can be pleuritic. Systemic mastocytosis, a disease characterized by mast cell proliferation in multiple organs, is usually associated with urticaria pigmentosa (brownish macules that transform into wheals upon stroking, called Darier's sign) and recurrent episodes of pruritus, flushing, tachycardia, abdominal pain, diarrhea, syncope, or headache. Mast cell activation syndrome (MCAS) is also associated with recurrent anaphylaxis; diagnostic algorithms for MCAS require three criteria including symptoms consistent with mast cell activation, biochemical markers such as tryptase, and response to medications that stabilize mast cells or inhibit mast cell mediators [52]. Neuroendocrine cell syndromes (e.g., carcinoid) may produce flushing and diarrhea. Other diagnostic considerations for children, in particular, include foreign-body aspiration, acute poisoning, and a seizure disorder. Diagnostic criteria for anaphylaxis in infants are published [90].

Signs and symptoms frequently observed in anaphylaxis may occur by themselves in other disorders. Subjects with hereditary angioedema, for example, experience episodes of nonpruritic, typically painless edema of the extremities with or without laryngeal edema and abdominal discomfort due to visceral involvement. Factitious anaphylaxis is characterized by repeated, self-induced episodes of anaphylaxis. Anaphylaxis alternatively may be surreptitiously inflicted upon a susceptible subject, an example of Munchausen syndrome by proxy. Undifferentiated somatoform idiopathic anaphylaxis likewise is a psychiatric disorder in which subjects report symptoms identical to those encountered in idiopathic anaphylaxis, but objective findings are absent [91].

38.5 VARIATIONS ON THE THEME

38.5.1 Exercise-induced anaphylaxis

Exercise-induced anaphylaxis (EIA) occurs with strenuous exercise, frequently in conditioned athletes, such as marathon runners, and is usually accompanied by a short prodrome of cutaneous warmth and generalized pruritus. Clinical manifestations may progress to generalized erythema and urticaria, angioedema, and vascular collapse [92]. Prophylaxis with antihistamines, a corticosteroid, or cromolyn sodium does not consistently prevent EIA, although some investigators suggest prophylaxis with these medications might be more successful in food-dependent EIA (see below) [94]. Case reports suggest that omalizumab and misoprostol may be helpful [94]. Episodes occur sporadically, which distinguishes EIA from other forms of physical urticaria in which exercise provocation invariably produces symptoms [92]. Some individuals may demonstrate symptoms during a controlled exercise challenge, but the test is often negative, despite a classic clinical history, likely due to unrecognized cofactors. Subjects with EIA should know how to administer epinephrine and preferably exercise with a partner educated about EIA and how to treat it.

Some subjects experience EIA only if they contemporaneously ingest specific foods and/or nonsteroidal anti-inflammatory drugs (NSAIDS). Foods, such as shrimp, celery, or wheat, or a medication, such as aspirin, are required to elicit symptoms in some subjects. Feldweg reviews the diagnosis and management of food-dependent exercise-induced anaphylaxis (FDEIA) [94]. Bartra reviews the relationship between EIA and cofactors including foods, NSAIDS, and alcohol [95].

Exercise avoidance remains the best treatment since the natural history of the syndrome is not fully understood. Shadick et al. surveyed 365 subjects with EIA over an average of 10.6 years [96]. Of survey respondents, 47% had fewer episodes and 46% had stabilized since diagnosis. Forty-one percent reported no episodes in the year preceding the survey. Successful respondents apparently had moderated their exercise programs and avoided provocative factors [96]. A European Academy of Allergy and Clinical Immunology (EAACI) position statement calls for increased research to elucidate the mechanism of EIA [97].

38.5.2 Cholinergic urticaria

Cholinergic urticaria, also called "heat urticaria," is caused by increased core body temperature due to fever, stress, environmental factors, or exercise. Skin lesions frequently appear as 2–4 mm pruritic wheals ("microhives") surrounded by erythema, which usually begin on the chest and spread over the body. Systemic manifestations, similar to those described for EIA, may also occur but are unusual. Subjects with this syndrome might develop wheals at the site where methacholine is injected or generalized urticaria when the body is warmed, as with a plastic occlusive suit [98].

38.5.3 Idiopathic anaphylaxis

Idiopathic anaphylaxis is a syndrome of repeated anaphylactic episodes for which no cause can be determined [91]. It may occur in children as well as adults [91,99], and fatalities are rare [91]. Within 1 year, almost all subjects enter a period of prolonged remission or have infrequent and less severe episodes [99]. Failure to respond to prednisone should prompt consideration of another diagnosis.

Serial histories and diagnostic tests for foods, spices, and vegetable gums have occasionally identified the culprit agent in subjects previously presumed to have idiopathic anaphylaxis [11]. The usefulness of skin prick testing for reactions to food allergens was tested in 102 subjects presumed to have idiopathic anaphylaxis [100]. One-third had positive tests to one or more foods from a battery of 79 food allergens. Five subjects experienced anaphylaxis after eating a food implicated by a positive skin test. Two subjects stopped having reactions after they eliminated the implicated food from their diet, but they refused a subsequent confirmatory oral food challenge. The 10 allergens that provoked anaphylaxis in these seven subjects were aniseed, cashew, celery, flaxseed, hops, mustard, mushroom, shrimp, sunflower, and walnut. The authors conclude that skin testing with selected foods may be useful to identify food allergens that cause anaphylaxis, since 7% of subjects in the reference group previously presumed to have idiopathic anaphylaxis had possible food-induced anaphylaxis.

However, the false-positive rate of indiscriminate food skin prick testing is high, especially in atopic individuals.

38.5.4 Anaphylaxis attributed to endogenous progesterone

A syndrome of recurrent anaphylaxis apparently triggered or exacerbated by progesterone is described in five female subjects [101,102]. Four of these subjects reported attacks that exacerbated during pregnancy, lessened during lactation, and increased when lactation ceased. Three of the five subjects experienced remission when treated with a luteinizing hormone-releasing hormone (LHRH) analogue, which apparently antagonizes LHRH and inhibits progesterone. Immediate skin test reactions to intradermal injection of 40–2000 µg of medroxyprogesterone were present in responders to LHRH analogue therapy. Systemic reactions characterized by urticaria and hypotension developed in two subjects after 100 µg of LHRH was administered intravenously during the luteal phase of their menstrual cycles. The authors postulated that progesterone, in some undefined way, facilitates mast cell mediator release. The three subjects whose anaphylactic symptoms were reduced by LHRH analogue therapy subsequently underwent oophorectomy with a long-lasting reduction in their symptoms. One subject, however, continued to require combined H_1 and H_2 antihistamine therapy to control attacks.

38.5.5 Recurrent and persistent anaphylaxis

The reported incidence of biphasic (recurrent) anaphylaxis varies from less than 1% to a maximum of 23% [103,104]. Additionally, the reported time of onset of the delayed phase may vary from 1 to 72 hours. Potential risk factors include severity of the initial phase, delayed or suboptimal doses of epinephrine during initial treatment, laryngeal edema or hypotension during the initial phase, delayed symptomatic onset after antigen exposure (often a food or insect sting), or prior history of biphasic anaphylaxis. It is unclear whether systemic corticosteroids administered in the initial phase can prevent or lessen delayed phase reactions [103,105].

Persistent anaphylaxis, which may last from 5 to 32 hours, occurred in 7 of 25 subjects (28%), with two fatalities, in the Stark and Sullivan report [106]. Of 13 subjects analyzed in a report on fatal or near-fatal anaphylaxis to foods, three (23%) similarly experienced persistent anaphylaxis [107]. Retrospective data from other investigators, however, suggest that persistent anaphylaxis is uncommon.

Neither biphasic nor persistent anaphylaxis can be predicted from the severity of the initial phase of an anaphylactic reaction, since they have occurred after what were perceived initially to be mild episodes. Since life-threatening manifestations of anaphylaxis may recur, it may be necessary to monitor selected subjects up to 24 hours after their apparent recovery from the initial phase.

38.6 MANAGEMENT OF ANAPHYLAXIS

38.6.1 General

Systematic reviews have noted the lack of optimal, randomized controlled trials of epinephrine, H_1-antihistamines, and corticosteroids in anaphylaxis [108–111]. Several ethical, clinical, and logistic considerations apply [112]. Pending a strengthening of the evidence basis for the treatment of anaphylaxis, practice parameters [2] and consensus emergency management guidelines [113,114] concerning anaphylaxis and its management are available. However, physicians and other healthcare professionals may not follow them. In a standardized clinical anaphylaxis scenario, as defined by UK Resuscitation Council guidelines, 5% of senior house officers would use the proper dose and/or route of administration for epinephrine [115]. Other reports examining treatment patterns for anaphylaxis in the emergency departments of civilian [116] and military hospitals [117] indicate that epinephrine is administered during anaphylaxis to 16% and 50% of patients, respectively. A systematic review of the medical literature identified over 200 gaps in management by physicians, patients, and community (parents, caregivers, teachers), with pervasive deficiencies noted in knowledge of anaphylaxis clinical features, treatment, and proper use of epinephrine auto-injector devices [118].

Clinicians who perform procedures and administer medications should have the appropriate medications and equipment available to treat anaphylaxis. The following equipment and supplies are recommended as bare essentials [119,120]: (1) stethoscope and sphygmomanometer; (2) injectable aqueous epinephrine 1:1000 (1 mg/mL); (3) intravenous (IV) fluids and needles; (4) equipment for administering oxygen by mask/cannula; and (5) airway adjuncts appropriate for the supervising physician's skill and expertise. The emergency kit should be up-to-date and complete. Everyone directly involved in patient care should be able to locate necessary supplies, rapidly assemble fluids for IV administration, and be aware of treatment guidelines for anaphylaxis.

A sequential approach to management is outlined in Table 38.3. The judicious use of epinephrine and maintenance of adequate oxygenation and an effective circulatory volume are the most important considerations. Assessment and maintenance of airway, breathing, circulation, and mentation are essential initial management steps. Altered mentation may reflect underlying hypoxia. Measurement of pulse oximetry and peak expiratory flow rate, where appropriate, may be useful to guide therapy. Patients should be monitored continuously to facilitate prompt detection of new clinical findings or treatment complications. A patient should be transferred to an emergency facility depending on the clinical severity of the reaction, response to treatment, and the likelihood that other complications will occur.

Anaphylactic shock, a form of distributive shock, may shift significant fluid volume from the central to the peripheral vascular compartment, potentially resulting in inadequate venous return to the heart [65,66]. Thus, the recumbent position with elevated lower extremities is strongly recommended, essential in the hypotensive subject, and provides autoinfusion (or preservation) of approximately 1–2 L of fluid into the central vascular compartment [121]. Patients with bronchospasm may be reticent to remain in the recumbent position but should be positioned as close to the horizontal as possible during treatment. Patients with anaphylaxis may rarely develop the "empty heart syndrome" with profound hypotension and heart failure from acute fluid shifts and require massive fluid resuscitation, inotropes, and even left ventricular assistive devices to maintain blood pressure [122].

Systemic absorption of the suspected culprit agent must be minimized by stopping IV infusion of offending medications or other biologic agents. Severe laryngeal edema may develop within 30–180 minutes [113]; therefore, an endotracheal tube should be inserted as soon as possible if laryngeal edema does not promptly

Table 38.3 Management of acute anaphylaxis

I. Immediate intervention
  a. Assessment of airway, breathing, circulation, and adequacy of mentation.
  b. Administer epinephrine intramuscularly, preferably in the anterolateral thigh, every 5–15 minutes or as often as necessary, in appropriate doses, depending on the presenting signs and symptoms of anaphylaxis, to control signs and symptoms and prevent progression to more severe symptoms such as respiratory distress, hypotension, shock and unconsciousness.
  c. Place patient in recumbent position and elevate lower extremities.

II. Appropriate subsequent measures depending on response to epinephrine
  a. Establish and maintain airway.
  b. Administer oxygen.
  c. Establish venous access.
  d. Use crystalloid (e.g., lactated Ringer's or normal saline) IV for fluid replacement.

III. Other measures to consider, where appropriate
  a. Dilute epinephrine infusion.
  b. H_1 and H_2 antihistamines.
  c. Nebulized β_2 agonist (e.g., albuterol) for bronchospasm resistant to epinephrine.
  d. Systemic glucocorticoid.
  e. Vasopressor (e.g., dopamine).
  f. Glucagon for patient on β-blocker.
  g. Atropine for symptomatic bradycardia.
  h. Transportation to an emergency department or an intensive care facility.

IV. Observation and subsequent outpatient follow-up
  a. Observation periods after apparent resolution must be individualized (see text for specific details).
  b. After recovery from the acute episode, consider self-injectable epinephrine.
  c. Postanaphylaxis evaluation by an allergist-immunologist.

Source: Modified from Lieberman P et al. *J Allergy Clin Immunol* 2010; 126: 477–480.e42.

reverse following parenteral administration of epinephrine. H_1 and H_2 antagonists, a corticosteroid, and volume expanders can be infused once IV access is established.

38.6.2 Epinephrine

38.6.2.1 HOW TO USE EPINEPHRINE

Epinephrine 0.3 mg (or 0.15 mg for subjects weighing 15 to 30 kg [33 pounds to 66 pounds]) administered intramuscularly is the treatment of choice for anaphylaxis [2,9,123]. It is important to note that *there are no absolute contraindications for epinephrine administration to treat anaphylaxis* [2,123]. It should be given as soon as any signs or symptoms of anaphylaxis appear. Data are limited concerning the frequency with which two or more doses

(reports range from 16% to 36%) of epinephrine are utilized to treat anaphylaxis [124]. Fatalities from anaphylaxis can result from delayed administration or inadequate doses of epinephrine and from severe respiratory and/or cardiovascular complications [2,13]. Factors associated with fatal anaphylaxis are reviewed by Golden [125]. Even with ideal treatment, patients still die from anaphylaxis [13,21,22,107,124,126]. All subsequent therapeutic interventions depend on the initial response to epinephrine. However, epinephrine toxicity or inadequate response to epinephrine indicates that additional therapeutic modalities are necessary [2,123].

IM epinephrine every 5–15 minutes, or as often as necessary, should be given to control symptoms and sustain blood pressure [2]. Comparisons of IM to subcutaneous injections have not been done during anaphylaxis. However, absorption is rapid and plasma levels higher in asymptomatic adults and children given epinephrine intramuscularly in the anterolateral thigh [127,128]. Obesity or other conditions that increase subcutaneous fat may prevent or complicate IM access [129].

The pharmacology of epinephrine is reviewed in detail by Westfall and Westfall [130]. The α-adrenergic, vasoconstrictive effects at recommended dosages given IM reverse peripheral vasodilation and alleviate hypotension and reduce generalized erythema, urticaria, and angioedema. Local injection of epinephrine may reduce further absorption of antigen from a sting or injection site, but this has not been studied systematically. The β-adrenergic properties of epinephrine cause bronchodilation, increase myocardial output and contractility, and suppress further mediator release from mast cells and basophils [123]. Epinephrine, administered in low concentrations (e.g., 0.1 µg/kg), can paradoxically produce vasodilation, produce hypotension, and increase the release of inflammatory mediators [123,130].

Epinephrine administration enhances coronary blood flow. Two mechanisms are probably responsible: an increased duration of myocardial diastole compared to systole and a coronary vasodilator effect due to increased contractility. These actions usually offset the vasoconstrictor effects of epinephrine on the coronary arteries [123,130].

Common pharmacologic effects of epinephrine that occur at recommended doses via any route of administration include agitation, anxiety, tremulousness, headache, dizziness, pallor, or palpitations [130]. Notably, none of the 69 subjects who accidentally self-administered epinephrine experienced long-term adverse effects [131]. Rarely, and usually associated with excessive doses, epinephrine administration might contribute to or cause myocardial ischemia or infarction, pulmonary edema, prolonged QTc interval, ventricular arrhythmias, accelerated or malignant hypertension, and intracranial hemorrhage in adults and children. Nonetheless, some patients have survived massive doses of epinephrine with no evidence of myocardial ischemia or residual complications [123].

38.6.2.2 INTRAVENOUS EPINEPHRINE

Because of the risk for potentially lethal arrhythmias, epinephrine, 1:10,000 (0.1 mg/mL) or 1:100,000 (0.01 mg/mL), characteristically is administered intravenously only in the presence of cardiac arrest or to unresponsive or hypotensive patients who fail to respond to IV volume replacement and multiple IM doses of epinephrine [2]. One group of investigators suggests that the early use of IV epinephrine is safe, effective, and well tolerated when the rate of administration is titrated to the clinical response, but this modality has not been compared systematically to intramuscular epinephrine [75]. Continuous hemodynamic monitoring with IV epinephrine is essential.

38.6.2.3 EPINEPHRINE ADMINISTRATION BY OTHER ROUTES

While IM administration of epinephrine is standard of care, intranasal administration of epinephrine may be another option in the future. Two devices that permit the administration of epinephrine intranasally have been given fast-track designation by the U.S. Food and Drug Administration [132,133]. In a small study on the pharmacokinetics of intranasal epinephrine, epinephrine was absorbed intranasally but required a higher dose (0.5 mg) than IM epinephrine (0.3 mg) to attain similar systemic absorption [134]. One of the intranasal formulations in development includes a technology called Intravail (Neurelis, Inc, San Diego, California) that increases intranasal absorption [132]. Anecdotally, alternative routes of administration have been reported for some time. These include, for example, inhaled epinephrine in the presence of laryngeal edema or sublingual injection if an IV route cannot be obtained. Intraosseous (IO) administration of epinephrine at doses equivalent to IV dosing have been recommended when IV access is not available and in instances where the clinician has proficiency in the technique [2]. Endotracheally administered dosages of epinephrine, previously proposed for use when IV access is not available in intubated patients experiencing cardiac arrest, are controversial. Further details can be found in the American Heart Association Guidelines for Cardiopulmonary Resuscitation (CPR) and Emergency Cardiovascular Care, which are regularly updated.

38.6.3 How to use ancillary medications

38.6.3.1 H_1 AND H_2 ANTIHISTAMINES

The standard treatment of anaphylaxis usually includes H_1 antihistamines and corticosteroids. However, antihistamines have a much slower onset of action than epinephrine, they exert minimal effect on blood pressure, and they should not be administered as treatment alone [2]. Even at maximum dosages, antihistamines cannot abort anaphylaxis if histamine already occupies its receptor. They do, however, attenuate cutaneous symptoms, such as urticaria or generalized pruritus, and they may help prevent recurrence. For example, diphenhydramine, 25–50 mg for adults and 12.5–25 mg for children, may be administered intravenously once the cardiovascular and respiratory conditions are stabilized by epinephrine and/or fluids. IV administration ensures effective dosing will not be impaired by hemodynamic compromise, which adversely affects gastrointestinal or IM absorption, but maximal effect may not be observed for 1 hour [135]. Oral or IM administration of antihistamines may suffice for milder anaphylaxis, but we recommend epinephrine first for all cases. A systemic review was unable to make any evidence-based recommendations for the use of H_1 antihistamines in the treatment of anaphylaxis [108].

A systematic review of the role of H_2 antihistamines, such as cimetidine and ranitidine, in anaphylaxis was unable to make evidence-based recommendations for their use in anaphylaxis [136]. According to the 2015 AAAAI/ACAAI/JCAAI practice parameter Update on Anaphylaxis, IV administration of some H_2 antihistamines (e.g., cimetidine) can potentiate hypotension [2]. The use of H_2

antihistamines is not supported by well-designed randomized controlled trials [2]. Nevertheless, the Practice Parameters provide the following doses for H_2 administration if administered intravenously, ranitidine, 1 mg/kg in adults and 12.5–50 mg in children, infused slowly or administered intramuscularly [2], is preferred over cimetidine. Since H_2 blockade without concomitant H_1 blockade could increase available histamine and H_1 receptor stimulation, H_2 antihistamines should not be administered prior to H_1 antihistamines.

38.6.3.2 CORTICOSTEROIDS

Systemic corticosteroids may not produce appreciable effects for several hours, but many clinicians believe that they may prevent persistent or biphasic reactions. Subjects with asthma or other conditions may be at increased risk for severe or fatal anaphylaxis and may receive additional benefit if corticosteroids are administered to them during anaphylaxis, but there is little evidence to support this claim. A review by Alqurashi and Ellis reported a lack of compelling evidence to support the claim that biphasic reactions are prevented by corticosteroid administration [137]. Similar conclusions were drawn by Sheikh [138]. The 2015 AAAAI/ACAAI/JCAAI Practice Parameter Update on Anaphylaxis states that corticosteroids may be given after epinephrine as adjunct treatment, but prompt epinephrine use is the standard of care [2]. Due to their delayed onset of action, corticosteroids do not prevent cardiorespiratory compromise in anaphylaxis. A Cochrane systemic review was unable to make any evidence-based recommendations for the use of corticosteroids in the treatment of anaphylaxis [110]. While "premedication protocols" for iodinated contrast media, snake antivenom therapy, and other agents often recommend high-dose corticosteroids, there is questionable evidence to support this concept [138].

38.6.3.3 OXYGEN AND β_2-AGONISTS

The use of oxygen and β_2-agonists in anaphylaxis is supported by practice parameters and international guidelines [2,3]. Oxygen should be administered and pulse oximetry monitored during anaphylaxis for those who require multiple doses of epinephrine, have protracted anaphylaxis, or have preexisting hypoxemia or myocardial dysfunction. Inhaled β_2-agonists, e.g., albuterol 2.5 mg, or 0.5 mL of 0.5% solution, diluted with normal saline to a total volume of 3 mL, may be administered for bronchospasm refractory to epinephrine.

38.6.3.4 PERSISTENT HYPOTENSION: APPROPRIATE ROLES OF VOLUME REPLACEMENT AND GLUCAGON

Treatment of refractory anaphylaxis is reviewed by Kemp and Kemp [111]. Usual doses of epinephrine administered during anaphylaxis to subjects taking β-adrenergic antagonists may not produce the desired clinical response and may instead cause predominantly α-adrenergic effects. In such situations, both isotonic volume expansion, in some circumstances up to 7 L of crystalloid are necessary, and glucagon administration are recommended [11]. Normal saline, 0.9%, is the crystalloid solution preferred in international guidelines, although there is little evidence to support its use instead of lactated Ringer's solution. If large volumes are necessary, consideration of 0.45%

normal saline ("half normal" saline) after infusion of several liters of normal saline may prevent hyperchloremic metabolic acidosis. Aggressive use of lactated Ringer's solution potentially risks respiratory acidosis [111]. A volume of 1–2 L of normal saline or lactated Ringer's solution is administered to adults at a rate of 5–10 mL/kg in the first 5 minutes. Children should receive up to 30 mL/kg in the first hour. Since glucagon directly activates adenyl cyclase and completely bypasses the β-adrenergic receptor, it may reverse refractory hypotension and bronchospasm associated with anaphylaxis, as demonstrated in case reports [139]. The recommended dosage for glucagon is 1–5 mg (in children, 20–30 μg/kg [maximum 1 mg]) administered intravenously over 5 minutes and followed by an infusion, 5–15 μg/min, titrated to clinical response. Protection of the airway is particularly important in severely drowsy or obtunded subjects since glucagon can cause emesis with the attendant risk for aspiration.

Some investigators report elevated endogenous levels of norepinephrine, epinephrine, and angiotensin II in individuals who experience hypotension during insect sting–induced anaphylaxis [74]. This may explain why more epinephrine fails to help some subjects with anaphylaxis. Subjects whose hypotension persists despite epinephrine and crystalloid fluid replacement may benefit from intravenous colloid solutions and volume expanders, such as hydroxyethyl starch (Hespan, B. Braun Medical, Bethlehem, Pennsylvania). Adults receiving colloid solution should receive 500 mL rapidly followed by slow infusion [11].

Clinicians proficient in establishing intraosseous (IO) access for either adults or children may consider it if attempts at IV access are unsuccessful. IO cannulation provides access to a noncollapsible venous plexus that is attainable in all age groups, and several studies have documented its safety and efficacy [113]. The technique requires a rigid needle, preferably a specially designed IO or bone marrow needle from an IO access kit [140]. Access often can be obtained in 30–60 seconds. Many sites may be used for IO infusions. For young children, the proximal tibia just distal to the growth plate is most commonly used. For older children and adults, appropriate IO insertion sites include the medial or lateral malleolus, the distal tibia just proximal to the medial malleolus, the distal femur, the anterior-superior iliac spine, the distal radius or ulna, and the sternum [140]. Fluids administered IO for volume replacement should be infused under pressure using an infusion pump, pressure bag, or manual pressure to overcome venous resistance [113]. Less than 1% of patients have complications after an IO infusion [140].

Vasopressors, such as dopamine, should be given if epinephrine ± antihistamines and volume expansion fail to alleviate hypotension. Dopamine, 400 mg in 500 mL of 5% dextrose, should be administered at 2–5 μg/kg/min and titrated to maintain systolic blood pressure. Central venous access is helpful to facilitate administration of fluids and to continue to assess intravascular volume status. Consultation with critical care specialist for subjects with intractable hypotension is prudent.

Seven case reports describe use of methylene blue for the treatment of anaphylactic shock refractory to epinephrine, intravenous fluids, vasoconstrictors, and intra-aortic balloon pump [141,142]. Methylene blue may exert its favorable effects by blocking NO-mediated vascular smooth muscle relaxation. However, methylene blue itself is capable of causing anaphylaxis in some subjects [143,144]. Methylene blue should be avoided in subjects with glucose-6 phosphate dehydrogenase deficiency, pulmonary hypertension, and acute lung injury [111].

38.7 SPECIAL MANAGEMENT PROBLEMS

38.7.1 Management of persistent airway obstruction

38.7.1.1 PERSISTENT UPPER AIRWAY OBSTRUCTION

Severe laryngeal edema may occur so quickly during anaphylaxis that endotracheal intubation becomes impossible. Therefore, an endotracheal tube should be quickly inserted if laryngeal edema is not reversed promptly with epinephrine. An endotracheal tube measuring at least 7.5 mm in diameter is preferred in adults since larger sizes reduce resistance to airflow. Aerosolized epinephrine, along with supplemental oxygen and extension of the neck, may be helpful for difficult endotracheal intubation. If intubation fails, a cricothyrotomy is next since it is more easily accomplished than is an emergency tracheostomy. To do so, the subject's neck is hyperextended, and the area of the cricothyroid membrane is palpated below the thyroid cartilage and above the cricoid cartilage. A small incision is made, the membrane is punctured, and the opening is enlarged with a blunt instrument such as a scalpel handle. Finally, a small diameter (4–5 mm) endotracheal tube is inserted. Alternatively, high-flow oxygen delivery through an 11-gauge needle or polyethylene catheter may suffice for the short term if an endotracheal tube is not available. Potential complications of cricothyrotomy include vocal cord injury, bleeding, and subcutaneous emphysema [122]. This procedure is not part of the training of allergy/immunology subspecialists and is performed in emergency/critical care units by specialists trained to do so.

38.7.1.2 PERSISTENT LOWER AIRWAY OBSTRUCTION

Epinephrine reduces bronchospasm associated with anaphylaxis, but ventilation and oxygenation may remain a problem despite an adequate airway. This persistent airway obstruction should be treated as status asthmaticus. Arterial blood gas determinations and continuous pulse oximetry help guide therapy. Subjects usually respond to inhaled β-agonists, such as albuterol 2.5 mg, or 0.5 mL of 0.5% solution diluted with normal saline to a total volume of 3 mL delivered via nebulization.

Since adequate oxygenation also depends on ventilation, it may be necessary to establish and maintain an airway and/or provide ventilatory assistance. One of the quickest, easiest, and most effective ways to support ventilation involves a one-way valve facemask with oxygen inlet port (e.g., Pocket-Mask [Laerdal Medical Corporation, Wappingers Falls, New York] or similar device). Oxygen saturations comparable to endotracheal intubation have been demonstrated in patients who require artificial ventilation via the mouth-to-mask technique with oxygen attached to the inlet port. Subjects with adequate, spontaneous respirations may breathe through the mask.

Ambu bags of less than 700 mL are not recommended in adults unless an endotracheal tube is in place since ventilated volume will not overcome the 150–200 mL of anatomic dead space and thus not provide effective tidal volumes. Recommended tidal volume during artificial ventilation is 6–7 mL/kg over 1.5–2 seconds. Ambu bags may be used in children if the reservoir volume of the device is sufficient. Endotracheal intubation or cricothyroidotomy may be considered where appropriate, depending on the skills of the physician and other healthcare professionals.

The rate of administered oxygen depends on the clinical response and the device used. A nasal cannula delivers 25%–40% oxygen with a 4–6 L/min flow. A simple plastic face mask delivers 50%–60% oxygen with an 8–12 L/min flow. By comparison, the one-way valve facemask with oxygen inlet valve (see earlier) permits ventilation with up to 50% oxygen at a flow rate of 10 L/min and approaches 90%–100% if the rescuer periodically occludes the opening of the mask with his or her tongue during mouth-to-mask ventilation.

Mechanical ventilation itself may present a danger for subjects requiring ventilator support during anaphylaxis. Frequent complications of mechanical ventilation include pulmonary barotrauma and hemodynamic compromise, which may result if extremely high inspiratory pressures are necessary to overcome airway obstruction. Mechanical ventilation may have serious consequences for subjects with persistent hypotension despite adequate ventilation. High inspiratory pressure and an inadequate internal diameter of the endotracheal tube also may decrease venous return and increase right ventricular afterload, which leads to inadequate oxygen delivery, arrhythmias, and possible cardiac arrest.

38.7.2 Problems posed by β-adrenergic antagonists during anaphylaxis

β-Adrenergic antagonists (β-blockers) are used to treat cardio-vascular disease, arrhythmias, hypertension, migraine headaches, anxiety, glaucoma, and thyrotoxicosis. Numerous cases of unusually severe or refractory anaphylaxis are reported in patients taking topical or oral β-adrenergic blockers [2]. Subjects taking β-adrenergic antagonists may be more likely to experience severe anaphylaxis characterized by paradoxical bradycardia, severe hypotension, and bronchospasm. These agents may also impede epinephrine treatment. Use of selective $β_1$-antagonists does not eliminate the risk for anaphylaxis [2,145]. The use of glucagon in subjects on β-blockers who experience anaphylaxis was discussed earlier.

38.7.3 Management of anaphylaxis in pregnancy

Anaphylaxis rarely occurs during pregnancy; therefore, data are insufficient to make recommendations for treatment. With a few modifications, however, consensus treatment modalities used are identical to those used for anaphylaxis occurring in nonpregnant subjects [146]. The utero-placental arteries are very responsive to α-adrenergic stimulation, and great care is necessary when epinephrine or other agents with α-adrenergic effects are utilized. There is no evidence that epinephrine or diphenhydramine causes teratogenicity in humans. Both drugs may be used during pregnancy for anaphylaxis as adequate oxygenation and intravascular volume are especially important to maintain and support fetal perfusion [146].

38.7.4 Management of idiopathic anaphylaxis

Treatment for subjects with idiopathic anaphylaxis depends on its frequency. The treatment of the acute episode is the same as for any other form of anaphylaxis. Various published protocols to prevent recurrent episodes recommend the administration of H_1 antagonists (including ketotifen, not commercially available in the United States), corticosteroids, with or without albuterol tablets/syrup, and possible consideration of leukotriene modifiers. The decision to begin preventive therapy should be individualized [2,91].

38.7.5 Self-treatment by subject

All subjects at risk for anaphylaxis should carry and know how to self-administer epinephrine. In one report, more than 80% of subjects who died from food anaphylaxis were not given appropriate information to avoid inadvertent food-induced reactions or self-administer epinephrine to treat such reactions [21]. Pumphrey determined that epinephrine was administered in 62% of fatal anaphylactic reactions in the United Kingdom, only 14% prior to cardiac arrest [147]. In a 10-country European Anaphylaxis Registry of 3333 severe allergic reactions, self-administered epinephrine was used by subjects with a recurrent reaction in 125/1013 (12.3%) compared to 78/1968 (4.0%) with no previous anaphylaxis to the same allergen [28]. Epinephrine treatment by healthcare professionals also was low; only 19.8% of subjects treated by healthcare professionals for first-time reactions received epinephrine; for recurrent reactions to the same antigen, 21.1% received epinephrine [28]. In an analysis of 48 cases of fatal food anaphylaxis from 1999 to 2006, Pumphrey and Gowland reported 19 (40%) received epinephrine auto-injectors, but over half of the fatalities occurred in patients whose previous clinical reactions were so mild that, in the opinion of the investigators, it was unlikely that a physician would have prescribed an epinephrine syringe for self-administration [126].

Demonstration of proper self-administration technique using a placebo trainer is recommended [123]. An EpiPen (Mylan, Canonsburg, Pennsylvania) auto-injector for adults is available with a single 0.3 mg epinephrine (USP, 1:1000, 0.3 mL) dose. Similarly, an EpiPen Jr., with a 0.15 mg epinephrine (USP, 1:2000, 0.3 mL) dose, is available for children weighing less than 30 kg. Auvi-Q (Kaléo, US, Richmond, Virginia) is an auto-injector device that is available in 0.1, 0.15, or 0.3 mg single dose. About the size of a credit card, it is equipped with blinking lights at the needle end and a voice recording that guides the user throughout administration. Other generic products enter and exit the market periodically.

Adherence with an action plan to keep epinephrine available at all times and to inject it during anaphylaxis is another concern. Kemp et al. [148] determined in a follow-up survey of patients that 32 (47%) of 68 did not have their epinephrine with them when they again experienced anaphylaxis from a previously identified allergen. In contrast, 31 (91%) of 34 patients with idiopathic anaphylaxis had epinephrine available at a subsequent episode. Implementation of an educational protocol with emphasis on carrying epinephrine increased the frequency of adherence from 53% to 92% over the ensuing 10 years [149]. Other studies indicate that 50%–75% of patients prescribed epinephrine will carry it with them; 30%–40% of them demonstrate proper administration technique [121]. Some carry the epinephrine kit but choose not to use it or prefer to seek emergency medical assistance with anaphylaxis [123].

The cost of epinephrine auto-injectors has progressively increased to a level that is an economic burden for some individuals [150,151]. Lower-cost alternatives include office-made kits of prefilled syringes or prescribed epinephrine ampules, syringes, and needles [150].

38.7.6 Observation after anaphylaxis

The best evidence suggests that observation periods after complete resolution of uniphasic anaphylaxis should be individualized, particularly since there are no reliable predictors of biphasic anaphylaxis. An observation period, based on the severity and response to treatment, is appropriate. Initial phases of anaphylaxis characterized by hypotension, respiratory failure or hypoxemia, repeated doses of epinephrine, poorly controlled asthma, or prior history of biphasic anaphylaxis are reasonable indications for a prolonged observation period of 24 hours or even longer. At discharge, all patients should be provided self-injectable epinephrine and receive proper instruction on how to self-administer it in case of a subsequent episode. Patients also should have ready and prompt access to emergency medical services for transportation to the closest emergency department for treatment. Further prospective studies on biphasic anaphylaxis are needed [105,152].

38.8 PREVENTION OF ANAPHYLAXIS

38.8.1 Certain anaphylactic reactions are preventable

Some anaphylactic reactions are so severe that treatment is unsuccessful and death occurs. This underscores the critical importance of education, avoidance, and prevention. Table 38.4 outlines basic principles for the prevention of future anaphylaxis. An allergist-immunologist can provide comprehensive professional advice on these matters.

Agents that cause anaphylaxis must be identified, whenever possible, and subjects should be instructed how to minimize future exposure. Prospective trials on the impact of concomitant β-blockers and angiotensin-converting enzyme (ACE) inhibitor use while on allergen immunotherapy are needed [153,154]. Traditionally, β-blockers have been discontinued where feasible, while subjects were on allergen immunotherapy. However, the evidence is inconclusive, and the dangers of poorly controlled cardiovascular disease must be weighed against the perceived likelihood of a systemic reaction. There is some preliminary evidence that ACE inhibitors may potentiate anaphylaxis by preventing compensatory angiotensin II mobilization during anaphylaxis [11]. One study determined that peanut- and nut-allergic subjects who experienced anaphylaxis characterized by severe pharyngeal angioedema have significantly lower serum ACE levels than those with no pharyngeal angioedema. None was taking an ACE inhibitor [155]. More clinical data are necessary to recommend that ACE inhibitors not be used when a patient is susceptible to anaphylaxis. Monoamine oxidase inhibitors and some tricyclic antidepressants render epinephrine usage more hazardous by interfering with its degradation.

Meals may deliver unsavory surprises for highly allergic individuals. A case report illustrates that anaphylaxis may occur in latex-allergic subjects whose food handlers wear latex gloves. Baked goods commonly contain peanuts and nuts, and accidental ingestion of these foods is common [149]. Pumphrey observed that commercial catering causes 76% of food-related anaphylaxis in the United Kingdom [147]. Education is of paramount importance, and Food Allergy Research and Education (FARE; https://www.foodallergy.org) is a helpful, nonprofit resource for many food-allergic individuals.

Table 38.4 Preventive measures for subjects with anaphylaxis

I. General measures
- Obtain thorough history to identify the cause(s) of anaphylaxis and those individuals at risk for future anaphylaxis.
- Provide instruction to read food and medication labels, as appropriate.
- Avoid exposure to causal agents and cross-reactive substances.
- Manage comorbid conditions.
- Implement a waiting period of 20–30 minutes after parenteral medications (30 minutes for SCIT[a]).
- Consider an observation period of up to 2 hours following first oral dose of a medication he or she has not previously taken.
- Consult allergist-immunologist for assistance.

II. Specific measures for high-risk patients
- Individuals at high risk for anaphylaxis should carry self-injectable syringes of epinephrine and receive instructions and demonstration in proper use.
- MedicAlert (MedicAlert Foundation, Turlock, California) or similar warning bracelet or chain when indicated.
- Avoid β-adrenergic antagonists, angiotensin-converting enzyme inhibitors, monoamine oxidase inhibitors, and tricyclic antidepressants, if possible.
- Supervised incremental administration of agents suspected of causing anaphylaxis, given orally, when necessary.
- Where appropriate, utilize specific preventative strategies, including pharmacologic prophylaxis, graded challenge, or desensitization.

[a] SCIT, subcutaneous allergen immunotherapy.
Source: Modified from Kemp SF. *Immunol Allergy Clin N Am* 2001; 21: 611–634.

The potential for anaphylaxis may be determined by skin tests in some circumstances (e.g., allergy to β-lactam antibiotics). However, the immunochemistry of most drugs and biologic agents is not well defined, and reliable *in vivo* or *in vitro* tests for most agents are unavailable.

Situations may arise for which it is necessary to administer a medication that previously caused anaphylaxis. Numerous protocols are available to assist in this process and decrease the risk of severe adverse reactions. Such "desensitization protocols" should only be conducted in clinical settings where anaphylaxis, if it occurs, can be properly managed. Techniques used in these protocols include antihistamine and corticosteroid prophylaxis to prevent or reduce the severity of IgE-independent reactions (e.g., radiocontrast media); administration of gradual incremental doses of medication over several hours (e.g., short-term desensitization to penicillin, carboplatin, etc.); or the highly effective, long-term desensitization with venom immunotherapy for stinging insect anaphylaxis (see Chapter 29).

SALIENT POINTS

1. Epinephrine is the most important therapeutic agent used to treat anaphylaxis. It must be used early and in appropriate doses to be effective.

2. Fatal anaphylaxis from subcutaneous allergen immunotherapy (SCIT) occurs at a rate of approximately 1 per 9,100,000 injection visits.
3. Anaphylaxis associated with SCIT occurs more frequently with accelerated dosage schedules than with traditional, more leisurely schedules.
4. The use of β-adrenergic antagonists (β-blockers) may increase the risk for refractory anaphylaxis.
5. Mast cell tryptase levels correlate with the severity of anaphylaxis in some instances. However, a normal tryptase level does not exclude anaphylaxis.
6. Some subjects with anaphylaxis have atypical findings such as bradycardia, vasomotor collapse without urticaria, or isolated gastrointestinal symptoms.
7. Myocardial dysfunction and arrhythmias may be prominent features of anaphylaxis.
8. Peanuts and tree nuts cause great concern in food-associated anaphylaxis. Peanuts and tree nuts are of special concern because of (1) the life-threatening severity of anaphylaxis to the peanut/tree nut, especially in subjects with concomitant asthma, and (2) the propensity for subjects to remain allergic for life.
9. Exercise avoidance remains the best treatment for exercise-induced anaphylaxis since medical prophylaxis is not very effective.
10. Glucagon may be considered for subjects on β-blockers not responding to epinephrine.
11. Intravenous epinephrine at dilute concentrations is a consideration when severe and life-threatening anaphylaxis is not responding to optimal therapy.

REFERENCES

1. Tanno LK, Simons FE, Annesi-Maesano I, Calderon MA, Ayme S, Demoly P. Fatal anaphylaxis registries data support changes in the who anaphylaxis mortality coding rules. *Orphanet J Rare Dis* 2017; 12(1): 8.
2. Lieberman P, Nicklas RA, Randolph C et al. Anaphylaxis—A practice parameter update 2015. *Ann Allergy Asthma Immunol* 2015; 115(5): 341–384.
3. Simons FE, Ardusso LR, Bilo MB et al. International consensus on (ICON) anaphylaxis. *World Allergy Organ J* 2014; 7(1): 9.
4. Cox L, Larenas-Linnemann D, Lockey RF, Passalacqua G. Speaking the same language: The world allergy organization subcutaneous immunotherapy systemic reaction grading system. *J Allergy Clin Immunol* 2010; 125(3): 569–574.e7.
5. Cox LS, Sanchez-Borges M, Lockey RF. World allergy organization systemic allergic reaction grading system: Is a modification needed? *J Allergy Clin Immunol Pract* 2017; 5(1): 58–62.e5.
6. Johansson SGO, Bieber T, Dahl R et al. Revised nomenclature for allergy for global use: Report of the Nomenclature Review Committee of the World Allergy Organization, October 2003. *J Allergy Clin Immunol* 2004; 113(5): 832–836.
7. Sampson HA, Munoz-Furlong A, Campbell RL et al. Second symposium on the definition and management of anaphylaxis: Summary report—Second National Institute of Allergy and Infectious Disease/Food Allergy and Anaphylaxis Network symposium. *Ann Emerg Med* 2006; 47(4): 373–380.
8. Greenberger PA, Ditto AM. Chapter 24: Anaphylaxis. *Allergy Asthma Proc* 2012; 33(Suppl 1): 80–83.
9. Sampson HA, Muñoz-Furlong A, Campbell RL et al. Second symposium on the definition and management of anaphylaxis: Summary Report—Second National Institute of Allergy and Infectious Disease/Food Allergy and Anaphylaxis Network Symposium. *Ann Emerg Med* 2006; 47(4): 373–380.
10. Simons FER, Ardusso LRF, Bilò MB et al. World Allergy Organization guidelines for the assessment and management of anaphylaxis. *World Allergy Organ J* 2011; 4(2): 13–36.
11. Lieberman PKS, Brown SA. Anaphylaxis. In: Adkinson NF BB, Burks W, Busse WW, editors. *Middleton's Allergy: Principles and Practice.* 8th ed. Mosby Elsevier, 2013.
12. Khan BQ, Kemp SF. Pathophysiology of anaphylaxis. *Curr Opin Allergy Clin Immunol* 2011; 11(4): 319–325.
13. Pumphrey R. Anaphylaxis: Can we tell who is at risk of a fatal reaction? *Curr Opin Allergy Clin Immunol* 2004; 4(4): 285–290.
14. Yocum MW, Butterfield JH, Klein JS, Volcheck GW, Schroeder DR, Silverstein MD. Epidemiology of anaphylaxis in Olmsted County: A population-based study. *J Allergy Clin Immunol* 1999; 104(2): 452–456.
15. Chinn DJ, Sheikh A. *Epidemiology of Anaphylaxis. Allergy Frontiers: Epigenetics, Allergens and Risk Factors* 2009. Japan: Springer, pp. 123–144.
16. Decker WW, Campbell RL, Manivannan V et al. The etiology and incidence of anaphylaxis in Rochester, Minnesota: A report from the Rochester Epidemiology Project. *J Allergy Clin Immunol* 2008; 122(6): 1161–1165.
17. Lieberman P, Camargo CA Jr, Bohlke K et al. Epidemiology of anaphylaxis: Findings of the American College of Allergy, Asthma and Immunology Epidemiology of Anaphylaxis Working Group. *Ann Allergy Asthma Immunol* 2006; 97(5): 596–602.
18. Neugut AI, Ghatak AT, Miller RL. Anaphylaxis in the United States. *Arch Intern Med* 2001; 161(1): 15.
19. Porter J, Jick H. Drug-induced anaphylaxis, convulsions, deafness, and extrapyramidal symptoms. *Lancet* 1977; 309(8011): 587–588.
20. Burks W, Bannon GA, Sicherer S, Sampson HA. Peanut-induced anaphylactic reactions. *Int Arch Allergy Immunol* 1999; 119(3): 165–172.
21. Bock SA, Munoz-Furlong A, Sampson HA. Fatalities due to anaphylactic reactions to foods. *J Allergy Clin Immunol* 2001; 107(1): 191–193.
22. Bock SA, Muñoz-Furlong A, Sampson HA. Further fatalities caused by anaphylactic reactions to food, 2001–2006. *J Allergy Clin Immunol* 2007; 119(4): 1016–1018.
23. Bernstein DI, Epstein T, Murphy-Berendts K, Liss GM. Surveillance of systemic reactions to subcutaneous immunotherapy injections: Year 1 outcomes of the ACAAI and AAAAI Collaborative Study. *Ann Allergy Asthma Immunol* 2010; 104(6): 530–535.
24. Bernstein DI, Epstein T. Systemic reactions to subcutaneous allergen immunotherapy. *Immunol Allergy Clinics North America* 2011; 31(2): 241–249.
25. Graft DF, Schuberth KC, Kagey-Sobotka A et al. A prospective study of the natural history of large local reactions after Hymenoptera stings in children. *J Pediatr* 1984; 104(5): 664–668.
26. Patterson R. Idiopathic anaphylaxis. *Arch Intern Med* 1995; 155(8): 869.
27. Yu JE, Lin RY. The epidemiology of anaphylaxis. *Clin Rev Allergy Immunol* 2018; 54(3): 366–374.

28. Worm M, Moneret-Vautrin A, Scherer K et al. First European data from the network of severe allergic reactions (NORA). *Allergy* 2014; 69(10): 1397–1404.

29. Turner PJ, Campbell DE. Epidemiology of severe anaphylaxis: Can we use population-based data to understand anaphylaxis? *Curr Opin Allergy Clin Immunol* 2016; 16(5): 441–450.

30. Grabenhenrich LB, Dolle S, Moneret-Vautrin A et al. Anaphylaxis in children and adolescents: The European Anaphylaxis Registry. *J Allergy Clin Immunol* 2016; 137(4): 1128–1137.e1.

31. Castells M. Diagnosis and management of anaphylaxis in precision medicine. *J Allergy Clin Immunol* 2017; 140(2): 321–333.

32. Levy JH, Bartz RR. Protamine, is something fishy about it? The spectre of anaphylaxis continues. *J Cardiothorac Vasc Anesth* 2019; 33(2): 487–488.

33. Lockey R, Benedict L, Turkeltaub P, Bukantz S. Fatalities from immunotherapy (IT) and skin testing (ST). *J Allergy Clin Immunol* 1987; 79(4): 660–677.

34. Reid M, Lockey R, Turkeltaub P, Plattsmills T. Survey of fatalities from skin testing and immunotherapy 1985–1989. *J Allergy Clini Immunol* 1993; 92(1): 6–15.

35. Epstein TG, Liss GM, Berendts KM, Bernstein DI. AAAAI/ACAAI Subcutaneous Immunotherapy Surveillance Study (2013–2017): Fatalities, infections, delayed reactions, and use of epinephrine autoinjectors. *J Allergy Clin Immunol Pract* 2019; 7(6): 1996–2003.

36. Bernstein DI, Wanner M, Borish L, Liss GM, Immunotherapy Committee AAoAA, Immunology. Twelve-year survey of fatal reactions to allergen injections and skin testing: 1990–2001. *J Allergy Clin Immunol* 2004; 113(6): 1129–1136.

37. Johnstone J, Hobbins S, Parekh D, O'Hickey S. Excess subcutaneous tissue may preclude intramuscular delivery when using adrenaline autoinjectors in patients with anaphylaxis. *Allergy* 2015; 70(6): 703–706.

38. Amin H, Liss G, Bernstein D. Evaluation of near-fatal reactions to allergen immunotherapy injections. *J Allergy Clin Immunol* 2006; 117(1): 169–175.

39. Stewart GE, Lockey RF. Systemic reactions from allergen immunotherapy. *J Allergy Clin Immunol* 1992; 90(4): 567–578.

40. Nolte H, Casale TB, Lockey RF et al. Epinephrine use in clinical trials of sublingual immunotherapy tablets. *J Allergy Clin Immunol Pract* 2017; 5(1):84–89.e3.

41. Calderon MA, Simons FE, Malling HJ, Lockey RF, Moingeon P, Demoly P. Sublingual allergen immunotherapy: Mode of action and its relationship with the safety profile. *Allergy* 2012; 67(3): 302–311.

42. Finkelman FD. Anaphylaxis: Lessons from mouse models. *J Allergy Clin Immunol* 2007; 120(3): 506–515.

43. Vadas P, Gold M, Perelman B et al. Platelet-activating factor, PAF acetylhydrolase, and severe anaphylaxis. *N Engl J Med* 2008; 358(1): 28–35.

44. Vadas P, Perelman B, Liss G. Platelet-activating factor, histamine, and tryptase levels in human anaphylaxis. *J Allergy Clin Immunol* 2013; 131(1): 144–149.

45. Erjefält JS, Korsgren M, Malm-Erjefält M, Conroy DM, Williams TJ, Persson CGA. Acute allergic responses induce a prompt luminal entry of airway tissue eosinophils. *Am J Respir Cell Mol Biol* 2003; 29(4): 439–448.

46. Kaliner M, Sigler R, Summers R, Shelhamer J. Effects of infused histamine: Analysis of the effects of H-1 and H-2 histamine receptor antagonists on cardiovascular and pulmonary responses. *J Allergy Clin Immunol* 1981; 68(5): 365–371.

47. Chrusch C, Sharma S, Unruh H et al. Histamine H3 receptor blockade improves cardiac function in canine anaphylaxis. *Am J Resp Crit Care* 1999; 160(4): 1142–1149.

48. Godot V, Arock M, Garcia G et al. H4 histamine receptor mediates optimal migration of mast cell precursors to CXCL12. *J Allergy Clin Immunol* 2007; 120(4): 827–834.

49. Yunginger JW, Nelson DR, Squillace DL et al. Laboratory investigation of deaths due to anaphylaxis. *J Forensic Sci* 1991; 36(3): 13095J.

50. Mertes PM, Laxenaire M-C, Alla F. Anaphylactic and anaphylactoid reactions occurring during anesthesia in France in 1999–2000. *Anesthesiology* 2003; 99(3): 536–545.

51. Valent P, Horny H-P, Triggiani M, Arock M. Clinical and laboratory parameters of mast cell activation as basis for the formulation of diagnostic criteria. *Int Arch Allergy Immunol* 2011; 156(2): 119–127.

52. Valent P, Akin C, Bonadonna P et al. Proposed diagnostic algorithm for patients with suspected mast cell activation syndrome. *J Allergy Clin Immunol Pract* 2019; 7(4): 1125–1133.e1.

53. Dua S, Dowey J, Foley L et al. Diagnostic value of tryptase in food allergic reactions: A prospective study of 160 adult peanut challenges. *J Allergy Clin Immunol Pract* 2018; 6(5): 1692–1698.e1.

54. Lin RY, Schwartz LB, Curry A et al. Histamine and tryptase levels in patients with acute allergic reactions: An emergency department–based study. *J Allergy Clin Immunol* 2000; 106(1): 65–71.

55. Smith PL, Kagey-Sobotka A, Bleecker ER et al. Physiologic manifestations of human anaphylaxis. *J Clin Invest* 1980; 66(5): 1072–1080.

56. Cauwels A. Nitric oxide in shock. *Kidney Int* 2007; 72(5): 557–565.

57. Rolla G, Nebiolo F, Guida G, Heffler E, Bommarito L, Bergia R. Level of exhaled nitric oxide during human anaphylaxis. *Ann Allergy Asthma Immunol* 2006; 97(2): 264–265.

58. Nakamura Y, Hashiba Y, Endo J, Furuie M, Isozaki A, Yagi K. Elevated exhaled nitric oxide in anaphylaxis with respiratory symptoms. *Allergol Int* 2015; 64(4): 359–363.

59. De Souza RL, Short T, Warman GR, Maclennan N, Young Y. Anaphylaxis with associated fibrinolysis, reversed with tranexamic acid and demonstrated by thrombelastography. *Anaesth Intens Care* 2004; 32(4): 580–587.

60. Reber LL, Hernandez JD, Galli SJ. The pathophysiology of anaphylaxis. *J Allergy Clin Immunol* 2017; 140(2): 335–348.

61. Marone G, Bova M, Detoraki A, Onorati AM, Rossi FW, Spadaro G. *The Human Heart as a Shock Organ in Anaphylaxis*. New York, NY: John Wiley & Sons, 2008: 133–156.

62. Raper RF, Fisher MM. Profound reversible myocardial depression after anaphylaxis. *Lancet* 1988; 331(8582): 386–388.

63. Wittstein IS, Thiemann DR, Lima JAC et al. Neurohumoral features of myocardial stunning due to sudden emotional stress. *N Engl J Med* 2005; 352(6): 539–548.

64. Bristow MR, Ginsburg R, Harrison DC. Histamine and the human heart: The other receptor system. *Am J Cardiol* 1982; 49(1): 249–251.

65. Fisher MM. Clinical observations on the pathophysiology and treatment of anaphylactic cardiovascular collapse. *Anaesth Intens Care* 1986; 14(1): 17–21.

66. Pumphrey RSH. Fatal posture in anaphylactic shock. *J Allergy Clin Immunol* 2003; 112(2): 451–452.

67. Kovanen PT, Kaartinen M, Paavonen T. Infiltrates of activated mast cells at the site of coronary atheromatous erosion or rupture in myocardial infarction. *Circulation* 1995; 92(5): 1084–1088.

68. Kounis NG. Kounis syndrome (allergic angina and allergic myocardial infarction): A natural paradigm? *Int J Cardiol* 2006; 110(1): 7–14.

69. Cevik C, Nugent K, Shome GP, Kounis NG. Treatment of Kounis syndrome. *Int J Cardiol* 2010; 143(3): 223–226.

70. Abela GS, Picon PD, Friedl SE et al. Triggering of plaque disruption and arterial thrombosis in an atherosclerotic rabbit model. *Circulation* 1995; 91(3): 776–784.

71. Steffel J, Akhmedov A, Greutert H, Lüscher TF, Tanner FC. Histamine induces tissue factor expression. *Circulation* 2005; 112(3): 341–941.

72. Schuligoi R, Amann R, Donnerer J, Peskar BA. Release of calcitonin gene-related peptide in cardiac anaphylaxis. *Naunyn-Schmiedeberg's Arch Pharmacol* 1997; 355(2): 224–229.

73. Rang W-Q, Du Y-H, Hu C-P et al. Protective effects of calcitonin gene-related peptide-mediated evodiamine on guinea-pig cardiac anaphylaxis. *Naunyn-Schmiedeberg's Arch Pharmacol* 2003; 367(3): 306–311.

74. van der Linden P-WG. Anaphylactic shock after insect-sting challenge in 138 persons with a previous insect-sting reaction. *Ann Int Med* 1993; 118(3): 161.

75. Brown SGA. Insect sting anaphylaxis; prospective evaluation of treatment with intravenous adrenaline and volume resuscitation. *Emerg Med J* 2004; 21(2): 149–154.

76. Schadt JC, Ludbrook J. Hemodynamic and neurohumoral responses to acute hypovolemia in conscious mammals. *Am J Physiol Heart Circ Physiol* 1991; 260(2): H305–HH18.

77. Demetriades D, Chan LS, Bhasin P et al. Relative bradycardia in patients with traumatic hypotension. *J Trauma* 1998; 45(3): 534–539.

78. Söreide E, Buxrud T, Harboe S. Severe anaphylactic reactions outside hospital: Etiology, symptoms and treatment. *Acta Anaesthesiologica Scandinavica* 1988; 32(4): 339–342.

79. Viner NA, Rhamy RK. Anaphylaxis manifested by hypotension alone. *J Urol* 1975; 113(1): 108–110.

80. Brown AFT, McKinnon D, Chu K. Emergency department anaphylaxis: A review of 142 patients in a single year. *J Allergy Clin Immunol* 2001; 108(5): 861–866.

81. Webb LM, Lieberman P. Anaphylaxis: A review of 601 cases. *Ann Allergy Asthma Immunol* 2006; 97(1): 39–43.

82. Commins SP, Jerath MR, Cox K, Erickson LD, Platts-Mills T. Delayed anaphylaxis to alpha-gal, an oligosaccharide in mammalian meat. *Allergol Int* 2016; 65(1): 16–20.

83. Cox L, Platts-Mills TAE, Finegold I, Schwartz LB, Simons FER, Wallace DV. American Academy of Allergy, Asthma and Immunology/American College of Allergy, Asthma and Immunology Joint Task Force Report on omalizumab-associated anaphylaxis. *J Allergy Clin Immunol* 2007; 120(6): 1373–1377.

84. Limb SL, Starke PR, Lee CE, Chowdhury BA. Delayed onset and protracted progression of anaphylaxis after omalizumab administration in patients with asthma. *J Allergy Clin Immunol* 2007; 120(6): 1378–1381.

85. Cheifetz A, Smedley M, Martin S et al. The incidence and management of infusion reactions to infliximab: A large center experience. *Am J Gastroenterol* 2003; 98(6): 1315–1324.

86. Stallmach A, Giese T, Schmidt C, Meuer SC, Zeuzem SS. Severe anaphylactic reaction to infliximab. *Eur J Gastroen Hepat* 2004; 16(6): 627–630.

87. Wong JT, Long A. Rituximab hypersensitivity: Evaluation, desensitization, and potential mechanisms. *J Allergy Clin Immunol Pract* 2017; 5(6): 1564–1571.

88. Ditto AM, Harris KE, Krasnick J, Miller MA, Patterson R. Idiopathic anaphylaxis: A series of 335 cases. *Ann Allergy Asthma Immunol* 1996; 77(4): 285–291.

89. James LP, Austen KF. Fatal systemic anaphylaxis in man. *N Engl J Med* 1964; 270(12): 597–603.

90. Greenhawt M, Gupta RS, Meadows JA et al. Guiding principles for the recognition, diagnosis, and management of infants with anaphylaxis: An expert panel consensus. *J Allergy Clin Immunol Pract* 2019; 7(4): 1148–1156.e5.

91. Greenberger PA. Idiopathic anaphylaxis. *Immunol Allergy Clin North Am* 2007; 27(2): 273–293.

92. Castells MC, Horan RF, Sheffer AL. Exercise-induced anaphylaxis. *Curr Allergy Asthma Rep* 2003; 3(1): 15–21.

93. Barg W, Medrala W, Wolanczyk-Medrala A. Exercise-induced anaphylaxis: An update on diagnosis and treatment. *Curr Allergy Asthma Rep* 2010; 11(1): 45–51.

94. Feldweg AM. Food-dependent, exercise-induced anaphylaxis: Diagnosis and management in the outpatient setting. *J Allergy Clin Immunol Pract* 2017; 5(2): 283–288.

95. Bartra J, Araujo G, Munoz-Cano R. Interaction between foods and nonsteroidal anti-inflammatory drugs and exercise in the induction of anaphylaxis. *Curr Opin Allergy Clin Immunol* 2018; 18(4): 310–316.

96. Shadick NA, Liang MH, Partridge AJ et al. The natural history of exercise-induced anaphylaxis: Survey results from a 10-year follow-up study. *J Allergy Clin Immunol* 1999; 104(1): 123–127.

97. Ansley L, Bonini M, Delgado L et al. Pathophysiological mechanisms of exercise-induced anaphylaxis: An EAACI position statement. *Allergy* 2015; 70(10): 1212–1221.

98. Feinberg JH, Toner CB. Successful treatment of disabling cholinergic urticaria. *Mil Med* 2008; 173(2): 217–220.

99. The International Collaborative Study of Severe Anaphylaxis. An epidemiologic study of severe anaphylactic and anaphylactoid reactions among hospital patients: Methods and overall risks. *Epidemiology* 1998; 9(2): 141–146.

100. Stricker W, Anorvelopez E, Reed C. Food skin testing in patients with idiopathic anaphylaxis. *J Allergy Clin Immunol* 1986; 77(3): 516–519.

101. Slater JE, Raphael G, Cutler GB, Loriaux LD, Meggs WJ, Kaliner M. Recurrent anaphylaxis in menstruating women. *Obstet Gynecol Surv* 1988; 43(4): 240–242.

102. Meggs WJ, Pescovitz OH, Metcalfe D, Loriaux DL, Cutler G, Kaliner M. Progesterone sensitivity as a cause of recurrent anaphylaxis. *N Engl J Med* 1984; 311(19): 1236–1238.

103. Kemp SF. The post-anaphylaxis dilemma: How long is long enough to observe a patient after resolution of symptoms? *Curr Allergy Asthma Rep* 2008; 8(1): 45–48.

104. Scranton SE, Gonzalez EG, Waibel KH. Incidence and characteristics of biphasic reactions after allergen immunotherapy. *J Allergy Clin Immunol* 2009; 123(2): 493–498.

105. Tole JW, Lieberman P. Biphasic anaphylaxis: Review of incidence, clinical predictors, and observation recommendations. *Immunol Allergy Clin North Am* 2007; 27(2): 309–326.

106. Stark B, Sullivan T. Biphasic and protracted anaphylaxis. *J Allergy Clin Immunol* 1986; 78(1): 76–83.

107. Sampson HA, Mendelson L, Rosen JP. Fatal and near-fatal anaphylactic reactions to food in children and adolescents. *N Engl J Med* 1992; 327(6): 380–384.

108. Sheikh A, ten Broek V, Brown SGA, Simons FER. H_1-antihistamines for the treatment of anaphylaxis: Cochrane systematic review. *Allergy* 2007; 62(8): 830–837.

109. Sheikh A, Shehata YA, Brown SG, Simons FE. *Adrenaline for the treatment of anaphylaxis with and without shock*. *Cochrane Database Syst Rev* 2008; (4): CD006312.

110. Choo KJL, Simons FER, Sheikh A. *Glucocorticoids for the treatment of anaphylaxis*. *Cochrane Database Syst Rev* 2010; (3): CD007596.

111. Kemp AM, Kemp SF. Pharmacotherapy in refractory anaphylaxis: When intramuscular epinephrine fails. *Curr Opin Allergy Clin Immunol* 2014; 14(4): 371–378.

112. Simons FER. Pharmacologic treatment of anaphylaxis: Can the evidence base be strengthened? *Curr Opin Allergy Clin Immunol* 2010; 10(4): 384–393.

113. 2005 American Heart Association (AHA) Guidelines for Cardiopulmonary Resuscitation (CPR) and Emergency Cardiovascular Care (ECC) of Pediatric and Neonatal Patients: Pediatric Advanced Life Support. *Pediatrics* 2006; 117(5): e989–1004.

114. Campbell RL, Li JT, Nicklas RA, Sadosty AT, Members of the Joint Task F, Practice Parameter W. Emergency department diagnosis and treatment of anaphylaxis: A practice parameter. *Ann Allergy Asthma Immunol* 2014;113 (6): 599–608.

115. Gompels LL. Proposed use of adrenaline (epinephrine) in anaphylaxis and related conditions: A study of senior house officers starting accident and emergency posts. *Postgraduate Med J* 2002; 78(921): 416–418.

116. Clark S, Bock SA, Gaeta TJ, Brenner BE, Cydulka RK, Camargo CA. Multicenter study of emergency department visits for food allergies. *J Allergy Clin Immunol* 2004; 113(2): 347–352.

117. Haymore BR, Carr WW, Frank WT. Anaphylaxis and epinephrine prescribing patterns in a military hospital: Underutilization of the intramuscular route. *Allergy Asthma Proc* 2005; 26(5): 361–365.

118. Kastner M, Harada L, Waserman S. Gaps in anaphylaxis management at the level of physicians, patients, and the community: A systematic review of the literature. *Allergy* 2010; 65(4): 435–444.

119. Lieberman P, Nicklas RA, Oppenheimer J et al. The diagnosis and management of anaphylaxis practice parameter: 2010 update. *J Allergy Clin Immunol* 2010; 126(3): 477–480. e1–42.

120. Cox L, Nelson H, Lockey R et al. Allergen immunotherapy: A practice parameter third update. *J Allergy Clin Immunol* 2011; 127(1): S1–S55.

121. Caroline NL. Medical care in the streets. *JAMA* 1977; 237(1): 43–46.

122. Soar J, Pumphrey R, Cant A et al. Emergency treatment of anaphylactic reactions—Guidelines for healthcare providers. *Resuscitation* 2008; 77(2): 157–169.

123. Kemp SF, Lockey RF, Simons FE. World Allergy Organization ad hoc Committee on Epinephrine in Anaphylaxis. Epinephrine: the drug of choice for anaphylaxis. A statement of the World Allergy Organization. *Allergy* 2008 Aug; 63(8): 1061–1070.

124. Yunginger JW. Fatal food-induced anaphylaxis. *J Am Med Assoc* 1988; 260(10): 1450.

125. Golden DBK. Anaphylaxis: Recognizing risk and targeting treatment. *J Allergy Clin Immunol Pract* 2017; 5(5): 1224–1226.

126. Pumphrey RSH, Gowland MH. Further fatal allergic reactions to food in the United Kingdom, 1999–2006. *J Allergy Clin Immunol* 2007; 119(4): 1018–1019.

127. Simons FER, Gu X, Simons KJ. Epinephrine absorption in adults: Intramuscular versus subcutaneous injection. *J Allergy Clin Immunol* 2001; 108(5): 871–873.

128. Simons FER, Roberts JR, Gu X, Simons KJ. Epinephrine absorption in children with a history of anaphylaxis. *J Allergy Clin Immunol* 1998; 101(1): 33–37.

129. Song TT, Nelson MR, Chang JH, Engler RJM, Chowdhury BA. Adequacy of the epinephrine autoinjector needle length in delivering epinephrine to the intramuscular tissues. *Ann Allergy Asthma Immunol* 2005; 94(5): 539–542.

130. Westfall TC WD. Adrenergic agonists and antagonists. In: Brunton LL CB, Knollman BC, editors. *The Pharmacological Basis of Therapeutics*. 12th ed. New York, NY: McGraw-Hill, 2011.

131. Simons FER, Lieberman PL, Read EJ, Edwards ES. Hazards of unintentional injection of epinephrine from autoinjectors: A systematic review. *Ann Allergy Asthma Immunol* 2009; 102(4): 282–287.

132. Pessoa Gingerich C. FDA tracks intranasal epinephrine spray. *MD*. https://www.mdmag.com/medical-news/fda-fast-tracks-intranasal-epinephrine-spray. Accessed April 14, 2019.

133. Insys' epinephrine nasal spray gets fast track status to treat anaphylaxis [updated August 31, 2018]. https://www.compelo.com/medical-devices/news/insys-epinephrine-nasal-spray-fast-track-status/

134. Srisawat C, Nakponetong K, Benjasupattananun P et al. A preliminary study of intranasal epinephrine administration as a potential route for anaphylaxis treatment. *Asian Pac J Allergy Immunol* 2016; 34(1): 38–43.

135. Simons FER. Advances in H_1-antihistamines. *N Engl J Med* 2004; 351(21): 2203–2217.

136. Nurmatov UB, Rhatigan E, Simons FE, Sheikh A. H_2-Antihistamines for the treatment of anaphylaxis with and without shock: A systematic review. *Ann Allergy Asthma Immunol* 2014; 112(2): 126–131.

137. Alqurashi W, Ellis AK. Do corticosteroids prevent biphasic anaphylaxis? *J Allergy Clin Immunol Pract* 2017; 5(5): 1194–1205.

138. Sheikh A. Glucocorticosteroids for the treatment and prevention of anaphylaxis. *Curr Opin Allergy Clin Immunol* 2013; 13(3): 263–267.

139. Thomas M, Crawford I. Glucagon infusion in refractory anaphylactic shock in patients on β-blockers. *Emerg Med J* 2005; 22(4): 272–273.

140. American Heart Association. Advanced Cardiovascular Support Provider Manual 2006. p. 48 and supplementary material pp. 1–86.

141. Evora PRB, Simon MR. Role of nitric oxide production in anaphylaxis and its relevance for the treatment of anaphylactic hypotension with methylene blue. *Ann Allergy Asthma Immunol* 2007; 99(4): 306–313.

142. Del Duca D, Sheth SS, Clarke AE, Lachapelle KJ, Ergina PL. Use of methylene blue for catecholamine-refractory vasoplegia from protamine and aprotinin. *Ann Thoracic Surg* 2009; 87(2): 640–642.

143. Dewachter P, Castro S, Nicaise-Roland P et al. Anaphylactic reaction after methylene blue-treated plasma transfusion. *Br J Anaesth* 2011; 106(5): 687–689.

144. Nubret K, Delhoume M, Orsel I, Laudy JS, Sellami M, Nathan N. Anaphylactic shock to fresh-frozen plasma inactivated with methylene blue. *Transfusion* 2011; 51(1): 125–128.

145. Benner S, Chen RJ, Wilson NA et al. Sequence-specific detection of individual DNA polymerase complexes in real time using a nanopore. *Nat Nanotechnol* 2007; 2(11): 718–724.

146. Schatz M, Zeiger RS, Falkoff R, Chambers C, Macy E, Mellon MH. *Asthma and Allergic Diseases during Pregnancy. Middleton's Allergy: Principles and Practice*. New York, NY: Elsevier, 2009: 1423–1444.

147. Pumphrey RS. Lessons for management of anaphylaxis from a study of fatal reactions. *Clin Exp Allergy* 2000; 30(8): 1144–1150.

148. Kemp SF, Lockey RF, Wolf BL, Lieberman P, Anaphylaxis. A review of 266 cases. *Arch Int Med* 1995; 155(16): 1749–1754.

149. Guidelines for the Diagnosis and Management of Food Allergy in the United States: Report of the NIAID-Sponsored Expert Panel. *J Allergy Clin Immunol* 2010; 126(6): S1–S58.

150. Westermann-Clark E, Fitzhugh DJ, Lockey RF. Increasing cost of epinephrine autoinjectors. *J Allergy Clin Immunol* 2012; 130(3): 822–823.

151. Pepper AN, Westermann-Clark E, Lockey RF. The high cost of epinephrine autoinjectors and possible alternatives. *J Allergy Clin Immunol Pract* 2017; 5(3): 665–668.e1.

152. Lee S, Sadosty AT, Campbell RL. Update on biphasic anaphylaxis. *Curr Opin Allergy Clin Immunol* 2016; 16(4): 346–351.

153. Carlson GS, Wong PH, White KM, Quinn JM. Evaluation of angiotensin-converting enzyme inhibitor and angiotensin receptor blocker therapy in immunotherapy-associated systemic reactions. *J Allergy Clin Immunol Pract* 2017; 5(5): 1430–1432.

154. Coop CA, Schapira RS, Freeman TM. Are ACE inhibitors and β-blockers dangerous in patients at risk for anaphylaxis? *J Allergy Clin Immunol Pract* 2017; 5(5): 1207–1211.

155. Summers CW, Pumphrey RS, Woods CN, McDowell G, Pemberton PW, Arkwright PD. Factors predicting anaphylaxis to peanuts and tree nuts in patients referred to a specialist center. *J Allergy Clin Immunol* 2008; 121(3):632–638.e2.

156. Lieberman P, Camargo CA, Bohlke K et al. Epidemiology of anaphylaxis: Findings of the American College of Allergy, Asthma and Immunology Epidemiology of Anaphylaxis Working Group. *Ann Allergy Asthma Immunol* 2006; 97(5): 596–602.

157. Simons FER, Ardusso LRF, Biló MB, El-Gamal Y, Ledford DK et al. World Allergy Organization Guidelines for the Assessment and Management of Anaphylaxis. *World Allergy Organization Journal* 2011; 4(2): 13–37. https://doi.org/10.1097/WOX.0b013e318211496c

Index

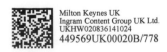

Milton Keynes UK
Ingram Content Group UK Ltd.
UKHW020836141024
449569UK00020B/778